2022

The Physicians' Guide

Medicare RBRVS

Sherry L. Smith, MS, CPA
Editor

Rebecca A. Gierhahn, MS
Michael J. Morrow, MBA, CPC
Managing Editors

AMA
AMERICAN MEDICAL ASSOCIATION

Executive Vice President, Chief Executive Officer: James L. Madara, MD
Senior Vice President, Health Solutions: Laurie McGraw
Vice President, Coding and Reimbursement Policy and Strategy: Jay Ahlman
Director, CPT Content Management and Development: Leslie W. Prellwitz
Director, CPT Editorial and Regulatory Services: Zachary Hochstetler
Vice President, Operations: Denise Foy
Manager, Publishing Operations: Elizabeth Goodman Duke
Manager, Developmental Editing: Lisa Chin-Johnson
Developmental Editor: Elizabeth Kennedy
Production Specialist: Mary Ann Albanese
Vice President, Sales: Lori Prestesater
Director, Channel Sales: Erin Kalitowski
Vice President, Product Development: Dave Sosnow
Marketing Manager: Vanessa Prieto

Printed in the United States of America. 21 22 23 24/BC-LSC/9 8 7 6 5 4 3 2 1

Additional copies of this book may be ordered by calling 612-435-6065. Refer to product number OP059622.

AMA publication and product updates, errata, and addendum can be found at amaproductupdates.org.

Internet address: www.ama-assn.org

For other correspondence, address inquiries to:

Medicare RBRVS
American Medical Association
330 N Wabash Avenue
Suite 39300
Chicago, IL 60611
ISBN: 978-1-64016-163-4
AC28: 02/22

Acknowledgments

The American Medical Association (AMA) is extremely grateful to the AMA staff and others who continue to make this book a reality.

The Department of Physician Payment Policy and Systems is responsible for the content of this publication and is staffed by Susan Clark, MJ, RHIA; Rebecca Gierhahn, MS; David Harms, MPA; Michael Morrow, MBA, CPC; Ruby Overton-Bridges, BA, CPC; Katlyn Palmer, MPH; and Sherry L. Smith, MS, CPA. The AMA thanks the following AMA/Specialty Society RVS Update Committee members, Advisory Committee members, Practice Expense Subcommittee members, and the Health Care Professionals Advisory Committee members for their efforts in advocating Resource-Based Relative Value Scale improvements to the Centers for Medicare & Medicaid Services.

AMA/Specialty Society RVS Update Committee (RUC)

Ezequiel Silva, III, MD
RUC Chair

Margie C. Andreae, MD
American Academy of Pediatrics

Amy Aronsky, MD
American Osteopathic Association

Sergio Bartakian, MD
The Society of Cardiovascular Angiography and Interventions

James Blankenship, MD
American College of Cardiology

R. Dale Blasier, MD
American Academy of Orthopaedic Surgeons

Kathleen K. Cain, MD
Primary Care Rotating Seat

Jim Clark, MD
College of American Pathologists

Joseph Cleveland, MD
Society of Thoracic Surgeons

Scott Collins, MD
American Academy of Dermatology

Daniel DeMarco, MD
American College of Gastroenterology

Gregory DeMeo, DO
American College of Obstetricians and Gynecologists

William D. Donovan, MD, MPH
American College of Radiology

Jeffrey P. Edelstein, MD
American Academy of Ophthalmology

Matthew J. Grierson, MD
American Academy of Physical Medicine & Rehabilitation

Gregory Harris, MD, MPH
American Psychiatric Association

Peter Hollmann, MD
American Medical Association

Timothy Laing, MD
American College of Rheumatology

Alan Lazaroff, MD
American Geriatrics Society

M. Douglas Leahy, MD
American College of Physicians

Scott Manaker, MD, PhD, FCCP
Practice Expense Subcommittee Chair

Bradley Marple, MD
American Academy of Otolaryngology–Head and Neck Surgery

Jordan Pritzker, MD
AMA CPT Editorial Panel

John H. Proctor, MD, MBA
American College of Emergency Physicians

Marc Raphaelson, MD
American Academy of Neurology

Richard Rausch, DPT, MBA
Health Care Professionals Advisory Committee (HCPAC) Co-Chair

Christopher K. Senkowski, MD
American College of Surgeons

Norman Smith, MD
American Urological Association

Stanley W. Stead, MD, MBA
American Society of Anesthesiologists

G. Edward Vates, MD
American Association of Neurological Surgeons

James C. Waldorf, MD
American Society of Plastic Surgeons

Thomas J. Weida, MD
American Academy of Family Physicians

RUC Advisory Committee

Megan Adamson, MD, MHS-CL
American Academy of Family Physicians

Curtis Anderson, MD
Society of Interventional Radiology

Sherry Barron-Seabrook, MD
American Academy of Child and Adolescent Psychiatry

Scott Bartley, MD
American College of Nuclear Medicine

Naveen D. Bhandarkar, MD
American Rhinologic Society

Elizabeth Blanchard, MD
American Society of Clinical Oncology

John Blebea, MD
American Vein and Lymphatic Society

Silvina Bocca, MD, PhD
American Society of Reproductive Medicine

Richard Bone, MD
American Medical Group Association

Michael Booker, MD, MBA
Radiological Society of North America

Matthew Brengman, MD
American Society of Metabolic and Bariatric Surgery

Joel V. Brill, MD
American Society of Addiction Medicine

Daniel Brown, MD, PhD, FCCM
Society of Critical Care Medicine

David Brown, MD, FAAAAI
American Academy of Allergy, Asthma & Immunology

R. Bruce Cameron, MD, FACG
American College of Gastroenterology

Lionel Candeleria, DDS
American Dental Association

Jordan Celeste, MD
American College of Emergency Physicians

Melissa Chen, MD
American Society of Neuroradiology

Audrey K. Chun, MD
American Geriatrics Society

William Creevy, MD
American Academy of Orthopaedic Surgeons

Melissa A. Davis, MD
Association of University Radiologists

Robert DeMarco, MD
American College of Chest Physicians

Gary Dillehay, MD
Society of Nuclear Medicine and Molecular Imaging

Paul T. Fass, MD
American Academy of Otolaryngic Allergy

Eddy Fraifeld, MD
American Academy of Pain Medicine

Demean Freas, MD
North American Neuromodulation Society

James L. Gajewski, MD
American Society for Transplantation and Cellular Therapy

Helen Gelly, MD
Underseas and Hyperbaric Medical Society

David B. Glasser, MD
American Academy of Ophthalmology

Lauren P. Golding, MD
American College of Radiology

Jay A. Gregory, MD
American Society of General Surgeons

Seth A. Gross, MD, FACG, FASGE
American Society for Gastrointestinal Endoscopy

Ryan Hakimi, DO, MS
American Society Neuroimaging

Charles J. Hamori, MD, FACP
American College of Physicians

Jon Kent Hathaway, MD, PhD
American College of Obstetricians and Gynecologists

Chase D. Hendrickson, MD
The Endocrine Society

Ryan Hick, MD
American Society of Dermatopathology

William Hickerson, MD
American Burn Association

Lee Hilborne, MD, MPH, DLM
American Society for Clinical Pathology

Wesley Ibazebo, MD
The Spine Intervention Society

Michelle A. Jorden, MD
National Association of Medical Examiners

Mark Kaufmann, MD
American Society for Dermatologic Surgery Association

Louise Perkins King, MD, JD, FACOG
American Association of Gynecologic Laparoscopists

Jeffrey Kozlow, MD
American Society of Plastic Surgeons

Steven E. Krug, MD
American Academy of Pediatrics

Michael Kuettel, MD, PhD, MBA, FACRO
American Society for Radiation Oncology

Stephen J. Lahey, MD, FACS
American Association for Thoracic Surgery

Dan Larriviere, MD, JD, FAAN
American Association of Neuromuscular & Electrodiagnostic Medicine

Ethan Lazarus, MD
Obesity Medicine Association

James Levett, MD
Society of Thoracic Surgeons

Howard Philip Levy, MD, PhD
American College of Medical Genetics

Morgan P. Lorio, MD
International Society for the Advancement of Spine Surgery

Michael C. Lubrano, MD
American Society of Interventional Pain Physicians

Charles D. Mabry, MD
American College of Surgeons

Dheeraj Mahajan, MD, CMD
AMDA-The Society for Post-Acute and Long-Term Care Medicine

Michael L. Main, MD
American Society of Echocardiography

R. Peter Manes, MD
American Academy of Otolaryngology–Head and Neck Surgery

Peter Mangone, MD
American Orthopaedic Foot and Ankle Society

Jeffrey McGovern, MD
American Academy of Sleep Medicine

Roger E. McLendon, MD, FCAP
College of American Pathologists

Daniel McQuillen, MD
Infectious Diseases Society of America

Swati Mehrotra, MD
American Society of Cytopathology

Shivan Mehta, MD
American Gastroenterological Association

Carlo Milani, MD
American Academy of Physical Medicine & Rehabilitation

Anne Miller-Breslow, MD
American Society for Surgery of the Hand

Jeremy S. Musher, MD
American Psychiatric Association

Kathrin Nicolacakis, MD, FCCP
American Thoracic Society

Marc R. Nuwer, MD, PhD
American Clinical Neurophysiology Society

Parag Parekh, MD
American Society of Cataract and Refractive Surgery

James J. Pomposelli, MD, PhD, FACS
American Society of Transplant Surgeons

John Ratliff, MD
American Association of Neurological Surgeons

Phillip E. Rodgers, MD, FAAHPM
American Academy of Hospice and Palliative Medicine

Howard Rogers, MD, PhD
American College of Mohs Surgery

Richard Rosenquist, MD
American Society of Anesthesiologists

Sharona B. Ross, MD, FACS
Society of Laparoscopic & Robotic Surgeons

Clemens Schirmer, MD, PhD
Congress of Neurological Surgeons

Joseph Schlecht, DO
American Osteopathic Association

Mark Schoenfeld, MD, FACC, FHRS
Heart Rhythm Society

Stephen Sentovich, MD
American Society of Colon and Rectal Surgeons

Ketan R. Sheth, MD, FACS
Society of American Gastrointestinal and Endoscopic Surgeons

Matthew Sideman, MD
Society for Vascular Surgery

Daniel M. Siegel, MD
American Academy of Dermatology

Samuel Silver, MD, PhD, MACP
American Society of Hematology

Fredrica Smith, MD
American College of Rheumatology

Marianna Spanaki, MD, PhD, MBA
American Academy of Neurology

James M. Startzell, DMD, MS
American Association of Oral and Maxillofacial Surgeons

James L. Sublett, MD
American College of Allergy, Asthma & Immunology

Karin Swartz, MD
North American Spine Association

Walton A. Taylor, MD
American Society of Breast Surgeons

Kim Temperton, MD, FAOA, FAMWA
American Medical Women's Association

Tarita Thomas, MD
American College of Radiation Oncology

John T. Thompson, MD
American Society of Retina Specialists

Edward Toggart, MD, FSCAI
The Society for Cardiovascular Angiography and Interventions

Raymond K. Tu, MD, FACR
American Roentgen Ray Society

Thomas Turk, MD
American Urological Association

Adam Weinstein, MD
Renal Physicians Association

Richard Weiss, MD
American Pediatric Surgical Association

Phillip Wise, MD, FACS
American Association of Clinical Urologist, Inc.

Richard F. Wright, MD
American College of Cardiology

Adolph J. Yates, MD, FAAOS, FAOA
American Association of Hip and Knee Surgeons

Robert Zipper, MD, MMM, SFHM
Society of Hospital Medicine

RUC Practice Expense Subcommittee

Scott Manaker, MD, PhD, FCCP
Chair

David C. Han, MD
Vice Chair

Amy Aronsky, DO
American Osteopathic Association

Gregory L. Barkley, MD
American Academy of Neurology

John Blebea, MD
American Vein and Lymphatic Society

Michael Booker, MD, MBA
Radiological Society of North America

Eileen D. Brewer, MD
American Academy of Pediatrics

Joseph Cleveland, MD
Society of Thoracic Surgeons

Neal H. Cohen, MD, MPH, MS
American Society of Anesthesiologists

RUC Health Care Professionals Advisory Committee

Contents

Foreword xv

Introduction: *A Guide to Medicare RBRVS: The Physicians' Guide* xvii

Part 1

The Roots of Medicare's RBRVS Payment System

1

Chapter 1

Development of the Resource-Based Relative Value Scale 2

The Profession's Interest in an RBRVS 2

The Government's Interest in an RBRVS 5

Harvard RBRVS Study 6

Reaction to the Completion of Phase I 8

Medicare Reform 9

Chapter 2

Legislation Creating the Medicare RBRVS Payment System 12

Prescription for Changing the Medicare Physician Payment System 12

OBRA 89 Physician Payment Reform Provisions 13

Changes in Law and Regulations 18

Chapter 3

The Scope of Medicare's RBRVS Payment System 22

Part 2

Major Components of the RBRVS Payment System

25

Chapter 4

The Physician Work Component 26

Harvard RBRVS Study 27

The 1992 RVS Refinement Process 30

The AMA/Specialty Society RVS Update Process 31

Five-Year Review 37

Chapter 5
Practice Expense Component 43
Data Used to Assign Charge-Based Practice Expense RVUs 43
OBRA 89 Method 43
OBRA 93 Revisions to the Practice Expense Component 46
Resource-Based Practice Expenses 47
The Bottom-Up Practice Expense RVU Methodology 57
Refinement of Resource-Based Practice Expenses 60

Chapter 6
Professional Liability Insurance Component 65
Data Used to Assign Charge-Based PLI RVUs 65
Creating Resource-Based PLI Relative Values 66
Major Improvements and Continued Concerns Regarding PLI Relative Value Methodology 68
Combining Work, Practice Expense, and PLI RVUs 70

Chapter 7
Geographic Variation in the Payment Schedule 71
OBRA 89 Provision for Geographic Adjustment 71
Geographic Practice Cost Index (GPCI) 72
Medicare Payment Localities 76

Chapter 8
Medicare Payment Schedule 79
Formula for Calculating the Payment Schedule 79
History of Budget Neutrality 80
Worksheets for Determining the Impact of Medicare Payment System on Individual Physician Practices 84

Chapter 9
Balance Billing Under the Payment Schedule 87
PAR Program 87
Limiting Charges 88
Monitoring Compliance 89

Part 3
The RBRVS Payment System in Operation
91

Chapter 10
Conversion Factor Updates 92
SGR Permanently Repealed 92
Medicare Economic Index 93
Expenditure Targets and Performance Adjustment 94
Budget Neutrality and Other Adjustments 98

Chapter 11
Standardizing Medicare Part B: RBRVS Payment Rules and Policies 101
Defining a Global Surgical Package: Major Surgical Procedures 102
Medically Unlikely Edits 104
Minor Surgery and Nonincisional Procedures (Endoscopies) 104
Moderate (Conscious) Sedation Services 105
Payment to Assistants-at-Surgery 106
CPT Modifiers 106
Telephone and Online Evaluation and Management Services 114
Telehealth 114
Medicare Expands Telehealth During COVID-19 PHE 115
AMA Tools and Resources 115
Remote Physiologic Monitoring 115
Remote Therapeutic Monitoring 116
Payment for "New" Physicians 117
Payment for Provider-Based and Teaching Physicians 117
Off-Campus Provider-Based Hospital Departments 118
Professional/Technical Component Services 119
Pathology Services 123

Payment for Supplies, Services, and Drugs Furnished Incident to a Physician's Service 124

Payment for Nonphysicians 127

Historical Information about E/M Codes 134

Interprofessional Telephone/Internet/Electronic Health Record Consultation 144

Psychiatric Collaborative Care Management Services 145

Other Primary Care Services 146

Legislative Initiatives to Detect Fraud and Abuse 151

Payment Policy Changes to Preventive Services Benefits 151

Other Payment Policy Changes Adopted Under the RBRVS 160

The AMA's Advocacy Efforts 161

Part 4

The RBRVS Payment System in Your Practice

167

Chapter 12

Practice Management Under the RBRVS: Implications for Physicians 168

Physician Payment Under the RBRVS 168

Practice Management Audit 170

Conducting Business Electronically 171

The 2009 Stimulus Law 171

Affordable Care Act 172

Privacy and Security of Health Information 172

ICD-10 172

Value-Based Health Care 173

Incentive Payments 174

Participation Decision 175

Private Contracting 176

Using the RBRVS to Establish Physician Charges 177

Chapter 13

Non-Medicare Use of the RBRVS: Survey Data 180

Survey Design 180

Characteristics of Respondents 181

Utilization of Medicare RBRVS 181

Use of Conversion Factors, All Payers 182
Determination of Conversion Factors 184
Use of RBRVS Payment Policies 185
Opinion of the RBRVS 186
Factors That Influence the Adoption of RBRVS 189
Other Uses of the RBRVS 189
Conclusion 190

Part 5

Reference Lists

191

List of Relative Value Units, Payment Schedule, and Payment Policy Indicators 192
National Place of Service Codes 194
Relative Value Units 200
List of Geographic Practice Cost Indices for Each Medicare Locality 521
RVUs for Anesthesiology Services 525
Anesthesia Base Units 525
Geographically Adjusted Dollar Anesthesia Conversion Factors, 2022 536

Appendices

539

A. Glossary 540
B. Directory of Resources 548

Index

561

Foreword

Medicare RBRVS: The Physicians' Guide 2022 is a result of the American Medical Association's (AMA's) commitment to provide its members and other physicians with timely and accurate information on the critical issues facing the medical profession. The 2022 *Guide* offers an updated overview of the resource-based relative value scale (RBRVS), including its components, operation, and applications, as well as new payment policies for the upcoming year and an explanation of how they may impact your practice.

The RBRVS, now in place for 31 years, reflects many policy objectives that the AMA sought in order to establish a fair and equitable system for physician payment. The RBRVS is based on the principle that payments for physician services should vary with the resource costs for providing those services and to improve and stabilize the payment system while providing physicians an avenue to continuously improve it. Since the introduction of the RBRVS, the AMA has worked with national medical specialty societies to provide recommended updates and changes to the RBRVS directly to the Centers for Medicare & Medicaid Services (CMS). The vehicle for this influence is the AMA/Specialty Society Relative Value Update Committee (RUC), which provides relative value unit (RVU) recommendations to CMS on an annual basis.

While the establishment and ongoing improvement of the RBRVS has been a great achievement for all of medicine, it has presented a unique set of challenges and exhibited some flaws. Congressionally mandated payment policies that add to the detrimental effects include annual targets for relative value adjustments for misvalued services, negative geographic adjustments, imaging cuts because of the Deficit Reduction Act, budget neutrality adjustments, and changes in the calculation of practice expenses.

The AMA worked to halt annual cuts to the conversion factor for more than a decade. These efforts, although victories for medicine, were only a temporary fix. Following years of extensive advocacy by the AMA and other physician organizations, Congress permanently repealed the sustainable growth rate (SGR) formula with the Medicare Access and Children's Health Insurance Program (CHIP) Reauthorization Act of 2015. Passage of this historic legislation finally brought an end to an era of uncertainty for Medicare beneficiaries and their physicians. The shortcomings of the SGR are well known. It threatened patients' access to health care; disrupted physician practice finances; and inhibited innovation in health care delivery.

It was a remarkable achievement during a time of political gridlock, when many other interest groups were struggling to reach legislative closure on their top issues. Over 700 physician organizations signed a letter urging Congress to support MACRA, and Congress responded with overwhelming bipartisan votes. On March 26, 2015, the US

House of Representatives voted 392-37 in support of H.R. 2 (MACRA), and on April 14, 2015, the Senate passed MACRA by a vote of 92-8. In a letter to the AMA Past-President, Robert M. Wah, MD, 46 state medical associations wrote, "Never before has the slogan 'Together We Are Stronger' been more true. It was the unity within organized medicine that brought us to this important victory."

The AMA remains committed to providing practicing physicians with the information they need to understand and deal with payment reform. *Medicare RBRVS: The Physicians' Guide 2022* is both a culmination of our work over the past years and the beginning of our efforts for the future. We sincerely hope that you find it useful as we continue to publish annual revisions with updated Medicare policies and payment schedule components. We urge you to send any suggestions or comments about this book to:

The Physicians' Guide
Physician Payment Policy and Systems
American Medical Association
330 N. Wabash Avenue
Suite 39300
Chicago, IL 60611

Introduction

A Guide to *Medicare RBRVS: The Physicians' Guide*

Medicare RBRVS: The Physicians' Guide 2022 has been developed as a comprehensive guide for physicians to Medicare's payment system for physicians' services that became effective January 1, 1992. In addition to providing detailed background information and explaining all features of the physician payment system, *The Physicians' Guide* is also a reference for physicians and their staff to use in answering specific questions about the system. The 31st edition of *The Physicians' Guide* reflects a detailed discussion of Medicare's payment policies, as well as 2022 relative values. It also provides updated information on new payment rules that took effect in 2022; more details are provided for each of the American Medical Association (AMA) Current Procedural Terminology (CPT®) codes on applicable payment policies and policy actions the AMA has taken since the enactment of payment system revisions. Finally, information on the use of resource-based relative value scale (RBRVS) by Medicaid programs and the private sector is described as well. To assist physicians to obtain answers to their questions as quickly as possible, *The Physicians' Guide* is organized into five parts:

- Part 1 introduces the RBRVS payment system. It provides a history and overview of the enabling legislation, explains the efforts of the government and the medical profession that led to the adoption of the RBRVS payment system and the introduction of its key components.
- Part 2 describes the RBRVS' key components, explains in detail RBRVS, geographic adjustments, conversion factor, and limits on physicians' charges.
- Part 3 explains the operation of the payment system, including the calculation of payments. This part describes all of the system's payment policies, including global surgical packages, modifiers, payment for assistants-at-surgery, evaluation and management codes, and other issues.
- Part 4 focuses on how the RBRVS payment system may affect physicians' practices. This part describes how private and public non-Medicare payers are changing their physician payment programs in response to the Medicare RBRVS and emerging forms of physician payment.
- Part 5 presents all the elements that are necessary to calculate the Medicare payment schedule: 2022 RVU and payment policy indicators for each physician service and geographic practice cost indices (GPCIs) for 2022 for each Medicare payment locality.

Physicians interested in understanding how and why Medicare's payment system was revised and how each of its components was established may wish to read Parts 1 through 4 in their entirety. Those interested only in understanding how payments are calculated and the effects on their practice may wish to skip Parts 1 and 2, and begin with Part 3.

Part 1

The Roots of Medicare's RBRVS Payment System

Part 1 provides an introduction to and an overview of the way Medicare pays for physicians' services under the resource-based relative value scale (RBRVS) payment system. Chapter 1 reviews the history of this approach to pay for physicians' services and explains why Medicare adopted this physician payment system. Chapter 2 summarizes the development of the RBRVS payment system legislation, including an overview of its major provisions. Chapter 3 briefly defines the scope of the RBRVS physician payment system and explains which Medicare-covered services are subject to the revised laws and regulations.

Chapter 1

Development of the Resource-Based Relative Value Scale

The resource-based relative value scale (RBRVS) payment schedule was fully phased in on January 1, 1996. The system's most significant changes to Medicare physician payment occurred during 1992, the first year of implementation; however, numerous legislative and regulatory provisions have been adopted since then that have had a major effect on the Medicare RBRVS. In addition, relative payment levels have continued to shift throughout the transition to the full-payment schedule. As a result, many physician practices have had to make major readjustments. This 31st revised edition of *The Physicians' Guide* describes the refinements and legislative changes made to the system during the last 31 years.

The transition to Medicare's RBRVS-based physician payment system began on January 1, 1992, culminating nearly a decade of effort by the medical profession and the government to change the way Medicare pays for physicians' services. Interest in changing the payment system for Part B of Medicare, which covers physicians' services, was initially motivated by steep annual increases in Medicare expenditures. Pressure to change the Part B payment system increased following the 1983 implementation of "prospective pricing" for the hospital portion of Part A, which covers inpatient hospital and nursing home services.

Three factors combined to heighten interest in physician payment reform between 1983 and the adoption of the 1989 payment reform legislation: rising dissatisfaction with Medicare's original payment system; continued escalation in Part B costs; and the promise of a credible basis for a new payment schedule-RBRVS. This chapter describes these three factors, including the rationale for organized medicine's involvement in RBRVS development, the alternative payment reform approaches considered by physicians and the federal government, Phase I of the Harvard University RBRVS study, and the events that followed publication of the Phase I Final Report in the autumn of 1988.

The Profession's Interest in an RBRVS

In 1992, payments for physicians' services comprised about 81% of expenditures for Medicare Part B, with the remainder divided among clinical laboratory services, durable medical equipment, hospital outpatient services, drugs, managed care services, and several other Medicare benefits.[1] The move to an RBRVS physician payment schedule (MFS*) represented the most significant change in Part B since Medicare's inception in 1966. (*Note: From the American Medical Association's [AMA's] perspective, the distinction between a "payment schedule" and a "fee schedule" is extremely important: a ***payment*** is what physicians establish as the fair price for the services they provide;

a *fee* is what Medicare approves as the payment level for the service. Therefore, the AMA has opted to use the term "payment" where appropriate, instead of "fee" in reference to the Medicare physician fee schedule [PFS] and has abbreviated the acronym to "MFS.") For 25 years, Medicare physician payment was based on a system of "customary, prevailing, and reasonable" (CPR) charges.

The CPR system (which will be referred to as the CPR henceforth) was designed to pay for physicians' services according to their actual payments, with some adjustments to keep government outlays predictable. It was based on the "usual, customary, and reasonable" (UCR) system used by many private health insurers. Medicare defined *customary charges* as the median of an individual physician's charges for a particular service for a defined period of time. The *prevailing charge* for this service was set at the 90th percentile of the customary charges of all peer physicians in a defined Medicare payment area. (The CPR was specialty specific.) The *reasonable charge* was defined as the lowest of the physician's actual payment for the service, that physician's customary charge, or the prevailing charge in the area.

Problems with CPR

Due to the diversity in physicians' payments for the same service, the CPR system allowed for wide variation in the amount Medicare paid for the same service. The insurance companies that process Medicare Part B claims, known as Medicare carriers, added to this diversity through their own policies. For example, some carriers paid only one prevailing charge per service, while others paid a different prevailing rate for each physician specialty providing the service. As a result, wide variations in Medicare payment levels developed among geographic areas and physician specialties.

Although these variations initially caused some dissatisfaction within the medical profession, the dissatisfaction reached a crescendo between the mid-1970s and the mid-1980s when Medicare placed a series of controls on the CPR payment levels. Designed to stem the growth in program costs, the first of these controls progressively reduced prevailing charges from the 90th to the 75th percentile. It was followed by an extension of the federal government's wage and price freeze on payments for physicians' services.

After lifting the freeze, the government implemented a new control in 1976, when it tied increases in prevailing charges to increases in the Medicare economic index (MEI). The MEI is intended to measure annual growth in physicians' practice costs since 1973 (prevailing charges in 1973 were in turn based on 1971 actual charges) as well as general earnings trends in the economy.

The major effect of the price controls and the MEI limit was to make permanent the basic pattern of Medicare prevailing charges that existed in the early 1970s. This pattern remained virtually unchanged until 1992. Payments per service were, therefore, unresponsive to changes in clinical practice and technology. Although compensation levels for new, high-technology procedures were generally commensurate with their high initial cost and limited availability, many physicians believed that payment increases for visits and consultations lagged far behind increases in the complexity and cost to diagnose and manage Medicare patients. Because compensation for new procedures remained relatively high even when their relative costs declined over time and compensation for visits remained relatively low while their relative costs increased, relative payment levels were thought to have become distorted.

Payment levels also remained stable across geographic areas. Consequently, as innovations in clinical practice and technology spread to rural and suburban areas, compensation did not increase. As a result, payment differences among Medicare localities, states, and regions remained, generally reflecting charge patterns that prevailed during the 1970s, despite changes in practice or demographics. Thus, Medicare often paid physicians in neighboring regions and states with similar costs of practice at very different levels for the same service.

As the prevailing charges became increasingly outdated, physicians in primary care specialties and rural areas, in particular, began to call for change. A new set of the CPR changes occurred in the 1980s. These included a second freeze on payment levels accompanied by limits on physicians' actual charges and reduced payments for surgical procedures deemed to be "overpriced." The CPR changes brought more calls for payment change to physicians in other specialties and geographic areas and accelerated interest in long-term, comprehensive physician payment reform. Because of the many constraints on the CPR, Medicare's physician payment system had become complex, confusing, unpredictable, and unrelated to physicians' actual payments, producing exactly the opposite result from what the CPR's architects had intended.

Options for Change

In the mid-1980s, as physician dissatisfaction with the CPR continued to grow and government policymakers produced several payment reform proposals, the medical profession faced several options for change:

- Modifying the CPR
- Extending the new approach introduced for hospitals under Part A of Medicare, diagnosis-related groups (DRGs), to physicians' services
- Mandating Medicare's health maintenance organization (HMO) program or other capitation approaches to be the dominant means of payment under Part B
- Replacing the CPR with a payment schedule based on a relative value scale (RVS)

Each option had its supporters and critics. Support was generally divided between physicians who wished to maintain the status quo by modifying the CPR and those seeking to develop a payment schedule based on an RVS. Under such a schedule, Medicare would pay a standardized "approved amount" for each service regardless of the physician's payment for the service, rather than basing payments on individual physician's payment as they originally had been under the CPR. (The Medicare "approved amount" includes both the 80% that Medicare pays and the 20% patient co-insurance.) Although Medicare would pay a standardized approved amount, physicians would still be able to charge patients their full payment. The difference between the Medicare-approved amount and the physician's payment is called the *balance bill.*

In an HMO-based system, HMOs receive a monthly Medicare payment for each beneficiary enrolled in the organization. The HMO pays physician and hospital services but usually limits patients' choices of physicians and hospitals.

Under the hospital DRG system, the hospital receives a standardized amount for each patient admitted with a particular diagnosis. The standardized amount represents the average hospital's cost to provide the average bundle of services required to treat patients with that diagnosis. Although a physician DRG system would vary from the hospital DRG system, the basic concept of bundling or packaging services covered by a single payment would be the same.

Of the four major payment reform options, only the CPR and a payment schedule are payment-for-service systems. Many medical professionals felt that preserving payment-for-service under Medicare was critical to protecting physicians' clinical and professional autonomy. Although the AMA supported a pluralistic payment system, it believed that adopting physician DRGs or mandatory capitation for Medicare, given the program's size, would severely threaten physicians' ability to use their own professional judgment in patient care decisions.

Historically, the AMA had also opposed policies to restrict or eliminate physicians' ability to charge patients the difference between their payment and the Medicare-approved amount. A DRG- or capitation-based system for physicians' services would, by definition, impose mandatory assignment, a policy requiring physicians to accept the Medicare-approved amount as payment in full, thereby prohibiting balance billing.

To preserve payment-for-service as a viable option under Medicare, the AMA pursued two parallel tracks. First, using lobbying efforts to influence legislation and litigation challenging the legality of various statutory provisions, the AMA tried to eliminate or mitigate the most onerous aspects of the CPR, including the payment limits, the Physician Participation Program (see Chapter 9), and the payment reductions. Second, it sought to develop a new RVS and the policy basis for its implementation, if appropriate. The first track achieved only limited success because Congress was reluctant to enact changes that would increase beneficiary expenses, and the courts upheld congressional authority to limit physicians' payments.[2]

The basis for the RVS. An RVS is a list of physicians' services ranked according to "value," with the value defined with respect to the basis for the scale. Using an RVS as a basis for determining payments and payments is a familiar concept for physicians and insurers. The California Medical Association (CMA) developed the first RVS in 1956 and updated it regularly until 1974. Beginning in 1969, the California relative value studies (CRVS) were based on median charges reported by California Blue Shield. Physicians used the CRVS to set payment schedules, and several state Medicaid programs, Blue Cross/Blue Shield plans, and commercial insurers used it to establish physician payment rates. In the late 1970s, however, Federal Trade Commission (FTC) actions raised concern that the CRVS might violate antitrust law, leading the CMA to suspend updating and distributing the CRVS.

Although many possible options existed for constructing a new RVS in the mid-1980s, the medical profession favored either a charge-based or a resource-based RVS. In a charge-based RVS, services are ranked according to the average payment for the service, the average Medicare prevailing charge, or some other charge basis. For example, if the average charges for service A is twice the charge for service B, the relative value for service A would be twice that of service B.

In a resource-based RVS, services are ranked according to the relative costs of the resources required to provide them. For example, suppose service A generally takes twice as long to provide, is twice as difficult, and requires twice as much overhead expense (such as nonphysician personnel, office space, and equipment) as service B. Then the relative value of service A in an RBRVS is twice that of service B.

An RVS must be multiplied by a dollar conversion factor (CF) to become a payment schedule. For example, if the relative value for service A is 200 and for service B is 100, a CF of $2 yields a payment of $400 for service A and $200 for service B. Likewise, a CF of $0.50 yields payments of $100 for A, $50 for B, and so on.

Most surgical specialty societies supported development of a charge-based RVS. These groups believed that physicians' payments provided the best basis for determining relative worth because payments reflected both the physician's cost of providing the service and the value of the service to patients. In addition, with readily available data, a charge-based RVS could easily become the basis for a payment schedule, thereby improving the degree of national standardization and eliminating the wide payment variations. However, experience with portions of the Harvard-RBRVS study that used charge data demonstrated that such data contained errors and often produced anomalous and unreasonable results.

Most nonprocedural specialty societies also considered these factors but reached a different conclusion, which the AMA shared. These groups believed that in a well-functioning market, physicians' relative charges would reflect their relative costs. In their view, however, Medicare payment levels did not reflect the prices that would emerge from a well-functioning market. They believed that the wide gap between payments for visits and payments for procedures, as well as the wide variations in payments for the same service between geographic areas and specialties, failed to reflect differences in the costs of the resources necessary to provide them. They also believed that the constraints on Medicare payments, including the freezes, reductions in prevailing charges, and tying annual updates to the MEI, had further distorted charges, so that Medicare charges would not provide an appropriate basis for a new RVS.

After weighing all of these factors, the AMA decided to drop a charge-based RVS, concluding that it was likely to preserve the same historical charge pattern that generated the dissatisfaction with the CPR. The AMA believed that an RVS based on relative resource costs was more likely to equitably cover physicians' costs of caring for Medicare patients. In choosing to pursue the development of an RBRVS, the AMA also emphasized the following:

- Any RVS-based payment system must reflect the often substantial variations in practice costs between geographic areas.
- Based on its long-standing policy, AMA would strongly oppose any newly developed payment system that required physicians to accept the Medicare-approved amount as payment in full.

The AMA proposal to develop an RBRVS. The AMA believed that organized medicine's participation in the development of an RBRVS was a key factor in physician acceptance of such a system. In January 1985, after discussing the issue with the national medical specialty societies, the AMA submitted a proposal to the Centers for Medicare & Medicaid Services (CMS, formerly known as the Health Care Financing Administration [HCFA]—the government agency responsible for administering the Medicare program) to develop a new RVS based on resource costs with extensive involvement of organized medicine and practicing physicians. Responding two months later, CMS said that despite its desire to involve organized medicine in developing an RBRVS, antitrust considerations raised by the FTC precluded a direct contract between CMS and a physicians' organization.

Because CMS had stated its intention to contract with a university or independent research center instead of a medical organization, the AMA discussed the possibility of jointly developing an RBRVS with several major universities. After careful consideration, the AMA accepted a Harvard University School of Public Health proposal for a "National Study of Resource-Based Relative Value Scales for Physician Services." It was similar to the AMA's earlier proposal and outlined an extensive role for the medical profession. With funding by CMS, Harvard began its study in December 1985.

The Government's Interest in an RBRVS

Through 1983, efforts to curtail the growth in Medicare spending focused principally on reducing expenditures for inpatient hospital care. Although Part B expenditures had been rising steeply each year, physicians' services accounted for only about 22% of Medicare spending, while hospital services accounted for about 70%. Hospital cost containment efforts, which curbed construction, admissions, length of stay, and intensity of services, had greater potential to reduce total Medicare spending than efforts to reduce spending on physicians' services.

The prospective payment system (PPS), introduced in 1983 to pay for Medicare patients' hospital costs, provides a standardized payment for each hospital admission, with variations to reflect geographic differences in wage rates and hospital location (urban or rural). The PPS authorized additional payment for "outlier" cases requiring exceptionally long stays or high costs. Admissions are categorized according to approximately 850 DRGs with payment based on the national average cost of hospital care for patients with a particular diagnosis.

The PPS assumes that hospitals care for patients whose severity levels range from mild to high within each DRG. While it is recognized that some patients' care will cost more than others, in the long run the cost of caring for all patients within a DRG is expected to equal the average approximate payment for the DRG. Because the DRG payment is the same regardless of the hospital's actual cost to provide care for a particular patient, prospective pricing provides an incentive for hospitals to improve their cost-efficiency.

Government policymakers view PPS as a success because the average annual growth rate in Medicare expenditures for inpatient hospital care decreased from 18% between 1975 and 1982 to 7% between 1983 and 1990. However, the extent to which PPS is solely responsible for this trend is unclear. In addition, those who believe that DRGs may adversely affect quality of care have been critical of PPS.

Governmental Options for Change

After the introduction of prospective payment, Congress and the Reagan administration turned their attention to reducing growth in Medicare spending for physicians' services, and the CPR system came under increasing attack. However, many physicians believed that CPR payments for primary care services and services provided in rural areas were inequitable. Although many members of Congress shared that view, other government and health policy officials criticized CPR as being inflationary. They argued that payment-for-service medicine encouraged overuse of services and that CPR encouraged overpricing of services, especially invasive and high-technology services.

Buoyed by the successful implementation of DRGs for hospitals, the government began exploring the feasibility of DRGs for physicians. In 1983, as part of the same law that created the prospective payment system for hospitals, Congress mandated that CMS study physician DRGs for Medicare and submit its report with recommendations by 1985.

In 1985, Congress also gave CMS authority to enroll Medicare beneficiaries in HMOs on a "risk-sharing" capitation basis. Previously, CMS could only enroll Medicare patients in HMOs using cost-based contracts, meaning that the HMO's capitation payment would rise or fall at year end depending on the actual cost of the services provided to Medicare enrollees. Under risk-sharing, if costs incurred by the HMO were less than the capitation payment, the HMO could retain up to 50% of the savings, but it would have to absorb 100% of any losses. By 1988, about 3% of Medicare beneficiaries had enrolled in HMOs and by 1999 that number had increased to more than 15% of Medicare beneficiaries. By 2005, this number had decreased to almost 12% enrolled in HMOs.

Expansion of HMOs for Medicare was partially a response to papers by health economists, published in the early 1980s, stating that the regulatory efforts of the 1970s had failed to control rising health care costs and calling instead for more competition in health care. The HMOs were viewed as the foundation of a more competitive system, in which employees and individuals enrolled in government entitlement programs could choose from a variety of HMO-type plans. Competition between these plans for enrollees would provide incentives for the plans to maintain low costs and premiums while providing high quality of care and amenities not offered by the Medicare payment-for-service program. CMS developed a strategy for increasing Medicare enrollment in HMOs and HMO-type plans, which it called the Private Health Plan Option. Despite strong support in Congress and the administration for mandating either DRG or HMO options for Medicare, the potential problems these options presented were also well known. For example, DRGs for physicians would be administratively complex and could produce serious inequities. In contrast to the approximately 579 DRGs for 5756 hospitals, more than 8000 codes describe the services that more than 800,000 physicians provide. Even if a DRG system could be developed for physicians' services, averaging DRG payments over the patient mix of a physician practice would be more difficult than it is for hospitals.

Recognizing these problems and responding to strong pressure from the AMA and organized medicine, Congress continued to explore payment-for-service options for Medicare physician payment reform. In the Consolidated Omnibus Budget Reconciliation Act of 1985 (COBRA, Public Law 99-272), Congress mandated that the secretary of Health and Human Services (HHS) develop an RBRVS and report on it to Congress by July 1, 1987. Simultaneously, however, legislation had been introduced in Congress to establish a DRG payment system for the major hospital-based physician specialties: radiologists, anesthesiologists, and pathologists.

Establishing the Physician Payment Review Commission

To evaluate the various physician payment reform options and to advise Congress, COBRA also created the Physician Payment Review Commission (PPRC). Composed of physicians, health policy researchers, and patient representatives, the PPRC's 13 members were nominated by the congressional Office of Technology Assessment. The PPRC's first meeting took place in November 1986.

The PPRC reviewed the options for Medicare payment reform, including changes in the CPR, physician DRGs, and expansion of capitation plans. It also studied international experience with physician payment, including the payment systems of Germany and Canada. The Commission's First Annual Report to Congress, submitted March 1, 1987, endorsed the concept of a payment schedule for Medicare. One year later, the PPRC recommended that the payment schedule be based on an RBRVS. A minority opinion signed by three commissioners endorsed the concept of a Medicare payment schedule but opposed the decision to base the schedule on relative resource costs because the RBRVS study had not yet been completed.

Harvard RBRVS Study

With Congress considering proposals for physician DRGs and the Reagan administration advocating its Private Health Plan Option for Medicare, the PPRC's 1987 endorsement of an RBRVS-based payment schedule gave a much-needed boost to the medical profession's efforts to preserve payment-for-service payment under Medicare. The other major factor that bolstered support for this payment reform alternative was the Harvard University RBRVS study. In addition to its intense lobbying and grassroots efforts, the AMA's argument that Congress should wait for results of the study before undertaking any major reform of Medicare's payment system was a crucial element in defeating proposals for physician DRGs.

The principal investigators in the Harvard study, William C. Hsiao, PhD, and Peter Braun, MD, had conducted previous studies that provided the foundation for the CMS-funded RBRVS study. In a 1979 exploratory study, Hsiao and William Stason, MD, attempted to rank 27 physicians' services provided by five specialties according to the time each service required and the complexity of each unit of time. Study results suggested that physicians had difficulty distinguishing between duration and complexity in ranking services. Consequently, the study results were considered unreliable. In a second study conducted by Hsiao and Braun in 1984, physicians directly ranked the overall work involved in their services without distinguishing between time and complexity. Although this study produced more consistent rankings, problems developed with the scale that was used (ie, the closed numeric scale, from 1 to 100, led to unreasonably low values for lengthy procedures).

In the national study, which began in 1985, CMS initially funded the Harvard team to develop an RBRVS for the following 12 physician specialties:

- Anesthesiology
- Family practice
- General surgery
- Internal medicine
- Obstetrics and gynecology
- Ophthalmology
- Orthopedic surgery
- Otolaryngology
- Pathology
- Radiology
- Thoracic and cardiovascular surgery
- Urology

The following six additional specialties were independently funded and included in the study at the request of the relevant national medical specialty societies:

- Allergy and immunology
- Dermatology
- Oral and maxillofacial surgery
- Pediatrics
- Psychiatry
- Rheumatology

The scope of what came to be known as Phase I of the study was considerably broader than previous studies. Its objectives were to develop an RBRVS for each of the 18 specialties included in the study and to combine the specialty-specific scales into a single cross-specialty RBRVS. Although COBRA required the secretary of HHS to report to Congress on the development of this cross-specialty RBRVS by July 1, 1987, the Omnibus Budget Reconciliation Act of 1986 (OBRA 86, PL 99-509) extended the report's submission date until July 1, 1989. The following year, Congress expanded the study mandate to include an additional 15 specialties, which became Phase II of the Harvard study. Phase III refined estimates from the earlier phases and expanded the RBRVS to include the remaining services coded by the Current Procedural Terminology (CPT®) system. Because Phase III was not completed by the January 1, 1992, implementation date, CMS established a process involving carrier medical directors (CMDs) to assign work relative value units (RVUs) to about 800 services for which Phase I and II data were not available. Phase III data were also used as part of CMS' refinement process for work RVUs first published in the 1992 Final Notice as part of the November 25, 1992, *Federal Register*. The study's methods and results are described in detail in Chapter 4.

The AMA's Role in the RBRVS Study

Under the terms of its subcontract from Harvard, the AMA's major role in the RBRVS study was to serve as a liaison between the Harvard researchers, organized medicine, and practicing physicians. The AMA worked with the national medical specialty societies representing the studied specialties to secure physician nominations to the project's Technical Consulting Groups. These groups studied specialty-provided advice to the researchers, helped to design the study's survey of practicing physicians, and reviewed and commented on its results.

Drawing on its Physician Masterfile, the AMA also supplied representative national samples of practicing physicians in each of the studied specialties. Throughout Phases I and II, the AMA advised the Harvard researchers, and an AMA representative attended every meeting of the Technical Consulting Groups.

The AMA's liaison role ensured that the RBRVS was based on the experience of a representative national sample of practicing physicians and that the specialty societies, through representation on the Technical Consulting Groups, were involved in important aspects of the development of relative values for their specialties. Involvement of both the AMA and the specialty societies also enhanced the study's credibility with practicing physicians and helped to increase its acceptance among physicians after results became available.

One additional benefit of organized medicine's involvement in the study was the high level of communication about the study, its results, and its policy implications. From 1985 to 1991, the front page of *American Medical News* covered this subject at least six times each year. Articles also appeared regularly in the *Journal of the American Medical Association (JAMA);* specialty journals such as the *Internist* and the *Bulletin of the American College of Surgeons;* state journals such as *Ohio Medicine;* and major newspapers, including *The New York Times*.

Reaction to the Completion of Phase I

On September 29, 1988, nearly three years after the study's inception, Harvard submitted its final report of Phase I of the RBRVS study to CMS. An overview of the study ran simultaneously in the *New England Journal of Medicine*. The entire October 28, 1988, issue of *JAMA* was devoted to the study. In addition to a series of articles on the study's methods and results, as well as simulations of the impact of a payment schedule based on the Phase I results, the *JAMA* issue included editorials by AMA, CMS, and PPRC leaders.

With completion of Phase I, the debate over whether Medicare should adopt an RBRVS-based payment schedule for Part B reached a pivotal moment. There were passionate views on all sides. Many rural and primary care physicians called for immediate adoption of a new Medicare payment system; surgeons viewed the study more cautiously. Even though CMS had funded the study, CMS' then-Administrator, William R. Roper, MD, expressed several reservations about continuing payment-for-service payment under Medicare:

. . . we face substantial problems in controlling the overall growth in expenditures for physicians. A payment schedule based on a relative value scale, no matter how carefully constructed, cannot be expected to address the growth in the volume and intensity of services. Whatever their merits, payment-for-service systems do not provide physicians with incentives to control this growth.[3]

The AMA's reaction to the study affirmed its belief that Medicare should adopt a payment schedule based on an appropriate RBRVS, but it reserved judgment about whether the Harvard study should serve that purpose. In his *JAMA* editorial on the subject, James S. Todd, MD, the AMA's then-Senior Deputy Executive Vice President, stated:

We went into this study with our eyes open. We have not wavered in our support for completing this study, or in our insistence that the AMA has no prior commitment to support its results or implementation.

. . . there must be external review and validation of the study's credibility, reliability, and validity. No less important will be the consideration of whether and how this academic research should be translated into the cold, hard realities of Medicare policy. The medical profession must and will assume a leading role in both of these endeavors.[4]

AMA Policy on the RBRVS Study

Immediately after the study's release, the AMA began an intensive evaluation to determine whether it could support the Harvard RBRVS as the basis for a Medicare payment schedule. It conducted an internal evaluation of the study's final report and retained the Consolidated Consulting Group, Inc, to provide an independent assessment of the RBRVS study. In November 1988, the AMA convened a meeting of 300 representatives of national medical specialty societies, state medical associations, and county medical societies to solicit their views on the study. To draft the AMA's policy positions on the RBRVS and related implementation issues, the AMA Board of Trustees appointed a physician payment task force, which comprised members of the Board and the AMA Councils on Medical Service and Legislation.

After considering the recommendations of this task force, findings from the internal and external reviews of the study, and the views of medical society representatives, the AMA Board of Trustees prepared a 40-page report containing its recommendations on the RBRVS, balance billing, geographic adjustments, and other policy issues. These recommendations became the focus of a hearing at the December 1988 meeting of the AMA's House of Delegates, at which more than 100 delegates testified.[i]

A principal theme of this testimony was the delegates' desire to maintain the AMA's leadership role in Medicare physician payment reform. Recognizing that change was coming, the key question was whether the change would be acceptable to the profession or a government-designed system without input from the medical profession would be enacted. They also recognized that organized medicine would need to remain unified for the AMA's policy proposals to be politically viable.

After a committee of the delegates amended the Board's recommendations to reflect the testimony presented at the hearing, the full House of Delegates unanimously adopted the revised recommendations. Unanimity was possible only because so many groups within the House agreed to compromise on policies that might concern their own specialty or locality, in order to create a new payment system that would serve the interests of the entire medical profession.

The key policy the AMA adopted at the December 1988 meeting was that the "Harvard RBRVS study and data, when sufficiently expanded, corrected, and refined, would provide an acceptable basis for a Medicare indemnity payment system." In addition, this policy specified which parts of the study needed improvement and acknowledged that specialties whose RBRVS data had significant, documented technical deficiencies needed to be restudied. The AMA committed itself to work with Harvard, the national medical specialty societies, CMS, Congress, and the PPRC to obtain the necessary refinements and modifications.

Besides these policies on the Harvard RBRVS study, the AMA's recommendations provided a blueprint for all the major features of a new Medicare physician payment system:

- Payment schedule amounts should be adjusted to reflect geographic differences in physicians' practice costs, such as office rent and wages of nonphysician personnel. Geographic differences in the costs of professional liability insurance (PLI) would be especially important, and these differences should be reflected separately from other practice costs.
- A transition period should be part of any new system to minimize disruptions in patient care and access.
- Organized medicine would seek to play a major role in updating the RBRVS.

The AMA reemphasized its long-standing policy on balance billing that physicians should have the right to decide on a claim-by-claim basis whether to accept the Medicare approved amount (including the patient's 20% coinsurance) as payment in full. The AMA also stated its intention to oppose any attempt to use implementation of an RBRVS-based system as a means to obtain federal budget savings, and to oppose "expenditure targets" for Medicare—a scheme that would automatically tie the payment schedule's monetary CF to projected increases in utilization of services. Finally, the AMA sought to eliminate differences between specialties in payment for the same service. Part 2 (Chapters 4–9) discusses each of these policy issues in greater detail.

The PPRC's Recommendations

Immediately after this momentous House of Delegates meeting, the AMA began advocating its Medicare physician payment reform policies before the PPRC, hoping to influence the recommendations the Commission would include in its 1989 Annual Report to Congress. These advocacy efforts were largely successful, and the Commission's recommendations, with several noteworthy exceptions, closely paralleled those of the AMA. Like the AMA, the PPRC endorsed the Harvard RBRVS study as the basis for a new Medicare payment schedule. Its list of necessary improvements was like those identified by the AMA. It also recommended using adjustment factors to reflect geographic differences in practice costs, eliminating specialty differentials, and opposing the use of the RBRVS's initial CF to obtain budget savings.

The views of organized medicine and those of the PPRC sharply diverged, however, on two policies: balance billing and expenditure targets. Given the widespread support for mandated assignment, which would have required physicians to accept the Medicare approved amount as payment in full, the AMA was pleased that the PPRC did not make such a recommendation. Against strong AMA opposition, however, the Commission did recommend placing percentage limits on the amount physicians could charge above the Medicare approved amount, although it did not specify a percentage. In contrast, the AMA believed that Medicare should establish only what it would pay and allow physicians to determine what they would charge.

The Commission's recommendation for a Medicare expenditure target was essentially its response to those who criticized payment-for-service payment systems because they did not control growth in costs or utilization. The AMA believed, in contrast, that an expenditure target could adversely affect patient access, and that profession-developed practice parameters held considerably more promise for reducing unnecessary utilization. Despite these differences, the AMA and PPRC core recommendations advanced the same fundamental reform: a Medicare payment schedule based on an expanded and refined Harvard RBRVS, with appropriate adjustments for geographic differences in practice costs and PLI costs. Congress had been under increasing pressure to take action to stem the flight of physicians from rural areas and primary care specialties and to change Medicare's physician payment system rather than continue its piecemeal, budget-driven approach. In early 1989, these factors heightened congressional interest in an RBRVS-based system, prompting initial legislative proposals from three different congressional subcommittees, which eventually became the foundation for the current payment-for-service payment system.

Medicare Reform

The Balanced Budget Act (BBA) of 1997 led to systemic Medicare program changes, including a wider array of health plan choices for beneficiaries, referred to as Medicare + Choice or Medicare Part C. It also altered the methodology for determining traditional payment-for-service payments under the Medicare RBRVS and permitted physicians to furnish health care services to Medicare patients on a private payment-for-service basis. Under the BBA, Medicare beneficiaries elected to receive benefits through either of two options: (1) the traditional Medicare payment-for-service program, or (2) Medicare + Choice plan.

On December 8, 2003, President George W. Bush signed into law the Medicare Prescription Drug, Improvement, and

Modernization Act (MMA). This legislation replaced the Medicare + Choice plan with Medicare Advantage.

Medicare Advantage (formerly Medicare + Choice) plans include the following:

- Private payment-for-service (PFFS)
- Health maintenance organizations (HMOs)
- Preferred provider organizations (PPOs)
- Special needs plans (SNPs)
- Medical savings account (MSA)

Under Medicare Advantage (MA), payments received by insurers to fund their MA plans are determined in part from insurer bids submitted to CMS. Bids reflect the amount for which an insurer believes it can provide standard Medicare benefits. Once CMS receives the bids, it creates benchmarks (target amounts) for each county across the nation. Each insurer's bid is then compared to the benchmark set for its county. If an insurer's bid is below the established benchmark, CMS will pay the insurer the benchmark. All payments to MA plans are risk adjusted, meaning that payment to plans is adjusted based on the relative health of the individual member. A brief description of traditional Medicare payment methodology, as well Medicare Advantage health plan options, follows:

Traditional payment-for-service. Physician payments under the Medicare RBRVS will be determined according to a single CF. Updates to the CF will be determined by a sustainable growth rate, which is described more fully in Chapter 10. The other elements of the RBRVS include the physician work relative values, the professional liability insurance (PLI) relative values, and the practice expense relative values. Practice expense relative values for 1999 and beyond include separate values depending on where the service is performed. Services provided in a physician's office are assigned a nonfacility practice expense RVU while services performed in a hospital and other settings are assigned a facility practice expense RVU. These and other changes to practice expense relative values are discussed in Chapter 5.

Private fee-for-service (PFFS). The MMA established a PFFS plan option. Under PFFS, physicians traditionally chose whether to provide care to PFFS enrollees on a case-by-case basis and agreed to the insurer's terms and conditions of service when treating enrollees. When a physician treated a PFFS patient, the physician was considered as deemed by the insurer. This deeming process only covered this single event, and the physician was under no obligation to treat that patient, or any other PFFS patient, in the future. In most cases, physicians would be reimbursed no less than the Medicare Payment Schedule. However, in 2011, the deeming authority for many PFFS plans was removed. Many PFFS plans (nonemployer-sponsored plans in areas where there are at least two other Medicare Advantage plans with contracted networks of providers) are now required to establish networks. Health insurers that intend to offer the network model must contract with a group of physicians or providers to provide health care services to their PFFS enrollees. The health insurers must also provide CMS with any categories of service for which they will be paying *less* than the Medicare allowable payment rates.

Health maintenance organizations (HMOs). Medicare Advantage HMOs contract with physician and provider networks to deliver Medicare services to beneficiaries. Beneficiaries with HMOs must see physicians in their networks.

Preferred provider organizations (PPOs). Medicare Advantage PPOs also contract with physician and provider networks to deliver Medicare services to beneficiaries. PPO beneficiaries may access physicians outside their plan's network but may pay more in co-insurance. Physicians without a contract may also bill patients for the difference between the plan's payment level and the allowed price the physician charges.

Special Needs Plans (SNPs). SNPs were created to improve access to MA plans for special needs individuals and allow health insurers to tailor programs to meet these beneficiaries' unique needs. SNPs differ from other Medicare Advantage plans in that they exclusively or disproportionately serve special needs individuals.

Medical Savings Account (MSA). An MSA is a high-deductible Medicare Advantage plan combined with a tax-free medical savings account that is funded by Medicare. The enrollee can use the money in the account to pay for his/her deductible expenses or other health care services not eligible for Medicare coverage. A medical savings account does not offer Part D drug coverage.

Private Contracting

In addition to these Medicare Advantage options, the BBA permits physicians and their Medicare patients to enter into private contracts to provide health care services. Private contracting arrangements are permitted only if certain conditions are met, including: (1) the physician does not receive Medicare payment for any items or services, either directly from Medicare or on a capitated basis; (2) inclusion in the contract of specified beneficiary protections, such as disclosure that Medicare balance billing requirements will not apply and the patient has the right to receive items and services offered by other physicians participating in Medicare; and (3) physician agreement through an affidavit filed with CMS to file no Medicare claims for any services provided to Medicare patients for a two-year period. Details on the private contracting provisions are provided in Chapter 12.

Congressional and Regulatory Commissions
In 1997, Congress merged two prior commissions to form the Medicare Payment Advisory Commission (MedPAC). The Commission is charged with advising Congress on payments to health plans, hospitals, physicians, and other Medicare provider groups. The Practicing Physician's Advisory Council (PPAC) was created by Congress as a federal advisory committee in the late 1980s in legislation backed by the AMA to provide physician input on prospective Medicare policies the Administration was considering. However, the Affordable Care Act discontinued PPAC in March 2010.

Note

i. The AMA's House of Delegates comprises voting representatives from all 50 states, as well as Puerto Rico, Guam, the Virgin Islands, and the District of Columbia; 124 national medical specialty societies; three professional interest medical associations; five Federal military service groups; and representatives of the AMA sections and special groups, such as the Medical Student Section, Organized Medical Staff Section, and the Young Physicians Section. The House is, therefore, an extremely democratic organization representing all types of physicians from all areas of the country.

References

1. Committee on Ways and Means. *Overview of Entitlement Programs: 1992 Green Book*. Washington, DC: Committee on Ways and Means. 1992:453.
2. *American Medical Association, et al v Bowen*, US Court of Appeals, Fifth Circuit, No. 87-1755, October 14, 1988. 857 FW 267 (5th Cir 1988).

   American Medical Association, et al v Bowen, US District Court, Northern District of Texas, Dallas Div, No. 3-86-3181-H, January 20, 1987. 659 FSupp 1143 (ND Tex 1987).

   Massachusetts Medical Society, et al v Dukakis, US District Court, District of Massachusetts, No. 85-4312-K, June 5, 1986. 637 FSupp 684 (DMass 1986).

   Massachusetts Medical Society, et al v Dukakis, US Court of Appeals, First Circuit, No. 86-1575, March 30, 1987. 815 FW 790 (1st Cir 1987), cert denied, 484 US 896 (1987).

   Whitney v Heckler, US Court of Appeals, 11th Circuit, No. 85-8129, January 22, 1986. 780 FW 963 (11th Cir 1986), cert denied, 479 US 813 (1986).

   Whitney v Heckler, US District Court, Northern District of Georgia, Atlanta Division, No. C84-1926, February 4, 1985. 603 FSupp 821 (ND Ga 1985).

   American Medical Association, et al v Heckler, US District Court, Southern District of Indiana, Indianapolis Division, No. IP 84-1317-C, April 18, 1985. 606 FSupp 1422 (SD Ind 1985).

   Pennsylvania Medical Society v Marconis, 755 FSupp 1305 (WD Pa), aff'd, 942 FW 842 (3rd Cir 1991).

   Medical Society of the State of New York v Cuomo, 1991 US Dist LEXIS 16405 (SDNY 1991).
3. Roper WR. Perspectives on physician payment reform. *N Engl J Med*. 1988;319:866.
4. Todd JS. At last, a rational way to pay for physicians' services? *JAMA*. 1988;260:2439–2440.

Chapter 2

Legislation Creating the Medicare RBRVS Payment System

In 1989, after years of debate within the medical profession about the distortions in historical charges, battles with Congress and the administration over rising expenditures, and a four-year wait for the results of the Harvard resource-based relative value scale (RBRVS) study, Congress finally enacted a new Medicare physician payment system. The process that led to enactment of the payment reform legislation was in many ways more historic than the law itself: the partnership forged between the medical profession, beneficiary groups, the Congress, and the Bush administration was unprecedented in the development of US health policy. The law resulting from this process gave participants a reasonable measure of what they had sought:

- An RBRVS-based payment schedule for physicians that narrowed specialty and geographic differences
- Continued balance billing limits for patients
- A system for monitoring expenditure increases for the government

This chapter provides a brief history and an overview of the physician payment reform legislation and the regulations promulgated since its enactment.

Prescription for Changing the Medicare Physician Payment System

During the spring of 1989, the American Medical Association (AMA), the Physician Payment Review Commission (PPRC), Centers for Medicare & Medicaid Services (CMS) (formerly the Health Care Financing Administration [HCFA]), and others presented their recommendations at several congressional hearings on Medicare physician payment reform. As the 1989 budget reconciliation process began, the following three congressional subcommittees with jurisdiction over the Medicare program presented proposals for such a reform for inclusion in what became the Omnibus Budget Reconciliation Act of 1989 (OBRA 89, PL 101-239):

- The Health Subcommittee of the House Ways and Means Committee
- The Subcommittee on Health and the Environment of the House Energy and Commerce Committee
- The Subcommittee on Medicare and Long-Term Care of the Senate Finance Committee

From the outset, the process of developing the payment reform legislation was controversial. The key parties to the legislative process presented markedly different initial proposals. Accepting the consensus between the AMA and the PPRC, however, all three included a geographically adjusted payment schedule based on an RBRVS.

The two most critical areas of contention for physicians were expenditure targets and balance billing limits. Although the AMA continued to oppose billing limits within Congress, balance billing limits were not an issue, only the specific percentage. Because Congress had enacted limits on Medicare balance billing under its "customary, prevailing, and reasonable" (CPR) payment system several years earlier (the maximum allowable actual charges [MAACs]), balance billing limits were considered a continuation of an existing policy rather than a completely new proposal. Moreover, balance billing limitations were necessary to obtain support for payment reform from beneficiary organizations, such as the American Association of Retired Persons (AARP).

The AMA opposed expenditure targets, believing they would simply reduce payment reform to another federal budget cutting tool. Under the Ways and Means provision, if the annual increase in Medicare expenditures exceeded a predetermined target increase, payments would automatically be reduced to recoup the overage. At the AMA's urging, the Energy and Commerce bill did not contain an expenditure target provision. Throughout the summer and fall of 1989, the AMA and the specialty societies worked closely with the three committees to forge a bill they all could support. As a result of this unprecedented joint effort by organized medicine, Congress, and the administration, the Senate finance bill emerged with a provision for a Medicare volume performance standard (MVPS), which addressed the difficult issue of increases in utilization but eliminated the most objectionable aspects of the expenditure target proposal.

OBRA 89 Physician Payment Reform Provisions

In December 1989, Congress passed and President Bush signed OBRA 89, which enacted the Medicare physician payment reform provisions into law. The legislation called for a payment schedule based on an RBRVS composed of the following three components:

- The relative physician work involved in providing a service
- Practice expenses (PE)
- Professional liability insurance (PLI) costs

The OBRA 89 defined the following key features of Medicare's new payment system for physicians' services:

- A five-year transition to the new system beginning on January 1, 1992
- Adjusting each component of the three RBRVS components for each service for geographic differences in resource costs
- Eliminating specialty differentials in payment for the same service
- Calculating a "budget neutral" conversion factor (CF) for 1992 that would neither increase nor decrease Medicare expenditures from what they would have been under a continuation of the CPR
- A process for determining the annual update in the CF
- Tighter limits on balance billing beginning in 1991
- An MVPS to help Congress understand and respond to increases in the volume and intensity of services provided to Medicare beneficiaries

Each of these key legislative provisions is described briefly in the following sections. The components of the payment system are described in greater detail in Parts 2 and 3 (Chapters 4 through 11).

RBRVS

As the AMA and PPRC had recommended, the physician work component of the RBRVS was to be based (implicitly) on data from the Harvard study, and the 1992 start date allowed Phase II of this study to be completed and reviewed prior to implementation. Physician work refers to the physician's individual effort in providing the service: the physician's time, the technical difficulty of the procedure, the average severity of the patient's medical problems, and the physical and mental effort required. A serious shortcoming in Phase I of the Harvard study was its approach to estimating physicians' relative practice costs. Therefore, the legislation provided a different method to determine the relative values for this component and for the PLI component.

In the Harvard study, the practice cost relative value of a service was related to the physician work relative value. In the transition to an RBRVS-based payment schedule, such an approach would mean that if the relative work of a service would lead to a reduction in its Medicare payment level, the relative practice costs would reduce the payment for the service even more. Both the AMA and the PPRC had identified this method as unfair and technically flawed. Their concern was that if physicians were not adequately compensated for their overhead costs, patient access would be impaired.

The practice cost method included in OBRA 89 separated practice costs from physician work and attempted to maintain the total practice cost revenue of a physician specialty at roughly the same as it had been under the CPR. Practice cost relative values were, therefore, based on the average proportion of a specialty's overall revenues devoted to practice expenses as a percentage of the average Medicare payment under the CPR. For example, if practice costs on average account for 45% of general surgeons' gross revenue for a service that is provided only by general surgeons and for which the average Medicare approved amount under the CPR was $1000, the practice cost component of the new payment schedule would be about $450. The actual calculation is a bit more complicated with other factors coming into play. However, the example illustrates the basic idea.

In response to these concerns, Congress adopted legislation in 1994 that required the development of resource-based practice expenses, with full implementation in 1998. Since that time, however, new legislation signed by President Clinton in August 1997 revised the implementation timeline. The Balanced Budget Act (BBA) of 1997 called for the CMS to collect additional data for use in developing the new practice expenses. Proposed values were published in May 1998, with a 60-day period for public comment. CMS received over 14,000 comments on its proposed rule and issued its Final Rule on November 2, 1998. CMS began implementation of the new practice expense values on January 1, 1999. The resource-based practice expense relative values became fully implemented on January 1, 2002. Chapter 5 describes these activities.

Initially, the PLI relative values were also determined in the same fashion as the practice expense relative values; they were based on the average proportion of a specialty's overall revenues that is devoted to PLI costs as a percentage of the average Medicare approved amount under the CPR. For instance, if the PLI cost percentage in the previous example was 5%, the PLI component of the new payment schedule would have been approximately $50. Although several concerns about this method have surfaced during the last six years, two factors account for the wide support it received when OBRA 89 was drafted. First, it was considered more equitable than the Harvard study's method; and second, no other alternatives would have been ready for 1992 implementation. In 2000, CMS implemented resource-based PLI relatives. The methodology used is described in Chapter 6.

Geographic Adjustments

Opinions varied on the degree to which the RBRVS should be geographically adjusted under the new system. Many physicians, especially those in rural areas, believed that Medicare should pay the same amount for a service regardless of where it was provided. Others believed that payments in a resource-based system should reflect geographic differences in physicians' resource costs, ie, differences in office rents, wages of nonphysician office staff, PLI costs, and cost of living.

The AMA's policy position represented one compromise on this issue, and the OBRA 89 method represented another. The AMA had stated that payments should be adjusted to reflect only differences in physicians' practice costs and PLI costs, and that geographic differences in costs of living should be ignored. Geographic differences in cost of living would be reflected in the physician work component of the payment schedule.

In the payment schedule, geographic differences in all three components are determined by three geographic cost indices known as geographic practice cost index (GPCIs). Under the OBRA 89 compromise, differences in cost of living are measured according to a geographic index of cost of living, but this index measures only one quarter of the geographic difference in cost of living. Practice cost differences are measured by a geographic index of overhead cost differences, and PLI differences by a geographic index of PLI costs.

In practice, the OBRA 89 compromise means that, if practice costs in a particular state are 10% higher than the national average, PLI costs are 12% higher, and costs of living are 8% higher, then the practice cost component of the payment will be increased by 10% above the national average payment and the PLI component will be increased by 12%, but the physician work component will be only 2% higher than the national average, because the cost-of-living index only reflects one quarter of the difference. The OBRA 89 provision substantially reduced the degree of geographic variation in payments. Whereas under the CPR, payments in one community could be three or four times greater than payments in another community for the same service, the RBRVS payment system reduced this variation to within 10% to 15% of the national average for most services.

The Medicare Prescription Drug, Improvement, and Modernization Act (MMA) of 2003 required that the physician work GPCIs cannot be less than 1.00, effective January 1, 2004, through December 31, 2006. This provision was extended through December 31, 2007, by the Tax Relief and Health Care Act of 2006 and extended once again through June 30, 2008, by the Medicare, Medicaid, and SCHIP Extension Act of 2007. On July 15, 2008, the Medicare Improvements for Patients and Providers Act of 2008 (MIPPA) was made into law and extended the 1.00 work GPCI floor from July 1, 2008, through December 31, 2009. In 2010, the work GPCI floor was extended by the Affordable Care Act of 2010 from January 1, 2010 through December 31, 2010. This work GPCI floor was extended once again through the passage of H.R. 4994 Medicare and Medicaid Extenders Act of 2010. This legislation extended the 1.00 work GPCI floor through December 31, 2011. On December 23, 2011, the Temporary Payroll Tax Cut Continuation Act of 2011 was signed into law, providing for a further extension through February 29, 2012. In addition, on February 22, 2012, the Middle Class Tax Relief and Job Creation Act of 2012 was signed into law, which provided a further extension through December 31, 2012. On January 2, 2013, the American Taxpayer Relief Act of 2012 was signed. As a result, the 2012 1.00 was extended through December 31, 2013. The Pathway for Sustainable Growth Rate (SGR) Reform Act of 2013 extended the 1.00 work GPCI floor through April 1, 2014. The Protecting Access to Medicare Act of 2014 (PAMA) again extended the 1.00 work GPCI floor, this time through March 31, 2015. The Medicare Access and Children's Health Insurance Program (CHIP) Reauthorization Act of 2015 (MACRA) extended the 1.00 work GPCI floor through December 31, 2017. Signed into law on February 9, 2018, the Bipartisan Budget Act of 2018 extended the 1.00 work GPCI floor through December 31, 2019. The Further Consolidated Appropriations Act, 2020, provided for extension of the work GCPI floor of 1.00 from January 1, 2020 through May 22, 2020. The Coronavirus Aid, Relief, and Economic Security (CARES) Act of 2020 further extended the work GPCI floor through November 30, 2020. The Continuing Appropriations Act, 2021, and Other Extensions Act included an extension of the work GPCI floor under the Medicare program through December 11, 2020, only. The Consolidated Appropriations Act, 2021 (the Act) that was signed into law on December 27, 2020, reinstated the 1.0 floor on the work GPCI through calendar year (CY) 2023.

Balance Billing Limits

Retaining the right to charge patients the difference between the Medicare approved amount and the physician's full payment for the service has been a cornerstone of AMA policy since the inception of the Medicare program. Under physician DRGs or HMOs, balance billing would not have been permitted given the nature of these payment approaches. Many physicians also feared that this right would be lost if an RBRVS-based payment schedule was adopted. The PPRC's decision not to recommend mandatory assignment and the absence of such a provision from all three legislative proposals was, therefore, a major victory for organized medicine.

In the late 1980s under the CPR, balance billing was limited by MAACs, which were different for each physician because they were based on each physician's customary charges in the second quarter of 1984. The OBRA 89 eliminated MAACs over a three-year transition period that began in 1991 and replaced them with "limiting charges." The major difference between limiting charges and MAACs is that limiting charges are a specified percentage above the Medicare approved amount (including the patient's 20% coinsurance), whereas MAACs were based on what physicians charged in a base period.

Since January 1, 1993, the limiting charge for a given service in each Medicare payment locality has been 15% greater than the Medicare approved amount for the service. It is the same for every physician who provides that service.

In addition, effective January 1, 1995, CMS has statutory authority to prohibit physicians and suppliers from billing Medicare patients, as well as supplemental insurers, above the limiting charge and to require that any excess charges be refunded or credited to the patient.

The OBRA 89 also retained the Participating Physician Program under the new Medicare payment system. "Participating" physicians are those who agree to accept assignment for all services that they provide to patients enrolled in the Medicare program. To give physicians an incentive to sign such an agreement, the full Medicare payment schedule amount for "nonparticipating" physicians is only 95% of the full payment schedule for participating physicians. Because the limiting charge is, in turn, based on the payment schedule for nonparticipating physicians, the effective limiting charge is 9.25% above the full Medicare payment schedule (ie, 115%, 95%, 109.25%).

Payment Updates and the Medicare Volume Performance Standard

A relative value scale can produce any level of payment for a given specialty or service; it all depends on the conversion factor.

James S. Todd, MD [1]

During the development of the OBRA 89 payment system provisions, much of the process for updating payments over time was widely debated. The problems caused by the historical charge patterns that developed under the CPR, the government's previous attempts to control Medicare's rising costs, and the PPRC's expenditure target proposal had combined to generate substantial interest in this aspect of the new payment system. In addition, physicians were skeptical that a Congress intent on reducing the federal budget deficit would all too willingly use the new payment schedule's dollar CF to achieve budget savings.

The OBRA 89 provisions that were ultimately adopted authorized Congress to annually update the CF based on the percentage increase in the Medicare Economic Index (MEI), a comparison of the MVPS with the actual increase in spending, and other factors. The MVPS is set annually, by either Congress or a statutory default formula, to reflect the expected growth rate in Medicare spending for physicians' services. It is supposed to encompass all the factors that contribute to this growth, including changes in payment levels, the size and age composition of the Medicare population, technology, utilization patterns, and access to care. The concept behind the CF updating process is that establishing a link between payment updates and increases in the volume of services provided to Medicare patients gives physicians an incentive to decrease unnecessary and inappropriate services. Enacting the MVPS instead of expenditure targets allowed the AMA and other physician organizations to relax that link.

The Balanced Budget Act of 1997, however, replaced the MVPS with a new sustainable growth rate (SGR) system to control Medicare expenditure growth. The SGR did not rely on historical patterns of growth in volume and intensity of physician services, as did the MVPS; rather, it used projected growth in real gross domestic product per capita. MACRA was signed into law on April 16, 2015. The legislation (P.L. 114-10) repealed the SGR update methodology for physicians' services, provided positive annual payment updates of 0.5% from July 1, 2015, through 2019, and required the Centers for Medicare & Medicaid Services

(CMS) to establish a merit-based incentive payment system (MIPS), under which MIPS-eligible professionals receive annual payment adjustments based on their performance in a prior period. CF updates and the sustainable growth rate are described in greater detail in Chapter 10.

Budget-Neutrality Adjustment

The OBRA 89 mandated that revisions to relative values resulting from changes in medical practice, coding, new data, or the addition of new services may not cause Part B expenditures to differ by more than $20 million from the spending level that would have occurred without these adjustments. Every year since 1993, CMS has projected net expenditure increases exceeding this limitation and, to limit the increase in Medicare expenditures, has made budget-neutrality adjustments to the payment schedule.

CMS has applied different types of "budget neutrality" adjustments. For the 1993 through 1995 payment schedules, CMS uniformly reduced all relative value units (RVUs) across all services; in 1996, it adjusted the CFs. For 1997, CMS made two separate adjustments: one to the physician work RVUs and another to the CFs. For 1998, it also made separate adjustments, including a –0.7% adjustment for increased work RVUs for global surgical services and –0.1% applied as a behavioral offset. The latter adjustment reflects CMS' belief that the volume and intensity of physician services will increase in response to payment schedule reductions, thus lessening their impact on overall Medicare expenditures.

Annually rescaling the RVUs created an administrative burden for physician practices and third-party payers in setting compensation levels, greatly impairing the usefulness of the RBRVS to these groups. In addition, the rescaling also masks any real changes in relative values due to changes in medical practice and refinements to the RBRVS. Beginning in 1999, CMS eliminated its separate adjustment to the work RVU and instead applied budget-neutrality adjustments directly to the CF. However, in 2003 CMS applied a volume and intensity offset by 0.49% to the practice expense relative values, rather than the CF. Despite comments from organized medicine requesting stability in the RVUs, CMS rescaled the work (–0.15%), practice expense (–1.320%), and professional liability insurance (+20.61%) relative values in 2004 to match the new Medicare economic index (MEI) weights. Chapter 10 explains these policies in detail.

In 2007, CMS returned to the use of a separate work adjustor applied directly to work RVUs to achieve budget neutrality. CMS estimated in the CY 2007 MFS Final Rule that the improvements resulting from the third Five-Year Review would account for an additional $4 billion in expenditures. Rather than achieve budget neutrality through a reduction in the CF, CMS introduced a 10.1% adjustment to all work RVUs. After this recommendation by CMS, the AMA RUC sent its recommendations on additional CPT codes from the Five-Year Review and recommendations for an increase in the work of anesthesia services. After these recommendations were reviewed, CMS determined that a revised work adjustor for 2008 would need to be implemented to account for the impact of these additional recommendations. CMS implemented a 11.94% adjustment to all work RVUs for 2008.

The AMA opposed the application of this separate work adjustor. Because the MFS is used widely by private and public payers to determine physician payment and physician group practices to determine compensation plans and/or to utilize as a benchmarking tool, adjusting work RVUs may compromise the integrity and relativity of the RBRVS. Since CMS first indicated that a work adjustor may be used, the AMA along with most specialty societies have advocated for the adjustment to be applied to the CF. Efforts included AMA and RUC comments to the June 29, 2006, August 22, 2006, and July 12, 2007, Proposed Rules, a joint letter from the AMA and 74 specialty societies, and numerous meetings with senior CMS officials. Despite these efforts, CMS moved forward with the separate work adjustor for 2008. However, because of these tremendous efforts made by the AMA, as well as the specialty societies, MIPPA was enacted on July 15, 2008, and required that the budget-neutrality adjustment be applied to the CF and not the work relative values for 2010 and subsequent years.

The annual determination of the CF accounts for both the statutory update factor and the budget-neutrality adjustment required by law, 0.00% and –0.10%, respectively, for 2022.

The CY 2022 CF will be reduced by approximately 0.8% from 34.8931 in 2021 to 34.6062. This reduction is due to the maintenance of a temporary 3.75% increase to the CF at a reduced 3%, stemming from Congressional action to temporarily avert a more significant cut for another year, as well as a budget-neutrality adjustment of – 0.10%.

The American Medical Association (AMA) strongly advocated for Congress to extend the 3.75% increase for CY 2022 as physician practices faced Medicare cuts amounting to a 9.71% overall decrease effective January 1, 2022, when factoring in sequestration reductions. Recognizing that these Medicare cuts would further compound the growing financial instability of physician practices due to the significant reduction in revenue caused by the continued severe acute respiratory syndrome coronavirus 2 (SARS-CoV-2) (coronavirus disease 2019 [COVID-19]) public health emergency (PHE), the cuts were diverted when President Biden signed S.610, Protecting Medicare and American Farmers from Sequester Cuts Act, into law on December 10, 2021. This law results in the following:

- A delay in resuming the 2% Medicare sequester for three months (January 1–March 31, 2022), followed by a reduction to 1% for three months (April 1–June 30, 2022).
- A 1-year increase in the MFS of 3% (0.75% less than the CF boost provided for 2021).

- A 1-year delay in the cuts to the clinical laboratory fee schedule.
- A 1-year delay in the Medicare radiation oncology demonstration.

In addition, the law will erase the 4% Medicare Pay-As-You-Go (PAYGO) cut and prevent any additional PAYGO cuts through 2022.

(See Chapters 8 and 10).

Transition to the New System

The OBRA 89 established a five-year transition to the new system, which began on January 1, 1992. The transition was consistent with the AMA's desire to postpone implementation until Phase II of the Harvard RBRVS study was completed, and then to proceed incrementally to avoid precipitous changes in payments and potential disruptions in patient care. In addition, the OBRA 89 transition method was intended to accelerate payment increases, principally for visits and consultations, while providing a slower transition for payment reductions.

Much of the change to the new payment levels occurred in the first year of the transition period. The first step in determining the 1992 payment levels was to adjust the CPR prevailing charges, thereby eliminating specialty differentials. The adjustment was essentially a weighted average that accounted for the frequency of each payment amount. In other words, if six different specialties in an area provided a service and six Medicare prevailing charge levels existed under the CPR, the averaging process would reflect the frequency of the service provided by physicians in each specialty. The averaging process also reflected the CPR customary charges of physicians who charged less than the prevailing charge. As a result, it was possible for an adjusted prevailing charge to be somewhat less than the average prevailing charge. CMS referred to this average charge as the "historical payment basis" for a service.

Eliminating specialty differentials placed no limit on the degree to which payments could change in 1992 because of this adjustment. For visit services formerly provided by both internists and family practitioners, for which the internists received higher payments, the adjustment created a double increase for the family practitioners: one because of the adjustment and one because of the transition to the RBRVS. For the internists, the adjustment would mean payments might be decreased and then increased in the process of calculating the 1992 payment, although the internist would only see the net effect. Medicare payments are now the same for all physicians who provide a service in a locality regardless of their specialty.

Many Medicare carriers did not recognize specialty differentials under the CPR, however, and maintained only one prevailing charge level for each service. In addition, because many services are only provided by physicians in one specialty, only one prevailing charge level existed in the area. Where there was only one CPR prevailing charge, the historical payment basis may have been closer to the 1991 prevailing charge for the service, although the presence of customary charges less than the prevailing charge, in general, would still have reduced the historical basis below the prevailing charge level.

Figure 2-1. OBRA 89 Transition Asymmetry: Percentage Change in Years 1 and 5

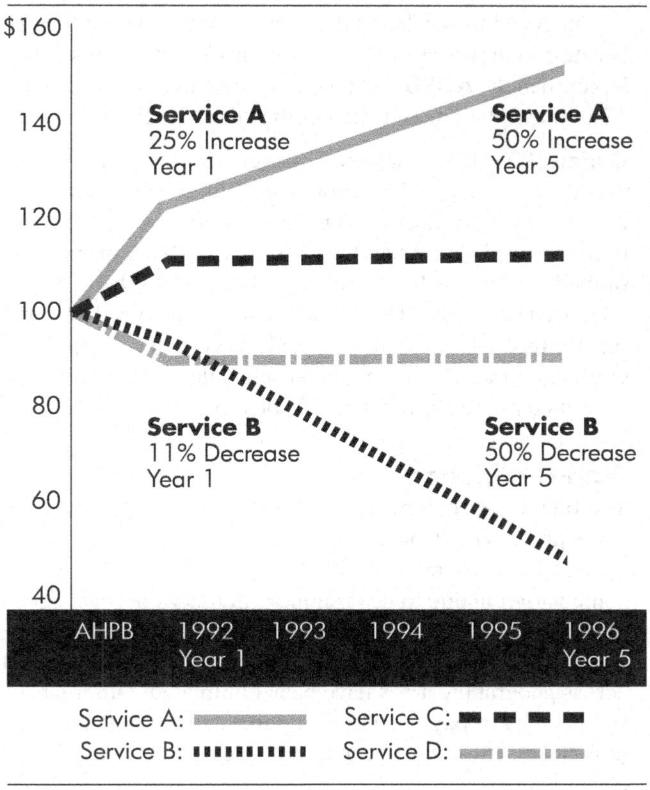

In calculating the CF for 1992, CMS determined that the historical payment basis for each service should be reduced by 5.5%. This reduction was intended to compensate for the fact that payments for visits were increasing faster than payments for procedures and other services were decreasing, thus increasing expenditures over what they otherwise would have been. Finally, the historical payment basis was increased by the payment update for 1992 of 1.9%. This 1.9% update was also applied to the CF for the RBRVS-based payment schedule. After the 5.5% reduction and the 1.9% increase were applied, the historical payment basis was referred to as the adjusted historical payment basis (AHPB).

The next step was the actual transition to the payment schedule. In this step, the statute required that services for which the AHPB was neither 15% higher nor 15% lower than the RBRVS payment schedule be paid entirely based on the new payment schedule. Services for which the schedule represented a change of more than 15% were increased or decreased from the AHPB by 15% of the full payment schedule amount in 1992. As Figure 2-1 illustrates, this process was intended to accelerate the change for payment increases because such increases were based on 15% of a dollar figure larger than the AHPB and payment decreases were based on 15% of a dollar amount smaller than the AHPB.

During 1993–1995, payments for services that did not move entirely to their RBRVS amounts in 1992 were incrementally increased or decreased using a blend of the 1992 transition approved amount and the RBRVS, with the proportion of the blend that is based on the full payment schedule increased each year. The annual payment update also is applied. Since 1996, payments for all services have been based entirely on the RBRVS payment schedule. The transition is described in greater detail in Chapter 10.

Standardization

The final major component of the RBRVS payment system is the process of standardization. The move to a nationally standardized payment schedule based on an RBRVS, with some variation due to geographic differences in practice costs, was a major change in Medicare's payment system. The twofold, threefold, and fourfold differences in payments across geographic areas have been eliminated. Differences by specialty in payments for the same service within a geographic area also have been eliminated.

Standardization of Medicare payment policies across local Medicare carriers also was initiated under the RBRVS payment system. Until 1992, each Medicare carrier had broad latitude to establish its own policies, including issues such as which services were included in the payment for a surgical procedure, local codes in addition to the national coding system, and policies for comparing Medicare payments to payments for privately insured patients.

One of the RBRVS payment system's most significant provisions substantially eliminated variation in national Medicare payment policies. Although the law did not spell out the details, it required CMS to adopt a uniform coding system for Medicare and a uniform global surgical policy and to standardize its approaches to payment for nonphysician providers, drugs and supplies, and other facets of Part B of Medicare. Chapter 11 describes all of these policies in detail.

Changes in Law and Regulations

In addition to defining these key components of the new Medicare payment system, OBRA 89 required CMS and PPRC to conduct a number of studies on issues related to the new physician payment system and make recommendations on these issues to Congress. One of these requirements directed the secretary of Health and Human Services (HHS) to publish a model payment schedule (ie, MFS) in September 1990.

The MFS, published in the *Federal Register* on September 4, 1990, provided an added step in CMS' normal regulatory process, giving physicians and their organizations an opportunity to review and comment on CMS' proposals for implementing the new payment system prior to a formal proposed rule. The MFS provided a detailed explanation of the new system; identified the options that CMS was considering on issues such as coding and site-of-service differentials in payment; and provided preliminary estimates of payment schedule amounts and geographic adjustments. In November 1990, Congress enacted the Omnibus Budget Reconciliation Act of 1990 (OBRA 90, PL 101-508), which changed some Medicare payment policies related to physician payment under the Medicare RBRVS. The three most significant changes:

- Sharply curtailed payments for interpreting electrocardiograms (ECGs)
- Reduced payments for assistants-at-surgery from 20% to 16% of the global payment for the surgery
- Extended payment reductions for "new" physicians from their first two years of providing Medicare services to their first four years

The legislation's ECG provision eliminated payment for interpreting ECGs whenever the ECG was provided as part of or in conjunction with a visit or consultation. Payment for these ECG services, however, as well as for "new" physicians, was restored in 1994 under provisions of Omnibus Budget Reconciliation Act of 1993 (OBRA 93).

Notice of Proposed Rule Making: 1991

On June 5, 1991, the payment reform process was almost derailed when CMS' publication of the *Notice of Proposed Rule Making (NPRM)* on Medicare physician payment in the *Federal Register* included a proposal to reduce the payment schedule's CF by 16% from an otherwise budget-neutral level. The proposed reduction was clearly at odds with congressional intent as described in OBRA 89 to maintain overall Medicare spending in 1992 at the level it would have been under a continuation of the CPR.

The NPRM prompted the AMA to initiate an extensive grassroots campaign to reverse the proposed cut before the Final Rule was issued. The campaign resulted in more than 100,000 comments on the *NPRM* and thousands of letters to Congress. Besides the campaign, the AMA testified before Congress and submitted detailed comments on the *NPRM*, including a legal analysis of the budget neutrality issue by the law firm of Sidley and Austin, which provided clear support for the AMA's position. As a result, 92 of the 99 members of the three congressional committees with authority over Medicare signed letters to Secretary Sullivan opposing the cuts, and 82% of the Congress indicated its support. In addition, two chairmen of the relevant subcommittees introduced legislation to prevent the reduction.

Although three factors contributed to the proposed reduction, the most offensive to physicians was CMS' "behavioral offset." Its premise was that physicians would increase the volume of their services in response to the payment reductions caused by the new payment system, and that payment levels must be reduced to compensate for this expected increase in utilization.

The AMA's comments on the *NPRM* provided a persuasive analysis opposing the proposed reduction in the CF, demonstrating that the cuts clearly violated the language and intent of the law, with potentially disastrous consequences for patient access. These comments also commended CMS for its decisions to adopt the AMA's coding system as its uniform system, to allow a major role for organized medicine in updating the RBRVS, and to eliminate several of the CPR policies that physicians had long opposed. Details of these comments and CMS' response are discussed in the relevant chapters of this book.

Final Rule: 1991

The Final Rule for the new Medicare physician payment system appeared in the *Federal Register* on November 25, 1991. It contained a summary of the regulation, an analysis of comments on the *NPRM* and CMS' responses, impact estimates for physicians and beneficiaries, and the regulations for the new system. It also listed the relative values for each service and geographic adjustment factors for each locality.

The Final Rule reflected several extremely positive changes from the *NPRM* that the AMA and other physician organizations had advocated. Most notable was the CF of $30.423, which exceeded the *NPRM* CF of $26.873 by 13.2%. This increase restored an estimated $10 billion to Medicare Part B over the period 1992 through 1996. CMS also announced the payment update for 1992 of 1.9%, thus making the 1992 CF $31.001.

Besides the CF, the Final Rule contained many other substantial changes compared to the *NPRM*, such as the following:

- In using a "baseline adjustment" to account for projected volume changes instead of the "behavioral offset," CMS acknowledged that volume increases result from many factors, including patient demand, rather than resulting from increases in unnecessary care.
- CMS further increased the CF consistent with AMA suggestions on several technical issues.
- Relative values for specific services were increased based on *NPRM* comments.
- CMS treated all relative values as "initial" for 1992 and allowed a 120-day period for public comment.
- Policies on global surgical packages were substantially improved.
- Medicare payments for drugs were limited to the average wholesale price, rather than to 85% of this price, as proposed in the *NPRM*.

Despite these changes, the AMA's House of Delegates called for substantial improvements in many important features of the payment system, including better data for the geographic indices and eliminating discriminatory payment limits for "new" physicians and for the services of assistants-at-surgery (see Chapter 11). To help identify problems arising during implementation of the new system, the AMA established a comprehensive program to monitor changes in patient access, physician practice patterns, and errors in carrier implementation, working closely with state and county medical societies.

During 1992, the first year of implementation, the AMA worked with CMS to make the system more responsive to physician needs:

- CMS enabled carriers to calculate transition amounts for about 50 new services that had dropped to full RBRVS amounts and increased about 150 technical components, which was consistent with the AMA's March 1992 comments on the 1991 Final Rule.
- CMS agreed to a grace period for the old system of visit codes, allowing physicians to use these codes for the first two months of 1992.
- CMS revised its definition of "new" patient for group practices to be consistent with the original intent of the CPT Editorial Panel. A "new patient" is one who has not been seen by a member of the group in the same specialty in the prior three-year period.
- CMS clarified several provisions of its global surgery, critical care, and other payment policies to reflect physician needs. Many of the problems identified in the first year of implementation have been resolved through either the legislative or the regulatory process, although the AMA continues to work with physicians and others in organized medicine for improvements to the Medicare RBRVS payment system.
- CMS converted the original Harvard scale to the same dollar scale as used for the practice expense and PLI RVUs, which aligned the three components on a common scale. It then assigned a total relative value of 1.00 to established patient office visit code 99213 and rescaled all other services accordingly. The common scale comprising the total RVUs for all services relative to 99213 is the complete Medicare RBRVS.

Legislative Activity

Several problems with Medicare's RBRVS payment system stemmed from statutory provisions of the Omnibus Budget Reconciliation Act (OBRA) of 1990 and could be corrected only through legislative action. These problems included payment reductions that further reduced Medicare payments to "new" physicians and eliminating payment for interpreting ECGs.

The AMA's legislative advocacy efforts led to the introduction in 1991 and 1992 of bills that would have restored payment for ECG interpretations, repealed payment reductions for new physicians, and required CMS to use the most recent data available for compiling the GPCIs. Many medical specialty societies supported these bills, even though their enactment would mean slight across-the-board reductions in physician payments pursuant to budget-neutrality requirements.

In August 1993, organized medicine won a substantial victory for physicians when provisions were included in OBRA 93 to restore payment for ECG interpretation and rescind payment reductions for "new" physicians. To ensure that these provisions were implemented in a budget-neutral manner, as required by OBRA 89, CMS reduced all RVUs in the 1994 payment schedule by 1.2%.

The Balanced Budget Act of 1997 gave physicians the right to contract privately with their Medicare patients for health care services, beginning in 1998. This new ability came with a heavy price, however. Physicians who contract with one or more of their Medicare patients for Medicare covered services may not bill the program for any Medicare services for two years. To correct this flaw, the AMA vigorously supported legislative proposals that would permit Medicare beneficiaries to pursue private contracts with their physicians, without isolating physicians from the Medicare program for two years.

Legislative Actions Impacting the Conversion Factor (CF)

The Consolidated Appropriations Resolution of 2003 (Pub. L. 108-7), signed into law on February 20, 2003, included language to allow CMS to correct mistakes in 1998 and 1999 SGR. This legislation resulted in a positive update in the 2003 CF of 1.6%, rather than the projected cut of 4.4%.

The MMA was signed by President George W. Bush on December 8, 2003. This legislation expanded Medicare to include prescription drug coverage. The law also included provisions related to the MFS. Most importantly, Congress halted another 4.5% cut to the 2004 CF, replacing it with 1.5% increases in both 2004 and 2005.

After a two-year respite following the MMA, the AMA faced a prospective cut to the CF in 2006 of 4.5%. The AMA's aggressive lobbying efforts, including an extensive grassroots network and broad media campaign, paid off in early 2006 as Congress passed the 2005 Deficit Reduction Act, which included a one-year freeze to the CF.

The AMA increased its lobbying efforts in 2006, knowing that January 1, 2007, would bring cuts to the CF of roughly 5% yet again. In addition to grassroots efforts and a media blitz, the AMA organized numerous physician fly-ins to Washington, DC. In deference to the collective voice of physicians, Congress passed the Tax Relief and Health Care Act of 2006. Not only did the new law contain a freeze to the CF for 2007, but it allowed a 1.5% increase for physicians who participated in a new quality reporting program.

On January 1, 2008, physicians faced a 10.1% reduction to the CF. Fortunately, the AMA succeeded in postponing this cut until July 1, 2008; Congress instead implemented a 0.5% increase to the Medicare CF from January 1 through June 30, 2008. By providing a temporary six-month reprieve from the 10% pay cut, the legislation passed by Congress left the outlook for the remainder of 2008 highly uncertain. The AMA mounted an aggressive effort in the beginning of 2008 to secure a longer-term solution to this continuing Medicare crisis. This hard work was rewarded through the passage of the Medicare Improvements for Patients and Providers Act of 2008 (MIPPA). MIPPA mandated an 18-month Medicare physician payment fix, stopping the 10.6% Medicare physician cut on July 1, 2008, and the 5.4% cut on January 1, 2009, continuing the June 2008 rates through December 31, 2008, and providing an additional 1.1% update for 2009. This triumph would not have been possible without the support of the AMA members.

The following legislative acts from 2009 through 2015, directly impacted the CFs and culminated with the repeal of the flawed Medicare sustainable growth rate (SGR) formula:

- **The Department of Defense Appropriation Act of 2010**—Signed into law on December 19, 2009; this Act applied a zero percent update to the 2010 CF from January 1, 2010, through February 28, 2010.
- **The Temporary Extension Act of 2010**—Signed into law on March 2, 2010; this Act further delayed the scheduled 21% Medicare payment reduction for physician services by applying a zero percent update to the 2010 CF from March 1-31, 2010.
- **The Continuing Extension Act of 2010**—Signed into law on April 15, 2010; this Act was the third time in 2010 that the 21% reduction to the CF was postponed. This Act extended the postponement of the reduction by again applying a zero percent update to the 2010 CF from April 1, 2010, through May 31, 2010.
- **The Preservation of Access to Care for Medicare Beneficiaries and Pension Relief Act of 2010**—Signed into law by President Barack Obama on June 25, 2010; this Act replaces the 21% Medicare physician payment cut to the 2010 CF that took effect June 1, 2010, with a retroactive 2.2% payment update to the 2010 CF from June 1, 2010, through November 30, 2010.
- **The Physician Payment and Therapy Relief Act of 2010**—Signed into law on November 30, 2010; this Act maintained the 2010 CF established by the Preservation of Access to Care for Medicare Beneficiaries and Pension

Relief Act from December 1-31, 2010. The cost ($1 billion over 10 years) of this one-month postponement will be paid for by changes in Medicare payment for outpatient therapy services.

- **The Medicare and Medicaid Extenders Act of 2010**—Signed into law December 15, 2010; this Act provides a one-year freeze on the Medicare CF for 2011 established by the Preservation of Access to Care for Medicare Beneficiaries and Pension Relief Act and avoided a 25% reduction to the CF that was set to take effect on January 1, 2011. Further provisions of this Act include: (1) extending the Work Geographic Practice Cost Indices (GPCI) floor of 1.00, created in the Medicare Prescription Drug, Improvement and Modernization Act of 2003 (MMA) through December 31, 2011; (2) extending the exceptions process for Medicare therapy caps through December 31, 2011; (3) extending the payment for the technical component of certain physician pathology services; and (4) extending the mental health add-on payment of 5% for certain mental health services through December 31, 2011.
- **The Temporary Payroll Tax Continuation Act of 2011**—Signed into law December 23, 2011; this Act delayed the 27.4% reduction to the CF that was to be implemented on January 1, 2012. Instead, a zero percent update to the CF and the other provisions listed above in the Medicare and Medicaid Extenders Act of 2010 were continued through February 29, 2012.
- **The Middle Class Tax Relief and Job Creation Act of 2012**—Signed into law on February 22, 2012; this Act further delayed the 27.4% reduction to the conversation factor and continued the zero percent update through December 31, 2012.
- **American Taxpayer Relief Act of 2012**—Signed into law on January 2, 2013; this Act prevented a scheduled payment cut of 25.5% from taking effect on January 1, 2013. This new law provides a zero percent update through December 31, 2013.
- **Pathway for SGR Reform**—Signed into law on December 26, 2013; this Act further delayed a scheduled payment cut of 24% and replaced it with a 0.5% increase until April 1, 2014.
- **Protecting Access to Medicare Act of 2014 (PAMA)**—On March 31, 2014, the Senate passed H.R. 4302, which postponed the imminent 24% Medicare physician payment cut for 12 months, until April 1, 2015. Section 220 of the Act established an annual target for reductions in the payment schedule expenditures that result from adjustments to relative values of misvalued codes. If the net reduction in expenditures for the year is equal to or greater than the target for the year, reduced expenditures attributable to such adjustments shall be redistributed in a budget-neutral manner within the payment schedule.
- **Achieving a Better Life Experience Act of 2014 (ABLE)**—Signed into law on December 19, 2014; this Act subsequently established the percent target recapture amount for the above provision in PAMA, setting a 1% target for reduced expenditures for CY 2016 and a 0.5% target for CYs 2017 and 2018. Physician payments must be reduced by the difference between the target for the year and the estimated net reduction in expenditures. For 2016 the target recapture amount produced a reduction to the CF of 0.77%. For 2017 the target recapture amount produced a reduction to the CF of 0.18%. For 2018 the target recapture amount produced a reduction to the CF of 0.09%.
- **Medicare Access and CHIP Reauthorization Act of 2015 (MACRA)**—Signed into law on April 16, 2015; this Act permanently repealed the flawed Medicare sustainable growth rate (SGR) formula, to provide positive annual payment updates of 0.5%, starting July 1, 2015, and lasting through 2019.

Following years of extensive advocacy by the AMA, Congress permanently repealed the SGR formula with MACRA. Passage of this historic legislation finally brought an end to an era of uncertainty for Medicare beneficiaries and their physicians.

The AMA believed that the previous short-term fixes to the annual CF exacerbated the problem. In 2005, the Congressional Budget Office (CBO) said that freezing physician payments would cost $48.6 billion over the next 10 years, and in 2011, the CBO estimated the cost at $245 billion. In March 2015, the CBO estimated the permanent repeal of the SGR to cost $141 billion.

Prior to the full repeal of the SGR, the AMA was also successful in advocating and achieving certain corrections within the SGR formula. These lobbying efforts resulted in CMS' determination to retroactively remove physician administered drugs from the SGR beginning January 1, 2010. In addition to the payments physicians receive for administering drugs, the cost of the drug itself had been included in the spending that is used to calculate the SGR. While the drug administration is a true physician service and should be included, the drug product is not a physician service and should not be included. As a result of CMS' agreement with the AMA's lobbying efforts to remove physician administered drugs from the SGR, the cost of eliminating the debt burden and freezing current payment rates fell by $50 billion over 10 years.

Reference

1. Todd JS. At last, a rational way to pay for physicians' services? *JAMA*. 1988;260:2439–2440.

Chapter 3

The Scope of Medicare's RBRVS Payment System

Medicare's resource-based relative value scale (RBRVS) physician payment system affects all services that were previously reimbursed according to the customary, prevailing, and reasonable (CPR) system. This means that all physicians' services are now paid according to a single cross-specialty RBRVS with payment determined by a single conversion factor (CF). The Medicare program applies the same payment schedule to every physician's service and every physician. (The only exception is anesthesia services, whose relative value guide is discussed in the Reference List section.) The payment system also encompasses the services of radiologists, replacing a separate payment schedule for radiology that began in 1989. Chapters 4 and 5 describe the Centers for Medicare & Medicaid Services' (CMS) process for integrating the radiology payment schedule into the cross-specialty RBRVS as required by the Omnibus Budget Reconciliation Act of 1989 (OBRA 89).

With the exception of physicians' services provided to Medicare patients enrolled in a Medicare HMO, the only physicians' services not included in the revision made to the payment system are some physicians' services provided in hospitals, skilled nursing facilities, comprehensive outpatient rehabilitation facilities, and some services provided by teaching physicians.

When a physician's service is defined as being part of the general patient care activities of a hospital or nursing facility, in contrast to a service provided for the benefit of an individual patient, that service is covered under Part A. When teaching physicians act as attending physicians for their patients, their direct patient care services are paid according to the Medicare payment schedule, but other services these physicians provide may be covered differently. Under the CPR, teaching physicians acting as attending physicians had separate customary charge profiles from other physicians, but these services are now all paid under the same payment schedule. CMS significantly revised the criteria for payment for services of teaching physicians, effective July 1, 1996. These rules and the special payment rules for "provider-based" physicians' services are covered in Chapter 11.

Medicare Part B encompasses a number of services in addition to those of physicians, and Medicare's RBRVS payment system applies to many of them. They include doctors of medicine (MDs) and osteopathy (DOs), optometrists, dentists, podiatrists, and chiropractors. Chapter 4 discusses assigning relative values for their services. Chapter 11 describes other features of Medicare's payment system, which may be especially relevant to their practices.

In addition to the non-MD/DO practitioners identified, Part B pays for the following categories of nonphysician practitioners' services:

- Physical and occupational therapists, speech language pathologists, and audiologists
- Physician assistants
- Nurse practitioners and clinical nurse specialists in certain settings
- Certified registered nurse anesthetists
- Certified nurse midwives
- Clinical psychologists
- Clinical social workers
- Registered dieticians

Each of these groups had its own coverage and payment rules under the CPR, based generally on payments for services provided by physicians, and this link continues under the RBRVS-based payment system's rules. Changes in physician payment, therefore, affect payment for nonphysicians' services. Chapter 11 describes the relationship between the Medicare RBRVS and the payment rates for each of the nonphysician categories and explains the standardization of payment practices for these services.

Frequently, nonphysicians provide their services "incident to," rather than independently of a physician's service. For example, "incident-to" services encompass services that nurses or physician assistants provide in a physician's office under the physician's supervision, such as an injection administered by a nurse. The CPR system did not require physicians to differentiate between claims for services they provided directly to patients and those that nonphysician personnel provided. The services of nonphysician personnel were compensated at the physician's CPR rate. The RBRVS-based payment system's rules do not affect "incident-to" services, which will continue to be reimbursed as if they have been furnished by physicians. In 1993, CMS broadened application of the "incident-to" provision to include services, such as physical exams, minor surgery, and setting simple fractures. This provision is discussed in more detail in Chapter 11. Payment rules were developed for drugs and supplies provided on an "incident-to" basis and are discussed in Chapter 11. For 2016, CMS amended the definition of "auxiliary personnel" who are permitted to provide "incident-to" services to exclude individuals who have been excluded from the Medicare program or have had their Medicare enrollment revoked. CMS also clarified that the physician (or other practitioner) directly supervising the auxiliary personnel does not have to be the same physician (or other practitioner) who is treating the patient more broadly, including adding a sentence to specify that only the physician (or other practitioner) that supervises the auxiliary personnel who provides incident-to services may bill Medicare Part B for those incident-to services.

The Balanced Budget Act of 1997 lifted some restrictions that were previously applicable to services furnished by certain categories of nonphysician practitioners. Effective January 1, 1998, nurse practitioners, clinical nurse specialists, and physician assistants are no longer required to practice under the direct, physical supervision of an MD/DO. Nurse practitioners and clinical nurse specialists may bill and receive direct payment from Medicare. Physician assistants maintain their relationships with physicians, although they may be considered independent contractors of physicians, which were not previously allowed. Payment continues to be made through the physician assistant's employer. Additional information on these provisions is available in Chapter 11.

The scope of the Medicare RBRVS payment system is quite comprehensive. The standardization of payment levels and diverse payment policies across different payment localities is an important, and often overlooked, aspect of the revisions made to Medicare physician payment. Chapters 4 through 8 describe the key components of this system, and Chapter 11 outlines many of the national policies enacted as part of the broad scope of the enabling legislation and regulations.

Part 2

Major Components of the RBRVS Payment System

From a practicing physician's perspective, the major components of Medicare's resource-based relative value scale (RBRVS) system include the following:

- Relative value scale
- Conversion factor
- Geographic adjustments
- Limits on balance billing

Although other aspects of the payment system figured prominently in the policy making process and are important to certain groups of physicians, these four components are the key determinants of a physician's Medicare payment for a service, comprising the "bread and butter" of the payment system.

Chapters 4, 5, and 6 discuss the physician work, the practice expense (PE) and professional liability insurance (PLI) components of the RBRVS; the actual relative values for each of these components are listed in Part 5. As Figure 4-1 illustrates, on average, the work component comprises 50.9% of the total relative value for a service, the practice expense component 44.8%, and the PLI component 4.3%.

The geographic practice cost indices (GPCIs) are described in Chapter 7, while a list of the indices appears in Part 5. Chapter 8 describes how the relative values, geographic adjustments, and conversion factors combine to determine the payment for a service in a locality. Part 2 concludes with Chapter 9, a description of the limits on balance billing.

Chapter 4

The Physician Work Component

Figure 4-1. Components of Medicare RBRVS

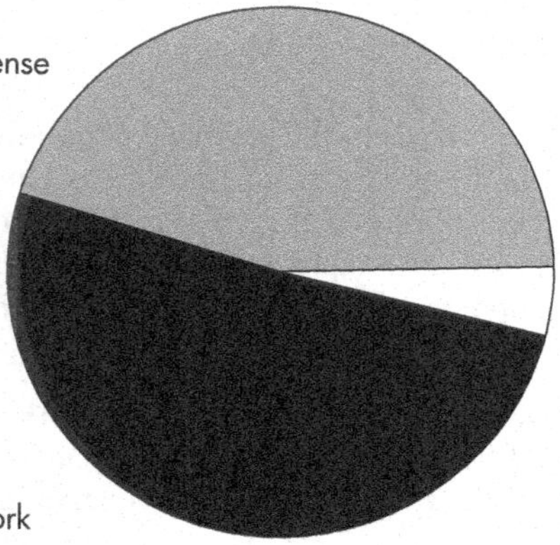

The greatest challenge in developing an RBRVS-based payment schedule was overcoming the lack of any available method or data for assigning specific values to physicians' work. The Harvard RBRVS study, therefore, played a critical role in the evolution of Medicare's payment system. Although the study contained several weaknesses, critical reviews of the data and methods concluded that it provided a reasonably valid basis for assigning relative values to the physician work component of the payment schedule. The physician work component now accounts for an average of 50.866% of the total relative value for a service because of the rebasing and revising of the Medicare economic index (MEI). (See Figure 4-1.) The MEI is an index intended to measure the annual growth in physicians' practice costs and general inflation in the cost of operating a medical practice. In 2011, the Centers for Medicare & Medicaid Services (CMS) announced their decision to rebase and revise the MEI to use a 2006 base year in place of a 2000 base year, which was the first time this was changed since 2004. CMS announced revisions to the MEI again in 2014. These changes were based on the recommendations of a technical advisory panel convened in 2012. These revisions included: moving payroll for nonphysician personnel who can bill independently from the PE portion to the physician work compensation (work) portion of the index; changing the price proxy for physician compensation to wages of professionals rather than of all private non-farm workers; creating new categories for clinical labor costs and for other professional services like billing; and changing the price proxy for fixed capital to business office space costs instead of residential costs. This change resulted in revised percentages for work, practice expense and professional liability insurance for the total relative value of a service, as listed below:

- Physician work percentage is 50.866%
- Practice expense percentage is 44.839%
- Professional liability insurance is 4.295%

Further, work relative value units (RVUs) were held constant, but these changes resulted in adjusted practice expense, and professional liability insurance RVUs to produce the appropriate balance in RVUs among components and payments.

The Harvard University School of Public Health, under a cooperative agreement CMS, conducted the study that led to the initial relative work values, which appeared in the November 1991 Final Rule. The core of Harvard's landmark study was a nationwide survey of physicians to determine the work involved in each of about 800 services. About 4300 relative value estimates of the nearly 6000 services included in the 1992 Medicare relative value scale (RVS) were based directly on findings from the Harvard RBRVS study. Besides the Harvard study, the 1992 Medicare RVS also relied on findings from CMS' "refinement process," which it developed in response to public comments on the 1992 values. This refinement process also has contributed to updating the payment schedule since 1993.

Finally, values for new and revised procedures in the American Medical Association's (AMA's) Current Procedural Terminology (CPT®) code set are also contained in the updated relative value scales for each year. To develop recommendations for CMS regarding relative values to be assigned to these new and revised codes, the AMA and the national medical specialty societies established the AMA/Specialty Society RVS Update Process.

This chapter describes the three major sources of the physician-work component relative values:

- The Harvard RBRVS study
- The 1992 RVS refinement process
- The AMA/Specialty Society RVS Update Process

The sources of relative values for anesthesiology services are discussed separately at the end of the chapter.

Harvard RBRVS Study

Phase I of the Harvard RBRVS study, completed in September 1988, provided relative value estimates for services provided by 18 medical and surgical specialties:

- Allergy and immunology
- Anesthesiology
- Dermatology
- Family practice
- General surgery
- Internal medicine
- Obstetrics and gynecology
- Ophthalmology
- Oral and maxillofacial surgery
- Orthopedic surgery
- Otolaryngology
- Pathology
- Pediatrics
- Psychiatry
- Radiology
- Rheumatology
- Thoracic and cardiovascular surgery
- Urology

Phase II, completed in December 1990, expanded the RBRVS to 15 additional specialties:

- Cardiology
- Emergency medicine
- Gastroenterology
- Hematology
- Infectious disease
- Nephrology
- Neurology
- Neurosurgery
- Nuclear medicine
- Oncology
- Osteopathic medicine
- Physical medicine and rehabilitation
- Plastic surgery
- Pulmonary medicine
- Radiation oncology

Phase II also reviewed four Phase I specialties (dermatology, ophthalmology, pathology, and psychiatry); expanded the study to include additional services provided by internists, general surgeons, and orthopedic surgeons; and included methodological refinements. Phase III, completed in August 1992, was primarily intended to revise problematic estimates from the earlier phases and expand the RBRVS to the remaining coded services. In particular, Phase III focused on a then-newly developed method for assigning relative value estimates to services closely related to those included in the Harvard study's national survey of physicians but that were not actually surveyed by the researchers.[1]

Phase IV, completed in July 1993, included research and policy recommendations regarding development of vignettes for services provided by two limited-license professions (optometry and podiatry) and one nonphysician profession (clinical psychology) and establishing work values for some psychology services; developing reference services for each major specialty; developing relative work values for services furnished on a "by-report" basis; and developing data to determine payment policies for multiple and bilateral procedures.[2]

Physician Work Defined

Before work on the RBRVS surveys could begin, the researchers needed to define physician work. The Harvard RBRVS study initially conceptualized work as the time a physician spends providing a service and the intensity with which the time is spent. To better define the non–time-related elements of work, the researchers interviewed physicians, including members of the study's Technical Consulting Groups (TCGs). The TCGs were small groups of physicians in each studied specialty who were nominated by national medical specialty societies in a process coordinated by the AMA. As a result of these interviews, the Harvard study defined the elements of physician work, as the following:

- Time required to perform the service
- Technical skill and physical effort
- Mental effort and judgment
- Psychological stress associated with the physician's concern about iatrogenic risk to the patient

This definition often caused confusion because some physicians thought that work RVUs are determined only by the time required to perform a service. Work RVUs are based on direct estimates of physician work; however, no separate measures of time are used. The Harvard study further divided physician work into the work involved before, during, and after a service.

The work involved in actually providing a service or performing a procedure is termed "intraservice work." For office visits, the intraservice period is defined as patient encounter time; for hospital visits, it is the time spent on the patient's floor; and for surgical procedures, it is the period from the initial incision to the closure of the incision (ie, "skin-to-skin" time).

Work prior to and following provision of a service, such as surgical preparation time, writing or reviewing records, or discussion with other physicians, is referred to as "preservice and postservice work." When preservice, intraservice, and postservice work are combined, the result is referred to as the "total work" involved in a service. For surgical procedures, the total work period is the same as the global surgical period, including recovery-room time, normal postoperative hospital care, and office visits after discharge, as well as preoperative and intraoperative work.

Although the Harvard study defined physician work according to these distinct components, it did not measure work in this manner. Earlier attempts to separately measure time and intensity had produced unsatisfactory results. Instead, the study directly measured the work involved in a service. The RBRVS study's definition of physician work is important because data from this study are the major basis for the physician work component of the Medicare payment schedule. A service on the schedule with more physician work–RVUs than another means that the former service involves more time, skill, effort, judgment, and stress than the latter. Efforts to refine and update the RBRVS have employed the same definition of work as the Harvard study.

Having defined and separated work into its component parts, the researchers then ensured that all surveyed physicians had the same basic service in mind when rating the work for value. The coding system used in the RBRVS is the AMA's CPT coding system. To allow physicians to rate the work of a service, the TCGs for each specialty developed "vignettes" for each coded service included in the survey of that specialty. In many cases, the vignette came directly from the CPT code, as in the following description (as described in CPT 1987) for CPT code 63017, a service surveyed for orthopedic surgery:

Laminectomy for decompression of spinal cord and/or cauda equina, more than two segments; lumbar.

In other cases, particularly for visits and consultations, the TCGs designed vignettes to be representative of an average patient for the particular service being rated by that specialty. For these services, the development of a vignette ensured that each surveyed physician had the same basic service in mind. For example, the neurology vignette for CPT code 99160 (this code was replaced by CPT code 99291 in CPT 1992) read:

Initial hour of critical care in the ICU (intensive care unit) for a 65-year-old male who presents with a fever and status epilepticus.

National Survey

Once the TCGs agreed on the descriptions, Harvard launched its national survey of physician work. In Phase I, researchers completed nearly 2000 telephone interviews with physicians in 18 specialties. In Phase II, they completed about 1900 interviews with physicians in 15 additional specialties.

To obtain work ratings for each of the vignettes, the study used a technique known as "magnitude estimation." Surveyed physicians were asked to use a particular service as a standard and to rate the intraservice work of about 25 other services relative to that standard.

The standard in each specialty was assigned an intraservice work value of 100. For a vignette that involved twice as much intraservice work as the standard, physicians were instructed to assign an intraservice work value of 200. Physicians would assign a value of 50 to a vignette that involved half as much intraservice work as the standard. Using this magnitude estimation method, physicians in each specialty assigned intraservice work relative values to all the vignettes on the survey for their specialty.

Cross-Specialty Process

Harvard researchers used the national survey to develop a relative value scale (RVS) for each specialty included in the study. The second step in constructing the RBRVS linked all of these specialty-specific scales onto a single scale.

The researchers organized cross-specialty panels to complete the second step. Panels consisted of about 10 physicians, each from a different specialty. The panel members, selected from the TCGs, considered potential specialty-to-specialty links, such as a single service that physicians in two or more different specialties were likely to provide. For example, the panelists determined that the following service had the same value in several different specialties:

Decompression of carpal tunnel in a 48-year-old female, unilateral, ambulatory surgery unit.

The panels also considered pairs of different services, which are typically performed by physicians in different specialties but appeared to involve equal amounts of work.

The following services, for example, served as a link between two specialties:

In nephrology, 'Insertion of a double-lumen femoral vein cannula for hemodialysis'; and, in general surgery, 'Excisional breast biopsy of a 2-centimeter lesion.'

The panels identified at least several specialty-to-specialty links for each of the studied specialties. Researchers then statistically analyzed the work ratings of the links obtained from the national survey for each specialty. This process linked all the specialty-specific scales to a common cross-specialty scale, while preserving, to the extent possible, the within specialty relationships of one service to another.

The cross-specialty process may have determined, for example, that two unilateral surgical procedures performed by different specialties, rated 80 and 120 in their respective specialty surveys, represented equal work. As a result, both might have been valued at 100 on the common scale. Assuming the magnitude estimation surveys for both services had rated the procedures as requiring 50% more work when done bilaterally, one would have been rated at 120, the other at 180 on their respective specialty scales. On the common scale, however, both bilateral procedures would be assigned a value of 150, preserving the values at 50% more than the unilateral procedures.

Preservice and Postservice Work

The RBRVS study employed several different methods to assign relative values to the preservice and postservice work involved in the surveyed services, depending on the type of service. Survey respondents rated both the intraservice work and the total work for visits and consultations in Phase II, for example, the difference being preservice and postservice work. For invasive procedures, surgeons were surveyed about the preservice and postservice time of specific components of procedures. For instance, general surgeons were surveyed about the time and work involved in a "hospital visit, three days post uncomplicated cholecystectomy with common bile duct exploration." Researchers then derived an "intensity per unit of time" factor from the survey data and used it to estimate preservice and postservice work from data on preservice and postservice time.

Assigning RVUs to Nonsurveyed Services

The researchers surveyed physicians about the work involved in 800 services and extrapolated work values for the remaining services. The extrapolation method grouped services into "families." For example, all coded services involving coronary artery bypass surgery became a family, as did all new patient office visits. The researchers theorized that the differences in average charges for services within a family would approximate the differences in physician work. Thus, if a nonsurveyed service in a family had a 20% higher average charge than the surveyed service, then the physician work involved in the former should be 20% higher than the latter. In practice, however, the extrapolation method often produced RVUs that seemed incongruous or paradoxical.

In Phase III of the study, the researchers developed a new extrapolation method using small groups of physicians. These groups established relationships between the surveyed and nonsurveyed services and assigned RVUs to them. The small-group process was also used to extend the RBRVS beyond the families of the surveyed services.

Phase IV, released in summer 1993, used the same small-group process to estimate work values for 227 by-report services. A review process was developed for 162 of these services, which previously had been studied in Phase III. Members of the TCG and assessment panels from Phase III were reassembled, and panelists reevaluated the existing work estimates. Researchers used a single survey of the assessment panels for each specialty for the review, which followed a two-step process: ranking the services by total and intraservice work, and then reviewing these values in the context of the specialty's reference services and suggesting changes where necessary. These assessments were compared with the original estimates of intraservice and total-service work from Phase III. Work value recommendations were made for 145 of the procedures, and these showed a high level of agreement with Phase III values. For services that were not previously studied, panelists rated the work of each service using magnitude estimation with multiple reference services. A total of 34 by-report services for oral and maxillofacial surgery, the major specialty studied, were reviewed.

Reviews of the RBRVS Study

After the final report of Phase I was released in September 1988, the AMA conducted an in-depth evaluation of the study's methods and results and contracted with the Consolidated Consulting Group, Inc., for an independent evaluation. The Physician Payment Review Commission (PPRC) also evaluated the Phase I results, as did CMS, which had provided the principal funding for the study.

These evaluations identified many flaws in the study, such as the inaccurate measurement of practice costs, but the reviewers' conclusions about the core of the study—measuring physicians' intraservice work—were very positive. The Consolidated Consulting Group report on the study concluded:

The RBRVS study's major effort—the measurement of physicians' intraservice work (ie, the work needed to perform specific services and procedures)—was successful. The RBRVS researchers . . . obtained generally accurate, reliable and consistent rankings of relative work from each of

18 specialties for about 22 representative services. These separate specialty-specific rankings were also successfully linked into a common scale. These results show that it is feasible to develop a work scale built on physicians' views about their work.

As a result of these reviews, the legislation that created the new Medicare payment system did not reflect two components of the RBRVS study: the study's method of assigning practice cost RVUs and its specialty training cost component. For the other components, the AMA and PPRC assessments recommended specific areas that needed refinement and correction.

Many of the national medical specialty societies also evaluated the study's data and results for their specialty's services. As a result, several societies requested that the Harvard researchers conduct a partial or complete restudy of their specialty's services. Some specialties turned to groups other than Harvard to reevaluate their services. For example, a group of specialty societies representing cardiovascular and thoracic surgeons jointly contracted with the consulting firm of Abt Associates for a separate study for their specialty. Finally, many of the specialty societies and individual physicians, as well as the AMA, commented on the work RVUs published in the *Notice of Proposed Rulemaking* (*NPRM*) and the November 1991 Final Rule.

The 1992 RVS Refinement Process

The 1992 Medicare RVS included RVUs for about 6000 CPT-coded services. Of these, about 1900 appeared for the first time in the 1991 Final Rule. Because there had been no opportunity for public review and comment on the RVUs for services that were excluded from the model payment schedule or the *NPRM*, all of the work RVUs in the 1991 Final Rule were published as "initial" RVUs.

In addition, the study was not completed in time for the January 1 implementation of the new system, although results for many of the services included in Phase III of the study had already been provided to CMS. Therefore, CMS established a process involving its carrier medical directors (CMDs) to assign work RVUs to about 800 services for which data were not available from the Harvard study. CMS also received comments on about 1000 proposed work RVUs included in the *NPRM* and used CMDs to review these RVUs prior to publishing the final 1992 RVS.

In the 1991 Final Rule, CMS was careful to state that the CMD process was not intended to be a short-term revision of the Harvard RBRVS. Instead, CMS used the process to assign RVUs to low-volume services, new services, and others that Harvard did not provide, and to refine some unreasonable estimates. For example, four-graft coronary artery bypass graft RVUs was adjusted to be greater than three-graft surgery.

CMS provided a 120-day period for public comment on the RVUs published in this first RBRVS Final Rule. During the comment period, CMS received about 7500 comments on the RVUs assigned to about 1000 services. Some specialty societies requested that CMS provide guidelines on how to prepare the comments, emphasizing the need for clinical arguments to support the comments.

In responding to the comments, CMS indicated that it considered principally those comments that followed its guidelines, rather than general comments regarding payment reductions. CMS also expanded its CMD process and developed an RVS refinement process, which involved 24 review panels, each with 13 members. Panel members included 33 CMDs and 127 physicians nominated by 42 specialty societies. The multidisciplinary panels included physicians from the specialty or specialties that most frequently provide the service, physicians in related specialties, primary care physicians, and CMDs.

The objective of the review process was to allow four different panels to review each of the services. The panels' ratings of physician work were statistically analyzed to assess the consistency of ratings across the four groups.

The panels reviewed the work RVUs assigned to 791 codes. The results from Phase III were used as one source of relevant data. CMS retained the 1992 value for about half of these codes in the 1993 Medicare RVS. The refinement process resulted in higher values for about 360 codes and lower values for 35 codes. Notable among the code groups increased by the refinement process were the following:

- Hernia repair
- Home visits
- Obstetrical care
- Electroencephalogram (EEG) and EEG monitoring
- Nursing facility care
- Coronary artery bypass graft surgery
- Removal of larynx

CMS also reviewed 120 codes published in the 1992 *Final Notice* as interim values and subject to comment in 1993. A multispecialty panel of physicians reviewed 42 of these codes and made final RVU determinations by comparing the interim values to "reference services" whose work RVUs had not been challenged in the comment process.

The 1992 RVU Refinement of Evaluation and Management Codes

Work RVUs were reviewed by CMS for the CPT evaluation and management codes for visit and consultation services, which had been introduced in *CPT 1992*. Conflicting comments on the values were made by various specialty societies. Some specialties argued that the values for the lower levels of service should have been increased to reflect higher intensity of service. Others argued that the higher levels of service failed to adequately reflect the greater intensity of providing these services. Still others argued for a more linear progression between levels 4 and 5 of each code group. In the 1992 *Final Notice*, CMS reported that the physician panel it convened on this issue could not reach a consensus. However, using data from Phase III, it increased mid- to upper- level visits to reflect a more linear progression of work and reduced some lower levels. This process also reduced the values of the follow-up inpatient consultation codes.

Work RVUs for Medicare Noncovered Services

For the 1995 RVS, as in previous years, CMS convened multispecialty panels of physicians to assist in the refinement process. The agency established final values for several carrier-priced and Medicare noncovered services for which it previously had published proposed values. CMS relied strongly on the AMA/Specialty Society RVS Update Committee's recommendations in establishing proposed and final values, as it has each year when developing the payment schedule.

In the Final Rule published on December 1, 2006, CMS accepted the AMA's and RUC's recommendation for noncovered and bundled services. CMS recognizes that the Medicare RBRVS is used widely now by private payers, Medicaid, and workers' compensation plans to determine physician payment. See Chapter 13 for more information related to the non-Medicare use of the RBRVS.

Completion of the Medicare RBRVS

In the 1994 Final Rule, CMS stated that with assignment of work RVUs for the 1995 RVS, it considered the RBRVS payment schedule to be "essentially" complete. Work relative value units were assigned to hundreds of codes that had been previously carrier-priced, for many commonly furnished services that were not covered by Medicare but paid by other payers, and for all pediatric services.

A mechanism to update the RBRVS on an ongoing basis was included as part of the Omnibus Budget Reconciliation Act of 1989 (OBRA 89). The statute requires that CMS conduct a comprehensive review of work relative values every five years. As part of this review process, all work RVUs on the 1995 and 2000 RVS were open for public comment. In the November 2004 Final Rule, CMS again opened the 2005 RVS for public comment for 60 days. The five-year review process and CMS' decisions are summarized later in this chapter.

The AMA/Specialty Society RVS Update Process[3]

Besides refinements to correct errors in the initial RVUs, the Medicare RVS also must be updated to reflect changes in practice and technology. The AMA updates the CPT coding system annually under an agreement with CMS to reflect such changes. The AMA maintains the coding system through the CPT Editorial Panel. Annual updates to the physician work relative values are based on recommendations from a committee involving the AMA and national medical specialty societies. The AMA/Specialty RVS Update Committee (RUC) was formed in 1991 to make recommendations to CMS on the relative values assigned to new or revised codes in CPT.

The core of the RVS Update Process is the RUC. During its first year, RUC established procedures for specialty societies to reconcile their different viewpoints and agree on relative value recommendations. RUC has now completed 31 cycles of recommendations for updating the physician work component of the RBRVS, demonstrating its commitment to developing objective measures of physician work for new and revised CPT codes. RUC has recently embarked on establishing recommendations on direct practice expense inputs for new and revised codes.

The AMA believes that updating and maintaining the Medicare RVS is a clinical and scientific activity that must remain in the hands of the medical profession and regards RUC as the principal vehicle for refining the work and practice expense components of the RBRVS. From the AMA's perspective, RUC provides a vital opportunity for the medical profession to continue to shape its own payment environment. For this reason, the AMA has strongly advocated that Medicare adopt RUC's recommendations.

Structure and Process

RUC represents the entire medical profession, with 22 of its 32 members appointed by major national specialty societies, including those recognized by the American Board of Medical Specialties, those with a large percentage of physicians in patient care, and those that account for high percentages of Medicare expenditures. Four seats rotate on a two-year basis, with one seat reserved for a primary care representative, two reserved for internal medicine subspecialty and one for any other specialty society not a member of RUC, except internal medicine subspecialties or primary care representatives. The RUC Chair, the co-chair of the RUC HCPAC Review Board (an advisory committee representing non-MD/DO health professionals); the chair of the Practice Expense Subcommittee; and representatives of the American Medical Association, American Osteopathic Association, and CPT Editorial Panel hold the remaining six seats.

The major source of specialty input for the updating process is RUC's Advisory Committee, which is open to all 124 specialty societies in the AMA House of Delegates. Specialty societies that are not in the House of Delegates also may be invited to participate in developing relative values for coding changes of particular relevance to their members. Advisory Committee members designate an *RVS Committee* for their specialty, which is responsible for generating relative value recommendations using a survey method developed by RUC. Advisors attend RUC meetings and present their societies' recommendations, which RUC evaluates. Specialties represented on both RUC and the Advisory Committee are required to appoint different physicians to each committee to distinguish the role of advocate from that of evaluator.

RUC refers procedural and methodological issues to the Research Subcommittee, which is composed of about one-third the members of the full RUC. This subcommittee's principal responsibility is to develop and refine RUC's methods and processes.

RUC also established the Practice Expense Subcommittee to examine the many issues relating to the development of practice expense relative values. This subcommittee also is composed of one-third of the members of the full RUC.

In 1999, RUC formed the Practice Expense Advisory Committee (PEAC) to review and suggest changes in the direct practice expense data, which was used to create practice expense relative values. The PEAC has completed its refinement activities. In 2005, RUC formed an ad hoc committee, the Practice Expense Review Committee (PERC) that reviewed any refinement issues that arose. This group assisted RUC in its review of practice expense inputs for new and revised codes. This group has since been disbanded, and RUC is now assisted by the Practice Expense (PE) Subcommittee for all practice expense refinement issues, as well as review of practice expense inputs for new, revised, and potentially misvalued codes.

The Administrative Subcommittee also includes one-third of RUC members and is primarily charged with the maintenance of the committee's procedural issues.

In 1992, the AMA recommended that a Health Care Professionals Advisory Committee (HCPAC) be established to allow for participation of limited license practitioners and allied health professionals in both RUC and CPT processes. All of these professionals use CPT to report the services they provide independently to Medicare patients, and they are paid for these services based on the RBRVS Medicare Physician Payment Schedule (MFS). Organizations representing physician assistants, nurses, occupational and physical therapists, optometrists, podiatrists, psychologists, registered dietitians, social workers, chiropractors, audiologists, and speech pathologists have been invited to nominate representatives to the CPT and RUC HCPACs. The CPT HCPAC fosters participation in and solicits comments from these professional organizations in coding changes affecting their members, while RUC HCPAC allows those organizations to participate in developing relative values for new and revised codes within their scope of practice.

To facilitate the decision-making process on issues of concern to both MDs/DOs and non-MDs/DOs, CPT and RUC HCPAC Review Boards were also formed. The review boards bring MDs/DOs and non-MDs/DOs together to discuss coding issues and relative value proposals. The RUC HCPAC Review Board comprises all 12 members of the current RUC HCPAC and three RUC members. For codes used by both MDs/DOs and non-MDs/DOs, the HCPAC Review Board acts much like a RUC facilitation committee. For codes used only by non-MDs/DOs, the RUC HCPAC Review Board replaces RUC as the body responsible for developing recommendations for CMS.

The Professional Liability Insurance (PLI) Workgroup was created in 2002 to review and suggest refinements to the PLI relative value methodology.

In 2006, RUC formed the Relativity Assessment Workgroup (formerly known as the Five-Year Identification Workgroup) to identify potentially misvalued services using objective mechanisms for reevaluation during the upcoming Five-Year Review. However, RUC determined in 2008 that this identification and review of potentially misvalued services will be conducted on an ongoing basis. The need for objective review of potential misvaluation has been a priority of RUC, CMS, and MedPAC. The Relativity Assessment Workgroup (RAW) has implemented a number of screens to identify potentially misvalued codes, including: site-of-service anomalies, high intensity anomalies, high-volume growth, CMS-identified high-volume growth, services surveyed by one specialty and now performed by a different specialty, Harvard-valued codes, CMS/Other source codes, codes inherently performed together, services with low-work RVUs but are high volume based on Medicare claims data, services with low-work RVUs that are commonly billed with multiple units in a single encounter, services on the Multi-Specialty Points of Comparison List, high-expenditure procedural codes, practice expense services in which the PE times are not based on physician-time assumptions, services with more pre-service time than the longest standardized pre-service package, services with more than six postoperative visits, services with a high-level evaluation and management (E/M) service included in the global period, services with a 000-day global period but reported with an E/M service, services with a negative intensity work per unit of time (IWPUT), contractor-priced services with high volume, services on the CPT modifier 51 exempt list, and services with more than one median unit of service reported and a direct PE supply item unit cost greater than $100 based on Medicare utilization. The Workgroup is also charged with developing and maintaining processes associated with the identification and reconsideration of the value of "new technology" services. To date, the Workgroup has identified 2,638 codes for review, of which 2,580 have been reviewed by RUC. RUC's efforts for years 2009–2022 have resulted in more than $5 billion in redistribution annually within the MFS.

Facilitation Committees are established as needed during RUC meetings to resolve differences of opinion about relative value recommendations before they are submitted to CMS.

Beginning with the release of the 2014 MFS in November 2013, RUC began publishing voting records of the RUC and RUC meeting minutes. The voting record will contain the RUC's aggregate vote for each issue.

RUC closely coordinates its annual cycle for developing recommendations with the CPT Editorial Panel's schedule for annual code revisions and with CMS' annual updates to the Medicare payment schedule.

The RUC process for developing relative value recommendations is as follows:

Step 1 The CPT Editorial Panel transmits its new and revised codes to RUC staff, which then prepares a "Level of Interest" form. The form summarizes the Panel's coding actions.

Step 2 Members of RUC and HCPAC Advisory Committee review the summary and indicate their societies' level of interest in developing a relative value recommendation. The societies have several options. They can:

A. Survey their members to obtain data on the amount of work involved in a service and develop recommendations based on the survey results.
B. Comment in writing on recommendations developed by other societies.
C. Decide, in the case of revised codes, that the coding change requires no action because it does not significantly alter the nature of the service.
D. Take no action because the codes are not used by physicians in their specialty.

Step 3 AMA staff develops survey instruments for the specialty societies. The specialty societies are required to survey at least 30 practicing physicians. For services with more than 100,000 claims, 50 surveys must be collected. For those with more than 1 million in claims, at least 75 physicians must respond. RUC survey instrument asks physicians to use a list of 10 to 20 services as reference points that have been selected by the specialty RVS committee.

Physicians receiving the survey are asked to evaluate the work involved in the new or revised code relative to the reference points. The survey data may be augmented by analysis of Medicare claims data and information from other studies of the procedure, such as the Harvard RBRVS study.

Step 4 The specialty RVS committees conduct the surveys, review the results, and prepare their recommendations to RUC. When two or more societies are involved in developing recommendations, RUC encourages them to coordinate their survey procedures and develop a consensus recommendation. The written recommendations are disseminated to RUC before the meeting.

Step 5 The specialty advisors present the recommendations at RUC meeting. The Advisory Committee members' presentations are followed by a thorough question-and-answer period during which the advisors must defend every aspect of their proposal(s).

Step 6 RUC may decide to adopt a specialty society's recommendation, refer it back to the specialty society, or modify it before submitting it to CMS. Final recommendations to CMS must be adopted by a two-thirds majority of RUC members. Recommendations that require additional evaluation by RUC are referred to a Facilitation Committee.

Step 7 RUC's recommendations are forwarded to CMS approximately one month after every RUC meeting.

Step 8 The MFS, which includes CMS' review of RUC recommendations, is published each July in the proposed rulemaking and is open for public comment. The final values are published each November in the Final Rule and are implemented each January 1, thereafter.

Updating Work Relative Values

Each year RUC submits recommendations to CMS for physician work relative values based on CPT coding changes to be included in the Medicare payment schedule. Over the last 31 years, RUC has reviewed nearly all services paid through the MFS, accounting for 98% of spending. In addition, RUC submitted hundreds of recommendations to CMS for contractor-priced or noncovered services, including preventive medicine services. Each year CMS has relied heavily upon these recommendations when establishing interim values for new and revised CPT codes. Key recommendations for each annual cycle are briefly summarized below.

RUC submitted its first recommendations to CMS in July 1992, based on 1993 CPT coding changes, to be included in the 1993 Medicare payment schedule. The recommendations addressed physician work relative values for new and revised codes spanning the entire range of physician services, including orthopedic trauma care; a new section of CPT for hospital observation care; critical care; cardiology; urology; and coronary artery bypass surgery.

RUC's second set of recommendations, included in the 1994 Medicare RVS, again encompassed coding changes for a wide range of physician services. These recommendations included physician work values for new primary care codes for prolonged physician services and care plan oversight; the initial recommendations for pediatric services, including new codes for neonatal intensive care; pediatric surgery; hospital observation care; general surgery; skull-based surgery; and magnetic resonance angiography.

In the November 1993 Final Rule, CMS stated that it would defer establishing relative values for pediatric services, transplant services, and other carrier-priced and noncovered services until RUC evaluated these codes and developed recommendations. During 1994, much of RUC's work was devoted to developing recommendations for these codes. In

May 1994, relative value recommendations were submitted for these services, including preventive medicine, newborn care, transplant surgery, and pediatric neurosurgery codes.

The third cycle of RUC recommendations for the 1995 Medicare RVS included values for orthopedic, esophageal, rectal, liver, bile duct, and endocrine surgery; neurology; and monthly end-stage renal disease. In addition, the RUC HCPAC Review Board developed its first set of work relative values, covering services for physical medicine and rehabilitation.

As previously discussed, OBRA 89 mandated that CMS conduct a comprehensive review of the RBRVS relative values on a five-year rolling basis. As part of this five-year review, RUC submitted work RVU recommendations for more than 1000 individual codes in September 1995. RUC activities related to this comprehensive review are detailed in the following section.

As a result of the Five-Year Review, RUC submitted relatively fewer recommendations for the 1996 RVS. RUC's relative value recommendations were reflected in the 1996 RVS for new CPT codes for trauma care and for new and revised codes for spinal procedures. Very few CPT coding changes were submitted for RUC's consideration for 1997. Extensive work RVU changes were implemented for the 1997 RVS, however, because of the five-year review. These changes are described in the "Five-Year Review" section.

RUC submitted its sixth year of work relative value recommendations for new and revised CPT codes in May 1997. The submission included recommendations on more than 200 CPT codes, including home care visits, observation same-day discharge services, various laparoscopic procedures, percutaneous abscess drainage procedures, and PET myocardial perfusion imaging. RUC also submitted recommendations for new CPT codes proposed by the American Academy of Pediatrics. The new codes better describe services provided to children, including conscious sedation, pediatric cardiac catheterization, and attendance at delivery. In addition, the RUC HCPAC Review Board developed recommendations in several areas, including paring, cutting, and trimming of nails; and occupational and physical therapy evaluation services.

RUC submitted work relative values for new and revised CPT codes in May of 1998, completing its seventh year of recommendations. RUC and the national medical specialty societies reviewed over 298 coding changes for CPT 1999 and submitted more than 100 recommendations to CMS. The remainder of the codes reviewed was editorial revisions or deletions. The recommendations included additions and revisions to the following services: inpatient and outpatient psychotherapy, hallux rigidus correction with cheilectomy, breast reconstruction, and radiologic examination of the knee. In addition, the RUC HCPAC Review Board also developed one recommendation for manual manipulative therapy techniques for CPT 1999.

In May 1999, RUC submitted its eighth year of work relative value recommendations to CMS. This year also marked the first submission of direct practice expense inputs (clinical staff, supplies, and equipment) to CMS for use in developing practice expense relative values for new and revised CPT codes. There were more than 300 coding changes for CPT 2000; however, most were considered editorial in nature or reflected laboratory services included on the Medicare clinical laboratory payment schedule. RUC submitted recommendations for more than 100 new and revised CPT codes, including: critical care, deep brain stimulation, spine injection procedures, integumentary system repair, and laparoscopic urological procedures.

RUC forwarded recommendations on 224 codes in May 2000 in its ninth submission of annual new and revised code recommendations. The major issues reviewed in this cycle included: GI endoscopy procedures; MRI procedures; anesthesia services; stereotactic breast biopsy; and endovascular graft for abdominal aortic aneurism. RUC also reviewed public comments and submitted recommendations on nearly 900 codes as part of the second five-year review of the RBRVS. This project is discussed in more detail in the next section.

In May 2001, RUC submitted its 10th year of work relative value recommendations to CMS. RUC reviewed 314 codes, including many codes describing anesthesia services, hand surgery, pediatric surgery, and urological procedures.

In May 2002, RUC submitted work relative value units and direct practice expense inputs for 350 new and revised CPT 2003 codes. This represented the 11th year of relative value submissions.

In May 2003, RUC submitted work and practice expense recommendations for 162 CPT codes, including a new CPT section for central venous procedures, fetal surgery, and a number of new vascular surgery services.

In May and October 2004, RUC submitted work relative values and direct practice expense inputs recommendations for 149 new/revised CPT codes, including bronchoscopy, carotid stenting, transplantation services, and flow cytometry. RUC also submitted suggestions regarding PLI relative value crosswalks for new CPT codes.

RUC, in its 14th year of existence, submitted work relative value recommendations, direct practice expense inputs, and PLI crosswalks for 283 new and revised CPT codes. The major issues reviewed in this cycle included: free skin grafts, nursing facility services, domiciliary care services, and drug administration. In addition, RUC reviewed public comments and made recommendations to over 700 existing procedures in the third Five-Year Review of the RBRVS. Additional discussion of the third Five-Year Review follows on page 37.

In May and October 2006, RUC submitted recommendations regarding the work, practice expense, and professional liability insurance information associated with 254 new and revised CPT codes. The major issues addressed in this cycle, include Mohs surgery, destruction of lesions, and various vascular surgery procedures. In addition, CMS accepted RUC's and the AMA's recommendation to publish RUC recommended values for 35 noncovered and bundled services in October 2006.

In May and October 2007, in its 16th submission of annual new and revised code recommendations, RUC forwarded recommendations on 266 codes. RUC reviewed many issues in 2007, including the clarification of the fracture treatment codes, alcohol/drug screening intervention, smoking cessation, telephone calls, and new hospital visits for infants aged 28 days or younger.

In its 17th year, RUC submitted work relative value recommendations, direct practice expense inputs, and PLI crosswalks for 233 new and revised CPT codes. This submission included recommendations for adult and pediatric end-stage renal disease services, as well as pediatric intensive care services. RUC also made recommendations on 204 potentially misvalued services as identified by RUC's RAW.

In May 2009, RUC forwarded recommendations on 216 CPT codes in its 18th submission of new and revised codes recommendations. In addition, RUC also made recommendations on 209 misvalued services as identified by RUC's RAW. This submission included recommendations for radical resection of soft tissue and bone tumor, myocardial perfusion, and urodynamic studies.

RUC in its 19th year submitted work relative value recommendations, direct practice expense input recommendations and PLI crosswalks for 204 new and revised CPT codes. This submission included recommendations for CT of the abdomen and pelvis, pathology consultation, diagnostic cardiac catheterization, excision and debridement, endovascular revascularization and subsequent observation visits. RUC also made recommendations on 88 potentially misvalued services as identified by RUC's RAW.

In May 2011, RUC submitted work relative value recommendations, direct practice expense input recommendations and PLI crosswalks for 252 new and revised CPT codes. More than 50% of the CPT code revisions for CPT 2012 originated from either the 4th Five-Year Review process or the potentially misvalued services process. This submission included recommendations for injection procedure for sacroiliac joint, molecular pathology services, pulmonary function testing and treatment of retinal lesion or choroid.

In May 2012, RUC submitted work relative value recommendations, direct practice expense input recommendations and PLI crosswalks for 204 new and revised CPT codes. Nearly 75% of the CPT code revisions for CPT 2013 originated from the potentially misvalued services process. This submission included recommendations for complex chronic care coordination (CCCC) services, transitional care management (TCM) services, psychotherapy and molecular pathology. CMS modified the interim work valuation for 17 CPT 2013 new/revised codes, by means of recommendations of the CMS organized refinement panel and comments submitted by the public to support RUC's data. Implementation of these new values for psychotherapy and other services increased the percentage or RUC 2013 work values accepted to 90%.

In November 2013, CMS announced acceptance of all RUC recommendations for psychotherapy services, leading to $150 million in improved payments for these services each year. Depending upon the individual physician's mix of services, Psychiatry, on average, will experience a six percent increase in Medicare payments. This results from a three-year effort by the CPT Editorial Panel, RUC, and organizations representing individuals providing mental health services to redefine and revalue these critical services. The CPT coding system implemented new codes on January 1, 2013. Some were surveyed in 2012, and others in 2013. CMS waited to implement the RUC recommendations for the entire family of codes as a group, for 2014.

In addition to the acceptance of the psychotherapy services, CMS reversed its positions on several other services (implemented in 2013) and will now accept the original RUC recommendations. As a result, the RUC acceptance rate for individual services for 2013 increased from 85% to 90%.

The CPT 2014 code set and the 2014 MFS included major changes for upper gastrointestinal (GI) endoscopy procedures. RUC reviewed and submitted recommendations for 65 individual upper GI endoscopy codes. Unfortunately, CMS only accepted 22 (34%) of these specific recommendations. CMS adopted the RUC-recommended time for GI endoscopy but felt that the intensity of the services was overstated and indicated that there is no differentiation in the intensity of the services within gastroenterology. CMS failed to recognize the appropriate coding and payment for immunohistochemistry, establishing payment per specimen, rather than per slide as defined by the CPT code set and valued by RUC. CMS accepted nearly 90% of the non-GI–related services.

In May 2014, RUC submitted work relative value recommendations, direct PE input recommendations, and PLI crosswalks for 350 new, revised or potentially misvalued CPT codes. This submission included recommendations for chronic care management services and lower GI endoscopy services. The chronic care management services recommendation was the result of a multi-year effort by the AMA, CPT Editorial Panel, RUC, and several national medical specialty societies. Starting on January 1, 2015, CMS established a payment rate of $42.91 for new CPT code 99490, which can be billed up to once per month per qualified patient. By adopting this RUC proposal, CMS is taking steps to improve Medicare beneficiaries' access to primary care.

In its 25th year, RUC submitted work relative value and direct PE input recommendations and PLI crosswalks for 278 new, revised, and potentially misvalued services. This submission for the 2016 MFS included recommendations for genitourinary catheter procedures, paravertebral block injection services, and percutaneous biliary procedures.

For CPT 2017, RUC submitted work relative value and direct PE input recommendations and PLI crosswalks for 200 new, revised, and potentially misvalued services. This submission for the 2017 MFS included recommendations for moderate sedation services, cognitive impairment assessment and care planning, and several other surgical and procedural services.

For CPT 2018, RUC submitted work relative value and direct PE input recommendations, as well as PLI crosswalks for 275 new, revised, and potentially misvalued services. This submission for the 2018 MFS included recommendations for psychiatric collaborative care management services, cognitive impairment assessment and care plan services, and several other surgical and procedural services.

For CPT 2019, RUC submitted work relative value and direct PE input recommendations, as well as PLI crosswalks for 182 new, revised, and potentially misvalued services. This submission for the 2019 MFS included recommendations for chronic care management services, chronic care remote physiologic monitoring, interprofessional Internet consultation, and several other surgical and procedural services.

For CPT 2020, RUC submitted work relative value and direct PE input recommendations, as well as PLI crosswalks for 301 new, revised, and potentially misvalued services. This submission for the 2020 MFS included recommendations for transitional care management services, emergency department visits, online digital evaluation service (e-visit), and several other surgical and procedural services.

During the public health emergency (PHE) in 2020, numerous new CPT codes were created for severe acute respiratory syndrome coronavirus 2 (SARS-CoV-2) (coronavirus 2019 [COVID-19]) testing, vaccines, immunization administration, and creation of CPT code 99072 to help practices pursue payment for additional supply and infection-control costs associated with caring for patients during the COVID-19 PHE.

For CPT 2021, RUC submitted work relative value and direct PE input recommendations, as well as PLI crosswalks for 154 new, revised, and potentially misvalued services. The submission for the 2021 MFS included recommendations for breast reconstruction, hip and knee arthroplasty, remote retinal imaging, and several other surgical and procedural services.

For CPT 2022, RUC submitted work relative value and direct PE input recommendations, as well as PLI crosswalks, for 185 new, revised, and potentially misvalued services. The submission for the 2022 MFS included recommendations for

Table 4-1. History of RUC Recommendations

Year	Recommendations Submitted (Number of CPT codes)	Work Relative Values at or Above RUC Recommendations (After Final Rule)
CPT 1993	253	79%
CPT 1994	561	89%
CPT 1995	339	90%
CPT 1996	196	90%
CPT 1997	90	96%
CPT 1998	208	96%
CPT 1999	70	93%
CPT 2000	130	88%
CPT 2001	224	95%
CPT 2002	314	95%
CPT 2003	350	96%
CPT 2004	162	96%
CPT 2005	149	99%
CPT 2006	283	97%
CPT 2007	254	98%
CPT 2008	266	100%
CPT 2009	233	97%
CPT 2010	216	98%
CPT 2011	292	82%*
CPT 2012	328	87%
CPT 2013	363	90%
CPT 2014	265	76%
CPT 2015	350	86%
CPT 2016	278	78%
CPT 2017	200	85%
CPT 2018	275	100%
CPT 2019	182	80%
CPT 2020	301	79%
CPT 2021	154	77%
CPT 2022	185	77%
First 5-Year Review (1997)	1118	96%
Second 5-Year Review (2002)	870	98%
Third 5-Year Review (2007)	751	97%
Fourth 5-Year Review (2012)	290	75%

*CMS applied a budget-neutrality adjustment for services in a way contrary to RUC recommendations.

principal care management and chronic care management, remote therapeutic monitoring, anesthesia services for image-guided spinal procedures, cataract surgery, and several other surgical and procedural services.

Table 4-1 summarizes all of RUC's recommendations to date and CMS' consideration of these recommendations.

Five-Year Review

In addition to annual updates reflecting changes in CPT, Section 1848(C)2(B) of the Omnibus Budget Reconciliation Act of 1990 requires CMS to comprehensively review all relative values at least every five years and make any needed adjustments. In November 1993, CMS began preparation for this project by inviting organized medicine to develop a proposal to participate in the review process.

RUC sought a significant role in this comprehensive review of physician work relative values and appointed a subcommittee on the Five-Year Review to develop this concept. To further expand organized medicine's participation in the five-year review process, the AMA solicited comments from the executive vice presidents of all the national medical specialty societies. Consensus emerged about how to conduct the five-year review and revolved around the following major points: (1) RUC should play a key role; (2) the refinement should focus on correcting errors and accounting for changes in medical practice, not the whole RVS; and (3) the methods should build upon the current RUC methodology for valuing codes. In March 1994, the AMA submitted a detailed plan to CMS, identifying medicines preferred approach to dealing with organizational and conceptual issues in the five-year review. The proposed plan incorporated much of RUC's current methodology and built upon the cooperative approach to review and refinement RUC and CMS had established. Furthermore, it was consistent with the AMA's policy goal that the medical profession should have the primary responsibility for long-term maintenance and refinement of the RBRVS.

The 1994 Final Rule described CMS' plans for conducting the five-year review. The agency indicated that RUC, based on its experience in developing relative values and its ability to involve a wide range of medical specialties in the refinement process, warranted a significant role in the five-year review.

All codes on the 1995 payment schedule were open for public comment as part of the first five-year review. Included was the development of relative values for pediatric services. The Social Security Amendments Act of 1994 required that RVUs be developed for the full range of pediatric services, as well as determining whether significant variations existed in the work required to furnish similar services to adult and pediatric patients.

In the 1999 Final Rule, CMS again invited the public to comment on the work relative value for any existing CPT code. RUC also proposed a major role in this second, five-year review of the RBRVS. The proposal and process were very similar to the first five-year review. CMS forwarded the public comments to RUC in March 2000.

In the November 15, 2004, Final Rule, CMS solicited comments from the public on misvalued codes. CMS also stated that the agency would also be identifying codes that were potentially misvalued. RUC Five-Year Review Compelling Evidence Standards were published in this Final Rule and CMS requested that those commenting considered these standards and reference them in their comment letters. As a result of these two processes, CMS identified 710 codes to be a part of the 2005 five-year review process and forwarded these comments to RUC in March 2005. RUC again used a similar process and procedure, as were utilized in the two previous five-year reviews. CMS and specialty societies identified 290 codes to be a part of the 2010 five-year review process.

In the 2012 Final Rule, CMS finalized a public nomination process for potentially misvalued codes. To allow for public input and to preserve the public's ability to identify and nominate potentially misvalued codes for review, CMS established a process by which the public can submit codes on an annual basis. This process has now replaced the traditional five-year review process.

Scope of the First Five-Year Review

The five-year review presented an unprecedented opportunity to improve the accuracy of the physician work component of the RBRVS, as well as a significant challenge to the medical community. During the public comment period, CMS received nearly 500 letters identifying about 1100 CPT codes for review. The Carrier Medical Directors, the American Academy of Pediatrics (AAP), and special studies conducted for three specialty societies identified additional codes for review. Following an initial review, in late February 1995, CMS referred to RUC comments on about 3500 codes. These comments fell into the following categories: public comments on 669 codes; Carrier Medical Director comments on 387 codes; the three special studies by Abt Associates, Inc; and comments submitted by the AAP.

In approaching its task, RUC determined that a high standard of proof would be required for all proposed changes in work values. For example, specialties were required to present a "compelling argument" to maintain current values for services that the comments had identified as overvalued. RUC's methodology for evaluating codes identified by public comment was similar to that used previously for the annual updates, with some innovations designed to require compelling arguments to support requested changes. The survey was modified to require additional information regarding comparisons with the key reference services selected, as well as the extent to which the service had changed over the previous five years.

RUC also established multidisciplinary work groups to help manage the large number of comments referred and to ensure objective review of potentially overvalued services. These workgroups evaluated the public and Carrier Medical Director comments and developed recommendations. The full RUC treated the recommendations as consent calendars, with other RUC members and specialty society representatives extracting for discussion any workgroup recommendations with which they disagreed.

RUC also considered comments on nearly 500 codes that the AAP submitted. The society believed that physician work differed, depending on whether children or adults were being treated. As a result, the AAP requested that appropriate new CPT codes be added to describe different age categories of patients and that relative values be assigned. RUC and the CPT Editorial Panel helped the AAP refine its proposal for new and revised codes, which became effective for CPT 1997.

Finally, RUC considered three studies Abt Associates conducted at the request of three medical specialty societies. RUC found that two of the studies correctly ranked ordered codes within the respective specialties but did not reach any conclusions about the third. Following these findings, however, the specialty societies each conducted further research on individually identified codes and submitted their recommendations to RUC.

Scope of the Second Five-Year Review

CMS received only 30 public comments in response to its solicitation of misvalued codes to be reviewed in the second five-year review. However, 870 codes were identified for review as several specialties (general surgery, vascular surgery, and cardiothoracic surgery) commented that nearly all of the services performed by their specialty were misvalued. In addition, RUC reviewed a number of codes performed by gastroenterology, obstetrics/gynecology, orthopaedic surgery, pediatric surgery, and radiology.

The process that RUC utilized in this five-year review was very similar to the process utilized in the first five-year review. Multidisciplinary workgroups were utilized to review the large number of codes. The full RUC then reviewed and discussed the reports of these work groups.

Scope of the Third Five-Year Review

In the November 15, 2004, Final Rule, CMS solicited comments from the public on misvalued codes. CMS also stated that the agency would also be identifying codes that they felt were potentially misvalued. RUC Five-Year Review Compelling Evidence Standards were published in this Final Rule and CMS requested that those commenting consider these standards and reference them in their comment letters. As a result of these two processes, 723 codes were identified by specialties and CMS to be a part of the 2005 five-year review process. These codes include services such as, but not limited to, dermatology, cardiothoracic surgery, and orthopaedic surgery, as well as the evaluation and management codes. CMS forwarded the comments pertaining to these codes to RUC in March 2005. RUC agreed that many of these recommendations met the compelling evidence standards as being misvalued. RUC again used a similar process and procedure as was used in the previous two five-year reviews to critically assess specialties' recommendations. This assessment included consideration of the comment letters, specialty society data, and other evidence provided throughout 2005.

Scope of the Fourth Five-Year Review

In the October 30, 2008, Final Rule, CMS solicited comments from the public on misvalued codes. RUC Five-Year Review Compelling Evidence Standards were published in this Final Rule, however, CMS announced that it would no longer recognize anomalous relationships between codes as a primary reason for specialty societies to submit codes for review. As a result of this solicitation, 290 codes were identified by specialties and CMS to be reviewed in the 2010 five-year review process. In October 2010 and February 2011, all RUC recommendations were submitted to CMS for consideration, with resulting changes effective January 1, 2012.

RUC Recommendations from the First Five-Year Review

In September 1995, RUC submitted to CMS relative value recommendations for more than 1,000 individual codes. These recommendations maintained values for about 60% of the codes reviewed, increased values for about one third, and decreased values for the remainder. CMS' proposed RVU changes were published in a May 1996 *Federal Register*. Overall, CMS accepted 93% of RUC's recommendations, including 100% acceptance for several specialties. Following a public comment period, final decisions were announced in the November 22, 1996, *Federal Register*. Summaries of the key results follow:

- *Evaluation and Management (E/M) Services.* CMS extended its review to include all 98 E/M codes that were assigned RVUs, although RUC submitted recommendations for only a portion of these codes. RUC asserted that the postservice work involved in E/M services had increased over the past five years and that the intraservice work was undervalued compared to other services on the RBRVS. CMS accepted the argument and increased work RVUs for most E/M services, including a 25% increase for *office visits* (CPT codes 99202–99215) and an average 16.6% increase for *emergency department services* (CPT codes 99281–99285). Work RVUs also were increased for *critical care, first hour* (CPT code 99291) and *office or other outpatient consultations* (CPT codes 99241–99245).

- *Anesthesia*. CMS accepted RUC's recommendation for a 22.76% increase to the work RVUs. CMS adopted the adjustment on an interim basis and opened it to public comment since it was not part of the proposed notice. RUC based its recommendation on results of a study conducted for the American Society of Anesthesiologists and on the expertise of RUC Research Subcommittee. There is no defined work RVU per code for anesthesia services, which required that the adjustment be made in the aggregate on the anesthesia conversion factor.
- *Psychiatry*. CMS accepted RUC's recommendation that the work RVUs should be increased for five psychotherapy services. The agency rejected the CPT code descriptors, however, stating that they did not sufficiently define physician work. For Medicare reporting and payment purposes, the CPT codes were replaced with 24 temporary alphanumeric codes. These codes were time-based and differentiated between office/outpatient psychotherapy and inpatient psychotherapy; insight-oriented, behavior modifying, and/or supportive psychotherapy and interactive psychotherapy; and psychotherapy furnished with and without medical evaluation and management. The 24 temporary codes were adopted by the CPT Editorial Panel for CPT 1998.
- *Routine Obstetric Care*. As part of the 1994 refinement process, CMS increased work values assigned to codes for routine obstetric care in response to a joint recommendation of the American College of Obstetricians and Gynecologists (ACOG) and the American Academy of Family Physicians (AAFP). The AMA had worked with ACOG and AAFP on this recommendation and urged CMS to adopt it. The ACOG-AAFP recommendation used a "building block" approach based on existing and RUC-proposed work values for the components of the obstetrical packages. The work values for CPT code 59400, *Routine obstetric care including antepartum care, vaginal delivery (with or without episiotomy, and/or forceps) and postpartum care*, were increased by 9% and for CPT code 59510, *Routine obstetric care including antepartum care, cesarean delivery, and postpartum care*, by 29%.

  The work values assigned to these codes equal the midrange joint recommendation. The overall RBRVS increase for these two codes (including practice expense and professional liability values and after applying the 1.3% reduction for budget neutrality) is 8% for 59400 and 27% for 59510. These increases enhanced the ability of non-Medicare RBRVS payment systems, such as state Medicaid programs, to ensure access to needed obstetrical services.
- *Global Surgical Services*. As part of the five-year review, RUC recommended that the relationship between E/M services and global surgical services be evaluated and that work RVUs for the latter services be increased consistent with the 1997 RVU increases for E/M services. CMS rejected RUC's views in its May 1996 *Proposed Rule*. The agency agreed, however, to reexamine the issue for the 1998 RVS in the November 1996 Final Rule.

Surgical specialty societies argued that E/M services related to a procedure were subject to the same increasing complexity as nonprocedural E/M services due to such factors as reduced inpatient lengths of stay and same-day admissions for major surgery. Another major contributing factor is the greater utilization of home health care services, requiring the surgeon to be more involved in postservice planning and management.

Following its evaluation, CMS concluded that the work RVUs associated with global surgical services should be increased to reflect the increased evaluation and management present in the preservice and postservice portions of these services. For 1998, CMS implemented an across-the-board increase to the work RVUs for global surgical services. The change produced an average increase of 4% in services with a 10-day global period and 7% for services with a 90-day global period. To maintain budget neutrality of physician payments under the payment schedule, CMS applied a –0.7% adjustment to the conversion factor.

Recommendations from the Second Five-Year Review

RUC found that several specialties presented compelling evidence that their services were indeed misvalued. As a result, RUC submitted recommendations to CMS in October 2000 to change the work relative value for many services. These recommendations may be summarized, as follows:

- Increase the work relative value for 469 CPT codes
- Decrease the work relative value for 27 CPT codes
- Maintain the work relative value for 311 CPT codes
- Refer 63 codes to the CPT Editorial Panel to consider coding changes prior to consideration of the work relative value

CMS published a *Proposed Rule* on June 8, 2001, and a Final Rule on November 1, 2001, announcing the agency's intention to accept and implement more than 95% of RUC's recommendations on January 1, 2002. Some of the important changes are as follows:

- *Vascular Surgery*. The American Association for Vascular Surgery and the Society for Vascular Surgery argued that vascular surgery services were historically undervalued dating back to the original Harvard studies. RUC reviewed detailed survey data for 95 codes. RUC recommended that 91 vascular surgical procedures be increased. CMS implemented 100% of these recommendations.

- *General Surgery*. The American College of Surgeons and the American Society for General Surgeons submitted comments related to more than 300 services performed predominately by general surgeons. Several rank order anomalies and historical undervalued codes were identified. RUC recommended that 242 codes be increased, 22 be decreased, and 50 be maintained. However, CMS was convinced that further increases were warranted and implemented further changes to the general surgery relative values.
- *Cardiothoracic Surgery*. The Society for Thoracic Surgery also commented that 89 codes describing services performed by cardiothoracic surgeons were undervalued. RUC recommended, and CMS implemented increases to 41 of these services. For example, RUC was convinced that the physician work related to congenital cardiac procedures has increased over the past five years.
- *Diagnostic Mammography*. RUC reviewed data submitted by the American College of Radiology (ACR) that indicated an increase in physician work created by the implementation of the Mammography Quality Standards Act of 1992 (MQSA). RUC agreed that these regulations and ACR standards did require more physician time and work. CMS implemented these increases on January 1, 2002.

Recommendations from the Third Five-Year Review

In October 2005, February 2006, and May 2007, RUC submitted recommendations on the work relative values for 751 CPT codes. Of the 751 codes in this review, RUC recommended:

- Increases in work RVUs for 285 CPT codes
- Decreases in work RVUs for 33 CPT codes
- Maintenance of the work RVUs for 294 CPT codes
- Reevaluation of 139 CPT codes by the CPT Editorial Panel

CMS published a *Proposed Notice* on June 29, 2006, and a Final Rule on December 1, 2006, stating that 95% of the recommendations submitted in October 2005 and February 2006 were accepted and would be implemented on January 1, 2007. Subsequently, CMS published a *Proposed Notice* on July 12, 2007, and Final Rule on November 27, 2007, stating that, including RUC's May 2007 submission to CMS, 97% of the recommendations were accepted by CMS and the remaining recommendations from the May 2007 submission would be implemented January 1, 2008. The following details some of the key changes announced by CMS:

- *Evaluation and Management Services*. This Five-Year Review included 35 evaluation and management (E/M) services. RUC agreed that incorrect assumptions were made in the previous valuation of E/M services. RUC recommended and CMS approved an increase in work RVUs for 28 services and maintained work RVUs for seven services. Furthermore, RUC also recommended and CMS accepted that the full increase of the E/M service be incorporated into the surgical global periods for each CPT code with global periods of 010 and 090.
- *Dermatology and Plastic Surgery*. Three significant dermatological issues—the excision of lesions, the destruction of lesions, and Mohs surgery—were addressed by RUC during the Five-Year Review. For these three groups of services, various issues had to be addressed including new Medicare coverage policies, the difference in work between treating a malignant or benign lesion, and potential changes in descriptors to reflect accurately where the service is being performed. RUC reaffirmed the relativity in payment for the excision of lesion codes and persuaded CMS that there is a difference in postoperative work in the excision of a benign and malignant lesion. RUC recommended relative value changes for destruction of lesion codes to reflect the change in the modality used. The CPT Editorial Panel considered major revisions to the Mohs surgery section prior to RUC review and development of recommendations. RUC recommendations for 100% of these dermatology and plastic surgery codes were accepted by CMS.
- *Orthopaedic Surgery*. The orthopaedic surgery community presented recommendations on 108 services that were identified as misvalued due to changes in the patient population and rank order anomalies. Of these services, 86 were referred to the CPT Editorial Panel to address various issues, eg, the differentiation between benign and malignant tumors, assignment of modifier 51, and clarification of any subjective terms within the existing descriptors. RUC recommendations for the remaining procedures were all approved by CMS, which included RUC's recommendation to retain relativity within the total joint codes (27130, 27236, and 27447).

Of these 86 codes that were referred to the CPT Editorial Panel, 64 fracture treatment procedures were reviewed by the Panel and subsequently RUC to clarify that external fixation should be an adjunctive procedure to these procedures. CMS has accepted all recommendations; however, CMS has applied a budget-neutrality adjustment for fracture treatment codes in a way contrary to RUC recommendations. In February 2009, the CPT Editorial Panel approved the coding proposal submitted by the Soft Tissue Tumor and Bone Workgroup which revised and expanded the soft tissue tumor and bone tumor sections to more accurately describe the services being provided and address the concerns raised by RUC during the Third Five-Year Review. CMS accepted these recommendations and agreed that RUC re-review these services in three years to determine the accuracy of the utilization assumptions.

- *Gynecology, Urology, and Neurosurgery*. RUC reviewed codes from gynecology, urology, and neurosurgery due to changes in the patient population, changes in technology, or an anomalous relationship between the code being valued and other codes. Of these 32 procedures, CMS implemented increases to 19 procedures. For example, RUC agreed that craniotomies with elevation of bone flap for lobectomy, temporal lobe with and without electrocorticography during surgery had, during the last five years, required additional physician work due to a change in the complexity of patient population.

- *Radiology, Pathology, and Other Miscellaneous Services*. RUC reviewed various procedures pertaining to radiology including maxillofacial X rays, radiation therapy, and general X rays. Of all the radiological procedures addressed by RUC during the Five-Year Review, 50 of these 80 procedures' work values were recommended by RUC and approved by CMS to be maintained.

- *Cardiothoracic Surgery*. RUC recommended increases to nine congenital cardiac surgery codes and 72 adult cardiac and general thoracic surgery codes, largely due to the increased complexity of the patient population to receive these services. CMS accepted 100% of RUC's recommendations for cardiothoracic surgery.

- *General Surgery, Colorectal Surgery, and Vascular Surgery*. RUC reviewed 116 recommendations for procedures predominately performed by general, colorectal, and vascular surgeons. These codes were identified to be a part of the Five-Year Review based on flawed crosswalk assumptions, rank-order anomalies, and, in the case of vascular surgery, the services were historically undervalued dating back to the original Harvard Studies. RUC recommended and CMS will implement increases in work RVUs associated with 58 out of 86 of the general surgical and vascular surgical services. CMS requested that new survey data for the colorectal surgery codes be reviewed by RUC at its February 2007 RUC meeting. This review resulted in recommendations being forwarded to CMS as part of RUC's May 2007 submission. All of these recommendations were accepted by CMS.

- *Otolaryngology and Ophthalmology*. There were two major issues identified by RUC pertaining to otolaryngology and ophthalmology. For otolaryngology, CMS identified a procedure—removal impacted cerumen—that had never been evaluated by RUC. RUC recommended and CMS implemented maintenance of the current value associated with this service as RUC felt the current value was justified based on a specialty society survey that indicated that 94% of respondents felt that the work in performing this service has not changed in the past five years. For ophthalmology, CMS identified cataract surgery as a procedure to be reviewed in the Five-Year Review because this procedure has experienced advances in technology that have likely resulted in a modification to the physician work. RUC recommended a slight decrease in physician work related to the intra-service portion of the procedure; however, the increase in the E/M component of the global period provided an overall increase to the physician work for this service.

- *Anesthesiology*. RUC convened a workgroup to consider the request from CMS to assign post-induction period procedure anesthesia (PIPPA) intensity. In addition, CMS referred to RUC the question of how and whether to apply the E/M Five-Year Review increases to the pre- and post-work of anesthesia services. (See *Federal Register*, Vol. 71, No. 231/December 1, 2006, page 69733.) Based on the extensive review of a building block approach that could be used to evaluate the work of all anesthesia service components other than the post-induction period time and validation of PIPPA work by the surgeons on RUC familiar with anesthesia services associated with their specialty, RUC reached agreement that anesthesia services are undervalued by 32%. CMS accepted these recommendations from RUC and will increase the work of anesthesia services by 32% on January 1, 2008.

Recommendations from the Fourth Five-Year Review

In October 2010 and February 2011, RUC submitted recommendations on the work relative values for 290 CPT codes culminating in the results of the fourth Five-Year Review of the RBRVS. The recommendations may be summarized as follows:

- Decreases in work RVUs for 41 CPT codes
- Maintenance of the work RVUs for 144 CPT codes
- Increases in work RVUs for 83 CPT codes
- Reevaluation of 52 CPT codes by the CPT Editorial Panel

On November 28, 2011, CMS published a Final Rule in the *Federal Register* announcing that 75% of RUC recommendations were accepted and would be implemented January 1, 2012. The most significant improvement that developed from RUC's recommendations, and continued advocacy, is the recognition that physician work in hospital observation visits is equivalent to hospital inpatient visits.

The Relativity Assessment Workgroup

As the trend continues toward adopting the Medicare RBRVS by non-Medicare payers, including state Medicaid programs, workers' compensation plans, TRICARE, and state health system reform plans, it is critical that the physician work component be complete and appropriate for all patient populations.

RUC is committed to improving and maintaining the validity of the RBRVS over time. The AMA, RUC, and the specialty societies have worked aggressively to identify and correct flaws and gaps in the RBRVS. RUC will continue to review all services considered to be inappropriately valued. CMS will now call for public comments on an annual basis, rather than in a five-year review, as part of the comment process on the MFS. Public nominations must be submitted to CMS no later than February 10 of each year.

In 2006, RUC formed the Relativity Assessment Workgroup (RAW) (originally called the Five-Year Review Identification Workgroup) to identify potentially misvalued services using objective mechanisms for reevaluation during each Five-Year Review. The need for objective review of potential misvaluation has been a priority of RUC, CMS, and MedPAC in recent years.

RUC will rely on the recommendations of the workgroup, based on established objective criteria, to identify codes that will be considered for reevaluation on an ongoing basis. The RAW also develops objective criteria to identify "new technology" services. The workgroup has established a review process and schedule for "new technology" services and will maintain the review process. In September 2010, the workgroup reviewed the first set of codes identified as "new technology." RUC will continue to identify new technology services as well as review and forward recommendations to CMS for necessary adjustments to recognize efficiencies.

RUC's efforts led to more than $100 million in annual work value redistribution, applied via a slight increase to the conversion factors in 2009 and 2010. In 2011, the redistribution was more substantial, with $400 million in work value decreases redistributed via a 0.4% increase to the 2011 conversion factor. RUC's efforts led to approximately $200 million in work value redistribution to the 2012 Medicare conversion factor (0.2% increase). In 2013, RUC's efforts resulted in approximately $600 million in work value redistribution. For the 2014 MFS, RUC efforts resulted in approximately $435 million in work value redistribution. In 2015, approximately $450 million in work and direct practice expense value redistribution occurred, largely in part of the film-to-digital direct practice expense inputs transition. For the 2016 MFS, RUC's review of potentially misvalued services led to $205 million in work-value redistribution, primarily due to the CPT/RUC efforts on bundling services that are typically performed together. For the 2017 MFS, RUC's review resulted in $500 million in total redistribution between work and practice expense revaluation. For the 2018 MFS, RUC's review resulted in approximately $400 million in total redistribution between work and practice expense revaluation. For the 2019 MFS, RUC's review resulted in approximately $100 million in total redistribution between work and practice expense revaluation. For the 2020 MFS, RUC's review resulted in approximately $250 million in total redistribution between work and practice expense revaluation. For the 2021 MFS, RUC's review resulted in approximately $50 million in total redistribution between work and practice expense revaluation. When combined with the PE and PLI changes resulting from this specific effort, over $5 billion has been redistributed annually within the MFS from 2009–2022. In total, RUC has identified 2,638 codes for review in this project.

The AMA strongly supports the RUC process as the principal method to provide recommendations to refine and maintain the Medicare RVS. RUC represents an important opportunity for the medical profession to retain input regarding the clinical practice of medicine. The AMA continues to support RUC in its efforts to secure CMS adoption of its relative value recommendations.

References

1. Department of Health Policy and Management, Harvard School of Public Health, and Department of Psychology. *A National Survey of Resource-Based Relative Value Scales for Physician Services: Phase III*. Revised. Harvard University. Boston, Mass: August 30, 1992.
2. Braun P, guest ed. The Resource-Based Relative Value Scale: its further development and reform of physician payment. *Med Care*. 1992;30.
3. Department of Health Policy and Management, Harvard School of Public Health, and Department of Psychology. *A National Study of Resource-Based Relative Value Scales for Physician Services: MFS Refinement*. Harvard University. Boston, Mass: July 30, 1993.

Chapter 5

Practice Expense Component

Beginning in January 1999, Medicare began a transition to resource-based practice expense relative values, which establish practice expense payment for each Current Procedural Terminology (CPT®) code that differs based on the site of service. Procedures that can be performed in a physician's office, as well as in a hospital have two practice expense relative values: facility and nonfacility practice expense relative values. The nonfacility setting includes physician offices, freestanding imaging centers, and independent pathology labs. Facility settings include all other settings, such as hospitals, ambulatory surgery centers, skilled nursing facilities, and partial hospitals. In 2002, practice expenses were fully transitioned and the practice-expense component of the resource-based relative value scale (RBRVS) is resource-based. In 2007, the Centers for Medicare & Medicaid Services (CMS) implemented a new practice expense methodology. This chapter describes the method that CMS used to assign practice expense in the 1991 Final Rule, as well as the history and methodology used to develop the current resource-based practice expense relative values.

Data Used to Assign Charge-Based Practice Expense RVUs

Most of the practice-expense data that CMS used to assign relative value units (RVUs) in the 1991 Final Rule were from the American Medical Association's (AMA's) Socioeconomic Monitoring System 1989 Core Survey, which reflects the responses of a nationally representative sample of 4000 physicians in 34 specialties. Because the Medicare payment schedule applies to several non-MD/DO practitioner groups, CMS also used data supplied by the American Association of Oral and Maxillofacial Surgeons, the American Optometric Association, the American Podiatric Medical Association, and the American Chiropractic Association. Data for clinics and other group practice arrangements were supplied by the Medical Group Management Association. When no other data was available, CMS used averages representing all physicians.

OBRA 89 Method

The fundamental approach used in developing the Medicare RBRVS measured the average resource costs involved in providing each physician service. The basis for the work component RVUs, therefore, measured the average work involved in a service by surveying randomly selected samples of practicing physicians.

The Omnibus Budget Reconciliation Act (OBRA) of 1989 approach to determine the practice expense component is similar to the work component because it relies, in part, on data from the AMA's national survey of physicians' average practice costs. However, physicians generally measure practice costs as a total sum, not service by service. Surveys of practicing physicians regarding their costs of practice, therefore, provided data on the average total amount that they spend on office rents, wages of nonphysician personnel, supplies, and equipment. The data did not provide the average office-rent expense, for example, related to a particular service or the average nursing time required for that service.

These surveys also indicated that average practice costs vary by specialty overall and as a percentage of gross revenue. Practice costs accounted for a higher proportion of general and family physicians' revenues (52.2%) than for cardiologists' (36.1%) or neurosurgeons' (38.9%), as shown in Table 5-1.

Table 5-1. Physician Practice Expense Ratios⁺ for 1989

⁺As a percentage of mean total revenue

Specialty	CMS Specialty	Mean Expenses Net PLI, %	Mean PLIAMA Expenses, %
All physicians		41.0	4.8
General/family practice	Family practice	52.2	3.9
	General practice	52.2	3.9
Internal medicine		46.4	2.8
General internal medicine	Internal medicine	46.4	2.8
Cardiovascular disease	Cardiovascular disease	36.1	2.7
Other	Allergy	40.5	2.6
	Gastroenterology	40.5	2.6
	Geriatrics	40.5	2.6
	Nephrology	40.5	2.6
	Pulmonary disease	40.5	2.6
Surgery		31.8	7.4
General surgery	General surgery	31.8	7.4
Otolaryngology	Otology, laryngology, rhinology	45.2	4.9
Orthopedic surgery	Orthopedic surgery	45.2	7.4
Ophthalmology	Ophthalmology	44.4	2.3
	Ophthalmology, otology, laryngology	44.4	2.3
Urological surgery	Urology	39.9	3.9
Other	Hand surgery	38.9	7.6
	Neurological surgery	38.9	7.6
	Peripheral vascular disease or surgery	38.9	7.6
	Plastic surgery	38.9	7.6
	Proctology	38.9	7.6
	Thoracic surgery	38.9	7.6
Pediatrics	Pediatrics	49.3	3.1
Obstetrics/gynecology	Gynecology	38.8	8.8
	Obstetrics	38.8	8.8
	Obstetrics/gynecology	38.8	8.8

Specialty	CMS Specialty	Mean Expenses Net PLI, %	Mean PLIAMA Expenses, %
Radiology*	Diagnostic X ray (groups)[1]	50.5	3.3
	Global for the radiology specialties that follow	37.2	3.0
	Radiation therapy (professional component)	22.9	3.3
	Radiology (professional component)	22.9	3.3
	Roentgenology, radiology (professional component)	22.9	3.3
	Radiation therapy (technical component)	94.1	5.9
	Radiology (technical component)	94.1	5.9
	Roentgenology, radiology (technical component)	94.1	5.9
Psychiatry	Psychiatry	26.4	3.7
	Psychiatry, neurology	26.4	3.7
Anesthesiology	Anesthesiology	23.2	7.3
Pathology	Diagnostic laboratory (groups)[1]	50.5	3.3
	Pathologic anatomy, clinical	28.5	1.9
	Pathology	28.5	1.9
Other specialty			
	Dermatology	40.3	3.0
	Occupational therapy (groups)[1]	50.5	3.3
	Other medical care (groups)[1]	50.5	3.3
	Neurology	40.3	3.0
	Nuclear medicine	40.3	3.0
	Physical medicine and rehabilitation	40.3	3.0
No AMA match	Clinic or other group practice (groups)[1]	50.5	3.0
No AMA match	Oral surgery[2]	54.7	4.4
No AMA match	Optometrist[3]	52.9	0.1
No AMA match	Podiatry[4]	47.8	4.2
No AMA match	Chiropractor, licensed[5]	58.4	1.8
No AMA match	Manipulative therapy[6]	41.0	4.8
	Miscellaneous[6]	41.0	4.8
	Physical therapy[6]	41.0	4.8
	Occupational therapist[6]	41.0	4.8
	Physiotherapy[6]	41.0	4.8

Sources: 1991 Final Rule, p 59868. American Medical Association, 1988–1990 Socioeconomic Monitoring System Core surveys, except where indicated.

[1]Source: Medical Group Management Association, 1990 Cost and Survey Production Report.

[2]Source: American Association of Oral and Maxillofacial Surgeons.

[3]Source: American Optometry Association.

[4]Source: American Podiatric Medical Association.

[5]Source: American Chiropractic Association.

[6]Source: For these remaining specialties, CMS used the practice cost percent from the AMA for all physicians.

*For radiology services, the professional component percentages were based on data for radiologists with equipment expenses of $5000 or less. The technical component percentages were based on data for radiologist with equipment expenses of more than $5000.

To distribute practice expense RVUs among the services each specialty provides, the OBRA 89 method applies the average practice cost percentage for each specialty to the 1991 average Medicare-approved amount for the service. (The average approved amount is initially expressed in dollars for this purpose and later put on the scale of RVUs, then converted back to dollars when the total RVUs for the service are multiplied by the monetary conversion factor.) For example:

- For a service that only family practitioners provide and for which the average Medicare payment in 1991 was $100, multiply the practice cost proportion (52.2%) by the $100 average approved amount. The practice expense component of the service would be assigned 52.2 (initial dollar) RVUs.
- For a service that only neurosurgeons provide and for which the average Medicare payment in 1991 was $1000, multiply the practice cost proportion (38.9%) by the $1000 average approved amount. The practice expense component of the service would be assigned 389.0 (initial dollar) RVUs.

For services provided by physicians in more than one specialty, each specialty's practice cost proportion is multiplied by the proportion of claims for the service that the specialty submits:

- For a service provided 70% of the time by family physicians and 30% of the time by internists and for which the average Medicare-approved amount in 1991 was $100, the family physicians' practice cost proportion (52.2%) is multiplied by 70% and the internal medicine practice cost proportion (46.4%) is multiplied by 30%. The sum of these two products becomes the practice cost proportion for the service:

$$(52.2\% \times 0.70) + (46.4\% \times 0.30) = 50.5\%$$

- This practice cost proportion is then multiplied by the $100 average approved amount:

$$(50.5\% \times 100) = 50.5$$

- The practice cost component of the service would be assigned 50.5 (initial dollar) RVUs.
- For a service that is provided 70% of the time by neurosurgeons and 30% of the time by orthopedic surgeons and for which the average Medicare-approved amount in 1991 was $1000, the neurosurgeons' practice cost proportion (38.9%) is multiplied by 70% and the orthopedic surgeons' practice cost proportion (45.2%) is multiplied by 30%. The sum of these two products becomes the practice cost proportion for the service:

$$(38.9\% \times 0.70) + (45.2\% \times 0.30) = 40.8\%$$

- This practice cost proportion is then multiplied by the $1000 average approved amount:

$$(40.8\% \times 1000) = 408$$

- The practice cost component of the service would be assigned 408 (initial dollar) RVUs.

The OBRA 89 method of assigning practice expense RVUs clearly provides a much rougher approximation of physicians' average resource-costs per service than does the method of assigning work component RVUs.

Because anesthesia services are not divided into work, practice expense, and professional liability insurance (PLI) cost RVUs, CMS computed the proportions of total payments for anesthesia that were comparable to these three components for other services. The portion of the anesthesiology conversion factor reflecting the work component was reduced by 42%. As for other services, to maintain a Medicare contribution comparable to the contribution under customary, prevailing, and reasonable (CPR), the portion of the conversion factor reflecting practice was not reduced.

CMS based the 1992 practice cost on 1989 charge data "aged" to reflect 1991 payment rules because those were the most recent data available. For the 1992 payment schedule, actual 1991 charge data were used to recalculate the practice cost for some codes for which CMS had imputed values the previous year. For services with insufficient charge data and for new codes, CMS developed crosswalks to predecessor codes, where possible. Since 1993, CMS has used a similar process to establish values for such codes.

In the years immediately following the implementation of the Medicare RBRVS, many organizations, especially the Physician Payment Review Commission (PPRC) and primary care specialties, expressed concern about the OBRA 89 method of calculating practice expenses. These organizations were concerned that practice expense relative values based on historical Medicare-allowed charges failed to reflect the relative resource costs of providing a service. They were also concerned that statutorily designated "overvalued procedure" reductions in 1990 and 1991 lowered the practice-cost RVUs to levels less than they would otherwise have been when OBRA 89 was enacted.

OBRA 93 Revisions to the Practice Expense Component

Congress adopted additional payment reductions to "overvalued" services under OBRA 93. The legislation called for reductions to the practice expense relative values for such "overvalued" procedure codes to be phased in over a three-year period, 1994–1996. The practice-expense RVUs of the affected services were reduced each year by 25% of the amount by which they exceeded the physician-work RVUs but could not fall below a floor of 128% of the work RVUs. Services performed at least 75% of the time in the physician office setting were exempt from the reductions, as were services without work RVUs (eg, diagnostic tests with only a technical component). In addition, practice-expense RVUs assigned to a global service were subject to the same reduction as its technical component.

Resource-Based Practice Expenses

Congress' interest in developing resource-based practice expense relative values goes back several years to 1992, when the PPRC published a report on resource-based practice expenses. Section 121 of the Social Security Act amendments, enacted in late 1994, required development of "resource-based" practice expense relative values for implementation in 1998. It required that the new resource-based methodology consider the staff, equipment, and supplies used to provide medical and surgical services in various settings.

Developing the Methodology

To respond to the Congressional mandate, CMS contracted with Abt Associates, Inc. for a national study of physicians' practice expenses. This study was designed to have three components: use of clinical practice expert panels (CPEPs) to estimate the direct costs associated with each CPT-coded service; use of a national mail survey of 5000 practices to obtain information on practice costs and service mix; and collection of data on the price of each input, such as equipment and disposable supplies. Because of delays in the Abt study at each step in the process and Congressional concern about the validity of CMS' methodology, Congress extended the implementation deadline by one year to January 1999.

CMS determined that the primary methodology for deriving resource-based practice expense values should incorporate microcosting, a cost accounting approach that identifies all direct costs associated with a particular service. This methodology was to produce a detailed database to support several analytical methods for estimating practice expense per service. Estimates for both direct and indirect practice expenses for all services under the RBRVS were to be included. Direct expenses are those for equipment, supplies, and clinical and administrative staff associated with providing a particular service to an individual patient. Indirect expenses include office rent and equipment, utilities, and staff and other costs not directly allocable to an individual service. Estimates would vary according to the site of service.

CMS began constructing the new database in March 1995. Data were to be collected from two types of expert panels and from a detailed practicing physician survey for distribution to 5000 physician offices.

The following two types of expert panels were formed:

- *Clinical Practice Expert Panels (CPEPs).* Fifteen CPEPs were formed, with membership based on nominations from medical associations. The role of the CPEPs was to produce data for Abt to use in constructing direct cost estimates. Each CPEP developed "resource profiles," a detailed list of direct cost elements associated with a service, for a selected group of reference procedures. The cost estimates were then extended to the rest of the codes in a family.
- *Clinical Practice Expert Panel Technical Expert Group (TEG).* The TEG's role was to monitor the data collection process to ensure that the data are usable by other researchers who might conduct further analyses for generating practice expense relative values. The TEG members include researchers in this area and representatives of organized medicine, including the AMA, American College of Physicians, American College of Surgeons, and American College of Radiologists. In addition, TEG meetings were attended by observers from the AMA/Specialty Society RVS Update Committee (RUC), American Hospital Association, and the PPRC.

The national mail survey was designed to collect detailed information on aggregate indirect and direct practice expenses and relate them to individual CPT codes. It also solicited information on the practice's case mix and general characteristics. The data compiled by the CPEPs and through the survey would be used by Abt to calculate indirect costs for individual services and validate direct cost estimates with review by the CPEPs. Two alternative CMS studies produced additional data to be used to allocate indirect costs across procedures. One study allocated indirect costs based on the physician time required for the service; the other set practice expense relative values so that they were the same proportion of relative value units as practice expenses are of total practice revenues within a specialty. Both studies relied on existing data, including that from the AMA's Socioeconomic Monitoring System (SMS), to determine the proportion of expenses that are direct and indirect.

The CPEPs and the national mail survey were designed to combine expert professional analysis and actual practice expense data, which could be used to develop relative values. The CPEPs were comprised of groups of physicians and other health care professionals who met to develop values for the direct cost component for each service. For each procedure on the RBRVS, the CPEPs developed lists of the practice resources required to provide the service, including the time of nonphysician clinical personnel, equipment, and supplies. The national mail survey would be used to validate the CPEP estimates, determine the proportions of practice expenses devoted to direct vs. indirect expenses, and indicate how indirect costs, which include rent, furnishings, computer equipment, office supplies, and other administrative overhead costs, could be appropriately allocated across procedures. However, in April 1996, CMS announced that, due to insufficient response rates to an initial survey, it could not use the results of the survey to develop the new relative values. In September 1996, CMS announced that it had cancelled all further work on the national mail survey. At the same time, however, CMS announced it would publish proposed practice expense RVUs in March 1997 to meet the implementation deadline of January 1, 1998.

CMS' decisions to cancel the mail survey and to proceed with plans for 1998 implementation heightened the level of concern about the process for developing resource-based practice expense relative values. In the absence of the mail survey, it was not clear where CMS would find data suitable for determining the split between indirect costs and direct costs; validating the results from the CPEP process; and allocating indirect costs among procedures. With estimates of the proportion of total costs that are direct costs ranging from 30% to 80% and the CPEP process relying on a very small number of physicians in each specialty, the lack of data on physicians' actual practice expenses made any assessment of the validity of the resource-based relative values extremely difficult.

Opposition to the Medicare Proposed Methodology

The AMA urged the Clinton administration to defer action on a Proposed Rule and to request Congress to adopt legislation extending the deadline for implementing practice expense changes. Deferment was necessary for several major reasons:

- The proposed relative values did not account for many practice expenses, including physician office staff, equipment utilization, and differences in actual practice costs of various specialties.
- A transition period and refinement process would not solve major problems with the practice expense proposal; rather, agreement must be reached on the basic methodology and the database before designing a transition and refinement process.
- Additional time was needed to allow physicians the opportunity to validate data and assumptions.
- Adopting the flawed proposed values would extend beyond the Medicare program, as some private sector payers had indicated they would implement payment cuts based on the CMS data.

In June 1997, CMS issued its proposed regulation, which included a practice expense methodology heavily dependent on the CPEP data. Instead of using actual practice expense data to verify the CPEP data, CMS used a number of assumptions and adjustments designed to improve data consistency among the expert panels. However, the AMA and some specialty societies were critical of the CMS methodology and called for a one-year delay in implementation. During the rule's public comment period, more than 8000 comments were submitted to CMS by individual physicians, professional societies, and others. Many groups, including the AMA, argued that CMS moved too quickly and without sufficient data to implement a resource-based methodology. The AMA submitted detailed comments for improving CMS' approach, including recommendations on the following issues:

- *Direct cost data.* (1) Per-procedure cost estimates the CPEPs developed should be reviewed and errors corrected. (2) CMS' assumptions regarding use of overhead and procedure-specific equipment greatly overstate its utilization, thus significantly undervaluing equipment costs. Data on actual equipment utilization rates should be collected and used in the relative values.
- *Indirect costs.* The methodology for assigning indirect cost RVUs should recognize all staff, equipment, supplies, and expenses, not just those that can be tied to specific procedures. CMS should evaluate the relationship between the proposed relative values and physicians' actual practice expenses and revise its methodology to account for specialty differences in the costs of operating a medical practice.
- *Multiple procedure reduction.* CMS should not apply the current multiple procedure rule for surgery to office procedures that are provided during the same encounter as a visit. Resource cost data are not available to demonstrate that physician work and practice expenses for office procedures are reduced by half when an office visit is also provided.

Legislation Revises Medicare's Proposal

Profound dissatisfaction with CMS' methodology and the proposed relative values led many physician groups, including the AMA, to work vigorously with members of Congress to enact needed legislative changes. Due to these concerns, Congress delayed the implementation of the new practice expense relative values until January 1999, and directed the General Accounting Office (GAO) to evaluate CMS' proposed methodology and data. Congress also adopted several provisions directed to improve the accuracy of the resource-based methodology. The provisions were included in the Balanced Budget Act of 1997. For example, it specified the data that must be used in developing the new values and required implementation over a four-year transition period.

As a first step toward implementing a resource-based system, the law called for adjusting the practice expense values for certain services for 1998. Services whose practice expense values were proposed for reduction by CMS in the June 1997 *Proposed Rule*, and that were not performed at least 75% of the time in an office setting, were reduced to be equivalent to 110% of the work RVUs for the service. The reduction was used to increase the practice expense RVUs for office visits.

The GAO issued its report in February 1998, and its recommendations were highly consistent with AMA policy. The GAO's review of CMS' methodology found that CMS' use of the CPEPs was reasonable but that many of CMS' adjustments to the data were questionable and may have biased the cost estimates. For example, the GAO reported that "CMS capped nonphysician clinical labor time at 1½ times the minutes used by a physician to perform a procedure. CMS has not, however, conducted tests or studies that validate these changes and thus cannot be assured that they are necessary or reasonable." The GAO recommended CMS collect additional data to validate its adjustments and assumptions and evaluate alternative methodologies for adjusting the CPEP data.

The 1999 Resource-Based Methodology

On June 5, 1998, CMS issued a new proposal that contained two options for a practice expense methodology. The first option was referred to as the "bottom-up" approach and was basically the same as the previously proposed methodology without many of the adjustments to the CPEP data. The second option was referred to as the "top-down" approach because it uses actual practice cost data developed by the AMA SMS data, which is allocated down to individual procedures using the data collected in the CPEP process. This methodology was significantly different from previous proposals.

On November 2, 1998, CMS issued its final proposal on the practice expense relative value methodology. CMS selected the new "top-down" approach published in June 1998 with only minor changes. CMS began it methodology by dividing practice costs into six categories: clinical labor, medical supplies, medical equipment, office expense, administrative labor, and all other expenses.

The SMS data consist of the average annual practice expense per average hours worked by physicians in a given specialty. These expense data are then multiplied by the total time spent treating Medicare patients, as determined by the RUC/Harvard physician-time data and Medicare-claims data. Each specialty cost pool is then allocated to procedures performed by that specialty using the CPEP data. This process can be broken down into six steps.

Step 1 Specialty Practice Expenses The AMA's SMS data provide the aggregate practice expense per hour (PE/HR) according to each specialty and cost category. This is obtained by dividing total practice expenses, as determined by the SMS survey, by total physician hours worked, which is also determined by the SMS survey. For those specialties not included in the SMS data, CMS crosswalked these specialties to specialties that were included in the SMS data. These data constitute the total practice expenses, which are allocated to specific codes according to the methodology discussed in Steps 2 through 5.

Step 2 Physician Time Spent Treating Medicare Patients The frequency with which each service is performed on Medicare patients by each specialty is multiplied by the estimated physician time required to perform each service. This results in the total physician time spent treating Medicare patients according to procedure. The physician time data were taken either from RUC surveys of new and revised codes or, for those codes that RUC has not examined, from the original Harvard RBRVS survey. The physician time data consists of all time involved in a procedure including pre, intra, and post service time.

Step 3 Specialty Practice Expense Cost Pools A practice expense pool for each specialty and cost category is calculated by multiplying the results of Step 1 by the results of Step 2. The practice expenses per hour multiplied by the total hours spent treating Medicare patients results in the total practice expenses, which will be allocated to codes according to specialty. For codes without a work relative value, CMS created a separate technical services cost pool that is not specialty specific. The costs for this technical pool were taken from specialty pools that have codes without a work RVU and allocated according to 1998 charge-based relative value units; therefore, these codes were not yet resource-based.

Step 4 Allocate Practice Expense Pools to Individual Codes As Figures 5-1 and 5-2 illustrate, each specialty's cost pool is divided into six categories: clinical labor, medical supplies, medical equipment, administrative labor, office expense, and all other expenses. These six categories are further separated into two groups, which can be considered direct and indirect costs. The first group of direct costs includes clinical labor, medical supplies, and medical equipment. The second group of indirect costs includes administrative labor, office expense, and all other expenses.

The practice expense cost pools are primarily allocated to individual codes using the CPEP cost per procedure data, which establishes the relativity among codes within each

Figure 5-1. Overall Allocation Approach

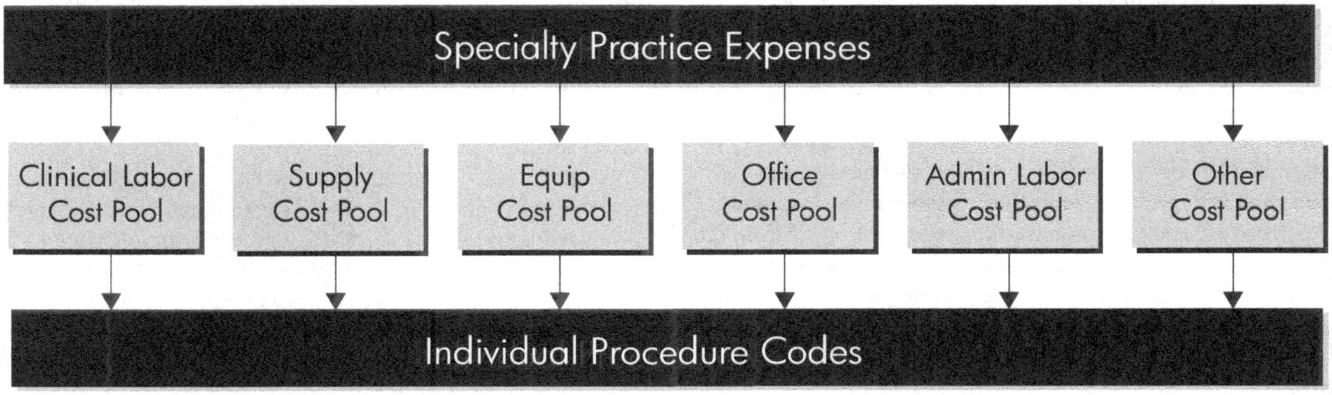

Figure 5-2. Cost Allocation Methodology

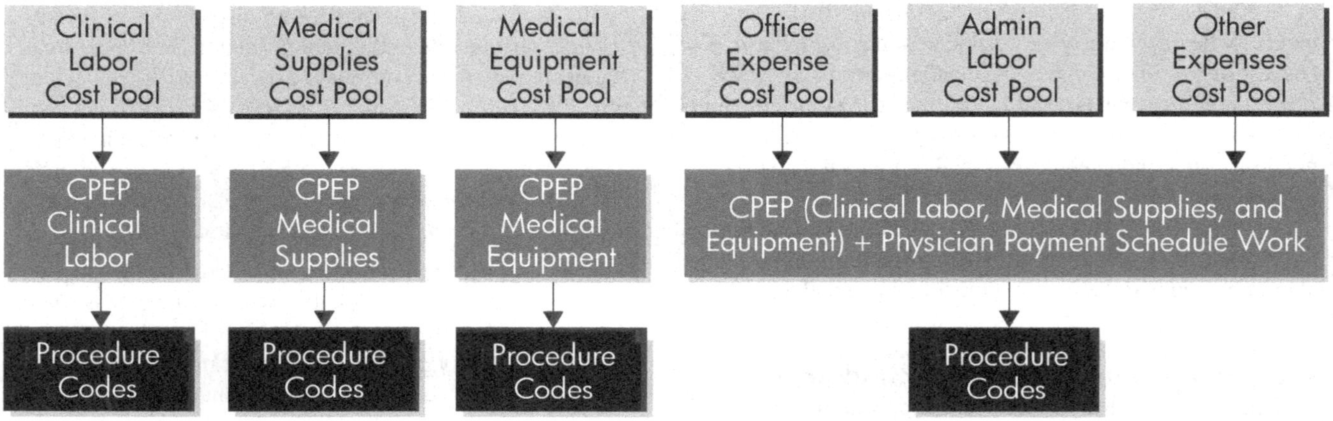

specialty. Unlike previous proposed methodologies, CMS used the original CPEP data without making any adjustments; however, CMS used a different allocation method for the direct and indirect categories.

The direct cost group consisting of clinical labor, medical supplies, and medical equipment was allocated by first multiplying the CPEP costs by the Medicare frequency data for each procedure. This produces a cost per procedure and category. These CPEP cost pools are then scaled to the SMS data so that the total CPEP costs for each specialty equal the total SMS cost by specialty. Changes to the CPEP values can change the total CPEP pool and the scaling factor resulting in the same size scaled pool but with different values assigned to individual codes. If, for example, one family of codes has the CPEP inputs reduced, then the total CPEP pool is reduced, creating a larger scaling factor. Therefore, this has the effect of increasing the scaled values of the remaining codes so that the scaled pool remains the same. This results in redistribution among codes for a specialty.

The second cost group consists of administrative labor, office expenses, and all other expenses. These costs are allocated by a combination of the direct costs calculated above and the work relative values. This methodology assumes a direct relationship between the work relative values and indirect expenses so that codes with higher work values will be assigned more indirect costs.

Step 5 Average the RVUs for Procedures Performed by More Than One Specialty For those codes performed by more than one specialty, CMS calculated a weighted average of the practice expenses based on Medicare frequency data. This weight averaging that occurs when services are provided by more than one specialty can sometimes have the effect of altering a specialty's payments when CPEP inputs are changed. When certain services have their CPEP inputs reduced, those expenses are then shifted to other services. As previously described, this only changes the allocation of costs but should not affect total payments for a specialty. However, when these inputs are weight averaged, a specialty can experience a decrease in costs if the specialty's costs for certain services are higher than costs in other specialties. The end result is sometimes a lower weighted average cost figure than the specialty's reported costs.

Step 6 Budget-neutrality Adjustment The final relative values are adjusted to match historical RVU totals to maintain budget neutrality.

During the transition period, practice expense relative value units were a combination of the 1998 charge-based value and the new resource value. In 1999, practice expense resource values were based on 75% of the 1998 charge-based relative value and 25% on the resource-based value. In 2000, the mix was equally weighted between the charge-based and resource-based values, and, in 2001, the practice expense relative values were 75% resource based and only 25% charged based. In 2002, the transition was completed with practice expense RVUs totally resource based.

SMS Data Used in CMS Methodology

The AMA's SMS specialty practice costs data plays a critical role in CMS' methodology for establishing practice expense relative values. The practice expense/hour data are based on the AMA SMS survey. The AMA has stated that these data were never collected for the purpose of developing relative values and has identified three potential problems with the use of these data for this purpose:

- The sample sizes for some specialties will be too small to permit separate calculation of expense data from SMS. Even among the larger specialties, the inherent variability of the expense data will mean that the average expense figures provided will be subject to significant sampling error.
- The response rates for the expense items tend to be low relative to other questions on the survey, leading to potential nonresponse bias.
- The SMS is a physician-level survey and physicians in group practices are asked for their share of expenses rather than the practice's expenses. Practice-level data may provide a better basis for constructing practice expense RVUs.

Although the SMS survey was not originally designed for the purpose of constructing practice expense RVUs, CMS made it clear that it intended to use the SMS and would look for improvements during the refinement process.

Example of Practice Expense-per-Hour Calculation

The SMS expense-per-hour data were calculated according to a formula specified by CMS. This formula adjusted the SMS expense data to obtain average hourly expenses per physician in the practice. These adjustments were necessary because physicians in groups are asked for their share of expenses on SMS (rather than the total for the practice) and because only self-employed physicians are asked the SMS expense questions. The expense per hour formula is:

$$\frac{X \times nown}{(ownhrs \times nown) + (emphrs \times nemp)}$$

in which:

X = the respondent's share of his or her practice's expenses for the previous year

$nown$ = the number of owner physicians in the respondent's practice

$nemp$ = the number of employee physicians in the respondent's practice

$ownhrs$ = an estimate of total hours worked in direct patient care by the respondent for the previous year

$emphrs$ = an estimate of average hours worked in direct patient care by employee physicians of the same specialty as the respondent for the previous year

The variable *ownhrs* is calculated as the product of the number of weeks the respondent reported practicing the previous year (*week*) and the number of hours the respondent reported spending in direct patient care activities in a typical week (*hours*). The same calculation for annual hours worked was performed for employee physicians, and the (weighted) mean of this amount was calculated for physicians of the same specialty as the respondent to obtain *emphrs*.

For solo physicians $nown = 1$ and $nemp = 0$, and the formula becomes:

$$\frac{X}{ownhrs}$$

or simply expenses divided by hours worked in direct patient care.

As an example of the expense per hour calculation for physicians in groups, suppose that a general surgeon reported that her share of the practice's office expenses was $100,000 for the previous year. Suppose she also reported that there were two owner physicians in the practice (including her) and two employee physicians, and that she worked 50 weeks the previous year and 60 hours per week in direct patient care in a typical week. Average annual hours worked for employee physicians in general surgery were 2381.8. The necessary data for calculating office expenses per hour for this respondent are:

$$X = \$100{,}000$$
$$nown = 2$$
$$nemp = 2$$
$$ownhrs = 50 \times 60 = 3000$$
$$emphrs = 2381.8$$

The numerator of the expense per hour formula will be $200,000 for this physician for office expenses. This is an estimate of the *practice's* total office expenses for the previous year, assuming physician owners share expenses equally.

The denominator of the expense-per-hour formula will be 10,763.8 hours for this physician. This is an estimate of total hours worked the previous year by all physicians (owners and employees) in the practice. It assumes that the average annual-hours worked among all owner physicians in the practice is equal to the annual-hours worked by the respondent. It also assumes that average annual-hours worked among all employee physicians in the practice is equal to average annual-hours worked among all employee physicians of that specialty.

Office expenses per hour for this respondent will be $18.58 ($200,000/10,763.8). This expense per hour amount were calculated for all self-employed physicians responding to the 1994–1998 SMS surveys subject to the edits specified by CMS. The weighted mean of this expense per hour amount was then calculated by specialty for each expense item to obtain the figures reported to CMS.

Table 5-2 contains the PE information that was provided to CMS for ongoing use in the Medicare Physician Payment Schedule (MFS). This table contains the information on the specialties that CMS had originally requested that use SMS data. In addition, through the rulemaking process, CMS establishes expense-per-hour (PE/HR) values for specialties without survey data from the SMS or the more recent Physician Practice Expense Information Survey by crosswalking them to other similar specialties to estimate a proxy PE/HR, as displayed in Table 5-3. All others are crosswalked to All Physician PE/HR, or they are not used in the development of PE RVUS. Note the data for the specialties that are crosswalked in Table 5-3 are de facto data based on the crosswalked specialty.

Table 5-2. Mean Practice Expenses per Hour Spent in Patient Care Activities (in 2006 Dollars)

Specialty	# of Cases	Nonphysician Clinical Staff	Clerical Payroll per Hour	Office Expense per Hour	Supplies Expense per Hour	Equipment Expense per Hour	Other Expense per Hour	Total Expense per Hour	Indirect Percentage
All Physicians	2,795	18.36	28.03	46.38	7.47	4.77	11.95	116.96	74%
Allergy and Immunology	100	50.56	53.17	91.56	21.51	6.33	17.95	241.08	67%
Anesthesiology	81	5.65	7.38	11.74	0.4	0.43	10.25	35.84	82%
Audiology	71	4.58	20.86	39.3	5.28	2.81	12.01	84.84	85%
Cardiology	55	31.07	30.09	47.83	5.63	10.82	10.12	135.56	65%
Cardiothoracic Surgery	84	8.98	22	33.15	3.09	1.51	12.68	81.4	83%
Chiropractor	120	5.02	15.7	40.38	1.64	4.04	9.25	76.03	86%
Clinical Psychology	56	0	1.65	14.64	0.07	1.38	3.78	21.52	93%
Clinical Social Work	127	0.21	2.26	10.82	0.19	0.13	4.72	18.33	97%
Colon and Rectal Surgery	93	13.38	23.66	55.27	6	2.66	11.92	112.88	80%
Dermatology	81	44.2	66.53	94.99	24.64	11.42	23.1	264.88	70%
Emergency Medicine	70	1.88	8.74	7.73	0.47	0.05	21.89	40.76	94%
Endocrinology	77	18.31	31.05	45.51	7.34	5.43	7.83	115.47	73%
Family Medicine	98	19.58	27.46	54.34	6.27	3.19	8.35	119.19	76%
Gastroenterology	57	17.11	35.18	50.68	9.04	5.42	10.92	128.34	75%
General Practice	30	16.43	25	47.47	16.24	3.39	6.12	114.65	69%
General Surgery	92	10.73	22.54	50.29	3.95	2.88	9.91	100.3	82%
Geriatrics	45	15.76	21.28	28.42	2.74	0.8	4.44	73.45	74%
Hand Surgery	73	26.23	54.47	73.08	8.42	9.65	21.23	193.08	77%

Specialty	# of Cases	Nonphysician Clinical Staff	Clerical Payroll per Hour	Office Expense per Hour	Supplies Expense per Hour	Equipment Expense per Hour	Other Expense per Hour	Total Expense per Hour	Indirect Percentage
Hematopoietic Cell Transplantation and Cellular Therapy	245	69.97	45.46	45.09	22.13	9.75	55.26	247.66	59%
Hospitalist	CW	1.88	8.74	7.73	0.47	0.05	21.89	40.76	94%
Independent Diagnostic Testing Facilities[1]	90	114.69	159.85	124.58	56.5	310.94	194.78	961.34	50%
Independent Lab[1]	90	87.17	26.49	19.63	20.4	9.08	22.21	184.97	37%
Internal Medicine	89	15.8	25.66	52.37	7.46	3.34	6	110.62	76%
Interventional Pain Management	52	37.28	54.89	78.22	18.77	11.07	23.68	223.91	70%
Interventional Radiology	33	9.02	24.81	15.93	5.92	4.05	41.81	101.55	81%
Medical Oncology[1]	245	69.97	45.46	45.09	22.13	9.75	55.26	247.66	59%
Medical Toxicology	70	1.88	8.74	7.73	0.47	0.05	21.89	40.76	94%
Nephrology	39	8.24	20.07	36.98	7.4	1.35	8.95	82.99	80%
Neurology	73	10.98	35.95	64.68	3.1	2.74	9.76	127.21	87%
Neurosurgery	81	9.35	41.29	62.69	1.75	5.66	11.78	132.52	87%
Nuclear Medicine	16	4.23	7.28	20.89	2.76	5.23	11.63	52.01	77%
Obstetrics/Gynecology	72	33.14	33.59	52.62	8.96	7.6	13.11	149.02	67%
Ophthalmology	80	45.7	54.66	92.21	13.77	13.14	23.21	242.68	70%
Optometry	106	15.79	23.44	52.35	4.62	6.35	12.23	114.78	77%
Oral Surgery (Dentists only)	70	40.34	50.65	102.78	35.4	16.81	19.76	265.74	65%
Orthopedic Surgery	66	21.35	46.13	69.45	5.27	4.92	15.82	162.94	81%
Osteopathic Manipulative Therapy	37	0.26	14.64	29.29	2.92	0.72	10	57.83	93%
Otolaryngology	72	30.38	50.71	76.96	7.82	9.95	13.86	189.69	75%
Pain Medicine	56	25.82	42.96	62.69	14.39	12.72	16.76	175.35	70%
Pathology	54	14.53	14.85	30.65	9.38	2.56	29.48	101.45	74%
Pediatrics	88	20.34	29.03	38.69	11.94	2.75	8.55	111.31	69%
Physical Medicine and Rehabilitation	69	8.11	46.65	52.82	5.7	7.05	10.66	130.98	84%
Physical Therapy	76	6.94	15.3	33.75	1.76	2.51	8.21	68.47	84%
Plastic Surgery	95	19.03	31.69	84.79	21.04	7.62	18.34	182.5	74%
Podiatry	99	7.07	20.9	45.68	6.69	2.51	8.18	91.03	82%
Psychiatry	86	1.54	8.88	16.11	0.13	0.34	5.1	32.1	94%
Pulmonary Disease	67	11.9	17.88	28.99	3.05	4.11	8.39	74.33	74%
Radiation Oncology (Hospital Based and Free Standing)	159	69.02	35.76	90.96	12.16	45.02	38.38	291.3	57%
Radiology	56	18.54	35.71	30.87	5.9	14.8	29.02	134.84	71%
Rheumatology	78	22.5	28.77	61.26	20.01	6.83	8.05	147.42	67%
Sleep Medicine	45	34.16	38.18	52.43	4.95	8.12	18.08	155.92	70%
Urology	80	16.75	30.81	51.2	11.69	7.69	15.01	133.14	73%
Vascular Surgery	74	15.95	28.11	43.31	6.55	8.22	12.56	114.69	73%

[1]Based on supplemental survey data.

Table 5-3. Specialty and Specialty Crosswalk Indirect Practice Expense per Hour Data

Specialty	Specialty Crosswalk	Clinical Labor	Supplies Expense	Equipment Expense	Direct PE/hr	Clerical Payroll	Office Expense	Other Expense	Indirect PE/hr	Total PE/hr
Addiction Medicine	Psychiatry	1.54	0.13	0.34	2.00	8.88	16.11	5.10	30.10	32.10
Advanced Heart Failure and Transplant Cardiology	Cardiology	31.07	5.63	10.82	47.52	30.09	47.83	10.12	88.04	135.56
Allergy/ Immunology		50.56	21.51	6.33	78.40	53.17	91.56	17.95	162.68	241.08
Anesthesiologist Assistants	Anesthesiology	5.65	0.40	0.43	6.47	7.38	11.74	10.25	29.36	35.84
Anesthesiology		5.65	0.40	0.43	6.47	7.38	11.74	10.25	29.36	35.84
Audiologist		4.58	5.28	2.81	12.67	20.86	39.30	12.01	72.17	84.84
Cardiac Electrophysiology	Cardiology	31.07	5.63	10.82	47.52	30.09	47.83	10.12	88.04	135.56
Cardiac Surgery		8.98	3.09	1.51	13.58	22.00	33.15	12.68	67.83	81.40
Cardiology		31.07	5.63	10.82	47.52	30.09	47.83	10.12	88.04	135.56
Certified Nurse Midwife	Obstetrics/ Gynecology	33.14	8.96	7.60	49.70	33.59	52.62	13.11	99.32	149.02
Chiropractic		5.02	1.64	4.04	10.70	15.70	40.38	9.25	65.33	76.03
Clinical Laboratory		87.17	20.40	9.08	116.65	26.49	19.63	22.21	68.32	184.97
Clinical Psychologist		0.00	0.07	1.38	1.45	1.65	14.64	3.78	20.07	21.52
Colorectal Surgery		13.38	6.00	2.66	22.04	23.66	55.27	11.92	90.84	112.88
CRNA	Anesthesiology	5.65	0.40	0.43	6.47	7.38	11.74	10.25	29.36	35.84
Dermatology		44.20	24.64	11.42	80.26	66.53	94.99	23.10	184.62	264.88
Diagnostic Radiology		18.54	5.90	14.80	39.24	35.71	30.87	29.02	95.60	134.84
Emergency Medicine		1.88	0.47	0.05	2.40	8.74	7.73	21.89	38.36	40.76
Endocrinology		18.31	7.34	5.43	31.08	31.05	45.51	7.83	84.39	115.47
Family Practice		19.58	6.27	3.19	29.04	27.46	54.34	8.35	90.15	119.19
Gastroenterology		17.11	9.04	5.42	31.56	35.18	50.68	10.92	96.78	128.34
General Practice		16.43	16.24	3.39	36.06	25.00	47.47	6.12	78.59	114.65
General Surgery		10.73	3.95	2.88	17.56	22.54	50.29	9.91	82.73	100.30
Geriatric Medicine		15.76	2.74	0.80	19.31	21.28	28.42	4.44	54.14	73.45
Geriatric Psychiatry	Psychiatry	1.54	0.13	0.34	2.00	8.88	16.11	5.10	30.10	32.10
Gynecologist/ Oncologist	Obstetrics/ Gynecology	33.14	8.96	7.60	49.70	33.59	52.62	13.11	99.32	149.02
Hand Surgery		26.23	8.42	9.65	44.29	54.47	73.08	21.23	148.78	193.08
Hematology/ Oncology[1]	Medical Oncology	69.97	22.13	9.75	101.85	45.46	45.09	55.26	145.81	247.66

Specialty	Specialty Crosswalk	Clinical Labor	Supplies Expense	Equipment Expense	Direct PE/hr	Clerical Payroll	Office Expense	Other Expense	Indirect PE/hr	Total PE/hr
Hematology[1]	Medical Oncology	69.97	22.13	9.75	101.85	45.46	45.09	55.26	145.81	247.66
Hematopoietic Cell Transplantation and Cellular Therapy	Medical Oncology	69.97	22.13	9.75	101.85	45.46	45.09	55.26	145.81	247.66
Hospitalist	Emergency Medicine	1.88	0.47	0.05	2.40	8.74	7.73	21.89	38.36	40.76
Independent Diagnostic Testing Facility[1]		114.69	56.50	310.94	482.13	159.85	124.58	194.78	479.21	961.34
Infectious Disease	Internal Medicine	15.80	7.46	3.34	26.60	25.66	52.37	6.00	84.02	110.62
Intensive Cardiac Rehab	Cardiology	31.07	5.63	10.82	47.52	30.09	47.83	10.12	88.04	135.56
Internal Medicine		15.80	7.46	3.34	26.60	25.66	52.37	6.00	84.02	110.62
Interventional Cardiology	Cardiology	31.07	5.63	10.82	47.52	30.09	47.83	10.12	88.04	135.56
Interventional Pain Management		37.28	18.77	11.07	67.12	54.89	78.22	23.68	156.79	223.91
Interventional Radiology		9.02	5.92	4.05	18.99	24.81	15.93	41.81	82.56	101.55
Licensed Clinical Social Worker		0.21	0.19	0.13	0.53	2.26	10.82	4.72	17.80	18.33
Mammography Screening Center	Independent Test Facility	114.69	56.50	310.94	482.13	159.85	124.58	194.78	479.21	961.34
Maxillofacial Surgery	Otolaryngology	30.38	7.82	9.95	48.15	50.71	76.96	13.86	141.54	189.69
Medical Oncology[1]		69.97	22.13	9.75	101.85	45.46	45.09	55.26	145.81	247.66
Medical Toxicology	Emergency Medicine	1.88	0.47	0.05	2.40	8.74	7.73	21.89	38.36	40.76
Nephrology		8.24	7.40	1.35	16.99	20.07	36.98	8.95	66.00	82.99
Neurology		10.98	3.10	2.74	16.82	35.95	64.68	9.76	110.39	127.21
Neuropsychiatry	Psychiatry	1.54	0.13	0.34	2.00	8.88	16.11	5.10	30.10	32.10
Neurosurgery		9.35	1.75	5.66	16.76	41.29	62.69	11.78	115.76	132.52
Nuclear Medicine		4.23	2.76	5.23	12.21	7.28	20.89	11.63	39.80	52.01
Obstetrics/ Gynecology		33.14	8.96	7.60	49.70	33.59	52.62	13.11	99.32	149.02
Occupational Therapist	Physical Therapy	6.94	1.76	2.51	11.21	15.30	33.75	8.21	57.26	68.47
Ophthalmology		45.70	13.77	13.14	72.61	54.66	92.21	23.21	170.07	242.68
Optometry		15.79	4.62	6.35	26.76	23.44	52.35	12.23	88.02	114.78
Oral Surgery		40.34	35.40	16.81	92.55	50.65	102.78	19.76	173.19	265.74
Orthopedic Surgery		21.35	5.27	4.92	31.54	46.13	69.45	15.82	131.40	162.94

(continued)

Table 5-3. Specialty and Specialty Crosswalk Indirect PE/HR Data (*continued*)

Specialty	Specialty Crosswalk	Clinical Labor	Supplies Expense	Equipment Expense	Direct PE/hr	Clerical Payroll	Office Expense	Other Expense	Indirect PE/hr	Total PE/hr
Osteopathic Manipulative Therapy		0.26	2.92	0.72	3.89	14.64	29.29	10.00	53.93	57.83
Otolaryngology		30.38	7.82	9.95	48.15	50.71	76.96	13.86	141.54	189.69
Pain Management		25.82	14.39	12.72	52.93	42.96	62.69	16.76	122.42	175.35
Pathology		14.53	9.38	2.56	26.47	14.85	30.65	29.48	74.98	101.45
Pediatric Medicine		20.34	11.94	2.75	35.04	29.03	38.69	8.55	76.27	111.31
Peripheral Vascular Disease	Vascular Surgery	15.95	6.55	8.22	30.72	28.11	43.31	12.56	83.98	114.69
Physical Medicine and Rehabilitation		8.11	5.70	7.05	20.85	46.65	52.82	10.66	110.13	130.98
Physical Therapist		6.94	1.76	2.51	11.21	15.30	33.75	8.21	57.26	68.47
Plastic and Reconstructive Surgery		19.03	21.04	7.62	47.69	31.69	84.79	18.34	134.81	182.50
Podiatry		7.07	6.69	2.51	16.27	20.90	45.68	8.18	74.76	91.03
Portable X-Ray Supplier	Independent Test Facility	114.69	56.50	310.94	482.13	159.85	124.58	194.78	479.21	961.34
Preventative Medicine	Internal Medicine	15.80	7.46	3.34	26.60	25.66	52.37	6.00	84.02	110.62
Psychiatry		1.54	0.13	0.34	2.00	8.88	16.11	5.10	30.10	32.10
Psychologist	Psychiatry	1.54	0.13	0.34	2.00	8.88	16.11	5.10	30.10	32.10
Pulmonary Disease		11.91	3.05	4.11	19.07	17.88	28.99	8.39	55.26	74.33
Radiation Oncology		69.02	12.16	45.02	126.20	35.76	90.96	38.38	165.10	291.30
Registered Dietician/Nutrition Professional	All Physicians	18.36	7.47	4.77	30.60	28.03	46.38	11.95	86.36	116.96
Rheumatology		22.50	20.01	6.83	49.34	28.77	61.26	8.05	98.08	147.42
Sleep Medicine	Sleep Medicine	34.16	4.95	8.12	47.23	38.18	52.43	18.08	108.69	155.92
Slide Preparation Facilities	Independent Laboratory	87.17	20.40	9.08	116.65	26.49	19.63	22.21	68.32	184.97
Speech Language Pathology	Physical Therapy	6.94	1.76	2.51	11.21	15.30	33.75	8.21	57.26	68.47
Sports Medicine	Family Practice	19.58	6.27	3.19	29.04	27.46	54.34	8.35	90.15	119.19
Thoracic Surgery		8.98	3.09	1.51	13.58	22.00	33.15	12.68	67.83	81.40
Urology		16.75	11.69	7.69	36.13	30.81	51.20	15.01	97.01	133.14
Vascular Surgery		15.95	6.55	8.22	30.72	28.11	43.31	12.56	83.98	114.69

[1]Based on supplemental survey data.

The Bottom-Up Practice Expense RVU Methodology

In the December 1, 2006, Final Rule, CMS revised the practice expense (PE) methodology to calculate direct PE RVUs from the existing top-down cost allocation methodology to a bottom-up methodology. Instead of using the top-down approach of calculating the direct PE RVUs, in which the aggregate practice expense input costs for each specialty are scaled to match the aggregate SMS costs, CMS has adopted a bottom-up method of determining the relative direct costs of each service. Under this method the direct costs would be determined by summing the costs of each of the resources typically required for the service. The clinical labor, medical supplies, and medical equipment costs would be summed from the refined PE inputs, reflected in the CMS direct PE input database. CMS has indicated that RUC-refined direct PE input data are "preferable to the SMS data for determining direct costs" and almost all of the comments received by CMS regarding this change in the PE methodology were supportive.

In the November 1, 2005, Final Rule, CMS made the following statement:

The bottom-up approach would be simple to understand—we merely sum the costs of the RUC/PEAC refined clinical staff, supply and equipment inputs that are assigned to each service. The bottom-up approach would be intuitive—any change in direct inputs would lead to a commensurate change in the direct PE RVUs. The bottom-up methodology should also be more stable—with no cost pools or scaling factors to complicate the computation, direct PE RVUs for a service would only change if there was a revision to the inputs assigned. It was the hard work put forth by the AMA, the PEAC, and RUC and specialty societies in refining the CPEP inputs that made it possible to propose using a bottom-up methodology.

However, the CMS bottom-up proposal was not implemented for CY 2006 because of an error in the PE program that resulted in a miscalculation of the indirect costs. This miscalculation resulted in almost all of the PE RVUs published in the August 8, 2005, Proposed Rule to be incorrect. CMS became concerned that interested parties were not provided with sufficient notification of the actual effect of the proposed changes in the PE methodology. The medical community and others, therefore, could not submit meaningful comments on the proposal. For 2006, CMS used the 2005 PE RVUs for all services, accounting for only two refinements for the year. These refinements included the application of the PE per hour data from the urology supplemental survey for urology drug administration codes. CMS also applied the savings from the multiple procedure reductions for certain imaging services across all PE RVUs. However, in 2007, this savings was removed due to a provision in the Deficit Reduction Act.

As previously explained, CMS did implement the bottom-up methodology in determining direct PE inputs in 2007. This change in methodology for calculating PE RVUs was implemented over a four-year period. During the transition period, the PE RVUs were based on a blend of RVUs weighted for the new method by 25% during 2007, 50% during 2008, 75% during 2009, and 100% thereinafter. It should be noted that the PE RVUs for codes that were new during this period were calculated using only the current PE methodology and were paid at the fully transitioned rate. In addition, CMS implemented a few other modifications to the indirect PE methodology, including:

- Elimination of the nonphysician work pool (NPWP). This pool had previously been created to allocate PE RVUs for technical component codes and other codes that did not have physician work RVUs. This methodology did not use the resource-based methodology but instead used the 1998 PE RVUs to allocate costs from a separate cost pool created for codes with no physician work. Now CMS has created "proxy work" RVUs for these services (and for services with minimal work), utilizing clinical staff costs or the Medicare conversion factor, and no longer applies this alternate methodology.
- An update of the utilization data used in the methodology.
- Acceptance of supplemental PE survey data for a number of specialties, including allergy, cardiology, dermatology, gastroenterology, radiology, radiation oncology, and urology. (Note: These data have now been replaced with the PPI survey data. See discussion on page 63.)
- Starting in 2016, CMS began using an average of three years of the most recent available Medicare-claims data to determine specialty mix. This change resulted in less fluctuation from year to year, especially for low-volume and new services.

The following is an example of how the PE RVUs for code 99213 will be calculated in 2022 using the 2007 ("bottom-up") PE methodology.

Step 1 Sum the direct costs of the clinical labor, medical supplies, and medical equipment for each service. The clinical labor cost is the sum of the total cost of all the staff types associated with the service (each staff type's cost is the product of the time for each staff type and the wage rate for the staff type). The medical supplies cost is the sum of the supplies associated with the service (each supplies' cost is the product of the quantity of each supply and the cost of the supply). The medical equipment cost is the sum of the equipment associated with the service (the product of the number of minutes each piece of equipment is used in the service and the equipment cost per minute).

$$\text{Direct Labor Cost} + \text{Direct Supply Cost} + \text{Direct Equipment Cost} = \text{Direct Costs}$$

$$\$14.87 + \$5.54 + \$0.34 = \$20.74$$

Step 2 Calculate the current aggregate pool of direct PE costs by multiplying the current aggregate pool of total direct and indirect PE costs (ie, the current aggregate PE RVUs multiplied by the conversion factor) by the average direct PE percentage from the physician practice information survey and supplementary specialty survey data.

Step 3 Calculate the aggregate pool of direct costs by summing the product of the direct costs for each service from Step 1 and the utilization data for that service.

Step 4 Using the results of Steps 2 and 3, calculate the direct adjustment and apply it to the direct costs from Step 1.

For 2022, CMS has computed this direct adjustment to be 0.5094.

$$\text{Labor Cost} \times \text{Direct Adjustment}$$

$$\$14.87 \times 0.5094 = \$7.57$$

$$\text{Supply Cost} \times \text{Direct Adjustment}$$

$$\$5.54 \times 0.5094 = \$2.82$$

$$\text{Equipment Cost} \times \text{Direct Adjustment}$$

$$\$0.34 \times 0.5094 = \$0.17$$

Step 5 Convert the products from Step 4 to an RVU by dividing them by the MFS conversion factor and sum these RVUs to obtain the adjusted direct RVUs. **Note that the actual value of the conversion factor (CF) used in this calculation does not influence the final direct cost PE RVUs, as long as the same CF amount is used in Step 4 and Step 5.** Different CFs would result in different direct PE scaling adjustments, but this has no effect on the final direct cost PE RVUs because changes in the CFs and changes in the associated direct scaling adjustments offset one another.

$$\text{Labor RVU}$$

$$\$7.57 \div \$33.6319 = 0.23 \text{ RVUs}$$

$$\text{Supply RVU}$$

$$\$2.82 \div \$33.6319 = 0.08 \text{ RVUs}$$

$$\text{Equipment RVU}$$

$$\$0.17 \div \$33.6319 = 0.01 \text{ RVUs}$$

$$\text{Labor RVU} + \text{Supply RVU} + \text{Equipment RVU} = \text{Adjusted Direct RVUs}$$

$$0.23 + 0.08 + 0.01 = 0.311$$

Note that CMS does not disclose how they handle rounding for each component for this step in the formula.

The computed direct PE RVU is 0.31

Step 6 Based on the physician practice information survey and supplementary specialty survey data, calculate direct and indirect PE percentage for each physician specialty.

Step 7 Calculate the direct and indirect PE percentages at the service level by taking a weighted average of the results of Step 6 for the specialties that provide the service. It should be noted that for services with technical components and professional components, the direct and indirect PE percentages are calculated across the global component.

In 2022, the direct percentage for CPT code 99213 is 25% and the indirect percentage is 75%.

Step 8 Calculate the service level allocators for the indirect PEs based on the percentages calculated in Step 7. The indirect PEs are allocated based on three components: the direct PE RVU, the clinical PE RVU, and the work RVU.

For most services, the formula is:

$$\text{Indirect Percentage} \times (\text{Direct PE RVU} \div \text{Direct Percentage}) + \text{Work RVU} = \text{Indirect Allocator}$$

In 2022, CPT code 99213 is computed as:

$$0.75 \times (0.31 \div 0.25) + 1.30 = 2.26$$

However, in two situations this formula would be altered. The first situation is when the service is a global service, and the indirect allocator is as follows:

$$\text{Indirect Percentage} \times (\text{Direct PE RVU} \div \text{Direct Percentage}) + \text{Clinical PE RVU} + \text{Work RVU}$$

The second situation is when the clinical labor PE RVU exceeds the work RVU; then the indirect allocator is as follows:

$$\text{Indirect Percentage} \times (\text{Direct PE RVU} \div \text{Direct Percentage}) + \text{Clinical PE RVU}$$

Step 9 Calculate the current aggregate pool of indirect PE RVUs by multiplying the current aggregate pool of PE RVUs by the average indirect PE percentage from the physician specialty survey data.

Step 10 Calculate the aggregate pool of proposed indirect PE RVUs for all MFS services by adding the product of the indirect PE allocators for a service from Step 8 and the utilization data for that service.

Step 11 Using the results of Steps 9 and 10, calculate an indirect PE adjustment so that the aggregate indirect allocation does not exceed the available aggregate indirect PE RVUs, and apply it to indirect allocators calculated in Step 8.

For 2022, the indirect adjustment is **0.3890**.

Code 99213: 2.26 (Step 8) $\times$ 0.3890 = 0.88

Step 12 Using the results of Step 11, calculate aggregate pools of specialty-specific adjusted indirect PE allocators for all MFS services for a specialty by adding the product of the adjusted indirect PE allocator for each service and the utilization data for that service.

Step 13 Using the specialty specific indirect PE/hour data, calculate specialty-specific aggregate pools of indirect PE for all MFS services for that specialty by adding the product of the indirect PE/hour for the specialty, the physician time for the service, and the specialty's utilization for the service.

Step 14 Using the results of Step 12 and Step 13, calculate the specialty specific indirect PE scaling factors as under the current methodology.

Step 15 Using the results of Step 14, calculate an indirect practice cost index at the specialty level by dividing each specialty-specific indirect scaling factor by the average indirect scaling factor for the entire MFS.

Step 16 Calculate the indirect practice cost index at the service level to ensure all of the indirect costs have been captured. Calculate a weighted average of the practice cost index values for the specialties that furnish the service. Note that for services with technical components and physician components, calculate the indirect practice cost index across the global components.

In 2022, the indirect practice cost index for code 99213 is 1.09.

Step 17 Apply the service level indirect practice cost index calculated in Step 16 to the service level adjusted indirect allocators calculated in Step 11 to obtain the indirect PE RVUs.

$$1.09 \times 0.88 = 0.96$$

Step 18 Add the direct PE RVUs from Step 5 to the indirect PE RVUs from Step 17 and apply the final PE budget-neutrality adjustment. The final PE budget-neutrality adjustment is calculated by comparing the aggregate work RVUs scaled by the ratio of current aggregate PE and work RVUs. This final PE budget-neutrality adjustment is required primarily because certain specialties are excluded from the PE RVU calculation for rate-setting purposes, but all specialties are included for purposes of calculating the final PE budget-neutrality adjustment.

0.31 (adjusted direct PE RVU) + 0.96 (adjusted indirect PE RVU) = 1.26

Note that CMS does not disclose how they handle rounding for each component for this step in the formula.

1.26 $\times$ 1.00 (budget-neutrality adjustment) = 1.26

Step 19 Apply the phase-in of significant RVU reductions and the associated adjustment.

This approach limits the year one reduction for the service to the maximum allowed amount (that is, 19%) and then phases in the remainder of the reduction. The PE RVUs are adjusted to ensure that the total RVUs for all services that are not new or revised codes decrease by no more than 19%, and then a relativity adjustment is applied to ensure that the total pool of aggregate PE RVUs remains relative to the pool of work and MP RVUs.

In 2022, the final PE RVU with phase-in for code 99213 is 1.26.

Adjustment to Allocation of Indirect PE for Some Office-Based Services

In the PE RVU calculation outlined above, CMS allocates indirect costs for each code based on the direct costs specifically associated with a code and the greater of either the clinical labor costs or the work RVUs. For MFS services priced in both the facility and nonfacility settings, the difference in indirect PE RVUs between the settings is driven by differences in direct PE inputs for those settings since the other allocator of indirect PE, the work RVU, does not differ between settings. Generally, the direct PE input costs are higher in the nonfacility setting than in the facility setting. As a result, indirect PE RVUs allocated to these services are higher in the nonfacility setting than in the facility setting. However, when direct PE inputs for a service are minimal, the allocation of indirect PE RVUs becomes almost entirely dependent on the work RVUs, causing the total PE RVUs in the facility and nonfacility settings to be almost the same. This allocation methodology does not allow for appropriate payment of the indirect costs involved in furnishing services in nonfacility setting. Among the services most affected by this anomaly are services for behavioral health.

Starting in 2018, CMS modified the existing methodology for allocating indirect PE RVUs to better reflect the relative indirect PE resources involved in furnishing behavioral health and other low direct PE inputs services in the nonfacility setting. CMS has used the following criteria to identify the services where an indirect PE adjustment will be applied: describe face-to-face services, have work RVUs greater than zero, and are priced in both the facility and nonfacility setting. From those codes CMS further narrowed the list by selecting those with the lowest ratio between nonfacility PE RVUs and work RVUs and selecting 0.4 as an appropriate threshold. There are fewer than 50 codes where the adjustment will be applied. CMS will address the anomaly by establishing a minimum nonfacility indirect PE RVU that would better reflect the resources involved in furnishing the identified services, using the indirect PE RVU to work RVU ratio for the most commonly furnished office-based, face-to-face service (CPT 99213). CMS has compared the ratio between indirect PE RVUs and work RVUs that result from the preliminary application of the standard methodology to the ratio for the marker code, CPT code 99213. This will increase the allocation of indirect PE RVUs to the anomalous codes to at least one quarter of the difference between the two ratios. Because the change in PE methodology has a significant impact on PE relativity across the MFS, CMS is phasing in the adjustment over four years, effectively implementing only one quarter of the minimum value for nonfacility indirect PE for the codes identified. The change in methodology will have an impact of approximately $40 million, or approximately 0.04% of total MFS allowed charges for each year of the proposed four-year transition. CY 2021 was the final year of the phase-in.

Computation of Medical Equipment Costs

In the November 1, 2012, Final Rule, CMS adopted a new approach to determine the interest rate used in the computation of medical equipment costs. The interest rate will vary based on a "sliding scale" determined by the equipment cost, useful life, and small business administration (SBA) maximum interest rates for different categories of loan size and maturity.

The equipment cost per minute is calculated as:

$$\left(1 \div \frac{\text{minutes}}{\text{per year}} \times \text{usage}\right) \times \text{price} \times \left[\frac{\text{Interest}}{\text{rate}} \div \left(1 - \left\{1 \div \left[1 + \frac{\text{interest}}{\text{rate}}\right]^{a}\right\}\right)\right] + \text{maintenance}$$

Minutes per year = maximum minutes per year if usage were continuous (that is, usage = 1); 150,000 minutes

Usage = equipment utilization assumption; 0.5*

Price = price of the particular piece of equipment

Interest rate = Sliding Scale (See table below)

^{a} = life of equipment, ie, useful life of the particular piece of equipment

Maintenance = factor for maintenance; 0.05

Medical Equipment Costs

		≤ $25,000	$25,000 – $50,000	≥ $50,000
Useful Life	< 7 years	7.5% (PR + 4.25)	6.5% (PR + 3.25)	5.5% (PR + 2.25)
	≥ 7 years	8.0% (PR + 4.75)	7.0% (PR + 3.75)	6.0% (PR + 2.75)

Abbreviation: PR indicates prime rate.

*Beginning in 2014, Section 1848(b)(4)(C) of the American Taxpayer Relief Act of 2012 (ATRA), as modified by section 635, indicates that expensive diagnostic imaging equipment, for example, MRI, CT, CTA and MRA services, the equipment utilization rate assumption of 0.90.

Refinement of Resource-Based Practice Expenses

The AMA closely monitored all phases in the development of the new relative values and advocated that they be based on valid physician practice expense data. Because there is not a single universally accepted cost allocation methodology, it is especially important that CMS continues to base its methodology on actual practice expense data. CMS' decisions not only affect Medicare payments, but because many other payment systems use the Medicare RBRVS, the change to resource-based practice expense relative values has broad implications for the entire health care system. Due to the significance of this issue, RUC established an advisory committee to assist in refining a portion of the data used to calculate practice expense relative values.

The transition period for practice expense relative value units reflected a combination of the 1998 charge-based value and the new resource value. The transition began in 1999 when practice expense resource values were based on 75% of the 1998 charge-based relative value and 25% on the resource-based value. In 2000, the mix was equally weighted between the charge-based and resource-based values, and in 2001, the practice expense relative values are 75% resource-based and only 25% charged-based. In 2002, the transition was completed with practice expense RVUs totally resource-based. In 2007, CMS implemented a new practice expense methodology.

The AMA advocated that the practice expense relative values remain interim during the refinement process and CMS has agreed to keep the values interim during the four-year transition to resource-based practice expense relative values. This interim period was necessary due to the amount of refinement work that needed to occur and so physicians would have had an opportunity to provide CMS with new data to be used in updating the practice expense relative values. In the November 1, 2001, Final Rule, CMS went further in offering to leave the practice expense values interim until refinement is complete.

The numerous issues that have been or will be addressed in refinement can be divided into the following six categories:

- Review and refine practice expense/hour data
- Obtain and review practice expense/hour data for specialties and practitioners not included in the SMS survey
- Address anomalies, if any, in code-specific Harvard/RUC physician time data
- Address anomalies, if any, in code-specific CPEP data on clinical staff types and times, quantity and cost of medical supplies, and quantity and cost of medical equipment
- Refine, as needed, the CMS process of developing practice expense RVUs for codes that were not addressed by the CPEP process, for example, codes that were new in 1996, 1997, 1998, and 1999
- Develop practice expense RVUs for codes that will be new in 2000 and beyond

RUC's Role in Refinement

RUC has played a key role in the refinement of practice expense relative values since first implemented in 1999. RUC is committed to providing CMS with recommendations that accurately reflect the resources required to perform the service. RUC has also agreed that as RUC reviews new or revised codes for the work component, the committee will also consider the direct practice expense inputs for these services.

When CMS published the details of its current practice expense methodology in June 1998, CMS stated:

There is much needed improvement in the CPEP data, and the identification and correction of any CPEP errors whether in staff times, supplies, equipment, or pricing will be a major focus of our refinement process.

In response to the need to update this set of data, RUC created a special advisory committee, the Practice Expense Advisory Committee (PEAC) to assist RUC in refining the direct input data CMS uses to calculate practice expense relative values. PEAC was charged to review direct expense inputs (ie, clinical time, supplies, and equipment) for individual CPT codes. PEAC held several meetings to develop a process for reviewing the direct inputs associated with CPT codes, and is working with CMS to develop clear definitions. In September 1999, RUC approved the first set of direct inputs reviewed by PEAC. These recommendations were forwarded to CMS, which then accepted a majority of the recommendations and incorporated these changes into the Medicare payment schedule for 2000. PEAC met several times in 2000, whereby it continued to review the direct input data and refine its methodology for code selection and analysis.

In May 2000, RUC submitted recommendations to CMS on direct practice expense inputs for new and revised CPT codes. PEAC and RUC also reviewed the Evaluation and Management codes and recommended new data be utilized to reflect clinical staff, medical supplies, and medical equipment. CMS accepted these recommendations and implemented the data on January 1, 2001. In addition, RUC recommended, and CMS has implemented, standardized medical supply packages for nearly 600 CPT codes. These revisions to medical supplies were based on recommendations from ophthalmology, neurosurgery, and obstetrics/gynecology.

The development of standardized medical supply packages and benchmarks of typical direct inputs contributed greatly to the refinement efforts, and 2001 was particularly successful with PEAC refining the inputs for over 1100 codes. Standardized medical supply packages and benchmarking allowed a few specialties including dermatology, orthopedic surgery, urology, pathology, ophthalmology, and physical medicine to refine large numbers of codes that were of importance to these specialties. CMS accepted virtually all recommendations with only minor revisions in that year.

In 2002, PEAC concentrated on each specialty's top 10 codes (per Medicare utilization), and refined the direct inputs for each. CMS accepted 100% of PEAC's recommendations on 1200 codes that year, and updated its clinical labor staff salary listing to reflect current wage data.

In 2003, PEAC reviewed and submitted standardized inputs for global surgical codes, as well as nearly 1000 individual codes. This submission included the remaining evaluation and management services. CMS also completed a major refinement of medical supply pricing.

In 2004, PEAC reviewed the direct practice expense inputs for most of the remaining CPT codes yet to be refined. PEAC made recommendations for these remaining 2200 codes and CMS accepted nearly all of them. In addition, CMS completed a major refinement of its medical equipment pricing in that year.

CMS has implemented practice expense refinements to all CPT codes, representing nearly all the MFS spending. PEAC concluded its work as a committee in March 2004, after CMS had implemented practice expense refinements to nearly all CPT codes, representing nearly all the MFS spending At that time, RUC created an ad hoc committee, the Practice Expense Review Committee (PERC), to assist RUC in refining the remaining few CPT codes not yet reviewed, and to offer advice on new/revised codes and other general refinement issues.

Throughout the PEAC/RUC process, practice expense standards and benchmarks were established which were not used when the data was originally collected. As a result, specialty societies have been able to refine their data using standards that apply to all specialties in a uniform manner. In addition, RUC has examined and made recommendations on other refinement issues involving the general methodology utilized to calculate practice expense RVUs.

In response to the 2012 Proposed Rule, RUC recommended that rather than applying the same interest rate across all equipment, CMS should consider a "sliding scale" approach to determine the interest rate utilized in computing equipment costs. Previously, CMS was using an interest rate of 11% and applied it across all equipment. RUC recommended a "sliding scale" approach that will account for changes in the prime rate or the SBA's formula for maximum allowed interest rates. In 2014, CMS adopted RUCs recommendation and implemented the "sliding scale" approach based on the current Small Business Administration (SBA) maximum interest rates for different categories of loan size (price of the equipment) and maturity (useful life of the equipment). In addition, CMS is updating this assumption through annual MFS rulemaking to account for fluctuations in the prime rate and/or changes to the SBA's formula to determine maximum allowed interest rates.

The maximum interest rates for SBA loans are as follows:

- Fixed rate loans of $50,000 or more must not exceed 5.50% if the maturity is less than 7 years, and 6.00% if the maturity is 7 years or more.
- For loans between $25,000 and $50,000, maximum rates must not exceed 6.50% if the maturity is less than 7 years, and 7.00% if the maturity is 7 years or more.
- For loans of $25,000 or less, the maximum interest rate must not exceed 7.50% if the maturity is less than 7 years, and 8.00%, if the maturity is 7 years or more.

Migration from Film to Digital Practice Expense Inputs

After two years of effort, the Practice Expense Subcommittee Migration from Film to Digital Imaging Workgroup completed their work and recommendations were submitted to CMS by RUC following the April 2013 RUC meeting. RUC recommended that for existing codes, CMS remove 21 supply items and nine equipment inputs from 604 imaging CPT codes and replace the film supplies and equipment with the recommended picture archiving and communication system (PACS) equipment. RUC recommended that there be no modifications to clinical labor activities for existing codes. RUC also recommended revised clinical labor activities and times for the new codes and codes that are being reviewed by RUC moving forward. CMS accepted the RUC recommendation to remove the identified supplies and equipment, however, they removed the supplies and equipment from the CMS direct PE input database entirely, including from 50 additional codes purposefully excluded from the RUC recommendation because digital technology is not yet typical or because the code describes a service that is not imaging, but does require one piece of equipment that is used to view past imaging studies. As a proxy for the PACS equipment recommended by RUC, CMS finalized its recommendation to allocate equipment minutes for a desktop computer (ED021). For 2016, as a proxy for the PACS equipment recommended by RUC and based on submitted invoices, CMS finalized its recommendation to allocate equipment minutes for a PACS workstation (ED050), representing more accurate pricing for the PACS equipment. In addition to the RUC recommendations that CMS approved regarding the migration from film to digital, CMS also agreed with RUC's recommendation to revise clinical labor time resulting from changes in film technology as CPT codes are reviewed and to make no modifications to clinical labor activities for existing codes. For 2016, CMS reported that the migration from film to digital technology accounts for $240 million in annual redistribution within the MFS.

For 2017, CMS finalized its recommendation to create a new equipment input for a professional PACS workstation (ED053), priced more than two and a half times higher than the less accurate proxy equipment input. The new input was incorporated into 513 CPT codes for 2017. CMS divided these 513 codes into diagnostic and therapeutic categories. For diagnostic codes, they assigned equipment minutes equal to half the preservice physician work time and the full intraservice physician work time. For the relatively smaller group of diagnostic codes with no service period time breakdown, CMS assigned equipment time equal to half of the total physician work time. For therapeutic codes, they allocated equipment minutes equal to half the preservice physician work time and half the post-service physician work time for the second group.

CMS' Efforts on Refinement

Since 1997, when CMS first proposed a resource-based PE methodology, CMS has had three major goals for this payment system and has encouraged input from the medical community regarding PE data and methodology. These three goals are:

- To ensure that the PE payments reflect, to the greatest extent possible, the actual relative resources required for each of the services on the MFS. This could only be accomplished by using the best available data to calculate the PE RVUs.
- To develop a payment system for PE that is understandable and at least somewhat intuitive, so that specialties could generally predict the impacts of changes in the PE data.
- To stabilize the PE payments so that there are not large fluctuations in the payment for given procedures from year-to-year.

Over the refinement period, CMS has made several broad-based changes in the practice expense data used to calculate resource-based practice expense relative value units. These are primarily "egregious errors and anomalies" that have been highlighted by specialties since the introduction of the new CMS methodology. In addition, CMS made a number of changes in CPEP data based on specific RUC recommendations. For example, a contractor examined criteria under which CMS would use survey (supplemental) data to improve specialty representation in CMS' calculation of the specialty specific PE/HR.

In 2001, CMS issued strict criteria that specialties would need to follow to submit supplemental practice expense data. CMS announced new criteria for supplemental survey data in the December 31, 2001, Final Rule. The criteria are as follows:

- Physician groups must draw their sample from the AMA Physician Masterfile to ensure a nationally representative sample that includes both members and nonmembers of a physician specialty group.
- Nonphysician specialties not included in the AMA's SMS must develop a method to draw a nationally representative sample of members and nonmembers.
- A group (or its contractors) must conduct the survey based on the SMS survey instruments and protocols. Physician groups must use a contractor that has experience with the SMS or a survey firm with experience successfully conducting national multispecialty surveys of physicians using nationally representative random samples.
- Physician groups or their contractors must submit raw survey data to CMS, including all complete and incomplete survey responses as well as any cover letters and instructions that accompanied the survey.
- Supplemental survey data must include data in the six practice expense categories: clinical labor, medical supplies, medical equipment, administrative labor, office overhead, and other.
- CMS requires a 90% confidence interval with a range of plus or minus 10% of the mean (ie, 1.645 times the standard error of the mean divided by the mean should be equal to or less than 10% of the mean).
- CMS has accepted supplemental data that meets the established criteria that they received by March 1, 2006, to determine calendar year (CY) 2006 practice expense relative values. CMS has stopped accepting supplemental survey data and has welcomed "comments on the most appropriate way to proceed to ensure the indirect PEs per hour are accurate and consistent across specialties."

Physician Practice Information Survey

As discussed earlier in this chapter, CMS implemented a change in its methodology for PE payments. As part of this change, both CMS and the Medicare Payment Advisory Commission (MedPAC) expressed interest in a multi-specialty PE survey to determine the current practice costs of physicians because the data they had been using was collected from 1995 through 1999. The AMA responded to this interest in March 2006, when more than 70 specialty societies and other health care professional organizations joined the AMA in a letter urging CMS to work with the entire physician community in a new multispecialty data collection effort.

The Physician Practice Information (PPI) Survey was conducted throughout 2007 and 2008 to collect data for the 2010 MFS including specialty-specific PE/hour data. CMS accepted and used the data collected from this survey effort to develop, starting in 2010, PE RVUs for those specialties that participated in the survey, excluding oncology in which CMS used the American Society of Clinical Oncology's supplemental survey data as mandated by the Medicare Prescription Drug, Improvement and Modernization Act (MMA) of 2003. This new specialty PE/hour data was incorporated into the new PE RVUs over a four-year transition period. However, practice expense relative values for new codes created during this four-year period were calculated using only the current practice expense method and were paid at the full transitioned rate. CY 2013 was the fourth and final year of the transition to new specialty practice expense data, collected in the PPI Survey.

One hundred percent of the practice expense relative values are now based on the PPI Survey data. The AMA and RUC continue to work with, and closely monitor, CMS' progress to ensure that the direct practice expense inputs assigned to each service are correct and that the overall methodology is appropriate. RUC also works to ensure that future data collection on physician's overall practice expense data is fair to all specialties.

2020 AMA Practice Expense Pilot Survey

A new PE data collection effort is underway. In March 2020, AMA staff conducted in-depth interviews with physicians and financial experts from several practices to help inform the planning of a PE pilot study. The practices represented varied specialties and practice characteristics. The interviews were encouraging and helpful in developing the study design. Improvements in information systems over the last decade, coupled with potential outreach to financial experts in each practice, indicate that a new data collection effort could be successful. A successful pilot survey was conducted in summer 2020. The pilot was administered to 32 physician practices. These practices represented 31 specialties of various practice types and sizes. Physicians were interviewed from various geographic regions throughout the United States. The AMA will convene meetings with CMS and national medical specialty societies and other health care organizations to share lessons learned from the pilot study and to discuss the potential for a large-scale survey. Because of the COVID-19 pandemic, the AMA Practice Expense Survey will be pursued for CY 2022.

Equipment Utilization Rate

As part of the PE methodology associated with the allocation of equipment costs for calculating PE RVUs, a 50% utilization assumption is currently used. In 2009, following MedPAC discussion, CMS announced that it would increase the equipment utilization rate to 90% for all CT and MRI services (ie, diagnostic equipment that cost in excess of $1 million). This new equipment-utilization rate assumption was to be transitioned into the new PE RVUs over four years beginning in 2010. However, from 2011-2013, CMS applied a 75% utilization rate for all diagnostic equipment in excess of $1 million assumption as mandated by the Affordable Care Act of 2010. In 2014 CMS applied a 90% utilization rate assumption to all the services to which the 75% equipment-utilization rate assumption applied in 2013. The equipment-utilization rate assumption for advanced imaging services furnished on or after January 1, 2014, is 90%. The equipment-utilization rate for services utilizing a linear accelerator on or after January 1, 2018, is 60%.

Supply, Equipment, and Clinical Labor Pricing Updates

The first comprehensive review of supply and equipment prices since 2004–2005 occurred with the Proposed Rule for CY 2019 when CMS used its authority under Section 220(a) of the Protecting Access to Medicare Act (PAMA) of 2014 to initiate a market research contract with a consulting firm, StrategyGen, to update the direct practice expense inputs for supply and equipment pricing. Based on the report from StrategyGen, CMS updated pricing for 2017 supply and equipment items used as direct PE inputs. Market research resources and methodologies included field surveys, aggregate databases, vendor resources, market scans, market analysis, physician substantiation, and statistical analysis. CMS transitioned the supply and equipment pricing update over a four-year phase-in. The RUC encouraged CMS to continue to consider all pricing data including invoices and other supporting evidence that they received from the specialty societies throughout the entirety of the four-year transition period. CY 2022 marks the final year of the four-year market-based transition for supply and equipment pricing.

Recognizing that the clinical labor pricing had not been updated since 2002, CMS began an update to the clinical labor pricing for CY 2022, in conjunction with the final year of its supply and equipment pricing update. The median Bureau of Labor Statistics (BLS) wage data will be used to calculate the clinical labor pricing updates because the BLS wage data continues to be the most accurate source to use as a basis for clinical labor pricing. The majority of the RBRVS data inputs are based on the median; therefore, using the median BLS data will appropriately reflect changes in clinical labor resource inputs for purposes of establishing practice expense relative values. In addition, CMS is updating the fringe benefit multiplier from 2002 to 1.296. There will be a four-year transition to the updated labor pricing, much like the transition used in updating the supply and equipment pricing. This transition will help account for the impact of the clinical labor rate update, thus recognizing that services with substantial direct costs attributable to clinical labor will experience increases while services with proportionally more supplies and equipment direct costs will experience declines.

The AMA understands that the update in clinical labor costs may result in a significant budget-neutrality adjustment to practice expense RVUs and will continue to advocate for Congress to provide a positive update to the Medicare conversion factor in 2022 and future years.

Chapter 6

Professional Liability Insurance Component

On January 1, 2000, the Centers for Medicare & Medicaid Services (CMS) implemented resource-based professional liability insurance (PLI) relative value units (RVUs). With this implementation and final transition of the resource-based practice expense relative values on January 1, 2002, components of the resource-based relative value scale (RBRVS) are no longer based on historical charges. This chapter explains the previous payment methodology for professional liability insurance expense and discusses the implementation of resource-based PLI relative values.

Data Used to Assign Charge-Based PLI RVUs

As explained in Chapter 5, the Omnibus Budget Reconciliation Act (OBRA) of 1989 approach to valuing the practice expense component was also utilized in creating PLI relative values. Table 2 in Chapter 5 illustrates the percentage of mean PLI expenses as a percentage of total revenue per specialty, based on data from the 1988–1990 American Medical Association (AMA) Socioeconomic Monitoring System Core Survey. To distribute PLI RVUs among services, the OBRA 89 method applies the average PLI expense percentage for each specialty to the 1991 average Medicare approved amount for each service. For example:

- For a service that only family practitioners provide and for which the average Medicare payment in 1991 was $100, the PLI proportion for family physicians (3.9%) is multiplied by the $100 average approved amount. The PLI expense component of the service would be assigned 3.9 (initial dollar) RVUs.
- For a service that only neurosurgeons provide and for which the average Medicare payment in 1991 was $1000, the PLI proportion for neurosurgeons (7.6%) is multiplied by the $1000 average approved amount. The PLI expense component of the service would be assigned 76 (initial dollar) RVUs.

For services provided by physicians in more than one specialty, each specialty's PLI expense proportion is multiplied by the proportion of claims for the service that the specialty submits, as follows:

- For a service that is provided 70% of the time by neurosurgeons and 30% of the time by orthopedic surgeons, the neurosurgeons' PLI proportion (7.6%) is multiplied by 70% and the orthopedic surgeons' PLI proportion (7.4%) is multiplied by 30%. The sum of these two products becomes the PLI proportion for the service:

$$(7.6\% \times 0.70) + (7.4\% \times 0.30) = 7.5\%$$

This PLI expense proportion is then multiplied by the $1000 average approved amount:

$$(7.5\% \times \$1000) = \$75$$

The PLI expense component of the service would be assigned 75 (initial dollar) RVUs.

Because anesthesia services are not divided into work, practice expense, and PLI RVUs, CMS computed the proportions of total payments for anesthesia that were comparable to these three components for other services. The portion of the anesthesiology conversion factor reflecting the work component was reduced by 42%. As for other services, to maintain a Medicare contribution comparable to the contribution under customary, prevailing, and reasonable (CPR), the portion of the conversion factor reflecting PLI was not reduced.

The CMS based the 1992 PLI RVUs on 1989 charge data "aged" to reflect 1991 payment rules because those were the most recent data available. For the 1992 payment schedule, actual 1991 charge data were used to recalculate the PLI RVUs for some codes for which CMS had imputed values the previous year. For services with insufficient charge data and for new codes, CMS developed crosswalks to predecessor codes, where possible. Since 1993, CMS has used a similar process to establish values for such codes.

Creating Resource-Based PLI Relative Values

In its 1996 and 1997 Annual Reports, the Physician Payment Review Commission (PPRC) called for Congress to revise current law to allow for the development of resource-based PLI RVUs. Further, the PPRC recommended that CMS be directed "to collect data on risk groups and relative insurance premiums across insurers" that could be used in the resource-based component. The AMA generally supported the PPRC's risk-of-service approach but identified a few issues that warrant further investigation. The AMA called for additional study to determine the extent to which relative premiums and classification methods differ across areas and insurers and to determine whether significant differences exist in liability premiums across physicians in a particular specialty resulting from differences in service mix. The Medicare Payment Advisory Commission (MedPAC) has also supported basing PLI RVUs not only on the physician specialty but also on the type of service. MedPAC contended that the research demonstrates that even within a specialty, the risk of malpractice claims varies according to procedure invasiveness.

The Balanced Budget Act of 1997 required the development of resource-based PLI RVUs by January 1, 2000. CMS contracted with KPMG Consulting to provide support in developing PLI RVUs and published their review of this report, along with proposed PLI RVUs, in their July 22, 1999, *Notice of Proposed Rule-making*. CMS finalized this proposal, with relatively few changes, in the November 2, 1999, Final Rule. In the November 1, 2000, Final Rule, CMS utilized updated premium data to derive new PLI RVUs.

CMS has computed the new resource-based PLI RVUs using actual professional liability premium data and current Medicare payment data on allowed services and charges, work relative value units, and specialty payment percentages. As stated, MedPAC had previously recommended that CMS base the new PLI RVUs on procedure-specific actual malpractice claims. CMS did not use this approach as this type of data was not available, and it is not possible to correlate claims paid to a specific Current Procedural Terminology (CPT®) code when a combination of services is performed. In the 1999 Final Rule, CMS encouraged MedPAC to further develop its idea, particularly as it relates to the statutory requirement to develop resource-based PLI RVUs, and submit its further analysis in comments to further Medicare Physician Payment Schedule (MFS) notices.

CMS is required to update the PLI relative values no less than every five years. The PLI RVUs were updated with new premium data in 2005, 2010, and 2015.

For CY 2020, the statutorily required five-year review of the PLI RVUs coincided with the required three-year review of the GPCIs. GPCIs are geographic practice cost indices that account for geographic differences in PLI costs. CMS adjusts the GPCIs every three years based on actual PLI premium data, so a sudden increase in PLI costs in a particular region of the country may not be reflected for several years. Considering that the PLI premium data used to update the GPCIs are the same data used to determine the specialty-level risk factors for the calculation of PLI RVUs, CMS finalized a proposal to align the update of PLI premium data with the update to the PLI GPCIs to every three years. Thus, the next mandated review and update of both PLI RVUs and the GPCIs will occur in 2023. See Chapter 7 for further details on GPCIs.

For 2017 and 2018, CMS determined it would not be appropriate to propose to update the specialty risk factors based on the updated PLI premium data that was reflected in the proposed CY 2017 and CY 2018 GPCI updates. Therefore, CMS did not update the specialty-risk factors based on the new premium data collected for the purposes of the three-year GPCI update for CY 2017, CY 2018 or CY 2019. For CY 2020, CMS finalized several refinements to the PLI

RVU methodology for premium data collection including using a broader set of state insurer filings beyond those listed as "physician" and "surgeon" and utilizing partial and total imputation when CMS specialty names are not distinctly identified in the insurer filings. The mappings for partial imputation utilize the longstanding mappings of the regulatory impact table included in all MFS *Federal Register* notices. The mappings for total imputation continue to crosswalk many nonphysician provider specialties to the lowest physician specialty. In previous years, CMS relied on a crosswalk methodology to develop PLI RVUs for any specialty without premium data from at least 35 states. For CY 2020, the methodological changes result in the Agency no longer using the crosswalk methodology since the 35-state threshold no longer has relevance. CMS will continue to work with RUC and interested stakeholders to improve the premium data collection process.

Aside from the refinements to data collection, the methodology used in the CY 2020 review of PLI RVUs essentially followed the same approach as the CY 2015 update. The steps in CMS' calculation of PLI RVUs are as follows:

Step 1 A preliminary national average professional liability premium is calculated for each specialty and mapped to the county level. In the CY 2016 MFS Final Rule, CMS adopted a weighting method based on share of total US population. Thus, the specialty premium for each county is multiplied by its share of the total US population, not by the total RVU per county as was the case in 2015. This calculation is then divided by the average PLI GPCI across all counties for each specialty to yield a normalized national average premium for each specialty. Premiums are for a $1 million/$3 million mature claims-made-policy (a policy covering claims made rather than services provided during the policy term).

Step 2 Risk factors (nonsurgical and surgical) are calculated for each specialty by dividing the national average premium for each specialty by the national average premium for the specialty with the lowest average premium, which remains allergy and immunology.

Premium service risk groups are utilized to subdivide some specialties that have premium rates that differ for surgery, surgery with obstetrics, and nonsurgery and therefore reflect differences in PLI risk within the specialty. For most specialties that do not clearly delineate into service risk groups, all services performed by the specialty receive the same risk factor.

CMS applied the surgical risk factors to CPT codes 10000 through 69999 and the nonsurgical risk factor to all others. In the November 2, 1999, Final Rule CMS acknowledged that certain codes in the "nonsurgical" section of CPT may indeed be invasive and, therefore, be valued based on the surgical risk factor. CMS changed the risk factor to surgical for the cardiology catheterization, angioplasty, and electrophysiology codes. Starting in 2015, this list of codes was updated to contain injection procedures used in conjunction with cardiac catheterization. In the case of OB/GYN services, the higher obstetric premiums and risk factors were used for services that were obstetrical services, while the lower gynecology risk factor was used for all other services. The complete CMS listing of Invasive Cardiology Services Outside of Surgical HCPCS Code Range Considered Surgery currently contains 81 codes and can be found on the CMS.gov website.

In CY 2020, CMS assigned a default minimum risk factor of 1.00—the lowest physician specialty-level risk factor—for Technical Component (TC) Only services, while working to acquire a broader set of data.

Step 3 PLI RVUs are calculated for each CPT code. The percentage of a specific service provided by each specialty is multiplied by the specialties' risk factor, and the product is then summed across specialties by service. This yields a specialty-weighted PLI RVU that is then multiplied by the physician work RVU for that code to account for differences in risk-of-service. In instances in which the work RVU equals zero, CMS retains the current professional liability RVUs. Beginning in 2016, CMS began using the last three years of an individual code's Medicare utilization to determine the specialty mix. However, there are still low-volume codes (Medicare utilization under 100) that CMS has identified as having an inappropriate specialty mix. Under these circumstances, CMS previously would identify an appropriate crosswalk. In CY 2018, CMS began to implement a long-sought RUC recommendation to use service-level overrides based on the expected specialty, instead of the claims-based specialty mix, to determine the specialty mix for low-volume procedures. These service-level overrides are used to determine the specialty for low-volume procedures for both PE and PLI. If a code has zero Medicare utilization in the last three years, the service will also be assigned a service-level override.

Step 4 The calculated PLI RVUs are then rescaled for budget neutrality as required by the statute. This final step adjusts for relativity by rescaling the proposed PLI RVUs so that the total proposed resource-based PLI RVUs are equal to the total current resource-based PLI RVUs. Scaling by the ratio of the pools of the proposed and current PLI and work RVUs is necessary to maintain the work RVUs for individual services from year to year while also maintaining the overall relationship between work, PE, and PLI RVUs.

In the CY 2011 Final Rule, CMS proceeded with rebasing the Medicare Economic Index (MEI) and adjusting the RVUs to align the RVU shares with the rebased MEI weights. CMS did not make an adjustment directly to the work RVUs; instead, the PE RVUs were increased by an adjustment factor of 1.181, and the malpractice RVUs were increased by an adjustment factor of 1.358. As the professional liability component is only 4.30% of the total payment amount, the initial impact in the 2011 MEI rebasing was minimal. Due to rebasing in 2011, many of the PLI RVUs increased to account for the increase in the cost-share weight percentage PLI received (3.90 to 4.30%). These increases were administered in a budget-neutral fashion. CMS again revised the MEI in the 2014 Final Rule. However, the PLI component maintained its total weight of total payment at 4.30%. This percentage is maintained in the Final Rule for 2020.

As explained in the previous methodology, the following is an example of how a PLI RVU will be calculated for a CPT code:

The percentage of a specific service to be performed by each specialty is determined from the Medicare utilization data. Except for E/M services, CMS only includes specialty premium data for those specialties that account for at least 5% of the total utilization for the past three years.

CPT Code X	Family practice	20%
	Dermatology	50%
	Plastic surgery	30%

This percentage is then multiplied by the specialty's risk factor.

CPT Code X (deemed to be "surgical")	
Family practice	0.20 × 3.62 = 0.72
Dermatology	0.50 × 2.63 = 1.32
Plastic surgery	0.30 × 4.98 = 1.49

The products for all specialties for the procedure are then summed, yielding a specialty-weighted PLI RVU reflecting the weighted professional liability costs across all specialties for that procedure.

CPT Code X 3.53

This number will then be multiplied by the procedure's work RVU to account for differences in risk-of-service.

CPT Code X 3.53 × 2.50 (work RVU) = 8.83

PLI RVU is adjusted for budget-neutrality factor (used in the initial implementation).

CPT Code X 8.83 × 0.025 = 0.22 PLI RVU

PLI RVU is adjusted for MEI rescaling factor.

CPT Code X 0.22 × 1.358 = 0.30 PLI RVU

The new resource-based PLI RVUs are available in Part 5, Reference Lists.

An increase in PLI expenses incurred by physicians can be reflected in Medicare payments in three different ways. For example, if PLI costs increase for most specialties, these increased expenses would be reflected in the annual update to the Medical Economic Index, which is used to update the Medicare conversion factor. These increased costs would have the potential to increase the conversion factor, which would then lead to increased payments for all physicians. (See Chapter 10 for an explanation of the conversion factor update.) Alternatively, if a particular specialty experiences increased PLI costs, those changes would most likely only be reflected in the relative values every three years when CMS updates the three-year average of professional liability premium data.

PLI RVUs for New and Revised Services

In the CY 2018 MFS Final Rule, CMS finalized a proposal to eliminate the general use of a PLI-specific specialty-mix crosswalk for new and revised codes. CMS will continue to consider specific recommendations regarding specialty mix assignments for new and revised codes, particularly in cases where coding changes are expected to result in differential reporting of services by specialty, or where the new or revised code is expected to be low volume. Absent such information, the specialty mix assumption for a new or revised code would derive from the analytic crosswalk in the first year, followed by the introduction of actual claims data, which is consistent with our approach for developing PE RVUs.

Major Improvements and Continued Concerns Regarding PLI Relative Value Methodology

In 2002, RUC created a new PLI workgroup to review the CMS methodology utilized to compute PLI relative values and to offer suggestions for improvement. The PLI workgroup has offered several suggestions for improvements, and CMS has adopted many of these recommendations to improve the PLI RVU methodology.

For example, during the mandated five-year reviews of the PLI RVUs, CMS has considered several recommendations submitted by RUC.

2005

- CMS improved the utilization data by removing assistant-at-surgery claims from the data set.
- RUC expressed concern that the PLI RVUs could inappropriately be inflated or deflated based on incorrectly reported specialty classifications listed for performing a particular service. In response to this recommendation, CMS implemented a 5% specialty threshold, in which liability data will be excluded for any specialty performing less than 5% of the service except for evaluation and management services, as all physicians report evaluation and management services.
- CMS revised the risk factor for several nonphysician provider specialties to a risk factor of 1.00 because of a recommendation made by RUC and its PLI workgroup. In 2019, CMS will continue to crosswalk non–MD/DO specialties to the lowest MD/DO risk factor specialty, Allergy Immunology. RUC maintains that a risk factor linked to a physician specialty is too high for many of the nonphysician health care professions.
- RUC and its PLI workgroup recommended, and CMS agreed, that a number of professions that were assigned to the average for the all physicians risk factor should be removed from the calculation of professional liability insurance RVUs.
- RUC began to include in its recommendations for new and revised codes recommended PLI relative value crosswalks.

2010

- As a result of RUC recommendations, CMS announced the implementation of the second review and update of the professional liability insurance RVUs. For 2010, PLI RVUs were based on actual CY 2006 and CY 2007 professional liability insurance premium data, CY 2008 Medicare payment data on allowed charges, and CY 2008 geographic adjustment data for professional liability insurance premiums. In the past, the premium data collected only included the top 20 physician specialties. For 2010, CMS included premium data for all physician specialties.
- CMS developed PLI RVUs for technical component services.
- CMS began assigning 0.01 PLI RVUs to physician services that currently have no PLI RVUs associated with them.
- CMS started crosswalking gynecological oncology to general surgery and surgical oncology, instead of medical oncology.
- CMS started crosswalking maxillofacial surgery and oral surgery to plastic surgery, instead of allergy/immunology.

2015

- CMS implemented the third review and update of the PLI RVUs. Beginning in 2015, CMS updated the PLI RVUs using actual 2011 and 2012 PLI premium data, 2013 Medicare payment and utilization data, and 2015 work RVUs and GPCIs.
- CMS implemented a RUC recommendation to assign for individual services with Medicare utilization under 100 a dominant specialty, consistent with a specialty that could be reasonably expected to furnish the service.
- CMS added injection procedures used in conjunction with cardiac catheterization as part of the class of nonsurgical services that receive surgical risk factors. The complete CMS listing of Invasive Cardiology Services Outside of Surgical HCPCS Code Range Considered Surgery currently contains 81 codes and can be found on the CMS.gov website

2020

- CMS implemented the fourth comprehensive review and update of PLI RVUs for CY 2020. PLI RVUs are based on actual CY 2017 PLI premium data; CY 2018 Medicare payment and utilization data; higher of the CY 2020 proposed work RVUs or the clinical labor portion of the direct PE RVUs); and CY 2019 GPCIs. As part of the review, the agency finalized a proposal to update the PLI RVUs every three years from this point forward to align with the required updates to the GPCIs.
- CMS made several refinements to its premium rate data collection process and therefore was able to finalize its proposal to use the most recent data for the CY 2020 PLI RVUs. This marked an improvement from CY 2018 when CMS did not finalize its proposal due to concerns expressed by RUC and others regarding sufficiency of the premium data. RUC continues to support improvements in data collection efforts such that updated premium data is obtained for all Medicare physician specialties, other health care professionals and facility providers, in all fifty states.
- CMS acquired premium data for five nonphysician health care professions that were formerly crosswalked, including anesthesiologist assistants, chiropractors, optometrists, certified nurse midwives, and certified registered nurse anesthetists (CRNAs). For all other non–MD/DO specialties, CMS continues to crosswalk to the lowest physician specialty risk factor of allergy/immunology. RUC has consistently maintained that a risk factor linked to a physician specialty is too high for many of the nonphysician health care professions.
- CMS finalized a proposal to assign a risk factor of 1.00, which corresponds to the lowest physician specialty risk factor of allergy/immunology, to TC-only services.

RUC is opposed to mapping these services to a physician specialty when the services are clearly not performed by a physician and conveys its continued concern with the data collection process.

- As recommended by RUC, CMS finalized a proposal in the CY 2018 Final Rule to use a list of expected specialties instead of the claims-based specialty mix for low volume services (fewer than 100 allowed services in the Medicare claims data), which also includes no volume services, and apply these overrides for both the PE and PLI valuation process. The complete Anticipated Specialty Assignment for Low Volume Services list is available for comment annually as part of the NPRM. RUC has encouraged CMS to ensure that the list of expected specialties is correctly and consistently applied for the low volume service-level overrides each year.

Combining Work, Practice Expense, and PLI RVUs

The sum of the work, practice expense, and PLI RVUs for each service is the total RVUs for the service. Adding the sum of the product of the work RVUs to the practice expense RVUs and PLI RVUs and then multiplying this sum for all of these services by the annual conversion factor yields the full unadjusted Medicare payment schedule. The unadjusted payment schedule is the full schedule with no geographic practice cost adjustment. It includes the 80% that Medicare pays and the 20% patient coinsurance. Part 5 lists the RVUs for each component and the unadjusted payment schedule for all of the CPT-coded services.

Chapter 7

Geographic Variation in the Payment Schedule

Support for adopting a nationally standardized payment schedule that would reduce geographic variation in Medicare payment levels developed independently of the movement for a resource-based relative value scale (RBRVS). The American Medical Association's (AMA's) House of Delegates adopted policy on reducing geographic variations before setting policy on an RBRVS-based Medicare payment schedule. Even after establishing its policy on the RBRVS, the House of Delegates sought to reduce geographic inequities before implementing the RBRVS. For example, at its December 1989 meeting, the AMA adopted policy to support pegging minimum Medicare prevailing charge levels at 80% of the national average prevailing charge level.

The Omnibus Budget Reconciliation Act of 1989 (OBRA 89) provision for and implementation of geographic adjustments often has drawn as much attention to the RBRVS payment system as did the relative values. This chapter describes the geographic adjustment provision in OBRA 89, revisions made to the geographic practice cost indices (GPCIs) in 1995, 1998, 2001, 2004, and 2005, and how and to what extent payments vary geographically under the Medicare RBRVS payment system. The chapter also explains a revised configuration of Medicare payment localities that became effective January 1, 1997. Finally, this chapter discusses the changes to the GPCIs resulting from federal legislation. A listing of all the GPCIs for 2022 may be found at the end of this publication.

OBRA 89 Provision for Geographic Adjustment

Most health policymakers understand rural communities face physician recruitment and retention problems and that people living in these communities find it difficult to obtain high-quality care. Many rural community hospitals have closed since Medicare implemented prospective pricing, emphasizing the impact that changes in government policy may have in rural areas and underscoring the health care needs of these communities.

Wide disparities in Medicare payments for the same service, with twofold to threefold differences in some cases, provoked physicians nationwide to call for a more equitable policy. For many physicians, the issue was not the wide variation in earnings, but whether Medicare payment levels were sufficient to even cover their costs of practicing in rural areas. Rural communities often have a higher proportion of Medicare and Medicaid patients, providing fewer opportunities for physicians to recover costs through higher charges to private sector patients.

In response, physicians in several predominantly rural states proposed a single national payment schedule with no geographic variation in payments. This proposal did not receive widespread support, however, because it would have merely shifted the underpayment problem to urban areas. In large cities where average Medicare payments based on customary, prevailing, and reasonable (CPR) exceeded the national average by 37%, overall shifting to a single national schedule would have reduced average payment levels by 27%.

Many other physicians believed that a policy adjusting the entire RBRVS to reflect geographic differences would be inequitable and provide insufficient relief for rural areas. Most physicians agreed that the practice expense and professional liability insurance (PLI) components of the RBRVS should be varied to reflect geographic differences, but they disagreed about whether the physician work component should be adjusted. While variation in the practice expense component would have reflected differences among localities in office rents and the wages of nonphysician office personnel in Medicare payments, variation in the work component would have reflected differences in physicians' costs of living.

Because the work component is valued according to the physician time and effort involved in a service, it may be viewed as the physician earnings component of the schedule. Earnings variations reflect costs of living and amenities. If costs of living and amenities are relatively high, then employers must pay higher wages to cover their employees' higher costs of living, but the amenities level will offset the degree to which wages must be higher. Likewise, professional workers such as lawyers, engineers, and physicians must charge higher payments to cover these higher costs, but the need for these higher payment levels is partially offset by the amenities.

Physicians who supported varying Medicare payments according to cost-of-living differences believed that higher payments were needed to offset these higher costs. Other physicians objected to variation based on cost-of-living differences, believing that the cultural, environmental, and other amenities of high-cost communities adequately compensated for their higher costs. Others objected because such variation would preserve existing payment disparities to a greater extent than variation based on overhead only.

OBRA 89 provided for adjusting the practice expense and PLI components of the payment schedule to fully reflect geographic differences in these costs, while adjusting the physician work component to reflect only one quarter of geographic differences in costs of living.

According to this provision, each component of each service provided in a locality is adjusted for geographic cost differences. Because the proportion of relative value units (RVUs) that comprise the work, practice expense, and PLI components are different for every service, the effect of this provision varies the amount of geographic adjustment for every service. For example, if the work adjustment in a state is 3% less than the national average, the practice expense adjustment is 10% less, and the PLI adjustment is 10% less, then, in that state, a service for which practice and PLI costs represent 75% of the total RVUs will be 8.5% less than the unadjusted payment schedule. In contrast, a service for which physician work RVUs represent 75% of the total RVUs will only be 5.5% less than the unadjusted schedule.

Geographic Practice Cost Index (GPCI)

The OBRA 89 legislation made three geographic adjustment factors the basis for the three geographic practice cost indices (GPCIs; pronounced "gypsies"), developed by researchers at the Urban Institute, the Center for Health Economics Research, and JIL Systems, Inc, with funding from the Centers for Medicare & Medicaid Services (CMS) (formerly known as the Health Care Financing Administration [HCFA]). The resources involved in operating a medical practice were identified by CMS as physician work or net income; employee wages; office rents; medical equipment, supplies, and other miscellaneous expenses; and professional liability insurance. Employee wages, office rents, medical equipment, medical supplies, and miscellaneous expenses are combined to comprise the practice expense GPCI. Each component within the practice expense GPCI is weighted according to its percentage of practice costs. These weights are obtained from the AMA's Socioeconomic Monitoring System Survey. The original GPCIs, in effect from 1992 through 1994, used practice cost weights from the AMA's 1987 survey.

The Omnibus Budget Reconciliation Act (OBRA) of 1990 requires that the GPCIs be updated at least every 3 years. Accordingly, CMS revised the GPCIs for 1995 to 1997, 1998 to 2000, 2001 to 2003, and 2004 to 2006. CMS worked with Acumen to revise the current GPCIs in accordance with legislation that GPCIs need to be reviewed every three years. For 2007, CMS used the fully implemented value of the practice expense and PLI GPCIs and reflected the 2007 budget neutral coefficients, as provided by the CMS Office of the Actuary. For 2008, CMS completed the review of GPCIs and proposed new GPCIs. The legislation specified that the updated GPCIs be phased in over a two-year period, with half of the overall adjustment occurring in 2008 and the other half of the adjustment in 2009. In 2010, the 6th GPCI update was completed. The new GPCIs were phased in over a two-year period using the following metric. For 2011, the work GPCIs represented half the difference between 2010 and 2012 work GPCIs. The practice expense (PE) GPCIs for

2011 represented the greater of half the difference between 2010 PE GPCI and 2012 PE GPCI with limited recognition of cost differences for the rent and employee compensation components, as mandated by the Affordability Care Act or half the difference between 2010 PE GPCI and 2012 PE GPCI without the limited recognition of cost differences for the rent and employee compensation components. For 2011, the professional liability insurance (PLI) GPCIs reflected half the difference between 2010 PLI GPCIs and 2012 GPCIs. For 2014, the GPCI updates were again phased in over two years, with final impacts realized in 2015. For 2020, CMS conducted its statutorily required three-year review of the GPCIs and is in the second year of phase-in. The data used to measure each of the three component GPCIs are more fully described in the following sections. The GPCIs for 2022 are included in the "Reference Lists" section.

Cost-of-Living GPCI

The physician work or cost-of-living GPCI is not based on differences in physicians' earnings, which some researchers and CMS argue have been affected by physicians' Medicare earnings under the previous CPR payment system. The 1995 to 1997 work GPCI measures geographic differences in the earnings of all college-educated workers, based on 1990 census data. In updating the work GPCIs for 1998 to 2000 and again for 2001 to 2004, no changes were made to the data sources. For the updates in 2005 and 2008, the physician work GPCIs were based on 2000 decennial US census data, by county, of seven professional occupations (architecture and engineering; computer, mathematical, and natural sciences; social scientists, social workers, and lawyers; education, library, and training; registered nurses; pharmacists; writers, artists, and editors). For the 2011 update, the physician work GPCIs were based on the 2006–2008 Bureau of Labor statistics (BLS) Occupational Employment Statistics (OES) data. CMS revaluated this data and stated that the agency continues to believe it is the best source of data for calculating GPCIs because of its reliability, public availability, level of detail and national scope. For the 2014 update, the physician work GPCIs were based on the 2009–2011 BLS OES data. The MMA required all work GPCIs in 2004 through 2006 to be set at least at the national average of 1.00. A provision to increase the work GCPI to 1.00 for any locality for which such work GCPI is less than 1.00 has been extended under Section 1848(e)(1)(E) of the Social Security Act (42 U.S.C.1395w–4(e)(1)(E)) through yearly legislation from 2004 to 2020. The Further Consolidated Appropriations Act, 2020, provided for extension of the work GCPI floor of 1.00 from January 1, 2020, through May 22, 2020. The Coronavirus Aid, Relief, and Economic Security (CARES) Act of 2020 further extended the work GPCI floor through November 30, 2020. The Continuing Appropriations Act, 2021, and Other Extensions Act included an extension of the work GPCI floor under the Medicare program through December 11, 2020, only. The Consolidated Appropriations Act, 2021, that was signed into law on December 27, 2020, reinstated the 1.0 floor on the work GPCI through CY 2023.

Practice Expense GPCI

The practice expense GPCI is designed to measure geographic variation in the prices of inputs to medical practice (eg, office rent per square foot and hourly wages of staff). While the physician work and PLI GPCIs are comprised of a single index, the practice expense GPCIs are comprised of four component indices: employee wages, purchased services, office rent and equipment, supplies and other miscellaneous expenses. It does not, therefore, reflect geographic differences in the amount of space that physicians rent or in the number of nonphysician personnel they employ. It is important to distinguish between the practice expense component of the relative value scale and the practice expense GPCI. The practice expense relative value reflects average direct and indirect expenses. The practice expense GPCI reflects only the differences in these costs across geographic areas relative to the national average.

Prior to 2012, the office rent portion of the practice expense GPCI was based on apartment rental data from the Department of Housing and Urban Development (HUD). CMS had concerns about the use of HUD rental data because it was not updated frequently, and the Census discontinued the collection of the necessary base year rents for the HUD Fair Market Rent (FMR) data in 2010. Therefore, CMS analyzed the US Census Bureau American Community Survey (ACS) rental data to replace the HUD data. For 2020, the office rent component of the PE GPCI was updated using 2013–2017 ACS five-year estimates. As it did in calculating the original GPCIs, CMS continues to use proxy data to update this index, stating that no national data for physician office rents are available. After reviewing alternative sources of commercial rental data, CMS does not believe that there are national data sources that would more accurately reflect rent costs, and CMS will continue to use the ACS five-year office rent data. The practice expense GPCI does not reflect geographic differences in medical equipment and supply costs. CMS has stated its belief that a national market exists for these components and that input prices do not vary specifically across geographic areas.

For 1995 to 1997, GPCIs were updated to reflect data from the 1990 census; the cost shares attributable to employee wages, rent, and miscellaneous expenses also were updated. The same 1990 census data sources were used to update GPCIs for 1998 to 2000 and 2001 to 2004, although updated (1996 and 2000, respectively) HUD fair market residential rent data were used. The 2000–2010 practice expense GPCIs were based on 2000 census data for employee wages and the residential apartment rental data produced annually by HUD as a proxy for physician office rents. For the 2011 update, the PE GPCIs were based on the AMA Physician Practice Information Survey data, Bureau of Labor and Statistics Occupational Employment Statistics data and American Community Survey (ACS) rental data. On January 1, 2011, the Affordable Care Act established a permanent 1.0 floor for the PE GPCI for frontier states which currently includes: Montana, Wyoming, Nevada, North Dakota, and South Dakota.

PLI GPCI

The PLI GPCIs (which Medicare regulations refer to as the "malpractice" GPCI) are geographic practice cost indices that account for geographic differences in PLI costs. They reflect geographic differences in premiums for mature claims made policy providing $1 million/$3 million of coverage. Adjustments are made for mandatory patient compensation funds.

Critics of the original GPCIs were particularly dissatisfied with CMS' calculations of the PLI GPCIs, which were based on outdated premium data drawn largely from a single nationwide carrier. Each of the subsequent updates, however, used more recent premium data, as well as data collected on 20 medical specialties and from insurers representing the majority of the market in each state. The 1995 to 1997 GPCIs were based on premium data for 1990 to 1992, while the 1998 to 2000 GPCIs were based on 1992 to 1994 data. The 2001 to 2003 PLI GPCIs were based on 1996 to 1998 data. A three-year average was used, rather than data from the most recent single year, to achieve a more accurate indication of historic PLI premium trends.

The 2004 to 2006 PLI GPCIs were based on actual premium data from 2001–2002 and projected data for 2003. The 2010 PLI GPCIs were based on actual premium data from 2004, 2005, and 2006. For the 2011 update, the PLI GPCIs were based on 2006 and 2007 premium data. For the 2014 update, CMS used 2011 and 2012 premium data. For the 2017 update, the PLI GPCIs were based on 2014 and 2015 premium data. For 2020, the update reflected premium data presumed in effect as of December 30, 2017.

CMS adjusts the GPCIs every three years based on actual PLI premium data, and so a sudden increase in PLI costs in a particular region of the country may not be reflected for several years. For CY 2020, this required three-year review of the GPCIs coincided with the statutorily required five-year review of the PLI RVUs. Considering that the PLI premium data used to update the GPCIs are the same data used to determine the specialty-level risk factors for the calculation of PLI RVUs, CMS finalized a proposal to align the update of PLI premium data with the update to the PLI GPCIs to every three years. Thus, neither the PLI risk premiums nor the PLI GPCIs changed for 2022. The next mandated review and update will occur in 2023.

Variation in the GPCIs

GPCIs allow for considerably less variation in physicians' costs of practice than under historic Medicare prevailing charges. The 2022 practice expense GPCIs range from 0.842 (Mississippi) to 1.383 (San Benito County and Santa Clara County, California). Because the cost-of-living GPCI (work) accounts for only one quarter of geographic differences, the range is even smaller. The 2022 work GPCI range encompasses the 1.00 work GPCI floor (as extended through December 31, 2023, by the Consolidated Appropriations Act, 2021) to the 1.5000 permanent–floor in Alaska (as established by MIPPA). The range is greatest with the PLI GPCI distribution: 0.235 (Nebraska) to 2.702 (NYC Suburbs/Long Island).

In an effort to provide greater consistency in the calculation of GPCIs in island territories, for 2017, CMS finalized a policy to treat the Caribbean Island territories (the Virgin Islands and Puerto Rico) in a consistent manner by assigning the national average of 1.0 to each GPCI index for both Puerto Rico and the Virgin Islands.

Because of this narrow range of variation, most Medicare payments under the fully transitioned RBRVS payment system are within 10% of the national average, rather than the twofold and threefold difference in payment common under CPR. For many areas in which physicians' payments were only 60% to 70% of the national average under CPR, payments increased to 80% to 90% of the national average under the payment schedule. Conversely, in areas in which Medicare's payments under CPR were twice the national average, payments declined to only 15% to 20% above the national average.

This pattern means that GPCIs do not necessarily indicate the impact of the payment schedule on Medicare payments in an area. In fact, the opposite may be true: many areas with the lowest GPCIs experienced the highest payment increases and many areas with the highest GPCIs experienced the most severe payment reductions.

Impact of the Revised GPCIs

The three GPCI components can be combined into a composite GPCI or geographic adjustment factor (GAF) by weighting each by the share of Medicare payments accounted for by the work, practice cost, and PLI components. The GAF indicates how Medicare payments in a locality differ from the national average (with the national average cost being 1.00).

Changes in the GPCIs do not affect total Medicare physician payments but redistribute payments among localities. The overall redistributive effects of the revisions to GPCIs for 1995 to 1997, as compared to the 1992 GPCIs, were modest. A CMS analysis indicated that 75% of localities experienced

GPCI changes of about 3% or less. An AMA analysis, comparing the GAFs for 1994 and 1996, showed that revisions in the practice cost GPCIs caused a variance of over 2% in the GAFs for about 60 localities. Revisions to the PLI GPCIs led to GAF changes of over 2% in 52 localities.

The impact of the GPCI revisions for 1998 to 2000 was even less pronounced than for the previous update, as the only data changes made were to the indices for office rent and PLI. Seventy-six of the 89 localities experience payment changes of less than 1% for the average service over the two-year transition period, while payment changes in 58 localities will be less than 0.5%. The largest gain for an area is 2.4% and the largest loss is 2.2% for the average service. Several localities experienced PLI GPCI changes of about 30%, reflecting the volatility in PLI premiums that occurs from year to year. Because the weight of the PLI GPCI is about 5% of the total GPCI, a 30% change in the PLI GPCI causes only a 1.5% change in payments. Two thirds of the localities, however, experience PLI GPCI changes of less than 10%.

The impacts were also minimal in 2001 to 2003 as CMS again only updated the indices for office rent and PLI. Only 14 of the 89 localities changed by at least 2%. Sixteen areas changed from 1% to 1.9%. The remaining 59 areas experienced payment changes of less than 1% under the revised GPCIs.

In 2004, CMS revised the PLI GPCIs. To account for the volatility in the PLI premium data, CMS reduced the change in the PLI GPCIs by 50%. Apart from Detroit, Michigan, no locality experienced an increase of more than 1% in total payments due to the revised PLI GPCIs in 2004. These revised GPCIs led to no decreases in payment greater than 1%. The MMA provisions to establish a floor of 1.00 in the work GPCIs and increase all Alaska GPCIs to 1.67 led to payment increases for 58 Medicare payment localities in 2005.

The 2005–2006 updates to the work and practice expense GPCIs resulted in an overall increase of no more than 3.5% or a decrease of no more than 1.6% for any locality. Only 10 of the 89 localities changed by more than 1% in 2005–2006.

The 2007 updates included the extension of the MMA established floor of 1.00. This established floor was further extended through June 30, 2008, by the Medicare, Medicaid, and SCHIP Extension Act of 2007.

The Medicare Improvements for Patients and Providers Act of 2008 (MIPPA) extended the 1.00 work GPCI floor from July 1, 2008, through December 31, 2009. Furthermore, MIPPA set a permanent 1.50 work GPCI floor in Alaska for all services beginning January 1, 2009. As a result of MIPPA, 55 out of 89 localities received an increase in their work GPCI. Alaska received the largest increase, 47.49%, followed by Puerto Rico, 10.62%. The estimated impact for this provision of MIPPA was $400 million for 2009. For 2010, the work GPCI floor was extended by the Affordable Care Act of 2010 from January 1, 2010, through December 31, 2010. For 2011, this work GPCI floor was extended once again through the passage of H.R. 4994 Medicare and Medicaid Extenders Act of 2010. The Temporary Payroll Tax Cut Continuation Act of 2011 extends the floor through February 29, 2012. The Middle Class Tax Relief and Job Creation Act of 2012 further extended the floor through December 31, 2012. The American Taxpayer Relief Act of 2012 further extended the 1.00 floor through December 31, 2013. The Pathway for SGR Reform Act extended the 1.00 floor through March 31, 2014. The Protecting Access to Medicare Act of 2014 (PAMA) again extended the 1.00 work GPCI floor through March 31, 2015. The Medicare Access and Children's Health Insurance Program (CHIP) Reauthorization Act of 2015 (MACRA) further extended the 1.00 work GPCI floor through December 31, 2017. The Bipartisan Budget Act of 2018 further extended the 1.00 work GPCI floor through December 31, 2019. The Further Consolidated Appropriations Act, 2020, provided for extension of the work GCPI floor of 1.00 from January 1, 2020, through May 22, 2020. The Coronavirus Aid, Relief, and Economic Security (CARES) Act of 2020 further extended the work GPCI floor through November 30, 2020. The Continuing Appropriations Act, 2021, and Other Extensions Act included an extension of the work GCPI floor under the Medicare program through December 11, 2020. The Consolidated Appropriations Act, 2021, that was signed into law on December 27, 2020, reinstated the 1.0 floor on the work GPCI through CY 2023.

Beginning January 1, 2011, the Affordable Care Act established a permanent 1.00 floor for the PE GPCI for frontier states which currently includes: Montana, Wyoming, Nevada, North Dakota and South Dakota.

As part of the seventh GPCI update for 2014, CMS finalized changes to the GPCI cost share weights consistent with the revised 2006-based MEI cost share weights finalized in the same year. Therefore, for the work GPCI the weight was increased from 48.27 to 50.87, the PE GPCI the weight was revised down from 47.44 to 44.84 and the PLI GPCI weight was unchanged at 4.30. For purposes of calculating GPCI values, the revised MEI weights only resulted in changes to the relative weighting within the PE GPCI (because there are no subcomponent cost share weights for the work GPCI or PLI GPCI). As CMS is statutorily required by law to do, if more than one year has elapsed since the date of the last adjustments to GPCIs, the current adjustments must be phased in over two years. Therefore, 2015 marked the second year of this transition to implement the 2014 GPCI changes as stated above. For the eight GPCI updates for 2017, CMS maintained the same work, PE, and PLI GPCI weights of 50.87, 44.84, and 4.30, respectively. These PLI GPCI weights remain the same for 2022.

Evaluating GPCIs

Because the geographic adjustments to the payment schedule and the resulting payment changes are such a critical part of Medicare's RBRVS payment system, GPCIs continue to be the focus of considerable debate and critical review. Physicians in places such as Puerto Rico, Texas, New York, and Florida have argued that GPCIs do not capture important dimensions of their practice costs, making the resulting adjustments too low.

The most serious charge leveled against the GPCIs, however, is that they fail to measure what they purport to measure. Physicians in several states argue that the GPCIs have no place in the RBRVS payment system because they do not accurately measure the geographic cost differences physicians face. Others feel that payments across geographic areas should be the same.

To assess how well GPCIs measure differences in physicians' practice costs, the AMA's Center for Health Policy Research compared data reported by physicians in its SMS surveys for 1991 and 1992 with the original GPCIs.[1]

The study found generally positive results:

- Although there is room for improvement, GPCIs do, in fact, measure a significant amount of the geographic difference in physicians' practice costs.
- The GPCIs measure variation in office expenses and personnel costs quite well, despite concerns about the representativeness and/or age of the data used to construct these GPCIs.
- Adjusting payments based on GPCIs reflects physicians' practice costs more accurately than a single national payment schedule.
- There are measurable geographic differences in the costs of supplies that should be reflected in the practice cost GPCI.

The study concluded that using GPCIs in the RBRVS payment system was appropriate but that improving the data sources as part of the updating process is critical, particularly the data used to construct the PLI GPCI. (The PLI GPCI was not highly correlated with physicians' reported PLI expenses.) The study recommended that with the collection of new data, the magnitude of changes in geographic cost differences over time should be determined to aid in assessing how frequently GPCIs should be updated.

The MMA required the General Accounting Office (GAO) to study GPCIs and issue a report by 2005. This study was published in March 2005. The GAO stated that the physician work GPCI, practice expense GPCI and professional liability insurance GPCI are valid in their fundamental design as tools to account for variations in geographic costs, however, the data used to calculate these indices needs to be refined due to the fact that the work and practice expense GPCIs are not current, and the data used in the PLI GPCI are incomplete. In addition, the GAO reported that GPCIs have a negligible impact on physicians' decisions to locate in rural areas citing that a spouse's employment opportunities, quality of local schools, and the availability of other physicians within the area to share in their delivery of care (ie, taking call) have just as much of an impact.

In 2013, the Institute of Medicine (IOM) completed a review of the GPCI methodology and underlying data and released two reports related to its work. Based in part on recommendations from the IOM, CMS finalized proposal to make certain modifications in 2013, including:

- Used the 2006 Medicare Economic Index (MEI) data to determine the relevant shares of work, practice expense, and PLI within the GPCI computation.
- Created a purchased services category within the practice expense GPCI to recognize that these costs vary regionally.
- Rental data from the 2006–2008 American Community Survey were used in lieu of the current US Department of Housing and Urban Development (HUD) data as a proxy for physician rental costs.
- Revised the nonphysician employee wage data using Bureau of Labor Statistics (BLS) with consistent occupations used in physicians' offices.

Medicare Payment Localities

Medicare payment localities are geographic areas defined by CMS for use in establishing payment amounts for physician services. Localities may be entire states, counties, or groups of counties. There were 240 localities prior to 1992, largely reflecting historic circumstances of the CPR payment system. The number dropped to 210 with RBRVS implementation, as a number of states with multiple localities converted to single payment areas. CMS implemented a more systematic approach to defining payment localities in 1997. The new policy achieved several goals, including administrative simplicity, reducing urban/rural payment differences among adjacent areas, and stabilizing payment updates resulting from periodic GPCI revisions.

The new policy increased the number of statewide payment localities to 34 from 22 and further reduced the overall number of localities to 89. To define the new payment localities, the CMS compared the GAF of a locality to the average GAF of lower-cost localities in the state in an iterative process.

If the difference exceeded 5%, the locality remained a distinct payment area. Otherwise, it was combined with other payment areas or the state converted to a single locality.

The 5% threshold automatically eliminated subcounty areas in all but three states, aggregating them into statewide or residual state localities. The subcounty approach, however, could not be applied in Pennsylvania, Massachusetts, and Missouri, wherein a major redesign to payment localities was required.

In addition to the new methodology for defining payment localities, CMS indicated that it would continue to consider physician requests for conversion to statewide localities. CMS has emphasized that such requests must demonstrate support for the change from both physicians whose payments would increase as well as those who would experience payment losses.

In the August 15, 2003, Proposed Rule, CMS indicated that it would consider comments on changes to the Medicare physician payment localities. CMS has indicated that it will continue to consider this issue as part of future rulemaking.

Beginning in CY 2017, PAMA required that the Medicare Physician Payment Schedule (MFS) areas used for payment in California be Metropolitan Statistical Areas (MSAs), as defined by the Office of Management and Budget (OMB) as of December 31 of the previous year, and that all areas not located in an MSA be treated as a single rest-of-state MFS area. The resulting modifications to California's locality structure increased its number of localities from 9 under the current locality structure to 27 under the MSA-based locality structure. PAMA defines transition areas as the MFS areas for 2013 that were the rest-of-state locality and locality 3, which was comprised of Marin County, Napa County, and Solano County. PAMA specifies that the GPCI values used for payment in a transition area be phased in over six years, from 2017 through 2021, using a weighted sum of the GPCIs calculated under the new MSA-based locality structure and the GPCIs calculated under the current MFS locality structure. That is, the GPCI values applicable for these areas during this transition period are a blend of what the GPCI values would have been under the current locality structure and what the GPCI values would be under the MSA-based locality structure. This incremental phase-in is only applicable to those counties that are in transition areas that are now in MSAs, which are only some of the counties in the 2013 California rest-of state locality and locality 3. Pursuant to implementation of the new MSA-based locality structure for California, the total number of MFS localities was increased from 89 to 112 in CY 2017.

PAMA established a hold harmless for transition areas beginning with CY 2017 whereby the applicable GPCI values for a year under the new MSA-based locality structure may not be less than what they would have been for the year under the current locality structure. Of the 58 counties in California, 50 are in transition areas and are subject to the hold-harmless provision. The eight counties that are not within transition areas are Orange, Los Angeles, Alameda, Contra Costa, San Francisco, San Mateo, Santa Clara, and Ventura.

Bonus Payments for Health Professional Shortage Areas

In addition to the geographic adjustment provision for all services, there are special payment provisions for physician services when provided in designated Health Professional Shortage Areas (HPSAs). The HPSAs are rural and inner-city areas, defined by the Public Health Service (PHS), as having a shortage of health care personnel. To help attract and retain physicians in HPSAs, Congress adopted a Medicare bonus payment program, effective in 1989. The program initially provided an incentive payment of 5% for all services furnished by physicians in rural HPSAs. In 1991, the bonus was increased to 10% and extended to services furnished by physicians in both urban and rural HPSAs.

The PHS identifies three separate types of HPSAs, each corresponding to shortages of three different categories of health personnel: primary medical care professionals, dental professionals, and mental health professionals. Separate sets of criteria are used to designate each type of HPSA. Only geographic areas with shortages of primary care physicians (defined as general or family practice, general internal medicine, pediatrics, and obstetrics and gynecology) are eligible for the Medicare bonus payments. Three criteria must be met for a geographic area to be designated as an HPSA with a shortage of primary care medical professionals:

- It must be a rational delivery area for primary medical care services.
- There must be at least 3500 people per full-time-equivalent primary care physician, or at least 3000 people per full-time equivalent primary care physician in areas with "unusually high needs for primary care services" or "insufficient capacity of existing primary care providers."
- Primary care physicians in contiguous areas must be overutilized, excessively distant, or inaccessible.

Although the ratio of primary care physicians to population is a criterion used to designate areas to receive the bonus payments, such payments are not restricted to primary care physicians or to primary care services. They apply to any Medicare covered service provided in a designated HPSA regardless of physician specialty.

Carriers make quarterly bonus payments to physicians in addition to the allowed amount under the payment schedule. To receive the bonus payment, prior to 2005, the claim form must have indicated that the service was provided in an HPSA. The MMA legislation shifts responsibility from the physicians to the secretary. Therefore, these 10% bonus payments will be made automatically.

The MMA legislation also added a bonus payment for services performed between 2005 and 2008 in newly established scarcity areas. CMS is required to calculate the ratios or primary and specialty care physicians to Medicare beneficiaries in each county. Physicians who provide care to beneficiaries in counties that fall in the bottom 20% of these ratios automatically qualify for the bonus. CMS has posted these scarcity areas on its Web site at www.cms.gov/Outreach-and-Education/Medicare-Learning-Network-MLN/MLNMattersArticles/downloads/MM3790.pdf. A service furnished in an area that qualifies for both the shortage bonus (10%) and scarcity bonus (5%) may receive both incentive bonuses.

The HPSA and scarcity bonus payments are calculated based on the amount Medicare paid for the covered physician service, and the beneficiary copayment is unaffected. When a physician furnishes a covered service in an area that is certified as a HPSA and scarcity bonus area, he or she will receive an additional payment of 15% based on what Medicare paid the physician for the service under the MFS. This program was extended through June 30, 2008, by the Medicare, Medicaid, and SCHIP Extension Act of 2007.

Beginning July 1, 2008, and extending through December 31, 2009, MIPPA provided for an additional 10% bonus payment for physician's services furnished in a year to a covered individual in an area that is designated as a geographic Health Professional Shortage Area (HPSA) prior to the beginning of such year. In the 2009 *Proposed Rule*, CMS clarified that physicians who furnish services in areas that are designated as geographic HPSAs as of December 31 of the prior year but not included on the list of zip codes for automated HPSA bonus payments should use the AQ modifier to receive the HPSA bonus payment.

The Affordable Care Act of 2010 created an incentive payment to general surgeons, who perform major procedures (with a 010- or 090-day global service period) and to primary care practitioners, who provide primary care services in a HPSA. These physicians were eligible for a bonus payment equal to 10% of the Medicare Payment Schedule payment for the surgical services furnished by the general surgeon for these services from January 1, 2011, to December 31, 2015.

Note

i. For example, the PPRC reported in its 1988 Annual Report that while the average prevailing charge in 1987 for a family practitioner for a comprehensive office visit was $64, 5% of these visits occurred in localities where the prevailing charge was less than $30, 5% in localities where the prevailing charge was more than $111—a more than threefold difference. Likewise, the average prevailing charge for a coronary artery bypass was $4385, but 5% of charges were less than $3092 and 5% were greater than $5919—a nearly twofold difference.

Reference

1. Gillis KD, Willke RJ, Reynolds RA. Assessing the validity of the geographic practice cost indices. *Inquiry*. Fall 1993;30:265–280.

Chapter 8

Medicare Payment Schedule

The Medicare Physician Payment Schedule's (MFS's) impact on a physician's Medicare payments is primarily a function of three key factors:

- The resource-based relative value scale (RBRVS)
- The geographic practice cost indices (GPCIs)
- The monetary conversion factor

This chapter briefly describes how these elements combine to form the payment schedule.

The enabling legislation and regulations, as well as Medicare carrier correspondence and forms, refer to the Medicare Physician Fee Schedule (MFS) as a "payment schedule." From the American Medical Association's (AMA's) perspective, the distinction between a payment schedule and a fee schedule is extremely important: a *payment* is what physicians establish as the fair price for the services they provide; a *fee* is what Medicare approves as the payment level for the service. Therefore, we have opted to use the term "payment" where appropriate, instead of "fee" in reference to the MFS. All references to the "full Medicare payment schedule" include the 80% that Medicare pays and the 20% patient coinsurance. Likewise, transition "approved amount" also includes the patient coinsurance.

Formula for Calculating the Payment Schedule

As discussed in Chapter 7, the Omnibus Budget Reconciliation Act of 1989 (OBRA 89) geographic adjustment provision requires all three components of the relative value for a service—physician work relative value units (RVUs), practice expense RVUs, and professional liability insurance (PLI) RVUs—to be adjusted by the corresponding GPCI for the locality. In effect, this provision increases the number of components in the payment schedule from three to the following six:

- Physician work RVUs
- Physician work GPCI
- Practice expense RVUs
- Practice expense GPCI
- PLI RVUs
- PLI GPCI

The formula for calculating payment schedule amounts entails adjusting RVUs, which correspond to services, by the GPCIs, which correspond to payment localities.

Table 8-1. Calculation of Locally Adjusted Payment Schedule

CPT Codes	Work RVU	Work GPCI	PE RVUs	PE GPCI	PLI RVUs	PLI GPCI	Total RVUs	Conversion Factor	Local Payment Schedule
99213	1.30	1.011	1.26	1.044	0.10	1.871	2.8064	33.5983	$94.64
27130	19.60	1.011	14.41	1.044	4.01	1.871	42.3623	33.5983	$1,423.30
33533	33.75	1.011	13.24	1.044	7.95	1.871	62.8181	33.5983	$2,110.58
71045-26	0.18	1.011	0.07	1.044	0.01	1.871	0.2738	33.5983	$9.20

The general formula for calculating Medicare payment amount is expressed as:

Total RVU = work RVU[1] × work GPCI[2]

+ practice expense RVU[1] × practice expense GPCI[2]

+ PLI RVU[1] × PLI GPCI[2]

Payment = Total RVU × conversion factor[3]

[1]The 2022 physician work, practice expenses, and PLI RVUs may be found in Part 5 of this guide (Reference Lists).

[2]The GPCIs for calendar year (CY) 2022 follow the Part 5 Reference Lists.

[3]This is an example using the 2022 conversion factor, 33.5983

Example = Payment for Current Procedural Terminology (CPT®) code 99213 is needed in the instance of an office/outpatient visit provided in a nonfacility (eg, in the physician's office) in Chicago, Illinois. The payment is calculated as follows:

Total RVU = 1.30 × 1.011 = 1.3143

+ 1.26 × 1.044 = 1.3154

+ 0.10 × 1.871 = 0.1871

= 2.8168 RVUs for CPT code 99213 in the Chicago locality

Payment = 2.8168 × $ 33.5983 = $94.64

Table 8-1 illustrates this calculation for four services in the Chicago locality using the 2022 conversion factor as an example. The first procedure is provided in a nonfacility and the subsequent procedures are in the facility.

History of Budget Neutrality

The Omnibus Budget Reconciliation Act of 1989 specifies that changes in RVUs resulting from changes in medical practice, coding, new data, or the addition of new services cannot cause Medicare Part B expenditures to differ by more than $20 million from the spending level that would occur in the absence of such changes. To limit the increases in Medicare expenditures as mandated by the statute, the Centers for Medicare & Medicaid Services (CMS) has applied various adjustments to the MFS to ensure budget neutrality. The following is a recap of the evolution of the measures implemented by CMS since the inception of the RBRVS in 1992 to address changes in physician work valuation.

1993–1995

For the 1993–1995 payment schedules, CMS achieved budget neutrality by uniformly reducing all work RVUs across all services. The work RVUs were reduced by 2.8% in 1993, 1.3% in 1994, and 1.1% in 1995. The AMA strongly objected to using work RVUs as a mechanism to preserve budget neutrality on the basis that such adjustments affect the relativity of the RBRVS and cause confusion among the many non-Medicare payers as well as physician practices that adopt the RBRVS payment system. Instead, the AMA and RUC advocated for budget-neutrality adjustments deemed necessary to be made to the conversion factor (CF) rather than the work RVUs.

1996

In the 1996 payment schedule, CMS discontinued its approach to preserving budget neutrality through reduction in work RVUs and instead applied a budget-neutrality adjustment to the multiple CFs in place at that time. In 1996, the CFs was reduced by 0.36% to account for the increases in Medicare Part B expenditures related to changes in physician work.

1997

CMS applied two separate budget-neutrality adjustments for the 1997 payment schedule. First, to adjust for changes in payments resulting from the first Five-Year Review of the RBRVS, CMS reduced work RVUs by 8.3% through a budget-neutrality adjuster. Rather than permanently alter the work RVUs or further reduce the CFs, this negative multiplier was applied directly to work RVUs. In addition, a separate budget-neutrality adjustment was made through a reduction to the CFs totaling 0.6%. This adjustment was due to new payment policies and annual CPT coding changes.

1998

Budget neutrality for 1998 was achieved by reducing the CF by 0.8%. The –8.3% budget-neutrality adjuster to all physician work RVUs continued through the calendar year.

1999

In 1999, CMS eliminated the separate 8.3% reduction in work RVUs. CMS stated, "We did not find the work adjustor to be desirable. It added an extra element to the MFS payment calculation and created confusion and questions among the public who had difficulty using the RVUs to determine a payment amount that matched the amount actually paid by Medicare" (*Federal Register*, Vol. 68, No. 216, p. 63246).

In this year, CMS also recalibrated the RBRVS to the Medicare economic index (MEI). As a result, work increased from 54.2% of the total to 54.5%, the practice expense portion increased from 41.0% to 42.3%, and the professional liability insurance portion decreased from 4.8% to 3.2%. The combined effects of this recalibration, the elimination of the work adjustor, and annual CPT coding changes resulted in a –7.5% budget-neutrality adjustment to the CF.

2000

In 2000, CMS continued to achieve budget neutrality through a change in the CF. The 2000 CF was increased by 0.07% to account for payment policy and annual CPT coding changes that would have accounted for a reduction in overall expenditures.

2001

In 2001, CMS again applied an adjustment to the CF to achieve budget neutrality. The 2001 CF was reduced 0.3% to account for payment policy and annual CPT coding changes.

2002

In 2002, following the second Five-Year Review of the RBRVS, CMS reduced the CF by 0.46% to achieve budget neutrality to account for the improvements resulting from the Five-Year Review.

2003

In 2003, CMS achieved budget neutrality through a 0.04% reduction in the CF to account for payment policy and annual CPT coding changes.

2004–2005

In 2004 and 2005, reductions in the CF were estimated to reach as high as 5% each year, partly due to the flawed sustainable growth rate. Through the Medicare Modernization Act, Congress acted to replace the predicted cuts with a mandatory 1.5% increase in the CF for both years. The 2004 CF did not include any adjustment for budget neutrality. However, CMS did re-weight the MEI, reducing work from 54.5% to 52.4% of the total and PE from 42.5% to 43.7% and increasing PLI from 3.1% to 3.9%. As a result, CMS reduced all work RVUs by 0.35%.

2006

In 2006, CMS achieved budget neutrality through a –0.15% reduction in the CF. On January 1, 2006, the CF was reduced by a total of 4.5%, but in March Congress acted to return the CF to its 2005 value. Following the CF freeze, the 0.15% reduction for budget neutrality was negated.

2007

In 2007, CMS returned to the application of a work RVU adjustor to achieve budget neutrality. Due to an estimated increase in expenditures from the third Five-Year Review of nearly $4 billion, CMS applied a –10.1% adjustor to all physician work RVUs.

2008

For 2008, CMS retained the budget neutrality work adjustor despite significant comment from the AMA and other national medical specialty societies that this was an inappropriate mechanism to achieve budget neutrality. The work adjustor increased from –10.10% to –11.94% because the Five-Year Review was finalized with the review of anesthesia services, eye exams, and other services.

2009

The budget-neutrality adjustor was removed for 2009 and applied to the CF as required by the Medicare Improvements for Patients and Providers Act of 2008 (MIPPA). The application of the adjustor to the CF would have reduced the CF by 6.41%. However, MIPPA also called for a 1.1% increase in the CF, and the efforts of RUC in reassessing several services resulted in a redistribution applied to the CF in the form of a 0.08% increase. The cumulative impact of these changes resulted in an overall reduction of the CF by 5.305%.

2010

CMS in calculating the 2010 CF could not consider the legislative mandated increases that were applied to the CF for 2007, 2008, and 2009. Thus, the 2010 conversion factor had to take into account the 5% cut in 2007, the 5.3% cut in

2008, and the 11.5% cut in 2009. Further adjustments were made based on the Medicare Economic Index (MEI) and the Update Adjustment Factor as well as a 0.103% increase because of RUC's work of evaluating potentially misvalued codes. The overall impact of these adjustments resulted in a 21.2% cut in the conversion factor. However, after Congress passed four legislative acts to postpone the scheduled 2010 conversion factor reduction, the Preservation of Access to Care for Medicare Beneficiaries and Pension Relief Act was signed into law by President Barack Obama on June 25, 2010. It replaced the 21% Medicare Physician Payment Cut that took effect June 1, 2010, with a 2.2% payment update that extended through November 2010. On November 30, 2010, President Obama signed HR 5712 Physician Payment and Therapy Relief Act of 2010. This Act maintained the 2010 conversion factor through December 31, 2010.

2011

RUC submitted recommendations to address misvaluation of the work values for 2011. This effort resulted in more than $400 million in redistribution and provides a positive adjustment to the 2011 CF of 0.4%.

2012

RUC submitted recommendations to address misvaluation of the work values for 2012. These efforts resulted in a positive update to the 2012 CF of 0.18%

2013

RUC submitted recommendations to address misvaluation of physician services again for 2013. These efforts resulted in approximately $1 billion in redistribution within the relative values. A small adjustment of –0.1% to the CF was also necessary to remain budget-neutral.

2014

RUC submitted recommendations to address misvaluation of physician services for 2014. These efforts resulted in approximately $435 million in redistribution within the relative values. In 2014, CMS increased the CF by 0.046% to offset the estimated decrease in Medicare physician expenditures. See Table 8-2 for a summary of this history.

2015

RUC submitted recommendations to address misvaluation of physician services for 2015, which resulted in approximately $450 million in redistribution within the relative values. However, implementation of a new chronic care management code and results of a CMS technical correction led to a budget-neutrality adjustment of 0.19%.

2016

RUC submitted recommendations to address misvaluation of physician services for 2016, which resulted in approximately $205 million in redistribution within the relative values (or a –0.23% redistribution). This redistribution offset a portion of the –1.00% adjustment due to the Achieving a Better Life Experience (ABLE) Act of 2014, resulting in a net change of –0.77%. There was also a –0.02% adjustment due to other work-neutrality adjustments. This collection of adjustments led to a total budget-neutrality adjustment of –0.79% for CY 2016.

2017

RUC submitted recommendations to address misvaluation of physician services for 2017, which resulted in approximately $288 million in redistribution within the relative values (or a –0.32% redistribution). This redistribution offset a portion of the –0.50% due to the ABLE Act of 2014, resulting in a net change of –0.18%. There was also a –0.013% adjustment due to budget-neutrality adjustment and –0.07% due to the imaging MPPR adjustment. Effective January 1, 2017, the Consolidated Appropriations Act, 2016 (Pub. L. 114–113, enacted on December 18, 2015) added a new section that revised the professional component (PC) of advanced imaging services MPPR reduction from 25% to 5%. This series of adjustments led to a total budget-neutrality adjustment of –0.263% for CY 2017.

2018

RUC submitted recommendations to address misvaluation of physician services for 2018, which resulted in approximately $400 million in redistribution within the relative values (or a –0.41% redistribution). This redistribution offset a portion of the –0.50% due to the ABLE Act of 2014, resulting in a net change of –0.09%. There was also a –0.1% adjustment due to a budget-neutrality adjustment to offset spending on new services, such as prolonged preventive services and new payment for CPT 99091.This series of adjustments led to a total budget-neutrality adjustment of –0.19% for CY 2018.

2019

The Bipartisan Budget Act of 2018 provided a positive payment update of 0.25% for 2019. To calculate the 2019 Medicare conversion factor, CMS applied the 0.25% update to the 2018 conversion factor as well as a budget-neutrality adjustment of –0.14%. Therefore, the increase, which was effective January 1, 2019, was 0.11%.

2020

To calculate the 2020 Medicare conversion factor, CMS applied the 0.00% update to the 2019 conversion factor as well as a budget-neutrality adjustment of 0.14%. Therefore, the increase, which was effective January 1, 2020, was 0.14%.

Table 8-2. 1992–2022 CMS Budget-Neutrality* Adjustments to Physician Work

**All work neutrality adjustments are related to annual payment policy and coding changes unless noted.*

Year	Work RVU Reduction	Work RVU Adjustor	Budget Neutrality—Applied to CF
1993	–2.80%[1]	—	—
1994	–1.30%	—	—
1995	–1.10%	—	—
1996	—	—	–0.36%
1997	—	–8.30%[2]	–0.60%
1998	—	–8.30%[2]	–0.80%
1999	—	Work adjuster eliminated	–7.50%[3]
2000	—	—	0.07%
2001	—	—	–0.30%
2002	—	—	–0.46%[4]
2003	—	—	–0.04%
2004	–0.35%[5]	—	—
2005	—	—	—
2006	—	—	20.15%[6]
2007	—	–10.10%[7]	—
2008	—	–11.94%[7]	—
2009	—	Work adjuster eliminated	–6.41%[8]
			0.08%[8]
2010	—	—	0.103%[9]
2011			–8.6%[5], 0.43%[9]
2012			0.18%[9]
2013			–0.1%[9]
2014			4.718%[5], 0.046%[9]
2015			–0.19%[10]
2016			–0.79%[11]
2017			–0.263%[12]
2018			–0.19%[13]
2019			–0.14%[14]
2020			–0.14%[15]
2021			–3.33%[16]
2022			–0.80%[17]

[1]Includes the CMS initial work refinement in additional to annual CPT coding changes.
[2]A result of the first Five-Year Review.
[3]Includes MEI re-weight, elimination of the work adjustor, and annual CPT coding changes.
[4]A result of the second Five-Year Review.
[5]A result of the MEI re-weight.
[6]Budget neutrality negated by CF freeze in 2006.
[7]A result of the third Five-Year Review.
[8]Includes the elimination of the work adjuster (–6.41%) and 0.08% savings from RUC review.
[9]Redistribution due to RUC review of misvalued codes.
[10]CMS technical corrections for 2015.
[11]Includes a –0.77% ABLE Act reduction (–0.23% redistribution from the RUC review offset a portion of the –1.00% change required from the ABLE Act) and –0.02% due to other CMS budget-neutrality adjustments.
[12]Includes a –0.18% ABLE Act reduction (–0.32% redistribution from the RUC review offset a portion of the –0.50% change required from the ABLE Act) and a –0.013% due to other CMS budget-neutrality adjustments. A –0.07% imaging MPPR adjustment was also implemented.
[13]Includes a –0.09% ABLE Act reduction (–0.41% redistribution from the RUC review offset a portion of the –0.50% change required from the ABLE Act) and a –0.10% due to other CMS budget-neutrality adjustments.
[14]–0.14% due to CMS budget-neutrality adjustment, which is largely to offset the cost of new payment for telemedicine services.
[15]–0.14% due to CMS budget-neutrality adjustment.
[16]For 2021, CMS finalized a profoundly steep budget-neutrality adjustment of –10.20% to the CF. However, the Consolidated Appropriations Act, 2021 (the Act) that was signed into law on December 27, 2020, included provisions that offset most of the –10.2% budget-neutrality adjustment that was slated to take effect for Medicare-covered services provided as of January 1, 2021. The Act delayed implementation of HCPCS add-on code G2211 (visit complexity inherent to evaluation and management services) until CY 2024. The Act also provided a 3.75% increase in MFS payments for CY 2021. As a result of these two actions, the CF was $34.8931 in 2021, a 3.3% decrease from 2020.
[17]–0.80% due to the maintenance of a temporary 3.75% increase to the CF at a reduced 3%, stemming from Congressional action to temporarily avert a more significant cut for another year, as well as a budget-neutrality adjustment of –0.10%.

2021

CMS adopted the significant changes in coding definitions and guidelines for office visits made by the CPT Editorial Panel, as well as the RUC-recommended relative value recommendations for implementation in 2021. These coding changes and payment increases represent a substantial improvement over the existing coding structure. Under current law, however, payment increases must be implemented in a budget-neutral manner, which would have led to steep negative adjustments for many physicians and other qualified health care professionals (QHPs) who report no or few office visits. Fortunately, the Consolidated Appropriations Act, 2021 (the Act), included provisions that offset most of the budget-neutrality adjustment that had been slated to take effect for Medicare-covered services provided as of January 1, 2021.

2022

On November 2, 2021, the Centers for Medicare & Medicaid Services (CMS) released the Final Rule for the calendar year (CY) 2022 Medicare Physician Payment Schedule (MFS). For 2022, the Medicare conversion factor (CF) will be reduced by approximately 0.8% from 34.8931 in 2021 to 34.6062. This reduction is due to the maintenance of a temporary 3.75% increase to the CF at a reduced 3%, stemming from Congressional action to temporarily avert a more significant cut for another year, as well as a budget-neutrality adjustment of – 0.10%.

The American Medical Association (AMA) strongly advocated for Congress to extend the 3.75% increase for CY 2022 as physician practices faced Medicare cuts amounting to a 9.71% overall decrease effective January 1, 2022, when factoring in sequestration reductions. Recognizing that these Medicare cuts would further compound the growing financial instability of physician practices due to the significant reduction in revenue caused by the continued severe acute respiratory syndrome coronavirus 2 (SARS-CoV-2) (coronavirus disease 2019 [COVID-19]) public health emergency (PHE), the cuts were diverted when President Biden signed S.610, Protecting Medicare and American Farmers from Sequester Cuts Act, into law on December 10, 2021. This law results in the following:

- A delay in resuming the 2% Medicare sequester for three months (January 1–March 31, 2022), followed by a reduction to 1% for three months (April 1–June 30, 2022).
- A 1-year increase in the MFS of 3% (0.75% less than the CF boost provided for 2021).
- A 1-year delay in the cuts to the clinical laboratory fee schedule.
- A 1-year delay in the Medicare radiation oncology demonstration.

In addition, the law will erase the 4% Medicare Pay-As-You-Go (PAYGO) cut and prevent any additional PAYGO cuts through 2022.

Effective January 1, 2022, the anesthesia CF is $21.5623 which reflects the same overall MFS adjustments with the addition of anesthesia-specific practice expense (PE) and malpractice (MP) adjustments.

Worksheets for Determining the Impact of Medicare Payment System on Individual Physician Practices

Physicians may use the CMS' November 2, 2021, publication of the Final Rule on the Medicare MFS to determine the impact that the Medicare MFS will have on their practices. The worksheet provided within this book will allow physicians to estimate their practice revenue under this payment system. In using the worksheet, the following factors and limitations should be closely noted:

- The mix and volume of, and assignment rate for, the services and procedures provided to Medicare patients, and the geographic location for the physician practice, are major factors determining the impact of the payment systems.
- The phrase "Medicare-approved amount" used throughout the worksheets includes 80% of the approved amount paid by Medicare and the 20% copayment collected from the patient.

Instructions for Worksheet A

The worksheet will enable physicians to calculate 2022 payment amounts for frequently provided procedures and services.

Step 1 Make as many copies of Worksheet A as needed for your personal use.

Step 2 Identify the most frequent services and procedures that you provide to Medicare patients by entering each CPT code (include a modifier if appropriate) and short descriptor in columns A and B, respectively.

Step 3 Using the List of Relative Value Units in Part 5 of the *Physicians' Guide*, find the RVUs for the work, practice expense (PE), and PLI components of the MFS and enter each RVU in column C. In selecting the practice expense relative values, make certain to select the appropriate site of service.

Step 4 Using the List of Geographic Practice Cost Indices for Each Medicare Locality, from Part 5 of the *Physicians' Guide*, find the work, practice expense, and PLI GPCIs for your payment locality. For each of the three RVUs that you recorded in column C, enter the three corresponding GPCIs.

Step 5 In column C, calculate the geographically adjusted RVU for the work, practice expense, and PLI components by multiplying each RVU by each GPCI.

Worksheet A

Calculating 2022 full Medicare payment schedule amounts for most frequently provided procedures

Column A	*Column B*		*Column C*		*Column D*	*Column E*
CPT	**Short Descriptor**	**RVU Components**	**RVU × GPCI =**	**Geographic Adjusted RVU**	**Conversion Factor**	**Full Payment Schedule Amount**
		Work RVU	×	=		
		PE	×	=		
		PLI	×	=		
		Total Adjusted RVU		=	×$34.6062	
		Work RVU	×	=		
		PE	×	=		
		PLI	×	=		
		Total Adjusted RVU		=	×$34.6062	
		Work RVU	×	=		
		PE	×	=		
		PLI	×	=		
		Total Adjusted RVU		=	×$34.6062	
		Work RVU	×	=		
		PE	×	=		
		PLI	×	=		
		Total Adjusted RVU		=	×$34.6062	
		Work RVU	×	=		
		PE	×	=		
		PLI	×	=		
		Total Adjusted RVU		=	×$34.6062	

Step 6 In the last box of column C, calculate the total geographically adjusted RVU by summing the three geographically adjusted RVUs.

Step 7 Multiply the total geographically adjusted RVU in column C by the conversion factor. For this example, the 2022 conversion factor, $34.6062, is used in column D to arrive at the full Medicare payment schedule amount and entered in column E.

Step 8 Repeat steps 3 through 7 to calculate full Medicare physician schedule amounts for each service and procedure that you provide most frequently to Medicare amounts.

Instructions for Worksheet B: "Nonparticipating" Physicians

Worksheet B will enable physicians to calculate 2022 payment amounts for frequently provided procedures and services.

Step 1 Make as many copies of Worksheet B as needed for your personal use.

Step 2 Identify the most frequent services and procedures that you provide to Medicare patients by entering each CPT code (include a modifier if appropriate).

Step 3 Using the List of Relative Units in Part 5 of the *Physicians' Guide*, find the RVUs for the work, PE, and PLI components of the MFS and enter each RVU in column B. In selecting the practice expense relative values, make certain to select the appropriate site of service.

Step 4 Using the List of Geographic Practice Cost Indices for Each Medicare Locality, from Part 5 of the *Physicians' Guide*, find the work, practice expense, and PLI GPCIs for your payment locality. For each of the three RVUs that you recorded in column B, enter the three corresponding GPCIs.

Step 5 In column B, calculate the geographically adjusted RVU for the work, PE, and PLI components by multiplying each RVU by each GPCI.

Step 6 In the last box of column B, calculate the total geographically adjusted RVU by summing the three geographically adjusted RVUs.

Step 7 Multiply the total geographically adjusted RVU in column B by the conversion factor. For this example, the 2022 conversion factor, $34.6062 is used in column C to arrive at the full Medicare payment schedule amount and entered in column D.

Step 8 Multiply the full Medicare payment schedule amount by 1.0925 to arrive at the nonparticipating amount. This adjustment corresponds to the Medicare approved amount for nonparticipating physicians of 95% of payment rated for participating physicians. Medicare then allows nonparticipating physicians to charge Medicare patients 15% more than the Medicare approved amount for nonparticipating physicians. This results in payments 9.25% greater than participating physician payments.

Step 9 Repeat steps 3 through 8 to calculate full Medicare physician schedule amounts for each service and procedure that you provide most frequently to Medicare patients.

Worksheet B

Calculating 2022 "nonparticipating" Medicare payment schedule amounts for most frequently provided procedures

Column A		*Column B*		*Column C*	*Column D*	*Column E*	*Column F*
CPT Code	**RVU Components**	**RVU 3 GPCI 5**	**Geographic Adjusted RVU**	**Conversion Factor**	**Full Payment Schedule Amount**	**Conversion Factor**	**Non-participating Amount**
	Work RVU	×	=				
	PE	×	=				
	PLI	×	=				
	Total Adjusted RVU		=	×$34.6062		×1.0925	
	Work RVU	×	=				
	PE	×	=				
	PLI	×	=				
	Total Adjusted RVU		=	×$34.6062		×1.0925	
	Work RVU	×	=				
	PE	×	=				
	PLI	×	=				
	Total Adjusted RVU		=	×$34.6062		×1.0925	
	Work RVU	×	=				
	PE	×	=				
	PLI	×	=				
	Total Adjusted RVU		=	×$34.6062		×1.0925	
	Work RVU	×	=				
	PE	×	=				
	PLI	×	=				
	Total Adjusted RVU		=	×$34.6062		×1.0925	

Chapter 9

Balance Billing Under the Payment Schedule

Two features of the Medicare program are designed to control the amount of money that patients pay out of pocket for Medicare-covered services: the physician participation (PAR) Program and the limiting charges. The purpose of the PAR Program is to encourage physicians to accept Medicare assignment for all claims, which means they accept the Medicare approved amount as payment in full (including the 80% that Medicare pays and the 20% coinsurance). Limiting charges restrict the amount that physicians who do not accept Medicare assignment may charge above the amount that Medicare approves.

The American Medical Association (AMA) has a long history of vigorously opposing any government policy that restricts physicians' ability to establish their own payments for the services they provide. The AMA believes that payments are a matter for discussion between patients and physicians, not a matter for government intervention. The AMA encourages physicians to consider patients' ability to pay when making payment decisions.

To facilitate assignment acceptance for low-income patients, several state and county medical societies have initiated voluntary assignment programs. Laws in several states limit the amounts physicians may bill patients to either the Medicare-approved amount or a percentage amount above the approved amount.

As Chapter 2 outlined, AMA opposed both the PAR Program and the earlier limits on balance billing, called maximum allowable actual charges (MAACs), which had been in place under the customary, prevailing, and reasonable (CPR) system for several years before Congress enacted the Omnibus Budget Reconciliation Act of 1989 (OBRA 89). Although the AMA continued its strong opposition during the drafting of the legislation, Chapter 2 explained why retaining the PAR Program and MAAC-type limits under the Medicare resource-based relative value system (RBRVS) payment system was unavoidable, with the larger battle being the one against mandated assignment. This chapter describes the PAR Program and the limiting charges.

PAR Program

Under Medicare law, Medicare patients must pay a $233 annual deductible in 2022 for Part B services and a 20% copayment on claims for Part B services that are submitted after meeting the deductible. Throughout this book, discussion of Medicare approved amounts and Medicare payment schedule amounts refers to 100% of the Medicare amount, for which the Medicare program pays 80% and patients 20%. The difference between the physician's actual charge and the Medicare allowed amount is known as "balance billing."

Most beneficiaries have Medicare supplemental insurance, such as that provided by an employer, or "Medigap," policies to cover the costs of the deductible and coinsurance; some of these policies also cover balance billing. Medicare beneficiaries who also qualify for state Medicaid programs have their deductibles and coinsurance covered by Medicaid; assignment is mandatory for these beneficiaries.

When a physician accepts Medicare assignment, the patient is still responsible for the 20% coinsurance. Assignment acceptance limits the patient's out-of-pocket financial responsibility to this 20% coinsurance, however, and precludes the physician from charging more than the Medicare approved amount.

The PAR Program was established in 1984 to provide incentives for physicians to accept Medicare assignment. A "participating" physician, or PAR physician, agrees to accept assignment for all services provided to Medicare patients. Physicians are invited to become PAR physicians in a "Medicare Participating Physician/Supplier Agreement" (formerly referred to as the "Dear Doctor" letter) from their Medicare carrier each fall. The deadline for physicians to change their Medicare participation or non-participation status was December 31, 2019. This decision is binding throughout the calendar year. For more information on this issue, please visit www.ama-assn.org/practice-management/medicare-participation-options-toolkit.

Failure to respond results in a continuation of the physician's current status. The agreement binds physicians to accept assignment for all Medicare claims during the calendar year in which the agreement is effective.

Medicare provides the following incentives for physicians to participate:

- The full payment schedule for "nonparticipating" (non-PAR) physicians is set at 95% of the full payment schedule for PAR physicians. Non-PAR approved amounts are 95% of PAR amounts for the same service.
- Directories of PAR physicians are provided to senior citizens groups and, upon request, to individual beneficiaries.
- Carriers provide toll-free claims processing lines to PAR physicians.
- PAR claims are processed more quickly than non-PAR claims.

The major incentive to participate in the PAR program is the payment differential. In 2009, 96.54% of MDs and DOs nationally were participating. In 2010, 95.8% of MDs and DOs were participating. In 2011, participation increased to 96.0%, and continued to increase in 2012 to 96.1%. A favorable trend continued in 2013 as participation reached 96.6%. In 2014, the physician participation rate increased to 97.5%. In 2015 and 2017, the physician participation rate rose to 97.9% and 98.3%, respectively. In 2019 and 2021, the physician participation rate increased further to 98.8% and 98.9%, respectively. Note that physician participation rates vary by specialty and practice location.

Limiting Charges

When established in 1986, MAACs were based on a complicated formula involving an individual physician's charges in the second quarter of 1984. As a result, the variation between physicians' MAACs was as wide as their individual payments for the services they provided. The change from MAACs to limiting charges, therefore, produced an effect like the geographic practice cost indices (GPCIs) because it eliminated much of the variation in payments (or, in this case, variation in charges) for the same service.

The RBRVS payment schedule compressed balance billing limits relative to their wide range under CPR. Since 1993, the limiting charge has been 115% of the Medicare approved amount for non-PAR physicians. Physicians whose MAACs were considerably higher than prevailing charges under CPR now have limiting charges that exceed the payment schedule amounts by a much lower percentage. Physicians whose MAACs were only 10% more than their prevailing charges generally experienced a slight increase in payments for visit services and services for which Medicare payments were not reduced under the Medicare RBRVS payment system.

Limiting charge information is provided in the annual "Medicare Participating Physician/Supplier Agreement," which the Medicare carrier sends to each physician. The letter must also include payment information on the PAR-approved amount, the non-PAR amount, and the limiting charge for all services paid under the RBRVS payment schedule.

The limiting charge provision has applied to drugs and biologicals provided "incident to" a physician's service since January 1, 1994. In addition, the limiting charge provisions apply to all nonparticipating providers and suppliers for services on the payment schedule. Prior to 1994, only services provided by nonparticipating physicians were subject to limiting charges.

In addition to controlling patient out-of-pocket payments, the limiting charges provide an additional incentive for physicians to participate. Medicare payment schedule amounts and transition approved amounts for non-PAR physicians are 95% of payment rates for PAR physicians. Therefore, the 15% limiting charge translates into only 9.25% more than the PAR approved amount for a service.

When considering whether to participate, physicians must determine whether their total revenues from balance billing would exceed their revenues as PAR physicians, particularly in light of collection costs, bad debts, and claims for which they do accept assignment. The 95% payment rate is not based on whether physicians accept assignment on the claim but whether they are PAR physicians; when non-PAR physicians accept assignment for their low-income or other patients, they still receive only 95% of the amount PAR physicians receive for the same service. A non-PAR physician would need to collect the full limiting charge amount roughly 35% of the time they provided the service for the revenues from the service to equal those of PAR physicians. In addition to payment considerations, other factors support the decision to participate.

Assignment acceptance, for either a PAR or a non-PAR physician, also means that the Medicare carrier pays the physician the 80% Medicare payment. For unassigned claims, even though the physician is required to submit the claim to Medicare, the program pays the patient, and the physician must then collect the entire amount for the service from the patient. Because PAR physicians receive 80% of their Medicare amounts directly from Medicare, they only need to collect the 20% coinsurance from patients. For assigned claims, non-PAR physicians receive 80% of the Medicare approved amount directly from Medicare but must bill patients for the 20% coinsurance. See Table 9-1 for an example showing the effect that participation has on payments.

Chapter 12 also discusses the options that physicians have regarding participation, nonparticipation, and private contracting.

Monitoring Compliance

The Centers for Medicare & Medicaid Services (CMS) received greater statutory authority to monitor compliance with Medicare balance billing limits through provisions contained in the Social Security Act Amendments of 1994. The legislation clarifies that nonparticipating physicians and suppliers may not bill patients more than the limiting charge and that patients, as well as supplemental insurers, are not liable for payment of any amount that exceeds the limiting charge. If billed charges exceed the limiting charge, carriers are required to notify the physician or other provider of the violation within 30 days. A refund or credit for the excess charges must be made to the patient within 30 days of carrier notification. Sanctions may be imposed for "knowingly and willfully" billing or collecting payments that exceed the limiting charge.

In addition, when an unassigned claim is submitted with charges that exceed the limiting charge, the law requires that limiting charge information be included on the explanation of Medicare benefits (EOMB), indicating the beneficiary's right to a refund if an excess charge has been collected. Information reflecting these changes appears on the EOMB and the limiting charge exception report (LCER).

To monitor physicians' and other providers' compliance with the limiting charges, carriers are required to screen all unassigned claims. Physicians and other providers who fail to adjust for overcharges as outlined in the LCER are subject to sanctions that can include fines and suspension from the Medicare program for up to five years. Finally, the law requires the Secretary of Health and Human Services (HHS) to report to Congress annually concerning the extent of limiting charge violations and the services involved.

Under CMS' comprehensive limiting charge compliance program (CLCCP) that took effect in mid-1992, carriers issue notifications to physicians when a violation of the limiting charge has occurred. Carriers send LCERs to those physicians and other Medicare providers whose unassigned claims include charges that exceed the limiting charge by $1.

Table 9-1. PAR/Non-PAR Table

Example: A service for which Medicare payment schedule amount is $100

Payment Arrangement	Total Payment Rate	Payment Amount from Medicare	Payment Amount for Patient
PAR Physician	100% Medicare payment Schedule = $100	$80 (80%) carrier direct to physician	$20 (20%) paid by patient or supplemental insurance (ie, Medigap)
Non-PAR/Assigned Claim	95% Medicare payment schedule = $95	$76 (80%) carrier direct to physician	$19 (20%) paid by patient or supplemental insurance (ie, Medigap)
Non-PAR/Unassigned Claim	Claim Limiting charge/ 109.25% Medicare payment schedule = $109.25	$0	$76 (80%) paid by carrier to patient + $19 (20%) paid by patient or supplemental insurance + $14.25 balance bill paid by patient

Part 3

The RBRVS Payment System in Operation

Part 3 addresses the operational details of Medicare's physician payment system. Chapter 10 explains the conversion factor and the methodology for updating physician payment. Chapter 11 describes all of the key features in the standardization of Medicare's payment system, including the policies on global surgical packages; visit coding; payments for assistants-at-surgery; nonphysicians; drugs, services, and supplies provided "incident to" a physician's service; and other issues.

Chapter 10

Conversion Factor Updates

The Medicare conversion factor (CF) is a scaling factor that converts the geographically adjusted number of relative value units (RVUs) for each service in the Medicare physician payment schedule into a dollar payment amount. The initial Medicare CF was set at $31.001 in 1992. Until 2015, subsequent default or current law CF updates were determined largely by an expenditure target formula. In 2015, the Medicare Access and Children's Health Insurance Program (CHIP) Reauthorization Act (MACRA) of 2015 permanently eliminated the existing expenditure target, ie, the sustainable growth rate (SGR), and replaced it with fixed updates that are specified in the legislation. The conversion factor update may also be affected by miscellaneous adjustments, including those for budget neutrality.

SGR Permanently Repealed

The SGR was enacted as part of the Balanced Budget Act of 1997, replacing the original Medicare physician payment schedule expenditure target, known as the Medicare volume performance standard (MVPS). Updates under the SGR formula were initially positive, but it turned negative beginning in 2002 in which payment cuts were allowed to go through, reducing the CF by about 5%. Subsequent cuts were blocked by legislation, using methods that, until recently, had resulted in ever-steeper cuts for the following years. In all, there were 17 temporary SGR fixes that blocked CF cuts that ranged from 4.4% in 2003 to 27.4% in 2012. The last temporary fix expired April 1, 2015, with a 21.2% CF cut, which was set to go into effect.

However, this cut was blocked by MACRA, which eliminated the SGR and, instead, specified updates for all future years. The update for April 1, 2015, was set at 0.0%; however, a 0.5% increase was provided on July 1, 2015. Updates for 2016 to 2019 were set at 0.5%, and for 2020 through 2025 were set at 0.0%. Beginning in 2016, MACRA specified that updates will differ depending on whether the provider is in an alternative payment model (APM). For providers in APMs, the annual CF update will be 0.75%. For others, the update will be 0.25%.

The impact of MACRA is enormous; with the SGR cut scheduled for April 1, 2015, the Medicare physician CF would have fallen from just under $36 to roughly $28.20. Instead, the CF was stabilized, and Medicare physician pay for the remainder of 2015 was 27% greater than it would have been under the SGR.

Projections of SGR updates provide an indication of future impacts. Although SGR updates beyond 2015 would have depended on a variety of factors, under reasonable assumptions Medicare physician pay under MACRA in 2024 is 12% greater than it would have been under the SGR. In addition, over the 10 years from 2015 to 2024, Medicare physician pay under MACRA is, on average, 17% greater than the projected pay under SGR (see Figure 10-1). Over the 10 years from 2015 to 2024, the update provisions of MACRA are projected to increase payments for Medicare physician services by roughly $150 billion, compared to what would have occurred under the SGR.

Figure 10-1. MACRA Stabilizes Medicare Physician Pay

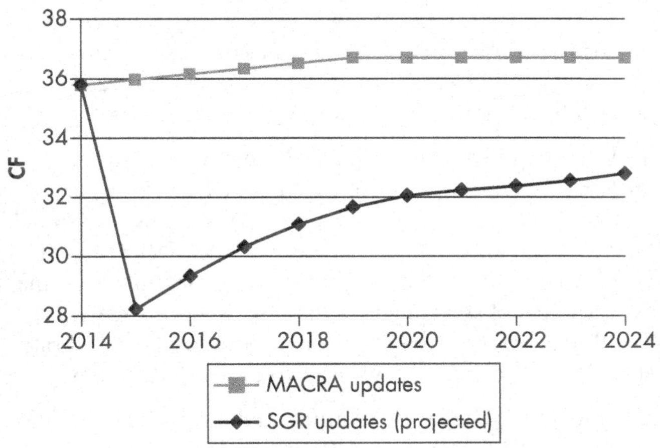

Note: MACRA and SGR updates exclude budget-neutrality and misvalued-code adjustments.

Medicare Economic Index

The Medicare economic index (MEI) is no longer part of the annual CF update process. The MEI is a measure of medical practice inflation; however, because CF updates are now set by MACRA, there is no longer an explicit inflation adjustment in the update.

The MEI was used between 1976 and 2015 as a proxy for inflation in the cost of operating a medical practice. The largest single determinant of changes in the MEI was the change in professional workers' earnings, which was the proxy for physicians' own time in the index. The index also included measures of changes in:

- Nonphysician compensation, including fringe benefits
- Expenses for office space and equipment
- Medical materials and supplies expenses
- Professional liability insurance
- Medical equipment expenses
- Other professional expenses

The Centers for Medicare & Medicaid Services (CMS) used data from the federal Bureau of Labor Statistics to measure changes in the prices of all these components of practice expense except professional liability insurance (PLI). CMS used its own survey data to measure changes in PLI premiums. These price changes are weighted by each component's share of total physician practice revenue. The revenue shares were based largely on data from the American Medical Association's (AMA's) physician practice information (PPI) survey, which was fielded in 2007 and collected practice expense information for 2006.

CMS convened a Technical Advisory Panel (Panel) in 2012 to review all aspects of the MEI. The Panel recommended several changes to the price proxies and cost components of the index, and CMS implemented most of the recommendations effective with the 2014 MEI. Key changes included:

- changing the price proxy for physician compensation from hourly earnings in the general economy to earnings of professional workers;
- using commercial rents in place of residential rents for the office space (fixed capital) portion of the index.
- moving payroll for nonphysician personnel who can bill independently from the practice expense portion to the physician compensation (work) portion of the index;
- creating new categories for clinical labor costs and for other professional services (eg, billing); and
- increasing the physician benefits share of the index.

The changes to the cost categories and weights are aimed at improving the accuracy of the MEI as a description of the cost structure of medical practice. Changes to the price proxies generally move away from broad price measures to those more closely associated with physicians. The revenue shares for the major MEI categories are shown in Table 10-1, along with the associated wage and price changes for the 2015 MEI.

The MEI includes an adjustment for productivity growth, ie, the MEI is reduced to account for potential improvement in the productivity of physician practices. Beginning with the 2003 MEI, the productivity adjustment is based on the 10-year average of economy-wide multifactor productivity growth. For 2015, the weighted average increase in input prices captured under the MEI was 1.7%, and the productivity adjustment was –0.9%, yielding a net change of 0.8% in the MEI.

Table 10-1. The 2015 MEI

Component	Weight	Wage/Price Change
Physicians' own time	50.9%	1.9%
Nonphysician payroll	16.6%	1.8%
Other practice expenses	32.6%	1.4%
Total (weighted average)		1.7%
Less productivity adjustment		–0.9%
2015 MEI		0.8%

Expenditure Targets and Performance Adjustment

Generally, the most important element in determining default or current law CF updates is the performance adjustment. The performance adjustment is based on a comparison of actual and target expenditures. The method of determining this factor has changed over time. Initially, the performance adjustment was based on the Medicare volume performance standard (MVPS). This formula, which had been altered under the Omnibus Budget Reconciliation Act of 1993 (OBRA 93), was projected to produce substantial long-term payment cuts.

In 1997, Congress enacted key changes to the conversion factor update process as part of the Balanced Budget Act (BBA), replacing the MVPS with the sustainable growth rate (SGR) system. This system was also seriously flawed, however, and further revisions that were advocated by AMA were adopted as part of the Balanced Budget Refinement Act (BBRA) of 1999. In 2015, MACRA legislation permanently repealed the SGR update methodology for physicians' services, which provides positive annual payment updates of 0.5%, beginning from July 1 and lasting through 2019, which requires that CMS establishes a merit-based incentive payment system (MIPS) under which MIPS eligible professionals receive annual payment adjustments based on their performance in a prior period. These and subsequent other changes to the expenditure target system are described in the remainder of this section.

The MVPS and Conversion Factor Updates Prior to 1998

Under the MVPS system, a target rate of fee-for-service Medicare physician spending growth was calculated each year. This target rate of growth was compared to actual spending growth for the year to determine the conversion factor update two years later. If actual spending growth exceeded the target in a given year, for example, physicians would be penalized with a below-inflation update two years later (in which MEI is the measure of inflation). If actual spending growth was below the target, then an above-inflation update would be awarded. The two-year lag was specified to allow for delays in claims processing.

This formula-driven approach to updating the conversion factor was not automatic, however. The Omnibus Budget Reconciliation Act of 1989 (OBRA 89) gave Congress the authority to set its own conversion factor updates and spending targets. As part of its deliberations, Congress was required to consider the recommendations submitted by CMS and the Physician Payment Review Commission (PPRC). If Congress failed to act on these recommendations, however, annual updates were set by the default (MVPS) formula, which had also been established under OBRA 89.

The default MVPS target rate of spending growth was based on the following factors:

- Changes in Medicare payment levels
- Changes in the size and age composition of the Medicare population
- The five-year historical average growth in the volume and intensity of physician services
- Changes in expenditures resulting from law and regulation

The target was then reduced by a legislatively determined number of percentage points known as the *performance standard factor*. The performance standard factor was increased from 2.0 to 4.0 percentage points by OBRA 93.

With the modifications to the MVPS formula specified in OBRA 93, Medicare payments were projected to decline steadily over time. Payments were virtually guaranteed to fall over the long term given the structure of the MVPS system, which essentially set the target rate of spending growth at the expected rate of spending growth minus 4 percentage points. The PPRC projected that the default formula would generate annual conversion factor cuts of 2% or more indefinitely.

Separate MVPS targets for surgical and nonsurgical services were also established under OBRA 89, allowing separate conversion factors for each service category. A third service category, for primary care services, was established in 1994 under provisions of OBRA 93. By 1997, the separate targets and updates under the MVPS system resulted in a surgical conversion factor that was 9% greater than that for primary care, and 14% greater than that for nonsurgical services. As the conversion factors diverged, interest grew among various groups to eliminate multiple MVPSs and return to a single conversion factor.

The Sustainable Growth Rate System and the BBA

The BBA of 1997 established a single conversion factor for all physician services excluding anesthesia as of January 1, 1998. The legislation also replaced the MVPS with the SGR expenditure target system. Under SGR, a target rate of spending growth is calculated each year based on changes in the following:

- Fees for physician services (in practice, primarily the MEI)
- Medicare fee-for-service enrollment
- Real (inflation-adjusted) per capita gross domestic product (GDP)
- Spending due to law and regulation

The factors that go into determining the SGR target (see Table 10-2) are like those used in the MVPS, with the major change being the use of real per capita GDP in place of

Table 10-2. SGR Targets for 2010–2014
Allowed Growth in Medicare Physician Spending as of November 2014

	2010	2011	2012	2013	2014
Payment (inflation), %	0.9	0.2	0.6	0.4	0.7
Fee-for-service enrollment, %	1.1	1.0	0.9	0.5	0.2
Real per-capita GDP growth, %	0.6	0.6	0.9	0.9	0.7
Law and regulation, %	6.1	2.8	2.6	0.5	2.4
Total	8.9	4.7	5.1	1.3	0.8

historical average volume growth. A second major change is that the SGR system is cumulative. The target growth rate is applied to the allowed amount of spending for the prior year to determine the (dollar amount of) allowed spending for the following year. Running totals of actual and allowed spending, beginning April 1, 1996, are kept, and the performance adjustment is based on the difference between cumulative allowed and actual spending. The performance adjustment is limited to a maximum bonus (if spending is below target) of 3% and a maximum penalty (if spending is above target) of –7%.

With the introduction of GDP to the target, funding for Medicare physician services was tied directly to the state of the US economy. In 1997, the Congressional Budget Office and others projected that the SGR would reduce physician payments even more than the MVPS. However, the system offered the opportunity for improved payment levels if growth in the utilization of Medicare physician services was relatively low.

The SGR system, as specified in the BBA, had several technical flaws. A key flaw was the lack of any specific provision regarding the correction of projection errors. CMS originally set a target rate of growth each fall for the coming fiscal year. This target rate of growth was based on projections of the components of the target for that year, including real per capita GDP growth and changes in fee-for-service enrollment. CMS underestimated these components for the fiscal year 1998 and 1999 targets, and this reduced target SGR spending relative to what it should have been.

Despite this shortfall, CMS estimated that actual spending was at or below the target amount for the first two years of SGR. The 1999 update, the first to be determined under the SGR system, was 2.3% (before budget-neutrality and other adjustments), and the 2000 update was 5.4%.

Congress corrected some of the SGR's technical flaws in the Balanced Budget Refinement Act of 1999 (BBRA). The BBRA did not, however, direct CMS to correct the fiscal year 1998 and 1999 projection errors (although it did allow CMS to correct projection errors going forward). Despite this, actual SGR spending appeared to be within the target amount as late as spring 2001. The 2001 update was 4.5%, which included the maximum 3% bonus performance adjustment. Then, US economic growth faltered, and the Commerce Department revised its official estimate of GDP growth in 2000 downward. These events reduced allowed or target spending. At the same time, utilization growth for SGR services increased, driven in part by rapid growth in the utilization of physician administered drugs, which were included in SGR at that time. Utilization of many diagnostic services also increased markedly. As a result, actual spending growth increased.

Combined, these changes would have resulted in a negative update in 2002. According to CMS, the update in 2002 would have been –3.8% based on these factors alone. In addition, CMS discovered it had undercounted actual SGR spending beginning in 1998. In all, actual spending was undercounted by $4.5 billion for 1998 through 2000, or roughly 3% of SGR spending over this period. Correcting this error further reduced the 2002 CF update to –5.4% and assured that another CF cut would be forthcoming in 2003.

Congress Acts on the 2003 Update . . .

In its December 31, 2002, Final Rule on the physician payment schedule, CMS announced that a 4.4% cut to the Medicare CF would take effect March 1, 2003. CMS also estimated that spending for SGR services for the period April 1, 1996, through December 31, 2002, exceeded the allowed or budgeted amount by $16.5 billion, an amount equal to roughly one-fourth of allowed spending for 2002. Barring any legislative or administrative action to correct this problem, the SGR "deficit" could easily have reached $20 billion through 2003. Another 4% to 5% pay cut in 2004 was a near certainty, and cuts would likely have extended out several years.

However, on February 13, 2003, after intense lobbying by the AMA and state and specialty societies, and with support from CMS, Congress passed an appropriations package (H. J. Res. 2) that included language authorizing CMS to correct the FY 1998 and 1999 SGR projection errors. Two weeks later, in a revised rule, CMS made the corrections to the targets. The fiscal 1998 target was increased from 1.5% to 3.2%, and the fiscal 1999 target was increased from –0.3% to 4.2%. As a result, the $16.5 billion shortfall in SGR funding through 2002 was eliminated (wiping out the huge "deficit" in the system) and allowed spending for SGR services was increased by 6.5% for 2003 and every subsequent year. With these changes, the 4.4% pay cut scheduled to go into effect March 1, 2003, was replaced with a 1.6% increase.

. . . but Deficits Quickly Return

Although the correction of the FY 1998 and FY 1999 projection errors had an estimated cost to the federal government of some $54 billion over 10 years and successfully reversed a Medicare pay cut in 2003, it did not eliminate the potential for future cuts. The bill restored money to the SGR budget, but it did not change the structure of a system with the potential to produce cuts in pay if GDP growth is slow or utilization growth for SGR services is high.

Both trends continued in 2002 and 2003. Real per capita GDP growth totaled less than 3% for 2001 through 2003 combined, averaging less than 1% annual growth. Utilization growth for Medicare physician payment schedule services accelerated from 2% to 3% per year in the late 1990s to roughly 5% in 2001 and 6% in 2002. Utilization of drugs, included in SGR spending, grew even faster. Medicare allowed charges for such drugs increased from $1.8 billion in 1996 to $8.6 billion in 2004, an average annual increase of 22%.

The combined effect of below-average growth in GDP and accelerating utilization growth for SGR services led to a quick return of an SGR deficit, projected in the fall of 2003 to total some $6 billion for CY 2003 alone. As a result, CMS announced in the November 7, 2003, final rule on the 2004 physician payment schedule that the 2004 update would be –4.5%.

. . . Cuts for 2004–2006 Are Blocked (Temporarily)

Congress blocked the 4.5% cut slated for 2004 and another likely cut in 2005 with a provision in the Medicare Prescription Drug, Improvement, and Modernization Act (MMA) that was enacted late in 2003. The provision replaced these cuts with updates of 1.5% for 2004 and 2005. The MMA also changed the real per capita GDP component of the SGR target from a single-year estimate to a 10-year moving average starting with the CY 2003 target.

Pay updates would have reverted to the SGR formula in 2006, with a resulting 4.4% cut, but Congress acted again, freezing the conversion factor at the 2005 level with a provision in the Deficit Reduction Act (DRA) of 2005. Although MMA and DRA prevented a steep decline in Medicare physician pay, no money was added to the SGR budget to accommodate the resulting increases in spending. The SGR provision of the MMA increased Medicare physician pay for 2004 alone by 6% (a 1.5% pay increase instead of a 4.5% pay cut), but no funds were added to the SGR budget for that provision. As a result, the SGR deficit ballooned, reaching $41 billion through 2006, or more than half of the $81.3 billion SGR budget for that year.

CMS announced a 5% CF cut for 2007 in its final rule for the 2007 physician payment schedule. This was the first of many predicted by CMS actuaries at that time. Medicare physician pay cuts of roughly 5% per year were projected out to at least 2015. The cuts were spread out due to the –7% limit on the performance adjustment.

These cuts were, in part, a consequence of not increasing the SGR budget to accommodate the 2004–2006 pay fixes. This approach kept the net federal cost of these provisions to a minimum. Given enough time, the SGR system will reclaim any unfunded increase in spending with future pay cuts. Funding the SGR pay fixes for 2004–2006 would have been expensive. In 2005, the Congressional Budget Office estimated that retroactively funding the 2004 and 2005 fixes would have cost $46 billion over 10 years. However, while less expensive in the short term, this approach of borrowing from future SGR budgets to fund current pay fixes greatly inflated the cost of subsequent attempts to block SGR cuts.

Temporary Fixes 2007–2015

Just prior to adjourning in December 2006, the 109th Congress passed HR 6111, which again included a stop gap measure to prevent the scheduled 5% CF cut for 2007. The bill again set the Medicare CF update at 0.0% for 2007, which froze the CF at the 2005 value of $37.8975. Cost was a major factor in the design of this provision, which differed in two important ways from the MMA and DRA update provisions.

First, unlike MMA and DRA, the Tax Relief and Health Care Act (TRHCA) of 2006 allowed funds to be added to the SGR budget for 2007 to accommodate the extra spending that occurred with a CF freeze instead of a 5% cut. According to the Congressional Budget Office, this would have increased net federal spending on Medicare by $11 billion over five years and $27 billion over 10, if not for the second unique feature of the TRHCA. Under the bill, the 2008 Medicare CF update was to start from the 2007 CF that would have been in place if not for the bill. That is, the 2008 CF update was to include both the 5% cut that would have occurred in 2007 and the 5.3% SGR cut for 2008, resulting in an actual CF cut for 2008 of 10.1%. This reduced the federal cost of this provision to roughly $3 billion over 10 years and did not increase the SGR deficit but, of course, greatly raised the stakes on fixing the 2008 CF update.

The 10.1% cut scheduled for January 1, 2008, was again postponed by a provision in the Medicare, Medicaid, and SCHIP Extension Act of 2007. This bill, passed in December 2007, replaced the cut with a 0.5% increase in the conversion factor for the first six months of 2008. However, the temporary nature of the fix would have resulted in a 10.6% cut on July 1, 2008, without further action. Congress did act, though, in July of 2008 to retroactively block the 10.6% cut and to further set the 2009 update at 1.1% with the Medicare Improvements for Patients and Providers Act (MIPPA) of 2008. The cuts were only postponed to 2010, though. Like the previous two fixes, the MIPPA rolled the cuts that would have occurred together in the subsequent update. Combining now four years of cuts (2007–2010), the January 1, 2010, SGR cut would have been 21.2%. Moreover, the Medicare actuaries projected additional cuts for 2011 through 2014 that would have put 2014 Medicare physician pay a further 20% below the 2010 level. Table 10-3 provides a summary of the SGR cuts that have been scheduled since 2002.

With cuts of this magnitude, the cost of SGR reform grew to substantial proportions. In April 2010, the Congressional Budget Office (CBO) estimated that to keep Medicare physician pay in line with medical-practice inflation would cost more than $330 billion over 10 years. CMS provided some relief in 2010 by proposing to remove drugs from their definition of allowed and actual SGR spending. CMS further decided to make this change effective for all years since the inception of SGR. Drugs accounted for about 4% of SGR allowed spending for any given year but accounted for as much as 10% of actual spending. As a result, this change greatly reduced the gap between target and actual spending in the SGR system. Before this change, the cumulative SGR deficit through 2009 was $72 billion, or more than 75% of allowed spending for 2009. With drugs removed, the cumulative SGR deficit through 2009 was $19 billion. This change fell short of affecting the huge cut for 2010 but reduced both the magnitude of SGR cuts under current law after 2010, and the cost of SGR reform.

The 21.2% cut for 2010 was blocked by months at a time. First, the Department of Defense Appropriations Act, the Temporary Extension Act, and the Continuing Extension Act froze pay at the 2009 level through May 31. Then, the Preservation of Access to Care for Medicare Beneficiaries and Pension Relief Act increased pay by 2.2% for June through November. Physicians were then facing a 23% cut December 1, 2010. This was blocked for one month by the Physician Payment and Therapy Relief Act of 2010, and physicians were facing a 25% cut on January 1, 2011 (the combination of the 23% that was postponed from December 1, and a further 2.5% cut scheduled for January 1, 2011). This in turn was blocked by the Medicare

Table 10-3. Dealing with SGR Cuts Since 2002

Date of Cut	Scheduled Cut	Replaced with	Legislation
Jan 1, 2002	5.4%		Not blocked
Mar 1, 2003	4.4%	1.6%	Consolidated Appropriations Resolution
Jan 1, 2004	4.5%	1.5%	Medicare Prescription Drug, Improvement, and Modernization Act (also set 2005 update of 1.5%)
Jan 1, 2006	4.4%	0.0%	Deficit Reduction Act
Jan 1, 2007	5.0%	0.0%	Tax Relief and Health Care Act
Jan 1, 2008	10.1%	0.5%	Medicare, Medicaid, and SCHIP Extension Act
Jul 1, 2008	10.6%	0.0%	Medicare Improvements for Patients and Providers Act (also set 2009 update of 1.1%)
Jan 1, 2010	21.2%	0.0%	Department of Defense Appropriations Act
Mar 1, 2010	21.2%	0.0%	Temporary Extension Act
Apr 1, 2010	21.2%	0.0%	Continuing Extension Act
Jun 1, 2010	21.2%	2.2%	Preservation of Access to Care for Medicare Beneficiaries and Pension Relief Act
Dec 1, 2010	23.0%	0.0%	Physician Payment and Therapy Relief Act
Jan 1, 2011	24.9%	0.0%	Medicare and Medicaid Extenders Act
Jan 1, 2012	27.4%	0.0%	Temporary Payroll Tax Cut Continuation Act of 2011
Mar 1, 2012	27.4%	0.0%	Middle Class Tax Relief and Job Creation Act of 2012
Jan 1, 2013	26.5%	0.0%	American Taxpayer Relief Act of 2012
Jan 1, 2014	23.7%	0.5%	Pathway for SGR Reform Act of 2013
Apr 1, 2014	24.1%	0.0%	Protecting Access to Medicare Act of 2014
Jul 1, 2015	21.2%	0.5%	Medicare Access and CHIP Reauthorization Act (MACRA) of 2015

and Medicaid Extenders Act of 2010, with the provision extending for the whole of 2011. Like the others, this bill only postponed the cut until January 1, 2012.

On December 23, 2011, President Obama signed the Temporary Payroll Tax Cut Continuation Act of 2011 into law, which in part provided for an additional two-month reprieve from the conversion factor cut, expiring after February 29, 2012. The cut was further postponed by the Middle Class Tax Relief and Job Creation Act of 2012, which provided a 0% update through December 31, 2012. A 26.5% cut would have taken effect on January 1, 2013. This cut was postponed for another year under the American Taxpayer Relief Act, which was signed into law just after this cut was scheduled to take effect. This once again set the update for 2013 at 0%.

In 2013, some positive news in the effort to do away with the SGR presented themselves. In response to the exceptionally low rates of growth in Medicare physician spending in recent years, the CBO cut its cost estimate for replacing SGR. The 10-year cost of replacing SGR updates with annual pay freezes, which stood at nearly $300 billion in 2011, fell from $244 billion in November 2012 to $117 billion as of December 2013 (it has since edged up somewhat). In 2013, both the Senate Finance and House Ways and Means committees overwhelmingly approved SGR repeal legislation. This repeal effort fell short, however, and a 3-month patch was implemented with the Pathway for SGR Reform Act of 2013, which included a 0.5% update.

Providers faced a 24.1% cut on April 1, 2014, but this was blocked for a year with another temporary fix in the Protecting Access to Medicare Act of 2014. In 2015, MACRA permanently eliminated the SGR and replaced it with fixed updates of 0.5%, which started on July 1, 2015, lasting through 2019.

Budget Neutrality and Other Adjustments

The OBRA 89 specified that changes in RVUs resulting from changes in medical practice, coding, new data, or addition of new services may not cause Part B expenditures to differ by more than $20 million from the spending level which would occur in the absence of these adjustments. To limit the increase in Medicare expenditures as mandated by the statute, CMS over the years has applied various adjustments to the payment schedule to ensure budget neutrality as evidenced in Table 10-4. For the 1993–1995 payment schedules, CMS achieved budget neutrality by uniformly reducing all RVUs across all services. The RVUs were reduced by 2.8% in 1993; 1.3% in 1994; and 1.1% in 1995. The AMA strongly objected to using the RVUs as a mechanism to preserve budget neutrality. Such annual budget-neutrality adjustments may cause confusion among physician practices and non-Medicare payers that adopt the resource-based relative value scale (RBRVS) payment system.

Since 1996, CMS has generally applied budget-neutrality adjustments to the conversion factor(s) rather than across RVUs. There have been exceptions, however. When the first Five-Year Review was implemented in 1997, CMS made two types of budget-neutrality adjustments. In addition to reducing the conversion factors by 1.5%, CMS made an across-the-board adjustment (8.3% reduction) to the physician work RVUs.

In 1999, CMS eliminated the work adjustor and applied this budget-neutrality adjustment directly to the CF. To ensure that the adjustment only applied to the work relative values, CMS then increased the practice expense and PLI RVUs by the same amount. As a result, there was a significant decline in the Medicare CF for 1999, but this decline was more than offset by the elimination of the work adjustor and increases in the practice expense and PLI RVUs. Overall, Medicare pay actually increased in 1999.

For the third Five-Year Review in 2007, CMS returned to the approach used with the first Five-Year Review, creating a separate work RVU adjustor of 10.1%. Despite strong objections from the AMA, this adjustment was not applied to the CF. In 2008, CMS continued to utilize the separate work adjustor, which increased to 11.94%. However, in 2009, the work adjustor was again eliminated with an offsetting reduction to the conversion factor of 6.4% under a provision in the Medicare Improvements for Patients and Providers Act of 2008. Again, despite the reduction in the CF, Medicare pay actually increased in 2009.

CMS has also adjusted the CF when rescaling the work, practice expense, and PLI RVU pools to match the weights in the MEI. The weights for the 2011 MEI were reduced for physician work and increased for practice expense and PLI. To make the RVU totals consistent with the MEI, CMS increased the practice expense RVUs across-the-board by 18% and the PLI RVUs by 36%, with an offsetting 8.2% reduction in the Medicare CF. This change was budget neutral overall, despite the reduction in the CF. The 2014 conversion factor update included a 4.7% budget-neutrality increase to offset decreases to the practice expense and PLI RVUs resulting from the rescaling of the RVU pools to match the revised 2014 MEI weights.

The 2022 Conversion Factor (CF) Update

On November 2, 2021, the Centers for Medicare & Medicaid Services (CMS) released the Final Rule for the calendar year (CY) 2022 Medicare Physician Payment Schedule (MFS). For 2022, the Medicare conversion factor (CF) will be reduced by approximately 0.8% from 34.8931 in 2021 to 34.6062. This reduction is due to the maintenance of a temporary 3.75% increase to the CF at a reduced 3%, stemming from Congressional action to temporarily avert a more significant cut for another year, as well as a budget-neutrality adjustment of – 0.10%.

The American Medical Association (AMA) strongly advocated for Congress to extend the 3.75% increase for CY 2022 as physician practices faced Medicare cuts amounting to a 9.71% overall decrease effective January 1, 2022, when factoring in sequestration reductions. Recognizing that these Medicare cuts would further compound the growing financial instability of physician practices due to the significant reduction in revenue caused by the continued severe acute respiratory syndrome coronavirus 2 (SARS-CoV-2) (coronavirus disease 2019 [COVID-19]) public health emergency (PHE), the cuts were diverted when President Biden signed S.610, Protecting Medicare and American Farmers from Sequester Cuts Act, into law on December 10, 2021. This law results in the following:

- A delay in resuming the 2% Medicare sequester for three months (January 1–March 31, 2022), followed by a reduction to 1% for three months (April 1–June 30, 2022).
- A 1-year increase in the MFS of 3% (0.75% less than the CF boost provided for 2021).
- A 1-year delay in the cuts to the clinical laboratory fee schedule.
- A 1-year delay in the Medicare radiation oncology demonstration.

In addition, the law will erase the 4% Medicare Pay-As-You-Go (PAYGO) cut and prevent any additional PAYGO cuts through 2022.

Effective January 1, 2022, the anesthesia CF is $21.5623 which reflects the same overall MFS adjustments with the addition of anesthesia-specific practice expense (PE) and malpractice (MP) adjustments.

Table 10-4. History of Medicare Conversion Factor(s)

Year	Conversion Factor	% Change	Primary Care Conversion Factor	% Change	Surgical Conversion Factor	% Change	Other Nonsurgical Conversion Factor	% Change
1992	$31.0010		N/A		N/A		N/A	
1993	N/A				$31.9620		$31.2490	
1994	**N/A**		**$33.7180**		**$35.1580**	**10.0**	**$32.9050**	**5.3**
1995	N/A		$36.3820	7.9	$39.4470	12.2	$34.6160	5.2
1996	N/A		$35.4173	–2.7	$40.7986	3.4	$34.6293	0.0
1997	N/A		$35.7671	1.0	$40.9603	0.4	$33.8454	–2.3
1998	$36.6873							
1999	$34.7315	–5.3						
2000	$36.6137	5.4						
2001	$38.2581	4.5						
2002	$36.1992	–5.4						
2003	$36.7856	1.6						
2004	$37.3374	1.5						
2005	$37.8975	1.5						
2006	$37.8975	0.0						
2007	$37.8975	0.0						
2008	$38.0870	0.5						
2009	$36.0666	–5.3						
1/1/10–5/31/10	$36.0791	0.03						
6/1/10–12/31/10	$36.8729	2.2						
2011	$33.9764	–7.9						
2012	$34.0376	0.18						
2013	$34.0230	–0.04						
2014	$35.8228	5.3						
1/1/15–6/30/15	$35.7547	–0.19						
7/1/15–12/31/15	$35.9335	0.50						
2016	$35.8043	–0.36						
2017	$35.8887	0.24						
2018	$35.9996	0.31						
2019	$36.0391	0.11						
2020	$36.0896	0.14						
2021	$34.8931	–3.3						
2022	$34.6062	–0.8						

Initially, the Medicare Physician Payment Schedule included distinct conversion factors for various categories of services. In 1998, a single conversion factor was implemented. The reduction in the 1999 conversion factor was offset by elimination of the work adjustor from the first Five-Year Review and increases in the practice expense and PLI RVUs. The reduction in the 2009 conversion factor was offset by elimination of the work adjustor from the third Five-Year Review. The reduction in the 2011 conversion factor was offset by increases to the practice expense and PLI RVUs resulting from the rescaling of those RVU pools to match the revised MEI weights. The 2014 conversion factor update included a budget-neutrality increase to offset decreases to the practice expense and PLI RVUs, which resulted from the rescaling of the RVU pools to match the revised MEI weights. For a number of years, the conversion factor was minimally changed to reflect budget neutrality. In 2021, the budget-neutrality reduction was more significant to reflect the increases in valuation of the office visit codes.

Chapter 11

Standardizing Medicare Part B: RBRVS Payment Rules and Policies

The resource-based relative value scale (RBRVS) payment system required the development of national payment policies and their uniform implementation by the Medicare carriers. As Chapter 2 described, under customary, prevailing, and reasonable payment (CPR), each Medicare carrier established its own policies, including issues such as which services were included in the payment for a surgical procedure. As with the elimination of specialty differentials and customary charges, there was no transition period for standardizing carrier payment policies under the RBRVS payment system. Standardization of payment policies became effective January 1, 1992. This revised edition of *The Physicians' Guide* reflects the Centers for Medicare & Medicaid Services' (CMS') clarifications and new policies issued since implementation, as well as new policies published in the November 2, 2021, Final Rule and effective for services provided January 1, 2022.

One of the most significant standardization provisions included in the Omnibus Budget Reconciliation Act of 1989 (OBRA 89) was the requirement that CMS adopt a uniform coding system for Medicare. In the June 1991 *Notice of Proposed Rulemaking (NPRM)*, CMS stated that the American Medical Association's (AMA's) *Current Procedural Terminology* (CPT®) would serve as that uniform system. The CPT 2022 code set includes more than 10,000 codes to describe physicians' services, including codes for evaluation and management (E/M), which originally became effective January 1, 1992. These codes are used to describe visit and consultation services and were developed for use under Medicare's RBRVS-based payment system. They are described briefly in this chapter.

The CPT code set is maintained and updated annually by the AMA's CPT Editorial Panel. To ensure that the CPT code set appropriately reflects the services provided by the broader spectrum of physician specialties, the CPT Advisory Committee assists the Editorial Panel in reviewing proposals for changes in codes and the addition of new codes. Currently, the Advisory Committee is limited to national medical specialty societies seated in the AMA House of Delegates and the AMA Health Care Professionals Advisory Committee (HCPAC), organizations representing limited-license practitioners and other allied health professionals.

In addition to the five-digit CPT codes, CMS recognizes other alphanumeric codes for some nonphysician services and supplier services, such as ambulances. Together, the CPT codes and the alphanumeric codes comprise the Healthcare Common Procedural Coding System (HCPCS).

As outlined in Chapter 3, besides coding, CMS also established a multitude of national policies as part of the revisions to the payment system, including uniform national policies on payment for the following:

- Global surgical packages
- Assistants-at-surgery
- "Incident-to" services
- Supplies and drugs
- Technical component–only services
- Diagnostic tests
- Nonphysicians' services
- Several other aspects of Medicare Part B

When reviewing this chapter, it is important for physicians to understand that the carriers are required to implement these policies in a uniform manner nationally. Carriers do not have an option to develop a different policy for their local area.

Defining a Global Surgical Package: Major Surgical Procedures

A global surgical package for major surgical procedures refers to a payment policy of bundling payment for the various services associated with an operation into a single payment covering the operation and these other services, such as postoperative hospital visits. It is common practice among surgeons to bill for such global surgical packages, which generally include the immediate preoperative care, the operation itself, and the normal, uncomplicated follow-up care. Under the CPR payment system, Medicare carriers were allowed wide latitude in establishing a global package, resulting in global surgery policies that varied from carrier to carrier and from service to service. (For a more detailed discussion of CPR, refer to Chapter l.) For example, about half of the carriers included preoperative care in their global surgery packages. In addition, carrier policies for the number of days included in postoperative care differed widely, from 0 to 270 days after surgery.

Revising Medicare's physician payment system required a nationally standardized definition of what constitutes the preoperative and postoperative time periods, as well as the specific services included in these periods. In the 1991 Final Rule, CMS identified specific services included in the global surgical package when provided by the physician who performs the surgery: preoperative visits the day before the surgery; intraoperative services that are normally a usual and necessary part of a surgical procedure; services provided by the surgeon within 90 days of the surgery that do not require a return trip to the operating room and follow-up visits provided during this time by the surgeon that are related to recovery from the surgery; and postsurgical pain management.

Each component of CMS' global surgical policy—evaluation or consultation, preoperative visits by the surgeon, intraoperative services, and postoperative period—is discussed below in further detail. Following the summary of the global surgery package is a discussion on using six coding modifiers (24, 25, 57, 58, 78, and 79) the CPT Editorial Panel established in 1992 and 1993, which CMS has adopted for payment purposes. These modifiers identify a service or procedure furnished during the global period that is not a usual part of the global surgical package and for which separate payment may be made. Also covered in this chapter in the section on modifiers are definitions for multiple procedures (51) and for physicians or other qualified health care professionals furnishing less than the full global package (54, 55, 56). Physician work relative value units (RVUs) for surgical services were generally based on the Harvard RBRVS study, which included the following:

- Preoperative visits on the day before surgery or the day of surgery
- The hospital admission workup
- The primary operation
- Immediate postoperative care, including dictating operative notes, talking with the family and other physicians
- Writing orders
- Evaluating the patient in the recovery room
- Postoperative follow-up on the day of surgery
- Postoperative hospital and office visits

Initial Evaluation or Consultation by the Surgeon

The surgeon's initial evaluation or consultation is considered a separate service from the surgery and is paid as a distinct service, even if the decision, based on the evaluation, is not to perform the surgery. Previously, some carriers bundled the initial evaluation or consultation into the global surgery payment if it occurred within the week prior to the surgery and, in some cases, even within 24 hours of surgery. If the decision to perform a major surgery (surgical procedures with a 090-day global period) is made on the day of or the day prior to the surgery, separate payment is allowed for the visit at which the decision is made if adequate documentation is submitted with the claim demonstrating that the decision for surgery was made during a specific visit. Modifier 57, *Decision for Surgery*, is used to indicate that an evaluation and management (E/M) service resulted in the initial decision to perform the surgery.

Preoperative Visits by the Surgeon

In the 1991 Final Rule, CMS adopted a preoperative period that included any visits by the surgeon, in or out of the hospital. For major procedures (090-day global), this includes preoperative visits before the day of surgery. For minor procedures (000- or 010-day global), this includes preoperative visits on the day of the surgery. It is important to note that CMS emphasized that preoperative billings are carefully monitored as part of carrier postpayment medical-necessity review, and a longer preoperative period may be adopted later.

Intraoperative Services

All intraoperative services that are normally included as a necessary part of a surgical procedure are included in the global package.

Complications Following Surgery

If a patient develops complications following surgery that require additional medical or surgical services, but do not require a return trip to the operating room (OR) (eg, a stitch pop), Medicare will include these services in the approved amount for the global surgery with no separate payment made. However, if the complications require the patient's return to the OR for care determined to be medically necessary, these services are paid separately from the global surgery amount. Modifier 78 is reported in this instance.

CMS defines *OR* as a:

Place of service specifically equipped and staffed for the sole purpose of performing procedures. The term includes a cardiac catheterization suite, a laser suite, and an endoscopy suite. It does not include a patient room, a minor treatment room, a recovery room, or an intensive care unit (unless the patient's condition was so critical there would be insufficient time for transportation to an OR).

Separate payment is allowed for treatment of complications requiring expertise beyond that of the surgeon. Full payment will be made to the physician who provides such treatment.

In addition, separate payment is allowed for the following tests when performed during the global period of a major surgery: visual field (92081-92083), fundus photography (92250), and fluorescein angiography (92235).

Postoperative Services by the Surgeon

Currently, the global period may include 0, 10, or 90 days of postoperative care, depending on the procedure.

Postoperative services specifically identified by CMS as part of the global package and not separately payable include:

- Dressing changes
- Local incisional care
- Removal of operative packs; removal of cutaneous sutures, staples, lines, wires, tubes, drains, casts, and splints
- Insertion, irrigation, and removal of urinary catheters
- Routine peripheral intravenous lines and nasogastric and rectal tubes
- Change and removal of tracheostomy tubes

Services that are unrelated to the diagnosis for which the surgery was performed are excluded from the global surgical payment. These services are separately paid by appending modifier 24 to the appropriate level of E/M service and submitting the appropriate documentation.

Services provided by the surgeon for the treatment of underlying conditions and for a subsequent course of treatment, which is not part of the normal surgery recovery period, are also paid separately. CMS provides an example of a urologist who performs surgery for prostate cancer and subsequently administers chemotherapy services. The chemotherapy services would not be part of the global surgery package. When reporting these circumstances, modifier 79 should be included.

Full payment for the procedure (not just the intraoperative services) is allowed for situations when distinctly separate but related procedures are performed during the global period of another surgery (eg, reconstructive and burn surgery) in which the patient is admitted to the hospital for treatment, discharged, and then readmitted for further treatment. When the decision is made prospectively or at the time of the first surgery to perform a second procedure (ie, to stage a procedure), modifier 58 *Staged or Related Procedure or Service by the Same Physician or Other Qualified Health Care Professional During the Postoperative Period*, should be reported.

When postoperative care following surgery is provided by a nonsurgeon for an underlying condition or medical complication, it is reported and will be considered as concurrent care and should be reported using the appropriate E/M code. The nonsurgeon should not append modifier 55 when reporting such services.

To determine if a procedure is part of a global package, refer to the List of Relative Value Units in Part 5 of this book. The column titled, "Global Period" indicates the appropriate global period (eg, 000) or one of the following alpha codes:

MMM	=	A service furnished in uncomplicated maternity cases including antepartum care, delivery, and postpartum care. The usual global surgical concept does not apply.
XXX	=	Global concept does not apply.
YYY	=	Global period is to be set by the carrier (eg, unlisted surgery code).
ZZZ	=	Code related to another service and is always included in the global period of the other service. (Note: Physician work is associated with intra-service time and in some instances the pre- and post-service time.)

Postoperative Pain Management

Payment for physician services related to patient-controlled analgesia is included in the surgeon's global payment. Pain management by continuous epidural is paid by reporting CPT code 62326 on the first day of service. This code includes the catheter and injection of the anesthetic substance. Payment will be allowed for CPT code 01996 for daily management of the epidural drug administration after the day on which the catheter was introduced. The global surgical payment will be reduced, if post-payment audits indicate that a surgeon's patients routinely receive pain management services from an anesthesiologist.

Duration of the Global Surgical Period

Currently, the preoperative period for major surgeries is the day immediately prior to the day of surgery, and the postoperative period is 90 days immediately following the day of surgery. Services provided on the day of surgery but before the surgery are considered preoperative, while services furnished on the same day but after the surgery are considered postoperative.

Rebundling of CPT-4 Codes

CMS implemented the first phase of a new correct coding initiative (CCI) January 1, 1996, with the stated goal to reduce program expenditures by detecting inappropriate coding on Medicare claims and denying payment for them. Code edits detect *unbundling* or reporting a CPT code for each component of a service rather than a single, comprehensive code for all services provided.

The coding matrix enables carriers to identify unbundled codes billed with a more comprehensive procedure code and "mutually exclusive" coding combinations. According to CMS, this CCI improves the carriers' ability to detect inappropriate billing code combinations, such as a comprehensive code with component code combinations and coding combinations that would not be performed at the same time. The bundling initiative seeks to eliminate carrier-specific interpretations of CMS' bundling policy.

The AMA and a number of medical specialty societies expressed concerns to CMS that the proposed coding edits contained many errors, and that implementation should be delayed until revisions were made. In response to these requests, CMS removed some edits and adopted other edit changes. CMS moved forward with the project, however, because of strong pressure from members of Congress to adopt more restrictive coding practices similar to coding rules that had been implemented by the private sector.

In response to widespread criticism about the coding edits, the AMA formed the Correct Coding Policy Committee (CCPC) to establish a process that would allow organized medicine to formally provide input to CMS on proposed code edits. The CCPC worked with specialty societies to evaluate proposed code edits and submit recommendations to CMS for revisions to improve appropriateness of the edits. In response to CCPC recommendations, CMS dropped or revised many proposed edits.

Medically Unlikely Edits

In early 2006, CMS announced that it would initiate a project called medically unlikely edits (MUEs). The purpose of the MUE project is to detect and deny Medicare claims on a prepayment basis to stop inappropriate payments in an effort to improve the accuracy of Medicare payments. According to CMS, the coding edits proposed prevent billing for items that are either (1) anatomically impossible (eg, more than one appendix cannot be removed), or (2) medically unreasonable (eg, implanting more than one pacemaker).

CMS indicated in mid-March 2006 that it planned to delay implementation of the MUE initiative until at least January 1, 2007, to allow the agency to revise the current proposal and re-release it for comment. This delay in implementation was an important win for the AMA and the physician community, which lobbied hard for the withdrawal of the MUE project. MUE implemented on January 1, 2007, consists of edits based on anatomic considerations that are determined by limitations based on anatomic structures. For example, the MUE for cataract surgical procedures would be two since there are two eyes. Phase II was implemented April 1, 2007, and included edits based on anatomic considerations, CPT code descriptors or coding instructions, CMS policies, nature of the procedure or service, nature of analyte, or nature or equipment. Future phases will be based on criteria other than claims data analysis.

In the Policy Narrative from the CCI Edits published October 1, 2007, CMS recognized modifiers in the MUE project and created an appeal process at the carrier level, if a unit of service is denied based on an MUE. As with National Correct Coding Initiative (NCCI) edits, proposed MUEs are sent to the AMA for distribution to the national medical specialty societies for review and comment.

Minor Surgery and Nonincisional Procedures (Endoscopies)

In 1992, a major revision was made in Medicare payment policy for endoscopic procedures and other minor surgeries for which global packages have generally not been established. No payment will be made for a visit on the same day a minor surgical or endoscopic procedure is performed, unless a separate, identifiable service is also provided. CMS provides the following example:

Payment for a visit would be allowed in addition to payment for suturing a scalp wound if, in addition, a full neurological exam is made for a patient with head trauma. If the physician only identified the need for sutures and confirmed allergy and immunization status, billing for a visit would not be appropriate.

Payment for the visit will be made by including modifier 25, when a separate, identifiable E/M service is provided. The carrier may contact those who bill extensively for visits on the same day as a minor surgery or endoscopy to request documentation for their billings.

There is no postoperative period for endoscopies performed through an existing body orifice. Endoscopic surgical procedures that require an incision for insertion of a scope will be covered under the appropriate major or minor surgical policy.

Currently, minor surgeries will include a postoperative period of either 0 or 10 days. For procedures with a 010-day global period, the global payment includes all postoperative services related to recovery from the surgery. Payment for unrelated E/M services provided during this time is allowed when billed with modifier 24. To determine the global period for a minor surgery, refer to the "Global Period" column included in the List of Relative Value Units in Part 5 of this book.

Multiple Endoscopic Procedures

Special rules apply to multiple endoscopic procedures and to some dermatologic procedures. In the case of multiple endoscopic procedures, the full value of the higher valued endoscopy will be recognized, plus the difference between the next highest endoscopy and the base endoscopy. CMS provides the following example:

In the course of performing a fiber optic colonoscopy (CPT code 45378), a physician performs a biopsy on a lesion (code 45380) and removes a polyp (code 45385) from a different part of the colon. The physician bills for codes 45380 and 45385. The value of code 45380 and code 45385 both have the value of the diagnostic colonoscopy (45378) built in. Rather than paying 100% for the highest valued procedure (45385) and 50% for the next (45380), the carrier pays the full value of the higher valued endoscopy (45385) plus the difference between the next highest endoscopy (45380) and the base endoscopy (45378).

In situations when two series of endoscopies are performed, the special endoscopy rules are applied to each series, followed by the multiple surgery rules of 100% and 50%. In the case of two unrelated endoscopic procedures (eg, 46606 and 43217), the usual multiple surgery rules apply. When two related endoscopies and a third unrelated endoscopy (eg, 43215, 43217, and 45305) are performed in the same operative session, the special endoscopic rules apply only to the related endoscopies. To determine payment for the unrelated endoscopy, the multiple surgery rules are applied. The total payments for the related endoscopies are considered one service and the unrelated endoscopy as another service.

For some dermatology services, the CPT descriptors contain language, such as "additional lesion," to indicate that multiple surgical procedures have been performed (eg, code 11201). The multiple procedures rules do not apply because the RVUs for these codes have been adjusted to reflect the multiple nature of the procedure. These services are paid according to the unit. A 50% reduction in value for the second procedure applies to dermatologic codes in the following series: 11400, 11600, 17260, 17270, 17280. If dermatologic procedures are billed with other procedures, the multiple surgery rules apply.

Moderate (Conscious) Sedation Services

Before CPT 2016, the CPT manual identified more than 400 diagnostic and therapeutic procedures, formerly listed in Appendix G of the CPT codebook, for which the CPT Editorial Panel had determined that moderate sedation is an inherent part of providing the procedure. The AMA/Specialty Society Relative Value Scale (RVS) Update Committee (RUC) and CMS previously bundled the relative resources associated with moderate sedation when valuing these procedures. Therefore, providers only reported the procedure code when furnishing a service that was listed in CPT Appendix G.

In the CY 2016 Medicare MFS proposed rule, CMS noted their understanding that practice patterns for endoscopic procedures, which made up a significant proportion of the Appendix G procedural codes, were changing. CMS observed that anesthesia was increasingly being separately reported for these procedures, indicating that the relative resources associated with sedation were no longer incurred by the practitioner reporting the Appendix G procedure. In response, the CPT Editorial Panel created CPT codes for separately reporting moderate sedation services in association with the elimination of Appendix G from the CPT codebook for CY 2017. In the CY 2016 MFS final rule, CMS finalized a proposal to unbundle moderate sedation services from all codes listed in Appendix G starting January 1, 2017. For the CY 2017 MFS final rule, CMS separately finalized a proposal to create a G code to separately report the first 15 minutes of moderate sedation for certain gastrointestinal endoscopic services.

The moderate sedation CPT codes and G code are as follows:

⊘ **99151** Moderate sedation services provided by the same physician or other qualified health care professional performing the diagnostic or therapeutic service that the sedation supports, requiring the presence of an independent trained observer to assist in the monitoring of the patient's level of consciousness and physiological status; initial 15 minutes of intraservice time, patient younger than 5 years of age

⊘ **99152** initial 15 minutes of intraservice time, patient age 5 years or older

+99153 each additional 15 minutes intraservice time (List separately in addition to code for primary service)
(Use 99153 in conjunction with 99151, 99152)
(Do not report 99153 in conjunction with 99155, 99156)

99155 Moderate sedation services provided by a physician or other qualified health care professional other than the physician or other qualified health care professional performing the diagnostic or therapeutic service that the sedation supports; initial 15 minutes of intraservice time, patient younger than 5 years of age

99156 initial 15 minutes intraservice time, patient age 5 years or older

+99157 each additional 15 minutes intraservice time (List separately in addition to code for primary service)
(Use 99157 in conjunction with 99155, 99156)
(Do not report 99157 in conjunction with 99151, 99152)

G0500 Moderate sedation services provided by the same physician or other qualified health care professional performing a gastrointestinal endoscopic service that sedation supports, requiring the presence of an independent trained observer to assist in the monitoring of the patient's level of consciousness and physiological status; initial 15 minutes of intra-service time; patient age 5 years or older (additional time may be reported with 99153, as appropriate)

Payment to Assistants-at-Surgery

By law, payment for services of assistants-at-surgery is the lower of the actual charge or 16% of the payment schedule amount for the global surgical service. (Before 1991, the law limited payment for assistant-at-surgery services to 20% of the prevailing charge for the surgical service.) In addition, the law provides that payment for services of assistants-at-surgery may be made only when the most recent national Medicare claims data indicate that a procedure has used assistants-at-surgery in at least 5% of cases based on a national average percentage. To determine when payment for an assistant-at-surgery is not allowed, refer to the List of Relative Value Units in Part 5 of this book under the "Payment Policy Indicators" column. The notation "A" indicates that CMS does not allow payment for a surgical assistant; "A+" indicates that payment is allowed when documentation is provided to establish that a surgical assistant was medically necessary.

In its comments to CMS on the 1991 Final Rule, the AMA opposed the arbitrary limits set by Congress for authorizing services of an assistant-at-surgery and cautioned that quality considerations may demand using an assistant even when the data indicate that an assistant is rarely required.

CPT Modifiers

Modifiers for CPT procedure codes are used to describe special circumstances under which the basic service was provided. With implementation of the Medicare RBRVS, the use of modifiers was standardized to establish national payment policies. The following sections describe reporting of the CPT modifiers and Medicare payment policies. The instructional notes pertaining to reporting five-digit modifiers have been deleted from the CPT code set to coincide with CMS-1500 claim form reporting instructions, as this conflicted with the previous instructions included in the CPT code set regarding the use of a separate five-digit modifier. According to the National Uniform Claim Committee (NUCC), the electronic claim format for CMS-1500 claim form, in compliance with the regulations that apply to the Health Insurance Portability and Accountability Act (HIPAA), will not accommodate a five-digit modifier. The current field-length of the electronic format that holds a modifier is limited to two characters. The CMS-1500 claim form can capture up to four modifiers.

Refer to the *CPT 2022* codebook for additional details on modifiers and their proper use.

Modifier 22, Increased Procedural Services

Modifier 22 is used when the work required to provide a service is substantially greater than is typically required. Documentation must support the substantial additional work and the reason for the additional work (ie, increased intensity, time, technical difficulty of procedure, severity of patient's condition, physician and mental effort required). **Note:** This modifier should not be appended to an E/M service.

Carriers continue to have authority to increase payment for increased services (22), based on review of medical records and other documentation. Modifier 22 may be reported when services provided are greater than what is usually required for the listed procedure. For CPT 2008, modifier 22 was revised to clarify that it is intended to identify physician work, not practice expense, and that it should not be reported with an E/M service. Documentation of the unusual circumstances must accompany the claim (eg, a copy of the operative report and a separate statement written by the physician explaining the unusual amount of work required).

Modifier 23, Unusual Anesthesia

Occasionally, a procedure that usually requires either no anesthesia or local anesthesia must be done under general anesthesia because of unusual circumstances. This change in procedure may be reported by adding modifier 23.

Modifier 24, Unrelated E/M Service by the Same Physician or Other Qualified Health Care Professional During a Postoperative Period

Modifier 24 indicates that an E/M service was provided by the surgeon during the postoperative period for reasons unrelated to the original procedure. It is added to the appropriate level of E/M service.

This modifier is primarily intended for use by the surgeon. In most circumstances, subsequent hospital care (99231-99233) provided by the surgeon during the same hospitalization as the surgery will be considered by the carrier to be related to the surgery. Separate payment for such visits will not be made, even if reported with modifier 24, unless documentation is submitted demonstrating that the care is unrelated to the surgery. Two exceptions to this policy are for treatment provided for immunotherapy management furnished by the transplant surgeon and critical care for a burn or trauma patient. Modifier 24 should be reported in these situations and appropriate documentation submitted with the claim.

When a visit is provided in the outpatient setting, an ICD-10-CM code indicating why the encounter is unrelated to the surgery may be sufficient documentation if it is clear the service is unrelated. If the ICD-10-CM code does not make this clear, a brief narrative explanation is required. Carriers will review all claims submitted with modifier 24.

Modifier 25, Significant, Separately Identifiable E/M Service by the Same Physician or Other Qualified Health Care Professional on the Same Day of the Procedure or Other Service

Modifier 25 was revised to indicate that on the day a procedure or service was performed the patient's condition required a significant, separately identifiable E/M service above and beyond the other service provided or beyond the usual preoperative and postoperative care associated with the procedure that was performed.

This modifier was further modified in 2006 to clearly define a significant, separately identifiable evaluation and management service. According to the *CPT 2006* codebook, "A significant, separately identifiable E/M service is defined or substantiated by documentation that satisfies the relevant criteria for the respective E/M service to be reported."

For example, the revised modifier 25 can be used with the preventive medicine codes. When a significant problem is encountered while performing a preventive medicine E/M service, requiring additional work to perform the key components of the E/M service, the appropriate office outpatient code also should be reported for that service with modifier 25 appended. Modifier 25 allows separate payment for these visits without requiring documentation with the claim form.

Another example relates to a gastroenterologist who examines an established patient on Monday and schedules the patient for an endoscopy on Tuesday. In this case, only the endoscopy can be billed for the Tuesday encounter because that was the sole purpose of the encounter.

Modifier 26, Professional Component

This modifier describes procedures that are a combination of a physician or other qualified health care professional component and a technical component. When the physician or other qualified health care professional component is reported separately, the service may be identified by adding modifier 26 to the usual procedure number.

Modifier 32, Mandated Services

Services related to mandated consultation and/or related services (eg, third-party payer, governmental, legislative, or regulatory requirement) may be identified by adding modifier 32 to the basic procedure.

Modifier 33, Preventive Services

In response to the Affordable Care Act, which requires all health care insurance plans to begin to cover preventative services and immunization without cost sharing, modifier 33 was created to allow providers to indicate to payers that the service performed was preventative under applicable laws and that the patient cost-sharing does not apply. In other words, this modifier indicates to payers where it is appropriate to waive deductibles or co-insurance payments. The definition of modifier 33 was changed for the CPT 2013 to indicate:

When the primary purpose of the service is the delivery of an evidence-based service in accordance with a US Preventative

Services Task Force A or B rating in effect and other preventive services identified in preventive mandates (legislative or regulatory), the service may be identified by adding 33 to the procedure. For separately reported services specifically identified as preventative, the modifier should not be used.

Modifier 47, Anesthesia by Surgeon

The CPT definition states regional or general anesthesia provided by the surgeon may be reported by adding modifier 47 to the basic service. (This does not include local anesthesia.) **Note:** Modifier 47 would not be used as a modifier for the anesthesia procedures.

Modifier 50, Bilateral Procedure

The bilateral modifier is used to indicate cases in which a procedure that is normally performed on only one side of the body was performed on both sides of the body. Unless otherwise identified in the listings, bilateral procedures that are performed at the same session should be identified by adding modifier 50 to the appropriate 5 digit code. **Note:** This modifier should not be appended to designated "add-on" codes (see Appendix D of the codebook). When identical procedures are performed by two different physicians on opposite sides of the body or when bilateral procedures requiring two surgical teams working during the same session are performed, the following rules apply:

- The surgery is considered co-surgery (see modifier 62), if the CPT code designates the procedure as bilateral (eg, 27395). CMS payment rules allow 125% of the procedure's payment amount divided equally between the two surgeons.
- If the CPT code set does not designate the procedure as bilateral, CMS payment rules first calculate 150% of the payment amount for the procedure. Then, the co-surgery rule is applied: split 125% of that amount between the two surgeons.

Modifier 51, Multiple Procedures

The definition of modifier 51 was changed for CPT 2008 to indicate:

When multiple procedures, other than E/M services, Physical Medicine and Rehabilitation services, or provision of supplies (eg, vaccines) are performed at the same session by the same individual, the primary procedure or service may be reported as listed. The additional procedure(s) or services(s) may be identified by appending modifier 51 to the additional procedure or service code(s). ***Note:*** *This modifier should not be appended to designated "add-on" codes (see Appendix D [of the codebook]).*

Medicare payment policy is based on the lesser of the actual charge or 100% of the payment schedule for the procedure with the highest payment, while payment for the second through fifth surgical procedures is based on the lesser of the actual charge or 50% of the payment schedule. Surgical procedures beyond the fifth are priced by carriers on a "by-report" basis. The payment adjustment rules do not apply, if two or more surgeons of different specialties (eg, multiple trauma cases) each perform distinctly different surgeries on the same patient on the same day. CMS has clarified that payment adjustment rules for multiple surgery, cosurgery, and team surgery do not apply to trauma surgery situations when multiple physicians from different specialties provide different surgical procedures. Modifier 51 is used only if one of the same surgeons individually performs multiple surgeries.

Under CMS' previous policy, carriers-based payment for the second procedure on the lesser of the actual charge or 50% of the payment schedule amount; the third, fourth, and fifth procedures were each based on 25%; any subsequent procedures were paid on a by-report basis.

For 2011, the criteria for procedures and service to be included on the modifier 51-exempt list were clearly defined. Firstly, all add-on codes, physical medicine and rehabilitation services, and vaccines were excluded from being coded with modifier 51. Secondly, the services on this list should have minimal preservice time and postservice time because these services are performed in addition to another service that has its own preservice and postservice time. Because the preservice and postservice activities of services performed together should not be replicated, only codes with minimal amounts of preservice and postservice time have been retained on this list. In addition, services that are currently subject to multiple-surgery reduction have been removed from the list to be consistent with Medicare payment policy.

Modifier 52, Reduced Services

Modifier 52 is used to indicate that a service or procedure is reduced or eliminated at the discretion of the physician or other qualified health care professional. The definition of modifier 52 was changed for CPT 2013 to indicate:

Under certain circumstances a service or procedure is partially reduced or eliminated at the discretion of the physician or other qualified health care professional. Under these circumstances the service provided can be identified by its usual procedure number and the addition of modifier 52, signifying that the service is reduced. This provides a means of reporting reduced services without disturbing the identification of the basic service. ***Note:*** *For hospital outpatient reporting of a previously scheduled procedure/service that is partially reduced or cancelled as a result of extenuating circumstances or those that threaten the well-being of the* *patient prior to or after administration of anesthesia, see modifiers 73 and 74 (see modifiers approved for ASC hospital outpatient use).*

Carriers continue to have authority to decrease payment for reduced services (52), based on review of medical records and other documentation. Documentation of the unusual circumstances must accompany the claim (eg, a copy of the operative report and a separate statement written by the physician explaining the unusual amount of work required).

Modifier 53, Discontinued Procedure

Modifier 53 is used to indicate that the physician elected to terminate a surgical or diagnostic procedure. In 1999, the CPT definition for this modifier was editorially revised to clarify its intent for outpatient physician reporting of this circumstance. The definition of modifier 53 was changed for CPT 2013 to indicate:

Under certain circumstances, the physician or other qualified health care professional may elect to terminate a surgical or diagnostic procedure. Due to extenuating circumstances or those that threaten the well-being of the patient, it may be necessary to indicate that a surgical or diagnostic procedure was started but discontinued. This circumstance may be reported by adding modifier 53 to the code reported by the individual for the discontinued procedure. ***Note:*** *This modifier is not used to report the elective cancellation of a procedure prior to the patient's anesthesia induction and/or surgical preparation in the operating suite. For outpatient hospital/ambulatory surgery center (ASC) reporting of a previously scheduled procedure/service that is partially reduced or cancelled as a result of extenuating circumstances or those that threaten the well-being of the patient prior to or after administration of anesthesia, see modifiers 73 and 74 (see modifiers approved for ASC hospital outpatient use).*

Modifiers 54, 55, and 56—Providers Furnishing Less Than the Global Package

When more than one physician provides services that are part of a global surgery package, the following modifiers are used to designate the scope of services:

- Modifier 54, Surgical Care Only
- Modifier 55, Postoperative Management Only
- Modifier 56, Preoperative Management Only (CMS does not recognize this modifier for payment purposes; it is reported for information purposes only.)

Questions arise about apportioning payment for global surgery packages in which more than one physician provides services. Examples include surgery by an itinerant surgeon with follow-up care provided by a local physician; cataract surgery by an ophthalmologist with follow-up care provided by an optometrist; and follow-up care provided by a cardiologist for cardiovascular surgery performed by a thoracic surgeon.

Under the CPR payment system, total payment for all parts of a surgical service furnished by several physicians could not exceed the amount paid if only one physician had provided all the services in the global package; although it appears that this policy was not uniformly implemented by carriers. This policy was adopted in the 1991 Final Rule.

The AMA objected to this policy because inequities result when an internist or other physician provides the preoperative or postoperative care. The Harvard RBRVS study surveyed only preoperative and postoperative care when provided by the surgeon who furnished the intraoperative care. The AMA believes that this is not an appropriate basis for determining payment when another physician, who must be familiar with the patient, furnishes some of the services.

Consistent with the AMA's objections, CMS revised its payment rules. This modified policy allows a physician who assumes postsurgical responsibility for a patient during the hospital stay to report subsequent hospital visits in addition to the postsurgery portion of the global payment, provided the appropriate modifiers are reported by both the physician assuming responsibility for the patient and also by the surgeon. Physicians assuming postsurgical responsibility should report appropriate subsequent hospital care codes for the inpatient hospital care and the surgical code with modifier 55 for the postdischarge care. The surgeon reports the appropriate surgery code with modifier 54.

The surgeon's payment, which includes preoperative, intraoperative, and postoperative hospital services, is based on the preoperative and intraoperative portions of the global payment. Where more than one physician bills for postoperative care, however, the postoperative percentage of the global payment is apportioned according to the number of days each physician was responsible for the patient's care.

When postoperative recovery care is split between several physicians, the physicians must agree on the transfer of care. The agreement may be in the form of a letter or an annotation in the discharge summary, hospital record, or ambulatory surgical center record. The physician assuming the patient's care reports the appropriate procedure code with modifier 55 but may not report any services included in the global period until at least one service has been provided. If the surgeon relinquishes care at the time of discharge, only the date of surgery needs to be indicated when billing with modifier 54.

However, if the surgeon provides care after the patient is discharged, it is necessary to show the date of surgery, date of discharge, and date on which postoperative care was relinquished to another physician.

When a physician other than the surgeon provides occasional postoperative services during the global period, separate payment is allowed. These services should be reported with the appropriate E/M codes. Physicians should code for services provided and should take particular care in using correct ICD-10-CM codes. Payment is not included in the global payment as long as these services are occasional and unusual and do not reflect a pattern of postoperative care. However, separate payment is not allowed if the physician is the covering physician (eg, locum tenens) or part of the same group as the surgeon who performed the procedure and provided most of the postoperative care included in the global package.

Modifier 54, Surgical Care Only

Modifier 54 indicates that the surgeon is billing the surgical care only. The definition of modifier 54 was changed for CPT 2013 to indicate:

When 1 physician or other qualified health care professional performs a surgical procedure and another provides preoperative and/or postoperative management, surgical services may be identified by adding modifier 54 to the usual procedure number.

Modifier 55, Postoperative Management Only

Modifier 55 indicates that a physician or other qualified health care professional, other than the surgeon, is billing for part of the outpatient postoperative care. It is also used by the surgeon when providing only a portion of the post-discharge and postoperative care. Append modifier 55 to the procedure code that describes the surgical procedure performed that has a 10- or 90-day postoperative period. The claim must show the date of surgery as the date of service. When two different physicians share in the postoperative care, each bills for their portion—reporting modifier 55 and indicating the assumed and relinquished dates on the claim.

Modifier 56, Preoperative Management Only

Modifier 56 is used when one physician or other qualified health care professional performs the preoperative care and evaluation and another performs the surgical procedure. The preoperative component may be identified by adding modifier 56 to the procedure code. Clinical documentation must support the use of this modifier.

Modifier 57, Decision for Surgery

Modifier 57 is used to indicate that an E/M service resulted in the initial decision to perform the surgery. It may be identified by adding modifier 57 to the appropriate level of E/M service. Use of modifier 57 is limited to operations with 90-day global periods. Modifier 57 allows separate payment for the visit at which the decision to perform the surgery was made, if adequate documentation is submitted demonstrating that the decision for surgery was made during a specific visit.

Modifier 58, Staged or Related Procedure or Service by the Same Physician or Other Qualified Health Care Professional During the Postoperative Period

Modifier 58 indicates a staged or related procedure or service by the same physician during the postoperative period. The definition of modifier 58 was changed for CPT 2013 to indicate:

It may be necessary to indicate that the performance of a procedure or service during the postoperative period was: (a) planned or anticipated (staged); (b) more extensive than the original procedure; or (c) for therapy following a surgical procedure. This circumstance may be reported by adding modifier 58 to the staged or related procedure. Note: For treatment of a problem that requires a return to the operating/procedure room (eg, unanticipated clinical condition), see modifier 78.

Modifier 59, Distinct Procedural Service

The definition of modifier 59 was changed for CPT 2015 to indicate:

Under certain circumstances, it may be necessary to indicate that a procedure or service was distinct or independent from other non-E/M services performed on the same day. Modifier 59 is used to identify procedures/services, other than E/M services, that are not normally reported together, but are appropriate under the circumstances. Documentation must support a different session, different procedure or surgery, different site or organ system, separate incision/excision, separate lesion, or separate injury (or area of injury in extensive injuries) not ordinarily encountered or performed on the same day by the same individual. However, when another already established modifier is appropriate it should be used rather than modifier 59. Only if no more descriptive modifier is available, and the use of modifier 59 best explains the circumstances, should modifier 59 be used. Note: Modifier 59 should not be appended to an E/M service. To report a separate and distinct E/M service with a non-E/M service performed on the same date, see modifier 25.

Modifier 62, Two Surgeons

Co-surgery or team surgery may be required because of the complexity of the procedure(s), the patient's condition, or both. The additional surgeon(s) is not acting as an assistant-at-surgery in these circumstances. The definition of modifier 62 was changed for CPT 2013 to indicate:

When 2 surgeons work together as primary surgeons performing distinct part(s) of a procedure, each surgeon should report his/her distinct operative work by adding modifier 62 to the procedure code and any associated add-on code(s) for that procedure as long as both surgeons continue to work together as primary surgeons. Each surgeon should report the co-surgery once using the same procedure code. If additional procedure(s) (including add-on procedure(s)) are performed during the same surgical session, separate code(s) may also be reported with modifier 62 added. ***Note:*** *If a co-surgeon acts as an assistant in the performance of additional procedure(s), other than those reported with the modifier 62, during the same surgical session, those services may be reported using separate procedure code(s) with modifier 80 or modifier 82 added, as appropriate.*

Payment is based on 125% of the global amount, which is divided equally between the two surgeons. Documentation to establish medical necessity for both surgeons is required for some services. Refer to the List of Relative Value Units in Part 5 of this book to determine if this requirement applies.

Modifier 63, Procedure Performed on Infants Less than 4 kg

Procedures performed on neonates and infants up to a present body weight of 4 kg may involve significantly increased complexity and physician or other qualified health care professional work commonly associated with these patients. This circumstance may be reported by adding modifier 63 to the procedure number unless designated otherwise.

Modifier 63 was established in 2003 to be appended only to invasive surgical procedures and reported only for those for neonates/infants up to the 4 kg cut-off. In this population of patients, there is a significant increase in work intensity specifically related to temperature control, obtaining IV access (which may require upwards of 45 minutes), and the operation itself, which is technically more difficult, especially with regard to maintenance of homeostasis.

Unless otherwise designated, this modifier may only be appended to procedures/services listed in the 20100-69990 code series and 92920, 92928, 92953, 92960, 92986, 92987, 92990, 92997, 92998, 93312, 93313, 93314, 93315, 93316, 93317, 93318, 93452, 93505, 93563, 93564, 93568, 93580, 93582, 93590, 93591, 93592, 93593, 93594, 93595, 93596, 93597, 93598, 93615, 93616 from the Medicine/Cardiovascular section. Modifier 63 should not be appended to any CPT codes listed in the Evaluation and Management Services, Anesthesia, Radiology, Pathology/Laboratory, or Medicine sections (other than those identified above from the Medicine/Cardiovascular section). It is not appropriate to report modifier 63 because the additional work that modifier 63 is intended to represent has been previously identified as an inherent element within the procedures in this list. When appended to a procedure, modifier 63 indicates the additional difficulty of performing a procedure, which may involve significantly increased complexity and physician work commonly associated with neonates and infants up to a body weight of 4 kg.

Modifier 66, Surgical Team

Team surgery involves a single procedure (reported with a single procedure code) that requires more than two surgeons of different specialties and is reported by each surgeon (with the same procedure code) with modifier 66. The definition of modifier 66 was changed for CPT 2013 to indicate:

Under some circumstances, highly complex procedures (requiring the concomitant services of several physicians or other qualified health care professionals, often of different specialties, plus other highly skilled, specially trained personnel, various types of complex equipment) are carried out under the "surgical team" concept. Such circumstances may be identified by each participating individual with the addition of modifier 66 to the basic procedure number used for reporting services.

Payment amounts are determined by contractor medical directors (CMDs) on an individual basis. Refer to the List of Relative Value Units in Part 5 of this book to determine if this requirement applies.

Modifier 76, Repeat Procedure or Service by Same Physician or Other Qualified Health Care Professional

Modifier 76 is used to indicate a repeat procedure by the same physician and is used when it is necessary to report repeat procedures performed on the same day. The definition of modifier 76 was changed for CPT 2013 to indicate:

It may be necessary to indicate that a procedure or service was repeated by the same physician or other qualified health care professional subsequent to the original procedure or service. This circumstance may be reported by adding modifier 76 to the repeated procedure or service. ***Note:*** *This modifier should not be appended to an E/M service.*

Modifier 77, Repeat Procedure by Another Physician or Other Qualified Health Care Professional

The definition of modifier 77 was changed for CPT 2013 to indicate:

It may be necessary to indicate that a basic procedure or service was repeated by another physician or other qualified health care professional subsequent to the original procedure or service. This circumstance may be reported by adding modifier 77 to the repeated procedure or service. ***Note:*** *This modifier should not be appended to an E/M service.*

Modifier 78, Unplanned Return to the Operating/Procedure Room by the Same Physician or Other Qualified Health Care Professional Following Initial Procedure for a Related Procedure During the Postoperative Period

The definition of modifier 78 was changed for CPT 2013 to indicate:

It may be necessary to indicate that another procedure was performed during the postoperative period of the initial procedure (unplanned procedure following initial procedure). When this procedure is related to the first, and requires the use of an operating/procedure room, it may be reported by adding modifier 78 to the related procedure. (For repeat procedures, see modifier 76.)

Payment for reoperations is made only for the intraoperative services. No additional payment is made for preoperative and postoperative care because CMS considers these services to be part of the original global surgery package. The approved amount will be set at the value of the intraoperative service the surgeon performed when an appropriate CPT code exists (eg, 32120, *Thoracotomy; for postoperative complications*). However, if no CPT code exists to describe the specific reoperation, the appropriate unlisted procedures code from the Surgery section of CPT would be used. Payment in these cases is based on up to 50% of the value of the intraoperative service that was originally provided.

Modifier 79, Unrelated Procedure or Service by the Same Physician or Other Qualified Health Care Professional During the Postoperative Period

Modifier 79 is used to indicate that the operating surgeon performed a procedure on a surgical patient during the postoperative period for problems unrelated to the original surgical procedure. Separate payment for the unrelated procedure is allowed under these circumstances and is reported by appending modifier 79 to the procedure code. Modifier 79 is used to report, for example, an appendectomy performed during the global period of a mastectomy by the same surgeon.

Modifiers 80 (Assistant Surgeon), 81 (Minimum Assistant Surgeon), and 82 (Assistant Surgeon [when qualified resident surgeon not available])

Modifier 80 is used to indicate surgical assistant services. The modifier would be appended to the usual procedure code. Modifier 81 is used to indicate services that require an assistant surgeon for a relatively short time. The primary surgeon may not append modifier 81 to the procedure code. Modifier 82 indicates the unavailability of a qualified resident surgeon. The modifier is appended to the usual procedure code.

Current law requires the approved amount for assistant surgeons to be set at the lower of the actual charge or 16% of the global surgical approved amount. In addition, the law requires that payment for services of assistant surgeons be made only when the most recent national Medicare claims data indicate that a procedure has involved assistants in at least 5% of cases based on a national average percentage. To determine if services are subject to this payment restriction, refer to the List of Relative Value Units in Part 5 under the "Payment Policy Indicator" column. Full payment for the assistant surgeon's services may be made for some procedures if documentation is provided establishing medical necessity. These procedures are indicated by an "A1" in the "Payment Policy Indicator" column. (Also see modifiers 50, 62, and 81.)

Modifier 90, Reference (Outside) Laboratory

This modifier is used to report laboratory procedures that are performed by a party other than the treating or reporting physician or other qualified health care professional.

Modifier 91, Repeat Clinical Diagnostic Laboratory Test

This modifier is used to indicate repeated laboratory tests on the same day. The definition of modifier 91 was changed for CPT 2013 to indicate:

In the course of treatment of the patient, it may be necessary to repeat the same laboratory test on the same day to obtain subsequent (multiple) test results. Under these circumstances, the laboratory test performed can be identified by its usual procedure number and the addition of modifier 91.
Note: *This modifier may not be used when tests are rerun to confirm initial results; due to testing problems with specimens or equipment; or for any other reason when a normal, one-time, reportable result is all that is required. This modifier may not be used when other code(s) describe a series of test results (eg, glucose tolerance tests, evocative/suppression testing). This modifier may only be used for laboratory*

test(s) performed more than once on the same day on the same patient.

Modifier 92, Alternative Laboratory Platform Testing

The definition of modifier 92 was changed for CPT 2013 to indicate:

When laboratory testing is being performed using a kit or transportable instrument that wholly or in part consists of a single use, disposable analytical chamber, the service may be identified by adding modifier 92 to the usual laboratory procedure code (HIV testing 86701-86703, and 87389). The test does not require permanent dedicated space, hence by its design may be hand carried or transported to the vicinity of the patient for immediate testing at that site, although location of the testing is not in itself determinative of the use of this modifier.

Modifier 93, Synchronous Telemedicine Service Rendered Via Telephone or Other Real-Time Interactive Audio-Only Telecommunications System

This audio-only telehealth modifier will be effective in the CPT 2022 code set and should be appended to codes when a service is provided via an audio-only technology (primarily via telephone). The definition of the modifier is as follows:

Synchronous telemedicine service is defined as a real-time interaction between a physician or other qualified health care professional and a patient who is located away at a distant site from the physician or other qualified health care professional. The totality of the communication of information exchanged between the physician or other qualified health care professional and the patient during the course of the synchronous telemedicine service must be of an amount and nature that is sufficient to meet the key components and/or requirements of the same service when rendered via a face-to-face interaction.

Modifier 95, Synchronous Telemedicine Service Rendered via a Real-Time Interactive Audio and Video Telecommunications System

This modifier was established for CPT 2017. The definition of modifier 95 is as follows:

Synchronous telemedicine service is defined as a ***real-time*** *interaction between a physician or other qualified health care professional and a patient who is located at a distant site from the physician or other qualified health care professional. The totality of the communication of information exchanged between the physician or other qualified health care professional and the patient during the course of the synchronous telemedicine service must be of an amount and nature that would be sufficient to meet the key components and/or requirements of the same service when rendered via a face-to-face interaction. Modifier 95 may only be appended to the services listed in Appendix P. Appendix P is the list of CPT codes for services that are typically performed face-to-face, but may be rendered via a real-time (synchronous) interactive audio and video telecommunications system.*

Modifier 96, Habilitative Services

This modifier was established for CPT 2018. The definition of modifier 96 is as follows:

When a service or procedure that may be either habilitative or rehabilitative in nature is provided for habilitative purposes, the physician or other qualified health care professional may add modifier 96 to the service or procedure code to indicate that the service or procedure provided was a habilitative service. Habilitative services help an individual learn skills and functioning for daily living that the individual has not yet developed, and then keep and/or improve those learned skills. Habilitative services also help an individual keep, learn, or improve skills and functioning for daily living.

Modifier 97, Rehabilitative Services

This modifier was established for CPT 2018. The definition of modifier 97 is as follows:

When a service or procedure that may be either habilitative or rehabilitative in nature is provided for rehabilitative purposes, the physician or other qualified health care professional may add modifier 97 to the service or procedure code to indicate that the service or procedure provided was a rehabilitative service. Rehabilitative services help an individual keep, get back, or improve skills and functioning for daily living that have been lost or impaired because the individual was sick, hurt, or disabled.

Modifier 99, Multiple Modifiers

This modifier is used to indicate the use of two or more modifiers. Claims for which additional modifiers may apply are manually priced by the carriers.

Payment Levels Unaffected by Modifiers

Contractors may continue to use CPT numeric and HCPCS alphanumeric modifiers and carrier unique local modifiers (HCPCS Level III modifiers beginning with the letters W through Z) that do not affect payment amounts. The local modifiers may be used for administrative purposes, such as utilization review, but they cannot be used to increase or decrease payment levels.

Telephone and Online Evaluation and Management Services

For CPT 2008, the CPT Editorial Panel created eight new codes for E/M services performed via telephone or online: codes 99441-99444 to describe E/M services performed by a physician and codes 98966-98969 to describe E/M services performed by a qualified health care professional (QHP). Typically, these calls involve the health care professional obtaining a history of the patient, assessing the patient's condition, making a medical decision, and communicating that decision via telephone or e-mail to the patient. Over the last two decades, medicine has seen a rapid increase of medical information and communications technology. Combined with changing consumer and health plan expectations for enhanced access to care, a new focus on chronic disease management, and continued pressure to reduce the codes of medical services, providers are delivering more care to patients in a nonface-to-face manner. In addition, these services describe work that is not currently captured in any other CPT codes. Throughout the coronavirus disease 2019 (COVID-19) public health emergency (PHE), CMS has been accepting and paying for E/M services via telephone with in-person office-visit rate. After the PHE ends, CMS will again modify the payment policy for telephone calls as a bundled service.

For CPT 2020, the CPT Editorial Panel deleted online E/M CPT codes 99444 and 98969 and replaced them with six new nonface-to-face codes for online digital evaluation services or e-visits. These services are nonface-to-face, patient-initiated communications using online patient portals. These digital assessment services are for established patients who require a clinical decision that would otherwise have been typically provided in the office. CMS finalized payment for these new online digital assessment services beginning in CY 2020 for practitioners reporting under the MFS. Three codes describe the physician e-visit (99421-99423) and three codes describe the qualified nonphysician health care professional e-visit (98970- 98972). CMS agreed to make separate payment for the physician e-visit services. However, it disagreed with the CPT Editorial Panel that services represented by codes 98970-98972 could be performed by qualified nonphysician health care professionals, based on the statutory requirements that govern the Medicare benefit and do not allow nonphysicians to report E/M services. Instead, CMS created parallel HCPCS G-codes (G2061-G2063) with descriptors that refer to the performance of an "assessment" rather than an "evaluation" and provided separate payment for the nonphysician online digital assessments. For CY 2021, the CPT Editorial Panel revised the CPT codes to refer to "assessment" and CMS replaced its e-visit G-codes (G2061-G2063) with corresponding revised CPT codes 98970-98972 for qualified nonphysician health care professional online digital E/M services.

Telehealth

Telehealth, telemedicine, and related terms generally refer to the exchange of medical information from one site or source to another through electronic communication. CMS defines telehealth as:

A two-way, real-time interactive communication between a patient and a physician or practitioner at a distant site through telecommunications equipment that includes, at a minimum, audio and visual equipment.

While *telemedicine* has historically referred to remote clinical services, *telehealth* can refer to broader services. The following definitions of synchronous vs asynchronous telehealth communications are also important:

Synchronous

- Real-time, audio-video communication that connect physicians and patients in different locations. (**Note:** This definition is used for telehealth for CMS coverage and payment.)
- Real-time audio and telephone communications.

Asynchronous

- Store-and-Forward technologies that collect images and data to be transmitted and interpreted later.
- Online digital visits and/or brief check-in services furnished using communication technology that are employed to evaluate whether an office visit is warranted (via patient portal, smartphone)
- Interprofessional Internet consultations between physicians and/or other qualified health care professionals to improve care coordination for patients by sharing verbal or written reports for further assessment and/or care management

There are over 250 services on the Medicare telehealth list effective January 1, 2022. The full list of these codes is available at https://www.cms.gov/Medicare/Medicare-General-Information/Telehealth/Telehealth-Codes. CMS selects telehealth services for the Medicare telehealth list using the following three categories:

- Category 1: Services that are similar to professional consultations, office visits, and office psychiatry services that are currently on the list of telehealth services.
- Category 2: Services that are not similar to the current list of telehealth services, but documentation has been accepted by CMS to add the codes permanently to the list.
- Category 3 (created for the COVID-19 PHE): Services that will be included on the Medicare telehealth services list on a temporary basis. These services will ultimately need to meet the criteria under Categories 1 or 2 to be permanently added to the Medicare telehealth services list. For CY 2022, CMS finalized its proposal to retain all services added to the Medicare telehealth services list on a Category 3 basis through the end of calendar year 2023.

Medicare Expands Telehealth During COVID-19 PHE

CMS lifted Medicare restrictions on the use of telehealth services during the COVID-19 PHE. Key changes include:

- Effective March 1, 2020, and throughout the national PHE, Medicare will pay physicians for telehealth services at the same rate as in-person visits for all diagnoses, not just services related to COVID-19.
- Medicare will pay physicians for audio-only telephone calls, also at the in-person rate through the end of the PHE. At the conclusion of the PHE, CMS will allow payment of phone calls as virtual check-ins using the rates of codes G2251 and G2252. In addition, CMS finalized its proposal to permanently establish separate coding and payment for the longer virtual check-in service, G2252, for CY 2022. This code can be reported by a physician or QHP for a virtual check-in of 11 to 20 minutes of clinical discussion for an established patient that does not originate from an E/M service. This code is in addition to the existing virtual check-in codes G2012 and G2251 for 5 to 10 minutes of clinical discussion.
- CMS expanded the list of covered telehealth services, creating a category for services that will be included on the Medicare telehealth services list on a temporary basis during the COVID-19 PHE.
- Physicians may utilize telehealth for both new and established patients.
- Reporting and documenting office visits performed via telehealth may be based on medical decision making (MDM) or time on date of encounter.
- Patients may receive telehealth services in all areas of the country and in all settings, including at their home.
- CMS will not enforce a requirement that patients have an established relationship with the physician providing telehealth.
- Consent for telehealth services may be obtained by staff or the practitioner at any time and this is required only once on an annual basis.
- Physicians may reduce or waive cost-sharing for telehealth visits.
- Physicians licensed in one state may provide services to Medicare beneficiaries in another state; however, state licensure laws still apply.
- Physicians may provide telehealth services from their home. Physicians **do not** have to add their home to their Medicare enrollment file.
- Health and Human Services (HHS) Office for Civil Rights (OCR) offers flexibility for telehealth via popular video-chat applications, such as FaceTime or Skype, during the pandemic.

In addition, telehealth has ensured access to valuable mental health services during the PHE. CMS acknowledges that there is not a "one size fits all" model in the management of mental health, and while some patients may benefit from more frequent in-person visits, some patients may require less. For CY 2022, CMS addresses the frequency with which a beneficiary receiving mental health services in their home through telehealth would need to receive an in-person, non-telehealth service. The Agency finalized that telehealth for mental health services will require in-person visits within 12 months of subsequent mental health telehealth services, instead of every six months.

AMA Tools and Resources

- Telehealth quick guide has detailed information to support physicians and practices in expediting implementation of telemedicine available at https://www.ama-assn.org/practice-management/digital/ama-telehealth-quick-guide.
- Coding scenarios with real-world examples of how to code for telehealth services available at https://www.ama-assn.org/system/files/2020-05/covid-19-coding-advice.pdf.
- Comparison of telehealth coding and payment policies between Medicare and commercial payers available at https://www.ama-assn.org/system/files/covid-19-telehealth-payment-policies.pdf.

Remote Physiologic Monitoring

Remote physiologic monitoring (RPM) refers to collecting and transmitting patient data outside of the office, mostly asynchronous, which results in clinical decision making and care management follow-up that may be provided in-person or virtually. For example, tools and wearable devices (which may involve the use of mobile health [mHealth] apps) that measure weight, blood pressure, pulse oximetry, respiratory flow rate, musculoskeletal system status, therapy adherence, therapy response, and other patient-generated data for review and treatment management. While many consider RPM services to be a subset of telehealth, CMS does not currently consider RPM as telehealth because it is inherently a nonface-to-face service.

Starting January 1, 2019, consistent with the AMA advocacy efforts and in response to work by the CPT Editorial Panel and RUC, CMS finalized new CPT codes for chronic care RPM.

Prior to 2019, the CPT code set had very general codes related to collection and analysis of electronic data. However, the new 2020 codes are specific to physiologic monitoring services (eg, weight, blood pressure, and pulse oximetry). The guidelines specify that the device used must be a medical device as defined by the US Food and Drug Administration (FDA) and ordered by the physician or other QHP. Code 99453 was added to report remote monitoring of the physiologic parameter(s) initial setup and patient education, specifically on the use of the device. It should be reported once for each episode of care, as defined in the new CPT guidelines. Code 99454 was established to report device supply for daily recordings or programmed alert transmissions for 30-day periods.

In addition, a new code (99457) was established to report RPM treatment management services for 20 minutes or more in a calendar month. Code 99457 requires interactive communication with the patient or caregiver during the month. As indicated in the guidelines, it is important to note that the device used to provide these services must be a medical device defined by the FDA, and it must be ordered by a physician or other QHP. For 2020, the CPT Editorial Panel revised the CPT code structure for code 99457 in which code 99457 remained as a parent code that describes the first 20 minutes of the treatment management services, while a new add-on code (99458) was added to describe subsequent 20-minute intervals of the service.

#99453 Remote monitoring of physiologic parameter(s) (eg, weight, blood pressure, pulse oximetry, respiratory flow rate), initial; set-up and patient education on use of equipment

#99454 device(s) supply with daily recording(s) or programmed alert(s) transmission, each 30 days

#▲99457 Remote physiologic monitoring treatment management services, clinical staff/physician/other qualified health care professional time in a calendar month requiring interactive communication with the patient/caregiver during the month; first 20 minutes.

#+99458 each additional 20 minutes (List separately in addition to code for primary procedure)

The AMA continues to work with CMS to further improve code refinements related to RPM.

During the COVID-19 PHE, CMS provided flexibilities to allow for timely delivery of reasonable and necessary health care. On an interim basis, CMS allowed RPM services to be furnished to new patients and established patients to reduce exposure and increase access to services. CMS has determined to allow RPM services only for established patients once the COVID-19 PHE ends. CMS will allow on a permanent basis for consent for RPM to be obtained at the time that the services are furnished and allow auxiliary personnel (eg, clinical staff) to furnish RPM under general supervision of the reporting physician or practitioner. CMS also will allow RPM to be reported for patients with either acute or chronic conditions.

Starting January 1, 2018, and in response to work by the CPT Editorial Panel and RUC, CMS established separate payment for the remote collection and interpretation of physiologic data using CPT code 99091. CPT code 99091 may not be reported in conjunction with RPM codes 99457 and 99458.

#99091 Collection and interpretation of physiologic data (eg, ECG, blood pressure, glucose monitoring) digitally stored and/or transmitted by the patient and/or caregiver to the physician or other qualified health care professional, qualified by education, training, licensure/regulation (when applicable) requiring a minimum of 30 minutes of time, each 30 days

Remote Therapeutic Monitoring

For CPT 2022, the CPT Editorial Panel created new codes to describe remote therapeutic monitoring (RTM) (CPT codes 98975, 98976, 98977, 98980, and 98981). These codes have the same structure as the remote physiological monitoring (RPM) codes and the services are similar in staff and physician work, although the specific equipment used is different because the data being monitored are nonphysiologic with RTM rather than physiologic as they are with

RPM. RPM services are considered to be E/M services. For example, physical therapists are not permitted to furnish E/M services. Similarly, the RTM codes are considered general medicine codes and, as such, CMS limits which qualified health care professionals may report them due to supervision requirements (eg, physical therapists may not supervise nursing staff). However, in the Final Rule for CY 2022, CMS finalized a policy permitting therapists and other qualified healthcare professionals to report the RTM codes. Thus, nonphysicians who cannot report E/M or general medicine services will be able to report and be paid for RTM services.

Payment for "New" Physicians

Prior to 1994, legislative requirements imposed lower payment schedule amounts on "new physicians," defined as those in their first through fourth years of submitting Medicare claims. Effective January 1, 1994, provisions contained in Omnibus Budget Reconciliation Act (OBRA) of 1993 repealed these payment reductions. As a result, payments to "new physicians" and other health care providers under the RBRVS payment system are no longer subject to these percentage reductions.

Payment for Provider-Based and Teaching Physicians

Medicare payment regulations distinguish between *direct* patient care services of hospital-based physicians and services related to *general* patient care. The latter category of services is payable to the facility as Part A services through the hospital prospective pricing system or on a reasonable cost basis.

Payment for direct patient care services is covered under Medicare Part B. Such payment may be made to the teaching hospital when it elects to be paid for physicians' direct medical and surgical services on a reasonable cost basis; otherwise, payment is made directly to the teaching physician who provided the services. CMS defines direct patient care as follows:

- The service is personally furnished by the physician.
- The service contributes directly to an individual patient's diagnosis or treatment.
- The service is ordinarily provided by a physician.

In the December 8, 1995, Final Rule, CMS described new payment rules for teaching physicians when services are provided by an intern or resident working under the supervision of the teaching physician. The regulations were developed with input from the AMA, national medical specialty societies, Association of American Medical Colleges, and Medical Group Management Association.

Before implementing the new rules, CMS required the attending physician to establish a professional relationship with the patient in order to bill for services provided by a resident or intern under the attending physician's supervision. The requirement and criteria defining such a relationship were eliminated in recognition of the fact that groups of physicians may share the teaching and supervision duties of residents, who provide care to individual patients. The new rules acknowledged that payable services provided by teaching physicians occur in a variety of circumstances not limited to the inpatient setting. Finally, in defining appropriate supervision of residents, the new rules gave the teaching physician greater flexibility to determine when "physical presence" is required.

The policy clarified that the teaching physician must be present only for the "key portion" of the time during which a resident performs a procedure. During a surgical or other complex procedure, the teaching physician must be present during all critical portions of the procedure and be immediately available during the entire service. The rules allow payment for supervision of two concurrent major surgical procedures, if the surgeon is physically present for the key portions of each procedure (ie, the key portions cannot take place at the same time) and another surgeon is standing by to assist in the first procedure. Only one surgeon can bill for each procedure concurrently. To receive payment for supervision of E/M services, the teaching physician must be physically present during that portion of the visit that determines the level of service billed. The teaching physician's presence must be documented in the patient's medical record.

CMS also recognized that requiring the teaching physician's physical presence is inherently incompatible with the nature of some residency training programs and acknowledged that, under certain circumstances, payment may be appropriate even though the teaching physician is not present to supervise the resident or intern. For family practice and other residency training programs that meet specified criteria, CMS established a limited exception to the physical presence requirement. Payment will be allowed for low- to mid-level E/M services (CPT codes 99202-99203 and 99211-99213) furnished by a resident without the presence of a teaching physician if specified criteria are met. Included among the criteria is a requirement that the teaching physician supervises no more than four residents at any given time and be immediately available to those residents. Other criteria set requirements are the entities in which the services are furnished, establish minimum training requirements for residents who provide services, and identify the range of services that residents must provide.

CMS indicated that the residency training programs most likely to meet the exception criteria are family practice and some programs in general internal medicine, geriatrics, and pediatrics. In the 1996 Final Rule, CMS clarified that obstetric and gynecologic residency programs or others focusing on women's health care would qualify for the exception, if all other criteria are met.

CMS also established an exception to the payment rules for services provided by residents in psychiatric programs. Under this exception, the physical presence requirement is satisfied, if the teaching physician observes services furnished to the patient by the resident (psychiatric as well as E/M services) through a one-way mirror or video equipment and meets with the patient following the visit.

Changes made in the carrier instructions in May 1996 clarified that it is appropriate to bill for qualified services performed by a teaching physician, when in the presence or with the assistance of a medical student.

On November 22, 2002, the *Medicare Carriers Manual* was modified to specifically state the following:

Any contribution and participation of a student to the performance of a billable service (other than the review of systems and/or past family/social history which are not separately billable, but are taken as part of an E/M service) must be performed in the physical presence of a teaching physician or physical presence of a resident in a service meeting the requirements set forth in this section for teaching physician billing. Students may document services in the medical record. However, the documentation of an E/M service by a student that may be referred to by the teaching physician is limited to documentation related to the review of systems and/or past family/social history. The teaching physician may not refer to a student's documentation of physical exam findings or medical decision making in his or her personal note. If the medical student documents E/M services, the teaching physician must verify and redocument the history of present illness as well as perform and redocument the physical exam and medical decision-making activities of the service.

In 2010, as requested by the AMA and the American Society of Anesthesiologists, in finalizing a new policy restoring full Medicare payment to academic anesthesiology programs, the final rule permits different anesthesiologists in the same anesthesia group practice to be considered the teaching physician, for purposes of being present at the key or critical portions of the case.

For anesthesia services furnished on or after January 1, 2010, payment may be made under the Medicare physician payment schedule at the regular payment schedule level if the teaching anesthesiologist is involved in the training of a resident in a single anesthesia case, two concurrent anesthesia cases involving residents, or a single anesthesia case involving a resident that is concurrent to another case paid under the medical direction rules. To qualify for payment, the teaching anesthesiologist, or different anesthesiologists in the same anesthesia group, must be present during all critical or key portions of the anesthesia service or procedure involved. The teaching anesthesiologist (or another anesthesiologist with whom the teaching physician has entered into an arrangement) must be immediately available to furnish anesthesia services during the entire procedure. The documentation in the patient's medical records must indicate the teaching physician's presence during all critical or key portions of the anesthesia procedure and the immediate availability of another teaching anesthesiologist as necessary.

If different teaching anesthesiologists are present with the resident during the key or critical periods of the resident case, the NPI of the teaching anesthesiologist who started the case must be indicated in the appropriate field on the claim form. The teaching anesthesiologist should use the "AA" modifier and the "GC" certification modifier to report such cases.

Off-Campus Provider-Based Hospital Departments

In the CY 2019 Hospital Outpatient Prospective Payment System (OPPS) final rule, CMS finalized a change in the clinical visit service payment, as described by HCPCS code G0463, *Hospital outpatient clinic visit for assessment and management of a patient*, for nonexcepted off-campus provider-based hospital departments (departments that bill the modifier "PO" on claim lines). CMS phased in the application of this reduction in payment for the clinic visit service described by HCPCS code G0463 over two years by paying 70% of the OPPS rate in CY 2019, then reducing payment to 40% of the OPPS rate for CY 2020 and future years. The rationale the Agency provided for this policy change in the CY 2020 MFS final rule was to "...control unnecessary increases in the volume of the clinic visit service furnished in excepted off-campus provider-based departments (PBDs) by removing the payment differential that drives the site-of-service decision and, as a result, unnecessarily increases service volume."

Professional/Technical Component Services

Professional and technical component modifiers were established for some services to distinguish the portion of a service furnished by a physician. The professional component includes the physician work and corresponding overhead and professional liability insurance (PLI) costs involved in three types of services:

- Diagnostic tests that involve a physician's interpretation, such as cardiac stress tests and electroencephalograms
- Physician diagnostic and therapeutic radiology services
- Physician pathology services

The technical component of a service includes the cost of equipment, supplies, technician salaries, PLI, etc. The global charge refers to both components when billed together. For services furnished to hospital outpatients or inpatients, the physician may bill only for the professional component, because the statute requires that payment for nonphysician services provided to hospital patients be paid only to the hospital. This requirement applies, even if the service for a hospital patient is performed in a physician's office.

Radiology Services

Before the introduction of the Medicare payment schedule in January 1992, payment for radiology services was based on a separate radiology payment schedule. Although this payment schedule had separate values for only professional component, only technical component, and global services, these relative values were not divided into work, practice expense, and PLI components. The professional component services on the radiology payment schedule were divided into these components and linked to the overall RBRVS payment schedule. Practice expense and PLI RVUs are calculated as they would be for other services. The RVUs for technical component–only radiology services are based on values for such services from the radiology payment schedule. CMS has indicated that it will consider developing new rules for reporting global radiology services by radiology groups under contract to a hospital.

The MFS established standardized payment practices for three types of radiological procedures, which were subject to carrier variations under the old payment schedule for radiologist services:

- Interventional radiological procedures
- Radiation therapy services
- Low-osmolar contrast media (LOCM)

The Protecting Access to Medicare Act (PAMA) of 2014, Section 218(b), established a program to apply appropriate use criteria (AUC) to advanced diagnostic imaging services such as computed tomography (CT), positron emission tomography (PET), nuclear medicine, and magnetic resonance imaging (MRI). CMS will require that when practitioners order an advanced diagnostic imaging service for a Medicare beneficiary, the practitioner or clinical staff acting under the practitioner's direction, will be required to consult a qualified Clinical Decision Support Mechanism (CDSM). CDSMs are electronic portals through which AUC is accessed. The CDSM provides a determination of whether the order adheres to AUC, or if the AUC consulted was not applicable. Ultimately, practitioners whose ordering patterns are considered outliers will be subject to prior authorization. The program is set to be fully implemented on January 1, 2021, which means AUC consultations with qualified CDSMs are required to occur along with reporting of consultation information on the furnishing professional and furnishing facility claim for the advanced diagnostic imaging service. Prior to this date, the program will operate in an Education and Operations Testing Period starting January 1, 2020, during which claims will not be denied for failing to include proper AUC consultation information.

Interventional radiological procedures. Separate payments are made, at the full approved amounts, for both the radiological portion (the supervision and interpretation code) of an interpretative radiologic service and for the primary medical-surgical service. Additional services associated with the procedure will be payable at reduced amounts: 50% of the otherwise payable approved amount for up to five additional procedures. Any additional procedures are payable by report.

Special payment rules apply to surgical intervention procedures for vascular studies: 100% to the first major family of vessels; 50% to the second through fifth; additional procedures are paid by report.

Radiation therapy services. The RVUs for the technical component of radiology services are generally based on the estimated average allowance for each technical component service based on the radiologist payment schedule. However, after analyzing the costs of free-standing radiation oncology centers, CMS indicated in the 1991 Final Rule that it had increased the RVUs to cover the costs of these centers. The RVUs for the technical component codes were, therefore, increased by 14.2%.

LOCM. In April 1989, carrier payment policies for LOCM (also known as low osmolar contrast material) were frozen, and CMS undertook a study to determine if the additional cost of using LOCM justified the benefits over using high osmolar contrast media. From January

1, 1992, through December 31, 2004, separate payment was made for LOCM for all intrathecal procedures and for intra-arterial and intravenous radiological procedures, when it is used for nonhospital patients with the following specified characteristics:

- A history of previous adverse reaction to contrast material, except for a sensation of heat, flushing, or a single episode of nausea or vomiting
- A history of asthma or allergy
- Significant cardiac dysfunction, including recent or imminent cardiac decompensation, severe arrhythmia, unstable angina pectoris, recent myocardial infarction, and pulmonary hypertension
- Generalized severe debilitation
- Sickle cell disease
- Effective January 1, 2005, CMS has eliminated the previously described restrictive criteria for the payment of LOCM. Effective April 1, 2005, payment for LOCM was based on average sales price (ASP) plus 6%.

Portable X Ray

With the elimination of specialty differentials, the payment policy for portable X-ray service suppliers was changed to make the technical, professional, and transportation components payable according to the MFS.

Recognizing the additional costs portable X-ray suppliers incur in setting up equipment and positioning patients, a Level II HCPCS code (Q0092) and national RVUs were established to reflect a per procedure equipment setup payment. Q0092 continues to be included in the zero-work pool and is assigned a total relative value of 0.33 in 2005. Carriers are instructed to continue pricing transportation costs locally.

Medicare allows separate payment for transporting equipment furnished by approved suppliers of portable X-ray services, which is used to perform X rays and diagnostic mammograms. These services are billed by reporting HCPCS code R0070. The Balanced Budget Act of 1997 reinstated payment for transporting ECG equipment for services furnished after December 31, 1997, and before January 1, 1999. These services are billed by reporting HCPCS code R0076 with CPT code 93000 (a 12-lead ECG with interpretation and report) or code 93005 (a 12-lead ECG, tracing only, without interpretation and report). In 2013, CMS revised regulations to allow limited-license and nonphysician practitioners to order portable X-ray services within the scope of their practice.

Diagnostic Tests

Under the RBRVS payment schedule, CMS established criteria to identify which services are considered diagnostic tests and include a technical component and a method to determine the technical component's relative value. Diagnostic tests are defined by the following two criteria:

- The service is diagnostic rather than therapeutic in nature.
- The physician's professional service is separable from the technical component of the test, ie, the professional diagnostic service is not so integrally related to performing the test, as to make separation a practical impossibility.

The professional component RVU is the physician work RVU plus practice expense and PLI RVUs, based on 1991 average allowed charges. The relative value for the technical component is based on the difference between the 1991 average approved-amount for the global service and the 1991 average approved-amount for the professional component. This formula will apply whenever a substantial volume of service is billed for either global or professional component services, and at least a 21% difference exists between the global and professional component average approved amount. An alternate formula for services not meeting these criteria is based on the actual charge-data for the component with the most charge-data, and an assumption that the technical component is 21% of the global services value.

For those services that do not have a professional component, RVUs are based on the 1991 average approved amount for the service itself. Diagnostic tests without a professional component are subject to the practice expense and PLI geographic practice cost index only.

Coverage Conditions for Diagnostic Tests

As noted in the ordering of diagnostic tests rule, Medicare payment policy for diagnostic tests, including radiologic procedures, covers such tests only when ordered by the physician responsible for a patient's treatment and when that physician will use the test results to manage the patient's specific medical problems. Coverage is also allowed when ordered by a physician who is consulting for another physician. Nonphysicians, such as physician assistants (PAs), nurse practitioners (NPs), clinical nurse specialists (CNPs), certified nurse midwives (CNMs), and clinical psychologists, would also be able to order these services if it is within their scope of practice. The ordering of diagnostics test rule does not apply to diagnostic tests furnished in the hospital setting.

It is recognized that a patient may have several treating physicians in various circumstances. CMS defined specific situations in which physicians will be recognized as the "treating physician":

- An on-call physician with responsibility for a patient's care during a period when the patient's physician is unavailable

- A patient's primary care physician who refers the patient to a specialist
- A specialist who is managing only one aspect of a patient's care
- Different members of a group practice who treat a patient at different times

CMS allows two exceptions to the above requirements:

- X rays ordered by a physician to be used by a chiropractor to demonstrate subluxation of the spine for a patient receiving manual manipulation treatments
- Diagnostic mammograms ordered by a physician based on the findings of a screening mammogram even though the physician does not treat the patient

Supervision Regulations

New requirements became effective January 1, 1998, for physician supervision of diagnostic X ray and other diagnostic tests. The new rules apply only to the technical component of diagnostic procedures that are paid under the Medicare RBRVS payment schedule. (They do not apply to diagnostic procedures furnished to hospital patients nor to diagnostic laboratory tests.) All such diagnostic tests would require one of the three levels of appropriate physician supervision that CMS adopted: general, direct, or personal.

Diagnostic procedures, such as magnetic resonance imaging, procedures in which contrast materials are used, and certain X rays, would require general or direct supervision. Cardiovascular stress tests, cardiac catheterization, and radiological supervision and interpretation procedures either would require general supervision or must be performed personally by the physician. The List of Relative Value Units in Part 5 includes an indicator denoting the required level of physician supervision, as assigned by CMS, for all relevant CPT codes.

The statute exempts several diagnostic tests that would otherwise meet CMS' physician supervision requirements. These exceptions are diagnostic mammography procedures; diagnostic tests personally furnished by a qualified audiologist; diagnostic psychological testing services personally furnished by a clinical psychologist or a qualified independent psychologist; and diagnostic tests personally performed by some physical therapists, as specified by regulations.

The Balanced Budget Act of 1997 also removed the restriction on the areas and settings in which NPs, CNSs, and PAs may be paid under the physician payment schedule for services if furnished by a physician. CMS will modify the exceptions for diagnostic X ray and other diagnostic tests to specify that no physician supervision of NPs and CNSs is required for diagnostic tests performed by NPs and CNSs, when they are authorized by the state to perform these tests. CMS also changed regulations to state that diagnostic p5eir state scope of practice and applicable state law, provided they maintain the required statutory relationships with supervising or collaborating physicians. CMS made this updated supervision policy permanent for 2021 and beyond.

Purchased Diagnostic Tests

In accordance with legislative requirements, CMS eliminated the physician markup for diagnostic tests performed by an outside supplier and purchased by a physician. When billing for a purchased diagnostic test, the physician must identify the supplier and the supplier's provider number and the amount the supplier charged the billing physician. Patients may be charged only the applicable deductible and coinsurance amounts. CMS applies these provisions to the technical component for all physician pathology services purchased from another laboratory. Beginning January 1, 2010, CMS will implement a requirement that suppliers of the technical component of advanced imaging services be accredited. The accreditation requirement will apply to mobile units physicians' offices and independent diagnostic testing facilities that produce the images but will not apply to the physician who interprets them.

In the 1995 Final Rule, CMS announced that it would no longer allow separate payment by the carriers for transporting diagnostic equipment, except under specified circumstances. The rule, which applies CMS' policy for travel expenses to transportation of diagnostic equipment, holds that any costs for travel associated with providing a particular service are included in the practice expense RVUs for that service. CMS will allow separate payment only for the transportation of equipment used to perform X rays and diagnostic mammograms furnished by approved suppliers of portable X-ray services. These services are reported by HCPCS Level II code R0070 or R0075 and are paid at the carrier's discretion. Effective January 1, 1996, payment for transportation of electrocardiographic equipment was bundled into payment for the ECG service. Other transportation services may be billed on a "by report" basis with CPT code 99082, *Unusual travel (eg, transportation and escort of patient).*

Multiple Procedure Payment Reduction for Diagnostic Imaging and Therapy Services

CMS implemented a multiple procedure payment reduction (MPPR) for therapy services in 2011. This policy reduced payment by 20% for the practice expense component of the second and subsequent therapy services furnished by a single provider to a patient on a single day of service. This policy applied to all "always" therapy services, as defined by CMS.

Furthermore, beginning July 1, 2010, the Affordable Care Act mandated that CMS increase the MPPR for the technical component of certain single session imaging services to consecutive body areas from 25% to 50% for the second and subsequent imaging procedures performed in the same session. CMS has expanded the imaging services for which this reduction will apply.

For 2012, CMS expanded its MPPR policy to include the professional component, as well as the technical component for certain advanced imaging services (CT, MRI, and ultrasound). Under this new policy, CMS will make full payment for the professional component for the highest valued service of those provided to the same patient in the same session. Payment will be reduced by 25% for each additional advanced imaging service furnished in the session.

For 2013, CMS expanded its MPPR policy to the technical component of certain diagnostic cardiovascular and ophthalmologic services. In addition, effective April 1, 2013, Congress included a provision in the American Taxpayer Relief Act of 2012 (HR 8) that applied a 50% MPPR to outpatient therapy services. This was an increase from the 20% MPPR reduction that applied to office settings and 25% MPPR reduction that applied to facilities. However, these increases were only included as part of the SGR patch for 2013 and will not be carried forward by CMS.

Effective January 1, 2017, the Consolidated Appropriations Act, 2016 (Pub. L. 114-113, enacted on December 18, 2015) added a new section that revises the professional component (PC) of advanced imaging services payment reduction from 25% to 5%.

The Medicare MPPR applies to the following circumstances:

- 50% reduction for the second and subsequent surgical procedure(s) furnished to the same patient by the same physician on the same day
- 50% reduction to the technical component for the second and subsequent advanced imaging service(s) furnished to a patient by the same physician in the same session
- 5% reduction to the professional component for the second and subsequent advanced imaging service(s) furnished to a patient by the same physician in the same session
- 25% reduction to the technical component for the second and subsequent diagnostic cardiovascular service(s) furnished to a patient by the same physician in the same session
- 20% reduction to the technical component for the second and subsequent diagnostic ophthalmology service(s) furnished to a patient by the same physician on the same day
- 20% reduction to the practice expense component for the second and subsequent "always therapy" service(s) furnished by a physician or members of the same group in an office or non-institutional setting on the same day
- 25% reduction to the practice expense component for the second and subsequent "always therapy" service(s) furnished by a physician or group in an institutional setting on the same day.

Deficit Reduction Act Imaging Caps to Outpatient Prospective Payment System

Effective January 1, 2007, CMS implemented the Deficit Reduction Act (DRA) that affected payment for various imaging services in the payment schedule, including X ray, ultrasound, nuclear medicine, magnetic resonance imaging, computed tomography, and fluoroscopy but excluding diagnostic and screening mammography (see Appendix D for a complete list of all affected services). Carrier priced services will be impacted also by the DRA since these services are within the statutory definition of imaging services and are also within the statutory definition of an MFS service. The DRA states that payment for the technical component of imaging services paid under the Medicare MFS should be capped at the outpatient prospective payment system (OPPS) payment amount for the same imaging services. It is important to note that payment for an individual service, which is affected by the DRA, will only be capped if the MFS technical component payment amount exceeds the OPPS payment amount.

Interaction of Multiple Imaging Payment Reduction and OPPS Cap

For procedures that would be affected by both the multiple imaging payment reduction and the OPPS cap, CMS will first apply the multiple imaging payment reduction and then apply the OPPS cap to the reduced amount, because the OPPS payment rates may implicitly include some multiple imaging discounts.

Payment Incentive for the Transition from Traditional X-Ray Imaging to Digital Radiography

The Consolidated Appropriations Act of 2016 requires a payment reduction of 7% for the technical component for X rays obtained using computed radiography technology (cassette-based imaging) rather than digital radiography technology. Effective January 1, 2018, CMS required the use of modifier FY to identify imaging services utilizing computed radiography technology.

Pathology Services

Physician pathology services were placed on the payment schedule effective January 1, 1992. These services are usually provided in a hospital or independent laboratory. The professional component of these services includes study of the specimen and interpretation of test results, while technician preparation of the material constitutes the technical component. When a physician performs these services in a hospital, only the professional component may be billed by the physician; the technical component costs are included in the hospital's payment. In addition, a hospital laboratory furnishing surgical pathology services to nonhospital patients is acting as an independent laboratory and is paid under the MFS for the technical component services.

The technical component of physician pathology services refers to the preparation of the slide involving tissue or cells, which a pathologist will interpret. In the 2000 Final Rule, CMS stated, "We would pay only the hospital for the TC of physician pathology services furnished to a hospital inpatient." BIPA allowed certain qualified independent laboratories to continue to bill the Medicare contractor under the MFS for the TC of physician pathology services furnished to a hospital inpatient. H.R. 4994 Medicare and Medicaid Extenders Act of 2010 extended this provision through December 31, 2011. If the independent laboratory did not qualify under this provision, then it must continue to bill the hospital and receive payment from that hospital. In the 2012 *Final Notice*, CMS concluded that independent laboratories may not bill Medicare Contractors for the TC of physician pathology services provided after June 30, 2012, to a hospital inpatient or outpatient.

In the 1992 *Final Notice*, in response to recommendations from the College of American Pathologists, CMS increased the payment for the technical component of physician pathology services to 30% of the professional component of these services. The payment increase was based on cost data for the technical component of anatomic pathology services furnished by hospital laboratories. In recent years, pathology technical components have been included in the resource-based refinement process and, as those changes have been implemented, the relationship of the technical components to the professional components has become service specific.

The geographic practice cost indices (GPCIs) are used to adjust the technical component RVUs in the same way as described above for radiology and diagnostic tests.

Molecular Pathology

The AMA CPT Editorial Panel (Editorial Panel) created new codes to replace the "stacking" codes that were previously used to bill for molecular pathology services, which were deleted at the end of 2012. The new codes describe distinct molecular pathology tests and test methods and were divided into two tiers. Tier 1 codes describe common gene-specific and genomic procedures. Tier 2 codes capture reporting for less common tests. Tier 2 codes represent tests that the Editorial Panel determined as tests that involve similar technical resources and interpretative work. The Editorial Panel created 101 new molecular pathology CPT codes for 2012 and 14 new molecular pathology codes for 2013. In 2014, the scope of the molecular pathology services codes has also been substantially broadened with the addition of 316 molecular tests for detection of genes, somatic disorders, and germlines to the nine molecular pathology resource–based Tier II codes. Molecular pathology tests were previously billed using a combination of CPT codes that describe each of the various steps required to perform a given test. This billing method was referred to as "stacking" because different "stacks" of codes were billed depending on the components of the furnished test. These stacking codes were paid through the clinical laboratory payment schedule (CLFS), and one stacking code, CPT code 83912, was paid on both the CLFS and MFS payment for the interpretation and report of a molecular pathology test when furnished and billed by a physician was made under the MFS using the professional component (PC) or modifier 26 (*Professional Component*) of the CPT code set in conjunction with code 83912. Beginning in 2013, CMS determined that the molecular pathology CPT codes will be paid under the CLFS, and HCPCS code + will be paid under the MFS. For 2015, the Editorial Panel created 21 new codes that describe Genomic Sequencing Procedures (GSP). For 2016, the CPT Editorial Panel continued defining new molecular pathology and created nine Tier 1 codes, eight multianalyte assays with algorithmic analyses (MAAA) codes, and six GSP codes. The CPT Editorial Panel continues to define new drug testing, Tier 1 codes, GSP, and MAAA codes. For 2017, the CPT Editorial Panel created a new section, Proprietary Laboratory Analyses (PLA), which includes Advanced Diagnostic Laboratory Tests (ADLTs) and Clinical Diagnostic Laboratory Tests (CDLTs) as defined under PAMA, sole source tests or kits from a sole source, MAAAs and GSPs that are performed on humans and requested by the clinical laboratory or manufacturer that offers the test.

Pathology Clinical Consultation Services

Pathology clinical consultation services codes (80503-80506) describe pathologist clinical consultation services provided at the request of another physician or other qualified health care professional at the same or another facility or institution. These services may be reported when the following conditions are met:

- The pathologist renders a pathology clinical consultation at the request of a physician or other qualified health care professional at the same or another institution.
- The pathology clinical consultation request is related to pathology and laboratory findings or other relevant clinical or diagnostic information (eg, radiology findings or operative/procedural notes) that require additional medical interpretive judgment.

A pathologist may also render a pathology clinical consultation when mandated by federal or state regulation. A standing order is no longer accepted by Medicare carriers as a substitute for an individual request by the patient's attending physician. CMS eliminated the standing order policy effective January 1, 1998, to address concerns that Medicare may be allowing payment for medically unnecessary services.

Advanced Diagnostic Laboratory Tests (ADLTs) and Clinical Diagnostic Laboratory Tests (CDLTs)

Medicare Part B pays for clinical laboratory diagnostic tests using a payment schedule established by the local Medicare carrier for each test or procedure. Each payment schedule is set at 60% of the prevailing charge level in each area, but payments are capped by a "national limitation amount." Effective January 1, 1998, this national limit became 74% of the median of all the payment schedules established for each test.

Payment is made at 100% of the payment schedule amount, with no deductible or coinsurance required. The laboratory must accept assignment for the services performed (unless the services are rendered in a rural health clinic). Physicians must accept assignment for tests in their offices, but are not required to accept assignment for other Medicare covered services furnished, even if the other services are billed together with the laboratory services.

Physicians are prohibited from purchasing these tests and billing Medicare or Medicare patients. The laboratory that performs the test must bill Medicare for the test.

The CPT Editorial Panel (Panel) established a new code section to provide an infrastructure in which a clinical laboratory or manufacturer that meets certain criteria may request a code to identify their test more specifically. This section is separate from the Category I Pathology and Laboratory section, and it will include ADLTs and CDLTs, as defined under PAMA. The clinical laboratory or manufacturer that offers the test must request the code. It is envisioned that the codes in this new section will be issued on a quarterly basis and effective the following quarter to allow payers time to load them into their systems. The Panel would be responsible for verification of the information submitted and codification of tests in this section. The Panel will not determine whether the test meets the criteria of an ADLT, which will be determined by CMS. This new section provides a sustainable coding infrastructure utilizing an established, transparent process that will ensure consistent national coding across Medicare and other public and private payers. This solution represents the longstanding commitment of the Panel to ensure the CPT code set provides a uniform language and meets the needs of a broad cross-section of stakeholders.

Clinical Laboratory Interpretation Services

The 1991 Final Rule created a new category of pathology service, clinical laboratory interpretation services. CMS has identified several clinical laboratory codes for which a separate payment under the payment schedule can be made. These codes are found in the Pathology and Laboratory section of the List of Relative Value Units.

The services are payable under the payment schedule if they are furnished to a patient by a hospital pathologist or independent laboratory. Payment criteria for these codes are as follows:

- The attending physician requests the interpretation service. (A hospital's standing order policy also fulfills this requirement.)
- The service results in a written report.
- The service requires the medical judgment of the pathologist.
- Modifier 26, *Professional Component*, should be included with the clinical laboratory test code.

Payment for Supplies, Services, and Drugs Furnished Incident to a Physician's Service

Separate payment is made for services that are incidental to a physician's service and for supplies for specified services, when provided in the office setting.

Supplies

Office medical supplies are generally considered by CMS to be practice expenses, and payment is included in the practice expense portion of the service or procedure for which they were provided. Such supplies are considered incident-to the physician's service. For example, surgical dressings are considered incident-to, when they are furnished during an office visit to treat a patient's accidental cut or scrape.

Separate payment is allowed for surgical dressings furnished to treat a wound resulting from a surgical procedure performed by the physician, or after debridement of a wound. CMS has clarified that primary surgical dressings are covered, as long as they are medically necessary.

CMS also allows separate payment for supplies used to treat fractures or dislocations. Separate payment is allowed for splints, casts, and other devices, if provided in the physician's office. These supplies are separately payable under the reasonable charge payment methodology.

Beginning in 2001, the casting supplies were removed from the practice expenses for all HCPCS codes, including the CPT codes for fracture management and for casts and splints. For settings in which CPT codes are used to pay for services that include the provision for a cast or splint, new temporary codes were established to pay physicians and other practitioners for the supplies used in creating casts. The work and practice expenses involved in the creation of the cast or splint should continue to be coded using the appropriate CPT code. The use of the temporary codes will replace less specific coding for the casting and splinting supplies.

Durable Medical Equipment

Durable medical equipment (DME) refers to such items as wheelchairs, crutches, and other equipment that is used repeatedly, as well as to such items as surgical dressings and urologic supplies. The DME is covered under Medicare Part B when furnished to a patient for use in the home if it is considered reasonable and medically necessary. Medicare payment for inexpensive and other routinely purchased DME is made according to a payment schedule, effective January 1993, which is based solely on CMS' estimate of the national cost for purchasing the item. Prior to 1994, physicians and other suppliers submitted claims for DME to the local Medicare Part B carrier. In response to Congressional concerns about fraud and abuse and to streamline administrative operations, however, CMS consolidated DME claims processing from local Medicare carriers into four DME regional carriers (DMERC).

Under the revised DMERC policies, physicians and suppliers, who sell or rent DME, prosthetics, orthotics, and other supplies (DMEPOS) must obtain a separate Medicare "supplier" identification number and submit claims to the appropriate DMERC. Jurisdiction for DMERC claims submission is based on the beneficiary's permanent address.

The AMA opposed this policy because its requirements add significantly to the administrative burden on physician practices. The AMA believes that low-cost supplies should be exempt from DME regulatory requirements. In response, CMS removed some of these supplies from the DME payment schedule.

Incident-to Services

Medicare covers services that are provided incident-to a physician's service by a nonphysician employee and pays for them under the payment schedule as if the physician performed the services. Coverage of incident-to services applies to part- and full-time nonphysician employees, such as nurses, psychologists, technicians, and therapists, and to licensed nonphysician practitioners. Services provided by leased employees may also be billed under the incident-to provision, effective October 1, 1996. Leased employees must work under a written agreement with the supervising physician or group practice.

Incident-to services must be provided in the physician's office under the direct personal supervision of the physician, although such supervision does not require the presence of the physician in the same room with the physician assistant or other nonphysician employee (unless otherwise provided by state law). CMS has indicated that to satisfy the direct supervision requirements, the physician must be immediately available to provide the nonphysician employee with assistance and directions, if needed. Furthermore, CMS guidelines state that patient contact is not required of the physician on each occasion that a nonphysician employee provides a service. According to CMS, the requirement would be met, if the physician initiates the course of treatment and provides subsequent services that reflect his or her active participation in managing the patient's treatment.

CMS broadened the application of the incident-to payment provision in 1993 to include services "ordinarily performed by the physician," such as physical exams, minor surgery, setting casts or simple fractures, and reading X rays. Before adopting this policy, CMS defined reimbursable incident-to services very narrowly, for example, administering injections, taking blood pressures and temperatures, and changing dressings.

The Balanced Budget Act of 1997 included changes to Medicare requirements for payment for services furnished by nurse practitioners, clinical nurse specialists, and physician assistants. Effective January 1, 1998, these practitioners are no longer required to work under the direct, personal supervision of an MD or DO. In addition, nurse practitioners and clinical nurse specialists may receive payment for services directly from Medicare at 85% of the MFS.

In the Final Rule for 2014, CMS adopted a new condition of payment imposing a requirement to comply with state laws for services furnished incident to a physician's or other practitioner's professional services. This requirement will protect the health and safety of Medicare beneficiaries and allow for the ability to recover federal dollars when care is not delivered in accordance with state laws. Further discussion of the changes made to payment for services of nonphysician practitioners under the Balanced Budget Act is available in "Payment for Nonphysicians." In the Final Rule for 2016, CMS amended the definition of the term, "auxiliary personnel" that are permitted to provide incident-to services to exclude individuals who have been excluded from the Medicare program or have had their Medicare enrollment revoked in §410.26(a)(1). CMS also amended §410.26(b)(5) by revising the final sentence to make clear that the physician (or other practitioner) directly supervising the auxiliary personnel need not be the same physician (or other practitioner) that is treating the patient more broadly and adding a sentence to specify that only the physician (or other practitioner) that supervises the auxiliary personnel that provide incident-to services may bill Medicare Part B for those incident-to services.

Drugs

Drugs provided on an outpatient basis are covered under Part B as incident-to a physician's service. Payment for drugs is limited to those that cannot be self-administered, generally drugs that must be administered by injection.

Prior to January 1, 1998, payment for drugs and biologicals not paid on a cost or prospective payment basis was based on the lower of the billed charge or the average wholesale price (AWP). The median of the average national wholesale generic prices was used for drugs with multiple sources.

Effective January 1, 1998, Medicare payment for such drugs is the lower of the actual charge or 95% of the AWP. Physician payments for drugs provided on an incident-to basis are subject to limiting charge restrictions.

Effective January 1, 2003, CMS implemented a new national Medicare payment system for drugs administered in physician offices. CMS contracted with one carrier to establish these rates on a quarterly basis. This new system is referred to as the "single drug pricer" (SDP) and is based on 95% AWP of the drug, as computed by this contracted carrier.

The Medicare Prescription Drug, Improvement, and Modernization Act (MMA) of 2003 modifies payment for drugs. Effective January 1, 2004, payment for Part B drugs is set at 85% of AWP from April 1, 2003. In 2005, a new payment system established drug payments at the average sales price plus 6%. There are some exceptions to this payment methodology (including blood clotting factors, certain vaccines, and ESRD drugs).

The MMA required CMS to evaluate the existing drug administration codes to ensure accurate reporting and payment for these services. All expenditure changes resulting from any coding review or relative value changes in 2005 and 2006 are exempt from budget-neutrality requirements.

The CPT Editorial Panel conducted an extensive effort, beginning in February 2004, to review the current coding structure for all drug administration services. This review process included the formation of a special workgroup, public meetings, and an extensive discussion by the Editorial Panel in finalizing changes at its August 2004 meeting. As the *CPT 2005* codebook had already been published by this date, the new CPT codes were not published. CMS, however, accepted these new codes and assigned temporary alphanumeric HCPCS "G" codes for use during 2005. In the *CPT 2006* codebook, these "G" codes were converted to Category I codes.

The AMA/Specialty Society RVS Update Committee (RUC) considered these new codes on an expedited basis and was able to submit recommendations to CMS in October 2004. CMS accepted 100% of RUC's recommendations related to all three categories of drug administration services: hydration; therapeutic or diagnostic injections and intravenous infusions; and chemotherapy injections and intravenous infusions. In addition, CMS agreed to assign physician work to the immunization administration codes.

In 2005, CMS also conducted a one-year demonstration project to identify and assess oncology services in an office-based oncology practice with the intent to positively affect outcomes in the Medicare population. Physicians who provide chemotherapy intravenous push or infusion services to oncology patients were allowed to automatically participate in this demonstration project by submitting three "G" codes, one for each assessment and intervention if appropriate, of the following patient status factors: nausea and/or vomiting, lack of energy (fatigue), and pain. Upon submission of these three "G" codes, the physician received an additional payment of $130 per patient encounter.

This demonstration project was modified and extended for 2006. The existing "G" codes associated with the 2005 demonstration project were deleted and new "G" codes were created. The 2006 demonstration project focused on the evaluation and management visits that a physician reported for an established patient with a specific form of cancer. When a physician reported one of the applicable "G" codes for each of the following three categories: (1) primary focus of the E/M service; (2) current disease state; and (3) whether current management adheres to clinical guidelines in coordination with an evaluation and management service, the physician qualified for a $23 oncology demonstration payment. This demonstration project ended December 31, 2006.

Vaccinations. Vaccinations and inoculations are covered if they are directly related to treatment of an injury or to direct exposure to a disease (for example, antirabies or tetanus); if furnished as preventive immunizations (for example, smallpox or polio), they are not covered. There are several exceptions to this limitation, however:

- *Blood clotting factors* for hemophilia are covered even when self-administered; supplies related to the administration of blood clotting factors are also covered.
- *Pneumococcal pneumonia and influenza* vaccines are covered for all patients. Hepatitis B vaccine is covered for patients at risk of contracting hepatitis B.
- *Immunosuppressive therapy* drugs are covered when administered to an organ transplant recipient within 36 months after the date of the transplant. (The "date of transplant" is defined by CMS as the date of discharge from the hospital.) Drugs not directly related to rejection control, such as antibiotics that can be self-administered, are not covered.
- *Osteoporosis drugs* and their administration, under certain conditions, are covered even if they may be self-administered. The drug must be injectable and used for treatment of a bone fracture related to postmenopausal osteoporosis.
- *Oral cancer* drugs are covered, effective January 1, 1994, even when self-administered, if they contain anticancer chemotherapeutic agents having the same active ingredients and are used for the same indications as anticancer drugs that are covered when administered intravenously. Four drugs currently meet the above requirements: cyclophosphamide tablets, etoposide capsules, methotrexate tablets, and melphalan tablets. Medicare allows individual carrier approval for "off-label" uses of oral anticancer drugs in an anticancer chemotherapy regimen, if the carrier determines that their use is generally considered medically acceptable. To reduce regional variations among carriers, OBRA 93 established specific criteria for medical acceptability of off-label uses: supported by at least one of the three major drug compendia; not listed as "not indicated" in any of the three compendia; or supported by clinical research that appears in peer-reviewed medical literature.

As part of the Tax Relief and Health Care Act of 2006, for 2007, the administration payment for Part D vaccines would be covered by Part B. Beginning January 1, 2008, the administration payment would be paid by the same Part D plan that pays for the vaccine itself.

Antigens. As a result of changes made in OBRA 93, antigen services are paid under the MFS, effective for services furnished on or after January 1, 1995. At the same time, CMS announced that it would delete the Level II HCPCS "J" codes for antigen services, and no longer recognize the complete service codes (CPT codes 95120-95134). Physicians may bill only CPT codes 95144-95149, 95165, and 95170 representing the antigen extract itself and the physician's professional service in creating the extract.

Vaccine Administration Services. In 2021, the AMA's CPT Editorial Panel (the Panel) created numerous new CPT codes for SARS-CoV-2 vaccines and immunization administration. The RUC developed recommendations related to the physician work and resource costs related to the provision of SARS-CoV-2 immunization administration.

CMS will maintain the current payment rate of $40 per dose for the administration of COVID-19 vaccines throughout the entire year in which the PHE ends. This value considers the approximate $10 increase for additional supplies, materials, and clinical staff time as encompassed in CPT code 99072, *Additional supplies, materials, and clinical staff time over and above those usually included in an office visit or other non-facility service(s), when performed during a Public Health Emergency, as defined by law, due to respiratory-transmitted infectious disease*, which CMS established as a bundled service on an interim basis in the CY 2021 Final Rule. The AMA continues to believe that payment for code 99072 should be fully funded, recognizing the additional supplies and new staff activities required to provide safe care during the PHE, and not be subject to budget neutrality. When the PHE ends, the payment rate for COVID-19 vaccine administration will be aligned with the $30 rate for other preventive vaccines. CMS also finalized a policy to continue the additional payment of $35.50 when a COVID-19 vaccine is administered in a beneficiary's home under certain circumstances until the end of the year in which the PHE ends.

In May 2021, the RUC submitted recommendations to CMS to increase payment for the administration of all other preventive vaccines for children and adults. CMS will defer the review of the RUC recommendations until the 2023 rulemaking process. However, CMS did consider the RUC recommendations in establishing a new payment rate for preventive immunization administration provided to Medicare patients. Therefore, in the Final Rule for CY 2022, CMS states its belief that "it is appropriate to finalize a payment rate that approximates the RUC's estimates of the costs involved in the typical case of COVID-19 vaccine administration after the PHE." Hence, beginning on January 1, 2022, payment will increase to $30 for the administration of an influenza, pneumococcal, or hepatitis B vaccine under the Medicare Part B vaccine benefit.

Payment for Nonphysicians

In addition to incident-to services, the Medicare program provides separate coverage and payment for limited license practitioners and eleven categories of nonphysician practitioners. The categories of nonphysician practitioners include the following:

- Chiropractors
- Physical/occupational therapists (PT/OTs)
- Speech language pathologists (SLPs)
- Audiologists
- Physician assistants (PAs)
- Nurse practitioners (NPs) and clinical nurse specialists (CNSs)
- Certified nurse midwives (CNMs)
- Certified registered nurse anesthetists (CRNAs)
- Clinical psychologists
- Clinical social workers (CSWs)
- Registered dietitians

As discussed in the next sections, the payment rules governing these services vary considerably according to such factors as site of service, medical supervision, and other circumstances.

Limited License Practitioners

The MFS applies to optometrists, chiropractors, dentists, oral and maxillofacial surgeons, and podiatrists when they furnish the specific services for which long-standing provisions of the Medicare law consider them to be physicians.

All carriers have implemented nationally standardized payment practices for nonphysician practitioners by using CPT codes for these services, where applicable; in all other instances, the appropriate HCPCS code is maintained. Payment amounts for each nonphysician category will be calculated by carriers. CMS uses the specialty designation of these nonphysician practitioners to collect and analyze data on the services they provide.

Approved amount for nonphysicians' services under the payment schedule are tied to approved amount for physicians' services in the locality. That is, the payment schedule for nonphysicians' services is implemented in the same manner as the payment schedule for physicians' services. In the section that follows, therefore, the term *payment schedule* refers to the full Medicare payment schedule amount for a particular physician's service in the locality.

Chiropractors

CPT codes for chiropractic manipulative treatment (CPT codes 98940-98943) were introduced in CPT 1997. In assigning work RVUs to these services, CMS accepted the recommendation of the RUC Health Care Professionals Advisory Committee (HCPAC) Review Board that these codes represented services and work essentially parallel to those of the osteopathic manipulation treatment (OMT) codes (CPT codes 98925-98929). Thus, the same RVUs were assigned to chiropractic manipulative treatment as for osteopathic manipulative treatment. In February 2011, RUC reviewed the OMT codes, which resulted in work RVUs increases. At that time, RUC and CMS agreed that there was compelling evidence that these services were based on flawed methodologies when established by Harvard. For CPT 2014, CMS again accepted the RUC recommendations that it is appropriate to crosswalk the CMT codes to the OMT codes. It is important to note that CPT code 98943 is not recognized for payment by Medicare.

Effective January 1, 2000, Medicare no longer required an X ray to show a subluxation of the spine for coverage of treatment. Medicare now pays for a chiropractic manual manipulation of the spine to correct a subluxation if the subluxation has resulted in a neuromusculoskeletal condition for which manipulation is appropriate treatment.

Currently, Medicare reimburses three CPT codes provided by chiropractors: 98940 for manipulative treatment of 1–2 regions of the spine; 98941, manipulative treatment of 3–4 regions of the spine; and 98942, manipulative treatment of 5 regions of the spine. In the November 21, 2005, Final Rule, CMS included a discussion of a two-year demonstration project authorized by the MMA, which would determine whether additional chiropractic services should be covered under Medicare, such as diagnostic and other services that a chiropractor is authorized to perform. This budget-neutral demonstration occurred at the following sites: Maine; New Mexico; Scott County, Iowa; 26 counties in Illinois; and 17 counties in central Virginia. This demonstration project ended March 31, 2007. In 2010, CMS announced that this demonstration project was not budget-neutral, and it cost the Agency $50 million. CMS recouped the cost of this demonstration project by reducing the payment of chiropractic CPT codes (98940, 98941 and 98942) by 2% between 2010 and 2014.

Physical/Occupational Therapists

The CPT codes for physical medicine services were substantially revised for the CPT 1995 and work RVU recommendations were developed according to RUC process. The 1995 work RVUs established for these codes represented the first time that work RVUs for physical medicine services had been based on the work associated with furnishing the service. Previously, work RVUs for the physical medicine codes were based on historic charges. CMS indicated in the 1995 Final Rule, however, that CPT codes 97545 and 97546 would continue to be carrier priced until better definitions for these services are developed.

The full range of CPT codes 97010 through 97799 may be reported by occupational and physical therapists in independent practice, if the service is within the scope of practice. Payment for these services is made according to the Medicare payment schedule. Physical and occupational therapy services must be furnished as part of a written treatment plan, which the physician or therapist caring for the patient establishes, and the provider of the services must be qualified within the state's scope-of-practice laws.

A new CPT code was established for CPT 1999 to describe manual therapy techniques, including mobilization and manipulation. It was expected that the primary users of new code 97140 would be physical and occupational therapists, as it was a better way to describe the spectrum of services they provide. This new code was developed after two years of discussion by the Manual Therapy Techniques Workgroup, which recommended distinct coding nomenclature for osteopathic manipulative treatment (OMT), chiropractic manipulative treatment (CMT), and manual therapy techniques performed by physical therapists and occupational therapists. The new code replaced five codes (97122, 97250, 97260, 97261, 97265).

Effective January 1, 1999, all outpatient physical therapy services including outpatient speech-language pathology were to be subject to an annual cap of $1500 per Medicare beneficiary according to the *Federal Register* published November 2, 1998. The cap would apply to all outpatient therapy except for therapy provided in hospital outpatient departments. The Balanced Budget Refinement Act placed a moratorium on Medicare Part B outpatient therapy caps until January 1, 2003. Litigation further delayed implementation.

In the December 31, 2002, Final Rule, CMS indicated that it would implement the outpatient rehabilitation therapy financial limitation via a program memorandum (AB-03-018) to carriers and fiscal intermediaries. Outpatient rehabilitation claims for services rendered on or after September 1, 2003, and before December 8, 2003, were subject to the payment limitation indexed to inflation at $1590 per year per patient.

The MMA, signed into law on December 8, re-established the moratorium on the therapy cap until December 31, 2005.

CMS announced in the November 21, 2005, Final Rule that an annual, per beneficiary combined cap on outpatient physical therapy, speech-language pathology, and occupational therapy services performed under Medicare Part B would be implemented January 1, 2006. The original cap for 1999–2001 was set at $1500. It was determined that for years after 2001, the therapy cap would be equal to the preceding year's cap increased by the percentage increase in the MEI. It should also be noted that physical therapy services performed by chiropractors under the chiropractor demonstration project were subject to the therapy cap as well.

The DRA of 2005 initiated an exceptions process for beneficiaries who exceed the therapy cap. Medically necessary therapy services beyond the therapy cap can be obtained in two ways: an automated exception or a manual exception. The automated exception process requires no specific or additional documentation, and no request is required on behalf of the beneficiary or provider. The automated exceptions process is designated using modifier KX to the claim. The manual exception process includes a manual application, which requires a written request by the beneficiary or provider for patients who do not qualify for an automated exception. This process will use medical review by the CMS contractor responsible for processing the claim. Originally, this exception process was to be employed only in 2006, but the utilization of this process was extended several times through subsequent legislation. Specifically, as part of the Tax Relief and Health Care Act of 2006, it was extended through 2007. The process was again extended through June 30, 2008, by the Medicare, Medicaid, and SCHIP Extension Act of 2007, and again from July 1, 2008, through December 31, 2009, by § 141 of the MIPPA of 2008. The Affordable Care Act extended the exception process from January 1, 2010, through December 31, 2010. The Medicare and Medicaid Extenders Act of 2010 extended the exceptions process from January 1, 2011, through December 31, 2011. An additional two-month extension, through February 29, 2012, was granted due to the Temporary Payroll Tax Cut Continuation Act of 2011. The exception process was extended through December 31, 2013, by the American Taxpayer Relief Act. Most recently, MACRA extended the therapy caps exceptions process through December 31, 2017, and modified the requirement for manual medical review for services over the $3700 therapy thresholds. MACRA also extended the application of the therapy caps and related provisions to outpatient hospitals until January 1, 2018. The Bipartisan Budget Act of 2018, effective January 1, 2018, repealed the application of the Medicare outpatient therapy caps and the therapy cap exceptions process while retaining and adding limitations to ensure therapy services are furnished when appropriate. After expenses for therapy service for the year have exceeded the previous therapy cap amounts, providers should continue to use the KX modifier on claims for subsequent services. For 2018-2028, the KX modifier threshold amount is $3000. A targeted medical review (MR) process (first established through MACRA at a threshold amount of $3700) may be initiated for claims over the threshold amount. For more information on the manual medical review process, please visit www.cms.gov/Research-Statistics-Data-and-Systems/Monitoring-Programs/Medical-Review/TherapyCap.html.

CMS implemented a multiple procedure payment reduction for therapy services beginning on January 1, 2011. This policy reduces payment by 20% for the practice expense component of the second and subsequent therapy services furnished by a single provider to a patient on a single day of service. This policy will be applied to all "always" therapy services, as defined by CMS.

The Bipartisan Budget Act of 2018 requires payment for services performed entirely or partially by a therapy assistant at 85% of the MFS payment starting on January 1, 2022. CMS created two new payment modifiers, CQ and CO, to be used with the current physical therapy and occupational therapy modifiers. Modifier CQ identifies services furnished in whole or in part by a physical therapist assistant (PTA) and modifier CO identifies services furnished in whole or in part by an occupational therapy assistant (OTA). As finalized, the modifiers are to be used when a therapy assistant performs more than 10% of a service (a 10% "*de minimis* standard"). These two modifiers are required starting January 2020 and CMS will apply the 15 percent payment reduction to therapy services provided by PTAs (using modifier CQ) or OTAs (using modifier CO), as required by statute effective January 1, 2022. In the CY 2022 final rule, CMS finalizes refinements to clarify the de minimis policy.

Requirements for these modifiers were revised and clarified in the CY 2020 Final Rule (CMS-1715-F). Modifiers CQ and CO are not required if a therapy assistant is involved in the entire duration of the service alongside a physical or occupational therapist. These modifiers will not be applied to the total time of the service, but rather to each 15-minute unit of codes.

For 2021, CMS permanently granted PTs and OTs the discretion to delegate the performance of maintenance therapy services, as clinically appropriate, to a therapy assistant, either a PTA or an OTA. This policy allows PTs or OTs to use the same discretion to delegate therapy-services maintenance to PTAs or OTAs that they utilize for rehabilitative services.

Speech Language Pathologists and Audiologists

Beginning July 15, 2008, Medicare no longer differentiates between audiologists and speech language pathologists, in that SLPs are now recognized by Medicare as independent practitioners who can independently bill for diagnostic audiologic tests. Section 143 of the MIPPA of 2008 specifies that SLPs may enroll independently as suppliers of Medicare services. Starting July 1, 2009, SLPs may begin independently report outpatient services they provide to Medicare patients. Amendments to §1848 of the Social Security Act do not create a separate therapy cap for SLP services. The therapy cap for 2018 is $2010 per beneficiary.

The American Speech-Language-Hearing Association (ASHA) met with CMS on September 8, 2006, and requested that CMS agree to consider establishing physician work relative values for services provided by audiologists. ASHA specifically requested that the professional work effort for audiologists providing these services be reflected in the work relative values, rather than in the practice expense relative values. CMS responded to ASHA on November 14, 2006, and indicated that they agree to further consider this possibility. CMS advised RUC and HCPAC that if the committee recommends the use of work values for the audiology services, CMS would consider their recommendations. RUC reviewed and accepted consensus recommendations for nine audiology services, as submitted by ASHA and the American Academy of Otolaryngology-Head and Neck Surgery (AAO-HNS). In the Final Rule, published on November 27, 2007, CMS assigned physician work RVUs to these nine audiology services. ASHA and AAO-HNS used the work RVUs assigned to these services as reference points, when establishing work RVUs for the remaining audiology services, which were reviewed for the CPT 2011 cycle. New, revised, and potentially misvalued audiology services continue to be valued with work RVUs today.

Physician Assistants

The Balanced Budget Act of 1997 eliminated the Medicare requirement that PAs practice under the direct, physical supervision of an MD/DO. The provision allows states to determine the required level of supervision; most states call for the physician to be accessible to the PA by electronic communication. The 2020 CMS Final Rule revised regulations on physician supervision for physician assistant services, so that the statutory physician supervision requirement for PA services is met when a PA furnishes their services in accordance with state law and state scope of practice rules for PAs in the state in which the services are furnished. If there is no state law governing physician supervision of PA services, Medicare will require documenting at the practice level the PA's scope of practice and the working relationship the PA has with the supervising physician/s when furnishing professional services.

PAs can maintain their relationships with physicians, but they can also be considered independent contractors of physicians, which previously was not allowed. Payment would continue to be made through the PA's employer, which could be a physician or medical group. Payment would be the lower of the 85% of the Medicare RBRVS or the actual charge. Medicare payment would be the same regardless of practice location. Previously, payment varied according to practice setting or whether performed in a rural Health Professional Shortage Area.

During the COVID-19 PHE, CMS allowed NPs, CNSs, PAs, and CNMs to supervise the performance of diagnostic tests, in addition to physicians, within their state scope of practice and applicable state law, provided they maintain the required statutory relationships with supervising or collaborating physicians. CMS made this updated supervision policy permanent for 2021 and beyond.

For CY 2022, CMS is implementing the change from the Consolidated Appropriations Act, 2021 (section 403), which removed the requirement to make payment for PA services only to the employer of a PA, effective January 1, 2022. This will allow PAs to bill the Medicare program, be paid directly for their services, reassign their rights to payment for their services, and incorporate as a group comprised solely of practitioners in their specialty and bill Medicare. This change impacts the statutory billing construct for PA services; however, it does not change the statutory benefit category for PA services, including the requirement that PA services are performed under physician supervision or collaboration and in accordance with state scope of practice laws, nor does it change the statutory payment percentage applicable to PA services.

Nurse Practitioners and Clinical Nurse Specialists

The Balanced Budget Act of 1997 also allows NPs and CNSs to practice without the direct, physical supervision of an MD/DO, and furthermore, allows these practitioners to receive direct Medicare payment. Medicare payment continues to be the lesser of the 85% of the Medicare RBRVS or the actual charge and does not vary by practice setting. However, as outlined in the November 2, 1998, *Federal Register*, beginning January 1, 1999, both NPs and CNSs must meet newly expanded certification requirements to be able to bill Medicare for their services.

A Nurse Practitioner must now meet the following qualifications: (1) Possess a master's degree in nursing; (2) Be a registered professional nurse who is authorized by the state in which the services are furnished to practice as a NP in accordance with state law, and; (3) Be certified as a nurse practitioner by the American Nurses Credentialing Center or other recognized national certifying bodies that have established standards for nurse practitioners.

Clinical Nurse Specialists must also meet similar qualifications to bill for Medicare Part B coverage of his or her services including: (1) Be a registered nurse who is currently licensed to practice in the state where he or she practices and be authorized to perform the services of a clinical nurse specialist in accordance with state law; (2) Have a master's degree in a defined clinical area of nursing from an accredited educational institution; and (3) Be certified as a clinical nurse specialist by the American Nurses Credentialing Center.

The new rules in the November 2, 1998, *Federal Register* also outlined the policy for NPs and CNSs in states with no regulations on their collaboration with a physician(s), as such that "NPs and CNSs must document their scope of practice and indicate the relationships that they have with physicians to deal with issues outside their scope of practice."

In the Final Rule for 2009, CMS announced that Medicare will recognize advanced practice nurses with more extensive education and experience (ie, Doctor of Nursing Practice [DNP] doctoral degree, which can be obtained without a master's degree in nursing), while continuing to recognize NPs and CNSs with a master's degree in nursing. NPs or CNSs with a doctoral degree in nursing practice will not be denied enrollment in the Medicare program because of the educational standard of a master's degree for NPs and CNSs.

During the COVID-19 PHE, CMS allowed NPs, CNSs, PAs, and CNMs to supervise the performance of diagnostic tests, in addition to physicians, within their state scope of practice and applicable state law, provided they maintain the required statutory relationships with supervising or collaborating physicians. CMS made this updated supervision policy permanent for 2021 and beyond.

Certified Nurse Midwives

Effective January 1, 1994, payment may be made for services provided by a nurse midwife as authorized by state law, including obstetric and gynecologic services, if otherwise covered when provided by a physician. Beginning January 1, 2011, the Affordable Care Act mandated that nurse midwives be paid at 100% of the MFS amount. Services must be provided on an assignment basis.

During the COVID-19 PHE, CMS allowed NPs, CNSs, PAs, and CNMs to supervise the performance of diagnostic tests, in addition to physicians, within their state scope of practice and applicable state law, provided they maintain the required statutory relationships with supervising or collaborating physicians. CMS made this updated supervision policy permanent for 2021 and beyond.

See Table 11-1 for a summary of nonphysician payment policies.

Certified Registered Nurse Anesthetists

The same relative value scale (RVS) is used to determine payment for both physician anesthesia services and certified registered nurse anesthetist services. The conversion factor for a nonmedically directed CRNA will be limited to the anesthesia CF applicable in that locality. All services must be furnished on an assignment basis. Beginning in 1998, Medicare pays on a uniform basis for the provision of anesthesia services, whether performed by a physician alone or with a team. For 2013, CMS clarified the definition of the Medicare benefit category for CRNAs, as including

Table 11-1. Nurse and Physician Assistant Payment

Practitioner	Medicare	Medicaid	Private Payers	Medicare Supervision Requirements
Nurse Practitioner (NP)	Pays 85% of the Medicare RBRVS, 100% if billed incident-to in a physician office or clinic	Pays in all states. Some states mandate payment at the physician rate. Some states pay at a reduced percentage of the physician rate.	Varies. Some states mandate payment at physician rate. Some payments made to the physician or employer. Twenty-nine states require insurers to reimburse directly.	Supervision requirements defer to state law for advance practice nurses. In most circumstances, NPs must collaborate with a physician, meaning that the NP works with a physician to deliver health care services within the scope of the practitioner's professional expertise, with medical direction and appropriate supervision as provided in jointly developed guidelines or other mechanism as defined by the law of the state in which the services are performed. They may supervise the performance of diagnostic tests, in addition to physicians, within their state scope of practice and applicable state law, provided they maintain the required statutory relationships with supervising or collaborating physicians.
Clinical Nurse Specialist (CNS)	Pays 85% of the Medicare RBRVS, 100% if billed incident-to in a physician office or clinic	Varies by state. CNSs treated as RNs in certain states and not eligible for reimbursement	Varies. Some states mandate payment at physician rate. Some payments made to the physician or employer. Thirty-seven states require insurers to reimburse directly.	Supervision requirements defer to state law for advance practice nurses. In most circumstances, CNSs must collaborate with a physician, meaning that the CNS works with a physician to deliver health care services within the scope of the practitioner's professional expertise, with medical direction and appropriate supervision as provided in jointly developed guidelines or other mechanism as defined by the law of the state in which the services are performed. They may supervise the performance of diagnostic tests, in addition to physicians, within their state scope of practice and applicable state law, provided they maintain the required statutory relationships with supervising or collaborating physicians.
Certified Nurse Midwife (CNM)	Pays 100% of the Medicare RBRVS	Pays in all states. Some states mandate payment at physician rate. Some states pay at a reduced percentage of the physician rate.	Varies. Some states mandate payment at physician rate. Some payments made to the physician or employer. Thirty-seven states require insurers to reimburse directly.	Supervision requirements defer to state law for advance practice nurses. CNMs may practice independently, but most state require some form of physician collaboration. They may supervise the performance of diagnostic tests, in addition to physicians, within their state scope of practice and applicable state law, provided they maintain the required statutory relationships with supervising or collaborating physicians.
Physician Assistant (PA)	Pays 85% of the Medicare RBRVS, 100% if billed incident to in a physician office or clinic	Pays in all states. Some states mandate payment at physician rate. Some states pay at a reduced percentage of the physician rate.	Varies. Payments are made to a PA's employer. Eleven states require insurers to cover services performed by a PA.	Supervision requirements for PA services is met when a PA furnishes services in accordance with state law and state scope of practice rules for PAs in the state in which the services are furnished. They may supervise the performance of diagnostic tests, in addition to physicians, within their state scope of practice and applicable state law, provided they maintain the required statutory relationships with supervising or collaborating physicians.

any services the CRNA is permitted to furnish under their state's scope of practice. In addition, this action resulted in CRNAs being treated similarly to other advanced practice nurses for Medicare purposes. This policy is consistent with the Institute of Medicine's recommendation that Medicare cover services provided by advanced practice nurses to the full extent of their state scope of practice. "Anesthesia and related care" under the statutory benefit for CRNA services is defined as follows: "Anesthesia and related care means those services that a certified registered nurse anesthetist is legally authorized to perform in the state in which the services are furnished." CMS will continue to monitor state scope of practice laws for CRNAs to ensure that they do not expand beyond the appropriate bounds of "anesthesia and related care" for purposes of the Medicare program. The aforementioned proposal does not address payment rates for anesthesiologists or CRNAs. The statutory provisions that establish payment rates for CRNAs at the same rate as anesthesiologists are relatively longstanding.

Clinical Psychologists

Medicare payment for diagnostic and therapeutic services provided by clinical psychologists was linked to the Medicare RBRVS payment schedule, effective January 1, 1997. Payment for such services is at 100% of the Medicare RBRVS. Previously, Medicare paid only for psychological testing services under the RBRVS payment schedule and paid for therapeutic services according to locality-based payment schedules determined by Medicare carriers. Diagnostic services provided by practitioners who do not meet the requirements for a clinical psychologist continue to be paid on a reasonable charge basis.

As part of the five-year review of the Medicare RBRVS, CMS developed 24 temporary HCPCS Level II codes for reporting psychotherapy services. These codes differentiate by the type of psychotherapy services provided, as well as the setting in which the service is furnished. They also allow psychotherapy services to be reported with and without medical evaluation and management services.

Only psychiatrists may perform and bill those codes that include medical evaluation and management. Clinical psychologists are not licensed to provide such services to Medicare patients, and therefore, may report only those codes involving nonmedical evaluation services. All services must be provided on an assignment basis. Diagnostic tests performed by an independently practicing psychologist (who is not a clinical psychologist) are paid, as are other diagnostic tests, if ordered by a physician. Clinical psychologist services, other than diagnostic services, furnished outside of the hospital inpatient setting are subject to the mental health services limitation (payment is limited to 62.5% of the payment schedule). However, beginning in January 1, 2010, the limitation on recognition of expenses incurred for outpatient mental health services will begin to be phased out by increasing the Medicare Part B payment for outpatient mental health services to 80% by 2014. Beginning in 2014, Medicare started paying for outpatient mental health services at the same level as other Part B services.

Beginning July 1, 2008, and ending December 31, 2009, MIPPA provided a 5% increase in the payment schedule for psychiatric therapeutic procedures, including insight oriented, behavior modifying, or supportive psychotherapy or interactive psychotherapy. This provision was extended by the Affordable Care Act from January 1, 2010–December 31, 2010, and further extended by the Medicare and Medicaid Extenders Act of 2010, from January 1, 2011–December 31, 2011.

Effective for CPT 1998, CPT codes for psychotherapy and psychological diagnostic testing replaced the HCPCS codes. The temporary HCPCS codes were crosswalked to the new CPT codes, as were the RVUs.

Effective for CPT 2013, a new coding structure was created for psychotherapy services, following three years of effort by the CPT Editorial Panel, RUC, several national specialty societies, and health care organizations. The new coding framework allows all codes to be used in all settings, instead of describing site-specific services. Psychotherapy is now being reported with either stand-alone codes without medical services (CPT codes 90832, 90834, and 90837) or with add-on codes, which are used only in conjunction with Evaluation and Management (E/M) services (90833, 90836, and 90838). When a medical service is provided with psychotherapy, the appropriate E/M service should be reported and then an add-on psychotherapy time-based code (30, 45, or 60 minutes) will be reported. For 2013, CMS assigned interim relative values for these services and requested that RUC review add-on codes for the interactive component of psychotherapy and for crisis services, before the full review of the recommendations for the entire family of psychotherapy services. For 2014, RUC submitted the remaining interactive complexity component add-on codes for psychotherapy and crisis services. CMS accepted 100% of the RUC recommendations for the psychotherapy services for 2014, leading to $150 million in improved payments for these services each year. Medicare payments for psychiatrists, psychologists and clinical social workers were expected to increase 6-8% for CY 2014.

Clinical Social Workers

The distinction that applies to clinical psychologists regarding diagnostic and therapeutic services is also applicable to clinical social workers. Payment for CSW therapeutic services will be limited to 75% of the clinical psychologist payment schedule amount, while payment for diagnostic services will be according to the MFS.

Registered Dietitians

Section 105 of the Medicare, Medicaid, and State Children's Health Insurance Program (SCHIP) Benefits Improvement and Protection Act of 2000 created a benefit for medical nutrition therapy (MNT) for certain Medicare patients who have diabetes or a renal disease. This benefit was implemented on January 1, 2002. Medicare Part B will pay for MNT services furnished by a registered dietitian or nutrition professional, when the beneficiary is referred for the service by the beneficiary's "treating physician." The *treating physician* is defined as the primary care physician or specialist coordinating care for the beneficiary with diabetes or renal disease. The statute specifies that the Medicare payment for MNT services must equal 80% of the lesser of the actual charge for the services, or 85% of the amount determined under the MFS for the same services, if furnished by a physician. The MNT services should be reported using CPT codes 97802-97804. CMS also clarified that medical nutrition therapy cannot be provided incident to a physician's service, unless the physician also meets the qualifications to bill Medicare as a registered dietitian or nutrition professional.

CMS proposed in its November 21, 2005, Final Rule to add individual medical nutrition therapy (HCPCS/CPT Codes G0720, 97802, and 97803) to the list of Medicare telemedicine services. Accordingly, because registered dietitians and nutrition professional are the primary providers of these services, they have been added to list of providers who are able to receive payment for telemedicine services.

In the Final Rule published on December 1, 2006, CMS announced that it will establish work RVUs for the medical nutrition therapy codes as recommended by RUC HCPAC for the 2001 MFS Final Rule. This action comes after much lobbying from the AMA and the American Dietetic Association.

In early 2008, CMS requested that the services described by CPT codes 97802 and 97803 be given the opportunity for consideration under the RUC process to help ensure that CMS payment for MNT services to nonphysician nutrition professionals is accurate. In the Final Rule published on November 25, 2008, CMS announced it accepted the new work RVUs for these services as recommended by RUC for the 2009 MFS. CMS has priced the work, practice expense, and professional liability insurance RVUs for MNT services as if they were performed by a physician. When registered dietitians perform these services, they are paid 85% of the amount that a physician performing these services would be paid.

Historical Information about E/M Codes

In 1989, the AMA's CPT Editorial Panel began revising the CPT coding system for visits and consultations. The panel developed new codes for visits and consultations in order to improve the coding uniformity for these services and to improve the codes' appropriateness for use in an RBRVS-based payment schedule. On a parallel track, CMS was required by law to establish a uniform procedure coding system for physician services, including visits and consultations, as part of the standardization of Medicare policies. There was considerable geographic variation in the use of CPT visit codes before 1992.

The CPT Editorial Panel developed new codes for office visits, hospital visits, and consultations, taking into account recommendations of the panel's Ad Hoc Committee on Visits and Levels of Service, a special AMA/Physician Payment Review Commission Consensus Panel, and research from Phases I, II, and III of the Harvard study. Issues that the panel considered included the appropriateness of using time in visit coding, the number of levels of service, the need for different codes for different sites of service, and the need for different codes for new and established patients.

The AMA and CMS conducted a two-part pilot test in January 1991. As the first phase, specialty societies developed clinical descriptions of typical patient visits; physicians from five specialties were then asked to select codes for the case studies. Discussions of the new codes' strengths and weaknesses followed. In the second phase—a field test conducted in California, Kentucky, New York, and South Carolina—physicians used the new codes in their clinical practices. Pilot test results indicated the proposed codes could be used reliably by practicing physicians.

Based on the pilot study results, the panel refined the proposed codes and implemented them in 1992. CMS accepted the proposed visit codes as developed by the CPT Editorial Panel. The new codes enabled physicians to select the proper CPT code more easily and help to assure that physicians receive the correct payment for the evaluation and management (E/M) services they provide. The 1992 CPT codes for E/M services adopted for use under the RBRVS payment system differ fundamentally from the previous version in the way they defined and categorized codes. The familiar levels of service were replaced by a more precise method of assigning codes based primarily on extent of history and examination and the complexity of medical decision making involved in diagnosing and treating a patient's problem(s). Four contributory components, usually less important, are counseling, coordination of care, nature of presenting illness, and time taken to perform the service.

The work RVUs for the E/M codes were revised by CMS for 1993, because of comments received from several specialty societies. The comments reflected widely differing views among specialty societies about the intensity of work involved in providing E/M services. CMS determined that, based on comments received and data from Phase III of the Harvard study, the RVUs for visits should increase in a linear fashion so that the work per unit of time is the same for every code within a given class, regardless of the duration of the visit. As a result, work RVUs were increased for the mid- to upper-level codes and slightly decreased for other E/M services.

CMS re-evaluated the work RVUs for all 98 E/M services as part of the 1995 five-year review of the RBRVS. The agency agreed with RUC's argument that these services were undervalued in relationship to other services, and that the preservice and postservice work involved had increased over time. As a result, work RVUs were increased in varying amounts for many of these services, including a 25% increase for office visits (CPT codes 99202-99215), an average 16.6% increase for emergency department services (CPT codes 99281-99285), and smaller increases for critical care, first hour (CPT code 99291), and office or other outpatient consultations (CPT codes 992241-99245).

Significant revisions were made to the CPT codes for 1998 for observation same-day discharge (99234-99236), nursing facility discharge (99315-99316), home care visits (99341-99350), and care plan oversight, including the addition of new codes. Work RVUs for many of the codes subsequently were changed. Coding changes and work RVUs for these codes are described more fully in the following section.

The 2005 Five-Year Review included 35 E/M services. RUC agreed that incorrect assumptions were made in the previous valuation of E/M services. RUC recommended and CMS approved an increase in work RVUs for 28 services and maintained work RVUs for seven services. Furthermore, RUC also recommended, and CMS accepted, that the full increase of the E/M service be incorporated into the surgical global periods for each CPT code with global periods of 010 and 090.

E/M Office Visit Revisions

On November 1, 2019, CMS finalized a historic provision in the 2020 MFS Final Rule. This provision includes revisions to the code descriptors and documentation standards E/M office visit CPT codes 99201-99215. These revisions directly address the continuing problem of administrative burden for physicians in nearly every specialty across the country. With these landmark changes, as approved by the CPT Editorial Panel, documentation for E/M office visits will now be centered around how physicians think and take care of patients and not on mandatory standards that encouraged re-recording information and checking boxes.

E/M Office Visit Revisions: A Background

For decades, the physician community has struggled with burdensome reporting guidelines for reporting office visits and other E/M codes. With the proliferation of electronic health records (EHRs) into physician practices, documentation requirements for office visits have moved toward increased "note bloat" within the patient record due to the largely check-box nature of meeting the current documentation requirements.

To address this, on February 9, 2019, the CPT Editorial Panel approved revisions to the CPT E/M office or other outpatient visit reporting guidelines and code descriptors. These revisions were in direct response to the leadership demonstrated by CMS Administrator, Seema Verma, to take on the challenge of revising the E/M office visit reporting guidelines.

Scope and Implementation Date

The scope of the AMA proposal was solely focused on revisions to the E/M office or other outpatient visits (CPT codes 99201-99215). The code set revisions will be effective January 1, 2021.

Administrative Burden

The AMA's proposal to reduce administrative burden achieves a shared goal with CMS, truly putting patients over paperwork and improving the healthcare system. These revisions work in lockstep with the already established administrative burden relief initiatives established by CMS for 2019:

- Eliminate the requirement to document medical necessity of furnishing visits in the home rather than office.
- Eliminate the requirement for clinicians to re-record elements of the history and physical examination when there is evidence that the information has been reviewed and updated. Physicians must only document that they reviewed and verified information regarding the chief complaint and history that are already recorded by ancillary staff or the patient.

Additional burden reduction will be seen through:

- Simplifying code selection criteria and making them more clinically relevant and intuitive
- Creating consistency across payers by adding detail within the CPT E/M Guidelines
- Alignment with current documentation guidelines from Medicare and the CPT code set to ensure minimal disruption to practices.

Summary of E/M Office Visit Revisions

See the following list for a summary of the revisions for E/M office visits that went into effect in 2021:

1. Eliminated the history and physical examination as elements for code selection: While the physician's work in capturing the patient's pertinent history and performing a relevant physical examination contributes to both the time and medical decision making (MDM), these elements alone should not determine the appropriate code level.
   - The code descriptors were revised to state that health care professionals should perform a "medically appropriate history and/or examination."
2. Allowed physicians to choose whether their documentation and code-selection level for E/M services provided is based on MDM or total time spent on the date of the patient encounter:
   - *MDM:* The three existing elements of MDM were not materially changed; however, edits were made to the elements for code selection and numerous clarifying definitions in the E/M guidelines were revised or created. (See below for additional discussion.)
   - *Time:* Definition of time was changed to total time spent on date of patient encounter, not typical time, and represents total physician or other qualified health care professional (QHP) time on the date of service. The use of date-of-service time builds on the movement over the last several years by Medicare to better recognize the work involved in nonface-to-face services such as care coordination. These definitions only apply when code selection is based primarily on time and not MDM.
3. Modified the criteria for MDM: The CPT Editorial Panel used the existing CMS Table of Risk as a foundation for designing the revised required elements for MDM. Existing CMS Contractor audit tools were also consulted to minimize disruption in MDM level criteria:
   - Removed ambiguous terms (eg, "mild") and defined previously ambiguous concepts (eg, "acute or chronic illness with systemic symptoms").
   - Defined important terms such as "independent historian."
   - Re-defined the data element to move away from simply adding up tasks to focus on tasks that affect the management of the patient (eg, independent interpretation of a test performed by another health care professional and/or discussion of test interpretation with an external physician or other QHP).
4. Deletion of code 99201: The CPT Editorial Panel agreed to eliminate code 99201 as codes 99201 and 99202 both had straightforward MDM and were only differentiated by history and examination elements.
5. Creation of a shorter prolonged services code: The CPT Editorial Panel created a shorter prolonged services code (99417) to capture physician or other QHP time in 15-minute increments. Code 99417 should only be reported with codes 99205 and 99215 and be used when time is the primary basis for code selection.

Primary Objectives of the CPT Editorial Panel Revisions

The CPT Editorial Panel took seriously the charge to create revisions to the E/M office visits and outlined four primary objectives to this important work:

1. Decrease the administrative burden of documentation and coding.
2. Decrease the need for audits through the addition and expansion of key definitions and guidelines.
3. Decrease unnecessary documentation in the medical record that is not needed for patient care.
4. Ensure that payment for E/M services is resource-based and that there is no direct goal for payment redistribution between specialties.

Collaboration for Revisions to Office Visit Codes

The AMA led a consensus-driven, open, and transparent workgroup process to ensure the reimagined approach to office visits represented input from the broad array of medical specialties that perform these visits. This workgroup was created with members who had both CPT Editorial Panel and RUC experience. In addition, the process engaged participants with diverse medical specialty backgrounds, including primary care, several surgical specialties (eg, general surgery, cardiology, and vascular surgery), private payers, and qualified healthcare professionals (eg, physician assistants).

The workgroup held numerous open conference calls, where on average, more than 300 individuals participated to provide direct input. Many of the major decisions made by the workgroup, including the definition of time and key definitions of MDM criteria, were based on targeted stakeholder survey results.

The workgroup brought its proposal to the CPT Editorial Panel as consensus recommendations and only minor modifications were made by the Panel prior to approving them.

For more details and the following valuable resources visit www.ama-assn.org/cpt-office-visits:

- CPT 2021 E/M office or other outpatient and prolonged services codes and guideline changes
- RUC recommendations on CPT E/M office visit codes
- Educational module providing an overview of the new E/M code revisions and details on how they will differ from current coding requirements and terminology
- A practice checklist and tips to help prepare for the 2021 transition
- Sign up for E/M code revision updates from the AMA

Historical Information about E/M Documentation Guidelines

In June 2000, CMS issued the draft *Evaluation and Management Documentation Guidelines* to serve as a potential replacement to the 1995 and 1997 *Documentation Guidelines for Evaluation and Management Services.* These guidelines were later revised in December 2000. They focused on correct documentation of E/M encounters with Medicare beneficiaries and offered an alternative approach through clinical examples. CMS contracted with Aspen Systems Corporation to develop clinical examples that were intended to illustrate acceptable E/M documentation practices, provide guidance for clinical practitioners, and promote consistent medical review of E/M claims by Medicare carriers. The clinical examples are meant to illustrate the guidelines for various levels of physical examination and MDM. Aspen developed clinical examples for 16 medical specialties from identification-stripped medical records obtained from Medicare carriers throughout the country. In May 2001, Aspen introduced the examples and their methods to organized medicine to begin an in-depth review by physicians and CMDs.

At the time of the introduction, specialty societies had many questions regarding how the clinical examples would be used in practice, the availability of carrier feedback to the specialties, coordination between carriers and specialty societies, and next steps. Also, the possibility that the clinical examples were based on medical records that were "down-coded" was raised as a serious concern. Because medical records were not available for some specialties, the issue about the ability to develop sufficient clinical examples for all E/M services for all specialties was raised. The participating specialty societies and carriers were given a short timeframe (60 days) to review a large volume of clinical examples.

On June 26, 2001, the AMA hosted a specialty society meeting designed to collect broad specialty society reaction to the CMS/Aspen clinical examples. This meeting resulted in a specialty sign-on letter to Thomas Scully, the then administrator of CMS. The letter attempted to capitalize on the Bush Administration's efforts to reduce the regulatory burden on physicians and called on CMS to re-examine the need for documentation guidelines and its commitment to the development of clinical examples. The letter made the point that it would be more appropriate for organized medicine to develop its own examples that accurately reflect appropriate levels of patient care, rather than use those suggested by the CMS contractor.

On July 19, 2001, the Department of Health and Human Services (HHS) responded to organized medicine's concerns indicating that the HHS was willing to address the E/M documentation burden. CMS stopped all work on the Aspen project and the 2000 *Documentation Guidelines.* (Carriers will continue to use either the 1995 or the 1997 *Documentation Guidelines.*) The announcement was a direct response to advocacy efforts by the AMA and the specialty societies, and it represents a significant concession to the physician community.

Over a three-year period, the CPT Editorial Panel worked with organized medicine and CMS to revise E/M code descriptors and guidelines to enhance the functionality and utility of CPT E/M codes so that physicians and payers can better apply and understand the codes and to decrease the need for extensive medical record documentation. The intention of E/M revisions was to make the codes more straightforward and simpler for physicians to implement, thus allowing physicians to practice medicine according to the needs of their patients.

In November 2002, the CPT Editorial Panel provisionally adopted new E/M code descriptors and instructions that maintained the same number of levels, but used descriptors that are less specific, and thus less susceptible for applying the detailed E/M documentation guideline. The proposed new E/M framework utilized code instructions and descriptors that focus on total physician work as the basis for selecting a code, rather than attempting to break this work down into detailed component parts (ie, history, physical, and MDM), as it is with the current E/M codes. To assist in code selection and to serve as a basis of comparison, specialty-oriented clinical examples would be used to describe reference services, Levels 3 and 5 for E/M code families that include five levels, and Level 2 for three-level E/M families. The clinical examples would be used to compare between the service just provided and the established reference levels. This is also called *magnitude estimation*.

The concept of total physician work and the use of reference services changed the nature of the E/M codes, leaving them much less open to carrier review based on checklists or documentation guidelines administered by nonphysicians. The new E/M framework would necessitate medical review based on the use of clinical examples, peer review of outliers, or other techniques not requiring checklists.

When the CPT Editorial Panel provisionally accepted the new E/M framework, all the states and specialty societies had the opportunity to review the proposed changes and to comment on them. When it accepted the new E/M framework, the Panel also appointed a Clinical Example Taskforce (Taskforce) to begin the process of developing and testing clinical examples, given their importance for illustrating the reference services and in providing a basis for code selection using magnitude estimation. The Taskforce worked with the federation of medicine and CMS on the development of a process for the creation of clinical examples by the national medical specialty societies and for the vetting of submitted examples for code level accuracy and for use by CMD in claims review. The Taskforce created a multipronged approach to develop and test the utility of clinical examples for use in E/M codes. It also developed comprehensive instructions to guide the process of developing clinical examples and to achieve some consistency.

The first phase of the project involved the development of clinical examples for Levels 3 and 5, new and established patient office visits, and Level 2, initial and subsequent hospital visits. The initial clinical examples were developed by 11 different specialty societies for five common clinical conditions encountered by the specialty. Three hundred and thirty clinical examples were collected from the 11 specialties. These examples were then tested for intraspecialty validity to ensure that physicians of the same specialty could accurately apply the examples. Physicians were asked to assign an E/M code level and type (ie, office or hospital visit) to each example reviewed.

Pilot studies on 330 clinical examples from each of the 11 initial specialty societies were conducted from December 2003 through February 2004. The AMA's Market Research and Analysis unit was asked to conduct an online survey and report the findings. E-mail addresses for a sample of 500 members of each of the participating specialties were obtained from the specialties and sent to the AMA. An e-mail message was sent to the sample physicians explaining the purpose of the study and providing a link to the survey. Sample members were sent two reminders to participate in the study.

Despite the AMA's best efforts to persuade physicians to participate, and, considering the importance of E/M to the physician community, the overall response rates were very low. Qualitative responses from several specialties raised concern about the time required to complete the survey, possibly explaining the low response rate. The practice experience of respondents was considerable; most respondents had been in practice more than 10 years and would be expected to have reasonable coding expertise.

In general, the results of the pilot study do not demonstrate that coding from clinical examples would be an improvement on the current system. Specialty physicians were only able to correctly assign the appropriate E/M code from the clinical examples with a maximum specialty accuracy of 44% and a minimum specialty accuracy of 26%. On a code-level basis, clinical examples for code 99213 were the most accurate with 54% correct, and clinical examples for code 99215 were the least accurate with 18% correct.

Based on a thorough analysis of the results of the pilot study, the E/M Clinical Example Taskforce recommended that the CPT Editorial Panel rescind its previous action to accept the new E/M descriptors.

At its May 2004 meeting, the CPT Editorial Panel reviewed the results of the clinical example pilot. Despite the low response rate, the Panel believed that the ability of physicians to use clinical examples to assign the correct code level was not an improvement over the current system of E/M assignment. Also, the new E/M coding system would have required significant physician education and changes in physician practices, as well as full CMS support and its development of new auditing and surveillance mechanisms. The poor pilot results made these investments in a new E/M coding system highly questionable. The CPT Editorial Panel voted to rescind the November 2002 adoption of E/M changes.

On January 1, 2019, CMS finalized the following changes to E/M documentation guidelines that were strongly supported by the AMA:

- The requirement to document medical necessity of providing visits in the home rather than office will be eliminated.
- Physicians will no longer be required to re-record elements of the history and physical examinations when there is evidence that the information has been reviewed and updated.
- Physicians must only document that they reviewed and verified information regarding the chief complaint and history that are already recorded by ancillary staff or the patient.

Additionally, for 2019, CMS revised federal regulations by allowing the presence of the teaching physician during E/M services to be demonstrated by notes in medical records made by a physician, resident, or nurse. CMS also revised federal regulations to provide that the medical record must document the extent of the teaching physician's participation in the review and direction of services furnished to each patient and that the extent of the teaching physician's participation may be demonstrated by the notes in the medical records made by a physician, resident, or nurse.

CMS announced that it would implement the AMA's recommendations to significantly modify the way physicians document and report Office Visits (CPT codes 99202-99215) beginning January 1, 2021. Detailed information on these changes is available at www.ama-assn.org/cpt-office-visits.

Accordingly, CMS implemented significant changes to CPT code descriptors and guidelines for office visits made by the CPT Editorial Panel and the corresponding RUC relative value recommendations in 2021. For 2022, the AMA continues to advocate for CMS to fully adopt the RUC recommendations for E/M office visit codes by applying the increased valuation of the E/M office visits to the postoperative office visits bundled into the global surgical packages.

Reporting E/M Codes

CMS reporting and payment guidelines differ in some respects from the CPT codes for certain E/M services. Coding changes and Medicare payment policies currently effective are described in the following sections.

Consultation services. CMS has finalized its proposal not to cover the office consultation services (99241-99245) or the inpatient consultation services (99251-99255) and redistribute the savings to the work RVUs, PE, and PLI of the new and established office visits, and the initial hospital and initial nursing facility visits. This redistribution of savings results in approximately a 6% increase in the new and established office visits and a 2% increase in the initial hospital and nursing facility visits. The increase in these services will be reflected in all procedures that have these services as part of their global period. Beginning in 2010, providers will report an initial hospital care or initial nursing facility care code for their first visit during a patient's admission to the hospital or nursing facility instead of a consultation code. Further, CMS will create a modifier to identify the admitting provider of record for hospital inpatient and nursing facility admission.

Physician care plan oversight services. Physician care plan oversight services were first recognized for Medicare payment in 1995, although on a more limited basis than described in CPT. For 1997, CMS eliminated for Medicare payment purposes the CPT definition of the care plan oversight code (99375) and replaced it with three temporary HCPCS codes (G0064-G0066) to eliminate confusion that the agency believed had arisen among physicians about proper reporting. The temporary codes specified the type of facility that provided care to the patient: home health agency, hospice, and nursing facility. Medicare allowed payment, however, only for physician oversight services provided to home health and hospice patients.

The CPT codes for care plan oversight services, as revised for the CPT 1998, retain the changes that CMS adopted in the 1997 HCPCS codes. The CPT Editorial Panel, however, adopted six codes for care plan oversight services (99374-99380), two for each facility, which differentiate between the amounts of physician time spent: 15 minutes to 29 minutes and 30 minutes or more. Although new work RVUs were assigned to each code in 1998, Medicare recognized payment for only CPT codes 99375 (home health care supervision, 30 minutes or more) and 99378 (hospice care supervision, 30 minutes or more).

For CPT 2001, the care plan oversight codes were revised to reflect the range of settings in which the services are applicable and to clarify that the time the physicians spends communicating with nonhealth professionals should also be included. CMS has stated that existing policy that this communication is included in the payment for evaluation and management services. CMS has, therefore, established new codes, G0181 and G0182, to describe the care-plan oversight codes that they will now cover. The AMA objected to this action and continues to work with specialty societies and CMS to resolve this issue.

The limitation of the existing care-plan oversight codes for children and adults with special health care needs is not in the definition of the service, but in the restriction on setting. Patients must be under the care of a home health agency, in hospice, or in a nursing facility. A significant number of children and adults with special health care needs and chronic medical conditions for the care model, and the care-plan oversight service code requirements that the patient be under the care of a multidisciplinary care modality are not under the care of a home health agency, in a hospice, or in a nursing facility. Thus, the limitation of the care plan oversight codes is not in the definition of the typical activities and services provided, but in the restriction on setting and circumstance. Therefore, the CPT Editorial Panel created two new timed codes for the CPT 2006 to address this limitation of the existing care-plan oversight codes: 99339 and 99340. CMS has bundled these services and will not allow separate reporting.

Home services. The CPT 2013 codebook included codes for new patient home visits (99341-99345) and established patient home visits (99347-99350). The home visit codes for new patients allow physicians to report comprehensive history and examination with medical decision making of moderate and high complexity. The home visit codes for established patients allow the physician to report services for those patients presenting with problems of moderate to high severity. For 2019 and beyond, CMS eliminated the requirement to document medical necessity of furnishing visits in the home rather than in the office.

Nursing facility services. For CPT 2006, revisions were made to the Nursing Facility Services codes by (1) revising the structure of the current Comprehensive Nursing Facility Assessment codes to create three levels of service for admissions, consistent with the structure of the three levels of service for admission in the Initial Hospital Care section of the CPT codebook; (2) adding a fourth level of service to the Subsequent Nursing Facility Care codes to allow the reporting of a comprehensive level of care (comprehensive history, comprehensive exam, high complexity decision making); (3) adding a new code in a new subsection (Other Nursing Facility Care) to allow the reporting of a comprehensive annual assessment; and (4) revising, renumbering, and deleting existing codes. CMS accepted RUC's work and practice expense for these services.

Domiciliary care services. For CPT 2006, the domiciliary codes were revised to reflect that congregate living facilities have changed dramatically over the past decade in size, scope of services, and the complexity of health concerns. The existing codes used to bill for visits by health care professionals were no longer descriptive of the range or intensity of services provided. Therefore, new codes were established, and revisions were made to codes 99324-99328 and 99334-99340 to permit the reporting of comprehensive levels of domiciliary rest home (eg, boarding home) and custodial services 99341-99345. RUC recommended that these codes be valued the same as the home care visit codes (CPT codes 99341-99350). CMS accepted RUC's work and practice expense for these services.

Prolonged physician services. Effective January 1, 1994, CMS adopted for payment a series of codes developed for the CPT 1994 to report prolonged physician services.

Prolonged physician service with direct (face-to-face) patient contact (CPT codes 99354-99357) is used when a physician or other qualified health care professional provides prolonged services that involve direct (face-to-face) patient contact beyond the usual service in either the outpatient (99354 and 99355) or inpatient (99356 and 99357) settings. These codes provide incentives for physicians or other health care professionals to furnish care in the most appropriate setting and reduce the incidence of more costly emergency department visits and hospital admissions. For guidance in selecting the appropriate prolonged service code, refer to the clinical examples in the CPT 2022 codebook.

In addition, CMS developed the following criteria to determine when payment will be allowed for these codes.

The physician or other qualified health care professional must furnish and bill one of the following CPT codes for the patient on the same day:

- To bill CPT code 99354: 90837, 90847, 99241-99245, 99324-99337, 99341-99350, 99483.
- To bill CPT code 99355: 99354.
- To bill CPT code 99356: 90837, 90847, 99218-99220, 99221-99223, 99224-99226, 99231-99233, 99234-99236, 99251-99255, 99304-99310.
- To bill CPT code 99357: 99356
- To bill CPT code 99417 (or G2212 for the Medicare program): 99205 or 99215

The time counted toward payment for prolonged E/M services includes only direct face-to-face contact between the physician or other qualified health care professional and the patient, even if the service is not continuous.

The medical record must document the content of the E/M service that was billed, and the duration and content of prolonged services personally furnished by the physician after the typical time of the E/M service was exceeded by 30 minutes.

CMS further specified that time counted toward the use of the prolonged services codes does not include "time that a patient spends occupying an examination or treatment room while there is no direct physician-patient contact," nor does it include time spent with a nonphysician practitioner for "incident-to" services.

The CPT codes 99354 and 99355 are considered primary care services for purposes of the payment schedule update, while CPT codes 99356 and 99357 are updated as nonsurgical services. Beginning in 2021, Medicare will not pay for CPT codes 99358-99359 in association with office/outpatient E/M visits. In addition, do not report 99358-99359 for time without direct patient contact reported in other services, such as care plan oversight services or chronic care management by a physician or other QHP.

Transitional Care Management Services (TCM)

In response to a CMS Proposal in 2011, to re-review the evaluation and management (E/M) services to ensure that care coordination was appropriately incorporated into E/M services, the AMA created the Chronic Care Coordination Workgroup (C3W). The C3W is a joint workgroup of the CPT Editorial Panel and RUC. This Workgroup immediately called upon CMS to begin payment for individual nonface-to-face services used to better coordinate care. At the same time, the C3W asked the CPT Editorial Panel to begin working on new code descriptors to describe transitional care management (TCM) and complex chronic care coordination services (CCCC). In 2012, the CPT Editorial Panel completed this work, and 14 organizations, including all the major primary care specialty societies completed a survey of several hundred physicians to determine the resources related to these new codes. CMS accepted RUC's recommendation for TCM, and effective January 1, 2013, will being paying for these services.

TCM describe services delivered to patients who are transitioning from a facility to a non-facility care setting. It is expected that TCM codes will be primarily reported by the primary care physician, CMS also acknowledges that specialists who provide these services may also report the new TCM codes. In addition, nonphysician qualified health care professional include nurse practitioners, physician assistants, clinical nurse specialists and certified nurse midwives can provide and bill for TCM services to the limit of their state's scope of practice. The reporting physician or qualified health care professional must have an established relationship with the patient. Under the CPT's TCM guidelines, an established patient relationship exists when a physician has billed a visit with the patient within the last three years. In addition, CMS accepted the AMA RUC's recommendation to allow a physician to report both TCM and the discharge management codes (99217, 99234-99236, 99238-99239, 99281-99285, or 99315-99316). However, the E/M service required for the CPT TCM codes cannot be furnished by the same physician or nonphysician practitioner on the same day as the discharge management service. The typical case is that of a patient transitioning from a hospital to home. Following a hospital discharge, TCM is a set of bundled face-to-face and nonface-to-face services performed by the physician or qualified health provider and clinical staff for the 30 days following discharge. The intent of TCM is to prevent re-hospitalization or emergency department visits. Therefore, TCM codes can be billed only once per patient within 30 days of discharge. TCM is targeted to moderately or highly complex patients, with multiple co-morbidities, who take multiple medications and who are at high risk of deterioration. The service requires early and frequent communication with the patient, family, other providers and agencies over the month following hospital discharge to ensure that the discharge summary and appropriate clinical information is obtained quickly and reviewed, that the patient's medication and therapeutic regimen is reconciled and optimized and that all necessary clinical and community services are coordinated and delivered. In addition to these nonface-to-face services, each code includes a timely face-to-face visit that typically occurs in the office but can also occur at home or other location where the patient resides.

The nonface-to-face services of TCM, include communication with the patient and caregivers; communication with home health agencies; education to support self-management and activities of daily living; assessment of medication adherence and management; identification of community resources; facilitating access to care and services needed; obtaining and reviewing discharge information as available; reviewing need for or follow up on pending diagnostic tests; interaction with other qualified health care professionals; and the establishment of referrals and arranging for community resources.

TCM codes 99495 and 99496 have an XXX global period. The TCM codes do not allow physicians reporting services with global periods of 010 and 090 days to report TCM. All physician and staff time appear in the intra-service time because any services provided during the 30-day service period are, by definition, intra-service time. The CPT introductory language specifically describes the physician and clinical staff activities included in these services. The two significant differences between codes 99495 and 99496 is that code 99496 **requires highly complex medical decision making** and a face-to-face visit must occur within 7 days of discharge, whereas, code 99495 requires **either moderate or highly complex medical decision making** and a face-to-face visit within **14 days** of discharge. It is important to note that the first face-to-face visit is part of the TCM service and not reported separately. However, E/M services following the initial face-to-face visit may be reported separately.

Code 99495, *Transitional Care Management Services with the following required elements:*

- *Communication (direct contact, telephone, electronic) with the patient and/or caregiver within 2 business days of discharge*
- *Medical decision making of at least moderate complexity during the service period*
- *Face-to-face visit, within 14 calendar days of discharge*

Code 99496, *Transitional Care Management Services with the following required elements:*

- *Communication (direct contact, telephone, electronic) with the patient and/or caregiver within 2 business days of discharge*
- *Medical decision making of high complexity during the service period*
- *Face-to-face visit, within 7 calendar days of discharge*

Studies have concluded that patients who receive TCM services have lower hospital readmission rates, lower mortality, and incur lower costs. Because of this success, CMS is exploring ways to increase utilization and improve payment for care management. To increase utilization, starting in 2020, CMS will ease restrictions so TCM services may be reported concurrently with other codes. CMS also finalized its proposal to increase payment for the services (99495 and 99496) codes as recommended by RUC. In 2021, CMS continues to enhance utilization of TCM services by allowing 15 additional codes to be reported concurrently with TCM services.

Chronic Care Management (CCM)

Resulting from a multi-year effort by the AMA, CPT Editorial Panel, RUC, and several national medical specialty societies, Medicare has paid for monthly chronic care management (CCM) services since January 1, 2015. The codes were originally created in response to the July 2011 Notice of Proposed Rulemaking. The CPT Editorial Panel and the AMA/Specialty Society RVS Update Committee created the Chronic Care Coordination Workgroup (C3W) to specifically address the CMS request to ensure that care coordination services were described and valued within the Evaluation and Management Services. The C3W requested that the CPT Editorial Panel consider creation of codes to describe transitional care management and monthly complex chronic care coordination services. These services are provided by physicians and other qualified health care professionals to an individual who resides at home or in a domiciliary, rest home, or assisted living facility, per calendar month.

For CPT 2021, the CPT Editorial Panel revised CPT code 99490 to describe the first 20 minutes of clinical staff time and created new add-on code 99439 to describe each additional 20 minutes of clinical staff time. The CPT Editorial Panel also revised codes 99487 and 99489 to eliminate the requirement to establish a care plan and revised the CCM services guidelines. For CPT 2022, the CPT Editorial Panel revised CPT code 99491 to describe the first 30 minutes of time provided personally by a physician or other QHP and created new add-on code 99439 to describe each additional 30 minutes of physician or other QHP time.

The coding structure is that CPT codes 99487 and 99489 exist as a family of two codes that describe *complex* CCM services. These services are provided during a calendar month that includes criteria for CCM services, including establishing, revising, implementing, or monitoring the care plan; medical, functional, and/or psychosocial problems requiring MDM of moderate or high complexity; and clinical staff care management services for at least 60 minutes, under the direction of a physician or other QHP

CPT codes 99439-99491 describe CCM services. These services are provided when medical and/or psychosocial needs of the patient require establishing, implementing, revising, or monitoring the care plan. Patients who receive CCM services have two or more chronic continuous or episodic health conditions that are expected to last at least 12 months, or until the death of the patient, and that place the patient at significant risk of death, acute exacerbation/decompensation, or functional decline.

#▲99490 Chronic care management services with the following required elements:

- multiple (two or more) chronic conditions expected to last at least 12 months, or until the death of the patient,
- chronic conditions that place the patient at significant risk of death, acute exacerbation/decompensation, or functional decline,
- comprehensive care plan established, implemented, revised, or monitored;

first 20 minutes of clinical staff time directed by a physician or other qualified health care professional, per calendar month.

#+▲99439 each additional 20 minutes of clinical staff time directed by a physician or other qualified health care professional, per calendar month (List separately in addition to code for primary procedure)

#▲99491 Chronic care management services with the following required elements:

- multiple (two or more) chronic conditions expected to last at least 12 months, or until the death of the patient,
- chronic conditions that place the patient at significant risk of death, acute exacerbation/decompensation, or functional decline,
- comprehensive care plan established, implemented, revised, or monitored;

first 30 minutes, provided personally by a physician or other qualified health care professional, per calendar month.

#+▲99437 each additional 30 minutes by a physician or other qualified health care professional, per calendar month (List separately in addition to code for primary procedure)

▲99487 Complex chronic care management services with the following required elements:

- multiple (two or more) chronic conditions expected to last at least 12 months, or until the death of the patient,
- chronic conditions place the patient at significant risk of death, acute exacerbation/decompensation, or functional decline,
- comprehensive care plan established, implemented, revised, or monitored,
- moderate or high complexity medical decision making;

first 60 minutes of clinical staff time directed by a physician or other qualified health care professional, per calendar month.

+▲99489 each additional 30 minutes of clinical staff time directed by a physician or other qualified health care professional, per calendar month (List separately in addition to code for primary procedure)

Principal Care Management (PCM) Services

For 2020, CMS created two G codes to make separate payment for care management for patients with one serious chronic condition. There was no review by the RUC for these services.

For CPT 2022, the CPT Editorial Panel created four new codes for principal care management (PCM). Two of the codes describe principal care management performed by clinical staff under the supervision of a physician or other QHP and the other two describe principal care management performed by the QHP. The PCM codes differ from the CCM codes in that they are to be reported by physicians or other QHPs when that professional is responsible for managing a patient's single chronic illness as opposed to being responsible for managing the entire care of a patient with two or more chronic illnesses. With the creation of the four new CPT codes, CMS deleted the two obsolete G codes.

#●99424 Principal care management services, for a single high-risk disease, with the following required elements:

- one complex chronic condition expected to last at least 3 months, and which places the patient at significant risk of hospitalization, acute exacerbation/decompensation, functional decline, or death,
- the condition requires development, monitoring, or revision of disease-specific care plan,
- the condition requires frequent adjustments in the medication regimen, and/or the management of the condition is unusually complex due to comorbidities
- ongoing communication and care coordination between relevant practitioners furnishing care;

first 30 minutes provided personally by a physician or other qualified health care professional, per calendar month

#+●99425 each additional 30 minutes provided personally by a physician or other qualified health care professional, per calendar month (List separately in addition to code for primary procedure)

#●99426 Principal care management services, for a single high-risk disease, with the following required elements;

- one complex chronic condition expected to last at least 3 months, and which places the patient at significant risk of hospitalization, acute exacerbation/decompensation, functional decline, or death,
- the condition requires development, monitoring, or revision of disease-specific care plan,
- the condition requires frequent adjustments in the medication regimen, and/or the management of the condition is unusually complex due to comorbidities,
- ongoing communication and care coordination between relevant practitioners furnishing care;

first 30 minutes of clinical staff time directed by physician or other qualified health care professional, per calendar month.

#+●99427 each additional 30 minutes of clinical staff time directed by a physician or other qualified health care professional, per calendar month (List separately in addition to code for primary procedure)

Advanced Care Planning

Starting on January 1, 2016, Medicare began paying for advanced care planning services. Two new CPT codes 99497 and 99498 were designed to capture the face-to-face encounter and time that a patient's treating physician spends with the patient, his or her family, or health care power of attorney to discuss advance directive planning. The factors considered in such discussions may include, but are not limited to, the patient's current disease state; disease progression; available treatments; cardiopulmonary resuscitation/life sustaining measures; do not resuscitate orders; life expectancy based on the patient's age and co-morbidities; and clinical recommendations of the treating physician, including reviews of patient's past medical history and medical documentation/reports, as well as response(s) to previous treatments.

Regular advanced directives are included as part of an E/M service; however, CPT codes 99497 and 99498 include separate advanced directive planning, palliative care, and detailed advance care planning determinations, as indicated in the code descriptors of both codes.

99497 Advance care planning including the explanation and discussion of advance directives such as standard forms (with completion of such forms, when performed), by the physician or other qualified health care professional; first 30 minutes, face-to-face with the patient, family member(s), and/or surrogate

+99498 each additional 30 minutes (List separately in addition to code for primary procedure)

Prolonged E/M Services

Starting on January 1, 2017, CMS provided separate payment for existing codes that describe prolonged E/M services without direct patient contact by the physician (or other billing practitioner) and increased payment for prolonged E/M services with direct patient contact by the physician (or other billing practitioner).

99358 Prolonged E/M service before and/or after direct patient care; first hour

99359 Prolonged E/M service before and/or after direct patient care; each additional 30 minutes (List separately in addition to code for prolonged service)

Beginning in 2021, CPT codes 99358-99359 will not be payable in association with office or other outpatient E/M visits. Along with the revisions to the E/M office or other outpatient visit services, new add-on code 99417 for prolonged E/M services was added to the CPT 2021 code set, effective January 1, 2021. In lieu of covering code 99417 for Medicare, CMS elected to create similar code G2212.

#★+●99417 Prolonged office or other outpatient evaluation and management service(s) beyond the minimum required time of the primary procedure which has been selected using total time, requiring total time with or without direct patient contact beyond the usual service, on the date of the primary service, each 15 minutes of total time (List separately in addition to codes 99205, 99215 for office or other outpatient Evaluation and Management services)

Interprofessional Telephone/ Internet/Electronic Health Record Consultation

Current codes 99446-99449 have been revised to include electronic health record and two new codes have been added to this subsection. Code 99451 has been established to report interprofessional consultation services provided by a consultative physician, and code 99452 has been established to report interprofessional referral services provided by a treating/requesting physician or other QHP. For 2019, in response to advocacy efforts by the AMA and other stakeholders, CMS will no longer consider 99446-99449 as bundled services and will begin pay for these services separately. Also, the CMS will cover 99451 and 99452 for Medicare beneficiaries.

Prior to 2019, codes 99446-99449 were available to report an assessment and management consultation service in which a patient's treating (eg, attending or primary) physician/QHP requests the opinion and/or treatment advice of a physician with specific specialty expertise (ie, the consultant) to assist the treating physician or other QHP in the diagnosis and/or management of the patient, with a verbal and written component as the vehicle for the consultant to convey the assessment. There were no codes for the consultant to report the service of sending the results of a consultation, without the additional verbal component. Therefore, code 99451 was established to allow reporting of telephone/Internet/electronic health record consultation services without a verbal component. The service described by code 99451 concludes with only a written report. Code 99452 should be reported for interprofessional telephone/Internet/electronic health record referral services provided either by a treating/requesting physician or other QHP. Report 16–30 minutes of a service day for time spent preparing for the referral and/or communicating with the consultant using code 99452. If the time spent exceeds 30 minutes, the treating/requesting physician or other QHP may report the prolonged services codes.

99446 Interprofessional telephone/Internet/electronic health record assessment and management service provided by a consultative physician including a verbal and written report to the patient's treating/requesting physician or other qualified health care professional; 5-10 minutes of medical consultative discussion and review

99447 Interprofessional telephone/Internet/electronic health record assessment and management service provided by a consultative physician including a verbal and written report to the patient's treating/requesting physician or other qualified health care professional; 11-20 minutes of medical consultative discussion and review

99448 Interprofessional telephone/Internet/electronic health record assessment and management service provided by a consultative physician including a verbal and written report to the patient's treating/requesting physician or other qualified health care professional; 21-30 minutes of medical consultative discussion and review

99449 Interprofessional telephone/Internet/electronic health record assessment and management service provided by a consultative physician including a verbal and written report to the patient's treating/requesting physician or other qualified health care professional; 31 minutes or more of medical consultative discussion and review

#99451 Interprofessional telephone/Internet/electronic health record assessment and management service provided by a consultative physician including a written report to the patient's treating/requesting physician or other qualified health care professional, 5 or more minutes of medical consultative time

#99452 Interprofessional telephone/Internet/electronic health record referral service(s) provided by a treating/requesting physician or qualified health care professional, 30 minutes

Psychiatric Collaborative Care Management Services

For 2017, CMS established new coding and payment mechanisms for behavioral health integration (BHI) services including substance use disorder treatment. CMS specifically created three codes to describe services furnished as part of psychiatric collaborative care management (CoCM) (G0502, G0503, and G0504) and one code to describe care management services for behavioral health conditions (G0507).

For 2018, the CPT Editorial Panel created CPT codes 99492, 99493, 99494, and 99484 to describe these services. Starting on January 1, 2018, CMS will pay for psychiatric CoCM services. This code set is one of several in response to a request from CMS to facilitate appropriate valuation of the services furnished under the Collaborative Care Model (CoCM). This CoCM is used to treat patients with common psychiatric conditions in the primary care setting through the provision of a defined set of services that operationalize the following core concepts: (1) Patient-Centered Team Care/Collaborative Care; (2) Population-Based Care; (3) Measurement-Based Treatment to Target; and (4) Evidence-Based Care.

99492 Initial psychiatric collaborative care management, first 70 minutes in the first calendar month of behavioral health care manager activities, in consultation with a psychiatric consultant, and directed by the treating physician or other qualified health care professional, with the following required elements:

- outreach to and engagement in treatment of a patient directed by the treating physician or other qualified health care professional;
- initial assessment of the patient, including administration of validated rating scales, with the development of an individualized treatment plan;
- review by the psychiatric consultant with modifications of the plan if recommended;
- entering patient in a registry and tracking patient follow-up and progress using the registry, with appropriate documentation, and participation in weekly caseload consultation with the psychiatric consultant; and
- provision of brief interventions using evidence-based techniques such as behavioral activation, motivational interviewing, and other focused treatment strategies.

99493 Subsequent psychiatric collaborative care management, first 60 minutes in a subsequent month of behavioral health care manager activities, in consultation with a psychiatric consultant, and directed by the treating physician or other qualified health care professional, with the following required elements:

- tracking patient follow-up and progress using the registry, with appropriate documentation;
- participation in weekly caseload consultation with the psychiatric consultant;
- ongoing collaboration with and coordination of the patient's mental health care with the treating physician or other qualified health care professional and any other treating mental health providers;
- additional review of progress and recommendations for changes in treatment, as indicated, including medications, based on recommendations provided by the psychiatric consultant;
- provision of brief interventions using evidence-based techniques such as behavioral activation, motivational interviewing, and other focused treatment strategies;
- monitoring of patient outcomes using validated rating scales; and
- relapse prevention planning with patients as they achieve remission of symptoms and/or other treatment goals and are prepared for discharge from active treatment.

+99494 Initial or subsequent psychiatric collaborative care management, each additional 30 minutes in a calendar month of behavioral health care manager activities, in consultation with a psychiatric consultant, and directed by the treating physician or other qualified health care professional (List separately in addition to code for primary procedure)

#99484 Care management services for behavioral health conditions, at least 20 minutes of clinical staff time, directed by a physician or other qualified health care professional, per calendar month, with the following required elements:

- initial assessment or follow-up monitoring, including the use of applicable validated rating scales;
- behavioral health care planning in relation to behavioral/psychiatric health problems, including revision for patients who are not progressing or whose status changes;
- facilitating and coordinating treatment such as psychotherapy, pharmacotherapy, counseling, and/or psychiatric consultation; and
- continuity of care with a designated member of the care team.

Other Primary Care Services

Starting on January 1, 2018, Medicare began paying for a new code describing an evidenced-based cognitive service. The CPT Editorial Panel created this code in response to a CMS request to capture cognitive service codes not currently described by E/M services. This service is provided when a comprehensive evaluation of a new or existing patient who exhibits signs of cognitive impairment is required to establish a diagnosis etiology and severity for the condition. The service includes a thorough evaluation of medical and psychosocial factors potentially contributing to increased morbidity. Typically, these patients are referred by a primary caregiver. There are 10 required elements for the service, and all 10 must be performed for the code to be reported. This service includes two distinct activities, assessment of the patient, and establishment of care plan that is shared with the patient and caregiver, along with education. It is important that all elements are performed to be able to report this code. Other face-to-face E/M codes cannot be reported on the same date as this service to prevent any overlap with E/M codes.

99483 Assessment of and care planning for a patient with cognitive impairment, requiring an independent historian, in the office or other outpatient, home or domiciliary or rest home, with all of the following required elements:

- Cognition-focused evaluation including a pertinent history and examination;
- Medical decision making of moderate or high complexity;
- Functional assessment (eg, basic and instrumental activities of daily living), including decision-making capacity;
- Use of standardized instruments for staging of dementia (eg, Functional Assessment Staging Test [FAST], Clinical Dementia Rating [CDR]);
- Medication reconciliation and review for high-risk medications;
- Evaluation for neuropsychiatric and behavioral symptoms, including depression, including use of standardized screening instrument(s);
- Evaluation of safety (eg, home), including motor vehicle operation;
- Identification of caregiver(s), caregiver knowledge, caregiver needs, social supports, and the willingness of caregiver to take on caregiving tasks;
- Development, updating or revision, or review of an Advance Care Plan;
- Creation of a written care plan, including initial plans to address any neuropsychiatric symptoms, neuro-cognitive symptoms, functional limitations, and referral to community resources as needed (eg, rehabilitation services, adult day programs, support groups) shared with the patient and/or caregiver with initial education and support.

Typically, 50 minutes are spent face-to-face with the patient and/or family or caregiver.

CMS established new coding and payment mechanisms for prolonged preventative services. CMS created two 30-minute add-on codes to report the additional time sometimes required to appropriately furnish care to a patient receiving a Medicare-covered preventive service. This will help ensure that the broad range of preventative services offered, ranging from wellness visits to cancer screenings, receive appropriate payment for preventative services that require more time. G0513 and G0514 can only be billed with Medicare-covered preventive services Coinsurance, and deductibles are not applicable as these codes will only be used to report prolonged portions of preventative services where beneficiary coinsurance and deductible are not applicable.

G0513 Prolonged preventive service(s) (beyond the typical service time of the primary procedure) in the office or other outpatient setting requiring direct patient contact beyond the usual service; first 30 minutes (List separately in addition to code for preventive service)

G0514 Prolonged preventive service(s) (beyond the typical service time of the primary procedure) in the office or other outpatient setting requiring direct patient contact beyond the usual service; each additional 30 minutes (List separately in addition to code for preventive service)

Other Issues for Reporting the E/M Codes

Since the implementation of Medicare RBRVS, CMS has issued many clarifications and policy changes concerning reporting of the E/M codes under specific circumstances. Descriptions of these reporting and coding issues follow.

Revised definition of new patient for selecting appropriate visit codes by group practices. In 1992, CMS revised its definition of *new patient* for group practices to be consistent with the original intent of the CPT Editorial Panel in developing the visit codes. *New patients* are those who have not been seen by a member of the group in the same specialty during the prior three-year period.

Annual routine (asymptomatic) exam in conjunction with a visit. CMS revised Medicare payment policy for routine physical exam, when performed at the same time as a medically necessary covered E/M service. Although Medicare does not cover routine physical exams, physicians generally were able to bill their patients at their regular payments for these services prior to May 1992.

In a May 29, 1992, in a memorandum issued to carriers, CMS stated that physicians could not divide the visit or consultation into covered and noncovered portions. Accordingly, if a symptom or medical condition was followed up during the annual exam, the physician was to report the visit with the appropriate level of E/M code. The visit was considered a covered E/M service and the limiting charge applied. The physician could not separately bill the patient for the *noncovered E/M services*. Variation in carrier interpretation of the CMS guidelines allowed some physicians to report a higher-level code appropriate for the overall encounter, while others were limited to reporting codes appropriate for the *covered services only*.

Revised CMS policy, for services rendered on or after October 30, 1993, allows physicians to bill the patient for noncovered-visit services provided as part of routine physical examinations. The preventive medicine services codes (99381-99397) should be reported for these services. The physician may continue to bill patients for noncovered *procedures*, such as routine chest X ray.

Payment for the covered visit services is the lesser of the physician's actual charge or the Medicare approved amount if the physician accepts assignment. If assignment is not accepted, Medicare bases its payment on the lesser of the physician's actual charge or 95% of the allowed amount. The physician, in addition to collecting the coinsurance, may bill up to his or her limiting charge. The physician's charge to the patient for the noncovered portion of the E/M service is the difference between the physician's usual payment for a routine physical exam and his or her usual payment (not the Medicare allowed amount) for the covered visit.

CMS' rationale for the revised policy is that the covered-visit services are provided in lieu of a part of the routine physical exam that is of equal value to the visit. Because the basis of noncoverage is a specific statutory exclusion rather than medical necessity, there is no statutory authority to preclude physicians from billing the patient for the noncovered portion of the E/M service. Therefore, the physician is not required to notify the patient in advance that the physical exam is a noncovered service.

Preoperative medical clearance by the primary care physician. Effective June 28, 1993, a primary care or specialist physician who performs a preoperative consultation or a postoperative evaluation for a new or established patient at the request of the surgeon may bill the appropriate consultation code. CMS' previous policy required the physician (if he or she had seen the patient within the previous three years) to report either an established patient office code or the appropriate subsequent hospital care code. All criteria for use of the consultation codes as identified in the CPT 1998 must be met. CMS has identified the following CPT requirements as the most relevant for reporting a preoperative consultation:

- The surgeon must request the opinion or advice of the physician regarding the evaluation and/or management of a specific problem.
- The surgeon's request for a consultation and the need for consultation must be documented in the patient's medical record.
- The consultant's opinion and any services ordered or performed must be documented in the patient's medical record and must be communicated to the surgeon.
- The physician must have provided all the services necessary to meet the CPT description of the level of service billed.

The patient's medical record should support these criteria. CMS provides these guidelines:

- In an inpatient setting, the request may be documented as part of a plan written in the requesting surgeon's progress note, an order in a hospital record, or a specific written request for the consultation.
- In an office or other outpatient setting, the request may be documented by specific written request for the consultation from the requesting surgeon, or the physician's records may reference the request.
- The medical record should identify the specific problem that was the reason for the consultation; describe the extent of history, physical, and decision making that supports the level of consultation code billed; and include the consultant's findings and recommendations to the requesting surgeon.

Postoperative consultations by nonsurgeons. A physician who performs a postoperative evaluation for a new or established patient at the request of the surgeon may bill the appropriate consultation code. However, if the physician had already provided the preoperative consultation, the same physician may not also bill for a postoperative consultation code. The same criteria as previously described for using the consultation codes must be met for a postoperative consultation.

CMS provides the following example:

... if the surgeon requests the opinion or advice of a physician regarding a specific problem that has arisen following the surgery and also requests that the physician assume responsibility for the management of that problem during the postoperative period, the physician may bill the initial encounter with the appropriate consultation code and subsequent encounters with the appropriate subsequent hospital care codes. This example applies whether the patient is new or established to the physician.

However, if the surgeon only refers the patient for the management of a specific condition during the postoperative period—and does not request specific advice from the physician—a consultation may not be billed. CMS considers these services as concurrent care. The services should be reported with the appropriate level of visit codes, not a consultation code.

In the CPT 2000, several changes have been made to the consultation notes to clarify any misinterpretation of the intent and use of the outpatient and inpatient consultation codes (99241-99255). The revisions clarify the following issues:

- A physician consultant may initiate diagnostic and/or therapeutic services at the same or subsequent visit.
- The written or verbal request for a consult may be made by a physician or other appropriate source and documented in the patient's medical record.
- The consultant's opinion and any services that were ordered or performed must also be documented in the patient's medical record and communicated by written report to the requesting physician or other appropriate source.
- In the hospital setting, the consulting physician should use the appropriate inpatient hospital consultation code for the initial encounter and then subsequent hospital care codes (not follow-up consultation codes). In the office setting, the appropriate established patient code should be used.

Critical care. In 1992, CMS issued a revised and reduced list of services bundled into critical care codes 99291 and 99292; this list of services was again revised for the CPT 2022 code set. The current list of codes includes: the interpretation of cardiac output measurements (93598); chest X rays (71045, 71046); pulse oximetry (94760, 94761, 94762); blood gases, and collection and interpretation of physiologic data (eg, ECGs, blood pressures, hematologic data); gastric intubation (43752, 43753); temporary transcutaneous pacing (92953); ventilatory management (94002-94004, 94660, 94662); and vascular access procedures (36000, 36410, 36415, 36591, 36600). Any services performed that are not included in this listing should be reported separately. Separate payments will be made, when services other than these are reported with the provision of critical care.

The critical care codes 99291 and 99292 should be reported when critical care is provided to a patient upon admission to the emergency department. If critical care is required upon admission to the emergency department, CMS has indicated that the physician should only report the appropriate critical care code. Payment will not be made for emergency department services reported for the same encounter as critical care, when provided by the same physician. However, if the physician provided emergency department services to a patient and later the same day provided critical care to the patient, each encounter should be reported, and separate payments would be made. Similarly, if the physician provides a hospital visit to a patient, who later that same day requires critical care, the physician should report both encounters and separate payments would be made. CMS has specified that documentation must be submitted when E/M services are reported on the same day as critical care.

Critical care services provided during the global period for a seriously injured or burned patient are not considered to be related to a surgical procedure and may be paid separately. CMS has indicated that preoperative and postoperative critical care may be paid separately from the global payment, if (1) the patient requires the physician's constant attendance, and (2) the critical care is unrelated to the specific anatomic injury, or the general surgical procedure performed. To report preoperative critical care, the appropriate critical care code and modifier 25, as well as supporting documentation, must be submitted. To report postoperative critical care, the appropriate critical care code and modifier 24, as well as supporting documentation, must be submitted.

In 2000, several important revisions were made to the critical care codes to clarify long-standing misinterpretations among Medicare carriers. These revisions, included (1) the elimination of the *word unstable*; (2) expansion of the definition of *critical care* to include care provided after the initial intervention; (3) replacing the term *constant attendance* to *constant attention*; (4) inclusion of language that critical care services include treatment and prevention of further deterioration; (5) inclusion of language making the determination of time for these codes consistent with the

CPT instructions for hospital inpatient E/M codes; and (6) inclusion of family discussion time as part of the intra-service work, which is consistent with the definition of work for E/M services in a hospital setting. In the CPT 2001 codebook, the CPT code set clarified that critical care services are those in which "there is a high probability of imminent or life-threatening deterioration in the patient's condition." The Panel also further clarified examples of vital organ system failure. For further detail on the new nomenclature for the critical care services, refer to the CPT 2004. RUC reviewed these changes and determined that the revisions were for clarification only and did not change the physician work required to perform the service. Unfortunately, CMS did not agree with RUC and decreased the work relative values for both codes 99291 and 99292 by 10%. The AMA, RUC, and several specialty societies objected to these decreases and argued that CMS should revert back to the 1999 work RVUs. In the November 1, 2000, Final Rule, CMS announced restoration of the work relative values for critical care, because of the further clarification in the CPT code set.

In 2022, CMS adopted the updated CPT guidelines for the reporting of critical care services (99291-99292) and the CPT listing of bundled services. When medically necessary, critical care services can be furnished concurrently to the same patient on the same day by more than one physician or other QHP representing more than one specialty. In the Final Rule for CY 2022, CMS did not finalize its proposal to always bundle critical care visits with procedure codes that have a global surgical period; it instead maintained its current policy that critical care visits may be paid separately in addition to a procedure with a global surgical period, as long as the critical care service is unrelated to the procedure. Physicians or other QHPs must document that the E/M service is medically necessary and separate and distinct from critical care services. Physicians must use modifier 25, *Significant, Separately Identifiable Evaluation and Management Service by the Same Physician or Other Qualified Health Care Professional on the Same Day of the Procedure or Other Service*, to report these services.

Emergency department services. The emergency department visit codes (99281-99285) should be reported whenever physicians, regardless of whether they are "assigned" to the emergency department, provide services to a patient registered in the emergency department. The emergency department codes may not be used for services provided in a physician's office, even though the services are for an emergency. Instead, critical care codes (99291 and 99292) may be reported for these circumstances. For 2020, CMS finalized its proposal to increase payment for the emergency department visit codes (99281-99284) as recommended by RUC. In addition, CMS issued the following guidelines for reporting emergency department services provided to the same patient by a primary care physician and an emergency department physician:

If a primary care physician advises his/her own patient to go to an emergency department of a hospital for care and subsequently is asked by the emergency department physician to come to the hospital to evaluate the patient and to advise the emergency department physician as to whether the patient should be admitted to the hospital or be sent home, the physicians should report the services as follows:

(a) If the patient is admitted to the hospital by the primary care physician, then that physician should report only the appropriate level of the initial hospital care codes (99221–99223) because all E/M services provided by that physician in conjunction with that admission are considered part of the initial hospital care when performed on the same date as the admission. The emergency department physician should report the appropriate level of the emergency department codes.

(b) If the emergency department physician sends the patient home, based on the advice of the primary care physician, then he/she should report the appropriate level of the emergency department codes. The primary care physician also should report the appropriate level of the emergency department codes. It would be inappropriate to report the consultation codes because the primary care physician is responsible for the overall management of the patient.

Observation care services. Observation care services codes (99217-99220 and 99234-99236) should be reported when E/M services are provided to patients designated/admitted as "observation status" in a hospital. It is not necessary that the patient be in an observation area designated by the hospital. In the November 1, 2000, Final Rule, CMS announced very specific policies for reporting these services. These policies are outlined as follows:

- When a patient is admitted to an observation status for less than 8 hours on the same date, CPT codes for initial observation care (99218 through 99220) should be used by the physician and no discharge code should be reported.
- When a patient is admitted to an observation status for more than 8 hours on the same calendar date, then CPT codes for observation or inpatient care services, including admission and discharge services (99234 through 99236), should be reported.
- When a patient is admitted for observation care and then discharged on a different calendar date, the physician should use CPT codes for initial observation care (99218 through 99220) and the CPT code for observation discharge (99217).

The physician must satisfy the document requirements for both admission to and discharge from inpatient or outpatient care to bill the codes 99234, 99235, and 99236. The length of time for observation care or treatment status also must be documented.

Subsequent observation care services. Shifts in practice and payment policy have made it increasingly common for patients to remain in a hospital for several days under observation or outpatient status, instead of being "admitted." Before 2011, there were only codes to report the initial day of observation service and discharge from observation in the CPT code set. Until 2011, the CPT guidelines for "subsequent" observation services were that code 99499, *Unlisted evaluation and management service*, should be reported for subsequent days. In response to the increase in the number of observation services that extend beyond the initial observation, three new codes (99224-99226) were approved to report subsequent observation services in a facility setting. RUC persuaded CMS that the physician work related to observation services is equivalent to inpatient hospital visits.

Psychotherapy. Beginning July 1, 2008, and ending December 31, 2009, MIPPA provided a 5% increase in the payment schedule for psychiatric therapeutic procedures including insight oriented, behavior modifying, or supportive psychotherapy or interactive psychotherapy. This provision was extended by the Affordable Care Act from January 1, 2010–December 31, 2010, and further extended by the Medicare and Medicaid Extenders Act of 2010 from January 1, 2011–December 31, 2011.

On January 1, 2010, the limitation on recognition of expenses incurred for outpatient mental health services began to be phased out by increasing the Medicare Part B payment for outpatient mental health services to 80%, the same level as other Part B services, by 2014. In the 4th Five-Year Review of the RBRVS, CMS identified CPT codes 90801–90880 as potentially misvalued and requested that the AMA RUC review these services. In response, the AMA concluded that the entire section of psychotherapy would benefit from restructuring. After a year of analysis, the CPT Editorial Panel created a new section, effective January 1, 2013, with a new structure to allow separate reporting of E/M codes, eliminating site of service differential, creation of CPT codes to describe crisis, and creation of add-on codes to describe interactive complexity and medication management. This revision was driven by the fact that the patient population receiving these services has dramatically changed.

The new coding framework allows all codes to be used in all settings, instead of describing site-specific services.

One major change involves psychotherapy services provided alongside an E/M service. For 2013, the CPT Editorial Panel created codes 90833, 90836, and 90838 to describe psychotherapy provided for 30 minutes, 45 minutes, and 60 minutes, performed with an E/M. Physicians and qualified nonphysician practitioners who can bill for E/M services will now bill for psychotherapy with evaluation and management using the existing E/M structure and a choice of one add-on psychotherapy time-based code. CMS determined that the work involved in providing the psychotherapy add-on codes is similar to the work of the stand-alone psychotherapy codes (CPT codes 90832, 90834, and 90837). RUC determined that the difference is related to the time involved rather than the intensity. The AMA RUC recommended, and CMS agreed, that the psychotherapy codes include 12 minutes less time than the stand-alone codes.

For 2013, CMS assigned interim relative values for these services and requested RUC review add-on codes for the interactive component of psychotherapy and crisis services (90839, 90840, and 90785) before the full review of the recommendations for the entire of family of psychotherapy services. For 2014, RUC submitted the remaining interactive complexity component add-on codes for psychotherapy and crisis services. CMS accepted 100% of the RUC recommendations for the psychotherapy services for 2014, leading to $150 million in improved payments for these services each year. Medicare payments for psychiatrists, psychologists, and clinical social workers increased 6%–8% in CY 2014.

Ventilator management on the same day as an E/M service. As part of RUC's recommendations for the 2005 Five-Year Review, the CPT Editorial Panel reviewed the ventilator management family of services to differentiate between those patients who received ventilation management services on an acute and those on long-term basis. CPT codes 94656 and 94657 have been replaced with four new codes (94002–94005) to differentiate between ventilation management in the acute care setting (initial and subsequent) and long-term care setting (nursing facility and home). CMS has assigned this service a status indicator of B (bundled), because they believe this service is captured in the E/M services despite RUC's objections.

Pulse oximetry. CMS will bundle payment for pulse oximetry services (CPT codes 94760 and 94761), when provided on the same date as other services. CMS implemented this policy on January 1, 2001, because as technology has progressed, and been simplified and reduced in cost, pulse oximetry is considered a routine minor part of a procedure or visit.

Payment for standby surgical team. CMS considers services furnished by the standby surgical team to be hospital services and paid by the hospital; consequently, physicians are precluded from billing the patient for these services.

Allergen immunotherapy. CMS clarified that it will not allow payment for an office visit provided on the same day as allergen immunotherapy (CPT codes 95115, 95117, 95144–95199), unless separate identifiable services are performed. This policy is consistent with CPT coding language: "Office visit codes may be used in addition to allergen immunotherapy, if and only if, other identifiable services are provided at that time."

Legislative Initiatives to Detect Fraud and Abuse

Under provisions of Health Insurance Portability and Accountability Act of 1996 (HIPAA), the secretary of Health and Human Services (HHS) and the attorney general are required to jointly establish a national health care fraud and abuse control program to coordinate federal, state, and local law enforcement to combat fraud related to health plans. The creation of a Health Care Fraud and Abuse Control (HCFAC) Account also was called for, whereby the assessment of civil money penalties and fines from court cases would be transferred into the Federal Hospital Insurance Trust Fund.

The law also authorizes CMS to contract with private entities to carry out certain review activities previously performed by local Medicare carriers. These private contractors, which may include carriers, will conduct medical and utilization review and fraud review, and determine when Medicare is the secondary payer. The legislation requires that Medicare adopts the commercial standards and claims processing software technology currently used by private insurers. CMS is expected to begin phasing in the new authority later this year.

Congressional members' continuing concerns about health fraud and abuse are reflected in the Balanced Budget Act (BBA) of 1997. The new law extends to 10 years or makes permanent Medicare and Medicaid program exclusion requirements for individuals convicted of a felony related to health care fraud and other specified offenses. Provisions are designed to identify beneficiaries and to report suspected Medicare fraud and abuse. These include requirements that the explanation of Medicare benefits (EOMB) form contain the toll-free telephone number for reporting complaints of suspected fraudulent activity, and that Medicare carriers and intermediaries give beneficiaries itemized bills for Medicare services within 30 days upon request. Other provisions target DME suppliers and home health agencies.

The AMA has consistently opposed the establishment of a fraud and abuse control account funded by fines and penalties collected from convictions for health care offenses. Such an account constitutes a bounty system and provides inappropriate incentives for objective implementation of the fraud and abuse program. The AMA will closely monitor government enforcement activities to ensure fairness.

The AMA is also concerned that CMS' current approach to waste, fraud, and abuse mixes two issues that should be separated: correct coding policy and fraud and abuse in Medicare claims. It is believed that only 1% to 2% of physicians are involved in filing fraudulent claims. Bad editing procedures, however, punish all physicians (and their Medicare patients) by denying payment and refusing coverage for medically necessary services. The AMA and CMS have worked cooperatively on CMS' correct coding initiative (CCI). The CCI, implemented by CMS in January 1996, is aimed at detecting and denying payment for inappropriate coding on Medicare claims.

The AMA believes that the problem of health care fraud is serious. At the same time, physicians cannot be expected to fulfill their obligations without standards to guide them. Therefore, the AMA has called for public and private payers and fraud enforcement agencies to work with the medical profession to clearly define the conduct that constitutes fraud and abuse.

Payment Policy Changes to Preventive Services Benefits

The BBA of 1997 expanded the Medicare benefits package to include coverage for some preventive medicine services. Effective January 1, 1998, Medicare covers an annual mammography screening for all women beneficiaries older than 39 years of age; colorectal cancer screening tests for beneficiaries 50 years of age and older; and screening pelvic examinations (including a clinical breast exam) for women beneficiaries. Frequency limits and coverage conditions for the new benefits are described in the following sections.

The Medicare, Medicaid, and SCHIP Benefits Improvement and Protection Act (BIPA) of 2000 was enacted on December 21, 2000, and provides for revisions to policies applicable to the MFS. This legislation created Medicare coverage changes for several services, including enhancements to screening mammography, pelvic examinations, colonoscopy, and telemedicine; new coverage for screening for glaucoma; and new coverage for medical nutrition therapy performed by registered dietitians and nutrition professionals.

The MMA further broadens the preventive benefits. Effective January 1, 2005, Medicare will pay for an initial preventive physical examination (IPPE) within the first six months a beneficiary begins Part B. The MMA also expands coverage to include cardiovascular and diabetes screening blood tests. The MIPPA mandates that Medicare will pay for an IPPE within the first 12 months a beneficiary begins Part B.

Beneficiary access to preventive services improved in 2011. In 2011, CMS removed the deductible and coinsurance for most of the preventive services including the initial preventive physician examination (IPPE) and waiving the deductible for tests that began as colorectal cancer screening tests, but during the test become diagnostic or therapeutic. For 2022, CMS finalized its proposal to implement the reduced beneficiary coinsurance phase-in for colorectal cancer screening tests as dictated by the Consolidated Appropriations Act, 2021 (section 122). Currently, the addition of any procedure beyond a planned colorectal cancer screening test (for which there is no coinsurance) results in the beneficiary having to pay coinsurance. The AMA supports the CMS proposal that between CYs 2022 and 2030, the coinsurance required of Medicare beneficiaries for planned colorectal cancer screening tests that result in additional procedures furnished in the same clinical encounter will be reduced over time from the current 20 or 25 percent to zero percent in CY 2030 and will remain at zero percent for these services furnished beginning in CY 2030 and thereafter.

CMS also covers an annual wellness visit (AWV), a service to be provided annually that augments the one-time IPPE service, which includes personalized prevention plan services. For 2012, CMS required physicians to incorporate the use and results of a health risk assessment (HRA) in the provision of personalized prevention plan services during the annual wellness visit. CMS also recognized the additional resources associated with adding an HRA to the service's requirements and increased the total RVUs for codes G0438 and G0439 for CY 2012. For 2014, CMS modified coverage of colorectal cancer screening. Specifically, coverage for "screening fecal occult blood test (FOBT)" was revised to allow an attending physician, physician assistant, nurse practitioner, or clinical nurse specialist to furnish written orders for screening FOBT. These modifications will allow for expanded coverage and access to screening FOBT, particularly in rural areas. In addition, coverage for abdominal aortic aneurysms (AAA) was revised to allow a one-time AAA screening without receiving a referral as part of the initial preventive physical examination for beneficiaries that meet certain criteria (a family history of AAA, or for men aged 65–75, a history of smoking).

Initial Preventive Physical Examination

The MMA provides for coverage for a Medicare beneficiaries' initial preventive physical examination (IPPE) effective January 1, 2005. MIPPA extended the enrollment of this "welcome to Medicare benefit" from six months to one year for an individual who elects to participate in Medicare Part B. This benefit includes all of the following:

- Review of the individual's comprehensive medical and social history
- Review of the individual's review of risk factors for depression
- Review of the individual's level of safety and functional ability and level of safety
- An examination to include measurement of height, weight, blood pressure, and visual acuity screen
- Performance and interpretation of an electrocardiogram
- Education, counseling, and referral as appropriate, based on the above five elements
- A written plan provided to the patient for obtaining the appropriate screening and other preventive services, which are separately covered under Medicare Part B benefits

The enactment of MIPPA revises this benefit by adding the following services:

- Measurement of an individual's body mass index
- End-of-life planning, upon individual's consent

However, MIPPA removed the electrocardiogram from the list of mandated services that must be included in this benefit, and made the IPPE an educational, counseling, and referral service to be discussed with the individual and ordered by the physician, if necessary.

G0402, *Initial preventive physical examination; face-to-face visit, services limited to new beneficiary during the first 12 months of Medicare enrollment*. The deductible and the coinsurance for code G0402 is waived.

Annual Wellness Visit

Beginning January 1, 2011, CMS covers an AWV, a service to be provided annually that augments the one-time IPPE service, which includes personalized prevention plan services. No coinsurance or deductible applies to this service. The AWV, as determined by law, may include at least the following six elements:

- Establish or update the individuals' current medical and family history
- List the individual's current medical providers and suppliers and all prescribed medications
- Record measurements of height, weight, body mass index, blood pressure, and other routine measurements
- Detect any cognitive impairment
- Establish or update a screening schedule for the next 5 to 10 years including screenings appropriate for the general population, and any additional screenings that may be appropriate because of the individual patient's risk factors
- Furnish personalized health advice and appropriate referrals to health education or preventative services

Cardiovascular Screening Blood Tests

The MMA provides for Medicare coverage of cardiovascular screening blood tests for the early detection of cardiovascular disease, effective January 1, 2005. CMS covers the total cholesterol, HDL cholesterol, and triglycerides tests performed after a 12-hour fast, for each patient every five years. LDL testing will only be covered, if the screening tests indicated an elevated triglyceride level, which would warrant obtaining a direct measurement LDL test.

Medicare will recognize CPT codes and the clinical lab payment schedule payments for these services, including codes 82465, *Cholesterol, serum or whole blood, total*; 83718, *Lipoprotein, direct measurement; high density cholesterol (HDL cholesterol)*; 84478, *Triglycerides;* and 80061, *Lipid panel.*

Diabetes Screening

The MMA requires coverage of diabetes screening tests effective January 1, 2005. CMS will cover a fasting blood glucose test and post-glucose challenge tests. Those patients diagnosed with pre-diabetes, defined as a previous fasting glucose level of 100–125 mg/dL or a two-hour post-glucose challenge of 140–199 mg/dL, are eligible for two screening tests per 12-month period. Those individuals who do not meet these criteria are eligible for one diabetes screening test per year.

Medicare will recognize CPT codes and the clinical lab payment schedule payments for these services, including codes 82947, *Glucose; quantitative, blood (except reagent strip);* 82950, *Glucose; post glucose dose (includes glucose)*; and 82951, *Glucose; tolerance test (GTT), 3 specimens (includes glucose).*

In 2017, CMS finalized an expansion of the duration and scope of the diabetes prevention program (DPP) model test. The Medicare DPP (MDPP) expanded model will be covered as a preventive service with no cost sharing under Medicare beginning January 1, 2018. The MDPP is a 12-month program that consists of at least 16 weekly core sessions during the first six months, followed by additional core maintenance sessions over the remaining six months.

Screening Mammography

Mammography screening is a covered benefit for all women beneficiaries older than 35 years of age. The BBA waived the Part B deductible. Further, beginning January 1, 2011, the coinsurance will be waived for screening mammography. The statute defines screening mammography as a radiologic procedure furnished to a woman, who does not have signs or symptoms of breast disease, for the purpose of early detection of breast cancer. It includes a physician's interpretation of the results of the procedure. Medicare will pay for one screening for women aged 35–39 and annually for women aged 40 and older.

Previously, the screening mammography benefit varied according to a woman's age and level of risk for developing breast cancer. Coverage for women 40 to 49 years of age was provided annually or twice per year for beneficiaries considered to be at high risk; coverage for women 50 to 64 years of age was annually; and coverage for women older than 64 years of age was biannually.

For medical purposes, the definition of diagnostic mammography was expanded beginning in January 1996, to include as candidates for this procedure "asymptomatic men or women who have a personal history of breast cancer or a personal history of biopsy-proven disease." The definition of biopsy-proven disease includes both benign and malignant neoplasms.

On January 1, 2002, payment for a screening mammography will no longer be established by statute. Instead, it will be based on the RBRVS and the MFS. BIPA also required CMS to pay for new digital technologies for both screening and diagnostic mammography beginning January 1, 2002.

Medicare will recognize the following code for this service: 77067, *Screening mammography, bilateral (2-view study of each breast), including computer-aided detection (CAD) when performed.*

Colorectal Cancer Screening

Colorectal cancer screening is covered for Medicare patients 50 years of age and older. Effective January 1, 2007, CMS exempted the colorectal cancer screening benefit from the Part B deductible. Further, beginning January 1, 2011, the coinsurance will be waived for fecal occult blood tests, flexible sigmoidoscopy and screening colonoscopy, eliminating a potential financial barrier to Medicare beneficiaries, who could use this benefit. The statute specified coverage for screening fecal occult blood tests, screening flexible sigmoidoscopy, and screening colonoscopy. Flexibility in the statute allowed CMS to expand the new benefit to include coverage for screening barium enema examinations.

The statute specified frequency limitations for Medicare coverage according to type of test. For 2014, CMS modified coverage for "screening fecal occult blood test (FOBT)" to allow an attending physician, physician assistant, nurse practitioner, or clinical nurse specialist to furnish written orders for screening FOBT. These modifications will allow for expanded coverage and access to screening FOBT, particularly in rural areas.

Screening flexible sigmoidoscopy examinations are covered once every 48 months. Screening colonoscopy examinations are covered once every 24 months for patients at high risk of developing colorectal cancer. The statute defines high-risk patients as those with a family history of such disease, prior experience of cancer or precursor neoplastic polyps, a history of chronic digestive disease condition (including inflammatory bowel disease, Crohn's disease, or ulcerative colitis), the presence of any appropriate recognized gene markers for colorectal cancer, or other predisposing factors. Medicare requires that an MD or DO performs screening flexible sigmoidoscopies and screening colonoscopies.

Screening barium enema examinations may be covered as an alternative to a flexible sigmoidoscopy once every 48 months for Medicare patients, who are not at high risk for developing colorectal cancer. For high-risk patients, screening barium enemas may be covered once every 24 months, as an alternative to a screening colonoscopy. (Current policy allows payment for diagnostic barium enemas, which are performed to evaluate a patient's specific complaint or to monitor an existing medical condition for patients with a history of colon cancer.) Screening barium enema exams are covered, only if ordered in writing by the patient's attending physician.

BIPA also added coverage of screening colonoscopies once every 10 years for individuals not at high risk for colorectal cancer. However, in the case of an individual who is not at high risk for colorectal cancer, but who has had a screening flexible sigmoidoscopy within the last four years, the statute provides that payment may be made for a screening colonoscopy only after at least 47 months have passed, following the month in which the last screening flexible sigmoidoscopy was performed. In addition, the statute provides that in the case of an individual, who is not at high risk for colorectal cancer but who does have a screening colonoscopy performed on or after July 1, 2001, payment may be made for a screening flexible sigmoidoscopy only after at least 120 months have passed, following the month in which the last screening colonoscopy was performed.

CMS developed new HCPCS codes for use in reporting the new services. The agency also developed relative values for the new codes, which are listed in the List of Relative Value Units in Part 5.

Payment for screening fecal occult blood tests (G0328) is at the same rate as diagnostic fecal occult blood tests (CPT code 82270) and is made under the clinical laboratory payment schedule.

Screening flexible sigmoidoscopies (HCPCS code G0104) are paid at rates consistent with payment for similar or related services under the MFS but may not exceed the rates for a diagnostic flexible sigmoidoscopy (CPT code 45330). If during the flexible sigmoidoscopy screening, a lesion or growth is detected that results in a biopsy or removal of the growth, the physician should bill for a flexible sigmoidoscopy with biopsy or removal, rather than use the new HCPCS code.

Payment for screening colonoscopy is made under HCPCS code G0121, *Colorectal cancer screening; colonoscopy on individual not meeting criteria for high risk*. Payment for screening colonoscopies (HCPCS code G0105) is consistent with that for similar or related services under the payment schedule but may not exceed that for a diagnostic colonoscopy (CPT code 45378). If during the colonoscopy screening, a lesion or growth is detected that results in a biopsy or removal of the growth, the physician should bill for a colonoscopy with biopsy or removal (45380), rather than codes G0105 or G0121.

HCPCS codes G0106, *Colorectal cancer screening*; alternative to G0104, *Screening sigmoidoscopy, barium enema*, and G0120, *Colorectal cancer screening*; alternative to G0105, *Screening colonoscopy, barium enema*, should be used to report the barium enema when it is substituted for either the sigmoidoscopy or the colonoscopy, as indicated by the code nomenclature. The RVUs for G0106 are the same as the diagnostic barium enema procedure (CPT code 74280). Physicians should use HCPCS codes G0121, *Colorectal cancer screening; colonoscopy on individual not meeting criteria for high risk (noncovered)*, and G0122, *Colorectal cancer screening; barium enema (noncovered)*, when the high-risk criteria are not met, or a barium enema is performed but not as a substitute for either a sigmoidoscopy or colonoscopy. Starting January 1, 2015, CMS waived the deductible and coinsurance for anesthesia service reported with screening colonoscopy.

For 2022, CMS finalized its proposal to implement the reduced beneficiary coinsurance phase-in for colorectal cancer screening tests as dictated by the Consolidated Appropriations Act, 2021 (section 122). Currently, the addition of any procedure beyond a planned colorectal cancer screening test (for which there is no coinsurance) results in the beneficiary having to pay coinsurance. The AMA supports the CMS proposal that between CYs 2022 and 2030, the coinsurance required of Medicare beneficiaries for planned colorectal cancer screening tests that result in additional procedures furnished in the same clinical encounter will be reduced over time from the current 20 or 25 percent to zero percent in CY 2030 and will remain at zero percent for these services furnished beginning in CY 2030 and thereafter.

Cervical and Vaginal Cancer Screenings

The BBA provided for Medicare coverage of screening pelvic examinations (including a clinical breast examination) for all women beneficiaries, subject to certain frequency and other limitations. The statute waived the Part B deductible requirement. Beginning January 1, 2011, the coinsurance for this service will not apply. Under the statute, the examination should include at least seven of the 11 elements listed for such an exam, as specified in the Documentation Guidelines for Evaluation and Management Services. Effective July 1, 2001, BIPA amended the coverage of pelvic examinations to provide that a woman qualifies for coverage of a screening pelvic examination (including a clinical breast examination) once every two years (rather than once every three years, as provided by the BBA of 1997). However, it would allow annual pelvic exams for certain women of childbearing age and for women at high risk for cervical or vaginal cancer.

Annual screening pelvic examinations would be covered, if one of the following conditions is met:

- The woman is of childbearing age and has had an examination indicating the presence of cervical or vaginal cancer or other abnormality during any of the preceding three years.
- The woman is considered by her physician or other practitioner to be at high risk of developing cervical or vaginal cancer.

Based on recommendations made by the National Cancer Institute and the Centers for Disease Control and Prevention, the Medicare program adopted the following as high-risk factors for cervical cancer:

- Early onset of sexual activity (younger than 16 years of age)
- Multiple sexual partners (five or more in a lifetime)
- History of a sexually transmitted disease (including the human immunodeficiency virus [HIV])
- Absence of three negative Pap smears or any Pap smears within the previous seven years

Prenatal exposure to diethylstilbestrol is considered the high-risk factor for development of vaginal cancer. Based on recommendations from the American College of Gynecologists and Obstetricians and other groups, a woman of childbearing age is considered to be a premenopausal woman and is considered by her physician or other practitioner to be of childbearing age, based on her medical history or other findings.

Medicare coverage requirements of the BBA specify that screening pelvic examinations must be performed by an MD or DO, or by a certified nurse midwife, physician assistant, nurse practitioner, or clinical nurse specialist, who is authorized by state law to perform the examination.

Medicare covers Pap tests and pelvic examinations to check for cervical and vaginal cancers. Medicare Part B also covers human papillomavirus (HPV) tests, included as part of Pap tests, once every 5 years if patients are age 30-65 without HPV symptoms.

Screening for Glaucoma

Section 102 of the BIPA provides for Medicare coverage under Part B for screening for glaucoma for individuals with diabetes, a family history of glaucoma, or others determined to be at "high risk" for glaucoma, effective for services furnished on or after January 1, 2002. Payment will be allowed for one glaucoma screening examination per year. Payment for glaucoma screening will be bundled, if provided on the same date as an E/M service or when it is provided as part of any ophthalmology service. When glaucoma screening is the only service provided, or when it is provided as part of an otherwise noncovered service (for example, preventive services visit), physicians should report either code G0117 (when performed directly by optometrist or ophthalmologist) or code G0118 (when performed under the supervision of an optometrist or ophthalmologist).

In the November 21, 2005, Final Rule, CMS announced it is expanding its definition of eligible beneficiary for glaucoma screening to include Hispanic Americans aged 65 or over, based on the review of current medical literature. Currently, the definition of eligible beneficiaries only includes individuals with diabetes mellitus, individuals with a family history of glaucoma, or African Americans aged 50 and over.

Medical Nutrition Therapy

Section 105 of BIPA created a benefit for medical nutrition therapy (MNT) for certain Medicare patients, who have diabetes or a renal disease or have received a kidney transplant within the last 3 years. This benefit was implemented on January 1, 2002. Medicare Part B will pay for 3 hours of one-on-one MNT counseling furnished by a registered dietitian or nutrition professional in the first year and 2 hours in subsequent years when these, when the beneficiary is referred for the service by the beneficiary's treating physician. The treating physician is defined as the primary care physician or specialist coordinating care for the beneficiary with diabetes or renal disease. The statute specifies that the Medicare payment for MNT services must equal 80% of the lesser of the actual charge for the services, or 85% of the amount determined under the MFS for the same services, if furnished by a physician. The MNT services should be reported using CPT codes 97802–97804. CMS also clarified that medical nutrition therapy cannot be provided incident to a physician's service unless the physician also meets the qualifications to bill Medicare as a registered dietitian or nutrition professional.

CMS proposed in its November 21, 2005, Final Rule to add individual medical nutrition therapy (HCPCS/CPT codes G0720, 97802, and 97803) to the list of Medicare telemedicine services. Subsequently, CMS proposed in its November 29, 2010, Final Rule to add group medical nutrition therapy (HCPAC/CPT code 97804) to the list of Medicare telemedicine services. Accordingly, because registered dietitians and nutrition professionals are the primary providers of these services, they have been added to the list of providers who are able to receive payment for telemedicine services. In the Final Rule published on December 1, 2006, CMS announced that it will establish work RVUs for the medical nutrition therapy codes, as recommended by RUC HCPAC for the 2001 MFS Final Rule. In early 2008, CMS requested that the services described by CPT codes 97802 and 97803 be given the opportunity for consideration under the RUC process, to help ensure that CMS payment for MNT services to nonphysician nutrition professionals is accurate. In the Final Rule published November 19, 2008, CMS announced it accepted the new work RVUs for these services, as recommended by RUC for the 2009 MFS.

In the CY 2022 Final Rule, CMS finalized its proposal to pay for MNT services at 100 percent (instead of 80 percent) of 85 percent of the Medicare PFS approved amount without cost sharing. Regulations continue to require that referrals for MNT services must be made by the treating physician—an MD or DO.

Ultrasound Abdominal Aortic Aneurysm

As part of the DRA, beginning January 1, 2005, Medicare will pay for preventative ultrasound screening for abdominal aortic aneurysms (AAA) (HCPCS/CPT codes G0389 and 76706) for at-risk beneficiaries. The screening will be available to men between the ages of 65 and 75, who have smoked at least 100 cigarettes in their lifetime, beneficiaries with a family history of AAAs, and any other individuals recommended for screening by the US Preventative Services Task Force. In 2014, coverage for abdominal aortic aneurysms (AAA) was revised to allow a one-time AAA screening without receiving a referral as part of the initial preventive physical examination for beneficiaries that meet certain criteria (a family history of AAA, or for men aged 65–75, a history of smoking).

For a complete listing of the preventive services covered by Medicare for 2022, see Table 11-2.

Table 11-2. Preventive Services Covered by Medicare for 2022

Service	Who and what is covered?	How often can I get this service?	Do I have to pay coinsurance or deductible?
Initial Preventive Physical Examination (IPPE) – The "Welcome to Medicare Preventive Visit"	All new enrollees in Medicare Part B may receive an examination that includes medical and social history review, physical examination with counseling about preventive services, and a written plan for additional preventive services that are needed.	One time only within the first 12 months of when an individual elects to participate in Medicare Part B	No coinsurance or deductible. Patient may have to pay coinsurance and deductible if the doctor or other health care professional performs additional tests or services during the same visit which are not covered under the preventive benefits; for example, electrocardiogram tests performed as a screening for the IPPE.
Annual Wellness Examination	People who have had Medicare Part B for longer than 12 months are eligible for a yearly "Wellness" visit.	An examination every 12 months to develop or update a personalized prevention plan.	No coinsurance or deductible Patient may have to pay coinsurance and deductible if the doctor or other health care professional performs additional tests or services during the same visit which are not covered under the preventive benefits.
Abdominal Aortic Aneurysm (AAA) Ultrasound Screening	People with Medicare who are at risk for AAAs may get a referral for a one-time screening ultrasound at their Welcome to Medicare Physical Examination.	Once in a lifetime	No coinsurance or deductible

Service	Who and what is covered?	How often can I get this service?	Do I have to pay coinsurance or deductible?
Alcohol Misuse Screenings and Counseling	Someone is considered to be misusing alcohol, if he or she is a: ■ Woman under the age of 65 who has more than three drinks at a time or seven drinks per week ■ Man under the age of 65 who has more than four drinks at a time or 14 drinks per week ■ Person over the age of 65 who has more than three drinks at a time or seven drinks per week Medicare will pay for annual alcohol misuse screenings for people with Medicare. You do not need to show any signs or symptoms of abuse to qualify for the preventive screening.	Screening once per year, if no alcohol dependency. Counseling: four counseling sessions with a primary care physician or qualified provider.	No coinsurance or deductible
Bone Mass Measurements (bone density)	People with Medicare whose physicians say they are at risk for osteoporosis.	Once every 24 months (more often if medically necessary) for people who have certain medical conditions or meet certain criteria	No coinsurance or deductible
Cardiovascular Disease Screenings	All people with Medicare Part B may receive cardiovascular screening blood tests for assessment of cholesterol, lipids, and triglyceride levels	Once every five years	No coinsurance or deductible
Cardiovascular Disease (behavioral therapy)	Covers a cardiovascular behavioral therapy visit for persons with Medicare	Once per year with a primary care physician or qualified health care professional.	No coinsurance or deductible
Cervical and Vaginal Cancer Screenings	All female Medicare beneficiaries are covered for Pap tests and pelvic exams to check for cervical and vaginal cancers. As part of the pelvic exam, Medicare also covers a clinical breast exam to check for breast cancer.	Once every 24 months. If high risk, Medicare covers these screening tests once every 12 months. Also covers human papillomavirus (HPV) tests, included as part of a Pap test, once every five years for age 30-65, without HPV symptoms.	No coinsurance or deductible
Colorectal Cancer Screenings	People with Medicare age 50 or older, except there is no minimum age for a screening colonoscopy. ■ Multi-target stool DNA tests ■ Screening barium enemas ■ Screening colonoscopies ■ Screening fecal occult blood tests ■ Screening flexible sigmoidoscopies	Varies depending on screening test provided.	Varies depending on screening test provided.

(continued)

Table 11-2. Preventive Services Covered by Medicare for 2022 (*continued*)

Service	Who and what is covered?	How often can I get this service?	Do I have to pay coinsurance or deductible?
COVID-19 Vaccine	All Medicare beneficiaries. Medicare covers a COVID-19 vaccine and booster shot at no cost. Medicare also covers COVID-19 tests, COVID-19 antibody tests, and COVID-19 monoclonal antibody treatments. For immunocompromised patients, Medicare will cover an additional vaccine dose of the COVID-19 vaccine, at least 28 days after a second dose, at no cost.	CMS has not mandated frequency limits for the COVID-19 vaccines.	No insurance or deductible for the vaccination and booster
Depression Screening	All Medicare beneficiaries	Once a year performed by primary care physician.	No insurance or deductible
Diabetes Screenings	Those individuals with Medicare who are at risk for diabetes or diagnosed with pre-diabetes. Risk factors include: ■ high blood pressure, dyslipidemia, ■ obesity, or ■ history of high blood sugar (glucose). Tests may also be covered if the patient is age 65 or older, overweight, or has a family history of diabetes.	Eligible for up to two screenings each year	No coinsurance or deductible
Diabetes Self-Management Training	Covers outpatient diabetes self-management training (DSMT) for Medicare beneficiaries who have been diagnosed with diabetes.	Up to 10 hours of initial DSMT (1 hour of individual training and 9 hours of group training) in the first year and up to 2 hours of follow-up training each subsequent year.	20% coinsurance and deductible apply
Flu Immunization	All Medicare beneficiaries	Once per influenza season	No coinsurance or deductible
Glaucoma Screening	People with Medicare who are at high risk for glaucoma. Patients who meet at least one high-risk criteria: ■ diabetes mellitus, ■ family history of glaucoma, ■ African-American aged 50 and older, ■ Hispanic-American aged 65 and older.	Once every 12 months	20% coinsurance and deductible apply
Hepatitis B Immunization	People with Medicare who are at medium or high risk, such as patients with hemophilia or end-stage renal disease.	One series (three shots) if ordered by the physician	No coinsurance or deductible

Service	Who and what is covered?	How often can I get this service?	Do I have to pay coinsurance or deductible?
Hepatitis B Virus (HBV) Infection Screening	Medicare covers HBV infection screenings for beneficiaries who are at high risk or pregnant.	Once a year if at continued high risk and do not get a hepatitis B shot	No coinsurance or deductible
Hepatitis C Virus (HCV) Screening	People with Medicare who are at high risk for HCV infection.	Yearly screenings for high-risk beneficiaries if ordered by primary care doctor or other primary care provider.	No coinsurance or deductible
HIV (Human Immunodeficiency Virus) Screenings	People with Medicare who are age 15-65. Or those younger than 15 or older than 65 and at an increased risk for HIV.	Once per year or up to 3 times during pregnancy	No coinsurance or deductible
Lung Cancer Screenings	Medicare covers lung cancer screenings with low dose computed tomography (LDCT) if all the following conditions are met: ■ Age 55-77, ■ No signs or symptoms of lung cancer (asymptomatic), ■ Current smoker or have quit smoking within the last 15 years, ■ A tobacco smoking history of at least 30 "pack years" (an average of one pack [20 cigarettes] per day for 30 years), and ■ Written doctor's order.	Once every 12 months	No coinsurance or deductible
Mammograms (screening)	Women with Medicare who are age 35 or older	One baseline for women aged 35–39 or annually for women aged 40 and older	No coinsurance or deductible
Medical Nutrition Therapy (MNT) Services	People with Medicare who have diabetes or renal disease or have had a kidney transplant in the last 36 months, and the physician refers the patient to the service. If a patient is receiving dialysis in a dialysis facility, Medicare covers MNT as part of overall dialysis care.	3 hours of counseling first year and 2 hours each subsequent year	No coinsurance or deductible
Medicare Diabetes Prevention Program	Medicare Part B beneficiaries who meet specific requirements are eligible for this proven health behavior change program to help prevent type 2 diabetes.	Once in a lifetime includes 16 core group sessions over a 6-month period, 6 months of monthly follow-up sessions, and an additional 12 months of ongoing maintenance sessions.	No cost for these services if eligible
Obesity Screenings and Counseling	All people with Medicare may be screened for obesity. Counseling is covered for anyone found to have a body mass index (BMI) of 30 or more.	An initial screening for BMI and behavioral therapy sessions to help lose weight by focusing on diet and exercise.	No coinsurance or deductible

(continued)

Table 11-2. Preventive Services Covered by Medicare for 2022 (*continued*)

Service	Who and what is covered?	How often can I get this service?	Do I have to pay coinsurance or deductible?
Pneumococcal Immunizations	All people with Medicare are covered for 2 different pneumococcal shots	Once in a lifetime; the first shot at any time and a different, second shot if it is given at least one year after the first shot.	No coinsurance or deductible
Prostate Cancer Screenings	All men with Medicare over the age of 50	Digital rectal exam: once every 12 months Prostate specific antigen (PSA) blood test: once every 12 months	20% coinsurance and deductible apply for digital rectal exam No coinsurance or deductible for PSA test
Sexually Transmitted Infections (STIs) Screening and Counseling	Medicare beneficiaries who are pregnant or at increased risk for an STI when a primary care doctor or other qualified primary care professional orders the screening tests and provides counseling.	Once every 12 months for STI screenings for chlamydia, gonorrhea, syphilis, and/or hepatitis B. Once each year for up to two 20-30 minute face-to-face high-intensity behavioral counseling (HIBC) sessions.	No coinsurance or deductible
Smoking and Tobacco Use Cessation Counseling	Any person with Medicare who uses tobacco can get counseling from a qualified doctor or other Medicare-recognized practitioner who can help them stop using tobacco.	This service includes 8 face-to-face visits in a 12-month period.	No coinsurance or deductible for counseling

Other Payment Policy Changes Adopted Under the RBRVS

In addition to the payment policy changes it has brought about due to legislation, CMS has also adopted other policies since implementing the payment schedule. These policies are explained in the following sections.

Emergency Department X rays and ECGs

CMS' policy generally allows for separate payment for only one interpretation, either by the radiologist/cardiologist or emergency department physician, of an ECG or X ray furnished to an emergency department patient. Payment for a second interpretation may be allowed in unusual circumstances, such as a "questionable finding," for which the physician performing the initial procedure believes another physician's expertise is needed. Previously, some Medicare carriers paid separately for an interpretation provided by the emergency department physician and a second interpretation by a hospital's radiologist or cardiologist.

Payment will be made for the interpretation that is used to diagnose and treat the patient. The criteria for reporting the applicable CPT code must be fully met, including written documentation of the interpretation that is prepared for the patient's medical record. Payment is allowed for a verbal interpretation furnished by the radiologist/cardiologist that is conveyed to the treating physician, which is later prepared as a written report. In this circumstance, the emergency department physician should not bill for the interpretation. In addition, interpretations furnished via teleradiology are payable interpretations, when used to diagnose and treat the patient.

Finally, CMS encourages hospitals to work with their medical staffs to establish guidelines for the billing of X-ray and ECG interpretations for emergency department patients, which will avoid multiple claims submission.

End-Stage Renal Disease

In the November 7, 2003, Final Rule, CMS announced that it will no longer recognize CPT codes 90918-90921 for reporting services provided to patients with end-stage renal disease (ESRD). Instead, CMS created new "G" codes to report these services, based on the number of physician visits provided each month to an ESRD patient. For 2009, codes 90918-90921 have been deleted and the existing "G" codes have been replaced with CPT codes 90951-90970, which describe adult and pediatric ESRD services. They are distinct codes—when the physician provides one visit per month, two to three visits per month, and four or more visits per month.

CMS has clarified that nonphysician practitioners (PAs, NPs, and clinical nurse specialists [CNS]) may provide care to ESRD patients using the incident-to rules for E/M services. The physician extender must be in the same group practice or employed by the same entity, and the physician must perform some portion of the face-to-face visit. To report the service utilizing the physician's identification number, the physician must perform the visit with the complete assessment and establish the patient's plan of care. If the nonphysician practitioner performs the complete assessment and establishes the plan of care, the service should be billed under the identification number of the PA, NP, or CNS.

Therapeutic Apheresis

Although payment is made for the physician work component of therapeutic apheresis in the hospital and nonhospital settings, CMS will not pay for both therapeutic apheresis and certain E/M codes on the same date. Separate payment is made for an initial hospital visit, initial consultations, and hospital discharge services. Separate payment is not allowed for established patient office visits, subsequent hospital care, or follow-up inpatient consultations, when furnished on the same date as therapeutic apheresis. Separate payment for services provided to establish the required vascular access will be allowed, if performed by the physician.

The policy was implemented in a budget-neutral manner by bundling the payment for the specified E/M codes performed on the same date, as therapeutic apheresis into the payment for the therapeutic apheresis service.

The AMA's Advocacy Efforts

Over the years, the AMA, working with state and specialty medical societies and other national organizations, has successfully advocated for physicians on a variety of issues related to Medicare law, regulation, and policy. In 2021, COVID-19 response efforts remained at the forefront of AMA advocacy, including assisting physician practices in mitigating the financial impact of the pandemic. There was also continuous activity on many other important issues for physicians and patients at the federal and state levels, such as access to care, the drug overdose epidemic, and immigration. These advocacy efforts included:

COVID-19

- Working at the federal and state levels to advocate for a comprehensive response to the PHE—including telehealth expansion, financial relief, testing, vaccination, and more (read the full AMA COVID-19 Advocacy efforts web page for details—highlights are included).
- Advocated that the American Rescue Plan Act include the following provisions: (a) added an additional $8.5 billion to the Provider Relief Fund; (b) directs the utilization of the Defense Production Act to boost domestic production of personal protective equipment (PPE), vaccines, and onshore production of rapid COVID-19 tests; and (c) adds $15 billion in new funding for Targeted Economic Injury Disaster Loan Grants to provide hard-hit, underserved small businesses with increased flexible monetary relief.
- The Biden Administration nearly doubled Medicare payment for administration of the COVID-19 vaccine, including administration of vaccines requiring two doses to $40 per administration.
- Successfully sought introduction of federal legislation to ensure Provider Relief Fund grants do not count as taxable income.
- The Centers for Disease Control and Prevention (CDC) announced new investments and activities aimed at improving health equity in response to the COVID-19 pandemic.
- The Biden Administration encouraged states to supply more vaccines to primary care physicians' offices to address immunization inequities and better reach patients who are hesitant to get vaccinated against COVID-19.
- Maintained enforcement discretion on Health Insurance Portability and Accountability Act (HIPAA) penalties for physicians using telehealth in the event of noncompliance with regulatory requirements.
- Successfully advocated for many services to be added to Medicare Telehealth List during the pandemic and for most to continue being covered through 2023. Obtained improved payment rates for telehealth services during the pandemic, with audio-video and audio-only services being equivalent to in-person office visits.

Access to Care

- The Biden Administration lifted the Title X "gag clause" rule.
- The Biden Administration has started to eliminate Medicaid work requirements.
- The American Rescue Plan Act of 2021 (ARPA) included provisions to extend postpartum coverage under Medicaid and The Children's Health Insurance Program (CHIP), increased premium subsidies for the Affordable Care Act (ACA) marketplace plans, and invested in trust and treaty obligations to provide essential safety-net programs that serve Native American communities.
- The American Families Plan announced by President Biden on April 28, 2021, would make ARPA's ACA subsidy enhancements permanent.
- An ACA special enrollment period was opened in 2021 to expand access to coverage.

Medicare Physician Payment

- Legislation signed into law that prevents a 2% sequester payment cut through 2021.
  - Grassroots campaign led by the AMA garnered over 133,000 emails to Congress and over 50,000 engagements.
- Physicians will be held harmless from the up to 9% Merit-based Incentive Payment System (MIPS) penalties due to the significant disruptions of the COVID-19 PHE on physician practices' performance in 2020 and 2021. Because of the concerns of the direct and indirect effects of the COVID-19 PHE, CMS will continue to double the complex patient bonus available for the 2021 MIPS performance year or 2023 MIPS payment year for physicians that chose to participate in MIPS.
- One year 3.75% increase in Medicare payments to offset impact of budget-neutrality adjustment.
- CMS reopened the hardship exception application for group practices, virtual groups, and alternative payment model entities who missed the previous 2020 deadline.
- Jointly with many specialty societies, the AMA made recommendations to CMS for improving design and implementation of alternative payment models, which are reflected in a new CMS strategy document.

Removing Obstacles to Patient Care

- Released 2020 prior authorization survey data that highlighted the continued negative impact of this onerous process on patients and physicians—even during the height of the COVID-19 pandemic.
  - The survey data also underscored the lack of progress by insurers on the prior authorization reforms agreed upon three-and-a-half years ago in the Consensus Statement on Improving the Prior Authorization Process.
- Advocated for federal and state prior authorization legislation as follows:
  - The AMA successfully pushed for reintroduction of the Improving Seniors' Timely Access to Care Act, which would require Medicare Advantage plans to follow many of the provisions of the Consensus Statement. In addition, the AMA sent a letter of support to the lead co-sponsors; this legislation now has bipartisan, majority support in the House and a Senate companion bill has been introduced.
  - Legislation to reform the prior authorization process, which was based on the AMA model bill, enacted in Georgia and Illinois. It is also being debated in Michigan, Pennsylvania, and other states.
  - Texas enacted legislation requiring state-regulated plans to offer prior authorization goldcards to physicians with 90% prior authorization approval ratings for a particular service under that plan. The AMA sought media promotion of the passage of this legislation, which resulted in interest from policymakers across the country in similar legislation to reduce the volume of prior authorizations.
- Facilitated a Federation sign-on letter which asked the Biden Administration to ensure that physicians have options to receive fee-free electronic funds transfer (EFT) payments and enforce regulations against payers not providing such options.
- Continued to build AMA's grassroots advocacy campaign with a dedicated website and associated social media presence around Fix Prior Authorization, which includes a toolkit for employers to leverage health plan negotiations and additional educational features.
- Joined the All Copays Count Coalition and supported model legislation to prohibit insurers' copay accumulator programs. More than a dozen bills based on the Coalition's model were introduced in various states. Arkansas, Connecticut, Louisiana, North Carolina, Kentucky, and Oklahoma have since enacted new laws around copay accumulator programs.
- Advocated for OptumPay to continue providing valuable revenue cycle functionalities for free vs assessing a percentage-based fee, as originally proposed.
- In response to AMA advocacy, UnitedHealthcare rescinded a policy that would have prohibited "incident-to billing" and would have financially harmed many physician practices.

Drug Overdose Epidemic

- The Biden Administration adopted policies to address overdose and substance use disorder in ways that will reduce stigma, more effectively prevent overdose deaths, and remove barriers to treatment—and in ways that are consistent with AMA policy recommendations.
- The Biden Administration waived burdensome administrative requirements so that all physicians will be able to prescribe buprenorphine for their patients with opioid use disorder.
- Using national principals and working with coalition partners, the AMA supported new laws in Virginia and Kentucky directing opioid litigation funds be earmarked for public health uses. In addition, the AMA influenced national policy and legislative model from a multi-stakeholder coalition led by the Johns Hopkins School of Public Health and Legislative Analysis and Public Policy Association, respectively.
- As part of a national coalition, the AMA helped support six new state mental health and substance use disorder parity laws that will help enhance oversight and enforcement to protect patients.
- Released the 2021 Overdose Epidemic Report, which highlighted the worsening epidemic (due primarily to illicit fentanyl, methamphetamine, and cocaine as well as polysubstance use of prescription opioids and heroin).

The Report also showed physicians' efforts to reduce opioid prescribing by 44.4%.

- Launched the AMA Substance Use and Pain Care Task Force to combine efforts and expertise from the Opioid and Pain Care task forces. The new task force and its member organizations released updated recommendations to address the worsening epidemic.
- Developed a new issue brief focused on actions employers can take to help improve access to evidence-based care for opioid use disorder and pain, as well as to support harm reduction efforts. In addition, the AMA presented the issue brief at multiple Drug Enforcement Administration-sponsored forums around the country organized by the Milken Institute.
- Held a national webinar with Manatt Health that featured medical, legal, and public health experts identifying ways to remove barriers to evidence-based treatment for opioid use disorder in justice-involved settings; other AMA-Manatt Health webinars focused on harm reduction and addiction medicine training in medical schools.
- Highlighted physician advocacy efforts to help their patients with a substance use disorder or chronic pain.
- AMA President Susan R. Bailey, MD, provided a keynote address at the National Rx Drug Abuse and Heroin Summit.

Immigration

- Helped to delay the implementation of a problematic Department of Homeland Security (DHS) final rule regarding cap-subject H-1B visa petitioners. However, the Biden Administration is now urging a Washington, DC, Federal Judge to uphold the rule, which would prioritize H-1B specialty occupation visas by salary, saying that they believe that the rule is valid.
- The Biden Administration continued Deferred Action for Childhood Arrivals (DACA) policy to defer the removal of certain undocumented immigrants who were brought to the United States as children. In an effort to buttress the program, the Administration is currently going through the rulemaking process to increase the stability of the program, and the AMA is drafting comments, despite a number of court cases opposing the rule.
- Consistent with AMA advocacy, the Biden administration lifted the immigration ban on Muslim countries and rescinded rules that would deem immigrants inadmissible on public charge grounds. In October 2021, in response to a Request for Information, the AMA submitted comments on the public charge grounds for inadmissibility.
- The AMA is currently advocating for a broad range of immigration and border security policy changes, including those that would ease visa restrictions for foreign-born physicians seeking to train or practice in the United States.

Preventing Gun Violence

- The Biden Administration issued rules to require background checks for "ghost guns."
- The House passed two bills supported by AMA that would:
  - Close the so-called "Charleston Loophole" by extending the time period the Federal Bureau of Investigation has to determine whether a buyer is qualified to purchase a gun.
  - Expand the existing background check system to cover all firearm sales, while providing exceptions for law enforcement and family and friend transfers.
- Helped to successfully secure FY 2021 federal appropriations of $25 million for the National Institutes of Health and $25 million for the CDC for research on gun violence.

Anti-Racism Efforts

- Applauded the CDC for recognizing racism as a "serious public health threat."
- Supported Asian American and Pacific Islander hate crime legislation, which was signed into law on May 20, 2021.
- Successfully opposed state legislation that would have barred state-funded entities from conducting trainings on diversity and inclusion.
- Responded to numerous requests for information from the federal government related to racism and bias in health care algorithms and recommended that clinicians and researchers focus on genetics and biology, structural racism, and other structural determinants; and collect, report, and use race data as a proxy for structural racism and not ancestry, when describing risk factors for disease and outcomes.
- Advocated to various stakeholders that more must be done to address why care experiences and clinical outcomes vary by race or ethnicity and encouraged additional efforts to improve outcomes and satisfaction for historically minoritized patients seen by nonracially concordant doctors.
- Engaged in a workgroup at the National Association of Insurance Commissioners (NAIC) which addressed race and ethnicity data in provider directories and network adequacy, urging careful consideration of implications and the use of appropriate safeguards and guardrails when data are collected and potentially published.

LGBTQ+ Health

- Supported H.R. 5, the Equality Act, passed by the House, which prohibits discrimination based on sex, sexual orientation, and gender identity in areas including public accommodations and facilities, education, federal funding, employment, housing, credit, and the jury system.
- The Biden Administration withdrew a previous Trump Administration proposal restricting transgender people

in homeless shelters. The AMA strongly opposed the proposal and urged the previous Trump and current Biden administrations to withdraw it.

- The Biden Administration announced it would provide protections against discrimination in health care based on gender identity and sexual orientation, reversing a rule issued by the previous Trump administration that allowed discrimination against transgender individuals. The AMA strongly opposed the previous policy and had urged the Biden Administration to reverse it.
- The Biden Administration withdrew the previous Trump administration's proposed rule that would have weakened the Equal Access Rule; this Rule ensures that all individuals—regardless of sexual orientation or gender identity—have equal access to the Office of Community Planning and Development programs, shelters, other buildings and facilities, benefits, services, and accommodations.
  - The AMA opposed the proposed rule and supports its withdrawal.
- Successfully defeated harmful anti-transgender legislation in over a dozen states that would have criminalized the provision of medically necessary gender-affirming care to minor patients, while work continues in other states.
- The AMA urged the nation's governors to reject legislation that would discriminate against transgender individuals in a letter to the National Governors Association.

Maternal Death

- Submitted an extensive statement for the record to the U.S. House of Representatives Committee on Oversight and Reform as part of the hearing entitled, "Birthing While Black: Examining America's Black Maternal Health Crisis."
- HHS approved a postpartum Medicaid expansion for Georgia, Illinois, Indiana, Missouri, and New Jersey. In turn, several state legislatures have also authorized coverage expansions for postpartum women.
- Successfully sought introduction of the "Mothers and Offspring Mortality and Morbidity Awareness Act," also known as the MOMMA Act, which would extend coverage for postpartum care from the existing 60 days to an expanded 12 months under Medicaid and CHIP. It would also support training clinicians on implicit bias and health equity issues.
- Supported the "Connected Maternal Online Monitoring (MOM) Act," which would require CMS to identify barriers to coverage of remote physiologic devices under state Medicaid programs to improve maternal and child health outcomes for pregnant and postpartum women.
- Supported the "Maternal Health Quality Improvement Act," which would provide grants to identify, develop, and disseminate best practices to improve maternal health care quality and outcomes; promote collaboration with state maternal mortality review committees to identify ways to reduce preventable maternal mortality and severe maternal morbidity; promote perinatal collaboration on quality; and implement integrated health care services for pregnant and postpartum women.
- Joined a second sign-on letter urging Congress to direct $20 million to the CDC Hospitals Promoting the Breastfeeding line item in the FY 2022 Labor, Health and Human Services, and Related Agencies appropriations bill, an increase of $10.5 million above the president's budget level.
- Supported a provision in the American Rescue Plan Act of 2021 that established a temporary, optional provision to assist states in expanding Medicaid and CHIP coverage opportunities to one year postpartum. The new option can take effect starting April 1, 2022, and would be available to states for five years.

Tobacco

- The Food and Drug Administration announced it will ban menthol-flavored cigarettes.
- Federal court upheld a ban on flavored tobacco products.

Privacy and Security of Health Data

- Federal Trade Commission (FTC) announced a new policy, Statement on Breaches by Health Apps and Other Connected Devices to clarify that the scope of its Health Breach Notification (HBN) rule includes "health apps and connected devices that collect or use consumers' health information." In addition, The AMA asked that the FTC "expand the HBN Rule's coverage to specifically include direct-to-consumer technologies and services such as mobile health apps, virtual assistants. and platforms' health tools."
- Developed guidance for health app developers to help implement the AMA's Privacy Principles.
- Advocated to Office of the National Coordinator for Health Information Technology (ONC) and the National Governors Association to develop, publicize, and enforce comprehensive guidelines related to the use of digital vaccine credential services.
- Encouraged National Institute of Standards and Technology (NIST) to provide guidance to physicians on which cybersecurity practices will be recognized by HHS during Office of Civil Rights (OCR) HIPAA investigations.
- Urged CDC and OCR to enforce their guidance prohibiting the use of patient/customer information collected by retail pharmacies for COVID-19 vaccination scheduling and/or the vaccine administration process for commercial marketing or future patient recruiting purposes, especially any targeting based on medical history or conditions.
- Recommended that OCR establish a 1-year glide path to HIPAA compliance for telemedicine technologies,

during which physicians and other affected parties shall not be subject to HIPAA audits and other HIPAA enforcement activity related to telemedicine.

Surprise Billing

- The Consolidated Appropriations Act, 2021, signed into law on December 27, 2020, included No Surprises Act (NSA) provisions that allow for price transparency, more accurate provider directories, and patient financial protections against "surprise medical bills" or unexpected gaps in health insurance coverage. The final provisions reflected significant advocacy by the AMA and Federation groups, which included an independent dispute resolution.
- Released the National Managed Care Legal Database, which pulled in over 1,000 patient and physician protections passed at the state and federal levels and sought to empower physicians, patients and their advocates in their dealings with health insurers and to inform policymakers, legislators and regulators about key issues—eg, surprise billing—involving health insurers, physicians, and patients.
- Lead an effort with national specialties and state medical associations to build consensus and impact the NSA regulations, which included developing common strategies and recommended revisions to eliminate increased leverage they provide for insurance companies. In addition, submitted numerous comment letters on various components of the law reflecting consensus among these groups. Worked with members of Congress to reemphasize their intent in drafting statutory provisions pertaining to the independent dispute resolution system.
- Worked with Federation members and outside stakeholders to address operationalization of the NSA requirements (eg, good faith estimates) and provide feedback to state and federal regulators.

Scope of Practice

- Successfully thwarted several attempts by the pharmacy community to advance legislation that would have recognized pharmacists as physicians in the Medicare program and allowed them to provide acute and chronic care.
- Launched new scope microsite providing an easier way for Federation colleagues and physician leaders to access AMA's scope materials, including geomaps, education and training modules, issue briefs, social media graphics, etc.
- Created a set of 2020 geomaps, which expanded the AMA's growing set of geomaps to 4500 giving key data to refute claims by nurse practitioners and others that scope expansions are necessary to increase access to care.
- Worked with 35 state medical associations on scope of practice legislation, resulting in key victories which include Alaska (naturopath), Alabama (optometrist, psychology), Colorado (PAs), Florida (optometry, APRN, PAs), Kansas (APRN), Louisiana (APRN), Maine (APRN), Maryland (podiatrist "physician" bill), Mississippi (APRN), South Dakota (PAs), Tennessee (APRN), Texas (APRN, optometrist, PA, and psychologist).
- AMA President Susan R. Bailey, MD, testified before the House Health & Human Services Committee in South Dakota on H.B. 1163 which would have expanded the scope of practice of physician assistants; however, the Committee voted against the bill.
- Sent 22 letters to lawmakers in 10 states expressing opposition to various scope of practice bills (Alaska, Colorado, Delaware, Kansas, Louisiana, Maryland, Maine, Mississippi, South Dakota, and Wisconsin).
- The Scope of Practice Partnership (SOPP) Steering Committee has approved nine grants so far in 2021 and welcomed American Academy of Otolaryngology–Head and Neck Surgery (AAO-HNS) to the SOPP, as well as American College of Emergency Physicians (ACEP) and American College of Radiology (ACR) to the SOPP Steering Committee.
- AMA and American Society of Anesthesiologists (ASA) co-hosted a Medical Title Misappropriation Summit with around 60 attendees representing the AMA, American Osteopathic Association (AOA), 11 national specialty societies, seven state medical associations, the American Board of Medical Specialties, AMA's Council on Legislation, AMA's Council on Medical Education, AMA's Academic Physicians Section, and AMA's Resident and Fellows Section.
- Conducted survey of U.S. voters' sentiment on scope of practice and created toolkit based on findings.
- Organized a letter with 102 national specialty and state medical associations to the Veterans Administration (VA) expressing strong concern with the VA Supremacy Project.
- Lead an effort to engage the VA, veterans groups, and leaders on Capitol Hill to raise awareness and impact the VA Supremacy Project.

Reducing Burnout and Improving Physician Wellness

- Sought introduction of the Dr. Lorna Breen Health Care Provider Protection Act to help reduce and prevent physician mental and behavioral health conditions, suicide and burnout, elements of which were included in the American Rescue Plan Act.
- Collaborated to ensure enactment of new laws in Indiana and South Dakota to provide for the confidentiality of physicians who sought care for wellness and related mental health concerns; AMA advocacy helped contribute to changes in medical licensing applications in Alaska, Minnesota, and Ohio to remove inappropriate questions related to past diagnosis rather than potential current impairment.

- Published an issue brief, "Confidential care to support physician health and wellness," that highlighted several different options for physicians seeking care and provided tangible legislative, regulatory, and other options for medical societies and other stakeholders to support those efforts. It sought to further the goals of balancing privacy and confidentiality while also reducing stigma and protecting public health.
- Planned an entire day at the annual American Bar Association Physician Legal Issues Conference dedicated to physician wellness. Speakers included Dr. Lorna Breen Foundation leadership, the AMA IPPS Section, and the AMA Advocacy Resource Center.
- Provided presentations to the Federation of State Physician Health Programs and Rush University.

Medical Liability reform

- Published the 2021 update to Medical Liability Reform NOW!
- Assisted the New Mexico Medical Society in successfully mitigating a plaintiff's trial bar bill that otherwise would have become law and have dire negative effects on both physicians and hospitals. This bill was the first major amendment to the 1976 New Mexico Malpractice Act and had widespread support in the New Mexico legislature.

Protecting Competition in Health Care and Health Care-Related Markets

- Presented to the Department of Justice (DOJ) a thorough written examination of significant competitive concerns that required the DOJ's investigation when Optum proposed to acquire Change HealthCare.
- Published the 20th edition of Competition in Health Insurance: A Comprehensive Study of U.S. Markets, which demonstrated that more than 70% of health insurance markets continue to be highly concentrated.

Reducing the Burden of Physician Health Information Technology (Health IT)

- Led efforts with the Federation to push back on federal information blocking requirements that force physicians to release medical information that can emotionally and mentally harm patients or their caregivers.
- Removed burdensome CMS requirements that would have required physicians to maintain the availability of electronic medical records indefinitely.
- Successfully added MIPS exceptions for physicians who do not have electronic health records certified to technical requirements needed to electronically report cases to their local public health departments.
- Successfully removed burdensome MIPS reporting requirements which could have complicated physicians' compliance with ONC's information blocking regulations.

Health Policy Research

Published five AMA Policy Research Perspectives:

- Demonstrated that the pandemic lowered Medicare fee schedule spending by 19% ($9.4 billion) in the first half of 2020.
- Called attention to the highest prevalence of medical liability premium increases in 15 years.
- Documented physician practice changes including that private practice dropped below 50% of physicians in 2020.
- Examined national health care spending in 2019 and included a first look at estimates for 2020.
- Documented the increased use of telehealth six months into the pandemic.

Part 4

The RBRVS Payment System in Your Practice

Part 4 describes how the resource-based relative value scale (RBRVS) payment system impacts physicians' practices and how other payers are utilizing the system. Chapter 12 provides information on electronic data interchange (EDI), the participation decision, and private contracting. Chapter 13 discusses the American Medical Association's (AMA's) survey of non-Medicare payers to determine the broader impact of the RBRVS.

Chapter 12

Practice Management Under the RBRVS: Implications for Physicians

In 1992, the Medicare Resource-Based Relative Value scale (RBRVS) payment system implemented fundamental changes in the way Medicare pays for physician services. The first year of RBRVS implementation, in particular, required substantial adjustments for the many physicians accustomed to Medicare's customary, prevailing, and reasonable (CPR) payment system. Although the complete transition to payments based fully on the RBRVS payment schedule occurred in 1996, the Medicare RBRVS payment system continues to evolve. For example, the relative value units (RVUs) assigned to the physician work component are adjusted each year in response to the American Medical Association's (AMA's) Current Procedural Terminology (CPT®) coding changes; and the original geographic practice cost indices have been updated in every three years. In addition, the Centers for Medicare & Medicaid Services (CMS) implemented a new resource-based methodology for assigning practice expense RVUs, which was fully implemented in 2002. Professional liability insurance (PLI) relative values became resource based in 2000.

This chapter briefly describes the fundamental elements of the RBRVS and suggests elements for consideration in an audit of basic practice management techniques. In addition, it reviews those aspects of the Medicare program that may significantly affect physician practices, including the Patient Activity Report (PAR) program, Medicare requirements related to electronic data interchange, and provisions related to private contracting with Medicare patients.

Physician Payment Under the RBRVS

The impact of the Medicare RBRVS payment system on a physician's practice is determined, in large part, by the volume of services the practice provides to Medicare patients, the mix of visit and procedural services it provides, and the geographic location of the practice. The following four basic elements of the Medicare RBRVS most greatly influence physician practices:

- Payment based on a national standard RBRVS payment schedule
- Payment adjustments for geographic differences in resource costs
- Balance billing limited to 115% of the Medicare allowed amount
- Standardization of Medicare carrier payment policies

RBRVS

The RBRVS pays for physicians' services according to a national standard payment schedule that is based on physicians' resource costs. As discussed in detail in Chapter 8, the major effect of the RBRVS is redistribution of payments among specialties by narrowing the gap between payments for visits and procedures. In general, the RBRVS has resulted in increased payments for visits, consultations, and other evaluation and management (E/M) services, and decreased payments for surgery, imaging, anesthesiology, and other procedural services.

Geographic Payment Variations

Payment based on a national standard payment schedule has narrowed considerably the wide range of geographic variation in payments that existed under the CPR. Payments in localities where practice costs are relatively high are greater than payments in lower-cost localities. Because there is less variation in costs than there was in Medicare prevailing charges, areas with low prevailing charges relative to the national average generally have experienced increased payments under the RBRVS; areas with very high prevailing charges relative to the national average generally have experienced decreased payments. These geographic payment variations are described in detail in Chapter 7.

Limiting Charges

Limiting charges apply to all nonparticipating physician payments and, generally, are more restrictive than those imposed prior to RBRVS implementation. The limiting charge since 1993 has been 15% more than the Medicare-approved amount (including the 80% that Medicare pays and patients' 20% coinsurance) for nonparticipating physicians. Nonparticipating physician payments are set at 95% of participating physician amounts. (For a detailed discussion of limiting charges, refer to Chapter 9.)

Medicare payment based on a national standard RBRVS payment schedule required that all carriers uniformly implement Medicare's payment rules. The shift to standardized payment policies across Medicare carriers resulted in payments that are more predictable and consistent than under the CPR.

Global Surgical Packages

The global surgery policy under the RBRVS resulted in major payment adjustments for some surgeons. For example, standardized policy under the RBRVS includes a postoperative period of 90 days. For surgeons accustomed to a postoperative period of 30 days or less, this longer postoperative period meant a decline in billing volume for follow-up visits. When other than normal surgical care is provided during this time, however, physicians may appropriately bill and receive separate payment for these services. Careful use of the appropriate CPT modifiers to indicate these services, as outlined in Chapter 11, will help avoid unnecessary claims denials. In addition, the global surgery policy specifically allows surgeons to bill for related services provided beyond the 90-day postoperative period.

Medicare RBRVS payment policy for minor surgeries and endoscopies eliminates payment for a visit on the same day unless a separate E/M service is also provided during the visit. Proper use of modifier 25 in these circumstances will help ensure that the claim is paid appropriately.

In 2015, CMS announced a major change for reporting global surgical packages. CMS would have begun transitioning all the 010-day and 090-day global periods to 000-day global periods, starting in 2017; however, on April 16, 2015, the Medicare Access and Children's Health Insurance Program (CHIP) Reauthorization Act (MACRA) legislation was enacted into law. Under the law, CMS is statutorily prohibited from implementing the transition policy. In its place, MACRA requires CMS to develop a process to gather information needed to value surgical services from a representative sample of physicians and that the data collection shall begin no later than January 1, 2017. The collected information must include the number and level of medical visits furnished during the global period and other items and services related to the surgery.

The initial CMS policy was based on a report from the HHS Office of Inspector General, which identified a few surgical procedures that include more visits in the global period than are being furnished. CMS was also concerned that post-surgical visits are valued higher than visits that were furnished and billed separately by other physicians, such as general internists or family physicians.

CMS originally proposed to collect data on the frequency of and inputs involved in global services through comprehensive claims-based reporting regarding the number and level of pre- and postoperative services furnished for 010-day and 090-day global services. Specifically, physicians would have been required to report a set of time-based G codes for every 10 minutes dedicated to a patient before and after a procedure or surgery. The AMA strongly opposed this proposal and provided alternative methodologies that would allow CMS to implement the MACRA statutory requirements with a minimal burden on physicians.

In response to significant advocacy from the AMA and other medical groups, CMS finalized a claims-based data collection process that was much less burdensome for physicians than CMS' proposal. Specifically, CMS finalized AMA's recommendations including:

- The use of CPT code 99024 for reporting postoperative services rather than the proposed set of time-based G codes.
- Reporting no longer required for preoperative visits included in the global package.
- Reporting was only required for services related to codes reported annually by more than 100 practitioners that

are reported more than 10,000 times or have allowed charges in excess of $10 million annually. For the CMS list of global codes for which reporting on postoperative visits is required from CY 2017 to CY 2021, information is available at https://www.cms.gov/Medicare/Medicare-Fee-for-Service-Payment/PhysicianFeeSched/Global-Surgery-Data-Collection-.

CMS also confirmed that only physicians in groups of 10 or more practitioners in the following nine states (Florida, Kentucky, Louisiana, Nevada, New Jersey, North Dakota, Ohio, Oregon, and Rhode Island) were required to report. Reporting for physicians in smaller groups or in other geographic areas was optional.

In addition, CMS implemented a delay in the requirement to report postoperative data. While physicians could begin reporting postoperative visits for procedures furnished starting January 1, 2017, the requirement to report began on July 1, 2017. Three years of claims data-based collection culminated in a 2021 RAND Report: "Using Claims-Based Estimates of Post-Operative Visits to Revalue Procedures with 10- and 90-Day Global Periods: Updated Results Using Calendar Year 2019 Data" (2021) available at https://www.cms.gov/Medicare/Medicare-Fee-for-Service-Payment/PhysicianFeeSched/Global-Surgery-Data-Collection-.

In CY 2021, CMS did not accept the RUC recommendation to apply the office visit payment increase to the postoperative office visits that are bundled into the surgical global period. The AMA continues to advocate for CMS to fully adopt the RUC recommendations for the office visit codes by including the payment increases to the postoperative office visits that are bundled in the global surgical packages.

Practice Management Audit

Physicians may want to consider conducting an audit of office management practices to ensure they reflect current RBRVS policies, as well as other Medicare requirements. The audit could be conducted by designated office staff or an outside consulting firm. Physician payment seminars sponsored by medical societies, carriers, and practice management consulting firms are available tools to medical practices, as an alternative to outside consultants.

The volume of Medicare services provided by the practice should determine how much time and expense to invest in an audit. If a practice treats a large number of Medicare patients, or if a previous financial analysis indicated that the RBRVS payment system significantly affects practice revenues, retaining a consultant may be a useful investment.

Office Management Practices

The practice management audit might include an evaluation of office management practices to ensure efficient operations. This evaluation should ensure that systems are in place to implement all aspects of the RBRVS payment system, as well as other Medicare requirements, as discussed in the following sections.

Educating office staff is important in adapting office management practices to changes in the RBRVS payment system. For example, appropriate staff should be knowledgeable about CPT coding changes, RVU revisions, and new Medicare payment policies, particularly for those services provided most frequently by the practice. Proficiency in using the new documentation guidelines for E/M services is also important for most practices. Numerous workshops and seminars are available for billing and other office staff, as well as physicians, through medical societies, hospitals, carriers, and practice management firms.

Medical practices should formalize their payment and collection procedures and communicate these policies to patients. Practices with a large Medicare patient base may want to collect payment when services are provided as a way to accelerate cash flow. This policy should be conveyed to patients during their initial visit. Information about patients' insurance plans should also be obtained at that time. The physician is required to file all Medicare claims for the patient, even if they are unassigned. Medicare prohibits any charge to the patient for this service. Statutes also prohibit Medicare carriers from imposing any payments on physicians related to claims filing, appeals, assigning unique provider identifier numbers, or for responding to inquiries on the status of pending claims.

Incomplete Claims

As part of efforts to streamline claims processing, CMS has developed a new policy to reduce the number of claims that enter the formal appeals process. Whereas previously carriers denied incomplete or invalid claims, which would start the appeals process, they must now return such claims to physicians as "unprocessable." Incomplete claims lack required information (eg, no provider number), while invalid claims contain complete and necessary information that is somehow illogical or incorrect. The claims are returned by the carrier with notification for correction and resubmission. No "initial determination" is made. Carriers must provide an explanation of errors and allow correction or resubmission of the claim.

Medigap and Other Supplemental Benefits

Billing procedures are simplified when Medicare patients assign their Medigap payments to a participating physician. When the participating physician submits a claim to the Medicare carrier for a patient with non–employment-related

Medigap coverage, the carrier automatically sends the claim to the Medigap insurer for payment of all coinsurance and deductible amounts due under the Medigap policy. The Medigap insurer must make payment directly to the physician.

Physicians and other providers are required to obtain information from their Medicare patients about coverage by other health benefit plans and to include this information on the claim form. It is important to maintain records of patients' health care coverage that may be primary to Medicare because carriers may search their records dating from January 1, 1983, to recover payments for which they believe Medicare may be the secondary payer. Supplemental claims are forwarded automatically to the private insurer if the insurer contracts with the Medicare carrier to send Medicare claim information electronically. Otherwise, the patient must file the supplemental claim.

In instances when another insurer is primary to Medicare, but pays only part of the doctor's bill, Medicare makes a supplemental payment. Total payment to the physician, however, may not exceed the 20% copayment or deductible on assigned claims. The physician should refund any excess payment to the supplemental insurer.

When assignment is not accepted, physicians may bill the supplemental insurer up to their limiting charge for the service. The Social Security Act Amendments of 1994 provide that supplemental insurers, as well as Medicare beneficiaries, are not liable for payment of any amount in excess of the limiting charge. Effective for services provided on or after January 1, 1995, nonparticipating physicians and suppliers may not bill supplemental insurers more than the limiting charge. Physicians and suppliers who collect payments from a Medicare beneficiary or supplemental insurer that exceed the limiting charge are required to refund the excess amount. Previously, many interpreted the statute to mean that billing and accepting payment from the supplemental insurer up to the private payer's allowed amount was an acceptable billing practice, even though this amount may have exceeded the physician's limiting charge for the service.

Conducting Business Electronically

Today, much effort and attention are placed on health information technology (health IT) and how to more widely use technology to support the business and clinical needs of health care. Health IT encompasses a broad range of software applications, hardware, and electronic devices used within a physician's practice to support administrative functions and clinical decision making, along with the collection, storage, and exchange of patient data. Examples of health IT applications include electronic health records (EHRs), e-prescribing systems (eRx), computerized provider order entry (CPOE), practice management systems (PMS), Picture Archiving & Communication System (PACS), and personal health records (PHRs).

The use of health IT has increased substantially in the past decade. In 2003, the health care industry moved from a largely paper environment to the first set of administrative health care standards. This move was prompted in large part by the Health Insurance Portability and Accountability Act (HIPAA) that passed into law in 1996. Among the requirements called for in HIPAA is the adoption of certain standards for health care administrative transactions, code sets, and identifiers related to the exchange of administrative information. The emphasis was placed on decreasing the administrative costs of health care through the standardization of data exchange. Collectively, these are known as HIPAA "Administrative Simplification" provisions. HIPAA Administrative Simplification provisions apply only to certain health care transactions conducted electronically. The most widely used HIPAA transaction standards are used for submitting claims and obtaining remittance advice. Several others, however, are not widely used for a variety of reasons including the fact that many physicians still do no find utility in them.

Three additional laws have enacted significant changes to HIPAA and to the exchange of clinical information electronically, and these are:

- Medicare Improvements for Patients and Providers Act (MIPPA) of 2008: MIPPA established the Medicare ePrescribing Incentive Program.
- American Recovery and Reinvestment Act (ARRA) of 2009: ARRA is commonly referred to as the "Stimulus law." This law created the Medicare/Medicaid Meaningful Use (MU) of Electronic Health Record (EHR) program and contained several changes to HIPAA privacy and security requirements.
- Affordable Care Act (ACA) of 2010: The ACA made changes to the HIPAA administrative standards by introducing new standards, operating rules for each adopted standard, and a compliance certification requirement for payers.

The 2009 Stimulus Law

The 2009 Stimulus law established an unprecedented program designed to help spur the purchase and use of EHRs by physicians, hospitals, and other eligible health care providers who deliver care to Medicare and Medicaid patients. Physicians participating in the Medicare incentive program were eligible for as much as $44,000, while those participating in the Medicaid incentive program were eligible for as much as $63,750. The programs (now known as the Promoting Interoperability Programs) began in 2011 with mixed success. On the one hand, the incentive programs have succeeded in achieving a higher rate of EHR use by health care providers. On the other hand, health care providers have been challenged by the requirement that they use a certified EHR and by the number and complexity of the requirements they must meet to demonstrate meaningful use to obtain the incentives. Medicare physicians began to experience a financial payment reduction in 2015 if they were not successful in meeting the program's criteria. The law also made a number of changes to HIPAA privacy requirements as discussed separately below. CMS renamed the EHR Incentive Programs to the Promoting Interoperability Programs in April 2018, marking a change that moved the programs to a new phase of EHR measurement with an increased focus on interoperability and improving patient access to health information.

Affordable Care Act

The ACA is considered to be a landmark legislation that is designed to, among other things, increase the number of Americans who have health insurance. The law also made several changes to HIPAA. Before the passage of the ACA, HIPAA only required that standards be named for the following business functions:

1. Health claims or equivalent encounter information
2. Enrollment and disenrollment in a health plan
3. Eligibility for a health plan
4. Health care payment and remittance advice
5. Health plan premium payments
6. Health claim status
7. Referral certification and authorization
8. Health claims attachments (Not yet adopted under HIPAA)
9. First report of injury (Not yet adopted under HIPAA)

While HIPAA also required naming standard code sets and identifiers, it did not require the Department of Health and Human Services (HHS) to adopt operating rules, which are rules that provide greater detail concerning how a standard is implemented. Below is a list of the HIPAA requirements added by the ACA:

- Standard for electronic funds transfer (EFT)
- Establishment of operating rules for all adopted HIPAA standards
- Health plan certification for meeting HIPAA standards
- Adoption of a health plan identifier
- Standard for claims attachments, which was named in HIPAA but no regulation was finalized for its adoption

To date, HHS has adopted a HIPAA standard and operating rules for EFT and operating rules for verification of eligibility, checking the status of a claim, and receiving an electronic remittance advice (ERA). Regulations for the other mandates are forthcoming.

Privacy and Security of Health Information

The HHS adopted new rules that made changes to existing requirements concerning privacy, security, and notifications that involve the breach of patient protected health information in what is often referred to as the final HIPAA Omnibus Rule. These new rules stemmed from changes made under ARRA. All covered physician practices—including physicians—must have updated their HIPAA policies and procedures and otherwise implemented the changes required by these regulations no later than the September 23, 2013, compliance date. These new rules meant that physicians had to update their business associate agreements (BAAs) and their notices of privacy practices (NPPs), and it will require that physicians understand the importance of encryption of electronic protected health information (ePHI).

Key provisions in the HIPAA Omnibus Rule cover:

- Extending the applicability of certain Privacy and Security Rule requirements to the business associate (BA) of the covered entities (CE)
- Requiring CEs and BAs to provide for notification of breaches of unsecured PHI
- Establishing new limitations on the use and disclosure of PHI for marketing and fundraising purposes
- Limiting circumstances on the sale of PHI
- Requiring the consideration of a limited data set as the minimum necessary amount of information for a particular use, disclosure, or request of PHI
- Expanding individuals' rights to obtain restrictions on certain disclosures of PHI to health plans
- Strengthening enforcement provisions

ICD-10

In addition to naming certain business functions, HIPAA also calls for HHS to name code sets to create greater uniformity and standardization for the way healthcare claims are processed by different payers. HIPAA initially named ICD-9 as the code set physicians and other providers must use to report diagnoses in the outpatient and inpatient settings and procedures in the inpatient setting. In 2009, a regulation that called for the replacement of ICD-9 with ICD-10 was promulgated. After several delays, ICD-10 went into effect on October 1, 2015.

Value-Based Health Care

In the current health reform environment, health care costs and quality remain an area of focus. As a result, health insurers and governmental bodies continue to examine and expand different strategies to slow the rise in the cost of health care.

The payment-for-performance (PFP) movement, now widely referred to as value-based care, is underway throughout the US health care system. The PFP incentive programs are designed to provide financial and/or nonfinancial incentives to improve the quality of care and/or reduce costs. The PFP incentive programs provide differentiated payments to providers based on their performance against a specific set of measures or benchmarks, typically reflecting some combination of clinical quality, patient experience, efficiency, and adoption of clinical information technology.

There are hundreds of PFP and other types of incentive programs currently being offered to physicians and other health care providers by health plans, coalitions, employers, and governmental entities. In Medicare, the movement has been spurred on over the last several years by the enactment of ACA and MACRA. In addition, an increasing number of incentives are now being offered directly to patients in an effort to influence their health care choices and pursuit of healthy lifestyles. The goal of value-based care is to promote changed behavior that will result in the desired clinical and business outcomes.

Value-Based Care and the AMA

The AMA continues to examine initiatives to improve quality and/or reduce costs, which are truly designed to support physician efforts to provide high-quality care more efficiently. These programs must be patient-centered, and link evidence-based performance measures developed by physicians in collaboration across specialties to financial incentives that are not takeaways from the system. The AMA's Principles and Guidelines for PFP, which was developed in 2005, provides a valuable backdrop for developing and accessing fair and ethical programs. These include:

1. Ensure quality of care
2. Foster the patient/physician relationship
3. Offer voluntary physician participation
4. Use accurate data and fair reporting
5. Provide fair and equitable program incentives

For information on available Medicare Alternative Payment Models, refer to the CMS Innovation website at https://innovation.cms.gov/.

CMS Quality Payment Program

Over the last decade, CMS has developed a variety of Congressionally mandated initiatives that are intended to incentivize higher quality and/or lower cost care across different settings, including physician offices, hospitals, skilled nursing facilities, home health agencies, and dialysis facilities for end-stage renal disease. Ultimately, the goal is to base payments on outcomes and resource use rather than the volume of services.

Movement toward a "value-based" system began in 2006 with the Tax Relief & Health Care Act, which included a requirement that led to the development of the Physician Quality Reporting System (PQRS). In 2009, the Health Information Technology for Economic and Clinical Health Act section of the American Recovery and Reinvestment Act provided financial incentives for physician purchase and "meaningful use" (MU) of electronic medical records. The value modifier (VM), which adjusted Medicare payments based on cost and quality comparisons, followed in 2010 as part of the Affordable Care Act. All three of these programs were then combined and revised in the Medicare Access and CHIP Reauthorization bill, which also permanently repealed the flawed sustainable growth rate (SGR) that had led to more than a decade of stagnant payment rates and annual threats of draconian pay cuts halted by last-minute Congressional action. Both ACA and MACRA also took steps to move more physicians out of fee-for-service payment and into new payment and delivery models that put more emphasis on team-based care, population health, and more coordination among physicians.

In the ACA, Congress created the Centers for Medicare & Medicaid Innovation and charged it with developing and testing new payment models that could be expanded without additional Congressional authority if they reduced costs and/or improved quality. MACRA built on this concept by providing physicians the option of either providing care to a significant percentage of their patients through an alternative payment model (APM) or participating in a modified fee-for-service program known as the merit-based incentive payment system (MIPS). Medicare officials are calling this two-pathway approach the Quality Payment Program (QPP). The new program provided several improvements over current law, including greater opportunities for achieving payment bonuses, lower potential penalties, and greater support for physicians who want to pursue new models.

Without the passage of MACRA, physicians could have been subject to negative payment adjustments of 11% or more in 2019 due to penalties associated with the existing PQRS, MU, and VM value-based payment programs—with even greater potential penalties in future years. Under MACRA, the largest penalty a physician could experience is 5% in 2020, 7% in 2021, and 9% in 2022 and later. In 2020–2022, physicians who meet the qualifying APM participation (QP) thresholds will receive a lump sum incentive payment equal to 5% of their total Medicare payments in the prior year. Partial QPs are participants in advanced APMs who do not reach the QP threshold for an APM bonus payment but who may opt out of MIPS. Those who do not qualify as an APM participant or partial QP will be judged on MIPS scores. In 2026 and later, physicians who meet the APM qualifications also will receive higher payment updates than those who remain in a fee-for-service model.

MACRA affects physicians' Medicare payments in 2022 with MIPS-related payment adjustments and identification of qualified advanced APM participants based on 2020 data. To qualify for the 5% bonus in 2022, physicians must have had at least 50% of their 2020 Medicare payments or 35% of their Medicare patients tied to an advanced APM that meets specific risk, electronic record, and quality criteria. To qualify as a partial QP, physicians must have at least 40% of their Medicare payments or 25% of their Medicare patients tied to an advanced APM. Additional physician-developed models are expected to become available in the next few years. See https://qpp.cms.gov for more information.

Until more APMs become available, most physicians are expected to take the MIPS pathway, which, in addition to the three existing value-based payment programs, also includes a fourth category that is intended to encourage a wide range of practice "improvement activities." When fully implemented, the categories will be blended into a single composite score weighted as follows:

- Quality (formerly PQRS)—30%
- Cost (formerly value-based modifier)—30%
- Promoting interoperability (formerly meaningful use)—25% with the potential of a reduction to 15%
- Improvement activities—15%

In the initial year, however, quality was worth 60% and cost was not to be counted in the score, though physicians received information on how they would have done on this component. In the second year, quality was worth 50% and cost was worth 10% of the physician's final score. In the third and fourth years, which were 2019 and 2020, quality was worth 45% and cost was worth 15% of the physician's final score. In 2021, which was the fifth year, quality was worth 40% and cost was worth 20% of the physician's final score. In 2022, the sixth year of the program, CMS is statutorily required to weight quality at 30% and cost at 30%.

Scores from each category are weighted, summed, and compared against a performance threshold determined by CMS. Payment adjustments applied two years later will be neutral for those at the threshold, negative for those below it, and positive for those above it. Maximum negative and positive adjustments are up to 5% in 2018–2020, up to 7% in 2019–2021, and up to 9% by 2020–2022 and thereafter. However, through 2022–2024, those who meet a higher threshold for exceptional performance can receive up to 10% in additional bonus money. See CMS' Quality Payment Program at https://qpp.cms.gov.

MIPS regulations for 2022 were issued on November 2, 2021, CMS set the 2022 performance threshold for determining bonuses or penalties in 2024 at 75 points and the additional exceptional performance threshold at 89 points. The 2022 performance year/2024 payment year is the final year for an additional performance threshold/additional MIPS adjustment for exceptional performance. This means that physicians who do not meet the participation thresholds to become a qualified participant of an Advanced Alternative Payment Model (AAPM) must achieve at least 75 points on their overall MIPS score to avoid a payment cut of up to 9% in 2024. However, the Bipartisan Budget Act of 2018, which was strongly supported by the AMA, gave CMS the flexibility to gradually increase the performance threshold over the next three years. CMS found that the mean final score in 2017 was 74.01 points, and the median final score was 88.97 points. In 2018, the mean final score was 86.96 and the median final score was 99.63.

CMS also responded to some of the recommendations made by the AMA and other physician representatives by outlining a new approach to MIPS—the MIPS Value Pathways (MVPs). MVPs would allow physicians to focus their MIPS reporting on a unified set of measures tailored to an episode of care or condition with the goal of reducing physician burden associated with the MIPS program. As a result of ongoing concerns with the MVP framework, CMS has finalized that MVPs would be available gradually, beginning with the 2023 performance year. For the 2023 and 2024 performance years, CMS has allowed individual clinicians, single specialty groups, multispecialty groups, subgroups, and APM Entities to report MVPs. As advocated by the AMA and specialty societies, CMS intends to provide more detailed and actionable data to MVP participants. CMS has also highlighted that it intends to work with specialty societies to further develop MVP.

In response to the coronavirus disease 2019 (COVID-19) Public Health Emergency (PHE), CMS extended the MIPS automatic extreme and uncontrollable circumstances (EUC) policy to all MIPS eligible clinicians in 2019 and has continued flexibility with MIPS due to the PHE into 2021.

Additional AMA resources on MACRA, including a decision tree to aid physicians in choosing among the various options, are available at www.ama-assn.org/qpp-specifics.

Incentive Payments

The ACA created an incentive payment to primary care physicians (PCPs), including family medicine, internal medicine, pediatric medicine, and geriatric medicine, as well as nurse practitioners, clinical nurse specialists, and physician assistants. To be eligible for this bonus payment, these practitioners' primary care percentage must be at least 60% of their Medicare allowed charges for services paid under the MFS. Primary care practitioners will be identified using the NPI number of the rendering practitioner on claims. If the claim is submitted by a practitioner's group practice, the rendering practitioner's NPI must be included on the line-item for the primary care service and reflect an eligible Healthcare Common Procedure Coding System (HCPCS) code as identified. To be eligible for the PCIP, physician assistants, clinical nurse specialists, and nurse practitioners must be billing for their services (and not furnishing services incident to physicians' services) under their own NPI.

Regardless of the specialty area in which they may be practicing, the specific nonphysician practitioners are eligible for the primary care incentive payment program (PCIP) based on their profession and historical percentage of allowed charges as primary care services that equals or exceeds the 60% threshold. Because of the AMA Advocacy efforts, CMS has announced that it will exclude Part B drugs and laboratory tests, and inpatient and outpatient hospital services from the denominator, as well as transitional care management (TCM) services from the numerator and denominator of this calculation. This modification will allow more PCP to qualify for the bonus payments. The calculation for the 2014 payments is based on allowed services in 2012 and is automatically applied by CMS, if the physician qualifies and has the correct specialty designation. No modifiers are required in reporting these services. Primary care services as defined by the Act are new and established patient office or other outpatient visits (CPT codes 99201–99215); nursing facility care visits, domiciliary, rest home or homecare plan oversight services (CPT codes 99304–99340); and patient home visits (CPT codes 99341–99350). These providers were eligible for a 10% bonus payment for these services from January 1, 2011, through December 31, 2015. No further legislation was enacted and the 10% incentives—section 5501(a) of the Affordable Care Act established for Part B services by primary care practitioners—ended on December 31, 2015.

Incentive Payments for Major Surgical Procedures in Health Professional Shortage Areas

The ACA created an incentive payment to general surgeons, who perform major procedures (with a 010- or 090-day global service period) in a health professional shortage area (HPSA). These physicians were eligible for a bonus payment equal to 10% of the Medicare Payment Schedule payment for the surgical services from January 1, 2011–December 31, 2015. The incentive payment was automatically applied to qualifying services performed by general surgeons, who were in zip codes already eligible for automatic HPSA physician bonus payment. Modifier AQ should be appended for these major surgical procedures, like claims for the Medicare original HPSA bonus when services are provided in zip code areas that do not fall entirely within a full or partial county HPSA.

Participation Decision

A medical practice should evaluate whether to sign a participation agreement with Medicare, along with other financial considerations. The advantages and disadvantages of each decision are discussed in the following sections.

- *Participation*

  Participation may present a significant advantage to a practice's cash flow, particularly if it has a substantial volume of Medicare claims. When 80% of the Medicare-approved amount is paid directly to the physician rather than to the patient, the payment collection process may be faster and completed with fewer administrative requirements than for nonparticipating claims. When selecting a physician, many Medicare patients consider participation an important advantage because they are responsible only for the annual deductible and 20% copayment for Medicare-covered services. Participating (PAR) physicians also benefit because their names are published in directories provided to senior citizen groups, and because they receive participation emblems from Medicare to display in their offices. Other benefits include the Medicare-approved payment amount for PAR physicians, which is 5% higher than the rate for non-PAR physicians, and toll-free claims processing lines provided to PAR physicians to process their claims more quickly.

  Participating physicians must agree to accept Medicare's approved amount as payment-in-full for all covered services for the duration of the calendar year. However, Medicare participation agreements do not require physician practices to accept every Medicare patient who seeks treatment.

- *Nonparticipation*

  Nonparticipating physicians have some advantages that are not available to participating physicians. They may choose to accept assignment on a claim-by-claim basis, and this freedom of choice may be an important philosophical consideration when making the participation decision. Nonparticipating physicians are allowed to bill Medicare patients for covered services above the Medicare-approved amount, which is referred to as "balance billing." Beginning in 1986, however, when maximum allowable actual charges (MAACs) were imposed, the amount a nonparticipating physician could bill a Medicare patient in excess of the approved amount was subject to limitations. In 1991, limiting charges replaced MAACs.

Since January 1993, the limiting charge has been 15% more than the Medicare-approved amount for nonparticipating physicians. Medicare payments for nonparticipating physicians are 95% of payment rates for participating physicians. As a result, the 15% limiting charge translates into only 9.25% more than the participating physician payment schedule. It should be further noted that the 95% payment rate received by non-PAR physicians is not based on whether physicians accept assignment on the claim, but is based on the physician's PAR or non-PAR designation. When non-PAR physicians accept assignment for their low-income or other patients, they still receive only 95% of the amount of the PAR physicians. Non-PAR physicians need to collect the full limiting-charge amount, roughly 35% of the time they provide a given service, in order for the revenues from that service to equal those of PAR physicians for providing the same service. Therefore, when considering whether to be non-PAR, a physician must determine whether his or her total revenues from Medicare, patient copayments, and balance billing would exceed his or her total revenues as a PAR physician, considering collection costs, bad debts, and claims for which he or she does not accept assignment.

As explained in Chapter 9, carriers closely monitor physician compliance with the limiting charges. Under CMS' Comprehensive Limiting Charge Compliance Program (CLCCP), when a physician bills a patient more than the limiting charge (by at least $1 or more), the physician is notified of the overcharges on a bi-weekly or case-by-case basis through a limiting charge–exception report. Patients are informed of overcharges on the explanation of Medicare benefits (EOMB). When limiting-charge violations occur, the physician must refund the patient any payment that exceeds the charge limit. The carrier may request that physicians provide documentation to verify that they have made the appropriate refunds to the patient.

The Social Security Act Amendments of 1994 gave CMS statutory authority to enforce Medicare balance billing limits for nonparticipating physicians and suppliers. Effective January 1, 1995, if billed charges exceed the limiting charge, carriers are required to notify the physician or other provider of the violation within 30 days. The physician or other provider must refund or credit the excess charges to the patient within 30 days of carrier notification. Sanctions may be imposed against physicians and other providers for "knowingly and willfully" billing or collecting payments that exceed the limiting charge.

The law also requires carriers to provide limiting-charge information on the EOMB form, following submission of an unassigned claim with charges, which exceed the limiting charge. The form must also indicate the beneficiary's right to a refund if an excess charge was collected. To monitor physicians' and other providers' compliance with the limiting charges, carriers are required to screen all unassigned claims.

The AMA urged Congress to ensure that due-process safeguards are applied in any enforcement process that is adopted. These safeguards should include the opportunity for physicians to protest a refund request in situations, such as "down-coding" by the carrier, which are beyond the physician's control. (For further details on the participation program, refer to Chapter 9.)

For those physicians who do not wish to change their PAR or non-PAR status, no action is required. For those considering a change in their PAR or non-PAR status, physicians should consider this decision carefully because it is binding throughout the calendar year, unless Congress modifies payment rules or the physician's practice changes significantly, eg, the physician relocates. In making this decision, physicians should determine if they are bound by any contractual arrangements with hospitals, health plans, or other entities that require PAR status. In addition, some states have legislation that prohibits physicians from balance billing their patients. The opportunity to change participation status is only offered once per year, usually during November when the carriers send the Medicare Participating Physicians/Supplier Agreement (formerly referred to as the Dear Doctor letters). Those physicians who wish to change their Medicare participation or nonparticipation status are required to do so before December 31. This decision is binding throughout the subsequent calendar year.

Prior to MACRA, physicians and practitioners that wished to renew their opt-out were required to file new valid affidavits with their Medicare administrative contractors (MACs) every two years. CMS clarified that under MACRA, physicians and practitioners that filed valid opt-out affidavits on or after June 16, 2015, were not required to file renewal affidavits. Such physicians and practitioners may cancel the renewal by notifying all MACs with which they have filed an affidavit in writing, at least 30 days prior to the beginning of the new two-year opt-out period.

Private Contracting

Physicians who wish to enter private contracts with Medicare patients may do so without fearing that such contracts would not be considered legally binding. Provisions in the Balanced Budget Act (BBA) of 1997, which became effective January 1, 1998, gave physicians and their Medicare patients the freedom to privately contract to provide health care services outside the Medicare system. These private contracts must meet the following specific requirements:

- Medicare does not pay the patient or the physician for the services provided or contracted.
- The contract is in writing and signed by the beneficiary before any item or service is provided.
- The contract is not entered into at a time when the beneficiary is facing an emergency or urgent health situation.
- The physician signs and files an affidavit agreeing to forgo receiving any payment from Medicare (either directly, on a capitated basis, or from an organization that receives Medicare payment directly or on a capitated basis) for items or services provided to any Medicare beneficiary for the following two-year period.

In other words, the new right comes with a hefty price; physicians who privately contract with even one Medicare patient cannot participate or receive any payment from Medicare for two years.

In addition, the contract must state unambiguously that by signing the private contract, the beneficiary gives up all Medicare payment for services furnished by the "opt out" physician; agrees not to bill Medicare or ask the physician to bill Medicare; is liable for all of the physician's charges, without any Medicare balance billing limits; acknowledges that Medigap or any other supplemental insurance will not pay toward the services; and acknowledges that he or she has the right to receive services from physicians for whom Medicare coverage and payment would be available. Nothing prohibits beneficiaries from seeing their physician for non-Medicare-covered services, such as routine annual physical exams, cosmetic surgery, hearing aids, and eye exams.

To opt out, a physician must file an affidavit that meets these criteria and received by the carrier at least 30 days before the first day of the next calendar quarter. There is a 90-day period after the effective date of the first opt-out affidavit, during which physicians may revoke the opt-out and return to Medicare as if they had never opted out. The physician must renew the opt-out every two years to continue to privately contract. A physician who "knowingly and willingly" submits a claim or receives any payment from Medicare during the affidavit's two-year period will lose the rights provided under the private contract provision and will not be eligible to receive Medicare payments for any service provided to any patient for the remainder of the period.

Several bills were introduced in Congress attempting to change the private contracting rules. For example, in 1998, the Medicare Beneficiary Freedom to Contract Act, also known as the Kyl-Archer Bill was introduced. The act would have repealed the requirement that physicians give up their Medicare payment for two years if they enter a private contract. The act would have also made it explicit that a patient could enter a private contract with their physicians on a case-by-case basis for any length of time, take steps to ensure that private contracting does not lead to fraud, and protected taxpayers from double payment for services rendered under private contracts. Further, in March 1999, the Medicare Preservation and Restoration Act was introduced in the US House of Representatives. This act sought to repeal the entire Medicare private contracting provision of the BBA, and clarify that private contracts are prohibited under Medicare for Medicare-covered services. The supposed reasoning behind the act was to retain Medicare's balance billing limits to guarantee beneficiaries reasonable and fair prices. Both bills have essentially died in committee.

The MACRA legislation signed into law on April 16, 2015, includes two provisions relevant to the current private contracting rules. Effective June 15, 2015, physicians who have opted out of Medicare no longer need to renew their opt-out status every two years. In addition, beginning on February 1, 2016, CMS is required to issue an annual list of physicians who have opted out of the program, including information on their specialty and region.

Using the RBRVS to Establish Physician Charges

The AMA believes that a strong payment-for-service sector is essential to patient choice and must be a central feature of the health care marketplace. To strengthen the viability of payment-for-service medicine in the current marketplace, the AMA developed a new approach to payment-for-service based on a national standard RBRVS. This approach, which is explained in Chapter 13, holds that RBRVS relative values could provide the basis for public and private physician payment and payment systems. Using RBRVS under this approach would apply only to the RBRVS relative values, not to Medicare's conversion factors, balance billing limits, geographic practice cost indices (GPCIs), or other inappropriate Medicare payment policies.

Using a National Standard RBRVS

A national standard RBRVS for physicians and payers would rely on advance disclosure of physician and other provider payments, hospital and facility charges, and health plan payments. Under this principle, payment-for-service physicians and health plans could offer the cost predictability that is often cited as a hallmark of managed care plans. Patients could use this information to help choose a physician, use plan payment levels to help choose a plan with the best coverage, and, through such comparisons, estimate out-of-pocket costs.

Table 12-1. Calculating a Conversion Factor Using the RBRVS: An Illustration

Service	RVUs/ Service	Service Frequency	Frequency × RVUs	Payments	Frequency × Payments
A	9	10	90	$500	$5,000
B	2	15	30	$90	$1,350
C	12	10	120	$600	$6,000
D	1	50	50	$60	$3,000
Total			290*		$15,350†

*Total RVUs = sum of RVUs for each service multiplied by frequency = 290

†Total payments = sum of payment per service multiplied by frequency = $15,350

Conversion factor = total payments divided by total RVUs = $52.93

A national standard RBRVS offers one method for physicians to establish their charges. Using the RBRVS, physicians can establish their payments based on a dollar-conversion factor that they select.[i]

Establishing the Conversion Factor

The following methodology offers one alternative to physicians for establishing a conversion factor (CF), which maintains current practice revenue. Other methods could also be used. The initial calculation of a CF provides the starting point for determining physician charges. Adjustments could then be made in accordance with other considerations, such as the local market for the physicians' services.

A CF using RBRVS relative values can be calculated with information on the types of physician services provided, utilization, and current billed charges. For the CF to accurately reflect the practice's charge levels, it is recommended that services representing 85% to 90% of the practice's volume be included in the calculations. As a result, determining a CF for a multispecialty group practice will be more complex than for a single specialty.

A CF is determined by dividing the total payments for all services provided (payment for each service multiplied by service frequency) by total RVUs (RVUs for each service multiplied by frequency). Total RVUs by CPT code can be found in Part 5, List of Relative Value Units. Table 12-1 illustrates how to set up the worksheet for calculating a CF. Physicians may want to consider developing an electronic spreadsheet to complete the calculations.

Copayments and Deductibles

Medicare beneficiaries are responsible for an annual deductible of $233 in 2022, an increase of $30 from the annual deductible of $203 in 2021, and 20% coinsurance for most services. In most cases, the physician (or other health care provider) must collect the deductible and coinsurance from the patient or the patient's Medigap insurer.

The HHS inspector general considers it fraudulent practice to routinely waive patients' Medicare copayments and deductibles. Under the RBRVS, if the copayments and/or deductibles are routinely waived, the charge minus this portion of the payment is the physician's actual charge. Medicare continues to pay at the lower of the actual charge or the approved amount. A physician's office must be able to demonstrate that it made a good faith effort to collect from the patient. Letters and records of phone calls that the physician's office or a collection agency makes to the patient would provide appropriate documentation that a good faith effort was made to collect from the patient.

Premiums

In 2022, the standard Medicare Part B monthly premium increased to $170.10 (or higher depending on the beneficiary's income), an increase of $21.60 from $148.50 in 2021. Part B coverage includes physician and nursing services; X rays; laboratory and diagnostic tests; influenza and pneumonia vaccinations; blood transfusions; renal dialysis; outpatient hospital procedures; limited ambulance transportation; immunosuppressive drugs for organ transplant recipients; chemotherapy; hormonal treatments, such as Lupron; and other outpatient medical treatments administered in a doctor's office. Medication administration is covered under Part B if it is administered by the physician during an office visit. In addition, Part B also helps with durable medical equipment (DME), including canes, walkers, wheelchairs, and mobility scooters for those with mobility impairments. Prosthetic devices, such as artificial limbs and breast prosthesis following mastectomy, as well as one pair of eyeglasses following cataract surgery, and oxygen for home use is also covered.

By law, the standard premium is set to cover one-fourth of the average cost of Part B services incurred by beneficiaries aged 65 and over, plus a contingency margin. The contingency margin is an amount to ensure that Part B has sufficient assets and income to (1) cover Part B expenditures

Table 12-2. The 2022 Medicare Part B Premiums

Beneficiaries Who File Individual Tax Returns with Modified Adjusted Gross Income	Beneficiaries Who File Joint Tax Returns with Modified Adjusted Gross Income	Total Monthly Premium Amount
≤$91,000	≤$182,000	$170.10
>$91,000 and ≤$114,000	>$182,000 and ≤$228,000	$238.10
>$114,000 and ≤$142,000	>$228,000 and ≤$284,000	$340.20
>$142,000 and ≤$170,000	>$284,000 and ≤$340,000	$442.30
>$170,000 and <$500,000	>$340,000 and <$750,000	$544.30
$500,000 and above	$750,000 and above	$578.30

during the year; (2) cover incurred-but-unpaid claims costs at the end of the year; (3) provide for possible variation between actual and projected costs; and (4) amortize any surplus assets. Most of the remaining Part B is financed through general revenues (72%), beneficiary premiums (25%), and interest and other sources (3%). Beneficiaries with annual incomes over $85,000/individual or $170,000/couple pay a higher, income-related Part B premium reflecting a larger share of total Part B spending, ranging from 35% to 80%; the ACA froze the income thresholds through 2019, which is expected to increase the share of beneficiaries paying the higher Part B premium. Each year from 2003 through 2014, Congress has acted to prevent physician payment reductions from occurring. PAMA postponed the 24% Medicare physician payment cut for 12 months, from March 31, 2014, until April 1, 2015. On April 16, 2015, MACRA was signed into law, eliminating the SGR. The legislation (P.L. 114-10) provides positive annual payment updates of 0.5%, starting July 1, 2015, and lasting through 2019. See Table 12-2 for the 2022 Medicare Part B individual and joint premiums, by annual income level.

For more information on the 2022 Medicare Parts A and B premiums and deductibles (CMS-8077-N, CMS-8078-N, CMS-8079-N), information is available at https://www.federalregister.gov/public-inspection.

Discussing Payments with Patients

The AMA policy supports disclosure by physicians, hospitals, and other health care providers of payments charged to patients before providing services. Such disclosure enables patients to make informed and cost-conscious health care choices. Physicians may provide this information to patients or prospective patients on request, or in the absence of a request, by volunteering the information. Physicians may volunteer payment information in a variety of ways: by posting payments in the office waiting area, by providing information for inclusion in directories, or through discussions with patients and families.

Medical practices should establish a specific policy for discussing charges with patients to ensure that they consistently observe patient concerns. Physicians and office staff should be familiar with this policy, which should be sensitive to patients' financial and family considerations. For example, the physician should first ask patients if they would like to discuss the physician's charges before initiating such a discussion, because the patient may want a spouse or other family member to participate. Such consideration is especially important, if a major surgical procedure is planned or when the physician anticipates that a service may not be a covered benefit. Before the discussion, the physician may want to obtain background information on the patient's insurance and have some knowledge about expected hospital expenses, if applicable.

When discussing charges, physicians may also want to explain their participation status and the concerns that influenced their decision. If possible, any discussion of payment policies with patients should take place in the business office or consultation room, rather than in the examining room.

Written information about charges and participation status may be very useful to Medicare patients. The information might be a simple list of charges for frequently provided services, which could include Medicare-approved amount, physician's actual charge, and an explanation of the limiting charge, if applicable. Other information could include the physician's participation status and the patient's responsibility for copayments and deductibles. A summary of charges and payment policies can be printed as a brochure and made available in the physician's waiting room or posted on the wall. Patients can then take home the information to review and share with family members, and they can refer to it for later discussions with the physician. The best opportunity to review the brochure or list of charges and payment policies with new patients, however, is during the initial office visit.

Note

i. Establishing a conversion factor is the equivalent of setting payments for antitrust purposes, and the law requires that this be done independently by each physician or physician group.

Chapter 13

Non-Medicare Use of the RBRVS: Survey Data

Since the adoption of Medicare's resource-based relative value scale (RBRVS) in 1992, the American Medical Association (AMA) has conducted national surveys of public and private payers to assess the effects of this payment method in non-Medicare health markets. The basis for these surveys is a persistent concern on the part of the AMA that policies implemented by the government could have consequences for non-Medicare payers. The AMA is committed to an RBRVS that will be an accurate, comprehensive standard uniformly covering all medical services nationwide. For this reason, it is important to understand the extent to which the RBRVS has been adopted outside of Medicare, the different payment policies used by payers, and the use of Medicare payment policies. While many payers may claim to use the RBRVS, adjustments to payment policies, large numbers of conversion factors, and other adjustments may result in a payment system that differs from Medicare's RBRVS system.

This chapter analyzes data collected in the summer of 2006 from 127 different public and private payers, representing 123 million covered lives. The survey showed that 77% of respondents use the RBRVS. This compares with a 74% adoption rate from the 2001 survey and 63% adoption rate from the 1998 survey. This also compares to two additional surveys: a 1993 Deloitte & Touche survey indicated an adoption rate of 32% and a Physician Payment Review Commission (PPRC) study for its 1995 Annual Report to Congress indicated a 28% adoption rate of the RBRVS.[1, 2] This suggests that non-Medicare use of the RBRVS continues to increase and is in wide use by a variety of payers.

Survey Design

The survey instrument was structured to capture data from a variety of different payers in both public and private sectors. In addition to collecting data on the use of the RBRVS, the survey also presented questions regarding conversion factors, payment policies used with the RBRVS, and the respondents' opinion of the RBRVS. In order to facilitate longitudinal analysis, the instrument contained some of the same questions as previous AMA surveys.

The survey sample contained Medicaid agencies, state workers' compensation plans, TRICARE (the US military health system), and a variety of private health insurance plans. A letter was sent to the medical directors of payers in the spring of 2006, a follow-up letter was sent in July to those plans whose directors had not responded, and additional follow-up telephone calls were made throughout the summer. The response rate was 80% of Medicaid plans, 54% of workers' compensation plans, one response from TRICARE (representing 100% of TRICARE), and 10% of private plans. However, the private plan responses represented 78.6 million covered lives, more than previous surveys had represented. Given a 10% response rate for private health plans, the survey runs the risk of introducing some possible selection bias where private health insurance plans that use the RBRVS may be more likely to respond to the survey. However, the survey results were consistent with anecdotal reports of private plan payer use of the RBRVS and, given the lack of other sources of data showing private payers' use of the RBRVS, no other benchmarks are available to determine the reasonableness of the data.

Characteristics of Respondents

Completed surveys were received from TRICARE, 45 Medicaid plans, 12 Blue Cross/Blue Shield plans, and 69 other private pay and workers' compensation plans. Respondents self-designated their primary payer type resulting in the following self-description:

- 38% Private insurers
- 38% Medicaid
- 24% Workers' compensation
- <1% TRICARE

In addition to the type of payer the respondents consider themselves, respondents can be described by the number of physicians they have under contract and the number of enrollees covered by their plan. Ranges that express these responses are compiled in Table 13-1.

The number of enrollees represented can be divided by four primary payer types (see Figure 13-1). The total number of covered lives represented in the survey is approximately 123 million. Private insurers accounted for 64% of enrollees represented, Medicaid accounted for 26% of enrollees, TRICARE accounted for 7% of enrollees, and workers' compensation plans accounted for 3% of enrollees represented. (Only 13% of workers' compensation plans indicated the number of total enrollees covered by their plan.)

Table 13-1. Payer Characteristics

	Percentage
Number of Contracted Physicians	
≤5,000	36%
5,001–10,000	14%
10,001–20,000	20%
≥$20,000	30%
Number of Enrollees	
≤100,000	27%
100,001–500,000	15%
500,001–1,000,000	35%
≥$1,000,000	23%

Figure 13-1. Number of Enrollees, by Payer Type

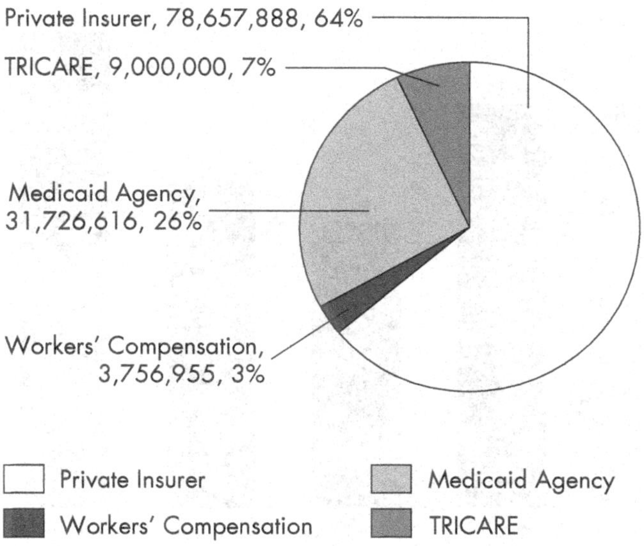

The number of enrollees represented in the last three AMA surveys on the non-Medicare use of the RBRVS were as follows:

Year	Enrollees Represented
2006	123,141,459
2001	87,908,525
1998	104,926,286

The US population was 300 million. The Kaiser Family Foundation 2004–2005 health insurance status for the US population indicated: 14% of individuals are covered by Medicaid, 12% by Medicare, and 58% by an employer or the individual; and 16% of individuals are uninsured.[3] By tying in the number of enrollees by payer based on the total population, the percentage of populations represented in the survey were 100% of TRICARE enrollees, 76% of Medicaid enrollees (45 out of 56 US states, territories, and DC), and 46% of private health plan enrollees.

Utilization of Medicare RBRVS

As previously mentioned, 77% of the respondents used the RBRVS. Of this group, 93% adopted and fully implemented it and 7% decided to adopt the system and were in the process of implementation. This has increased since 2001, where previously 83% indicated they had adopted and fully implemented the RBRVS and 17% were deciding to adopt the system. Additionally, 8% are examined the potential use

Figure 13-2. Utilization of Medicare RBRVS by Payer Type, by Respondent

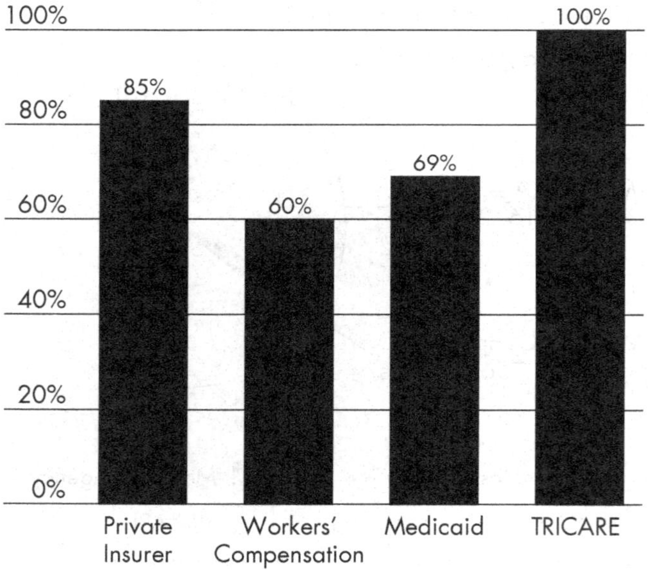

Figure 13-3. Utilization of Medicare RBRVS by Payer Type, by Enrollee

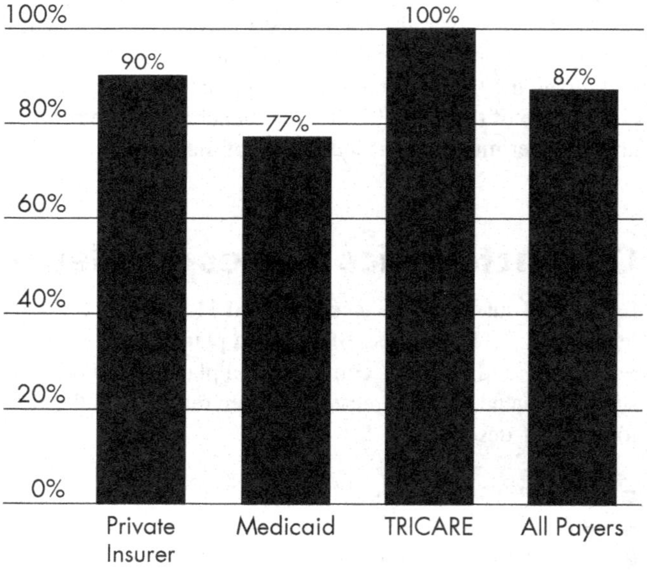

of the Medicare RBRVS. This indicated that 85% of respondents either used the RBRVS or considered its use. Alternatively, only 11% considered using the RBRVS but decided not to adopt, and 4% have not considered using the RBRVS.

Also, of those using the RBRVS, 91% use all three components (work, practice expense [PE], and professional liability insurance), while only 6% use work RVUs only, 1% use only PE RVUs only, and 2% use a combination of work and PE RVUs.

In examining the utilization of the RBRVS further by payer type, based on the number of respondents, 85% of private insurers, 60% of workers' compensation plans, 69% of Medicaid plans and 100% of TRICARE use the Medicare RBRVS (see Figure 13-2).

In analyzing the utilization of the RBRVS by payer type based on the number of enrollees represented, it has been determined that 87%, or approximately 107 million enrollees, use the RBRVS. Ninety percent of private insurers, 77% of Medicaid, and 100% of TRICARE enrollees are covered under a plan that uses the RBRVS (see Figure 13-3).

Use of Conversion Factors, All Payers

While the RBRVS establishes the relativity among procedures, it is the conversion factor that also determines the final payment amount. The AMA has been concerned that private payers would use the conversion factors and associated payment policies only to contain costs. Such an inappropriate use of the RBRVS could have negative consequences for patient access. The survey showed that with the exception of Medicaid, the conversion factor amounts were generally in excess of Medicare.

Fifty-seven percent of survey respondents had more than one conversion factor. The distribution of the number of conversion factors was as follows:

No. of Conversion Factors	Percentage of Payers
1	43%
2	16%
3–5	15%
6 or more	26%

The majority of payers use one or two conversion factors. As Figure 13-4 illustrates, 81% of Medicaid plans and 50% of private plans use one or two conversion factors.

While Medicare switched to a single conversion factor in 1998, the survey data indicate that a majority of the respondents continue to use multiple conversion factors. Most frequently the conversion factors were arranged by surgical, nonsurgical, or primary care.

A range of conversion factors was provided for payers who use a single conversion factor. The minimum was $19.99 and the maximum was $76.31. For payers using multiple

Figure 13-4. Number of Conversion Factors Used, by Payer

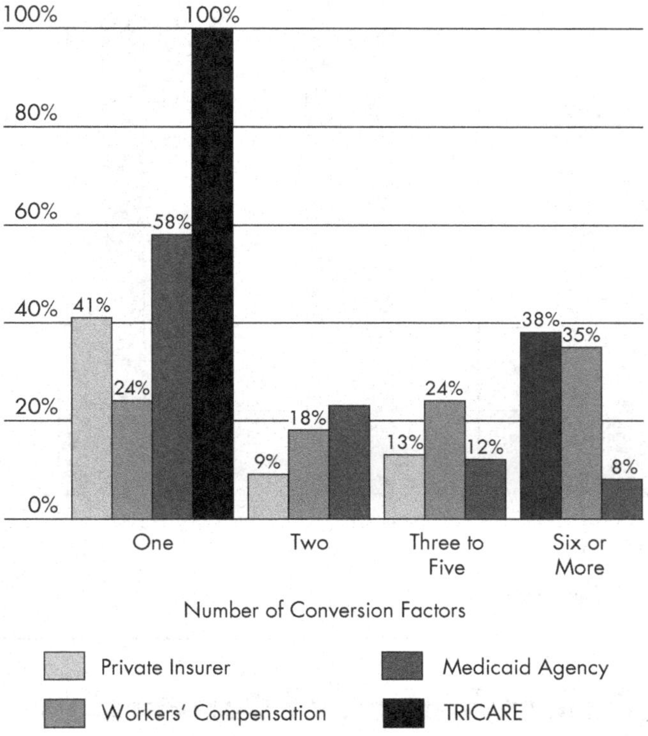

Figure 13-5. Average Conversion Factor by Payer Type (2006)

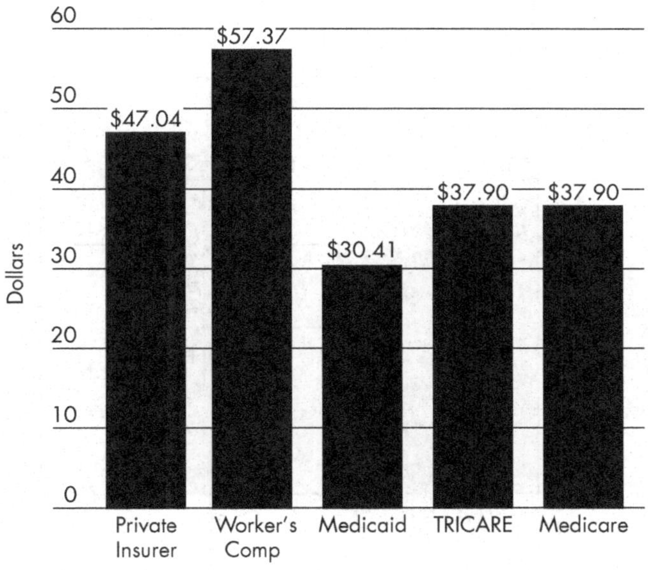

conversion factors, the minimum was $25.28 and the maximum was $79.80. At the time of the survey, Medicare had a single conversion factor of $37.90.

The average conversion factor by payer type (see Figure 13-5), taking the average of the single and multiple conversion factor plans were both higher and lower than the 2006 Medicare conversion factor of $37.90. TRICARE maintained the same conversion factor as Medicare; whereas, Medicaid had a slightly lower average conversion factor of $30.41. Private insurers' average conversion factor was $47.04 and the highest average conversion factor of $57.37 was from the workers' compensation plans.

To obtain a better understanding of how the payers varied conversion factors among specialties, respondents were asked to provide the conversion factor for a number of specialties. As seen in Figure 13-6, payers that differentiated conversion factors among specialties remained relatively consistent when comparing current conversion factors to the responses from the 2001 survey. Payers applied the highest conversion factor to surgery and the lowest to primary care. For those payers that did not differentiate among specialties, the average single conversion factor was $38.04 in 2006, slightly greater than the 2006 Medicare conversion factor of $37.90.

Eighty-five percent of respondents indicated that their organization uses the anesthesia base unit methodology. Figure 13-7 shows the conversion factor for anesthesia services by payer type compared to the 2006 Medicare conversion factor. Medicaid established an anesthesia conversion factor relatively similar to the Medicare anesthesia conversion factor and TRICARE used the same anesthesia conversion factor as Medicare. On the other hand, private insurers and workers' compensation plans maintained an anesthesia conversion factor that was more than double the 2006 Medicare anesthesia conversion factor.

Anesthesia services are reimbursed according to a different methodology than other physician services. This methodology is based on base units and time units. See Part 5 for a description of anesthesiology payments.

- For payers that used a single conversion factor for all physicians who receive payment under the RBRVS, the average conversion factor was $38.04, with a minimum of $19.99 and a maximum of $76.31. In 2006, the Medicare conversion factor was $37.90.
- For payers that used multiple conversion factors, for primary care services the average conversion factor was $44.78, with a minimum of $25.28 and a maximum of $68.40.
- For payers that used multiple conversion factors, for radiology services the average conversion factor was $48.91, with a minimum of $27.23 and a maximum of $79.80.

Figure 13-6. Average Conversion Factor by Specialty, 2001 vs 2006

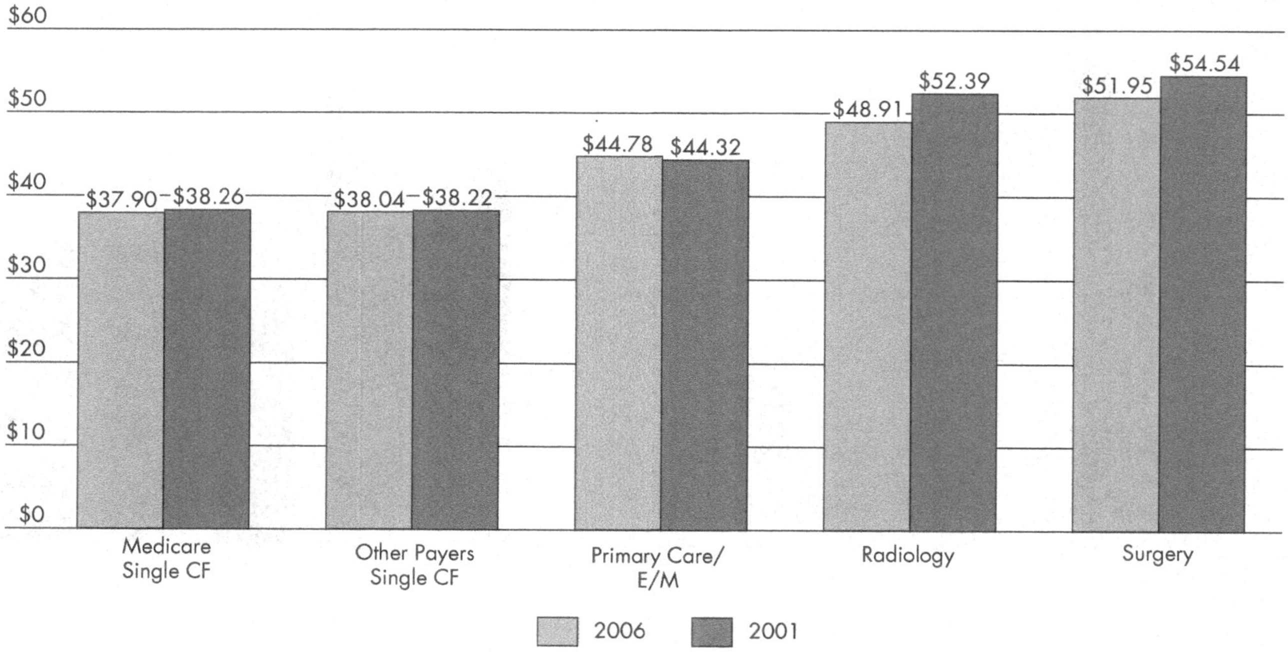

- For payers that used multiple conversion factors, for surgical services the average conversion factor was $51.95, with a minimum of $25.28 and a maximum of $79.10.
- For anesthesia services, the average conversion factor was $31.84, with a minimum of $10 and a maximum of $58.19. In 2006, the Medicare anesthesia conversion factor was $17.76.

Figure 13-7. Average Anesthesia Conversion Factor by Payer Type (2006)

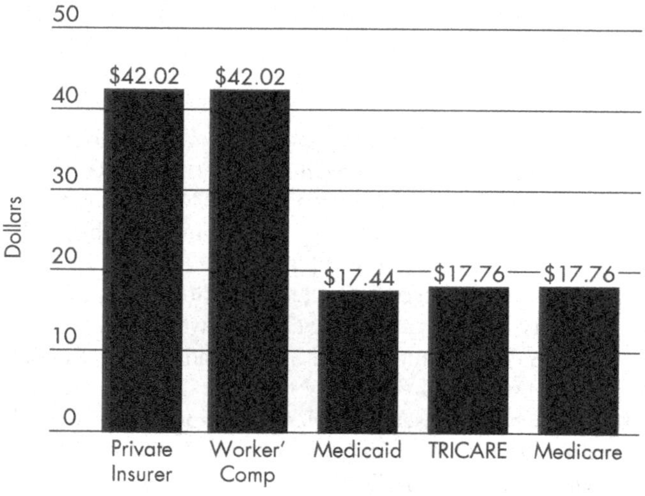

Determination of Conversion Factors

Respondents were asked how their organization determines their conversion factor(s). Fifty-one percent of respondents indicated that they use the Medicare conversion factor as the basis for determining their own conversion factor (by using the Medicare conversion factor or using a percentage of the Medicare payment [eg, 125% of Medicare]). The payers who indicated they use the Medicare conversion factor as a benchmark had a combined enrollment of 50 million individuals.

When examining the number of patients covered by health plans where the physician payment is linked to the Medicare conversion factor, the direct data from the survey indicated that 86 million patients or at least 34% of the insured population may have been directly affected by Medicare conversion factor cuts. When broken down by payer, the raw survey data indicated that 36 million Medicare patients, 9 million TRICARE patients, 10 million Medicaid patients, and 31 million patients covered by a private insurer were affected by Medicare conversion factor cuts.

If the survey sample data are extrapolated and tied to the entire US population, as many as 174 million patients or nearly 70% of the insured population may have been directly affected by Medicare conversion factor cuts. When broken down by payer, the extrapolated data indicated that

36 million Medicare patients, 9 million TRICARE patients, 14 million Medicaid patients, and 115 million patients covered by a private insurer may have been affected by Medicare conversion factor cuts.

Use of RBRVS Payment Policies

Respondents were asked the extent to which they have adopted a variety of Medicare payment policies. The acceptance of these policies was an important aspect of correctly implementing the RBRVS system. Based on data collected in 1998, 2001, and 2006, the acceptance rates appeared to be consistently high for the global surgical periods and the multiple surgery reduction. The increase in acceptance of the Medicare site-of-services differential since 1998 was most likely due to payers gaining a better understanding of this policy, which had been in use for almost a decade. The site-of-service differential related to the difference in practice expenses between services provided in a facility, such as a hospital, and a nonfacility, such as a physician's office. The Centers for Medicare & Medicaid Services (CMS) structured the PE methodology to recognize more physician costs when services were provided in the office as compared to when services are performed in the hospital. The reasoning behind this policy was that physicians incurred more expenses, such as staff and supplies, when they perform services in their office as opposed to in the hospital where staff and supply expenses are incurred by the hospital. The hospital then receives separate payment through Medicare Part A (see Table 13-2).

Respondents who used the RBRVS were also asked which of the following eight modifiers they accept. The 1998 and 2001 surveys asked if respondents used six specific modifiers. In 2006, modifiers 24 and 79 were added to this question. In 2006, 64% of the respondents indicated that they accept all eight of the modifiers. In the 2001 survey, 35% of respondents indicated that they accepted all six modifiers listed on the survey. Overall, the use of modifiers has continued to increase since 1998 (see Table 13-3).

Table 13-2. Acceptance Rates for Respondents Who Use the RBRVS

	2006	2001	1998
Global surgical periods	72%	73%	74%
Multiple surgery reduction	79%	85%	84%
Medicare site service differentials	72%	55%	26%
Geographic practice cost indices (GPCIs)	55%	51%	45%

Table 13-3. Acceptance Rates of Modifiers by Respondents Who Use the RBRVS

Modifier	2006	2001	1998
22, Unusual procedural services	79%	68%	81%
24, Unrelated evaluation and management services by the same physician during a postoperative period	78%	N/A	N/A
25, Significant, separately identifiable E/M service by the same physician on the same day of the procedure	81%	79%	75%
26, Professional component	96%	95%	92%
51, Multiple procedures	89%	90%	89%
57, Decision for surgery	69%	48%	64%
59, Distinct procedural service	76%	50%	63%
79, Unrelated procedure or service by the same physician during the postoperative period	72%	N/A	N/A

While respondents indicated their acceptance of modifiers, the use of claims-editing software may affect the acceptance of modifiers. Sixty-eight percent of the respondents indicated that they use a commercial or internally developed claims-editing package or a combination of commercial and internally developed systems. Therefore, if a particular claims-editing package does not recognize certain modifiers, then most likely payers' use of the software will result in certain modifiers automatically recognized or rejected. Only 24% of respondents do not use such software to process claims.

While AMA's primary interest rests in learning the extent to which payers who use the RBRVS recognize modifiers, the AMA studies are also meant to compare RBRVS user responses with those of payers who do not use the RBRVS. It is important to remember that payers' acceptance of modifiers is not reliant on payers' use of the RBRVS because Current Procedural Terminology (CPT®) modifiers can be used in a variety of payment systems. AMA found that generally payers who do not use the RBRVS are slightly less likely to recognize the eight modifiers surveyed, with the exception of modifier 26, Professional component. Forty-seven percent of the respondents who do not use the RBRVS indicated that they recognize all eight modifiers compared to 64% for those payers that use the RBRVS.

However, even for those respondents who do not use the RBRVS, a high rate of acceptance was found for some modifiers (see Table 13-4).

Figure 13-8 indicates that, regardless of payer type, 20% of payers use Medicare CCI edits. Medicaid plans primarily develop claims editing packages internally, private payers

Table 13-4. Acceptance of Modifiers by Nonusers of the RBRVS

Modifier	2006	2001	1998
22, Unusual procedural services	77%	68%	68%
24, Unrelated evaluation and management services by the same physician during a postoperative period	65%	N/A	N/A
25, Significant, separately identifiable E/M service by the same physician on the same day of the procedure	65%	68%	62%
26, Professional component	100%	90%	80%
51, Multiple procedures	81%	83%	80%
57, Decision for surgery	65%	35%	52%
59, Distinct procedural service	73%	53%	54%
79, Unrelated procedure or service by the same physician during the postoperative period	65%	N/A	N/A

primarily use commercial claims editing packages, TRICARE uses a commercial-claims editing package, and workers' compensation plans primarily do not use editing packages.

Figure 13-8. Code Editing Packages Utilized, by Payer Type 2006

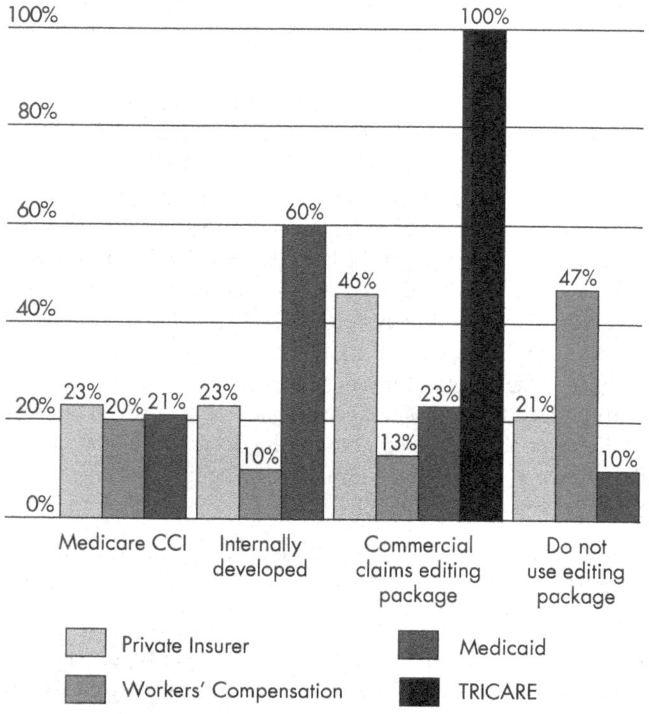

The responses to the policy questions indicated that payers continued to be likely to implement Medicare payment policies. Payers' acceptance of these policies was critical to properly implementing the RBRVS system. It is not sufficient to use only the Medicare established RVUs and then not recognize modifiers. Such a system would resemble Medicare's RBRVS in name only because the actual implementation of the system would be quite different. One important facet of the RBRVS methodology that non-Medicare payers should implement is the use of current CPT codes and relative values. Each year, new services are assigned relative values and existing codes receive revised relative values. Therefore, it is important that payers continually update their payment schedule so physicians and other health care providers are reimbursed according to the most recent relative value and payment policies. Seventy-five percent of respondents indicated that they update their conversion factor at least annually. While users of the RBRVS seem to accept many of the Medicare payment policies, a majority of respondents, 57%, continue to use multiple conversion factors that differentiate among specialties and health plans.

Medicare publishes its revised payment schedule on November 1 each year, with implementation on January 1. Respondents were further queried about the specific date in which they implement payment schedule changes (see Figure 13-9). Forty-one percent indicated that they implement their payment schedule changes on January 1, the same as Medicare; 16% indicated April 1; 20% indicated July 1; and 24% indicated "other." Respondents who indicated "other" generally indicated that they implemented their payment schedule based on legislation, as needed, or less than annually.

Respondents were asked how they provide their payment schedule to contracted physicians (see Figure 13-10). Ninety-two percent of respondents indicated the method in which they provide their payment schedule. Only one respondent indicated that it does not provide its payment schedule. Respondents may have indicated more than one method of providing a payment schedule to contracted physicians.

Opinion of the RBRVS

In addition to questions on the use of the RBRVS, conversion factors, and payment policies, payers' opinions of the RBRVS were surveyed by asking a series of questions related to possible benefits and drawbacks of the RBRVS system. These questions were asked of all respondents, both those that use the RBRVS and those that do not. Respondents could select from five categories: strongly agree, agree, neither agree or disagree, disagree, or strongly disagree. The questions were divided into positive and negative issues that could be associated with the RBRVS.

Figure 13-9. How Frequently Respondents Update Their Payment Schedule

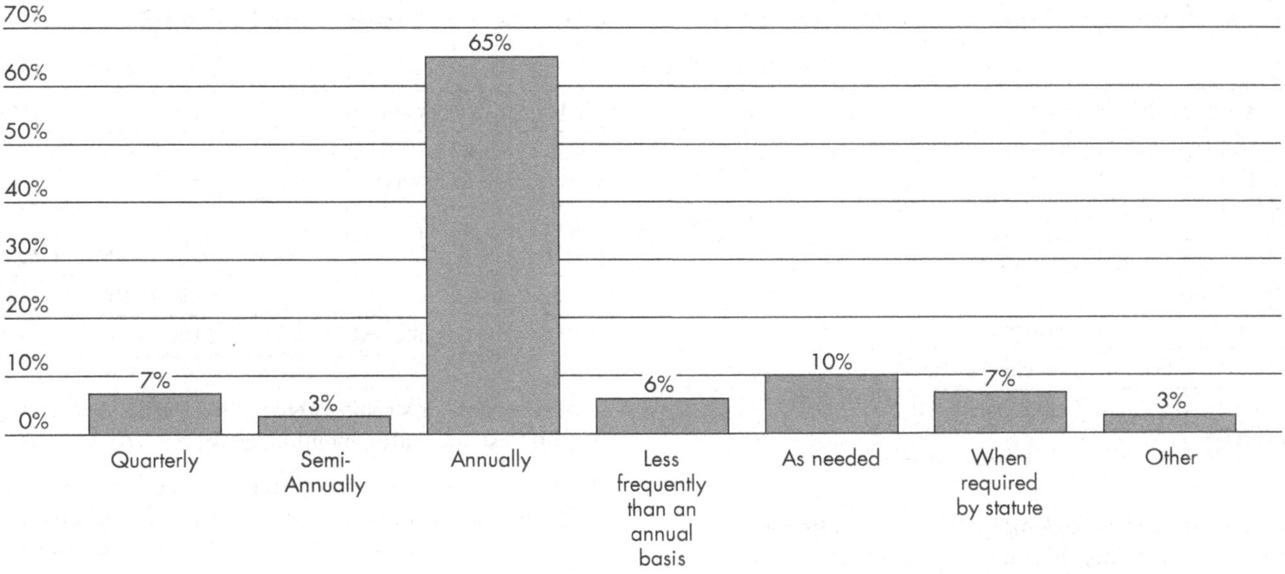

It is apparent from the data in Table 13-5 that respondents' positive opinions of the RBRVS have increased or remained consistent each time this survey has been conducted. At least 64% of the respondents agreed or strongly agreed that the RBRVS successfully addresses all of the aforementioned issues (except the ability of the RBRVS to control costs, 48%). However, it is important to note that this data include respondents who do not incorporate RBRVS into their payment policies. When the same responses are divided into RBRVS and non-RBRVS users, the results are quite different.

Figure 13-10. How Payment Schedules Are Provided to Contracted Physicians

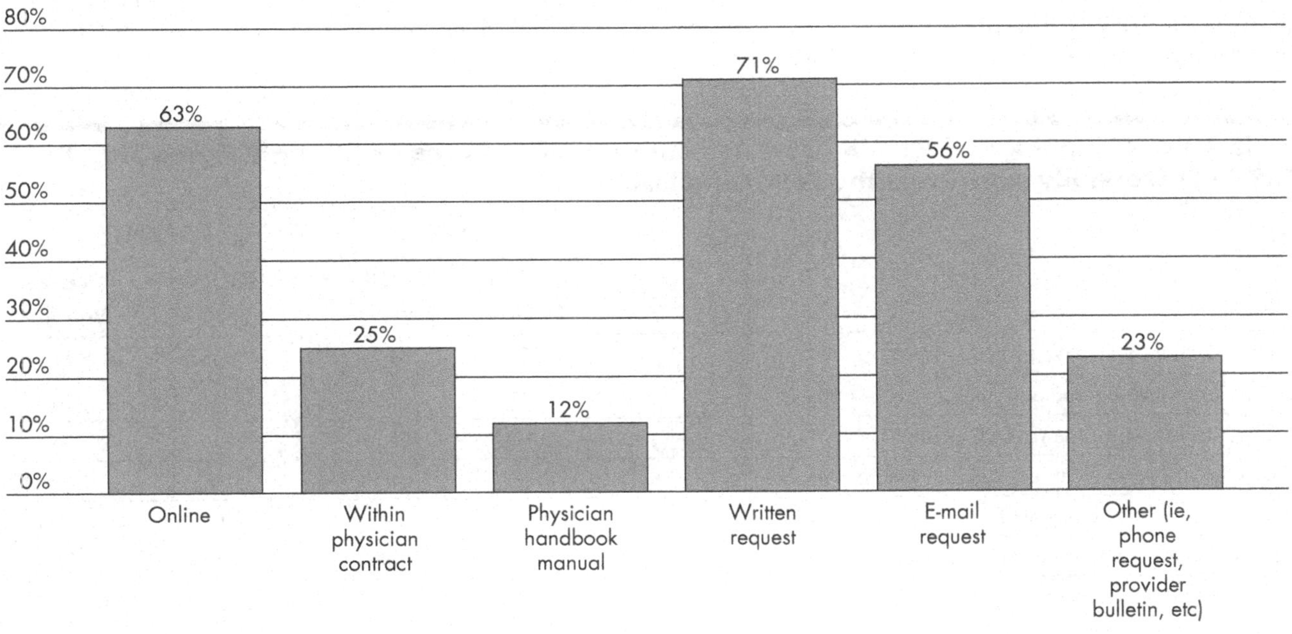

Table 13-5. Percentage of Respondents Who Agree or Strongly Agree That the RBRVS Successfully Addresses the Following Issues

	2006	2001	1998
Controls health care costs	**48%**	**39%**	**37%**
Allows for payment based on actual resources utilized	70%	68%	67%
Makes system compatible with Medicare	76%	66%	68%
Makes physician payment more equitable across specialties	64%	66%	70%
Rationalizes physician payment	74%	71%	74%
Increases control over physician payment	64%	54%	53%
Makes it easy to implement and update each year	72%	70%	69%

The data in Table 13-6 demonstrate a clear difference in opinion of the perceived benefits of the RBRVS system among RBRVS users and non-users. For example, 81% of the RBRVS users agreed or strongly agreed that the RBRVS allows for payment based on actual resources used while only 39% of non-RBRVS users concur. According to this table, at least 70% of RBRVS users, up from 61% in 2001, agreed that the RBRVS system successfully addresses all the aforementioned issues (except the RBRVS ability to control costs, 52%). The ability to rationalize payment, allowance of payment to be based on actual resources used, ease of implementing and updating, and compatibility with Medicare are the major perceived benefits among the RBRVS users. However, the ability to make payments more equitable across specialties and the control over physician payment ranked at least 70%. When comparing 2001 results to 2006, the data shows a steady increase that both RBRVS users and non-users agree or strongly agree that the RBRVS successfully addresses the aforementioned issues.

Table 13-7. Percentage of Respondents Who Agree or Strongly Agree That the Following Are Potential Drawbacks to the RBRVS System

	2006	2001	1998
Problems with methodology	30%	30%	26%
Potential to disrupt beneficiary access to physician services	27%	17%	32%
Potential to disrupt physician relations	30%	30%	12%
Current system is better	14%	10%	6%
RBRVS is too complicated	13%	13%	10%

The data in Table 13-7 demonstrates that no more than 30% of the respondents agreed or strongly agreed with any of the aforementioned potential drawbacks. The greatest drawbacks appear to be the potential to disrupt physician relations and problems associated with the methodology, both at 30% and exactly the same as respondents had indicated in 2001. However, only 13% and 14% agreed or strongly agreed that the RBRVS Is too complicated and that their current system is better.

When comparing the responses of the RBRVS users and non-users (see Table 13-8) to these questions, it was discovered, as expected, that the non-users had a higher percentage of respondents agreeing or strongly agreeing with the aforementioned potential drawbacks to the RBRVS system. Specifically, the non-users' express concern that the RBRVS has potential to disrupt physician relations and potential problems with its methodology, which were also the highest drawbacks among RBRVS users.

Table 13-6. Percentage of RBRVS Users vs Nonusers Who Agree or Strongly Agree That the RBRVS Successfully Addresses the Following Issues

	2006		2001	
	RBRVS Users	RBRVS Non-Users	RBRVS Users	RBRVS Non-Users
Controls health care costs	52%	35%	46%	21%
Allows for payment based on actual resources utilized	81%	39%	74%	46%
Makes system compatible with Medicare	80%	65%	74%	46%
Makes physician payment more equitable across specialties	71%	45%	71%	41%
Rationalizes physician payment	84%	48%	80%	38%
Increases control over physician payment	70%	48%	61%	31%
Makes it easy to implement and update each year	80%	52%	76%	50%

Table 13-8. Percentage of RBRVS Users vs Nonusers Who Agree or Strongly Agree That the Following Are Potential Drawbacks to the RBRVS System

	2006	
	RBRVS Users	RBRVS Non-Users
Problems with methodology	26%	39%
Potential to disrupt beneficiary access to physician services	21%	42%
Potential to disrupt physician relations	26%	39%
Current system is better	8%	29%
RBRVS is too complicated	11%	19%

Factors That Influence the Adoption of RBRVS

The AMA survey asked a question regarding the factors that influence an organization's adoption of the RBRVS. This was an attempt to examine the elements that contributed to adoption. In essence, it is another measure of the payers' perception of the RBRVS, this time in terms of application of the RBRVS to their individual needs.

The factors that influence adoption (see Table 13-9) can be divided into those that are internal forces to the system and those that are driven by external forces. The purpose of this division is to distinguish those that organized medicine, payers, and the government may be able to control and those that are determined by market forces. From these responses it is evident that payers are primarily concerned about the same issues that concern the AMA. Both seek to maintain the soundness and effectiveness of the RBRVS system. This is a factor that is internal to the system but can be affected by the care and maintenance provided by the medical community and CMS. Other factors internal to the system are physician participation in setting values for work and PE and that all three components of the RBRVS are resource based. Several of these factors, such as physician participation and making all three components resource based, have already been achieved. It is interesting to note that physician participation in setting the values has increased in importance, while the assurances that Medicare adjustments will not negatively affect the accuracy of the RBRVS has remained low as an influence. This could be a recognition of a greater understanding of the important role that physicians play in maintaining the RBRVS, in spite of inappropriate payment policies instituted by CMS that sometimes may affect the accuracy of the RBRVS.

Several factors listed by the respondents are outside of the RBRVS system and subject to the control of other forces, such as the market. These external influences over adoption include competitors' adoption of the RBRVS, physicians' demand of payment under the RBRVS, and the affect and effectiveness of RBRVS under Medicare. Some of these external factors, especially the effectiveness of the Medicare RBRVS, are highly ranked influences.

None of the respondents rated the factors influencing adoption very highly; all but one are less than 50% and most are lower than the 1998 and 2001 survey responses. This suggests that there are other factors affecting a payers' decision. Some of these may be specific to the health care market the payer serves, part of the organizational structure of the payer, or contingent on political decisions of state legislatures.

Table 13-9. Percentage of Respondents Who Selected the Following as an Influence Over Their Adoption of the RBRVS

	2006	2001	1998
Physicians in plan demand payment under the RBRVS	27%	35%	29%
Medicare has effectively used the RBRVS	52%	51%	48%
There is physician participation in setting relative values for work and practice expense	47%	35%	28%
Competitors have adopted a RBRVS	30%	44%	45%
Assurances have been made that Medicare adjustments to the RBRVS will not negatively affect its accuracy and/or its consistency	28%	23%	37%

Other Uses of the RBRVS

In addition to using the RBRVS for its primary purpose as a payment mechanism for specific procedures, payers have begun to use the RBRVS for other purposes. Using RVUs is a primary measure to determine physician productivity. For example, if a group of physicians wanted to examine its collective as well as its individual physician performance it would need to collect RVU data for a period of time. First, the group would compile the total work RVUs associated with individual physicians by multiplying the frequency associated with each CPT code billed during a period of time by the work RVU for each code. This would allow the physicians to examine the total work RVUs associated for each physician and the group as a whole. Physicians could use these data as one method for beginning to assess physician performance, identify variations and causes for the

Figure 13-11. Use of RVUs for Physician Productivity/Compensation 1997–2006

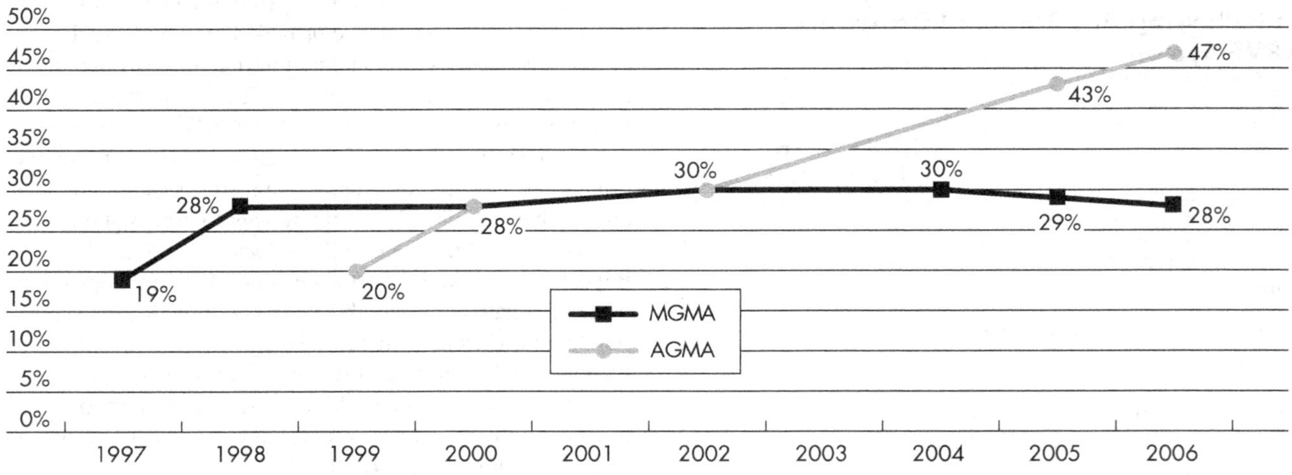

variations, and possibly make adjustments to the group's remuneration policies.

Physician compensation and productivity surveys conducted by the Medical Group Management Association (MGMA) and the American Medical Group Association (AMGA) examine the use of the RVUs to determine physician productivity and compensation.

The MGMA data (see Figure 13-11) show an increase in the use of RVUs to determine productivity and compensation between 1997 and 2000, which has since plateaued. On the other hand, the AGMA data continues to show a steady increase of linking physician productivity and compensation to RVUs.[4, 5]

Conclusion

The three AMA surveys and comparisons with other past surveys, such as the 1993 Deloitte & Touche and 1994 PPRC studies, revealed a continuing increase in non-Medicare use of the RBRVS.[4, 5] The 2006 study also showed that all non-Medicare users of the RBRVS had a high rate of adoption of Medicare payment policies, indicating a high probability of incorporating new policies. These results confirm the necessity of maintaining the RBRVS as an accurate, comprehensive standard, uniformly containing all medical services nationwide.

The RBRVS is not simply Medicare's method of physician payment. This AMA study showed that multiple payers are using the RBRVS. Although the RBRVS is maintained by and for Medicare, it has evolved into a payment mechanism that is well beyond the Medicare program.

Part of the reason for such extensive and diverse utilization is the perception that the RBRVS is a rational system, easy to implement and update, and its relativity is based on actual resources used. This is not to say that problems do not exist or that RBRVS is viewed favorably by all parties. It is clear that those that employ the RBRVS have a more favorable view of the RBRVS as compared to those that have not adopted the RBRVS. The critical task is to continue cooperative efforts at maintaining the relativity and accuracy of the RBRVS system.

References

1. Physician Payment Review Commission. Annual Report to Congress. The Commission. 1995:399–408.
2. Swem RT. How and why private payers are using the RBRVS: 1993 Deloitte & Touche survey of physician payment methods. Presented at the Non-Medicare Adoption of the RBRVS Plenary Session III, May 5, 1994.
3. Henry J. Kaiser Family Foundation. State Medicaid fact sheets (2004–2005). www.kff.org/mfs/medicaid.jsp?r1=AL&r2=US.
4. American Medical Group Association. Compensation and Productivity Survey. American RSM McGladrey, Inc. 1999, 2000, 2002, 2005, and 2006.
5. Medical Group Management Association. Physician Compensation and Production Survey. 1997, 1998, 2000, 2004, 2005, and 2006.

Part 5

Reference Lists

Part 5 presents all the elements that are necessary to calculate the Medicare payment schedule, including the 2022 relative value units (RVUs), payment policy indicators, and geographic practice cost indices (GPCIs).

List of Relative Value Units, Payment Schedule, and Payment Policy Indicators

This list presents:

- The RVUs for the three components of each physician's service covered by the Medicare program
- The unadjusted payment Medicare amount for each service (including the 80% that Medicare pays and the 20% patient coinsurance)
- The global period covered by the payment
- Applicable payment policy indicators for assistant surgeon, co-surgeon, and team surgeon; multiple and bilateral surgery

The RVUs are listed according to either their numeric five-digit codes in the American Medical Association's Current Procedural Terminology (CPT®) coding system for physicians' services or their alphanumeric five-digit Healthcare Common Procedural Coding System (HCPCS) codes. The CPT code set comprises level I of the Medicare HCPCS. Alphanumeric HCPCS codes consist of level II of HCPCS and are presented at the end of the list.

In this list, each CPT code is also identified by a brief description (eg, Revision of Knee Joint, Removal of Lung). These descriptions are included to help physicians identify the services they provide, but they do not contain sufficient information to code a service. For example, six codes (27440, 27441, 27442, 27443, 27445, and 27446) are described as "Revision of Knee Joint." Full descriptions of each of the CPT-coded services are available in the *CPT 2022* codebook, which can be purchased by calling 800-621-8335 or visit https://www.ama-assn.org/practice-management/cpt/need-coding-resources.

Codes describing a professional component—only or technical component—only service are also accompanied by modifiers 26 (Professional only) and TC (Technical component). If the physician provides both the technical and professional components of a service (which is called the "global service"), no modifier should be used.

The RVU schedule contains all coded services included in the Medicare physician payment schedule. Several categories of codes that were included in the November 2, 2021, *Federal Register* have been omitted from this list:

- Services not covered by Medicare without assigned RVUs
- Deleted codes
- Codes that are covered by Medicare but not included in the physician payment schedule, and for which payment continues under the previous rules, ie, clinical diagnostic laboratory services, ambulance services
- Bundled codes, which are services or supplies that are only payable as part of another service, ie, a telephone call from a hospital nurse regarding care of a patient is not separately payable because it is included in the payment for other services such as hospital visits

For over 100 services not covered by the Medicare program, but for which payment is frequently allowed by other payers, the Centers for Medicare & Medicaid Services (CMS) has assigned relative values. These services are included in the table and are denoted by a section symbol (§) immediately to the right of the CPT code.

Where no RVUs have been assigned, "0.00" appears in each of the RVU columns. These services are priced by the carrier. Carriers will generally establish payment amounts for these services on an individual-case basis after reviewing documentation, such as an operative report. The designation "CP" appears immediately to the right of the CPT code.

For the CPT and HCPCS-coded services included in the list of RVUs, the following information is provided:

- **Work RVUs.** RVUs for the physician work component of the service. Chapter 4 provides an explanation of the resource-based relative value scale (RBRVS) and the physician work component.
- **Practice expense RVUs.** RVUs for the practice expense component of the service are explained in Chapter 5. The practice expense RVUs are fully resource-based, and CMS assigned two different levels (nonfacility or facility) of practice-expense RVUs to each code, depending on the site of service. Facility includes hospitals (inpatient, outpatient, and emergency department), ambulatory surgical centers (ASCs), and skilled nursing facilities (SNFs). Nonfacility includes all other settings.
- **Professional Liability Insurance (PLI) RVUs.** RVUs for the PLI component of the service. The *Federal Register* refers to this component as the "malpractice" component or the "malpractice" RVUs. Chapter 6 explains the PLI component.
- **Medicare payment schedule.** This column is the full payment amount for a service under the Medicare RBRVS, excluding the adjustment for geographic location. It includes both the 80% that Medicare pays and the

20% patient coinsurance. The limiting charge for a service is 109.25% of the payment-schedule amount. There are separate payment totals according to whether the service was provided in a facility or nonfacility.

For the year 2022, Medicare payment amounts are calculated by summing the RVUs for all three components of a service and multiplying the sum by the 2022 Medicare conversion factor.

In addition, Section 5102(b) of the Deficit Reduction Act (DRA) of 2005 requires a payment cap on the technical component (TC) of certain diagnostic imaging procedures and the TC portions of the global diagnostic imaging services. This cap is based on the outpatient prospective payment system (OPPS) payment. To implement this provision, the physician payment schedule amount is compared to the OPPS payment amount, and the lower amount is paid. The following OPPS formula is used to calculate payment.

2022 OPPS nonfacility payment amount
= [work RVU × work GPCI)
+ (OPPS nonfacility PE RVU × PE GPCI)
+ (OPPS MP RVU × MP GPCI)]
× conversion factor

2022 OPPS facility payment amount
= [work RVU × work GPCI)
+ (OPPS facility PE RVU × PE GPCI)
+ (OPPS MP RVU × MP GPCI)]
× conversion factor

To calculate the full 2022 payment schedule amount for a locality, refer to Chapter 8 and to the List of Geographic Practice Cost Indices for each Medicare Locality in this section.

- **Global period.** The global period refers to the number of postoperative days of care that are included in the payment for a global surgical package, ie, a 090 in the column means that 90 days of postoperative care is included in the payment. Medicare policies on global packages are described in Chapter 11. The following alpha codes also appear in this column:

XXX = The global concept does not apply to the code.

YYY = The global period is to be set by the carrier.

ZZZ = Code is related to another service and always included in the global period of the other service. (Note: Physician work is associated with intra-service time and in some instances the pre- and post-service time.)

MMM = A service that is furnished in uncomplicated maternity cases, including antepartum care, delivery, and postpartum care. The usual global surgical concept does not apply.

- The payment policy indicators include Medicare's supervision requirements, including:

  General supervision (GS): The physician is not required to be on premises but is responsible for overall quality of the service performed.

  Direct supervision (DS): The physician is required to be on premises and be immediately available in the office suite but is not required to have direct contact with the patient.

  Personal supervision (PS): The physician must be in direct contact with the patient.

  Assistant-at-surgery services are not payable for those codes in which an **A** appears in the Payment Policies Indicator–column. An **A+** indicates this payment restriction applies unless medical necessity is established.

  A **B** indicates that the 150% payment adjustment for a bilateral procedure does apply. A procedure can be based on a bilateral procedure, if (1) the code descriptor specifically states that the procedure is bilateral; (2) the code descriptor states that the procedure may be performed either unilaterally or bilaterally; or (3) the procedure is usually performed as a bilateral procedure.

  A **C** indicates that payment for a co-surgeon is allowed, while a **C1** indicates that documentation establishing medical necessity is required before payment for the co-surgeon would be allowed.

  A **T** indicates that payment for a surgical team is allowed and paid on a by-report basis. A **T+** indicates team surgeons are payable if medical necessity is established and are paid on a by-report basis.

  An **M** indicates that Medicare's standard multiple surgery rule applies, which allows 100% of the global payment schedule for the highest valued procedure, and 50% of the global payment schedule for the second through fifth procedures. Subsequent procedures are priced by the carrier.

  An **Mt** indicates that Medicare's 20% payment reduction applies to the practice expense component of the second and subsequent physical therapy services billed by the same practitioner or facility on the same date of service for the same patient.

  An **Me** indicates that special Medicare rules apply, if the procedure is billed with another endoscopy in the same family (ie, another endoscopy that has the same base procedure). Under **Me**, Medicare pays the full value of the highest valued endoscopy, plus the difference between the next highest valued procedure and the base endoscopy. For example, in the course of performing a fiberoptic colonoscopy in the nonfacility setting (CPT code

45378), a physician performs a biopsy on a lesion (code 45380) and removes a polyp (code 45385) from a different part of the colon. The physician bills for codes 45380 and 45385. The value of codes 45380 and 45385 have the value of the diagnostic colonoscopy in the nonfacility setting (code 45378) built in. Rather than paying 100% for the highest valued procedure (code 45385) and 50% for the next (code 45380), Medicare pays the full value of the highest valued endoscopy (code 45385), plus the difference between the next highest endoscopy (code 45380) and the base endoscopy procedure (code 45378). Assuming the following are the payment schedule amounts for these codes (this example uses the 2022 conversion factor):

Code 45378	Diagnostic colonoscopy	$357.14
Code 45380	Colonoscopy with biopsy	$460.26
Code 45385	Colonoscopy with polypectomy	$478.60

Medicare would pay the full value of code 45385 ($478.60) plus the difference between codes 45380 and 45378 ($103.12) for a total of $581.72. If an endoscopic procedure with an **Me** is billed with modifier 51 with other procedures that are not endoscopies, then the standard rules for multiple surgeries apply.

An **Mtc** indicates that special Medicare rules apply if the procedure is billed with another diagnostic imaging procedure. If the procedure is reported in the same session on the same day as another procedure, Medicare ranks the procedures by payment-schedule amount for the TC and pays 100% for the highest priced procedure and 50% for each subsequent procedure. Medicare bases the payment for subsequent procedures on the lower of (a) the actual charge, or (b) the payment schedule amount reduced by the appropriate percentage. The professional component (PC) is paid at 100% for all procedures.

A **DRA** indicates the service is subjected to the Deficit Reduction Act payment limit. Codes with these initials are capped at the OPPS rate if the normal payment exceeds this rate for the technical portion of the service.

National Place of Service Codes

National place of service (POS) codes are two-digit codes placed on health care professional claims to indicate the setting in which a service was provided. CMS maintains POS codes throughout the health care industry.

This code set is required for use in the implementation guide adopted as the national standard for electronic transmission of professional health care claims under the provisions of the Health Insurance Portability and Accountability Act (HIPAA) of 1996. HIPAA directed the Secretary of Health and Human Services (HHS) to adopt national standards for electronic transactions. These standard transactions require all health plans and providers to use standard code sets to populate data elements in each transaction. The Transaction and Code Set Rule adopted the ASC X12-837 Health Care Claim: Professional, volumes 1 and 2, version 4010, as the standard for electronic submission of professional claims. This standard was later updated by CMS to version 5010, with a compliance date of January 1, 2012. This standard selected the POS code set, currently maintained by CMS, as the code set to be used for describing sites of service in such claims. POS information is often needed to determine the acceptability of direct billing of Medicare, Medicaid, and private insurance services provided by a given provider.

National Place of Service Definitions

The following is the current national place of service (POS) code set with facility and nonfacility designations noted for Medicare payment for services on the Physician Payment Schedule:

POS Code/Name Description	**Payment Rate** Facility = F Nonfacility = NF
01/Pharmacy A facility or location where drugs and other medically related items and services are sold, dispensed, or otherwise provided directly to patients.	**NF**
02/Telehealth Provided Other than in Patient's Home The location where health services and health-related services are provided or received through telecommunication technology. Patient is not located in their home when receiving health services or health-related services through telecommunication technology. (Effective January 1, 2017) (Description change effective January 1, 2022, and applicable for Medicare April 1, 2022.)	**F**
03/School A facility whose primary purpose is education.	**NF**
04/Homeless Shelter A facility or location whose primary purpose is to provide temporary housing to homeless individuals (eg, emergency shelters, individual or family shelters).	**NF**
05/Indian Health Service Free-standing Facility A facility or location, owned and operated by the Indian Health Service, which provides diagnostic, therapeutic (surgical and nonsurgical), and rehabilitation services to American Indians and Alaska Natives who do not require hospitalization.	Not applicable for adjudication of Medicare claims; systems must recognize for HIPAA
06/Indian Health Service Provider-based Facility A facility or location, owned and operated by the Indian Health Service, which provides diagnostic, therapeutic (surgical and non-surgical), and rehabilitation services rendered by, or under the supervision of, physicians to American Indians and Alaska Natives admitted as inpatients or outpatients.	Not applicable for adjudication of Medicare claims; systems must recognize for HIPAA
07/Tribal 638 Free-standing Facility A facility or location owned and operated by a federally recognized American Indian or Alaska Native tribe or tribal organization under a 638 agreement, which provides diagnostic, therapeutic (surgical and nonsurgical), and rehabilitation services to tribal members who do not require hospitalization.	Not applicable for adjudication of Medicare claims; systems must recognize for HIPAA
08/Tribal 638 Provider-based Facility A facility or location owned and operated by a federally recognized American Indian or Alaska Native tribe or tribal organization under a 638 agreement, which provides diagnostic, therapeutic (surgical and nonsurgical), and rehabilitation services to tribal members admitted as inpatients or outpatients.	Not applicable for adjudication of Medicare claims; systems must recognize for HIPAA
09/Prison—Correctional Facility A prison, jail, reformatory, work farm, detention center, or any other similar facility maintained by either federal, state, or local authorities for the purpose of confinement or rehabilitation of adult or juvenile criminal offenders.	**NF**
10/Telehealth Provided in Patient's Home The location where health services and health-related services are provided or received through telecommunication technology. Patient is located in their home (which is a location other than a hospital or other facility where the patient receives care in a private residence) when receiving health services or health-related services through telecommunication technology. (This code is effective January 1, 2022, and available to Medicare April 1, 2022.)	**F**

(continued)

National Place of Service Definitions

The following is the current national place of service (POS) code set with facility and nonfacility designations noted for Medicare payment for services on the Physician Payment Schedule:

POS Code/Name Description	**Payment Rate** Facility = F Nonfacility = NF
11/Office Location, other than a hospital, skilled nursing facility (SNF), military treatment facility, community health center, state or local public health clinic, or intermediate care facility (ICF), where the health professional routinely provides health examinations, diagnosis, and treatment of illness or injury on an ambulatory basis.	**NF**
12/Home Location, other than a hospital or other facility, where the patient receives care in a private residence.	**NF**
13/Assisted Living Facility Congregate residential facility with self-contained living units providing assessment of each resident's needs and on-site support 24 hours a day, 7 days a week, with the capacity to deliver or arrange for services, including some health care and other services.	**NF**
14/Group Home A residence, with shared living areas, where clients receive supervision and other services, such as social and/or behavioral services, custodial service, and minimal services (eg, medication administration).	**NF**
15/Mobile Unit A facility/unit that moves from place-to-place, equipped to provide preventive, screening, diagnostic, and/or treatment services.	**NF**
16/Temporary Lodging A short-term accommodation, such as a hotel, camp ground, hostel, cruise ship, or resort, where the patient receives care and that is not identified by any other POS code.	**NF**
17/Walk-in Retail Health Clinic A walk-in health clinic, other than an office, urgent care facility, pharmacy, or independent clinic and not described by any other POS code, that is located within a retail operation and provides, on an ambulatory basis, preventive and primary care services.	**NF**
18/Place of Employment Worksite A location, not described by any other POS code, owned or operated by a public or private entity where the patient is employed, and where a health professional provides ongoing or episodic occupational medical, therapeutic or rehabilitative services to the individual.	**NF**
19/Off-Campus Outpatient Hospital A portion of an off-campus hospital provider-based department that provides diagnostic, therapeutic (both surgical and nonsurgical), and rehabilitation services to sick or injured persons, who do not require hospitalization or institutionalization.	**F**
20/Urgent Care Facility Location, distinct from a hospital emergency room, an office, or a clinic, whose purpose is to diagnose and treat illness or injury for unscheduled, ambulatory patients seeking immediate medical attention.	**NF**
21/Inpatient Hospital A facility, other than psychiatric, that primarily provides diagnostic, therapeutic (both surgical and nonsurgical), and rehabilitation services by, or under, the supervision of physicians to patients admitted for a variety of medical conditions.	**F**
22/On-Campus Outpatient Hospital A portion of a hospital's main campus that provides diagnostic, therapeutic (both surgical and nonsurgical), and rehabilitation services to sick or injured persons who do not require hospitalization or institutionalization.	**F**

National Place of Service Definitions

The following is the current national place of service (POS) code set with facility and nonfacility designations noted for Medicare payment for services on the Physician Payment Schedule:

POS Code/Name Description	**Payment Rate** Facility = F Nonfacility = NF
23/Emergency Room Hospital A portion of a hospital where emergency diagnosis and treatment of illness or injury is provided.	**F**
24/Ambulatory Surgical Center A free-standing facility, other than a physician's office, where surgical and diagnostic services are provided on an ambulatory basis.	**F (Note: Pay at nonfacility rate for payable procedures not on the ASC list)**
25/Birthing Center A facility, other than a hospital's maternity facilities or a physician's office, which provides a setting for labor, delivery, and immediate postpartum care as well as immediate care of newborn infants.	**NF**
26/Military Treatment Facility A medical facility operated by one or more of the Uniformed Services. Military Treatment Facility (MTF) also refers to certain former US Public Health Service (USPHS) facilities now designated as Uniformed Service Treatment Facilities (USTF).	**F**
27–30/Unassigned	—
31/Skilled Nursing Facility A facility that primarily provides inpatient skilled nursing care and related services to patients who require medical, nursing, or rehabilitative services but does not provide the level of care or treatment available in a hospital.	**F**
32/Nursing Facility A facility that primarily provides to residents skilled nursing care and related services for the rehabilitation of injured, disabled, or sick persons, or, on a regular basis, health-related care services above the level of custodial care to other than individuals with intellectual disabilities.	**NF**
33/Custodial Care Facility A facility that provides room, board, and other personal assistance services, generally on a long-term basis, and that does not include a medical component.	**NF**
34/Hospice A facility, other than a patient's home, in which palliative and supportive care for terminally ill patients and their families are provided.	**F**
35–40/Unassigned	—
41/Ambulance—Land A land vehicle specifically designed, equipped, and staffed for lifesaving and transporting the sick or injured.	**F**
42/Ambulance—Air or Water An air or water vehicle specifically designed, equipped, and staffed for lifesaving and transporting the sick or injured.	**F**
43–48/Unassigned	—
49/Independent Clinic A location, not part of a hospital and not described by any other POS code, that is organized and operated to provide preventive, diagnostic, therapeutic, rehabilitative, or palliative services to outpatients only.	**NF**
50/Federally Qualified Health Center A facility located in a medically underserved area that provides Medicare beneficiaries preventive primary medical care under the general direction of a physician.	**NF**

(continued)

National Place of Service Definitions

The following is the current national place of service (POS) code set with facility and nonfacility designations noted for Medicare payment for services on the Physician Payment Schedule:

POS Code/Name Description	**Payment Rate** Facility = F Nonfacility = NF
51/Inpatient Psychiatric Facility A facility that provides inpatient psychiatric services for the diagnosis and treatment of mental illness on a 24-hour basis, by or under the supervision of a physician.	**F**
52/Psychiatric Facility—Partial Hospitalization A facility for the diagnosis and treatment of mental illness that provides a planned therapeutic program for patients who do not require full time hospitalization, but who need broader programs than are possible from outpatient visits to a hospital-based or hospital-affiliated facility.	**F**
53/Community Mental Health Center A facility that provides the following services: outpatient services, including specialized outpatient services for children, the elderly, individuals who are chronically ill, and residents of the CMHC's mental health services area who have been discharged from inpatient treatment at a mental health facility; 24 hour a day emergency care services; day treatment, other partial hospitalization services, or psychosocial rehabilitation services; screening for patients being considered for admission to state mental health facilities to determine the appropriateness of such admission; and consultation and education services.	**F**
54/Intermediate Care Facility/Individuals with Intellectual Disabilities A facility that primarily provides health-related care and services above the level of custodial care to individuals with intellectual disabilities but does not provide the level of care or treatment available in a hospital or SNF.	**NF**
55/Residential Substance Abuse Treatment Facility A facility that provides treatment for substance (alcohol and drug) abuse to live-in residents who do not require acute medical care. Services include individual and group therapy and counseling, family counseling, laboratory tests, drugs and supplies, psychological testing, and room and board.	**NF**
56/Psychiatric Residential Treatment Center A facility or distinct part of a facility for psychiatric care that provides a total 24-hour therapeutically planned and professionally staffed group living and learning environment.	**F**
57/Non-residential Substance Abuse Treatment Facility A location which provides treatment for substance (alcohol and drug) abuse on an ambulatory basis. Services include individual and group therapy and counseling, family counseling, laboratory tests, drugs and supplies, and psychological testing.	**NF**
58/Non-residential Opioid Treatment Facility A location that provides treatment for opioid use disorder on an ambulatory basis. Services include methadone and other forms of medication assisted treatment (MAT). (Effective January 1, 2020)	**NF**
59/Unassigned	—
60/Mass Immunization Center A location where providers administer pneumococcal pneumonia and influenza virus vaccinations and submit these services as electronic media claims, paper claims, or using the roster billing method. This generally takes place in a mass immunization setting, such as a public health center, pharmacy, or mall but may include a physician office setting.	**NF**
61/Comprehensive Inpatient Rehabilitation Facility A facility that provides comprehensive rehabilitation services under the supervision of a physician to inpatients with physical disabilities. Services include physical therapy, occupational therapy, speech pathology, social or psychological services, and orthotics and prosthetics services.	**F**

National Place of Service Definitions

The following is the current national place of service (POS) code set with facility and nonfacility designations noted for Medicare payment for services on the Physician Payment Schedule:

POS Code/Name Description	**Payment Rate** Facility = F Nonfacility = NF
62/Comprehensive Outpatient Rehabilitation Facility A facility that provides comprehensive rehabilitation services under the supervision of a physician to outpatients with physical disabilities. Services include physical therapy, occupational therapy, and speech pathology services.	**NF**
63–64/Unassigned	—
65/End-Stage Renal Disease Treatment Facility A facility other than a hospital, which provides dialysis treatment, maintenance, and/or training to patients or caregivers on an ambulatory or home-care basis.	**NF**
66–70/Unassigned	—
71/Public Health Clinic A facility maintained by either state or local health departments that provides ambulatory primary medical care under the general direction of a physician.	**NF**
72/Rural Health Clinic A certified facility, which is located in a rural medically underserved area, that provides ambulatory primary medical care under the general direction of a physician.	**NF**
73–80/Unassigned	—
81/Independent Laboratory A laboratory certified to perform diagnostic and/or clinical tests independent of an institution or a physician's office.	**NF**
82–98/Unassigned	—
99/Other Place of Service Other place of service not identified above.	**NF**

Relative Value Units

CPT Code and Modifier		Description	Work RVU	Nonfacility Practice Expense RVU	Facility Practice Expense RVU	PLI RVU	Total Non-facility RVUs	Medicare Payment Nonfacility	Total Facility RVUs	Medicare Payment Facility	Global Period	Payment Policy Indicators
10004		Fna bx w/o img gdn ea addl	0.80	0.60	0.35	0.11	1.51	$52.26	1.26	$43.60	ZZZ	A+
10005		Fna bx w/us gdn 1st les	1.46	2.48	0.54	0.17	4.11	$142.23	2.17	$75.10	XXX	A+ M
10006		Fna bx w/us gdn ea addl	1.00	0.68	0.38	0.10	1.78	$61.60	1.48	$51.22	ZZZ	A+
10007		Fna bx w/fluor gdn 1st les	1.81	7.01	0.66	0.20	9.02	$312.15	2.67	$92.40	XXX	A+ M
10008		Fna bx w/fluor gdn ea addl	1.18	3.63	0.39	0.11	4.92	$170.26	1.68	$58.14	ZZZ	A+
10009		Fna bx w/ct gdn 1st les	2.26	11.09	0.77	0.22	13.57	$469.61	3.25	$112.47	XXX	A+ M
10010		Fna bx w/ct gdn ea addl	1.65	6.17	0.54	0.14	7.96	$275.47	2.33	$80.63	ZZZ	A+
10011	CP	Fna bx w/mr gdn 1st les	0.00	0.00	0.00	0.00	0.00	$0.00	0.00	$0.00	XXX	A+ M
10012	CP	Fna bx w/mr gdn ea addl	0.00	0.00	0.00	0.00	0.00	$0.00	0.00	$0.00	ZZZ	A+
10021		Fna bx w/o img gdn 1st les	1.03	1.87	0.45	0.12	3.02	$104.51	1.60	$55.37	XXX	A+ M
10030		Guide cathet fluid drainage	2.75	16.91	0.94	0.25	19.91	$689.01	3.94	$136.35	000	A+ M
10035		Perq dev soft tiss 1st imag	1.70	9.51	0.61	0.17	11.38	$393.82	2.48	$85.82	000	A+ B M
10036		Perq dev soft tiss add imag	0.85	8.55	0.30	0.10	9.50	$328.76	1.25	$43.26	ZZZ	A+
10040		Acne surgery	0.91	2.45	0.52	0.09	3.45	$119.39	1.52	$52.60	010	A M
10060		Drainage of skin abscess	1.22	2.35	1.74	0.12	3.69	$127.70	3.08	$106.59	010	A M
10061		Drainage of skin abscess	2.45	3.55	2.63	0.32	6.32	$218.71	5.40	$186.87	010	A M
10080		Drainage of pilonidal cyst	1.22	6.29	1.67	0.20	7.71	$266.81	3.09	$106.93	010	A M
10081		Drainage of pilonidal cyst	2.50	7.56	2.14	0.41	10.47	$362.33	5.05	$174.76	010	A M
10120		Remove foreign body	1.22	3.12	1.70	0.12	4.46	$154.34	3.04	$105.20	010	A M
10121		Remove foreign body	2.74	4.76	2.28	0.39	7.89	$273.04	5.41	$187.22	010	A M
10140		Drainage of hematoma/fluid	1.58	3.28	1.68	0.21	5.07	$175.45	3.47	$120.08	010	A M
10160		Puncture drainage of lesion	1.25	2.45	1.40	0.14	3.84	$132.89	2.79	$96.55	010	A M
10180		Complex drainage wound	2.30	5.08	2.46	0.50	7.88	$272.70	5.26	$182.03	010	A M
11000		Debride infected skin	0.60	1.08	0.16	0.05	1.73	$59.87	0.81	$28.03	000	A M
11001		Debride infected skin add-on	0.30	0.45	0.08	0.04	0.79	$27.34	0.42	$14.53	ZZZ	A
11004		Debride genitalia & perineum	10.80	NA	3.95	2.04	NA	NA	16.79	$581.04	000	A M
11005		Debride abdom wall	14.24	NA	5.37	3.33	NA	NA	22.94	$793.87	000	A+
11006		Debride genit/per/abdom wall	13.10	NA	4.87	2.73	NA	NA	20.70	$716.35	000	A M
11008		Remove mesh from abd wall	5.00	NA	1.89	1.20	NA	NA	8.09	$279.96	ZZZ	A+
11010		Debride skin at fx site	4.19	8.63	3.18	0.76	13.58	$469.95	8.13	$281.35	010	A M
11011		Debride skin musc at fx site	4.94	9.04	2.84	0.95	14.93	$516.67	8.73	$302.11	000	A M
11012		Deb skin bone at fx site	6.87	11.18	4.04	1.33	19.38	$670.67	12.24	$423.58	000	A M
11042		Deb subq tissue 20 sq cm/<	1.01	2.74	0.63	0.12	3.87	$133.93	1.76	$60.91	000	A M

11043	Deb musc/fascia 20 sq cm/<	2.70	3.81	1.40	0.41	6.92	$239.47	4.51	$156.07	000	A M
11044	Deb bone 20 sq cm/<	4.10	4.44	1.85	0.65	9.19	$318.03	6.60	$228.40	000	A M
11045	Deb subq tissue add-on	0.50	0.62	0.18	0.09	1.21	$41.87	0.77	$26.65	ZZZ	A+
11046	Deb musc/fascia add-on	1.03	0.95	0.40	0.20	2.18	$75.44	1.63	$56.41	ZZZ	A+
11047	Deb bone add-on	1.80	1.43	0.71	0.34	3.57	$123.54	2.85	$98.63	ZZZ	A+
11055	Trim skin lesion	0.35	1.77	0.08	0.04	2.16	$74.75	0.47	$16.26	000	A M
11056	Trim skin lesions 2 to 4	0.50	1.93	0.11	0.04	2.47	$85.48	0.65	$22.49	000	A M
11057	Trim skin lesions over 4	0.65	2.01	0.14	0.05	2.71	$93.78	0.84	$29.07	000	A M
11102	Tangntl bx skin single les	0.66	2.32	0.37	0.07	3.05	$105.55	1.10	$38.07	000	A M
11103	Tangntl bx skin ea sep/addl	0.38	1.10	0.22	0.04	1.52	$52.60	0.64	$22.15	ZZZ	A
11104	Punch bx skin single lesion	0.83	2.87	0.45	0.09	3.79	$131.16	1.37	$47.41	000	A M
11105	Punch bx skin ea sep/addl	0.45	1.27	0.25	0.05	1.77	$61.25	0.75	$25.95	ZZZ	A
11106	Incal bx skn single les	1.01	3.57	0.54	0.11	4.69	$162.30	1.66	$57.45	000	A M
11107	Incal bx skn ea sep/addl	0.54	1.53	0.30	0.07	2.14	$74.06	0.91	$31.49	ZZZ	A
11200	Removal of skin tags <w/15	0.82	1.76	1.31	0.09	2.67	$92.40	2.22	$76.83	010	A M
11201	Remove skin tags add-on	0.29	0.21	0.15	0.04	0.54	$18.69	0.48	$16.61	ZZZ	A
11300	Shave skin lesion 0.5 cm/<	0.60	2.39	0.33	0.07	3.06	$105.89	1.00	$34.61	000	A+ M
11301	Shave skin lesion 0.6-1.0 cm	0.90	2.67	0.50	0.09	3.66	$126.66	1.49	$51.56	000	A+ M
11302	Shave skin lesion 1.1-2.0 cm	1.05	2.98	0.59	0.11	4.14	$143.27	1.75	$60.56	000	A+ M
11303	Shave skin lesion >2.0 cm	1.25	3.19	0.69	0.12	4.56	$157.80	2.06	$71.29	000	A+ M
11305	Shave skin lesion 0.5 cm/<	0.80	2.33	0.24	0.08	3.21	$111.09	1.12	$38.76	000	A+ M
11306	Shave skin lesion 0.6-1.0 cm	0.96	2.63	0.39	0.09	3.68	$127.35	1.44	$49.83	000	A+ M
11307	Shave skin lesion 1.1-2.0 cm	1.20	2.90	0.53	0.11	4.21	$145.69	1.84	$63.68	000	A+ M
11308	Shave skin lesion >2.0 cm	1.46	2.88	0.49	0.12	4.46	$154.34	2.07	$71.63	000	A+ M
11310	Shave skin lesion 0.5 cm/<	0.80	2.60	0.44	0.09	3.49	$120.78	1.33	$46.03	000	A+ M
11311	Shave skin lesion 0.6-1.0 cm	1.10	2.90	0.61	0.11	4.11	$142.23	1.82	$62.98	000	A+ M
11312	Shave skin lesion 1.1-2.0 cm	1.30	3.23	0.73	0.12	4.65	$160.92	2.15	$74.40	000	A+ M
11313	Shave skin lesion >2.0 cm	1.68	3.56	0.94	0.19	5.43	$187.91	2.81	$97.24	000	A+ M

*Please note that these calculations are based on the Medicare 2022 Conversion Factor of $34.6062 and the DRA RVU cap rates at time of publication.

A = assistant-at-surgery restriction
A+ = assistant-at-surgery restriction unless medical necessity established with documentation
B = bilateral surgery adjustment applies
C = cosurgeons payable
C+ = cosurgeons payable if medical necessity established with documentation
CP = carriers may establish RVUs and payment amounts for these services, generally on an individual basis following review of documentation such as an operative report
M = multiple surgery adjustment applies
Me = multiple endoscopy rules may apply
M+ = multiple therapy rules apply
Mtc = multiple diagnostic imaging rules apply
T = team surgeons permitted
T+ = team surgeons payable if medical necessity established with documentation
§ = indicates code is not covered by Medicare
GS = procedure must be performed under the general supervision of a physician
DS = procedure must be performed under the direct supervision of a physician
PS = procedure must be performed under the personal supervision of a physician
DRA = procedure subject to DRA limitation

Relative Value Units

CPT Code and Modifier	Description	Work RVU	Nonfacility Practice Expense RVU	Facility Practice Expense RVU	PLI RVU	Total Non-facility RVUs	Medicare Payment Nonfacility	Total Facility RVUs	Medicare Payment Facility	Global Period	Payment Policy Indicators
11400	Exc tr-ext b9+marg 0.5 cm<	0.90	2.81	1.44	0.11	3.82	$132.20	2.45	$84.79	010	A M
11401	Exc tr-ext b9+marg 0.6-1 cm	1.28	3.22	1.65	0.17	4.67	$161.61	3.10	$107.28	010	A M
11402	Exc tr-ext b9+marg 1.1-2 cm	1.45	3.49	1.75	0.20	5.14	$177.88	3.40	$117.66	010	A M
11403	Exc tr-ext b9+marg 2.1-3cm	1.84	3.80	2.26	0.25	5.89	$203.83	4.35	$150.54	010	A M
11404	Exc tr-ext b9+marg 3.1-4 cm	2.11	4.25	2.37	0.34	6.70	$231.86	4.82	$166.80	010	A M
11406	Exc tr-ext b9+marg >4.0 cm	3.52	5.34	3.14	0.65	9.51	$329.10	7.31	$252.97	010	A M
11420	Exc h-f-nk-sp b9+marg 0.5/<	1.03	2.68	1.28	0.10	3.81	$131.85	2.41	$83.40	010	A M
11421	Exc h-f-nk-sp b9+marg 0.6-1	1.47	3.13	1.56	0.17	4.77	$165.07	3.20	$110.74	010	A M
11422	Exc h-f-nk-sp b9+marg 1.1-2	1.68	3.46	2.08	0.21	5.35	$185.14	3.97	$137.39	010	A M
11423	Exc h-f-nk-sp b9+marg 2.1-3	2.06	3.77	2.23	0.27	6.10	$211.10	4.56	$157.80	010	A M
11424	Exc h-f-nk-sp b9+marg 3.1-4	2.48	4.16	2.38	0.35	6.99	$241.90	5.21	$180.30	010	A M
11426	Exc h-f-nk-sp b9+marg >4 cm	4.09	5.18	3.26	0.65	9.92	$343.29	8.00	$276.85	010	A M
11440	Exc face-mm b9+marg 0.5 cm/<	1.05	3.12	1.93	0.11	4.28	$148.11	3.09	$106.93	010	A M
11441	Exc face-mm b9+marg 0.6-1 cm	1.53	3.47	2.16	0.20	5.20	$179.95	3.89	$134.62	010	A M
11442	Exc face-mm b9+marg 1.1-2 cm	1.77	3.75	2.28	0.24	5.76	$199.33	4.29	$148.46	010	A M
11443	Exc face-mm b9+marg 2.1-3 cm	2.34	4.13	2.58	0.32	6.79	$234.98	5.24	$181.34	010	A M
11444	Exc face-mm b9+marg 3.1-4 cm	3.19	4.82	3.01	0.43	8.44	$292.08	6.63	$229.44	010	A M
11446	Exc face-mm b9+marg >4 cm	4.80	6.02	3.93	0.66	11.48	$397.28	9.39	$324.95	010	A M
11450	Removal sweat gland lesion	3.22	9.15	3.81	0.75	13.12	$454.03	7.78	$269.24	090	A B M
11451	Removal sweat gland lesion	4.43	10.53	4.42	0.94	15.90	$550.24	9.79	$338.79	090	A+ B M
11462	Removal sweat gland lesion	3.00	9.07	3.73	0.66	12.73	$440.54	7.39	$255.74	090	A+ B M
11463	Removal sweat gland lesion	4.43	10.79	4.51	0.95	16.17	$559.58	9.89	$342.26	090	A+ B M
11470	Removal sweat gland lesion	3.74	9.25	3.98	0.75	13.74	$475.49	8.47	$293.11	090	A M
11471	Removal sweat gland lesion	4.89	10.55	4.54	1.00	16.44	$568.93	10.43	$360.94	090	A+ M
11600	Exc tr-ext mal+marg 0.5 cm/<	1.63	4.07	1.74	0.21	5.91	$204.52	3.58	$123.89	010	A M
11601	Exc tr-ext mal+marg 0.6-1 cm	2.07	4.49	2.02	0.25	6.81	$235.67	4.34	$150.19	010	A M
11602	Exc tr-ext mal+marg 1.1-2 cm	2.27	4.74	2.19	0.25	7.26	$251.24	4.71	$163.00	010	A M
11603	Exc tr-ext mal+marg 2.1-3 cm	2.82	5.11	2.48	0.33	8.26	$285.85	5.63	$194.83	010	A M
11604	Exc tr-ext mal+marg 3.1-4 cm	3.17	5.64	2.64	0.40	9.21	$318.72	6.21	$214.90	010	A M
11606	Exc tr-ext mal+marg >4 cm	5.02	7.42	3.46	0.84	13.28	$459.57	9.32	$322.53	010	A M
11620	Exc h-f-nk-sp mal+marg 0.5/<	1.64	4.08	1.75	0.21	5.93	$205.21	3.60	$124.58	010	A M
11621	Exc s/n/h/f/g mal+mrg 0.6-1	2.08	4.50	2.03	0.25	6.83	$236.36	4.36	$150.88	010	A M
11622	Exc s/n/h/f/g mal+mrg 1.1-2	2.41	4.82	2.25	0.27	7.50	$259.55	4.93	$170.61	010	A M

11623	Exc s/n/h/f/g mal+mrg 2.1-3	3.11	5.29	2.61	0.39	8.79	$304.19	6.11	$211.44	010	A M
11624	Exc s/n/h/f/g mal+mrg 3.1-4	3.62	5.89	2.84	0.50	10.01	$346.41	6.96	$240.86	010	A M
11626	Exc s/n/h/f/g mal+mrg >4 cm	4.61	6.73	3.22	0.76	12.10	$418.74	8.59	$297.27	010	A M
11640	Exc f/e/e/n/l mal+mrg 0.5cm<	1.67	4.19	1.82	0.21	6.07	$210.06	3.70	$128.04	010	A M
11641	Exc f/e/e/n/l mal+mrg 0.6-1	2.17	4.62	2.11	0.25	7.04	$243.63	4.53	$156.77	010	A M
11642	Exc f/e/e/n/l mal+mrg 1.1-2	2.62	5.02	2.37	0.32	7.96	$275.47	5.31	$183.76	010	A M
11643	Exc f/e/e/n/l mal+mrg 2.1-3	3.42	5.50	2.79	0.43	9.35	$323.57	6.64	$229.79	010	A M
11644	Exc f/e/e/n/l mal+mrg 3.1-4	4.34	6.59	3.32	0.60	11.53	$399.01	8.26	$285.85	010	A M
11646	Exc f/e/e/n/l mal+mrg >4 cm	6.26	7.79	4.25	0.95	15.00	$519.09	11.46	$396.59	010	A M
11719	Trim nail(s) any number	0.17	0.23	0.04	0.01	0.41	$14.19	0.22	$7.61	000	A M
11720	Debride nail 1-5	0.32	0.60	0.07	0.04	0.96	$33.22	0.43	$14.88	000	A
11721	Debride nail 6 or more	0.54	0.72	0.12	0.04	1.30	$44.99	0.70	$24.22	000	A
11730	Removal of nail plate	1.05	2.29	0.43	0.09	3.43	$118.70	1.57	$54.33	000	A M
11732	Remove nail plate add-on	0.38	0.58	0.09	0.04	1.00	$34.61	0.51	$17.65	ZZZ	A
11740	Drain blood from under nail	0.37	1.29	0.51	0.04	1.70	$58.83	0.92	$31.84	000	A M
11750	Removal of nail bed	1.58	3.06	1.27	0.12	4.76	$164.73	2.97	$102.78	010	A M
11755	Biopsy nail unit	1.25	2.32	0.42	0.10	3.67	$127.00	1.77	$61.25	000	A+ M
11760	Repair of nail bed	1.63	3.80	1.44	0.20	5.63	$194.83	3.27	$113.16	010	A M
11762	Reconstruction of nail bed	2.94	5.38	2.27	0.34	8.66	$299.69	5.55	$192.06	010	A M
11765	Excision of nail fold toe	1.22	3.63	1.37	0.10	4.95	$171.30	2.69	$93.09	010	A M
11770	Remove pilonidal cyst simple	2.66	7.66	2.27	0.60	10.92	$377.90	5.53	$191.37	010	A M
11771	Remove pilonidal cyst exten	6.09	11.53	5.91	1.40	19.02	$658.21	13.40	$463.72	090	A M
11772	Remove pilonidal cyst compl	7.35	14.40	8.34	1.65	23.40	$809.79	17.34	$600.07	090	A M
11900	Inject skin lesions </w 7	0.52	1.11	0.29	0.05	1.68	$58.14	0.86	$29.76	000	A M
11901	Inject skin lesions >7	0.80	1.20	0.45	0.09	2.09	$72.33	1.34	$46.37	000	A M
11920	Correct skin color 6.0 cm/<	1.61	3.92	1.34	0.27	5.80	$200.72	3.22	$111.43	000	A+ M
11921	Correct skn color 6.1-20.0cm	1.93	4.33	1.54	0.34	6.60	$228.40	3.81	$131.85	000	A+ M
11922	Correct skin color ea 20.0cm	0.49	1.20	0.28	0.09	1.78	$61.60	0.86	$29.76	ZZZ	A+

*Please note that these calculations are based on the Medicare 2022 Conversion Factor of $34.6062 and the DRA RVU cap rates at time of publication.

A = assistant-at-surgery restriction
A+ = assistant-at-surgery restriction unless medical necessity established with documentation
B = bilateral surgery adjustment applies
C = cosurgeons payable
C+ = cosurgeons payable if medical necessity established with documentation
CP = carriers may establish RVUs and payment amounts for these services, generally on an individual basis following review of documentation such as an operative report
M = multiple surgery adjustment applies
Me = multiple endoscopy rules may apply
M+ = multiple therapy rules apply
Mtc = multiple diagnostic imaging rules apply
T = team surgeons permitted
T+ = team surgeons payable if medical necessity established with documentation
§ = indicates code is not covered by Medicare
GS = procedure must be performed under the general supervision of a physician
DS = procedure must be performed under the direct supervision of a physician
PS = procedure must be performed under the personal supervision of a physician
DRA = procedure subject to DRA limitation

Relative Value Units

CPT Code and Modifier	Description	Work RVU	Nonfacility Practice Expense RVU	Facility Practice Expense RVU	PLI RVU	Total Non-facility RVUs	Medicare Payment Nonfacility	Total Facility RVUs	Medicare Payment Facility	Global Period	Payment Policy Indicators
11950	Tx contour defects 1 cc/<	0.84	1.39	0.54	0.14	2.37	$82.02	1.52	$52.60	000	A+ M
11951	Tx contour defects 1.1-5.0cc	1.19	1.77	0.74	0.22	3.18	$110.05	2.15	$74.40	000	A+ M
11952	Tx contour defects 5.1-10cc	1.69	2.25	1.03	0.31	4.25	$147.08	3.03	$104.86	000	A+ M
11954	Tx contour defects >10.0 cc	1.85	2.49	1.12	0.34	4.68	$161.96	3.31	$114.55	000	A+ M
11960	Insert tissue expander(s)	11.49	NA	16.49	2.04	NA	NA	30.02	$1038.88	090	A M
11970	Rplcmt tiss xpndr perm implt	7.49	NA	7.74	1.38	NA	NA	16.61	$574.81	090	A B M
11971	Rmvl tis xpndr wo insj implt	7.02	NA	7.94	1.28	NA	NA	16.24	$562.00	090	A+ B M
11976	Remove contraceptive capsule	1.78	2.23	0.68	0.28	4.29	$148.46	2.74	$94.82	000	A+ M
11980	Implant hormone pellet(s)	1.10	1.52	0.38	0.12	2.74	$94.82	1.60	$55.37	000	A M
11981	Insertion drug dlvr implant	1.14	1.65	0.51	0.22	3.01	$104.16	1.87	$64.71	000	A+ M
11982	Remove drug implant device	1.34	1.78	0.60	0.25	3.37	$116.62	2.19	$75.79	000	A+ M
11983	Remove/insert drug implant	1.91	1.99	0.81	0.33	4.23	$146.38	3.05	$105.55	000	A+ M
12001	Rpr s/n/ax/gen/trnk 2.5cm/<	0.84	1.79	0.32	0.17	2.80	$96.90	1.33	$46.03	000	A M
12002	Rpr s/n/ax/gen/trnk2.6-7.5cm	1.14	2.01	0.38	0.22	3.37	$116.62	1.74	$60.21	000	A M
12004	Rpr s/n/ax/gen/trk7.6-12.5cm	1.44	2.20	0.44	0.27	3.91	$135.31	2.15	$74.40	000	A M
12005	Rpr s/n/a/gen/trk12.6-20.0cm	1.97	2.92	0.45	0.39	5.28	$182.72	2.81	$97.24	000	A M
12006	Rpr s/n/a/gen/trk20.1-30.0cm	2.39	3.31	0.59	0.47	6.17	$213.52	3.45	$119.39	000	A M
12007	Rpr s/n/ax/gen/trnk >30.0 cm	2.90	3.48	0.84	0.56	6.94	$240.17	4.30	$148.81	000	A C+ M
12011	Rpr f/e/e/n/l/m 2.5 cm/<	1.07	2.07	0.35	0.21	3.35	$115.93	1.63	$56.41	000	A M
12013	Rpr f/e/e/n/l/m 2.6-5.0 cm	1.22	2.03	0.26	0.24	3.49	$120.78	1.72	$59.52	000	A M
12014	Rpr f/e/e/n/l/m 5.1-7.5 cm	1.57	2.40	0.33	0.31	4.28	$148.11	2.21	$76.48	000	A M
12015	Rpr f/e/e/n/l/m 7.6-12.5 cm	1.98	2.76	0.42	0.39	5.13	$177.53	2.79	$96.55	000	A M
12016	Rpr fe/e/en/l/m 12.6-20.0 cm	2.68	3.36	0.61	0.52	6.56	$227.02	3.81	$131.85	000	A M
12017	Rpr fe/e/en/l/m 20.1-30.0 cm	3.18	NA	0.67	0.66	NA	NA	4.51	$156.07	000	A+ M
12018	Rpr f/e/e/n/l/m >30.0 cm	3.61	NA	0.74	0.77	NA	NA	5.12	$177.18	000	M
12020	Closure of split wound	2.67	5.90	2.44	0.41	8.98	$310.76	5.52	$191.03	010	A M
12021	Closure of split wound	1.89	3.08	1.95	0.31	5.28	$182.72	4.15	$143.62	010	A M
12031	Intmd rpr s/a/t/ext 2.5 cm/<	2.00	5.65	2.17	0.25	7.90	$273.39	4.42	$152.96	010	A M
12032	Intmd rpr s/a/t/ext 2.6-7.5	2.52	6.24	2.73	0.27	9.03	$312.49	5.52	$191.03	010	A M
12034	Intmd rpr s/tr/ext 7.6-12.5	2.97	6.63	2.63	0.40	10.00	$346.06	6.00	$207.64	010	A M
12035	Intmd rpr s/a/t/ext 12.6-20	3.50	7.51	2.95	0.64	11.65	$403.16	7.09	$245.36	010	A M
12036	Intmd rpr s/a/t/ext 20.1-30	4.23	7.87	3.24	0.89	12.99	$449.53	8.36	$289.31	010	A M
12037	Intmd rpr s/tr/ext >30.0 cm	5.00	8.46	3.64	1.04	14.50	$501.79	9.68	$334.99	010	A+ C+ M

12041	Intmd rpr n-hf/genit 2.5cm/<	2.10	5.58	1.86	0.25	7.93	$274.43	4.21	$145.69	010	A M
12042	Intmd rpr n-hf/genit2.6-7.5	2.79	6.16	2.60	0.32	9.27	$320.80	5.71	$197.60	010	A M
12044	Intmd rpr n-hf/genit7.6-12.5	3.19	7.77	2.62	0.43	11.39	$394.16	6.24	$215.94	010	A M
12045	Intmd rpr n-hf/genit12.6-20	3.75	7.80	3.58	0.65	12.20	$422.20	7.98	$276.16	010	A M
12046	Intmd rpr n-hf/genit20.1-30	4.30	9.72	4.07	1.09	15.11	$522.90	9.46	$327.37	010	A+ M
12047	Intmd rpr n-hf/genit >30.0cm	4.95	10.32	4.31	1.25	16.52	$571.69	10.51	$363.71	010	C+ M
12051	Intmd rpr face/mm 2.5 cm/<	2.33	5.88	2.32	0.29	8.50	$294.15	4.94	$170.95	010	A M
12052	Intmd rpr face/mm 2.6-5.0 cm	2.87	6.22	2.60	0.34	9.43	$326.34	5.81	$201.06	010	A M
12053	Intmd rpr face/mm 5.1-7.5 cm	3.17	7.33	2.69	0.40	10.90	$377.21	6.26	$216.63	010	A M
12054	Intmd rpr face/mm 7.6-12.5cm	3.50	7.50	2.35	0.56	11.56	$400.05	6.41	$221.83	010	A M
12055	Intmd rpr face/mm 12.6-20 cm	4.50	9.82	3.48	0.79	15.11	$522.90	8.77	$303.50	010	A M
12056	Intmd rpr face/mm 20.1-30.0	5.30	11.11	5.06	0.96	17.37	$601.11	11.32	$391.74	010	A+ M
12057	Intmd rpr face/mm >30.0 cm	6.00	11.25	5.25	1.09	18.34	$634.68	12.34	$427.04	010	C+ M
13100	Cmplx rpr trunk 1.1-2.5 cm	3.00	6.85	2.50	0.35	10.20	$352.98	5.85	$202.45	010	A M
13101	Cmplx rpr trunk 2.6-7.5 cm	3.50	8.00	3.35	0.40	11.90	$411.81	7.25	$250.89	010	A M
13102	Cmplx rpr trunk addl 5cm/<	1.24	2.05	0.68	0.20	3.49	$120.78	2.12	$73.37	ZZZ	A
13120	Cmplx rpr s/a/l 1.1-2.5 cm	3.23	7.02	3.20	0.39	10.64	$368.21	6.82	$236.01	010	A M
13121	Cmplx rpr s/a/l 2.6-7.5 cm	4.00	8.29	3.08	0.42	12.71	$439.84	7.50	$259.55	010	A M
13122	Cmplx rpr s/a/l addl 5 cm/>	1.44	2.14	0.77	0.20	3.78	$130.81	2.41	$83.40	ZZZ	A
13131	Cmplx rpr f/c/c/m/n/ax/g/h/f	3.73	7.44	2.91	0.42	11.59	$401.09	7.06	$244.32	010	A M
13132	Cmplx rpr f/c/c/m/n/ax/g/h/f	4.78	8.77	3.53	0.52	14.07	$486.91	8.83	$305.57	010	A M
13133	Cmplx rpr f/c/c/m/n/ax/g/h/f	2.19	2.54	1.21	0.25	4.98	$172.34	3.65	$126.31	ZZZ	A
13151	Cmplx rpr e/n/e/l 1.1-2.5 cm	4.34	7.77	3.27	0.52	12.63	$437.08	8.13	$281.35	010	A M
13152	Cmplx rpr e/n/e/l 2.6-7.5 cm	5.34	8.87	3.84	0.61	14.82	$512.86	9.79	$338.79	010	A M
13153	Cmplx rpr e/n/e/l addl 5cm/<	2.38	2.77	1.28	0.34	5.49	$189.99	4.00	$138.42	ZZZ	A
13160	Late closure of wound	12.04	NA	9.43	2.09	NA	NA	23.56	$815.32	090	A M
14000	Tis trnfr trunk 10 sq cm/<	6.37	11.36	7.30	1.09	18.82	$651.29	14.76	$510.79	090	A M
14001	Tis trnfr trunk 10.1-30sqcm	8.78	13.62	8.83	1.57	23.97	$829.51	19.18	$663.75	090	A M

*Please note that these calculations are based on the Medicare 2022 Conversion Factor of $34.6062 and the DRA RVU cap rates at time of publication.

A = assistant-at-surgery restriction

A+ = assistant-at-surgery restriction unless medical necessity established with documentation

B = bilateral surgery adjustment applies

C = cosurgeons payable

C+ = cosurgeons payable if medical necessity established with documentation

CP = carriers may establish RVUs and payment amounts for these services, generally on an individual basis following review of documentation such as an operative report

M = multiple surgery adjustment applies

Me = multiple endoscopy rules may apply

M+ = multiple therapy rules apply

Mtc = multiple diagnostic imaging rules apply

T = team surgeons permitted

T+ = team surgeons payable if medical necessity established with documentation

§ = indicates code is not covered by Medicare

GS = procedure must be performed under the general supervision of a physician

DS = procedure must be performed under the direct supervision of a physician

PS = procedure must be performed under the personal supervision of a physician

DRA = procedure subject to DRA limitation

Relative Value Units

CPT Code and Modifier	Description	Work RVU	Nonfacility Practice Expense RVU	Facility Practice Expense RVU	PLI RVU	Total Non-facility RVUs	Medicare Payment Nonfacility	Total Facility RVUs	Medicare Payment Facility	Global Period	Payment Policy Indicators
14020	Tis trnfr s/a/l 10 sq cm/<	7.22	12.49	8.30	1.01	20.72	$717.04	16.53	$572.04	090	A M
14021	Tis trnfr s/a/l 10.1-30 sqcm	9.72	14.48	9.67	1.32	25.52	$883.15	20.71	$716.69	090	A M
14040	Tis trnfr f/c/c/m/n/a/g/h/f	8.60	12.68	8.53	1.06	22.34	$773.10	18.19	$629.49	090	A M
14041	Tis trnfr f/c/c/m/n/a/g/h/f	10.83	14.97	10.10	1.28	27.08	$937.14	22.21	$768.60	090	A M
14060	Tis trnfr e/n/e/l 10 sq cm/<	9.23	12.26	9.07	1.09	22.58	$781.41	19.39	$671.01	090	A M
14061	Tis trnfr e/n/e/l10.1-30sqcm	11.48	16.35	11.02	1.34	29.17	$1009.46	23.84	$825.01	090	A M
14301	Tis trnfr any 30.1-60 sq cm	12.65	17.51	10.88	1.94	32.10	$1110.86	25.47	$881.42	090	M
14302	Tis trnfr addl 30 sq cm	3.73	1.96	1.96	0.65	6.34	$219.40	6.34	$219.40	ZZZ	
14350	Filleted finger/toe flap	11.05	NA	7.80	1.16	NA	NA	20.01	$692.47	090	A+ M
15002	Wound prep trk/arm/leg	3.65	6.10	2.15	0.65	10.40	$359.90	6.45	$223.21	000	A+
15003	Wound prep addl 100 cm	0.80	1.11	0.36	0.18	2.09	$72.33	1.34	$46.37	ZZZ	A+
15004	Wound prep f/n/hf/g	4.58	6.58	2.44	0.65	11.81	$408.70	7.67	$265.43	000	A+
15005	Wnd prep f/n/hf/g addl cm	1.60	1.57	0.75	0.33	3.50	$121.12	2.68	$92.74	ZZZ	A+
15040	Harvest cultured skin graft	2.00	5.54	1.25	0.39	7.93	$274.43	3.64	$125.97	000	A
15050	Skin pinch graft	5.57	11.15	7.06	1.04	17.76	$614.61	13.67	$473.07	090	A M
15100	Skin splt grft trnk/arm/leg	9.90	14.08	9.32	1.93	25.91	$896.65	21.15	$731.92	090	A M
15101	Skin splt grft t/a/l add-on	1.72	3.58	1.24	0.35	5.65	$195.53	3.31	$114.55	ZZZ	A
15110	Epidrm autogrft trnk/arm/leg	10.97	11.60	7.85	2.17	24.74	$856.16	20.99	$726.38	090	A M
15111	Epidrm autogrft t/a/l add-on	1.85	1.09	0.75	0.41	3.35	$115.93	3.01	$104.16	ZZZ	A
15115	Epidrm a-grft face/nck/hf/g	11.28	10.82	7.27	1.78	23.88	$826.40	20.33	$703.54	090	A M
15116	Epidrm a-grft f/n/hf/g addl	2.50	1.89	1.44	0.44	4.83	$167.15	4.38	$151.58	ZZZ	A C+
15120	Skn splt a-grft fac/nck/hf/g	10.15	13.29	8.51	1.64	25.08	$867.92	20.30	$702.51	090	A M
15121	Skn splt a-grft f/n/hf/g add	2.00	3.94	1.59	0.40	6.34	$219.40	3.99	$138.08	ZZZ	A C+
15130	Derm autograft trnk/arm/leg	7.53	12.63	8.70	1.38	21.54	$745.42	17.61	$609.42	090	A M
15131	Derm autograft t/a/l add-on	1.50	1.10	0.87	0.27	2.87	$99.32	2.64	$91.36	ZZZ	A C+
15135	Derm autograft face/nck/hf/g	11.03	13.40	9.65	1.60	26.03	$900.80	22.28	$771.03	090	A M
15136	Derm autograft f/n/hf/g add	1.50	1.07	0.87	0.27	2.84	$98.28	2.64	$91.36	ZZZ	A C+
15150	Cult skin grft t/arm/leg	9.39	9.48	7.34	2.37	21.24	$735.04	19.10	$660.98	090	A M
15151	Cult skin grft t/a/l addl	2.00	1.03	0.75	0.51	3.54	$122.51	3.26	$112.82	ZZZ	A
15152	Cult skin graft t/a/l +%	2.50	1.38	1.13	0.47	4.35	$150.54	4.10	$141.89	ZZZ	A
15155	Cult skin graft f/n/hf/g	10.14	11.66	9.53	1.84	23.64	$818.09	21.51	$744.38	090	A M
15156	Cult skin grft f/n/hfg add	2.75	1.31	1.03	0.70	4.76	$164.73	4.48	$155.04	ZZZ	A C+
15157	Cult epiderm grft f/n/hfg +%	3.00	1.52	1.12	0.76	5.28	$182.72	4.88	$168.88	ZZZ	A C+

15200	Skin full graft trunk	9.15	14.09	9.00	1.63	24.87	$860.66	19.78	$684.51	090	A M
15201	Skin full graft trunk add on	1.32	2.64	0.67	0.25	4.21	$145.69	2.24	$77.52	ZZZ	A
15220	Skin full graft sclp/arm/leg	8.09	13.51	8.63	1.11	22.71	$785.91	17.83	$617.03	090	A M
15221	Skin full graft add-on	1.19	2.53	0.64	0.20	3.92	$135.66	2.03	$70.25	ZZZ	A
15240	Skin full grft face/genit/hf	10.41	15.60	11.45	1.38	27.39	$947.86	23.24	$804.25	090	A M
15241	Skin full graft add-on	1.86	3.03	0.95	0.28	5.17	$178.91	3.09	$106.93	ZZZ	A
15260	Skin full graft een & lips	11.64	16.38	11.69	1.32	29.34	$1015.35	24.65	$853.04	090	A M
15261	Skin full graft add-on	2.23	3.59	1.45	0.31	6.13	$212.14	3.99	$138.08	ZZZ	A
15271	Skin sub graft trnk/arm/leg	1.50	2.90	0.74	0.22	4.62	$159.88	2.46	$85.13	000	A M
15272	Skin sub graft t/a/l add-on	0.33	0.35	0.12	0.07	0.75	$25.95	0.52	$18.00	ZZZ	A
15273	Skin sub grft t/arm/lg child	3.50	5.32	1.67	0.65	9.47	$327.72	5.82	$201.41	000	A M
15274	Skn sub grft t/a/l child add	0.80	1.53	0.36	0.18	2.51	$86.86	1.34	$46.37	ZZZ	A
15275	Skin sub graft face/nk/hf/g	1.83	2.72	0.71	0.20	4.75	$164.38	2.74	$94.82	000	A M
15276	Skin sub graft f/n/hf/g addl	0.50	0.39	0.17	0.08	0.97	$33.57	0.75	$25.95	ZZZ	A
15277	Skn sub grft f/n/hf/g child	4.00	5.66	1.90	0.73	10.39	$359.56	6.63	$229.44	000	A C+ M
15278	Skn sub grft f/n/hf/g ch add	1.00	1.70	0.47	0.20	2.90	$100.36	1.67	$57.79	ZZZ	A C+
15570	Skin pedicle flap trunk	10.21	14.93	9.47	1.94	27.08	$937.14	21.62	$748.19	090	A M
15572	Skin pedicle flap arms/legs	10.12	14.10	9.73	1.71	25.93	$897.34	21.56	$746.11	090	A M
15574	Pedcle fh/ch/ch/m/n/ax/g/h/f	10.70	13.77	9.42	1.63	26.10	$903.22	21.75	$752.68	090	A M
15576	Pedicle e/n/e/l/ntroral	9.37	12.72	8.61	1.11	23.20	$802.86	19.09	$660.63	090	A M
15600	Delay flap trunk	2.01	7.70	3.84	0.37	10.08	$348.83	6.22	$215.25	090	A+ M
15610	Delay flap arms/legs	2.52	7.98	4.20	0.42	10.92	$377.90	7.14	$247.09	090	A+ M
15620	Delay flap f/c/c/n/ax/g/h/f	3.75	8.94	5.25	0.60	13.29	$459.92	9.60	$332.22	090	A M
15630	Delay flap eye/nos/ear/lip	4.08	9.04	5.42	0.56	13.68	$473.41	10.06	$348.14	090	A M
15650	Transfer skin pedicle flap	4.77	9.67	5.71	0.73	15.17	$524.98	11.21	$387.94	090	A+ M
15730	Mdfc flap w/prsrv vasc pedcl	13.50	27.61	11.82	1.47	42.58	$1473.53	26.79	$927.10	090	A C+ M
15731	Forehead flap w/vasc pedicle	14.38	16.69	12.82	2.17	33.24	$1150.31	29.37	$1016.38	090	A+ M
15733	Musc myoq/fscq flp h&n pedcl	15.68	NA	12.24	2.49	NA	NA	30.41	$1052.37	090	A C+ M

*Please note that these calculations are based on the Medicare 2022 Conversion Factor of $34.6062 and the DRA RVU cap rates at time of publication.

A = assistant-at-surgery restriction

A+ = assistant-at-surgery restriction unless medical necessity established with documentation

B = bilateral surgery adjustment applies

C = cosurgeons payable

C+ = cosurgeons payable if medical necessity established with documentation

CP = carriers may establish RVUs and payment amounts for these services, generally on an individual basis following review of documentation such as an operative report

M = multiple surgery adjustment applies

Me = multiple endoscopy rules may apply

M+ = multiple therapy rules apply

Mtc = multiple diagnostic imaging rules apply

T = team surgeons permitted

T+ = team surgeons payable if medical necessity established with documentation

§ = indicates code is not covered by Medicare

GS = procedure must be performed under the general supervision of a physician

DS = procedure must be performed under the direct supervision of a physician

PS = procedure must be performed under the personal supervision of a physician

DRA = procedure subject to DRA limitation

Relative Value Units

CPT Code and Modifier	Description	Work RVU	Nonfacility Practice Expense RVU	Facility Practice Expense RVU	PLI RVU	Total Non-facility RVUs	Medicare Payment Nonfacility	Total Facility RVUs	Medicare Payment Facility	Global Period	Payment Policy Indicators
15734	Muscle-skin graft trunk	23.00	NA	16.61	4.90	NA	NA	44.51	$1540.32	090	C+ M
15736	Muscle-skin graft arm	17.04	NA	15.64	3.27	NA	NA	35.95	$1244.09	090	A C+ M
15738	Muscle-skin graft leg	19.04	NA	15.04	3.61	NA	NA	37.69	$1304.31	090	C+ M
15740	Island pedicle flap graft	11.80	16.23	11.09	1.72	29.75	$1029.53	24.61	$851.66	090	A M
15750	Neurovascular pedicle flap	12.96	NA	12.12	2.43	NA	NA	27.51	$952.02	090	M
15756	Free myo/skin flap microvasc	36.94	NA	24.65	5.96	NA	NA	67.55	$2337.65	090	C M
15757	Free skin flap microvasc	37.15	NA	24.21	5.81	NA	NA	67.17	$2324.50	090	C M
15758	Free fascial flap microvasc	36.90	NA	24.50	5.68	NA	NA	67.08	$2321.38	090	C M
15760	Composite skin graft	9.86	13.76	9.33	1.33	24.95	$863.42	20.52	$710.12	090	A M
15769	Grfg autol soft tiss dir exc	6.68	NA	6.23	1.24	NA	NA	14.15	$489.68	090	A M
15770	Derma-fat-fascia graft	8.96	NA	9.47	1.36	NA	NA	19.79	$684.86	090	C+ M
15771	Grfg autol fat lipo 50 cc/<	6.73	9.56	6.68	1.18	17.47	$604.57	14.59	$504.90	090	A M
15772	Grfg autol fat lipo ea addl	2.50	2.66	1.40	0.44	5.60	$193.79	4.34	$150.19	ZZZ	A
15773	Grfg autol fat lipo 25 cc/<	6.83	9.73	6.81	1.33	17.89	$619.10	14.97	$518.05	090	A M
15774	Gfrg autol fat lipo ea addl	2.41	2.66	1.39	0.42	5.49	$189.99	4.22	$146.04	ZZZ	A
15775	Hair trnspl 1-15 punch grfts	3.95	6.58	2.83	0.73	11.26	$389.67	7.51	$259.89	000	A+ M
15776	Hair trnspl >15 punch grafts	5.53	8.67	3.74	1.00	15.20	$526.01	10.27	$355.41	000	A+ M
15777	Acellular derm matrix implt	3.65	1.97	1.97	0.72	6.34	$219.40	6.34	$219.40	ZZZ	A B
15780	Dermabrasion total face	8.73	15.35	9.68	0.85	24.93	$862.73	19.26	$666.52	090	A+ M
15781	Dermabrasion segmental face	5.02	10.25	6.81	0.79	16.06	$555.78	12.62	$436.73	090	A M
15782	Dermabrasion other than face	4.44	9.45	5.87	0.42	14.31	$495.21	10.73	$371.32	090	A+ M
15783	Dermabrasion suprfl any site	4.41	8.38	5.45	0.42	13.21	$457.15	10.28	$355.75	090	A+ M
15786	Abrasion lesion single	2.08	4.60	1.61	0.21	6.89	$238.44	3.90	$134.96	010	A M
15787	Abrasion lesions add-on	0.33	0.57	0.15	0.02	0.92	$31.84	0.50	$17.30	ZZZ	A
15788	Chemical peel face epiderm	2.09	9.33	3.94	0.24	11.66	$403.51	6.27	$216.98	090	A M
15789	Chemical peel face dermal	4.91	10.18	6.44	0.56	15.65	$541.59	11.91	$412.16	090	A M
15792	Chemical peel nonfacial	1.86	7.84	4.02	0.21	9.91	$342.95	6.09	$210.75	090	A+ M
15793	Chemical peel nonfacial	3.96	9.55	5.92	0.50	14.01	$484.83	10.38	$359.21	090	A+ M
15819	Plastic surgery neck	10.65	NA	11.01	1.94	NA	NA	23.60	$816.71	090	A+ M
15820	Revision of lower eyelid	6.27	10.25	8.31	0.47	16.99	$587.96	15.05	$520.82	090	A+ B M
15821	Revision of lower eyelid	6.84	10.76	8.63	0.68	18.28	$632.60	16.15	$558.89	090	A+ B M
15822	Revision of upper eyelid	4.62	8.51	6.60	0.54	13.67	$473.07	11.76	$406.97	090	A B M
15823	Revision of upper eyelid	6.81	10.86	8.71	0.60	18.27	$632.26	16.12	$557.85	090	A B M

15824		Removal of forehead wrinkles	0.00	0.00	0.00	0.00	0.00	$0.00	0.00	$0.00	000	A+ B M
15825		Removal of neck wrinkles	0.00	0.00	0.00	0.00	0.00	$0.00	0.00	$0.00	000	A+ B M
15826		Removal of brow wrinkles	0.00	0.00	0.00	0.00	0.00	$0.00	0.00	$0.00	000	A+ B M
15828		Removal of face wrinkles	0.00	0.00	0.00	0.00	0.00	$0.00	0.00	$0.00	000	A+ B M
15829		Removal of skin wrinkles	0.00	0.00	0.00	0.00	0.00	$0.00	0.00	$0.00	000	A+ B M
15830		Exc skin abd	17.11	NA	14.17	3.38	NA	NA	34.66	$1199.45	090	C+ M
15832		Excise excessive skin thigh	12.85	NA	11.81	2.46	NA	NA	27.12	$938.52	090	B C+ M
15833		Excise excessive skin leg	11.90	NA	11.83	2.17	NA	NA	25.90	$896.30	090	A+ B M
15834		Excise excessive skin hip	12.17	NA	11.99	2.22	NA	NA	26.38	$912.91	090	A+ B M
15835		Excise excessive skin buttck	12.99	NA	12.12	2.37	NA	NA	27.48	$950.98	090	A+ M
15836		Excise excessive skin arm	10.61	NA	10.99	1.94	NA	NA	23.54	$814.63	090	A+ B M
15837		Excise excess skin arm/hand	9.55	14.41	9.86	1.73	25.69	$889.03	21.14	$731.58	090	A+ M
15838		Excise excess skin fat pad	8.25	NA	9.42	1.50	NA	NA	19.17	$663.40	090	A+ M
15839		Excise excess skin & tissue	10.50	14.05	9.43	1.93	26.48	$916.37	21.86	$756.49	090	A+ M
15840		Nerve palsy fascial graft	14.99	NA	12.70	2.33	NA	NA	30.02	$1038.88	090	A M
15841		Nerve palsy muscle graft	25.99	NA	21.82	4.76	NA	NA	52.57	$1819.25	090	C+ M
15842		Nerve palsy microsurg graft	41.01	NA	31.17	7.50	NA	NA	79.68	$2757.42	090	C+ M
15845		Skin and muscle repair face	14.32	NA	14.40	2.62	NA	NA	31.34	$1084.56	090	M
15847	CP	Exc skin abd add-on	0.00	0.00	0.00	0.00	0.00	$0.00	0.00	$0.00	YYY	C+
15850	§	Remove sutures same surgeon	0.78	1.94	0.30	0.07	2.79	$96.55	1.15	$39.80	XXX	
15851		Remove sutures diff surgeon	0.86	2.25	0.37	0.09	3.20	$110.74	1.32	$45.68	000	A M
15852		Dressing change not for burn	0.86	NA	0.35	0.17	NA	NA	1.38	$47.76	000	A M
15860		Test for blood flow in graft	1.95	NA	0.84	0.35	NA	NA	3.14	$108.66	000	A+ M
15876		Suction lipectomy head&neck	0.00	0.00	0.00	0.00	0.00	$0.00	0.00	$0.00	000	A+ M
15877		Suction lipectomy trunk	0.00	0.00	0.00	0.00	0.00	$0.00	0.00	$0.00	000	A+ M
15878		Suction lipectomy upr extrem	0.00	0.00	0.00	0.00	0.00	$0.00	0.00	$0.00	000	A+ B M
15879		Suction lipectomy lwr extrem	0.00	0.00	0.00	0.00	0.00	$0.00	0.00	$0.00	000	A+ B M
15920		Removal of tail bone ulcer	8.29	NA	8.91	1.86	NA	NA	19.06	$659.59	090	A+ M

*Please note that these calculations are based on the Medicare 2022 Conversion Factor of $34.6062 and the DRA RVU cap rates at time of publication.

A = assistant-at-surgery restriction

A+ = assistant-at-surgery restriction unless medical necessity established with documentation

B = bilateral surgery adjustment applies

C = cosurgeons payable

C+ = cosurgeons payable if medical necessity established with documentation

CP = carriers may establish RVUs and payment amounts for these services, generally on an individual basis following review of documentation such as an operative report

M = multiple surgery adjustment applies

Me = multiple endoscopy rules may apply

M+ = multiple therapy rules apply

Mtc = multiple diagnostic imaging rules apply

T = team surgeons permitted

T+ = team surgeons payable if medical necessity established with documentation

§ = indicates code is not covered by Medicare

GS = procedure must be performed under the general supervision of a physician

DS = procedure must be performed under the direct supervision of a physician

PS = procedure must be performed under the personal supervision of a physician

DRA = procedure subject to DRA limitation

Relative Value Units

CPT Code and Modifier		Description	Work RVU	Nonfacility Practice Expense RVU	Facility Practice Expense RVU	PLI RVU	Total Non-facility RVUs	Medicare Payment Nonfacility	Total Facility RVUs	Medicare Payment Facility	Global Period	Payment Policy Indicators
15922		Removal of tail bone ulcer	10.38	NA	11.33	1.90	NA	NA	23.61	$817.05	090	C+ M
15931		Remove sacrum pressure sore	10.07	NA	8.51	2.26	NA	NA	20.84	$721.19	090	A M
15933		Remove sacrum pressure sore	11.77	NA	11.55	2.62	NA	NA	25.94	$897.68	090	A+ M
15934		Remove sacrum pressure sore	13.68	NA	11.66	2.84	NA	NA	28.18	$975.20	090	A M
15935		Remove sacrum pressure sore	15.78	NA	15.54	2.89	NA	NA	34.21	$1183.88	090	C+ M
15936		Remove sacrum pressure sore	13.16	NA	10.94	2.78	NA	NA	26.88	$930.21	090	A C+ M
15937		Remove sacrum pressure sore	15.14	NA	12.91	3.01	NA	NA	31.06	$1074.87	090	A C+ M
15940		Remove hip pressure sore	10.20	NA	8.49	2.18	NA	NA	20.87	$722.23	090	A M
15941		Remove hip pressure sore	12.41	NA	12.76	2.50	NA	NA	27.67	$957.55	090	A+ M
15944		Remove hip pressure sore	12.44	NA	12.95	2.27	NA	NA	27.66	$957.21	090	A+ M
15945		Remove hip pressure sore	13.75	NA	13.93	2.50	NA	NA	30.18	$1044.42	090	A+ M
15946		Remove hip pressure sore	24.12	NA	19.15	4.76	NA	NA	48.03	$1662.14	090	A C+ M
15950		Remove thigh pressure sore	8.03	NA	9.36	1.47	NA	NA	18.86	$652.67	090	A M
15951		Remove thigh pressure sore	11.58	NA	12.95	2.13	NA	NA	26.66	$922.60	090	A+ C+ M
15952		Remove thigh pressure sore	12.31	NA	12.55	2.25	NA	NA	27.11	$938.17	090	C+ M
15953		Remove thigh pressure sore	13.57	NA	13.83	2.49	NA	NA	29.89	$1034.38	090	A C+ M
15956		Remove thigh pressure sore	16.79	NA	14.64	3.36	NA	NA	34.79	$1203.95	090	A C+ M
15958		Remove thigh pressure sore	16.75	NA	15.39	3.22	NA	NA	35.36	$1223.68	090	A C+ M
15999	CP	Removal of pressure sore	0.00	0.00	0.00	0.00	0.00	$0.00	0.00	$0.00	YYY	A+ C+ M T+
16000		Initial treatment of burn(s)	0.89	1.24	0.31	0.12	2.25	$77.86	1.32	$45.68	000	A M
16020		Dress/debrid p-thick burn s	0.71	1.69	0.78	0.11	2.51	$86.86	1.60	$55.37	000	A M
16025		Dress/debrid p-thick burn m	1.74	2.67	1.26	0.27	4.68	$161.96	3.27	$113.16	000	A M
16030		Dress/debrid p-thick burn l	2.08	3.40	1.40	0.39	5.87	$203.14	3.87	$133.93	000	A M
16035		Incision of burn scab initi	3.74	NA	1.35	0.56	NA	NA	5.65	$195.53	000	A M
16036		Escharotomy addl incision	1.50	NA	0.56	0.25	NA	NA	2.31	$79.94	ZZZ	A
17000		Destruct premalg lesion	0.61	1.31	0.93	0.07	1.99	$68.87	1.61	$55.72	010	A M
17003		Destruct premalg les 2-14	0.04	0.16	0.02	0.00	0.20	$6.92	0.06	$2.08	ZZZ	A
17004		Destroy premal lesions 15/>	1.37	3.51	1.35	0.12	5.00	$173.03	2.84	$98.28	010	A
17106		Destruction of skin lesions	3.69	6.00	3.94	0.40	10.09	$349.18	8.03	$277.89	090	A M
17107		Destruction of skin lesions	4.79	7.80	5.12	0.56	13.15	$455.07	10.47	$362.33	090	A M
17108		Destruction of skin lesions	7.49	10.13	6.88	0.94	18.56	$642.29	15.31	$529.82	090	A+ M
17110		Destruct b9 lesion 1-14	0.70	2.59	1.17	0.08	3.37	$116.62	1.95	$67.48	010	A M
17111		Destruct lesion 15 or more	0.97	2.87	1.31	0.10	3.94	$136.35	2.38	$82.36	010	A M

17250		Chem caut of granltj tissue	0.50	2.09	0.51	0.09	2.68	$92.74	1.10	$38.07	000	A M
17260		Destruction of skin lesions	0.96	1.91	1.01	0.09	2.96	$102.43	2.06	$71.29	010	A M
17261		Destruction of skin lesions	1.22	3.05	1.18	0.11	4.38	$151.58	2.51	$86.86	010	A M
17262		Destruction of skin lesions	1.63	3.50	1.40	0.17	5.30	$183.41	3.20	$110.74	010	A M
17263		Destruction of skin lesions	1.84	3.70	1.52	0.19	5.73	$198.29	3.55	$122.85	010	A M
17264		Destruction of skin lesions	1.99	3.94	1.60	0.20	6.13	$212.14	3.79	$131.16	010	A M
17266		Destruction of skin lesions	2.39	4.34	1.82	0.24	6.97	$241.21	4.45	$154.00	010	A M
17270		Destruction of skin lesions	1.37	2.91	1.25	0.12	4.40	$152.27	2.74	$94.82	010	A M
17271		Destruction of skin lesions	1.54	3.23	1.35	0.14	4.91	$169.92	3.03	$104.86	010	A M
17272		Destruction of skin lesions	1.82	3.59	1.51	0.19	5.60	$193.79	3.52	$121.81	010	A M
17273		Destruction of skin lesions	2.10	3.88	1.67	0.21	6.19	$214.21	3.98	$137.73	010	A M
17274		Destruction of skin lesions	2.64	4.34	1.97	0.25	7.23	$250.20	4.86	$168.19	010	A M
17276		Destruction of skin lesions	3.25	4.83	2.28	0.33	8.41	$291.04	5.86	$202.79	010	A M
17280		Destruction of skin lesions	1.22	2.81	1.17	0.11	4.14	$143.27	2.50	$86.52	010	A M
17281		Destruction of skin lesions	1.77	3.38	1.48	0.18	5.33	$184.45	3.43	$118.70	010	A M
17282		Destruction of skin lesions	2.09	3.79	1.66	0.21	6.09	$210.75	3.96	$137.04	010	A M
17283		Destruction of skin lesions	2.69	4.23	1.99	0.25	7.17	$248.13	4.93	$170.61	010	A M
17284		Destruction of skin lesions	3.20	4.65	2.26	0.32	8.17	$282.73	5.78	$200.02	010	A M
17286		Destruction of skin lesions	4.48	5.54	2.90	0.43	10.45	$361.63	7.81	$270.27	010	A M
17311		Mohs 1 stage h/n/hf/g	6.20	13.07	3.54	0.60	19.87	$687.63	10.34	$357.83	000	A M
17312		Mohs addl stage	3.30	8.49	1.88	0.32	12.11	$419.08	5.50	$190.33	ZZZ	A
17313		Mohs 1 stage t/a/l	5.56	12.56	3.18	0.55	18.67	$646.10	9.29	$321.49	000	A M
17314		Mohs addl stage t/a/l	3.06	8.24	1.74	0.29	11.59	$401.09	5.09	$176.15	ZZZ	A
17315		Mohs surg addl block	0.87	1.31	0.50	0.09	2.27	$78.56	1.46	$50.53	ZZZ	A
17340		Cryotherapy of skin	0.77	0.68	0.58	0.09	1.54	$53.29	1.44	$49.83	010	A M
17360		Skin peel therapy	1.46	2.01	1.08	0.12	3.59	$124.24	2.66	$92.05	010	A M
17380		Hair removal by electrolysis	0.00	0.00	0.00	0.00	0.00	$0.00	0.00	$0.00	000	A+ M
17999	CP	Skin tissue procedure	0.00	0.00	0.00	0.00	0.00	$0.00	0.00	$0.00	YYY	A+ C+ M T+

*Please note that these calculations are based on the Medicare 2022 Conversion Factor of $34.6062 and the DRA RVU cap rates at time of publication.

A = assistant-at-surgery restriction
A+ = assistant-at-surgery restriction unless medical necessity established with documentation
B = bilateral surgery adjustment applies
C = cosurgeons payable
C+ = cosurgeons payable if medical necessity established with documentation
CP = carriers may establish RVUs and payment amounts for these services, generally on an individual basis following review of documentation such as an operative report
M = multiple surgery adjustment applies
Me = multiple endoscopy rules may apply
M+ = multiple therapy rules apply
Mtc = multiple diagnostic imaging rules apply
T = team surgeons permitted
T+ = team surgeons payable if medical necessity established with documentation
§ = indicates code is not covered by Medicare
GS = procedure must be performed under the general supervision of a physician
DS = procedure must be performed under the direct supervision of a physician
PS = procedure must be performed under the personal supervision of a physician
DRA = procedure subject to DRA limitation

Relative Value Units

CPT Code and Modifier	Description	Work RVU	Nonfacility Practice Expense RVU	Facility Practice Expense RVU	PLI RVU	Total Non-facility RVUs	Medicare Payment Nonfacility	Total Facility RVUs	Medicare Payment Facility	Global Period	Payment Policy Indicators
19000	Drainage of breast lesion	0.84	2.14	0.31	0.10	3.08	$106.59	1.25	$43.26	000	A M
19001	Drain breast lesion add-on	0.42	0.32	0.15	0.05	0.79	$27.34	0.62	$21.46	ZZZ	A
19020	Incision of breast lesion	3.83	9.45	4.59	0.89	14.17	$490.37	9.31	$322.18	090	A B M
19030	Injection for breast x-ray	1.53	3.29	0.55	0.12	4.94	$170.95	2.20	$76.13	000	A B M
19081	Bx breast 1st lesion strtctc	3.29	11.72	1.19	0.33	15.34	$530.86	4.81	$166.46	000	A+ B M
19082	Bx breast add lesion strtctc	1.65	10.20	0.60	0.17	12.02	$415.97	2.42	$83.75	ZZZ	A+
19083	Bx breast 1st lesion us imag	3.10	12.11	1.12	0.32	15.53	$537.43	4.54	$157.11	000	A+ B M
19084	Bx breast add lesion us imag	1.55	10.20	0.56	0.14	11.89	$411.47	2.25	$77.86	ZZZ	A+
19085	Bx breast 1st lesion mr imag	3.64	19.92	1.31	0.31	23.87	$826.05	5.26	$182.03	000	A+ B M
19086	Bx breast add lesion mr imag	1.82	16.66	0.66	0.14	18.62	$644.37	2.62	$90.67	ZZZ	A+
19100	Bx breast percut w/o image	1.27	3.07	0.48	0.31	4.65	$160.92	2.06	$71.29	000	A B M
19101	Biopsy of breast open	3.23	6.00	2.68	0.77	10.00	$346.06	6.68	$231.17	010	A B M
19105	Cryosurg ablate fa each	3.69	68.61	1.63	0.94	73.24	$2534.56	6.26	$216.63	000	A B M
19110	Nipple exploration	4.44	9.18	4.96	1.10	14.72	$509.40	10.50	$363.37	090	A B M
19112	Excise breast duct fistula	3.81	9.21	4.87	0.95	13.97	$483.45	9.63	$333.26	090	A+ B M
19120	Removal of breast lesion	5.92	8.19	5.08	1.43	15.54	$537.78	12.43	$430.16	090	A B M
19125	Excision breast lesion	6.69	8.79	5.44	1.66	17.14	$593.15	13.79	$477.22	090	A B C+ M
19126	Excision addl breast lesion	2.93	NA	1.11	0.73	NA	NA	4.77	$165.07	ZZZ	A C+
19281	Perq device breast 1st imag	2.00	4.99	0.72	0.18	7.17	$248.13	2.90	$100.36	000	A+ B M
19282	Perq device breast ea imag	1.00	4.02	0.36	0.09	5.11	$176.84	1.45	$50.18	ZZZ	A+
19283	Perq dev breast 1st strtctc	2.00	5.62	0.72	0.20	7.82	$270.62	2.92	$101.05	000	A+ B M
19284	Perq dev breast add strtctc	1.00	4.74	0.36	0.11	5.85	$202.45	1.47	$50.87	ZZZ	A+
19285	Perq dev breast 1st us imag	1.70	9.60	0.61	0.17	11.47	$396.93	2.48	$85.82	000	A+ B M
19286	Perq dev breast add us imag	0.85	8.53	0.31	0.09	9.47	$327.72	1.25	$43.26	ZZZ	A+
19287	Perq dev breast 1st mr guide	2.55	17.09	0.92	0.21	19.85	$686.93	3.68	$127.35	000	A+ B M
19288	Perq dev breast add mr guide	1.28	14.04	0.46	0.11	15.43	$533.97	1.85	$64.02	ZZZ	A+
19294	Prep tum cav iort prtl mast	3.00	NA	1.14	0.75	NA	NA	4.89	$169.22	ZZZ	A+
19296	Place po breast cath for rad	3.63	112.73	1.71	0.89	117.25	$4057.58	6.23	$215.60	000	A+ B M
19297	Place breast cath for rad	1.72	NA	0.65	0.42	NA	NA	2.79	$96.55	ZZZ	A+
19298	Place breast rad tube/caths	5.75	20.31	3.06	0.42	26.48	$916.37	9.23	$319.42	000	A+ B M
19300	Removal of breast tissue	5.31	11.02	6.36	1.24	17.57	$608.03	12.91	$446.77	090	A B M
19301	Partial mastectomy	10.13	NA	7.11	2.50	NA	NA	19.74	$683.13	090	A+ B M
19302	P-mastectomy w/ln removal	13.99	NA	9.64	3.48	NA	NA	27.11	$938.17	090	B C+ M

19303		Mast simple complete	15.00	NA	9.88	3.73	NA	NA	28.61	$990.08	090	B C+ M
19305		Mast radical	17.46	NA	12.51	4.33	NA	NA	34.30	$1186.99	090	B C+ M
19306		Mast rad urban type	18.13	NA	13.85	4.60	NA	NA	36.58	$1265.89	090	B C+ M
19307		Mast mod rad	17.99	NA	12.83	4.47	NA	NA	35.29	$1221.25	090	B C+ M
19316		Suspension of breast	11.09	NA	10.16	2.18	NA	NA	23.43	$810.82	090	B C+ M
19318		Breast reduction	16.03	NA	13.31	2.99	NA	NA	32.33	$1118.82	090	B C+ M
19325		Breast augmentation w/implt	8.12	NA	8.57	1.49	NA	NA	18.18	$629.14	090	A+ B M
19328		Rmvl intact breast implant	7.44	NA	7.56	1.40	NA	NA	16.40	$567.54	090	A B M
19330		Rmvl ruptured breast implant	9.00	NA	8.45	1.68	NA	NA	19.13	$662.02	090	A B M
19340		Insj breast implt sm d mast	10.48	NA	9.93	2.03	NA	NA	22.44	$776.56	090	A B C+ M
19342		Insj/rplcmt brst implt sep d	10.48	NA	10.10	1.94	NA	NA	22.52	$779.33	090	A+ B C+ M
19350		Breast reconstruction	9.11	13.86	9.11	1.68	24.65	$853.04	19.90	$688.66	090	A B M
19355		Correct inverted nipple(s)	8.52	12.38	8.17	1.55	22.45	$776.91	18.24	$631.22	090	A+ B M
19357		Tiss xpndr plmt brst rcnstj	14.84	NA	16.66	2.82	NA	NA	34.32	$1187.68	090	B C+ M
19361		Brst rcnstj latsms drsi flap	23.36	NA	18.39	4.31	NA	NA	46.06	$1593.96	090	B C+ M
19364		Brst rcnstj free flap	42.58	NA	30.02	7.87	NA	NA	80.47	$2784.76	090	B C+ M
19367		Brst rcnstj 1 pdcl tram flap	26.80	NA	20.63	4.91	NA	NA	52.34	$1811.29	090	B C+ M
19368		Brst rcnstj 1pdcl tram anast	33.90	NA	24.10	6.21	NA	NA	64.21	$2222.06	090	B C+ M
19369		Brst rcnstj 2 pdcl tram flap	31.31	NA	22.61	5.74	NA	NA	59.66	$2064.61	090	B C+ M
19370		Revj peri-implt capsule brst	9.17	NA	8.99	1.69	NA	NA	19.85	$686.93	090	A B M
19371		Peri-implt capslc brst compl	9.98	NA	9.24	1.84	NA	NA	21.06	$728.81	090	A B M
19380		Revj reconstructed breast	11.17	NA	10.65	2.05	NA	NA	23.87	$826.05	090	A B M
19396		Design custom breast implant	2.17	5.72	1.63	0.40	8.29	$286.89	4.20	$145.35	000	A+ B M
19499	CP	Breast surgery procedure	0.00	0.00	0.00	0.00	0.00	$0.00	0.00	$0.00	YYY	A+ B C+ M T+
20100		Explore wound neck	10.38	NA	5.38	2.13	NA	NA	17.89	$619.10	010	B M
20101		Explore wound chest	3.23	14.00	2.23	0.83	18.06	$624.99	6.29	$217.67	010	A M
20102		Explore wound abdomen	3.98	13.91	2.69	0.94	18.83	$651.63	7.61	$263.35	010	A M
20103		Explore wound extremity	5.34	10.62	3.87	0.99	16.95	$586.58	10.20	$352.98	010	A+ M

*Please note that these calculations are based on the Medicare 2022 Conversion Factor of $34.6062 and the DRA RVU cap rates at time of publication.

A = assistant-at-surgery restriction
A+ = assistant-at-surgery restriction unless medical necessity established with documentation
B = bilateral surgery adjustment applies
C = cosurgeons payable
C+ = cosurgeons payable if medical necessity established with documentation
CP = carriers may establish RVUs and payment amounts for these services, generally on an individual basis following review of documentation such as an operative report
M = multiple surgery adjustment applies
Me = multiple endoscopy rules may apply
M+ = multiple therapy rules apply
Mtc = multiple diagnostic imaging rules apply
T = team surgeons permitted
T+ = team surgeons payable if medical necessity established with documentation
§ = indicates code is not covered by Medicare
GS = procedure must be performed under the general supervision of a physician
DS = procedure must be performed under the direct supervision of a physician
PS = procedure must be performed under the personal supervision of a physician
DRA = procedure subject to DRA limitation

Relative Value Units

CPT Code and Modifier	Description	Work RVU	Nonfacility Practice Expense RVU	Facility Practice Expense RVU	PLI RVU	Total Non-facility RVUs	Medicare Payment Nonfacility	Total Facility RVUs	Medicare Payment Facility	Global Period	Payment Policy Indicators
20150	Excise epiphyseal bar	14.75	NA	11.96	3.03	NA	NA	29.74	$1029.19	090	B C+ M
20200	Muscle biopsy	1.46	4.83	0.98	0.35	6.64	$229.79	2.79	$96.55	000	A M
20205	Deep muscle biopsy	2.35	6.23	1.58	0.62	9.20	$318.38	4.55	$157.46	000	A M
20206	Needle biopsy muscle	0.99	5.82	0.59	0.09	6.90	$238.78	1.67	$57.79	000	A M
20220	Bone biopsy trocar/needle	1.65	5.39	0.75	0.14	7.18	$248.47	2.54	$87.90	000	A M
20225	Bone biopsy trocar/needle	2.45	9.17	1.11	0.23	11.85	$410.08	3.79	$131.16	000	A M
20240	Bone biopsy open superficial	2.61	NA	1.23	0.31	NA	NA	4.15	$143.62	000	A M
20245	Bone biopsy open deep	6.00	NA	3.17	1.05	NA	NA	10.22	$353.68	000	A M
20250	Open bone biopsy	5.19	NA	4.95	1.33	NA	NA	11.47	$396.93	010	A M
20251	Open bone biopsy	5.72	NA	5.29	1.53	NA	NA	12.54	$433.96	010	M
20500	Injection of sinus tract	1.28	2.19	1.16	0.12	3.59	$124.24	2.56	$88.59	010	A M
20501	Inject sinus tract for x-ray	0.76	3.58	0.25	0.08	4.42	$152.96	1.09	$37.72	000	A M
20520	Removal of foreign body	1.90	4.33	2.18	0.27	6.50	$224.94	4.35	$150.54	010	A M
20525	Removal of foreign body	3.54	9.83	3.12	0.64	14.01	$484.83	7.30	$252.63	010	A M
20526	Ther injection carp tunnel	0.94	1.32	0.57	0.18	2.44	$84.44	1.69	$58.48	000	A B M
20527	Inj dupuytren cord w/enzyme	1.00	1.39	0.74	0.19	2.58	$89.28	1.93	$66.79	000	A B M
20550	Inj tendon sheath/ligament	0.75	0.85	0.30	0.10	1.70	$58.83	1.15	$39.80	000	A B M
20551	Inj tendon origin/insertion	0.75	0.88	0.31	0.09	1.72	$59.52	1.15	$39.80	000	A M
20552	Inj trigger point 1/2 muscl	0.66	0.84	0.36	0.09	1.59	$55.02	1.11	$38.41	000	A M
20553	Inject trigger points 3/>	0.75	0.98	0.41	0.10	1.83	$63.33	1.26	$43.60	000	A M
20555	Place ndl musc/tis for rt	6.00	NA	3.31	0.43	NA	NA	9.74	$337.06	000	A+ M
20560	Ndl insj w/o njx 1 or 2 musc	0.32	0.44	0.10	0.02	0.78	$26.99	0.44	$15.23	XXX	A
20561	Ndl insj w/o njx 3+ musc	0.48	0.61	0.15	0.02	1.11	$38.41	0.65	$22.49	XXX	A
20600	Drain/inj joint/bursa w/o us	0.66	0.82	0.30	0.09	1.57	$54.33	1.05	$36.34	000	A B M
20604	Drain/inj joint/bursa w/us	0.89	1.44	0.36	0.10	2.43	$84.09	1.35	$46.72	000	A B M
20605	Drain/inj joint/bursa w/o us	0.68	0.85	0.32	0.09	1.62	$56.06	1.09	$37.72	000	A B M
20606	Drain/inj joint/bursa w/us	1.00	1.53	0.41	0.11	2.64	$91.36	1.52	$52.60	000	A B M
20610	Drain/inj joint/bursa w/o us	0.79	1.01	0.42	0.12	1.92	$66.44	1.33	$46.03	000	A B M
20611	Drain/inj joint/bursa w/us	1.10	1.71	0.50	0.14	2.95	$102.09	1.74	$60.21	000	A B M
20612	Aspirate/inj ganglion cyst	0.70	1.10	0.41	0.10	1.90	$65.75	1.21	$41.87	000	A M
20615	Treatment of bone cyst	2.33	4.90	2.11	0.27	7.50	$259.55	4.71	$163.00	010	A M
20650	Insert and remove bone pin	2.28	4.01	2.14	0.34	6.63	$229.44	4.76	$164.73	010	A C+ M
20660	Apply rem fixation device	4.00	NA	1.90	1.22	NA	NA	7.12	$246.40	000	A M

20661	Application of head brace	5.26	NA	8.22	1.70	NA	NA	15.18	$525.32	090	A M
20662	Application of pelvis brace	6.38	NA	7.77	1.32	NA	NA	15.47	$535.36	090	A+ M
20663	Application of thigh brace	5.74	NA	7.33	1.18	NA	NA	14.25	$493.14	090	A+ B M
20664	Application of halo	10.06	NA	12.39	3.85	NA	NA	26.30	$910.14	090	A M
20665	Removal of fixation device	1.36	1.96	1.36	0.10	3.42	$118.35	2.82	$97.59	010	A+ M
20670	Removal of support implant	1.79	8.75	2.19	0.27	10.81	$374.09	4.25	$147.08	010	A M
20680	Removal of support implant	5.96	10.98	5.39	1.04	17.98	$622.22	12.39	$428.77	090	A+ M
20690	Apply bone fixation device	8.78	NA	7.20	1.70	NA	NA	17.68	$611.84	090	A M
20692	Apply bone fixation device	16.27	NA	14.01	2.85	NA	NA	33.13	$1146.50	090	C+ M
20693	Adjust bone fixation device	6.06	NA	6.07	1.00	NA	NA	13.13	$454.38	090	A M
20694	Remove bone fixation device	4.28	7.74	5.02	0.77	12.79	$442.61	10.07	$348.48	090	A M
20696	Comp multiplane ext fixation	17.56	NA	14.22	3.22	NA	NA	35.00	$1211.22	090	C+ M
20697	Comp ext fixate strut change	0.00	56.46	NA	0.04	56.50	$1955.25	NA	NA	000	C+
20700	Mnl prep&insj dp rx dlvr dev	1.50	0.72	0.72	0.29	2.51	$86.86	2.51	$86.86	ZZZ	A+
20701	Rmvl deep rx delivery device	1.13	0.55	0.55	0.23	1.91	$66.10	1.91	$66.10	ZZZ	A+
20702	Mnl prep&insj imed rx dev	2.50	1.23	1.23	0.50	4.23	$146.38	4.23	$146.38	ZZZ	A+
20703	Rmvl imed rx delivery device	1.80	0.91	0.91	0.37	3.08	$106.59	3.08	$106.59	ZZZ	A+
20704	Mnl prep&insj i-artic rx dev	2.60	1.33	1.33	0.54	4.47	$154.69	4.47	$154.69	ZZZ	A+
20705	Rmvl i-artic rx delivery dev	2.15	1.09	1.09	0.42	3.66	$126.66	3.66	$126.66	ZZZ	A+
20802	Replantation arm complete	42.62	NA	29.68	8.78	NA	NA	81.08	$2805.87	090	B C+ M
20805	Replant forearm complete	51.46	NA	34.28	10.61	NA	NA	96.35	$3334.31	090	B C+ M
20808	Replantation hand complete	63.09	NA	40.18	13.03	NA	NA	116.30	$4024.70	090	B C+ M
20816	Replantation digit complete	31.95	NA	22.18	6.58	NA	NA	60.71	$2100.94	090	C+ M
20822	Replantation digit complete	26.66	NA	20.27	5.50	NA	NA	52.43	$1814.40	090	C+ M
20824	Replantation thumb complete	31.95	NA	22.29	6.58	NA	NA	60.82	$2104.75	090	B C+ M
20827	Replantation thumb complete	27.48	NA	20.68	5.65	NA	NA	53.81	$1862.16	090	B C+ M
20838	Replantation foot complete	42.88	NA	30.65	8.85	NA	NA	82.38	$2850.86	090	B C+ M
20900	Removal of bone for graft	3.00	8.27	1.83	0.52	11.79	$408.01	5.35	$185.14	000	C+ M

*Please note that these calculations are based on the Medicare 2022 Conversion Factor of $34.6062 and the DRA RVU cap rates at time of publication.

A = assistant-at-surgery restriction
A+ = assistant-at-surgery restriction unless medical necessity established with documentation
B = bilateral surgery adjustment applies
C = cosurgeons payable
C+ = cosurgeons payable if medical necessity established with documentation
CP = carriers may establish RVUs and payment amounts for these services, generally on an individual basis following review of documentation such as an operative report
M = multiple surgery adjustment applies
Me = multiple endoscopy rules may apply
M+ = multiple therapy rules apply
Mtc = multiple diagnostic imaging rules apply
T = team surgeons permitted
T+ = team surgeons payable if medical necessity established with documentation
§ = indicates code is not covered by Medicare
GS = procedure must be performed under the general supervision of a physician
DS = procedure must be performed under the direct supervision of a physician
PS = procedure must be performed under the personal supervision of a physician
DRA = procedure subject to DRA limitation

Relative Value Units

CPT Code and Modifier		Description	Work RVU	Nonfacility Practice Expense RVU	Facility Practice Expense RVU	PLI RVU	Total Non-facility RVUs	Medicare Payment Nonfacility	Total Facility RVUs	Medicare Payment Facility	Global Period	Payment Policy Indicators
20902		Removal of bone for graft	4.58	NA	2.72	0.87	NA	NA	8.17	$282.73	000	C+ M
20910		Remove cartilage for graft	5.53	NA	7.44	1.12	NA	NA	14.09	$487.60	090	A+ M
20912		Remove cartilage for graft	6.54	NA	6.73	0.99	NA	NA	14.26	$493.48	090	A+ M
20920		Removal of fascia for graft	5.51	NA	5.50	0.77	NA	NA	11.78	$407.66	090	A C+ M
20922		Removal of fascia for graft	6.93	9.60	6.14	1.37	17.90	$619.45	14.44	$499.71	090	C+ M
20924		Removal of tendon for graft	6.68	NA	7.06	1.25	NA	NA	14.99	$518.75	090	C+ M
20931		Sp bone algrft struct add-on	1.81	NA	0.89	0.56	NA	NA	3.26	$112.82	ZZZ	A C+
20932		Osteoart algrft w/surf & b1	13.01	NA	6.60	2.68	NA	NA	22.29	$771.37	ZZZ	C+
20933		Hemicrt intrclry algrft prtl	11.94	NA	6.06	2.47	NA	NA	20.47	$708.39	ZZZ	C+
20934		Intercalary algrft compl	13.00	NA	6.59	2.68	NA	NA	22.27	$770.68	ZZZ	C+
20937		Sp bone agrft morsel add-on	2.79	NA	1.38	0.75	NA	NA	4.92	$170.26	ZZZ	C+
20938		Sp bone agrft struct add-on	3.02	NA	1.48	0.93	NA	NA	5.43	$187.91	ZZZ	C+
20939		Bone marrow aspir bone grfg	1.16	NA	0.57	0.32	NA	NA	2.05	$70.94	ZZZ	A+ B
20950		Fluid pressure muscle	1.26	6.53	1.09	0.24	8.03	$277.89	2.59	$89.63	000	A+ M
20955		Fibula bone graft microvasc	40.26	NA	26.24	6.27	NA	NA	72.77	$2518.29	090	C+ M
20956		Iliac bone graft microvasc	41.18	NA	28.35	8.50	NA	NA	78.03	$2700.32	090	C+ M
20957		Mt bone graft microvasc	42.61	NA	29.86	8.77	NA	NA	81.24	$2811.41	090	C+ M
20962		Other bone graft microvasc	39.21	NA	31.39	8.09	NA	NA	78.69	$2723.16	090	C+ M
20969		Bone/skin graft microvasc	45.43	NA	27.98	6.62	NA	NA	80.03	$2769.53	090	C+ M
20970		Bone/skin graft iliac crest	44.58	NA	30.36	9.18	NA	NA	84.12	$2911.07	090	C+ M
20972		Bone/skin graft metatarsal	44.51	NA	30.19	9.17	NA	NA	83.87	$2902.42	090	M
20973		Bone/skin graft great toe	47.27	NA	31.59	9.77	NA	NA	88.63	$3067.15	090	B C+ M
20974		Electrical bone stimulation	0.62	1.66	0.71	0.12	2.40	$83.05	1.45	$50.18	000	A
20975		Electrical bone stimulation	2.60	NA	1.89	0.61	NA	NA	5.10	$176.49	000	C+
20979		Us bone stimulation	0.62	0.93	0.22	0.09	1.64	$56.75	0.93	$32.18	000	A
20982		Ablate bone tumor(s) perq	7.02	100.41	2.70	0.95	108.38	$3750.62	10.67	$369.25	000	A B M
20983		Ablate bone tumor(s) perq	6.88	151.07	2.34	0.66	158.61	$5488.89	9.88	$341.91	000	A B M
20985		Cptr-asst dir ms px	2.50	NA	1.27	0.51	NA	NA	4.28	$148.11	ZZZ	A+
20999	CP	Musculoskeletal surgery	0.00	0.00	0.00	0.00	0.00	$0.00	0.00	$0.00	YYY	A+ C+ M T+
21010		Incision of jaw joint	11.04	NA	9.78	1.05	NA	NA	21.87	$756.84	090	A+ B M
21011		Exc face les sc <2 cm	2.99	7.65	4.13	0.54	11.18	$386.90	7.66	$265.08	090	M
21012		Exc face les sbq 2 cm/>	4.45	NA	4.72	0.90	NA	NA	10.07	$348.48	090	M
21013		Exc face tum deep < 2 cm	5.42	9.64	5.51	0.96	16.02	$554.39	11.89	$411.47	090	M

21014	Exc face tum deep 2 cm/>	7.13	NA	7.00	1.33	NA	NA	15.46	$535.01	090	M
21015	Resect face/scalp tum < 2 cm	9.89	NA	9.11	1.70	NA	NA	20.70	$716.35	090	A M
21016	Resect face/scalp tum 2 cm/>	15.26	NA	11.68	2.89	NA	NA	29.83	$1032.30	090	M
21025	Excision of bone lower jaw	10.03	12.32	8.40	0.99	23.34	$807.71	19.42	$672.05	090	A M
21026	Excision of facial bone(s)	5.70	9.58	6.33	0.56	15.84	$548.16	12.59	$435.69	090	A M
21029	Contour of face bone lesion	8.39	13.18	8.71	1.12	22.69	$785.21	18.22	$630.52	090	A+ M
21030	Excise max/zygoma b9 tumor	4.91	8.37	5.31	0.44	13.72	$474.80	10.66	$368.90	090	A B M
21031	Remove exostosis mandible	3.30	7.84	4.40	0.31	11.45	$396.24	8.01	$277.20	090	A B M
21032	Remove exostosis maxilla	3.34	7.40	4.00	0.32	11.06	$382.74	7.66	$265.08	090	A M
21034	Excise max/zygoma mal tumor	17.38	18.79	13.58	2.38	38.55	$1334.07	33.34	$1153.77	090	C+ M
21040	Excise mandible lesion	4.91	8.57	5.40	0.44	13.92	$481.72	10.75	$372.02	090	A M
21044	Removal of jaw bone lesion	12.80	NA	11.06	1.71	NA	NA	25.57	$884.88	090	C+ M
21045	Extensive jaw surgery	18.37	NA	14.58	2.48	NA	NA	35.43	$1226.10	090	C+ M
21046	Remove mandible cyst complex	14.21	NA	14.03	1.37	NA	NA	29.61	$1024.69	090	A+ C+ M
21047	Excise lwr jaw cyst w/repair	20.07	NA	14.53	2.33	NA	NA	36.93	$1278.01	090	C+ M
21048	Remove maxilla cyst complex	14.71	NA	13.73	1.41	NA	NA	29.85	$1033.00	090	A+ C+ M
21049	Excis uppr jaw cyst w/repair	19.32	NA	14.02	2.73	NA	NA	36.07	$1248.25	090	C+ M
21050	Removal of jaw joint	11.76	NA	12.68	1.11	NA	NA	25.55	$884.19	090	A+ B M
21060	Remove jaw joint cartilage	11.07	NA	11.06	1.06	NA	NA	23.19	$802.52	090	B C+ M
21070	Remove coronoid process	8.62	NA	8.36	1.02	NA	NA	18.00	$622.91	090	A+ B M
21073	Mnpj of tmj w/anesth	3.45	7.37	3.45	0.35	11.17	$386.55	7.25	$250.89	090	A+ B M
21076	Prepare face/oral prosthesis	13.40	10.63	6.09	1.22	25.25	$873.81	20.71	$716.69	010	A+ M
21077	Prepare face/oral prosthesis	33.70	25.35	14.33	2.99	62.04	$2146.97	51.02	$1765.61	090	A+ B M
21079	Prepare face/oral prosthesis	22.31	18.24	10.02	1.99	42.54	$1472.15	34.32	$1187.68	090	A M
21080	Prepare face/oral prosthesis	25.06	21.91	11.83	2.25	49.22	$1703.32	39.14	$1354.49	090	A M
21081	Prepare face/oral prosthesis	22.85	20.26	10.81	2.07	45.18	$1563.51	35.73	$1236.48	090	A+ M
21082	Prepare face/oral prosthesis	20.84	18.78	9.83	1.84	41.46	$1434.77	32.51	$1125.05	090	A+ M
21083	Prepare face/oral prosthesis	19.27	18.61	9.22	1.70	39.58	$1369.71	30.19	$1044.76	090	A+ M

*Please note that these calculations are based on the Medicare 2022 Conversion Factor of $34.6062 and the DRA RVU cap rates at time of publication.

A = assistant-at-surgery restriction
A+ = assistant-at-surgery restriction unless medical necessity established with documentation
B = bilateral surgery adjustment applies
C = cosurgeons payable
C+ = cosurgeons payable if medical necessity established with documentation
CP = carriers may establish RVUs and payment amounts for these services, generally on an individual basis following review of documentation such as an operative report
M = multiple surgery adjustment applies
Me = multiple endoscopy rules may apply
M+ = multiple therapy rules apply
Mtc = multiple diagnostic imaging rules apply
T = team surgeons permitted
T+ = team surgeons payable if medical necessity established with documentation
§ = indicates code is not covered by Medicare
GS = procedure must be performed under the general supervision of a physician
DS = procedure must be performed under the direct supervision of a physician
PS = procedure must be performed under the personal supervision of a physician
DRA = procedure subject to DRA limitation

Relative Value Units

CPT Code and Modifier		Description	Work RVU	Nonfacility Practice Expense RVU	Facility Practice Expense RVU	PLI RVU	Total Non-facility RVUs	Medicare Payment Nonfacility	Total Facility RVUs	Medicare Payment Facility	Global Period	Payment Policy Indicators
21084		Prepare face/oral prosthesis	22.48	20.72	10.47	1.99	45.19	$1563.85	34.94	$1209.14	090	A+ M
21085		Prepare face/oral prosthesis	8.99	9.99	4.33	0.85	19.83	$686.24	14.17	$490.37	010	A+ M
21086		Prepare face/oral prosthesis	24.88	19.12	10.54	2.20	46.20	$1598.81	37.62	$1301.89	090	A+ B M
21087		Prepare face/oral prosthesis	24.88	19.12	10.54	2.20	46.20	$1598.81	37.62	$1301.89	090	A+ M
21088	CP	Prepare face/oral prosthesis	0.00	0.00	0.00	0.00	0.00	$0.00	0.00	$0.00	090	A+
21089	CP	Prepare face/oral prosthesis	0.00	0.00	0.00	0.00	0.00	$0.00	0.00	$0.00	YYY	A C+ T+
21100		Maxillofacial fixation	4.73	13.45	5.26	0.41	18.59	$643.33	10.40	$359.90	090	A+ M
21110		Interdental fixation	5.99	19.57	15.11	0.56	26.12	$903.91	21.66	$749.57	090	A M
21116		Injection jaw joint x-ray	0.81	5.75	0.43	0.09	6.65	$230.13	1.33	$46.03	000	A B M
21120		Reconstruction of chin	5.10	13.82	9.11	0.95	19.87	$687.63	15.16	$524.63	090	A C+ M
21121		Reconstruction of chin	7.81	10.29	7.15	0.68	18.78	$649.90	15.64	$541.24	090	M
21122		Reconstruction of chin	8.71	NA	11.99	1.60	NA	NA	22.30	$771.72	090	M
21123		Reconstruction of chin	11.34	NA	12.77	1.09	NA	NA	25.20	$872.08	090	C+ M
21125		Augmentation lower jaw bone	10.80	68.92	7.87	0.95	80.67	$2791.68	19.62	$678.97	090	M
21127		Augmentation lower jaw bone	12.44	110.11	8.96	1.09	123.64	$4278.71	22.49	$778.29	090	C+ M
21137		Reduction of forehead	10.24	NA	10.11	1.86	NA	NA	22.21	$768.60	090	M
21138		Reduction of forehead	12.87	NA	11.84	2.34	NA	NA	27.05	$936.10	090	C+ M
21139		Reduction of forehead	15.02	NA	14.60	2.76	NA	NA	32.38	$1120.55	090	C+ M
21141		Lefort i-1 piece w/o graft	19.57	NA	17.88	1.87	NA	NA	39.32	$1360.72	090	C+ M
21142		Lefort i-2 piece w/o graft	20.28	NA	18.15	1.94	NA	NA	40.37	$1397.05	090	C+ M
21143		Lefort i-3/> piece w/o graft	21.05	NA	18.53	2.01	NA	NA	41.59	$1439.27	090	C+ M
21145		Lefort i-1 piece w/ graft	23.94	NA	19.51	2.31	NA	NA	45.76	$1583.58	090	M
21146		Lefort i-2 piece w/ graft	24.87	NA	20.51	2.38	NA	NA	47.76	$1652.79	090	C+ M
21147		Lefort i-3/> piece w/ graft	26.47	NA	21.26	2.55	NA	NA	50.28	$1740.00	090	M
21150		Lefort ii anterior intrusion	25.96	NA	18.99	3.70	NA	NA	48.65	$1683.59	090	M
21151		Lefort ii w/bone grafts	29.02	NA	20.38	4.12	NA	NA	53.52	$1852.12	090	M
21154		Lefort iii w/o lefort i	31.29	NA	21.85	4.45	NA	NA	57.59	$1992.97	090	C+ M
21155		Lefort iii w/ lefort i	35.22	NA	23.64	5.00	NA	NA	63.86	$2209.95	090	M
21159		Lefort iii w/fhdw/o lefort i	43.14	NA	27.25	6.13	NA	NA	76.52	$2648.07	090	C+ M
21160		Lefort iii w/fhd w/ lefort i	47.19	NA	29.09	6.70	NA	NA	82.98	$2871.62	090	M
21172		Reconstruct orbit/forehead	28.20	NA	24.09	10.82	NA	NA	63.11	$2184.00	090	C+ M
21175		Reconstruct orbit/forehead	33.56	NA	25.78	6.15	NA	NA	65.49	$2266.36	090	M
21179		Reconstruct entire forehead	22.65	NA	18.24	4.14	NA	NA	45.03	$1558.32	090	M

21180	Reconstruct entire forehead	25.58	NA	20.04	4.67	NA	NA	50.29	$1740.35	090	C+ M
21181	Contour cranial bone lesion	10.28	NA	9.78	1.87	NA	NA	21.93	$758.91	090	A+ M
21182	Reconstruct cranial bone	32.58	NA	24.02	5.96	NA	NA	62.56	$2164.96	090	C+ M
21183	Reconstruct cranial bone	35.70	NA	25.82	6.54	NA	NA	68.06	$2355.30	090	C+ M
21184	Reconstruct cranial bone	38.62	NA	27.51	7.07	NA	NA	73.20	$2533.17	090	M
21188	Reconstruction of midface	23.15	NA	21.39	2.22	NA	NA	46.76	$1618.19	090	M
21193	Reconst lwr jaw w/o graft	18.90	NA	15.59	1.81	NA	NA	36.30	$1256.21	090	C+ M
21194	Reconst lwr jaw w/graft	21.82	NA	18.13	2.09	NA	NA	42.04	$1454.84	090	M
21195	Reconst lwr jaw w/o fixation	19.16	NA	18.71	1.84	NA	NA	39.71	$1374.21	090	M
21196	Reconst lwr jaw w/fixation	20.83	NA	19.59	2.01	NA	NA	42.43	$1468.34	090	C+ M
21198	Reconstr lwr jaw segment	15.71	NA	12.98	1.94	NA	NA	30.63	$1059.99	090	C+ M
21199	Reconstr lwr jaw w/advance	16.73	NA	11.63	1.61	NA	NA	29.97	$1037.15	090	C+ M
21206	Reconstruct upper jaw bone	15.59	NA	11.59	1.43	NA	NA	28.61	$990.08	090	C+ M
21208	Augmentation of facial bones	11.42	37.46	9.20	1.04	49.92	$1727.54	21.66	$749.57	090	A+ M
21209	Reduction of facial bones	7.82	15.70	9.62	0.85	24.37	$843.35	18.29	$632.95	090	M
21210	Face bone graft	11.69	40.75	9.50	1.04	53.48	$1850.74	22.23	$769.30	090	A M
21215	Lower jaw bone graft	12.23	112.77	9.76	1.09	126.09	$4363.50	23.08	$798.71	090	A C+ M
21230	Rib cartilage graft	11.17	NA	9.24	1.81	NA	NA	22.22	$768.95	090	A+ M
21235	Ear cartilage graft	7.50	13.23	8.25	1.00	21.73	$751.99	16.75	$579.65	090	A M
21240	Reconstruction of jaw joint	16.07	NA	13.23	1.51	NA	NA	30.81	$1066.22	090	B C+ M
21242	Reconstruction of jaw joint	14.59	NA	13.82	1.40	NA	NA	29.81	$1031.61	090	B C+ M
21243	Reconstruction of jaw joint	24.53	NA	20.29	2.45	NA	NA	47.27	$1635.84	090	B C+ M
21244	Reconstruction of lower jaw	13.62	NA	14.48	1.68	NA	NA	29.78	$1030.57	090	C+ M
21245	Reconstruction of jaw	13.12	20.17	12.35	1.68	34.97	$1210.18	27.15	$939.56	090	M
21246	Reconstruction of jaw	12.92	NA	10.89	1.25	NA	NA	25.06	$867.23	090	M
21247	Reconstruct lower jaw bone	24.37	NA	19.88	2.33	NA	NA	46.58	$1611.96	090	B C+ M
21248	Reconstruction of jaw	12.74	15.15	9.34	1.16	29.05	$1005.31	23.24	$804.25	090	A M
21249	Reconstruction of jaw	18.77	19.05	12.18	1.72	39.54	$1368.33	32.67	$1130.58	090	A+ M

*Please note that these calculations are based on the Medicare 2022 Conversion Factor of $34.6062 and the DRA RVU cap rates at time of publication.

A = assistant-at-surgery restriction
A+ = assistant-at-surgery restriction unless medical necessity established with documentation
B = bilateral surgery adjustment applies
C = cosurgeons payable
C+ = cosurgeons payable if medical necessity established with documentation
CP = carriers may establish RVUs and payment amounts for these services, generally on an individual basis following review of documentation such as an operative report
M = multiple surgery adjustment applies
Me = multiple endoscopy rules may apply
M+ = multiple therapy rules apply
Mtc = multiple diagnostic imaging rules apply
T = team surgeons permitted
T+ = team surgeons payable if medical necessity established with documentation
§ = indicates code is not covered by Medicare
GS = procedure must be performed under the general supervision of a physician
DS = procedure must be performed under the direct supervision of a physician
PS = procedure must be performed under the personal supervision of a physician
DRA = procedure subject to DRA limitation

Relative Value Units

CPT Code and Modifier		Description	Work RVU	Nonfacility Practice Expense RVU	Facility Practice Expense RVU	PLI RVU	Total Non-facility RVUs	Medicare Payment Nonfacility	Total Facility RVUs	Medicare Payment Facility	Global Period	Payment Policy Indicators
21255		Reconstruct lower jaw bone	18.46	NA	19.34	1.78	NA	NA	39.58	$1369.71	090	B C+ M
21256		Reconstruction of orbit	17.66	NA	15.74	3.23	NA	NA	36.63	$1267.63	090	B C+ M
21260		Revise eye sockets	17.90	NA	19.54	3.28	NA	NA	40.72	$1409.16	090	C+ M
21261		Revise eye sockets	34.07	NA	31.68	6.23	NA	NA	71.98	$2490.95	090	C+ M
21263		Revise eye sockets	31.01	NA	29.92	5.68	NA	NA	66.61	$2305.12	090	C+ M
21267		Revise eye sockets	20.69	NA	23.11	3.79	NA	NA	47.59	$1646.91	090	B C+ M
21268		Revise eye sockets	27.07	NA	27.64	4.96	NA	NA	59.67	$2064.95	090	B C+ M
21270		Augmentation cheek bone	10.63	17.43	9.54	1.94	30.00	$1038.19	22.11	$765.14	090	B C+ M
21275		Revision orbitofacial bones	11.76	NA	11.12	2.17	NA	NA	25.05	$866.89	090	C+ M
21280		Revision of eyelid	7.13	NA	9.32	0.70	NA	NA	17.15	$593.50	090	A+ B M
21282		Revision of eyelid	4.27	NA	6.87	0.54	NA	NA	11.68	$404.20	090	A B M
21295		Revision of jaw muscle/bone	1.90	NA	3.60	0.25	NA	NA	5.75	$198.99	090	A+ B M
21296		Revision of jaw muscle/bone	4.78	NA	6.64	0.67	NA	NA	12.09	$418.39	090	A+ B M
21299	CP	Cranio/maxillofacial surgery	0.00	0.00	0.00	0.00	0.00	$0.00	0.00	$0.00	YYY	A+ C+ M T+
21315		Clsd tx nsl fx mnpj wo stblj	0.96	3.41	0.64	0.14	4.51	$156.07	1.74	$60.21	000	A M
21320		Clsd tx nsl fx w/mnpj&stablj	1.59	4.72	0.98	0.24	6.55	$226.67	2.81	$97.24	000	A M
21325		Open tx nose fx uncomplicatd	4.18	NA	8.52	0.60	NA	NA	13.30	$460.26	090	A+ M
21330		Open tx nose fx w/skele fixj	5.79	NA	9.34	0.83	NA	NA	15.96	$552.31	090	A+ M
21335		Open tx nose & septal fx	9.02	NA	10.97	1.30	NA	NA	21.29	$736.77	090	A M
21336		Open tx septal fx w/wo stabj	6.77	NA	11.45	1.00	NA	NA	19.22	$665.13	090	A+ M
21337		Closed tx septal&nose fx	3.39	8.63	4.97	0.52	12.54	$433.96	8.88	$307.30	090	A+ M
21338		Open nasoethmoid fx w/o fixj	6.87	NA	12.24	0.98	NA	NA	20.09	$695.24	090	A+ M
21339		Open nasoethmoid fx w/ fixj	8.50	NA	12.99	1.20	NA	NA	22.69	$785.21	090	C+ M
21340		Perq tx nasoethmoid fx	11.49	NA	9.13	1.64	NA	NA	22.26	$770.33	090	A+ M
21343		Open tx dprsd front sinus fx	14.32	NA	16.00	2.03	NA	NA	32.35	$1119.51	090	C+ M
21344		Open tx compl front sinus fx	21.57	NA	16.81	3.05	NA	NA	41.43	$1433.73	090	C M
21345		Closed tx nose/jaw fx	9.06	13.45	8.54	1.29	23.80	$823.63	18.89	$653.71	090	A+ M
21346		Opn tx nasomax fx w/fixj	11.45	NA	17.65	1.63	NA	NA	30.73	$1063.45	090	A C+ M
21347		Opn tx nasomax fx multple	13.53	NA	15.57	1.94	NA	NA	31.04	$1074.18	090	C+ M
21348		Opn tx nasomax fx w/graft	17.52	NA	12.35	2.49	NA	NA	32.36	$1119.86	090	C M
21355		Perq tx malar fracture	4.45	8.21	4.63	0.62	13.28	$459.57	9.70	$335.68	010	A+ B M
21356		Opn tx dprsd zygomatic arch	4.83	10.51	6.26	0.89	16.23	$561.66	11.98	$414.58	010	A+ B M
21360		Opn tx dprsd malar fracture	7.19	NA	7.27	1.01	NA	NA	15.47	$535.36	090	B M

21365	Opn tx complx malar fx	16.77	NA	12.85	2.39	NA	NA	32.01	$1107.74	090	B C+ M
21366	Opn tx complx malar w/grft	18.60	NA	15.77	3.41	NA	NA	37.78	$1307.42	090	B C M
21385	Opn tx orbit fx transantral	9.57	NA	10.46	1.75	NA	NA	21.78	$753.72	090	B C+ M
21386	Opn tx orbit fx periorbital	9.57	NA	9.16	1.75	NA	NA	20.48	$708.73	090	B M
21387	Opn tx orbit fx combined	10.11	NA	10.77	1.84	NA	NA	22.72	$786.25	090	B M
21390	Opn tx orbit periorbtl implt	11.23	NA	10.99	1.48	NA	NA	23.70	$820.17	090	B C+ M
21395	Opn tx orbit periorbt w/grft	14.70	NA	12.52	2.69	NA	NA	29.91	$1035.07	090	B C+ M
21400	Closed tx orbit w/o manipulj	1.50	4.52	3.13	0.25	6.27	$216.98	4.88	$168.88	090	A+ B M
21401	Closed tx orbit w/manipulj	3.68	10.87	5.34	0.67	15.22	$526.71	9.69	$335.33	090	B M
21406	Opn tx orbit fx w/o implant	7.42	NA	8.54	1.36	NA	NA	17.32	$599.38	090	B C+ M
21407	Opn tx orbit fx w/implant	9.02	NA	8.81	1.12	NA	NA	18.95	$655.79	090	B C+ M
21408	Opn tx orbit fx w/bone grft	12.78	NA	11.64	2.33	NA	NA	26.75	$925.72	090	B C M
21421	Treat mouth roof fracture	6.02	12.69	9.65	0.54	19.25	$666.17	16.21	$560.97	090	A+ M
21422	Treat mouth roof fracture	8.73	NA	8.63	1.16	NA	NA	18.52	$640.91	090	C+ M
21423	Treat mouth roof fracture	10.85	NA	10.89	1.99	NA	NA	23.73	$821.21	090	C M
21431	Treat craniofacial fracture	7.90	NA	12.16	0.70	NA	NA	20.76	$718.42	090	M
21432	Treat craniofacial fracture	8.82	NA	10.98	1.62	NA	NA	21.42	$741.26	090	M
21433	Treat craniofacial fracture	26.29	NA	20.20	4.82	NA	NA	51.31	$1775.64	090	C+ M
21435	Treat craniofacial fracture	20.26	NA	17.63	3.73	NA	NA	41.62	$1440.31	090	M
21436	Treat craniofacial fracture	30.30	NA	24.35	5.54	NA	NA	60.19	$2082.95	090	C M
21440	Treat dental ridge fracture	3.44	16.94	12.83	0.39	20.77	$718.77	16.66	$576.54	090	A+ M
21445	Treat dental ridge fracture	6.26	17.24	12.53	0.66	24.16	$836.09	19.45	$673.09	090	M
21450	Treat lower jaw fracture	3.71	13.85	10.46	0.33	17.89	$619.10	14.50	$501.79	090	A+ M
21451	Treat lower jaw fracture	5.65	17.05	13.19	0.50	23.20	$802.86	19.34	$669.28	090	A+ M
21452	Treat lower jaw fracture	2.40	20.16	11.42	0.23	22.79	$788.68	14.05	$486.22	090	A+ M
21453	Treat lower jaw fracture	6.64	25.55	20.61	0.86	33.05	$1143.73	28.11	$972.78	090	A+ M
21454	Treat lower jaw fracture	7.36	NA	6.30	0.65	NA	NA	14.31	$495.21	090	A+ C+ M
21461	Treat lower jaw fracture	9.31	44.99	21.17	1.21	55.51	$1920.99	31.69	$1096.67	090	A C+ M

*Please note that these calculations are based on the Medicare 2022 Conversion Factor of $34.6062 and the DRA RVU cap rates at time of publication.

A = assistant-at-surgery restriction

A+ = assistant-at-surgery restriction unless medical necessity established with documentation

B = bilateral surgery adjustment applies

C = cosurgeons payable

C+ = cosurgeons payable if medical necessity established with documentation

CP = carriers may establish RVUs and payment amounts for these services, generally on an individual basis following review of documentation such as an operative report

M = multiple surgery adjustment applies

Me = multiple endoscopy rules may apply

M+ = multiple therapy rules apply

Mtc = multiple diagnostic imaging rules apply

T = team surgeons permitted

T+ = team surgeons payable if medical necessity established with documentation

§ = indicates code is not covered by Medicare

GS = procedure must be performed under the general supervision of a physician

DS = procedure must be performed under the direct supervision of a physician

PS = procedure must be performed under the personal supervision of a physician

DRA = procedure subject to DRA limitation

Relative Value Units

CPT Code and Modifier		Description	Work RVU	Nonfacility Practice Expense RVU	Facility Practice Expense RVU	PLI RVU	Total Non-facility RVUs	Medicare Payment Nonfacility	Total Facility RVUs	Medicare Payment Facility	Global Period	Payment Policy Indicators
21462		Treat lower jaw fracture	11.01	48.32	22.92	1.39	60.72	$2101.29	35.32	$1222.29	090	C+ M
21465		Treat lower jaw fracture	13.12	NA	9.10	1.17	NA	NA	23.39	$809.44	090	B C+ M
21470		Treat lower jaw fracture	17.54	NA	14.47	2.28	NA	NA	34.29	$1186.65	090	C+ M
21480		Reset dislocated jaw	0.61	3.50	0.19	0.11	4.22	$146.04	0.91	$31.49	000	A B M
21485		Reset dislocated jaw	4.77	24.26	18.83	0.44	29.47	$1019.84	24.04	$831.93	090	A+ B M
21490		Repair dislocated jaw	12.95	NA	8.93	1.16	NA	NA	23.04	$797.33	090	B C+ M
21497		Interdental wiring	4.64	16.36	12.73	0.40	21.40	$740.57	17.77	$614.95	090	A+ M
21499	CP	Head surgery procedure	0.00	0.00	0.00	0.00	0.00	$0.00	0.00	$0.00	YYY	A+ C+ M T+
21501		Drain neck/chest lesion	3.98	9.81	5.13	0.79	14.58	$504.56	9.90	$342.60	090	A M
21502		Drain chest lesion	7.55	NA	5.83	1.78	NA	NA	15.16	$524.63	090	M
21510		Drainage of bone lesion	6.20	NA	5.84	1.47	NA	NA	13.51	$467.53	090	A+ M
21550		Biopsy of neck/chest	2.11	5.62	2.20	0.29	8.02	$277.54	4.60	$159.19	010	A M
21552		Exc neck les sc 3 cm/>	6.49	NA	5.36	1.48	NA	NA	13.33	$461.30	090	M
21554		Exc neck tum deep 5 cm/>	11.13	NA	8.24	2.38	NA	NA	21.75	$752.68	090	M
21555		Exc neck les sc < 3 cm	3.96	8.33	4.37	0.79	13.08	$452.65	9.12	$315.61	090	A M
21556		Exc neck tum deep < 5 cm	7.66	NA	6.66	1.48	NA	NA	15.80	$546.78	090	A M
21557		Resect neck thorax tumor<5cm	14.75	NA	10.55	3.03	NA	NA	28.33	$980.39	090	C+ M
21558		Resect neck tumor 5 cm/>	21.58	NA	13.64	4.62	NA	NA	39.84	$1378.71	090	C+ M
21600		Partial removal of rib	7.26	NA	7.77	1.63	NA	NA	16.66	$576.54	090	C+ M
21601		Exc chest wall tumor w/ribs	17.78	NA	12.11	4.32	NA	NA	34.21	$1183.88	090	C+ M
21602		Exc ch wal tum w/o lymphadec	22.19	NA	18.64	5.23	NA	NA	46.06	$1593.96	090	C+ M
21603		Exc ch wal tum w/lymphadec	25.17	NA	18.93	5.96	NA	NA	50.06	$1732.39	090	C+ M
21610		Partial removal of rib	15.91	NA	13.82	6.11	NA	NA	35.84	$1240.29	090	M
21615		Removal of rib	10.45	NA	5.23	2.55	NA	NA	18.23	$630.87	090	B C+ M
21616		Removal of rib and nerves	12.69	NA	5.26	3.18	NA	NA	21.13	$731.23	090	B M
21620		Partial removal of sternum	7.28	NA	6.09	1.68	NA	NA	15.05	$520.82	090	C+ M
21627		Sternal debridement	7.30	NA	7.20	1.64	NA	NA	16.14	$558.54	090	M
21630		Extensive sternum surgery	19.18	NA	16.17	3.52	NA	NA	38.87	$1345.14	090	C+ M
21632		Extensive sternum surgery	19.68	NA	11.58	4.67	NA	NA	35.93	$1243.40	090	C+ M
21685		Hyoid myotomy & suspension	15.26	NA	11.75	2.17	NA	NA	29.18	$1009.81	090	C+ M
21700		Revision of neck muscle	6.31	NA	2.67	1.57	NA	NA	10.55	$365.10	090	B M
21705		Revision of neck muscle/rib	9.92	NA	3.40	2.48	NA	NA	15.80	$546.78	090	B M
21720		Revision of neck muscle	5.80	NA	7.78	2.22	NA	NA	15.80	$546.78	090	M

21725		Revision of neck muscle	7.19	NA	7.48	1.48	NA	NA	16.15	$558.89	090	C+ M
21740		Reconstruction of sternum	17.57	NA	8.60	4.17	NA	NA	30.34	$1049.95	090	C+ M
21742	CP	Repair stern/nuss w/o scope	0.00	0.00	0.00	0.00	0.00	$0.00	0.00	$0.00	090	C+ M
21743	CP	Repair sternum/nuss w/scope	0.00	0.00	0.00	0.00	0.00	$0.00	0.00	$0.00	090	C+ M
21750		Repair of sternum separation	11.40	NA	5.99	2.67	NA	NA	20.06	$694.20	090	C+ M
21811		Optx of rib fx w/fixj scope	10.79	NA	4.27	2.50	NA	NA	17.56	$607.68	000	B M
21812		Treatment of rib fracture	13.00	NA	5.29	3.00	NA	NA	21.29	$736.77	000	B M
21813		Treatment of rib fracture	17.61	NA	7.12	4.45	NA	NA	29.18	$1009.81	000	B M
21820		Treat sternum fracture	1.36	2.82	2.73	0.27	4.45	$154.00	4.36	$150.88	090	A M
21825		Treat sternum fracture	7.76	NA	6.79	1.81	NA	NA	16.36	$566.16	090	C+ M
21899	CP	Neck/chest surgery procedure	0.00	0.00	0.00	0.00	0.00	$0.00	0.00	$0.00	YYY	A+ C+ M T+
21920		Biopsy soft tissue of back	2.11	5.36	2.19	0.29	7.76	$268.54	4.59	$158.84	010	A M
21925		Biopsy soft tissue of back	4.63	9.20	5.58	1.00	14.83	$513.21	11.21	$387.94	090	A M
21930		Exc back les sc < 3 cm	4.94	9.14	4.84	1.04	15.12	$523.25	10.82	$374.44	090	A M
21931		Exc back les sc 3 cm/>	6.88	NA	5.53	1.61	NA	NA	14.02	$485.18	090	M
21932		Exc back tum deep < 5 cm	9.82	NA	7.72	2.23	NA	NA	19.77	$684.16	090	M
21933		Exc back tum deep 5 cm/>	11.13	NA	8.30	2.60	NA	NA	22.03	$762.37	090	M
21935		Resect back tum < 5 cm	15.72	NA	11.21	3.55	NA	NA	30.48	$1054.80	090	A C+ M
21936		Resect back tum 5 cm/>	22.55	NA	14.15	5.29	NA	NA	41.99	$1453.11	090	C+ M
22010		I&d p-spine c/t/cerv-thor	12.75	NA	12.26	3.78	NA	NA	28.79	$996.31	090	A+ M
22015		I&d abscess p-spine l/s/ls	12.64	NA	12.14	3.48	NA	NA	28.26	$977.97	090	A M
22100		Remove part of neck vertebra	11.00	NA	11.63	3.06	NA	NA	25.69	$889.03	090	C+ M
22101		Remove part thorax vertebra	11.08	NA	11.48	2.97	NA	NA	25.53	$883.50	090	C+ M
22102		Remove part lumbar vertebra	11.08	NA	9.86	2.17	NA	NA	23.11	$799.75	090	C+ M
22103		Remove extra spine segment	2.34	NA	1.10	0.55	NA	NA	3.99	$138.08	ZZZ	C+
22110		Remove part of neck vertebra	14.00	NA	13.03	4.32	NA	NA	31.35	$1084.90	090	C+ M
22112		Remove part thorax vertebra	14.07	NA	14.28	5.40	NA	NA	33.75	$1167.96	090	C+ M
22114		Remove part lumbar vertebra	14.07	NA	14.28	5.40	NA	NA	33.75	$1167.96	090	C+ M

*Please note that these calculations are based on the Medicare 2022 Conversion Factor of $34.6062 and the DRA RVU cap rates at time of publication.

A = assistant-at-surgery restriction
A+ = assistant-at-surgery restriction unless medical necessity established with documentation
B = bilateral surgery adjustment applies
C = cosurgeons payable
C+ = cosurgeons payable if medical necessity established with documentation
CP = carriers may establish RVUs and payment amounts for these services, generally on an individual basis following review of documentation such as an operative report
M = multiple surgery adjustment applies
Me = multiple endoscopy rules may apply
M+ = multiple therapy rules apply
Mtc = multiple diagnostic imaging rules apply
T = team surgeons permitted
T+ = team surgeons payable if medical necessity established with documentation
§ = indicates code is not covered by Medicare
GS = procedure must be performed under the general supervision of a physician
DS = procedure must be performed under the direct supervision of a physician
PS = procedure must be performed under the personal supervision of a physician
DRA = procedure subject to DRA limitation

Relative Value Units

CPT Code and Modifier		Description	Work RVU	Nonfacility Practice Expense RVU	Facility Practice Expense RVU	PLI RVU	Total Non-facility RVUs	Medicare Payment Nonfacility	Total Facility RVUs	Medicare Payment Facility	Global Period	Payment Policy Indicators
22116		Remove extra spine segment	2.32	NA	1.13	0.73	NA	NA	4.18	$144.65	ZZZ	C+
22206		Incis spine 3 column thorac	37.18	NA	24.39	11.00	NA	NA	72.57	$2511.37	090	C+ M
22207		Incis spine 3 column lumbar	36.68	NA	24.12	10.23	NA	NA	71.03	$2458.08	090	C+ M
22208		Incis spine 3 column adl seg	9.66	NA	4.72	3.02	NA	NA	17.40	$602.15	ZZZ	C+
22210		Incis 1 vertebral seg cerv	25.38	NA	20.15	7.51	NA	NA	53.04	$1835.51	090	C+ M
22212		Incis 1 vertebral seg thorac	20.99	NA	17.88	5.96	NA	NA	44.83	$1551.40	090	C+ M
22214		Incis 1 vertebral seg lumbar	21.02	NA	17.88	5.94	NA	NA	44.84	$1551.74	090	C+ M
22216		Incis addl spine segment	6.03	NA	2.98	1.69	NA	NA	10.70	$370.29	ZZZ	C+
22220		Osteot dsc ant 1 vrt sgm crv	22.94	NA	18.57	6.56	NA	NA	48.07	$1663.52	090	C+ M
22222		Osteot dsc ant 1vrt sgm thrc	23.09	NA	20.31	8.85	NA	NA	52.25	$1808.17	090	C+ M
22224		Osteot dsc ant 1vrt sgm lmbr	23.09	NA	18.47	5.53	NA	NA	47.09	$1629.61	090	C+ M
22226		Osteot dsc ant 1vrt sgm ea	6.03	NA	2.98	1.61	NA	NA	10.62	$367.52	ZZZ	C+
22310		Closed tx vert fx w/o manj	3.45	5.06	4.64	0.75	9.26	$320.45	8.84	$305.92	090	A M
22315		Closed tx vert fx w/manj	10.11	13.76	10.44	2.33	26.20	$906.68	22.88	$791.79	090	A M
22318		Treat odontoid fx w/o graft	22.72	NA	17.89	8.24	NA	NA	48.85	$1690.51	090	C M
22319		Treat odontoid fx w/graft	25.33	NA	19.40	9.72	NA	NA	54.45	$1884.31	090	C M
22325		Treat spine fracture	19.87	NA	17.51	6.26	NA	NA	43.64	$1510.21	090	C+ M
22326		Treat neck spine fracture	20.84	NA	17.05	6.92	NA	NA	44.81	$1550.70	090	C+ M
22327		Treat thorax spine fracture	20.77	NA	18.03	6.65	NA	NA	45.45	$1572.85	090	C+ M
22328		Treat each add spine fx	4.60	NA	2.25	1.43	NA	NA	8.28	$286.54	ZZZ	C+
22505		Manipulation of spine	1.87	NA	1.57	0.39	NA	NA	3.83	$132.54	010	A M
22510		Perq cervicothoracic inject	7.90	47.24	3.75	1.00	56.14	$1942.79	12.65	$437.77	010	A M
22511		Perq lumbosacral injection	7.33	47.76	3.63	0.96	56.05	$1939.68	11.92	$412.51	010	A M
22512		Vertebroplasty addl inject	4.00	17.90	1.42	0.64	22.54	$780.02	6.06	$209.71	ZZZ	A
22513		Perq vertebral augmentation	8.65	169.35	4.81	1.55	179.55	$6213.54	15.01	$519.44	010	A M
22514		Perq vertebral augmentation	7.99	169.26	4.56	1.42	178.67	$6183.09	13.97	$483.45	010	A M
22515		Perq vertebral augmentation	4.00	87.68	1.65	0.77	92.45	$3199.34	6.42	$222.17	ZZZ	A
22526	§	Idet single level	5.85	55.69	3.24	0.47	62.01	$2145.93	9.56	$330.84	010	
22527	§	Idet 1 or more levels	3.03	47.97	1.17	0.25	51.25	$1773.57	4.45	$154.00	ZZZ	
22532		Arthrd lat xtrcvtry tq thrc	25.99	NA	19.36	8.16	NA	NA	53.51	$1851.78	090	C M
22533		Arthrd lat xtrcvtry tq lmbr	24.79	NA	18.16	6.11	NA	NA	49.06	$1697.78	090	C M
22534		Arthrd lat xtrcvtry tq ea ad	5.99	NA	2.94	1.66	NA	NA	10.59	$366.48	ZZZ	C
22548		Arthrd ant toral/xoral c1-c2	27.06	NA	20.91	10.37	NA	NA	58.34	$2018.93	090	C M

22551	Arthrd ant ntrbdy cervical	25.00	NA	17.63	7.87	NA	NA	50.50	$1747.61	090	C M
22552	Arthrd ant ntrbd cervical ea	6.50	NA	3.18	2.01	NA	NA	11.69	$404.55	ZZZ	C
22554	Arthrd ant ntrbd min dsc crv	17.69	NA	14.26	5.43	NA	NA	37.38	$1293.58	090	C M
22556	Arthrd ant ntrbd min dsc thc	24.70	NA	17.58	7.13	NA	NA	49.41	$1709.89	090	C M
22558	Arthrd ant ntrbd min dsc lum	23.53	NA	15.57	6.24	NA	NA	45.34	$1569.05	090	C M
22585	Arthrd ant ntrbd min dsc ea	5.52	NA	2.54	1.54	NA	NA	9.60	$332.22	ZZZ	C
22586	Arthrd pre-sac ntrbdy l5-s1	28.12	NA	21.46	10.78	NA	NA	60.36	$2088.83	090	C M
22590	Arthrd pst tq craniocervical	21.76	NA	17.84	7.51	NA	NA	47.11	$1630.30	090	C M
22595	Arthrd pst tq atlas-axis	20.64	NA	17.29	7.10	NA	NA	45.03	$1558.32	090	C M
22600	Arthrd pst tq 1ntrspc crv	17.40	NA	15.51	5.69	NA	NA	38.60	$1335.80	090	C M
22610	Arthrd pst tq 1ntrspc thrc	17.28	NA	15.27	5.38	NA	NA	37.93	$1312.61	090	C M
22612	Arthrd pst tq 1ntrspc lumbar	23.53	NA	17.02	6.51	NA	NA	47.06	$1628.57	090	C M
22614	Arthrd pst tq 1ntrspc ea add	6.43	NA	3.16	1.94	NA	NA	11.53	$399.01	ZZZ	C
22630	Arthrd pst tq 1ntrspc lum	22.09	NA	17.52	7.35	NA	NA	46.96	$1625.11	090	C M
22632	Arthrd pst tq 1ntrspc lm ea	5.22	NA	2.54	1.70	NA	NA	9.46	$327.37	ZZZ	C
22633	Arthrd cmbn 1ntrspc lumbar	27.75	NA	18.90	8.24	NA	NA	54.89	$1899.53	090	C M
22634	Arthrd cmbn 1ntrspc ea addl	8.16	NA	4.01	2.47	NA	NA	14.64	$506.63	ZZZ	C
22800	Arthrd pst dfrm<6 vrt sgm	19.50	NA	15.64	5.15	NA	NA	40.29	$1394.28	090	C+ M
22802	Arthrd pst dfrm 7-12 vrt sgm	32.11	NA	21.91	8.70	NA	NA	62.72	$2170.50	090	C+ M
22804	Arthrd pst dfrm 13+ vrt sgm	37.50	NA	24.62	9.83	NA	NA	71.95	$2489.92	090	C+ M
22808	Arthrd ant dfrm 2-3 vrt sgm	27.51	NA	19.13	7.53	NA	NA	54.17	$1874.62	090	C+ M
22810	Arthrd ant dfrm 4-7 vrt sgm	31.50	NA	21.44	6.50	NA	NA	59.44	$2056.99	090	C+ M
22812	Arthrd ant dfrm 8+ vrt sgm	34.25	NA	23.80	7.07	NA	NA	65.12	$2253.56	090	C+ M
22818	Kyphectomy 1-2 segments	34.33	NA	22.21	7.08	NA	NA	63.62	$2201.65	090	C M T
22819	Kyphectomy 3 or more	39.38	NA	25.73	8.12	NA	NA	73.23	$2534.21	090	C M T
22830	Exploration of spinal fusion	11.22	NA	9.99	3.22	NA	NA	24.43	$845.43	090	C+ M
22840	Insert spine fixation device	12.52	NA	6.16	3.70	NA	NA	22.38	$774.49	ZZZ	C+
22842	Insert spine fixation device	12.56	NA	6.17	3.77	NA	NA	22.50	$778.64	ZZZ	C

*Please note that these calculations are based on the Medicare 2022 Conversion Factor of $34.6062 and the DRA RVU cap rates at time of publication.

A = assistant-at-surgery restriction

A+ = assistant-at-surgery restriction unless medical necessity established with documentation

B = bilateral surgery adjustment applies

C = cosurgeons payable

C+ = cosurgeons payable if medical necessity established with documentation

CP = carriers may establish RVUs and payment amounts for these services, generally on an individual basis following review of documentation such as an operative report

M = multiple surgery adjustment applies

Me = multiple endoscopy rules may apply

M+ = multiple therapy rules apply

Mtc = multiple diagnostic imaging rules apply

T = team surgeons permitted

T+ = team surgeons payable if medical necessity established with documentation

§ = indicates code is not covered by Medicare

GS = procedure must be performed under the general supervision of a physician

DS = procedure must be performed under the direct supervision of a physician

PS = procedure must be performed under the personal supervision of a physician

DRA = procedure subject to DRA limitation

Relative Value Units

CPT Code and Modifier		Description	Work RVU	Nonfacility Practice Expense RVU	Facility Practice Expense RVU	PLI RVU	Total Non-facility RVUs	Medicare Payment Nonfacility	Total Facility RVUs	Medicare Payment Facility	Global Period	Payment Policy Indicators
22843		Insert spine fixation device	13.44	NA	6.61	4.01	NA	NA	24.06	$832.63	ZZZ	C
22844		Insert spine fixation device	16.42	NA	8.15	4.45	NA	NA	29.02	$1004.27	ZZZ	C
22845		Insert spine fixation device	11.94	NA	5.83	3.69	NA	NA	21.46	$742.65	ZZZ	C
22846		Insert spine fixation device	12.40	NA	6.07	3.84	NA	NA	22.31	$772.06	ZZZ	C
22847		Insert spine fixation device	13.78	NA	6.98	2.85	NA	NA	23.61	$817.05	ZZZ	C
22848		Insert pelv fixation device	5.99	NA	2.97	1.64	NA	NA	10.60	$366.83	ZZZ	C
22849		Reinsert spinal fixation	19.17	NA	14.12	5.50	NA	NA	38.79	$1342.37	090	C+ M
22850		Remove spine fixation device	9.82	NA	9.24	2.85	NA	NA	21.91	$758.22	090	C+ M
22852		Remove spine fixation device	9.37	NA	8.99	2.68	NA	NA	21.04	$728.11	090	C+ M
22853		Insj biomechanical device	4.25	NA	2.08	1.28	NA	NA	7.61	$263.35	ZZZ	C
22854		Insj biomechanical device	5.50	NA	2.68	1.70	NA	NA	9.88	$341.91	ZZZ	C
22855		Remove spine fixation device	15.86	NA	12.38	4.67	NA	NA	32.91	$1138.89	090	C+ M
22856		Tot disc arthrp ant 1ntrspc	24.05	NA	17.06	7.25	NA	NA	48.36	$1673.56	090	C M
22857		Tot disc arthrp ant lumbar	27.13	NA	19.55	5.59	NA	NA	52.27	$1808.87	090	C M
22858		Tot disc arthrp ant 2nd lvl	8.40	NA	4.13	2.40	NA	NA	14.93	$516.67	ZZZ	C
22859		Insj biomechanical device	5.50	NA	2.70	1.62	NA	NA	9.82	$339.83	ZZZ	C
22861		Revise cerv artific disc	33.36	NA	22.64	12.78	NA	NA	68.78	$2380.21	090	C M
22862		Revise lumbar artif disc	32.63	NA	23.61	12.51	NA	NA	68.75	$2379.18	090	C M T
22864		Remove cerv artif disc	29.40	NA	20.74	11.28	NA	NA	61.42	$2125.51	090	C M
22865		Remove lumb artif disc	31.75	NA	23.19	12.18	NA	NA	67.12	$2322.77	090	C M T
22867		Insj stablj dev w/dcmprn	15.00	NA	12.35	4.55	NA	NA	31.90	$1103.94	090	M
22868		Insj stablj dev w/dcmprn	4.00	NA	1.93	1.25	NA	NA	7.18	$248.47	ZZZ	C
22869		Insj stablj dev w/o dcmprn	7.03	NA	5.07	0.72	NA	NA	12.82	$443.65	090	M
22870		Insj stablj dev w/o dcmprn	2.34	NA	0.92	0.24	NA	NA	3.50	$121.12	ZZZ	C
22899	CP	Spine surgery procedure	0.00	0.00	0.00	0.00	0.00	$0.00	0.00	$0.00	YYY	C+ M T+
22900		Exc abdl tum deep < 5 cm	8.32	NA	6.64	1.90	NA	NA	16.86	$583.46	090	C+ M
22901		Exc abdl tum deep 5 cm/>	10.11	NA	7.44	2.39	NA	NA	19.94	$690.05	090	C+ M
22902		Exc abd les sc < 3 cm	4.42	8.81	4.49	1.04	14.27	$493.83	9.95	$344.33	090	C+ M
22903		Exc abd les sc 3 cm/>	6.39	NA	5.24	1.52	NA	NA	13.15	$455.07	090	C+ M
22904		Radical resect abd tumor<5cm	16.69	NA	10.83	3.85	NA	NA	31.37	$1085.60	090	C+ M T+
22905		Rad resect abd tumor 5 cm/>	21.58	NA	12.88	4.99	NA	NA	39.45	$1365.21	090	C+ M T+
22999	CP	Abdomen surgery procedure	0.00	0.00	0.00	0.00	0.00	$0.00	0.00	$0.00	YYY	A+ C+ M T+
23000		Removal of calcium deposits	4.48	11.94	5.63	0.89	17.31	$599.03	11.00	$380.67	090	B C+ M

23020	Release shoulder joint	9.36	NA	9.33	1.86	NA	NA	20.55	$711.16	090	B M
23030	Drain shoulder lesion	3.47	9.13	3.40	0.72	13.32	$460.95	7.59	$262.66	010	A M
23031	Drain shoulder bursa	2.79	9.44	3.15	0.57	12.80	$442.96	6.51	$225.29	010	A B M
23035	Drain shoulder bone lesion	9.16	NA	9.32	1.87	NA	NA	20.35	$704.24	090	B M
23040	Exploratory shoulder surgery	9.75	NA	9.70	1.98	NA	NA	21.43	$741.61	090	B C+ M
23044	Exploratory shoulder surgery	7.59	NA	7.76	1.55	NA	NA	16.90	$584.84	090	A B C+ M
23065	Biopsy shoulder tissues	2.30	4.14	2.11	0.33	6.77	$234.28	4.74	$164.03	010	A B M
23066	Biopsy shoulder tissues	4.30	11.75	5.66	0.89	16.94	$586.23	10.85	$375.48	090	A B M
23071	Exc shoulder les sc 3 cm/>	5.91	NA	5.27	1.36	NA	NA	12.54	$433.96	090	B M
23073	Exc shoulder tum deep 5 cm/>	10.13	NA	8.36	2.26	NA	NA	20.75	$718.08	090	B M
23075	Exc shoulder les sc < 3 cm	4.21	10.58	4.70	0.90	15.69	$542.97	9.81	$339.49	090	A B M
23076	Exc shoulder tum deep < 5 cm	7.41	NA	7.15	1.64	NA	NA	16.20	$560.62	090	A B M
23077	Resect shoulder tumor < 5 cm	17.66	NA	11.72	4.23	NA	NA	33.61	$1163.11	090	B C+ M
23078	Resect shoulder tumor 5 cm/>	22.55	NA	14.85	5.06	NA	NA	42.46	$1469.38	090	B C+ M
23100	Biopsy of shoulder joint	6.20	NA	7.64	1.28	NA	NA	15.12	$523.25	090	B C+ M
23101	Shoulder joint surgery	5.72	NA	6.76	1.18	NA	NA	13.66	$472.72	090	A B C+ M
23105	Remove shoulder joint lining	8.48	NA	8.90	1.70	NA	NA	19.08	$660.29	090	B C+ M
23106	Incision of collarbone joint	6.13	NA	7.61	1.27	NA	NA	15.01	$519.44	090	A B C+ M
23107	Explore treat shoulder joint	8.87	NA	9.04	1.78	NA	NA	19.69	$681.40	090	B C+ M
23120	Partial removal collar bone	7.39	NA	8.63	1.49	NA	NA	17.51	$605.95	090	B C+ M
23125	Removal of collar bone	9.64	NA	9.53	1.99	NA	NA	21.16	$732.27	090	B C+ M
23130	Remove shoulder bone part	7.77	NA	9.11	1.60	NA	NA	18.48	$639.52	090	A B C+ M
23140	Removal of bone lesion	7.12	NA	7.99	1.47	NA	NA	16.58	$573.77	090	A B M
23145	Removal of bone lesion	9.40	NA	9.42	1.94	NA	NA	20.76	$718.42	090	B C+ M
23146	Removal of bone lesion	8.08	NA	8.86	1.66	NA	NA	18.60	$643.68	090	A+ B M
23150	Removal of humerus lesion	8.91	NA	9.03	1.80	NA	NA	19.74	$683.13	090	B C+ M
23155	Removal of humerus lesion	10.86	NA	10.67	2.23	NA	NA	23.76	$822.24	090	B C+ M
23156	Removal of humerus lesion	9.11	NA	9.27	1.86	NA	NA	20.24	$700.43	090	B M

*Please note that these calculations are based on the Medicare 2022 Conversion Factor of $34.6062 and the DRA RVU cap rates at time of publication.

A = assistant-at-surgery restriction
A+ = assistant-at-surgery restriction unless medical necessity established with documentation
B = bilateral surgery adjustment applies
C = cosurgeons payable
C+ = cosurgeons payable if medical necessity established with documentation
CP = carriers may establish RVUs and payment amounts for these services, generally on an individual basis following review of documentation such as an operative report
M = multiple surgery adjustment applies
Me = multiple endoscopy rules may apply
M+ = multiple therapy rules apply
Mtc = multiple diagnostic imaging rules apply
T = team surgeons permitted
T+ = team surgeons payable if medical necessity established with documentation
§ = indicates code is not covered by Medicare
GS = procedure must be performed under the general supervision of a physician
DS = procedure must be performed under the direct supervision of a physician
PS = procedure must be performed under the personal supervision of a physician
DRA = procedure subject to DRA limitation

Relative Value Units

CPT Code and Modifier	Description	Work RVU	Nonfacility Practice Expense RVU	Facility Practice Expense RVU	PLI RVU	Total Non-facility RVUs	Medicare Payment Nonfacility	Total Facility RVUs	Medicare Payment Facility	Global Period	Payment Policy Indicators
23170	Remove collar bone lesion	7.21	NA	8.16	1.48	NA	NA	16.85	$583.11	090	A B M
23172	Remove shoulder blade lesion	7.31	NA	8.21	1.50	NA	NA	17.02	$589.00	090	B M
23174	Remove humerus lesion	10.05	NA	10.64	2.07	NA	NA	22.76	$787.64	090	B C+ M
23180	Remove collar bone lesion	8.99	NA	8.92	1.94	NA	NA	19.85	$686.93	090	A B C+ M
23182	Remove shoulder blade lesion	8.61	NA	9.65	1.78	NA	NA	20.04	$693.51	090	B M
23184	Remove humerus lesion	9.90	NA	10.13	1.98	NA	NA	22.01	$761.68	090	B C+ M
23190	Partial removal of scapula	7.47	NA	8.17	1.53	NA	NA	17.17	$594.19	090	B C+ M
23195	Removal of head of humerus	10.36	NA	9.73	2.01	NA	NA	22.10	$764.80	090	B C+ M
23200	Resect clavicle tumor	22.71	NA	17.16	4.67	NA	NA	44.54	$1541.36	090	B C+ M
23210	Resect scapula tumor	27.21	NA	19.44	5.60	NA	NA	52.25	$1808.17	090	B C+ M
23220	Resect prox humerus tumor	30.21	NA	20.91	6.23	NA	NA	57.35	$1984.67	090	B C+ M
23330	Remove shoulder foreign body	1.90	6.78	2.66	0.39	9.07	$313.88	4.95	$171.30	010	A+ B M
23333	Remove shoulder fb deep	6.00	NA	6.85	1.24	NA	NA	14.09	$487.60	090	A+ B M
23334	Shoulder prosthesis removal	15.50	NA	12.95	3.02	NA	NA	31.47	$1089.06	090	A B C+ M
23335	Shoulder prosthesis removal	19.00	NA	14.77	3.76	NA	NA	37.53	$1298.77	090	A B C+ M
23350	Injection for shoulder x-ray	1.00	3.98	0.37	0.09	5.07	$175.45	1.46	$50.53	000	A B M
23395	Muscle transfer shoulder/arm	18.54	NA	15.73	3.63	NA	NA	37.90	$1311.57	090	C+ M
23397	Muscle transfers	16.76	NA	13.57	3.41	NA	NA	33.74	$1167.61	090	C+ M
23400	Fixation of shoulder blade	13.87	NA	12.19	2.85	NA	NA	28.91	$1000.47	090	B C+ M
23405	Incision of tendon & muscle	8.54	NA	8.33	1.57	NA	NA	18.44	$638.14	090	C+ M
23406	Incise tendon(s) & muscle(s)	11.01	NA	9.28	1.84	NA	NA	22.13	$765.84	090	M
23410	Repair rotator cuff acute	11.39	NA	10.70	2.29	NA	NA	24.38	$843.70	090	B C+ M
23412	Repair rotator cuff chronic	11.93	NA	11.00	2.40	NA	NA	25.33	$876.58	090	B C+ M
23415	Release of shoulder ligament	9.23	NA	9.69	1.90	NA	NA	20.82	$720.50	090	A B C+ M
23420	Repair of shoulder	13.54	NA	12.63	2.78	NA	NA	28.95	$1001.85	090	B C+ M
23430	Repair biceps tendon	10.17	NA	9.98	2.01	NA	NA	22.16	$766.87	090	B C+ M
23440	Remove/transplant tendon	10.64	NA	9.71	2.17	NA	NA	22.52	$779.33	090	B C+ M
23450	Repair shoulder capsule	13.70	NA	11.60	2.83	NA	NA	28.13	$973.47	090	B C+ M
23455	Repair shoulder capsule	14.67	NA	11.88	2.94	NA	NA	29.49	$1020.54	090	B C+ M
23460	Repair shoulder capsule	15.82	NA	13.30	3.27	NA	NA	32.39	$1120.89	090	B C+ M
23462	Repair shoulder capsule	15.72	NA	12.73	3.24	NA	NA	31.69	$1096.67	090	B C+ M
23465	Repair shoulder capsule	16.30	NA	13.55	3.38	NA	NA	33.23	$1149.96	090	B C+ M
23466	Repair shoulder capsule	15.80	NA	14.23	3.22	NA	NA	33.25	$1150.66	090	B C+ M

23470	Reconstruct shoulder joint	17.89	NA	14.11	3.55	NA	NA	35.55	$1230.25	090	B C+ M
23472	Reconstruct shoulder joint	22.13	NA	16.31	4.39	NA	NA	42.83	$1482.18	090	B C+ M
23473	Revis reconst shoulder joint	25.00	NA	17.75	4.97	NA	NA	47.72	$1651.41	090	B C+ M
23474	Revis reconst shoulder joint	27.21	NA	18.88	5.40	NA	NA	51.49	$1781.87	090	B C+ M
23480	Revision of collar bone	11.54	NA	10.50	2.37	NA	NA	24.41	$844.74	090	A B C+ M
23485	Revision of collar bone	13.91	NA	11.54	2.79	NA	NA	28.24	$977.28	090	B C+ M
23490	Reinforce clavicle	12.16	NA	10.94	2.50	NA	NA	25.60	$885.92	090	B M
23491	Reinforce shoulder bones	14.54	NA	12.65	3.00	NA	NA	30.19	$1044.76	090	B C+ M
23500	Treat clavicle fracture	2.21	4.06	4.20	0.42	6.69	$231.52	6.83	$236.36	090	A B M
23505	Treat clavicle fracture	3.83	6.23	5.46	0.77	10.83	$374.79	10.06	$348.14	090	A B M
23515	Treat clavicle fracture	9.69	NA	9.80	1.94	NA	NA	21.43	$741.61	090	B C+ M
23520	Treat clavicle dislocation	2.29	4.51	4.41	0.45	7.25	$250.89	7.15	$247.43	090	A+ B M
23525	Treat clavicle dislocation	3.79	7.35	6.34	0.77	11.91	$412.16	10.90	$377.21	090	A+ B M
23530	Treat clavicle dislocation	7.48	NA	8.18	1.54	NA	NA	17.20	$595.23	090	B M
23532	Treat clavicle dislocation	8.20	NA	8.81	1.68	NA	NA	18.69	$646.79	090	B M
23540	Treat clavicle dislocation	2.36	4.36	4.25	0.47	7.19	$248.82	7.08	$245.01	090	A B M
23545	Treat clavicle dislocation	3.43	6.42	5.34	0.73	10.58	$366.13	9.50	$328.76	090	A+ B M
23550	Treat clavicle dislocation	7.59	NA	8.01	1.47	NA	NA	17.07	$590.73	090	B C+ M
23552	Treat clavicle dislocation	8.82	NA	8.95	1.73	NA	NA	19.50	$674.82	090	B C+ M
23570	Treat shoulder blade fx	2.36	4.26	4.47	0.45	7.07	$244.67	7.28	$251.93	090	A B M
23575	Treat shoulder blade fx	4.23	7.24	6.30	0.89	12.36	$427.73	11.42	$395.20	090	A+ B M
23585	Treat scapula fracture	14.23	NA	11.99	2.85	NA	NA	29.07	$1006.00	090	B C+ M
23600	Treat humerus fracture	3.00	6.44	5.91	0.60	10.04	$347.45	9.51	$329.10	090	A B M
23605	Treat humerus fracture	5.06	8.04	6.74	1.02	14.12	$488.64	12.82	$443.65	090	A B M
23615	Treat humerus fracture	12.30	NA	11.47	2.49	NA	NA	26.26	$908.76	090	B C+ M
23616	Treat humerus fracture	18.37	NA	14.53	3.70	NA	NA	36.60	$1266.59	090	B C M
23620	Treat humerus fracture	2.55	5.10	4.78	0.51	8.16	$282.39	7.84	$271.31	090	A B M
23625	Treat humerus fracture	4.10	6.63	5.65	0.84	11.57	$400.39	10.59	$366.48	090	A B M

*Please note that these calculations are based on the Medicare 2022 Conversion Factor of $34.6062 and the DRA RVU cap rates at time of publication.

A = assistant-at-surgery restriction
A+ = assistant-at-surgery restriction unless medical necessity established with documentation
B = bilateral surgery adjustment applies
C = cosurgeons payable
C+ = cosurgeons payable if medical necessity established with documentation
CP = carriers may establish RVUs and payment amounts for these services, generally on an individual basis following review of documentation such as an operative report
M = multiple surgery adjustment applies
Me = multiple endoscopy rules may apply
M+ = multiple therapy rules apply
Mtc = multiple diagnostic imaging rules apply
T = team surgeons permitted
T+ = team surgeons payable if medical necessity established with documentation
§ = indicates code is not covered by Medicare
GS = procedure must be performed under the general supervision of a physician
DS = procedure must be performed under the direct supervision of a physician
PS = procedure must be performed under the personal supervision of a physician
DRA = procedure subject to DRA limitation

Relative Value Units

CPT Code and Modifier		Description	Work RVU	Nonfacility Practice Expense RVU	Facility Practice Expense RVU	PLI RVU	Total Non-facility RVUs	Medicare Payment Nonfacility	Total Facility RVUs	Medicare Payment Facility	Global Period	Payment Policy Indicators
23630		Treat humerus fracture	10.57	NA	10.50	2.09	NA	NA	23.16	$801.48	090	B C+ M
23650		Treat shoulder dislocation	3.53	5.58	4.63	0.73	9.84	$340.53	8.89	$307.65	090	A B M
23655		Treat shoulder dislocation	4.76	NA	6.56	0.95	NA	NA	12.27	$424.62	090	A B M
23660		Treat shoulder dislocation	7.66	NA	8.25	1.52	NA	NA	17.43	$603.19	090	B C+ M
23665		Treat dislocation/fracture	4.66	7.43	6.40	0.95	13.04	$451.26	12.01	$415.62	090	A B M
23670		Treat dislocation/fracture	12.28	NA	11.16	2.38	NA	NA	25.82	$893.53	090	B C+ M
23675		Treat dislocation/fracture	6.27	9.03	7.48	1.25	16.55	$572.73	15.00	$519.09	090	A B M
23680		Treat dislocation/fracture	13.15	NA	11.74	2.66	NA	NA	27.55	$953.40	090	B C+ M
23700		Fixation of shoulder	2.57	NA	2.75	0.51	NA	NA	5.83	$201.75	010	A B M
23800		Fusion of shoulder joint	14.73	NA	12.75	3.02	NA	NA	30.50	$1055.49	090	B C+ M
23802		Fusion of shoulder joint	18.42	NA	15.80	3.80	NA	NA	38.02	$1315.73	090	B C+ M
23900		Amputation of arm & girdle	20.72	NA	16.05	4.26	NA	NA	41.03	$1419.89	090	M
23920		Amputation at shoulder joint	16.23	NA	13.72	3.35	NA	NA	33.30	$1152.39	090	B C+ M
23921		Amputation follow-up surgery	5.72	NA	7.15	1.18	NA	NA	14.05	$486.22	090	A B M
23929	CP	Shoulder surgery procedure	0.00	0.00	0.00	0.00	0.00	$0.00	0.00	$0.00	YYY	C+ M T+
23930		Drainage of arm lesion	2.99	7.30	2.79	0.62	10.91	$377.55	6.40	$221.48	010	A B M
23931		Drainage of arm bursa	1.84	6.98	2.58	0.34	9.16	$316.99	4.76	$164.73	010	A B M
23935		Drain arm/elbow bone lesion	6.38	NA	7.58	1.25	NA	NA	15.21	$526.36	090	A+ B M
24000		Exploratory elbow surgery	6.08	NA	6.84	1.21	NA	NA	14.13	$488.99	090	A+ B C+ M
24006		Release elbow joint	9.74	NA	9.62	1.85	NA	NA	21.21	$734.00	090	B C M
24065		Biopsy arm/elbow soft tissue	2.13	5.40	2.40	0.31	7.84	$271.31	4.84	$167.49	010	A B M
24066		Biopsy arm/elbow soft tissue	5.35	12.13	5.98	1.16	18.64	$645.06	12.49	$432.23	090	A B M
24071		Exc arm/elbow les sc 3 cm/>	5.70	NA	5.12	1.29	NA	NA	12.11	$419.08	090	B M
24073		Ex arm/elbow tum deep 5 cm/>	10.13	NA	8.30	2.20	NA	NA	20.63	$713.93	090	B M
24075		Exc arm/elbow les sc < 3 cm	4.24	11.05	4.69	0.90	16.19	$560.27	9.83	$340.18	090	A B M
24076		Ex arm/elbow tum deep < 5 cm	7.41	NA	7.29	1.55	NA	NA	16.25	$562.35	090	A B M
24077		Resect arm/elbow tum < 5 cm	15.72	NA	11.51	3.45	NA	NA	30.68	$1061.72	090	A B C+ M
24079		Resect arm/elbow tum 5 cm/>	20.61	NA	14.07	4.61	NA	NA	39.29	$1359.68	090	B C+ M
24100		Biopsy elbow joint lining	5.07	NA	6.44	1.04	NA	NA	12.55	$434.31	090	B C+ M
24101		Explore/treat elbow joint	6.30	NA	7.53	1.22	NA	NA	15.05	$520.82	090	B M
24102		Remove elbow joint lining	8.26	NA	8.59	1.61	NA	NA	18.46	$638.83	090	B C+ M
24105		Removal of elbow bursa	3.78	NA	6.22	0.75	NA	NA	10.75	$372.02	090	A B M
24110		Remove humerus lesion	7.58	NA	8.49	1.55	NA	NA	17.62	$609.76	090	A B C+ M

24115	Remove/graft bone lesion	10.12	NA	9.77	2.08	NA	NA	21.97	$760.30	090	B C+ M
24116	Remove/graft bone lesion	12.23	NA	10.85	2.51	NA	NA	25.59	$885.57	090	B M
24120	Remove elbow lesion	6.82	NA	7.76	1.33	NA	NA	15.91	$550.58	090	A+ B M
24125	Remove/graft bone lesion	8.14	NA	8.78	1.68	NA	NA	18.60	$643.68	090	B C+ M
24126	Remove/graft bone lesion	8.62	NA	9.02	1.78	NA	NA	19.42	$672.05	090	B M
24130	Removal of head of radius	6.42	NA	7.58	1.22	NA	NA	15.22	$526.71	090	A B C+ M
24134	Removal of arm bone lesion	10.22	NA	9.94	2.11	NA	NA	22.27	$770.68	090	B M
24136	Remove radius bone lesion	8.40	NA	8.76	1.72	NA	NA	18.88	$653.37	090	A B M
24138	Remove elbow bone lesion	8.50	NA	10.26	1.75	NA	NA	20.51	$709.77	090	B M
24140	Partial removal of arm bone	9.55	NA	9.51	1.90	NA	NA	20.96	$725.35	090	B M
24145	Partial removal of radius	7.81	NA	8.34	1.61	NA	NA	17.76	$614.61	090	A B C+ M
24147	Partial removal of elbow	7.84	NA	9.38	1.54	NA	NA	18.76	$649.21	090	A B C+ M
24149	Radical resection of elbow	16.22	NA	15.60	3.11	NA	NA	34.93	$1208.79	090	B C+ M
24150	Resect distal humerus tumor	23.46	NA	17.43	4.84	NA	NA	45.73	$1582.54	090	B C+ M
24152	Resect radius tumor	19.99	NA	15.66	4.12	NA	NA	39.77	$1376.29	090	B C+ M
24155	Removal of elbow joint	12.09	NA	10.77	2.49	NA	NA	25.35	$877.27	090	B C+ M
24160	Remove elbow joint implant	18.63	NA	14.86	3.58	NA	NA	37.07	$1282.85	090	A B C+ M
24164	Remove radius head implant	10.00	NA	9.51	2.06	NA	NA	21.57	$746.46	090	A B C+ M
24200	Removal of arm foreign body	1.81	4.46	2.07	0.32	6.59	$228.05	4.20	$145.35	010	A+ B M
24201	Removal of arm foreign body	4.70	10.76	5.20	1.02	16.48	$570.31	10.92	$377.90	090	A B M
24220	Injection for elbow x-ray	1.31	4.40	0.51	0.12	5.83	$201.75	1.94	$67.14	000	A+ B M
24300	Manipulate elbow w/anesth	4.04	NA	8.21	0.77	NA	NA	13.02	$450.57	090	A B M
24301	Muscle/tendon transfer	10.38	NA	9.87	2.09	NA	NA	22.34	$773.10	090	C+ M
24305	Arm tendon lengthening	7.62	NA	8.24	1.41	NA	NA	17.27	$597.65	090	A+ M
24310	Revision of arm tendon	6.12	NA	6.92	1.18	NA	NA	14.22	$492.10	090	A+ M
24320	Repair of arm tendon	10.86	NA	10.14	2.23	NA	NA	23.23	$803.90	090	C+ M
24330	Revision of arm muscles	9.79	NA	9.60	2.01	NA	NA	21.40	$740.57	090	B M
24331	Revision of arm muscles	10.95	NA	10.19	2.25	NA	NA	23.39	$809.44	090	B M

*Please note that these calculations are based on the Medicare 2022 Conversion Factor of $34.6062 and the DRA RVU cap rates at time of publication.

A = assistant-at-surgery restriction
A+ = assistant-at-surgery restriction unless medical necessity established with documentation
B = bilateral surgery adjustment applies
C = cosurgeons payable
C+ = cosurgeons payable if medical necessity established with documentation
CP = carriers may establish RVUs and payment amounts for these services, generally on an individual basis following review of documentation such as an operative report
M = multiple surgery adjustment applies
Me = multiple endoscopy rules may apply
M+ = multiple therapy rules apply
Mtc = multiple diagnostic imaging rules apply
T = team surgeons permitted
T+ = team surgeons payable if medical necessity established with documentation
§ = indicates code is not covered by Medicare
GS = procedure must be performed under the general supervision of a physician
DS = procedure must be performed under the direct supervision of a physician
PS = procedure must be performed under the personal supervision of a physician
DRA = procedure subject to DRA limitation

Relative Value Units

CPT Code and Modifier	Description	Work RVU	Nonfacility Practice Expense RVU	Facility Practice Expense RVU	PLI RVU	Total Non-facility RVUs	Medicare Payment Nonfacility	Total Facility RVUs	Medicare Payment Facility	Global Period	Payment Policy Indicators
24332	Tenolysis triceps	7.91	NA	8.83	1.63	NA	NA	18.37	$635.72	090	A B M
24340	Repair of biceps tendon	8.08	NA	8.73	1.64	NA	NA	18.45	$638.48	090	B C+ M
24341	Repair arm tendon/muscle	9.49	NA	10.82	1.84	NA	NA	22.15	$766.53	090	B C+ M
24342	Repair of ruptured tendon	10.86	NA	10.08	2.13	NA	NA	23.07	$798.37	090	B C+ M
24343	Repr elbow lat ligmnt w/tiss	9.16	NA	10.33	1.78	NA	NA	21.27	$736.07	090	B C+ M
24344	Reconstruct elbow lat ligmnt	15.21	NA	14.30	2.98	NA	NA	32.49	$1124.36	090	B C+ M
24345	Repr elbw med ligmnt w/tissu	9.16	NA	10.21	1.80	NA	NA	21.17	$732.61	090	B C+ M
24346	Reconstruct elbow med ligmnt	15.21	NA	14.45	3.13	NA	NA	32.79	$1134.74	090	B C+ M
24357	Repair elbow perc	5.44	NA	6.33	0.73	NA	NA	12.50	$432.58	090	A+ B M
24358	Repair elbow w/deb open	6.66	NA	7.85	1.28	NA	NA	15.79	$546.43	090	A+ B M
24359	Repair elbow deb/attch open	8.98	NA	9.03	1.72	NA	NA	19.73	$682.78	090	A+ B M
24360	Reconstruct elbow joint	12.67	NA	11.58	2.62	NA	NA	26.87	$929.87	090	B C+ M
24361	Reconstruct elbow joint	14.41	NA	12.57	2.98	NA	NA	29.96	$1036.80	090	B C+ M
24362	Reconstruct elbow joint	15.32	NA	13.03	3.17	NA	NA	31.52	$1090.79	090	B M
24363	Replace elbow joint	22.00	NA	16.54	4.28	NA	NA	42.82	$1481.84	090	B M
24365	Reconstruct head of radius	8.62	NA	8.74	1.78	NA	NA	19.14	$662.36	090	B C+ M
24366	Reconstruct head of radius	9.36	NA	9.12	1.82	NA	NA	20.30	$702.51	090	B C+ M
24370	Revise reconst elbow joint	23.55	NA	17.38	4.57	NA	NA	45.50	$1574.58	090	B M
24371	Revise reconst elbow joint	27.50	NA	19.42	5.35	NA	NA	52.27	$1808.87	090	B M
24400	Revision of humerus	11.33	NA	10.95	2.28	NA	NA	24.56	$849.93	090	B C+ M
24410	Revision of humerus	15.11	NA	13.20	3.12	NA	NA	31.43	$1087.67	090	B C+ M
24420	Revision of humerus	13.73	NA	15.27	2.84	NA	NA	31.84	$1101.86	090	B C+ M
24430	Repair of humerus	15.25	NA	13.01	3.04	NA	NA	31.30	$1083.17	090	B C+ M
24435	Repair humerus with graft	14.99	NA	14.05	3.02	NA	NA	32.06	$1109.47	090	B C+ M
24470	Revision of elbow joint	8.93	NA	9.29	1.84	NA	NA	20.06	$694.20	090	B M
24495	Decompression of forearm	8.41	NA	13.97	1.85	NA	NA	24.23	$838.51	090	A+ B M
24498	Reinforce humerus	12.28	NA	10.99	2.50	NA	NA	25.77	$891.80	090	B C+ M
24500	Treat humerus fracture	3.41	6.81	5.97	0.67	10.89	$376.86	10.05	$347.79	090	A B M
24505	Treat humerus fracture	5.39	8.65	7.10	1.10	15.14	$523.94	13.59	$470.30	090	A B M
24515	Treat humerus fracture	12.12	NA	11.64	2.45	NA	NA	26.21	$907.03	090	B C+ M
24516	Treat humerus fracture	12.19	NA	10.88	2.48	NA	NA	25.55	$884.19	090	B C M
24530	Treat humerus fracture	3.69	7.08	6.14	0.73	11.50	$397.97	10.56	$365.44	090	A B M
24535	Treat humerus fracture	7.11	10.00	8.49	1.43	18.54	$641.60	17.03	$589.34	090	A B M

24538	Treat humerus fracture	9.77	NA	11.86	2.01	NA	NA	23.64	$818.09	090	A B M
24545	Treat humerus fracturc	13.15	NA	11.77	2.66	NA	NA	27.58	$954.44	090	B C+ M
24546	Treat humerus fracture	14.91	NA	12.86	3.00	NA	NA	30.77	$1064.83	090	B C M
24560	Treat humerus fracture	2.98	6.45	5.30	0.60	10.03	$347.10	8.88	$307.30	090	A B M
24565	Treat humerus fracture	5.78	9.29	7.87	1.18	16.25	$562.35	14.83	$513.21	090	A B M
24566	Treat humerus fracture	9.06	NA	10.57	1.85	NA	NA	21.48	$743.34	090	A B M
24575	Treat humerus fracture	9.71	NA	10.15	1.94	NA	NA	21.80	$754.42	090	B C+ M
24576	Treat humerus fracture	3.06	6.92	5.77	0.60	10.58	$366.13	9.43	$326.34	090	A B M
24577	Treat humerus fracture	6.01	9.46	7.99	1.24	16.71	$578.27	15.24	$527.40	090	A B M
24579	Treat humerus fracture	11.44	NA	11.08	2.26	NA	NA	24.78	$857.54	090	B C+ M
24582	Treat humerus fracture	10.14	NA	12.09	2.09	NA	NA	24.32	$841.62	090	A B M
24586	Treat elbow fracture	15.78	NA	13.34	3.13	NA	NA	32.25	$1116.05	090	B C+ M
24587	Treat elbow fracture	15.79	NA	13.28	3.26	NA	NA	32.33	$1118.82	090	B C+ M
24600	Treat elbow dislocation	4.37	6.00	4.93	0.90	11.27	$390.01	10.20	$352.98	090	A B M
24605	Treat elbow dislocation	5.64	NA	7.57	1.12	NA	NA	14.33	$495.91	090	A B M
24615	Treat elbow dislocation	9.83	NA	9.48	1.94	NA	NA	21.25	$735.38	090	B C+ M
24620	Treat elbow fracture	7.22	NA	8.18	1.47	NA	NA	16.87	$583.81	090	A+ B M
24635	Treat elbow fracture	8.80	NA	9.57	1.73	NA	NA	20.10	$695.58	090	B C+ M
24640	Treat elbow dislocation	1.25	1.77	1.04	0.09	3.11	$107.63	2.38	$82.36	010	A+ B M
24650	Treat radius fracture	2.31	5.19	4.63	0.43	7.93	$274.43	7.37	$255.05	090	A B M
24655	Treat radius fracture	4.62	7.90	6.58	0.93	13.45	$465.45	12.13	$419.77	090	A B M
24665	Treat radius fracture	8.36	NA	9.61	1.64	NA	NA	19.61	$678.63	090	B C+ M
24666	Treat radius fracture	9.86	NA	9.99	1.94	NA	NA	21.79	$754.07	090	B C+ M
24670	Treat ulnar fracture	2.69	5.59	4.84	0.54	8.82	$305.23	8.07	$279.27	090	A B M
24675	Treat ulnar fracture	4.91	8.06	6.74	1.00	13.97	$483.45	12.65	$437.77	090	A B M
24685	Treat ulnar fracture	8.37	NA	9.45	1.66	NA	NA	19.48	$674.13	090	B C+ M
24800	Fusion of elbow joint	11.41	NA	11.06	2.34	NA	NA	24.81	$858.58	090	B C+ M
24802	Fusion/graft of elbow joint	14.32	NA	12.53	2.96	NA	NA	29.81	$1031.61	090	B M

*Please note that these calculations are based on the Medicare 2022 Conversion Factor of $34.6062 and the DRA RVU cap rates at time of publication.

A = assistant-at-surgery restriction

A+ = assistant-at-surgery restriction unless medical necessity established with documentation

B = bilateral surgery adjustment applies

C = cosurgeons payable

C+ = cosurgeons payable if medical necessity established with documentation

CP = carriers may establish RVUs and payment amounts for these services, generally on an individual basis following review of documentation such as an operative report

M = multiple surgery adjustment applies

Me = multiple endoscopy rules may apply

M+ = multiple therapy rules apply

Mtc = multiple diagnostic imaging rules apply

T = team surgeons permitted

T+ = team surgeons payable if medical necessity established with documentation

§ = indicates code is not covered by Medicare

GS = procedure must be performed under the general supervision of a physician

DS = procedure must be performed under the direct supervision of a physician

PS = procedure must be performed under the personal supervision of a physician

DRA = procedure subject to DRA limitation

Relative Value Units

CPT Code and Modifier		Description	Work RVU	Nonfacility Practice Expense RVU	Facility Practice Expense RVU	PLI RVU	Total Non-facility RVUs	Medicare Payment Nonfacility	Total Facility RVUs	Medicare Payment Facility	Global Period	Payment Policy Indicators
24900		Amputation of upper arm	10.18	NA	9.71	2.09	NA	NA	21.98	$760.64	090	B C+ M
24920		Amputation of upper arm	10.13	NA	9.62	2.08	NA	NA	21.83	$755.45	090	B C+ M
24925		Amputation follow-up surgery	7.30	NA	8.19	1.50	NA	NA	16.99	$587.96	090	B M
24930		Amputation follow-up surgery	10.83	NA	9.98	2.23	NA	NA	23.04	$797.33	090	B M
24931		Amputate upper arm & implant	13.44	NA	11.45	2.78	NA	NA	27.67	$957.55	090	B M
24935		Revision of amputation	16.45	NA	16.65	3.39	NA	NA	36.49	$1262.78	090	A+ B M
24940	CP	Revision of upper arm	0.00	0.00	0.00	0.00	0.00	$0.00	0.00	$0.00	090	B M
24999	CP	Upper arm/elbow surgery	0.00	0.00	0.00	0.00	0.00	$0.00	0.00	$0.00	YYY	A+ B C+ M T+
25000		Incision of tendon sheath	3.55	NA	6.09	0.66	NA	NA	10.30	$356.44	090	A B M
25001		Incise flexor carpi radialis	3.79	NA	5.87	0.68	NA	NA	10.34	$357.83	090	A B M
25020		Decompress forearm 1 space	6.06	NA	15.36	1.11	NA	NA	22.53	$779.68	090	A B M
25023		Decompress forearm 1 space	13.83	NA	23.04	2.79	NA	NA	39.66	$1372.48	090	A+ B M
25024		Decompress forearm 2 spaces	10.79	NA	10.32	2.17	NA	NA	23.28	$805.63	090	A B M
25025		Decompress forearm 2 spaces	17.94	NA	13.51	3.54	NA	NA	34.99	$1210.87	090	A+ B M
25028		Drainage of forearm lesion	5.39	NA	14.69	1.07	NA	NA	21.15	$731.92	090	A B M
25031		Drainage of forearm bursa	4.26	NA	5.88	0.89	NA	NA	11.03	$381.71	090	A+ B M
25035		Treat forearm bone lesion	7.65	NA	8.35	1.47	NA	NA	17.47	$604.57	090	A+ B M
25040		Explore/treat wrist joint	7.50	NA	7.76	1.41	NA	NA	16.67	$576.89	090	A+ B M
25065		Biopsy forearm soft tissues	2.04	5.40	2.36	0.28	7.72	$267.16	4.68	$161.96	010	A B M
25066		Biopsy forearm soft tissues	4.27	NA	5.80	0.85	NA	NA	10.92	$377.90	090	A B M
25071		Exc forearm les sc 3 cm/>	5.91	NA	5.46	1.27	NA	NA	12.64	$437.42	090	B M
25073		Exc forearm tum deep 3 cm/>	7.13	NA	7.38	1.42	NA	NA	15.93	$551.28	090	B M
25075		Exc forearm les sc < 3 cm	3.96	11.02	4.66	0.78	15.76	$545.39	9.40	$325.30	090	A B M
25076		Exc forearm tum deep < 3 cm	6.74	NA	7.37	1.29	NA	NA	15.40	$532.94	090	A B M
25077		Resect forearm/wrist tum<3cm	12.93	NA	10.78	2.78	NA	NA	26.49	$916.72	090	A B M
25078		Resect forarm/wrist tum 3cm>	17.69	NA	12.90	3.92	NA	NA	34.51	$1194.26	090	B M
25085		Incision of wrist capsule	5.64	NA	6.70	1.04	NA	NA	13.38	$463.03	090	B M
25100		Biopsy of wrist joint	4.02	NA	5.63	0.84	NA	NA	10.49	$363.02	090	A+ B M
25101		Explore/treat wrist joint	4.83	NA	6.34	0.94	NA	NA	12.11	$419.08	090	A+ B M
25105		Remove wrist joint lining	6.02	NA	7.38	1.12	NA	NA	14.52	$502.48	090	A+ B C+ M
25107		Remove wrist joint cartilage	7.70	NA	9.23	1.44	NA	NA	18.37	$635.72	090	B C+ M
25109		Excise tendon forearm/wrist	6.94	NA	7.75	1.27	NA	NA	15.96	$552.31	090	A B M
25110		Remove wrist tendon lesion	4.04	NA	5.56	0.77	NA	NA	10.37	$358.87	090	A B M

25111	Remove wrist tendon lesion	3.53	NA	5.49	0.66	NA	NA	9.68	$334.99	090	A B M
25112	Reremove wrist tendon lesion	4.67	NA	6.09	0.89	NA	NA	11.65	$403.16	090	A B M
25115	Remove wrist/forearm lesion	10.09	NA	10.51	1.84	NA	NA	22.44	$776.56	090	A B M
25116	Remove wrist/forearm lesion	7.56	NA	8.99	1.40	NA	NA	17.95	$621.18	090	A+ B C+ M
25118	Excise wrist tendon sheath	4.51	NA	6.08	0.84	NA	NA	11.43	$395.55	090	A B M
25119	Partial removal of ulna	6.21	NA	7.53	1.28	NA	NA	15.02	$519.79	090	B C+ M
25120	Removal of forearm lesion	6.27	NA	7.52	1.18	NA	NA	14.97	$518.05	090	A+ B C+ M
25125	Remove/graft forearm lesion	7.67	NA	8.54	1.57	NA	NA	17.78	$615.30	090	A+ B M
25126	Remove/graft forearm lesion	7.74	NA	8.57	1.60	NA	NA	17.91	$619.80	090	B M
25130	Removal of wrist lesion	5.43	NA	7.05	0.99	NA	NA	13.47	$466.15	090	A+ B M
25135	Remove & graft wrist lesion	7.08	NA	8.23	1.44	NA	NA	16.75	$579.65	090	B C+ M
25136	Remove & graft wrist lesion	6.14	NA	7.49	1.27	NA	NA	14.90	$515.63	090	B C+ M
25145	Remove forearm bone lesion	6.54	NA	7.70	1.34	NA	NA	15.58	$539.16	090	B M
25150	Partial removal of ulna	7.38	NA	8.13	1.43	NA	NA	16.94	$586.23	090	A B C+ M
25151	Partial removal of radius	7.68	NA	8.28	1.47	NA	NA	17.43	$603.19	090	B C+ M
25170	Resect radius/ulnar tumor	22.21	NA	16.68	4.60	NA	NA	43.49	$1505.02	090	B C+ M
25210	Removal of wrist bone	6.12	NA	7.45	1.11	NA	NA	14.68	$508.02	090	A+ C+ M
25215	Removal of wrist bones	8.14	NA	8.79	1.50	NA	NA	18.43	$637.79	090	B C+ M
25230	Partial removal of radius	5.37	NA	6.56	0.99	NA	NA	12.92	$447.11	090	A B C+ M
25240	Partial removal of ulna	5.31	NA	6.53	0.98	NA	NA	12.82	$443.65	090	A+ B C+ M
25246	Injection for wrist x-ray	1.45	4.44	0.56	0.12	6.01	$207.98	2.13	$73.71	000	A B M
25248	Remove forearm foreign body	5.31	NA	6.15	1.09	NA	NA	12.55	$434.31	090	A B M
25250	Removal of wrist prosthesis	6.77	NA	7.80	1.40	NA	NA	15.97	$552.66	090	B M
25251	Removal of wrist prosthesis	9.82	NA	9.61	2.01	NA	NA	21.44	$741.96	090	B M
25259	Manipulate wrist w/anesthes	4.04	NA	8.08	0.75	NA	NA	12.87	$445.38	090	A B M
25260	Repair forearm tendon/muscle	8.04	NA	9.36	1.51	NA	NA	18.91	$654.40	090	A M
25263	Repair forearm tendon/muscle	8.04	NA	9.25	1.65	NA	NA	18.94	$655.44	090	M
25265	Repair forearm tendon/muscle	10.10	NA	10.34	1.90	NA	NA	22.34	$773.10	090	M

*Please note that these calculations are based on the Medicare 2022 Conversion Factor of $34.6062 and the DRA RVU cap rates at time of publication.

A = assistant-at-surgery restriction
A+ = assistant-at-surgery restriction unless medical necessity established with documentation
B = bilateral surgery adjustment applies
C = cosurgeons payable
C+ = cosurgeons payable if medical necessity established with documentation
CP = carriers may establish RVUs and payment amounts for these services, generally on an individual basis following review of documentation such as an operative report
M = multiple surgery adjustment applies
Me = multiple endoscopy rules may apply
M+ = multiple therapy rules apply
Mtc = multiple diagnostic imaging rules apply
T = team surgeons permitted
T+ = team surgeons payable if medical necessity established with documentation
§ = indicates code is not covered by Medicare
GS = procedure must be performed under the general supervision of a physician
DS = procedure must be performed under the direct supervision of a physician
PS = procedure must be performed under the personal supervision of a physician
DRA = procedure subject to DRA limitation

Relative Value Units

CPT Code and Modifier	Description	Work RVU	Nonfacility Practice Expense RVU	Facility Practice Expense RVU	PLI RVU	Total Non-facility RVUs	Medicare Payment Nonfacility	Total Facility RVUs	Medicare Payment Facility	Global Period	Payment Policy Indicators
25270	Repair forearm tendon/muscle	6.17	NA	7.41	1.16	NA	NA	14.74	$510.10	090	A+ M
25272	Repair forearm tendon/muscle	7.21	NA	8.04	1.48	NA	NA	16.73	$578.96	090	A+ M
25274	Repair forearm tendon/muscle	8.94	NA	9.20	1.65	NA	NA	19.79	$684.86	090	A+ C+ M
25275	Repair forearm tendon sheath	8.96	NA	9.37	1.68	NA	NA	20.01	$692.47	090	A+ B C+ M
25280	Revise wrist/forearm tendon	7.39	NA	8.12	1.38	NA	NA	16.89	$584.50	090	A+ C+ M
25290	Incise wrist/forearm tendon	5.43	NA	6.59	1.00	NA	NA	13.02	$450.57	090	A M
25295	Release wrist/forearm tendon	6.72	NA	7.75	1.25	NA	NA	15.72	$544.01	090	A M
25300	Fusion of tendons at wrist	9.02	NA	9.73	1.84	NA	NA	20.59	$712.54	090	B M
25301	Fusion of tendons at wrist	8.59	NA	8.95	1.60	NA	NA	19.14	$662.36	090	B M
25310	Transplant forearm tendon	8.08	NA	8.91	1.48	NA	NA	18.47	$639.18	090	C+ M
25312	Transplant forearm tendon	9.82	NA	9.63	1.84	NA	NA	21.29	$736.77	090	C+ M
25315	Revise palsy hand tendon(s)	10.68	NA	10.05	2.20	NA	NA	22.93	$793.52	090	B M
25316	Revise palsy hand tendon(s)	12.90	NA	11.70	2.67	NA	NA	27.27	$943.71	090	B M
25320	Repair/revise wrist joint	12.75	NA	14.09	2.37	NA	NA	29.21	$1010.85	090	B M
25332	Revise wrist joint	11.74	NA	11.13	2.23	NA	NA	25.10	$868.62	090	B M
25335	Realignment of hand	13.39	NA	11.95	2.78	NA	NA	28.12	$973.13	090	B M
25337	Reconstruct ulna/radioulnar	11.73	NA	12.39	2.17	NA	NA	26.29	$909.80	090	A B M
25350	Revision of radius	9.09	NA	9.29	1.70	NA	NA	20.08	$694.89	090	B M
25355	Revision of radius	10.53	NA	10.10	2.17	NA	NA	22.80	$789.02	090	B M
25360	Revision of ulna	8.74	NA	9.11	1.68	NA	NA	19.53	$675.86	090	B C+ M
25365	Revise radius & ulna	12.91	NA	11.72	2.67	NA	NA	27.30	$944.75	090	B M
25370	Revise radius or ulna	14.10	NA	13.10	2.91	NA	NA	30.11	$1041.99	090	B M
25375	Revise radius & ulna	13.55	NA	12.04	2.80	NA	NA	28.39	$982.47	090	B C+ M
25390	Shorten radius or ulna	10.70	NA	10.17	1.99	NA	NA	22.86	$791.10	090	B C+ M
25391	Lengthen radius or ulna	14.28	NA	12.40	2.95	NA	NA	29.63	$1025.38	090	B C+ M
25392	Shorten radius & ulna	14.58	NA	12.56	3.00	NA	NA	30.14	$1043.03	090	B M
25393	Lengthen radius & ulna	16.56	NA	13.56	3.42	NA	NA	33.54	$1160.69	090	B M
25394	Repair carpal bone shorten	10.85	NA	10.28	2.23	NA	NA	23.36	$808.40	090	B C+ M
25400	Repair radius or ulna	11.28	NA	10.41	2.17	NA	NA	23.86	$825.70	090	B C+ M
25405	Repair/graft radius or ulna	15.01	NA	12.91	2.89	NA	NA	30.81	$1066.22	090	B C+ M
25415	Repair radius & ulna	13.80	NA	12.16	2.85	NA	NA	28.81	$997.00	090	B C+ M
25420	Repair/graft radius & ulna	17.04	NA	14.07	3.52	NA	NA	34.63	$1198.41	090	B C+ M
25425	Repair/graft radius or ulna	13.72	NA	12.13	2.84	NA	NA	28.69	$992.85	090	B C+ M

25426	Repair/graft radius & ulna	16.45	NA	13.51	3.39	NA	NA	33.35	$1154.12	090	B C+ M
25430	Vasc graft into carpal bone	9.71	NA	10.08	2.01	NA	NA	21.80	$754.42	090	A B M
25431	Repair nonunion carpal bone	10.89	NA	10.33	2.23	NA	NA	23.45	$811.52	090	B C+ M
25440	Repair/graft wrist bone	10.68	NA	10.18	1.96	NA	NA	22.82	$789.71	090	B C+ M
25441	Reconstruct wrist joint	13.29	NA	11.89	2.73	NA	NA	27.91	$965.86	090	B C+ M
25442	Reconstruct wrist joint	11.12	NA	10.89	2.06	NA	NA	24.07	$832.97	090	B C+ M
25443	Reconstruct wrist joint	10.66	NA	10.55	2.18	NA	NA	23.39	$809.44	090	B C+ M
25444	Reconstruct wrist joint	11.42	NA	11.05	2.17	NA	NA	24.64	$852.70	090	B M
25445	Reconstruct wrist joint	9.88	NA	9.67	1.84	NA	NA	21.39	$740.23	090	A B C+ M
25446	Wrist replacement	17.30	NA	14.14	3.24	NA	NA	34.68	$1200.14	090	B C+ M
25447	Repair wrist joints	11.14	NA	11.48	2.06	NA	NA	24.68	$854.08	090	B C+ M
25449	Remove wrist joint implant	14.94	NA	12.93	2.79	NA	NA	30.66	$1061.03	090	B C+ M
25450	Revision of wrist joint	8.06	NA	8.73	1.66	NA	NA	18.45	$638.48	090	A B M
25455	Revision of wrist joint	9.71	NA	10.08	2.01	NA	NA	21.80	$754.42	090	A B M
25490	Reinforce radius	9.73	NA	9.69	2.01	NA	NA	21.43	$741.61	090	B M
25491	Reinforce ulna	10.15	NA	9.79	2.09	NA	NA	22.03	$762.37	090	B M
25492	Reinforce radius and ulna	12.66	NA	11.71	2.62	NA	NA	26.99	$934.02	090	B M
25500	Treat fracture of radius	2.60	5.47	4.64	0.50	8.57	$296.58	7.74	$267.85	090	A B M
25505	Treat fracture of radius	5.45	8.64	7.23	1.09	15.18	$525.32	13.77	$476.53	090	A B M
25515	Treat fracture of radius	8.80	NA	9.43	1.72	NA	NA	19.95	$690.39	090	B C+ M
25520	Treat fracture of radius	6.50	9.50	8.50	1.33	17.33	$599.73	16.33	$565.12	090	A B M
25525	Treat fracture of radius	10.55	NA	10.83	2.07	NA	NA	23.45	$811.52	090	B C M
25526	Treat fracture of radius	13.15	NA	12.58	2.71	NA	NA	28.44	$984.20	090	B C M
25530	Treat fracture of ulna	2.24	5.27	4.62	0.42	7.93	$274.43	7.28	$251.93	090	A B M
25535	Treat fracture of ulna	5.36	8.50	7.33	1.04	14.90	$515.63	13.73	$475.14	090	A B M
25545	Treat fracture of ulna	7.94	NA	9.13	1.55	NA	NA	18.62	$644.37	090	B C+ M
25560	Treat fracture radius & ulna	2.59	5.64	4.69	0.51	8.74	$302.46	7.79	$269.58	090	A B M
25565	Treat fracture radius & ulna	5.85	8.57	6.94	1.20	15.62	$540.55	13.99	$484.14	090	A B M

*Please note that these calculations are based on the Medicare 2022 Conversion Factor of $34.6062 and the DRA RVU cap rates at time of publication.

A = assistant-at-surgery restriction

A+ = assistant-at-surgery restriction unless medical necessity established with documentation

B = bilateral surgery adjustment applies

C = cosurgeons payable

C+ = cosurgeons payable if medical necessity established with documentation

CP = carriers may establish RVUs and payment amounts for these services, generally on an individual basis following review of documentation such as an operative report

M = multiple surgery adjustment applies

Me = multiple endoscopy rules may apply

M+ = multiple therapy rules apply

Mtc = multiple diagnostic imaging rules apply

T = team surgeons permitted

T+ = team surgeons payable if medical necessity established with documentation

§ = indicates code is not covered by Medicare

GS = procedure must be performed under the general supervision of a physician

DS = procedure must be performed under the direct supervision of a physician

PS = procedure must be performed under the personal supervision of a physician

DRA = procedure subject to DRA limitation

Relative Value Units

CPT Code and Modifier	Description	Work RVU	Nonfacility Practice Expense RVU	Facility Practice Expense RVU	PLI RVU	Total Non-facility RVUs	Medicare Payment Nonfacility	Total Facility RVUs	Medicare Payment Facility	Global Period	Payment Policy Indicators
25574	Treat fracture radius & ulna	8.80	NA	9.55	1.75	NA	NA	20.10	$695.58	090	B C M
25575	Treat fracture radius/ulna	12.29	NA	12.12	2.47	NA	NA	26.88	$930.21	090	B C+ M
25600	Treat fracture radius/ulna	2.78	6.86	6.42	0.55	10.19	$352.64	9.75	$337.41	090	A B M
25605	Treat fracture radius/ulna	6.25	8.71	7.82	1.27	16.23	$561.66	15.34	$530.86	090	A B M
25606	Treat fx distal radial	8.31	NA	9.92	1.68	NA	NA	19.91	$689.01	090	A B M
25607	Treat fx rad extra-articul	9.56	NA	10.57	1.85	NA	NA	21.98	$760.64	090	B M
25608	Treat fx rad intra-articul	11.07	NA	11.36	2.17	NA	NA	24.60	$851.31	090	B M
25609	Treat fx radial 3+ frag	14.38	NA	14.06	2.78	NA	NA	31.22	$1080.41	090	B M
25622	Treat wrist bone fracture	2.79	5.93	5.22	0.54	9.26	$320.45	8.55	$295.88	090	A B M
25624	Treat wrist bone fracture	4.77	9.01	7.62	0.99	14.77	$511.13	13.38	$463.03	090	A+ B M
25628	Treat wrist bone fracture	9.67	NA	9.95	1.81	NA	NA	21.43	$741.61	090	B M
25630	Treat wrist bone fracture	3.03	5.60	4.95	0.57	9.20	$318.38	8.55	$295.88	090	A B M
25635	Treat wrist bone fracture	4.61	8.46	7.16	0.95	14.02	$485.18	12.72	$440.19	090	A+ B M
25645	Treat wrist bone fracture	7.42	NA	8.14	1.52	NA	NA	17.08	$591.07	090	B M
25650	Treat wrist bone fracture	3.23	6.11	5.36	0.61	9.95	$344.33	9.20	$318.38	090	A B M
25651	Pin ulnar styloid fracture	5.82	NA	7.67	1.11	NA	NA	14.60	$505.25	090	A+ B M
25652	Treat fracture ulnar styloid	8.06	NA	8.96	1.55	NA	NA	18.57	$642.64	090	A B C+ M
25660	Treat wrist dislocation	4.98	NA	7.46	1.02	NA	NA	13.46	$465.80	090	A+ B M
25670	Treat wrist dislocation	8.09	NA	8.46	1.62	NA	NA	18.17	$628.79	090	B C+ M
25671	Pin radioulnar dislocation	6.46	NA	8.09	1.28	NA	NA	15.83	$547.82	090	A B M
25675	Treat wrist dislocation	4.89	7.64	6.33	0.99	13.52	$467.88	12.21	$422.54	090	A+ B M
25676	Treat wrist dislocation	8.29	NA	8.91	1.61	NA	NA	18.81	$650.94	090	B M
25680	Treat wrist fracture	6.23	NA	8.37	1.29	NA	NA	15.89	$549.89	090	A+ B M
25685	Treat wrist fracture	10.09	NA	9.75	2.07	NA	NA	21.91	$758.22	090	B M
25690	Treat wrist dislocation	5.72	NA	7.84	1.18	NA	NA	14.74	$510.10	090	A+ B M
25695	Treat wrist dislocation	8.51	NA	8.69	1.75	NA	NA	18.95	$655.79	090	B C+ M
25800	Fusion of wrist joint	10.07	NA	9.80	1.90	NA	NA	21.77	$753.38	090	B C+ M
25805	Fusion/graft of wrist joint	11.73	NA	11.11	2.40	NA	NA	25.24	$873.46	090	B C+ M
25810	Fusion/graft of wrist joint	11.95	NA	11.51	2.20	NA	NA	25.66	$888.00	090	B C+ M
25820	Fusion of hand bones	7.64	NA	10.37	1.42	NA	NA	19.43	$672.40	090	B C+ M
25825	Fuse hand bones with graft	9.69	NA	12.22	1.78	NA	NA	23.69	$819.82	090	B C+ M
25830	Fusion radioulnar jnt/ulna	10.88	NA	17.98	2.23	NA	NA	31.09	$1075.91	090	B C+ M
25900	Amputation of forearm	9.61	NA	9.84	1.87	NA	NA	21.32	$737.80	090	A+ B M

25905		Amputation of forearm	9.59	NA	9.37	1.98	NA	NA	20.94	$724.65	090	B M
25907		Amputation follow-up surgery	8.09	NA	8.60	1.66	NA	NA	18.35	$635.02	090	B M
25909		Amputation follow-up surgery	9.31	NA	9.22	1.93	NA	NA	20.46	$708.04	090	B M
25915		Amputation of forearm	17.52	NA	13.49	3.61	NA	NA	34.62	$1198.07	090	B M
25920		Amputate hand at wrist	9.03	NA	11.01	1.85	NA	NA	21.89	$757.53	090	A+ B M
25922		Amputate hand at wrist	7.65	NA	10.19	1.57	NA	NA	19.41	$671.71	090	B M
25924		Amputation follow-up surgery	8.81	NA	10.78	1.81	NA	NA	21.40	$740.57	090	B M
25927		Amputation of hand	9.09	NA	15.15	1.86	NA	NA	26.10	$903.22	090	A+ B M
25929		Amputation follow-up surgery	7.82	NA	8.46	1.62	NA	NA	17.90	$619.45	090	B M
25931		Amputation follow-up surgery	8.04	NA	14.51	1.65	NA	NA	24.20	$837.47	090	A B M
25999	CP	Forearm or wrist surgery	0.00	0.00	0.00	0.00	0.00	$0.00	0.00	$0.00	YYY	A+ B C+ M T+
26010		Drainage of finger abscess	1.59	8.69	2.32	0.27	10.55	$365.10	4.18	$144.65	010	A M
26011		Drainage of finger abscess	2.24	12.09	2.87	0.40	14.73	$509.75	5.51	$190.68	010	A M
26020		Drain hand tendon sheath	6.84	NA	8.45	1.30	NA	NA	16.59	$574.12	090	A M
26025		Drainage of palm bursa	5.08	NA	6.49	0.99	NA	NA	12.56	$434.65	090	A+ B M
26030		Drainage of palm bursas	6.25	NA	7.20	1.18	NA	NA	14.63	$506.29	090	A+ B M
26034		Treat hand bone lesion	6.63	NA	8.57	1.26	NA	NA	16.46	$569.62	090	A M
26035		Decompress fingers/hand	11.37	NA	11.91	2.33	NA	NA	25.61	$886.26	090	A+ M
26037		Decompress fingers/hand	7.57	NA	7.70	1.42	NA	NA	16.69	$577.58	090	A+ B M
26040		Release palm contracture	3.46	NA	5.35	0.62	NA	NA	9.43	$326.34	090	A B M
26045		Release palm contracture	5.73	NA	7.27	1.10	NA	NA	14.10	$487.95	090	A B M
26055		Incise finger tendon sheath	3.11	14.24	4.98	0.60	17.95	$621.18	8.69	$300.73	090	A M
26060		Incision of finger tendon	2.91	NA	4.32	0.43	NA	NA	7.66	$265.08	090	A+ M
26070		Explore/treat hand joint	3.81	NA	5.11	0.66	NA	NA	9.58	$331.53	090	A B M
26075		Explore/treat finger joint	3.91	NA	5.45	0.73	NA	NA	10.09	$349.18	090	A B M
26080		Explore/treat finger joint	4.47	NA	6.60	0.84	NA	NA	11.91	$412.16	090	A M
26100		Biopsy hand joint lining	3.79	NA	5.60	0.77	NA	NA	10.16	$351.60	090	A+ B M
26105		Biopsy finger joint lining	3.83	NA	5.62	0.78	NA	NA	10.23	$354.02	090	A+ B M

*Please note that these calculations are based on the Medicare 2022 Conversion Factor of $34.6062 and the DRA RVU cap rates at time of publication.

A = assistant-at-surgery restriction
A+ = assistant-at-surgery restriction unless medical necessity established with documentation
B = bilateral surgery adjustment applies
C = cosurgeons payable
C+ = cosurgeons payable if medical necessity established with documentation
CP = carriers may establish RVUs and payment amounts for these services, generally on an individual basis following review of documentation such as an operative report
M = multiple surgery adjustment applies
Me = multiple endoscopy rules may apply
M+ = multiple therapy rules apply
Mtc = multiple diagnostic imaging rules apply
T = team surgeons permitted
T+ = team surgeons payable if medical necessity established with documentation
§ = indicates code is not covered by Medicare
GS = procedure must be performed under the general supervision of a physician
DS = procedure must be performed under the direct supervision of a physician
PS = procedure must be performed under the personal supervision of a physician
DRA = procedure subject to DRA limitation

Relative Value Units

CPT Code and Modifier	Description	Work RVU	Nonfacility Practice Expense RVU	Facility Practice Expense RVU	PLI RVU	Total Non-facility RVUs	Medicare Payment Nonfacility	Total Facility RVUs	Medicare Payment Facility	Global Period	Payment Policy Indicators
26110	Biopsy finger joint lining	3.65	NA	5.40	0.68	NA	NA	9.73	$336.72	090	A M
26111	Exc hand les sc 1.5 cm/>	5.42	NA	5.91	1.02	NA	NA	12.35	$427.39	090	M
26113	Exc hand tum deep 1.5 cm/>	7.13	NA	7.79	1.32	NA	NA	16.24	$562.00	090	M
26115	Exc hand les sc < 1.5 cm	3.96	11.88	5.16	0.73	16.57	$573.42	9.85	$340.87	090	A M
26116	Exc hand tum deep < 1.5 cm	6.74	NA	7.62	1.25	NA	NA	15.61	$540.20	090	A M
26117	Rad resect hand tumor < 3 cm	10.13	NA	9.86	1.93	NA	NA	21.92	$758.57	090	A M
26118	Rad resect hand tumor 3 cm/>	14.81	NA	13.58	2.93	NA	NA	31.32	$1083.87	090	M
26121	Release palm contracture	7.73	NA	8.69	1.43	NA	NA	17.85	$617.72	090	A B M
26123	Release palm contracture	10.88	NA	11.97	2.01	NA	NA	24.86	$860.31	090	A B M
26125	Release palm contracture	4.60	NA	2.47	0.86	NA	NA	7.93	$274.43	ZZZ	A
26130	Remove wrist joint lining	5.59	NA	7.29	1.16	NA	NA	14.04	$485.87	090	A B M
26135	Revise finger joint each	7.13	NA	8.08	1.33	NA	NA	16.54	$572.39	090	A+ M
26140	Revise finger joint each	6.34	NA	7.65	1.16	NA	NA	15.15	$524.28	090	A M
26145	Tendon excision palm/finger	6.49	NA	7.68	1.21	NA	NA	15.38	$532.24	090	A M
26160	Remove tendon sheath lesion	3.57	14.44	5.18	0.66	18.67	$646.10	9.41	$325.64	090	A M
26170	Removal of palm tendon each	4.91	NA	6.38	0.90	NA	NA	12.19	$421.85	090	A+ M
26180	Removal of finger tendon	5.35	NA	7.09	0.96	NA	NA	13.40	$463.72	090	A+ M
26185	Remove finger bone	6.52	NA	8.75	1.34	NA	NA	16.61	$574.81	090	B C+ M
26200	Remove hand bone lesion	5.65	NA	6.71	1.04	NA	NA	13.40	$463.72	090	A+ M
26205	Remove/graft bone lesion	7.93	NA	8.53	1.64	NA	NA	18.10	$626.37	090	A M
26210	Removal of finger lesion	5.32	NA	7.06	0.96	NA	NA	13.34	$461.65	090	A M
26215	Remove/graft finger lesion	7.27	NA	8.19	1.49	NA	NA	16.95	$586.58	090	A M
26230	Partial removal of hand bone	6.47	NA	7.24	1.20	NA	NA	14.91	$515.98	090	A+ M
26235	Partial removal finger bone	6.33	NA	7.17	1.17	NA	NA	14.67	$507.67	090	A+ M
26236	Partial removal finger bone	5.46	NA	6.69	1.04	NA	NA	13.19	$456.46	090	A M
26250	Extensive hand surgery	15.21	NA	13.24	3.13	NA	NA	31.58	$1092.86	090	A+ M
26260	Resect prox finger tumor	11.16	NA	10.22	2.31	NA	NA	23.69	$819.82	090	M
26262	Resect distal finger tumor	8.29	NA	8.77	1.70	NA	NA	18.76	$649.21	090	M
26320	Removal of implant from hand	4.10	NA	5.60	0.76	NA	NA	10.46	$361.98	090	A M
26340	Manipulate finger w/anesth	2.80	NA	7.21	0.52	NA	NA	10.53	$364.40	090	A B M
26341	Manipulat palm cord post inj	0.91	2.41	1.24	0.18	3.50	$121.12	2.33	$80.63	010	A B M
26350	Repair finger/hand tendon	6.21	NA	15.29	1.17	NA	NA	22.67	$784.52	090	A M
26352	Repair/graft hand tendon	7.87	NA	15.94	1.44	NA	NA	25.25	$873.81	090	C+ M

26356	Repair finger/hand tendon	9.56	NA	12.35	1.78	NA	NA	23.69	$819.82	090	A M
26357	Repair finger/hand tendon	11.00	NA	13.33	2.26	NA	NA	26.59	$920.18	090	M
26358	Repair/graft hand tendon	12.60	NA	14.15	2.61	NA	NA	29.36	$1016.04	090	M
26370	Repair finger/hand tendon	7.28	NA	15.20	1.36	NA	NA	23.84	$825.01	090	A+ M
26372	Repair/graft hand tendon	9.01	NA	16.94	1.84	NA	NA	27.79	$961.71	090	M
26373	Repair finger/hand tendon	8.41	NA	16.63	1.72	NA	NA	26.76	$926.06	090	M
26390	Revise hand/finger tendon	9.43	NA	15.21	1.94	NA	NA	26.58	$919.83	090	C+ M
26392	Repair/graft hand tendon	10.50	NA	17.69	2.17	NA	NA	30.36	$1050.64	090	C+ M
26410	Repair hand tendon	4.77	NA	12.63	0.90	NA	NA	18.30	$633.29	090	A M
26412	Repair/graft hand tendon	6.48	NA	14.09	1.20	NA	NA	21.77	$753.38	090	A+ M
26415	Excision hand/finger tendon	8.51	NA	15.58	1.75	NA	NA	25.84	$894.22	090	A+ M
26416	Graft hand or finger tendon	9.56	NA	16.38	1.98	NA	NA	27.92	$966.21	090	A M
26418	Repair finger tendon	4.47	NA	13.65	0.85	NA	NA	18.97	$656.48	090	A M
26420	Repair/graft finger tendon	6.94	NA	14.37	1.29	NA	NA	22.60	$782.10	090	M
26426	Repair finger/hand tendon	6.32	NA	7.52	1.18	NA	NA	15.02	$519.79	090	A M
26428	Repair/graft finger tendon	7.40	NA	15.28	1.52	NA	NA	24.20	$837.47	090	A+ M
26432	Repair finger tendon	4.16	NA	11.63	0.77	NA	NA	16.56	$573.08	090	A M
26433	Repair finger tendon	4.70	NA	11.82	0.89	NA	NA	17.41	$602.49	090	A M
26434	Repair/graft finger tendon	6.26	NA	13.61	1.29	NA	NA	21.16	$732.27	090	M
26437	Realignment of tendons	5.99	NA	13.13	1.11	NA	NA	20.23	$700.08	090	A M
26440	Release palm/finger tendon	5.16	NA	13.72	0.94	NA	NA	19.82	$685.89	090	A M
26442	Release palm & finger tendon	9.75	NA	18.31	1.78	NA	NA	29.84	$1032.65	090	A M
26445	Release hand/finger tendon	4.45	NA	13.25	0.83	NA	NA	18.53	$641.25	090	A M
26449	Release forearm/hand tendon	8.59	NA	10.53	1.61	NA	NA	20.73	$717.39	090	A+ M
26450	Incision of palm tendon	3.79	NA	9.58	0.72	NA	NA	14.09	$487.60	090	A+ M
26455	Incision of finger tendon	3.76	NA	9.49	0.68	NA	NA	13.93	$482.06	090	A+ M
26460	Incise hand/finger tendon	3.58	NA	9.48	0.65	NA	NA	13.71	$474.45	090	A M
26471	Fusion of finger tendons	5.90	NA	13.06	1.07	NA	NA	20.03	$693.16	090	A+ M

*Please note that these calculations are based on the Medicare 2022 Conversion Factor of $34.6062 and the DRA RVU cap rates at time of publication.

A = assistant-at-surgery restriction
A+ = assistant-at-surgery restriction unless medical necessity established with documentation
B = bilateral surgery adjustment applies
C = cosurgeons payable
C+ = cosurgeons payable if medical necessity established with documentation
CP = carriers may establish RVUs and payment amounts for these services, generally on an individual basis following review of documentation such as an operative report
M = multiple surgery adjustment applies
Me = multiple endoscopy rules may apply
M+ = multiple therapy rules apply
Mtc = multiple diagnostic imaging rules apply
T = team surgeons permitted
T+ = team surgeons payable if medical necessity established with documentation
§ = indicates code is not covered by Medicare
GS = procedure must be performed under the general supervision of a physician
DS = procedure must be performed under the direct supervision of a physician
PS = procedure must be performed under the personal supervision of a physician
DRA = procedure subject to DRA limitation

Relative Value Units

CPT Code and Modifier	Description	Work RVU	Nonfacility Practice Expense RVU	Facility Practice Expense RVU	PLI RVU	Total Non-facility RVUs	Medicare Payment Nonfacility	Total Facility RVUs	Medicare Payment Facility	Global Period	Payment Policy Indicators
26474	Fusion of finger tendons	5.49	NA	13.22	1.11	NA	NA	19.82	$685.89	090	M
26476	Tendon lengthening	5.35	NA	13.14	1.10	NA	NA	19.59	$677.94	090	A M
26477	Tendon shortening	5.32	NA	12.71	0.96	NA	NA	18.99	$657.17	090	A C+ M
26478	Lengthening of hand tendon	5.97	NA	13.06	1.10	NA	NA	20.13	$696.62	090	A+ M
26479	Shortening of hand tendon	5.91	NA	13.43	1.21	NA	NA	20.55	$711.16	090	M
26480	Transplant hand tendon	6.90	NA	15.65	1.27	NA	NA	23.82	$824.32	090	A+ M
26483	Transplant/graft hand tendon	8.48	NA	16.33	1.55	NA	NA	26.36	$912.22	090	C+ M
26485	Transplant palm tendon	7.89	NA	15.96	1.44	NA	NA	25.29	$875.19	090	C+ M
26489	Transplant/graft palm tendon	9.86	NA	17.37	2.03	NA	NA	29.26	$1012.58	090	A+ M
26490	Revise thumb tendon	8.60	NA	15.05	1.78	NA	NA	25.43	$880.04	090	A+ M
26492	Tendon transfer with graft	9.84	NA	16.21	2.01	NA	NA	28.06	$971.05	090	C+ M
26494	Hand tendon/muscle transfer	8.66	NA	15.08	1.78	NA	NA	25.52	$883.15	090	C+ M
26496	Revise thumb tendon	9.78	NA	15.65	2.01	NA	NA	27.44	$949.59	090	A+ M
26497	Finger tendon transfer	9.76	NA	15.64	2.01	NA	NA	27.41	$948.56	090	M
26498	Finger tendon transfer	14.21	NA	18.42	2.94	NA	NA	35.57	$1230.94	090	C+ M
26499	Revision of finger	9.17	NA	15.34	1.87	NA	NA	26.38	$912.91	090	C+ M
26500	Hand tendon reconstruction	6.13	NA	13.04	1.12	NA	NA	20.29	$702.16	090	A+ M
26502	Hand tendon reconstruction	7.31	NA	14.14	1.50	NA	NA	22.95	$794.21	090	M
26508	Release thumb contracture	6.18	NA	13.23	1.10	NA	NA	20.51	$709.77	090	A+ B M
26510	Thumb tendon transfer	5.60	NA	12.83	1.06	NA	NA	19.49	$674.47	090	A+ M
26516	Fusion of knuckle joint	7.32	NA	13.85	1.37	NA	NA	22.54	$780.02	090	A+ B M
26517	Fusion of knuckle joints	9.08	NA	15.30	1.86	NA	NA	26.24	$908.07	090	B M
26518	Fusion of knuckle joints	9.27	NA	15.39	1.93	NA	NA	26.59	$920.18	090	B C+ M
26520	Release knuckle contracture	5.47	NA	14.30	1.00	NA	NA	20.77	$718.77	090	A M
26525	Release finger contracture	5.50	NA	14.33	1.01	NA	NA	20.84	$721.19	090	A C+ M
26530	Revise knuckle joint	6.88	NA	7.96	1.30	NA	NA	16.14	$558.54	090	M
26531	Revise knuckle with implant	8.13	NA	9.17	1.50	NA	NA	18.80	$650.60	090	C+ M
26535	Revise finger joint	5.41	NA	6.66	0.95	NA	NA	13.02	$450.57	090	A M
26536	Revise/implant finger joint	6.56	NA	14.96	1.20	NA	NA	22.72	$786.25	090	A+ M
26540	Repair hand joint	6.60	NA	13.40	1.22	NA	NA	21.22	$734.34	090	A+ C+ M
26541	Repair hand joint with graft	8.81	NA	14.75	1.65	NA	NA	25.21	$872.42	090	C+ M
26542	Repair hand joint with graft	6.95	NA	13.66	1.29	NA	NA	21.90	$757.88	090	A+ M
26545	Reconstruct finger joint	7.11	NA	13.76	1.29	NA	NA	22.16	$766.87	090	A+ M

26546	Repair nonunion hand	10.83	NA	18.33	2.01	NA	NA	31.17	$1078.68	090	B M
26548	Reconstruct finger joint	8.22	NA	14.42	1.52	NA	NA	24.16	$836.09	090	A+ M
26550	Construct thumb replacement	21.68	NA	23.54	4.47	NA	NA	49.69	$1719.58	090	B M
26551	Great toe-hand transfer	48.48	NA	39.72	10.00	NA	NA	98.20	$3398.33	090	B M
26553	Single transfer toe-hand	48.17	NA	39.44	9.93	NA	NA	97.54	$3375.49	090	B C+ M
26554	Double transfer toe-hand	57.01	NA	44.71	11.75	NA	NA	113.47	$3926.77	090	B C+ M
26555	Positional change of finger	17.08	NA	21.21	3.53	NA	NA	41.82	$1447.23	090	M
26556	Toe joint transfer	49.75	NA	41.40	10.26	NA	NA	101.41	$3509.41	090	C+ M
26560	Repair of web finger	5.52	NA	12.71	1.12	NA	NA	19.35	$669.63	090	M
26561	Repair of web finger	11.10	NA	16.33	2.28	NA	NA	29.71	$1028.15	090	C+ M
26562	Repair of web finger	16.68	NA	21.20	3.46	NA	NA	41.34	$1430.62	090	M
26565	Correct metacarpal flaw	6.91	NA	13.56	1.29	NA	NA	21.76	$753.03	090	M
26567	Correct finger deformity	6.99	NA	13.54	1.29	NA	NA	21.82	$755.11	090	A+ M
26568	Lengthen metacarpal/finger	9.27	NA	17.07	1.93	NA	NA	28.27	$978.32	090	M
26580	Repair hand deformity	19.75	NA	22.41	4.06	NA	NA	46.22	$1599.50	090	B M
26587	Reconstruct extra finger	14.50	NA	13.54	3.00	NA	NA	31.04	$1074.18	090	M
26590	Repair finger deformity	18.67	NA	20.52	3.85	NA	NA	43.04	$1489.45	090	M
26591	Repair muscles of hand	3.38	NA	10.79	0.64	NA	NA	14.81	$512.52	090	A+ M
26593	Release muscles of hand	5.50	NA	13.06	1.01	NA	NA	19.57	$677.24	090	A M
26596	Excision constricting tissue	9.14	NA	13.66	1.87	NA	NA	24.67	$853.73	090	M
26600	Treat metacarpal fracture	2.60	5.96	5.52	0.50	9.06	$313.53	8.62	$298.31	090	A M
26605	Treat metacarpal fracture	3.03	6.35	5.35	0.60	9.98	$345.37	8.98	$310.76	090	A M
26607	Treat metacarpal fracture	5.48	NA	8.76	1.11	NA	NA	15.35	$531.21	090	A+ M
26608	Treat metacarpal fracture	5.55	NA	7.82	1.05	NA	NA	14.42	$499.02	090	A+ M
26615	Treat metacarpal fracture	7.07	NA	8.75	1.33	NA	NA	17.15	$593.50	090	A M
26641	Treat thumb dislocation	4.13	7.64	6.52	0.86	12.63	$437.08	11.51	$398.32	090	A+ B M
26645	Treat thumb fracture	4.58	7.53	6.36	0.95	13.06	$451.96	11.89	$411.47	090	A+ B M
26650	Treat thumb fracture	5.35	NA	8.05	1.01	NA	NA	14.41	$498.68	090	A B M

*Please note that these calculations are based on the Medicare 2022 Conversion Factor of $34.6062 and the DRA RVU cap rates at time of publication.

A = assistant-at-surgery restriction

A+ = assistant-at-surgery restriction unless medical necessity established with documentation

B = bilateral surgery adjustment applies

C = cosurgeons payable

C+ = cosurgeons payable if medical necessity established with documentation

CP = carriers may establish RVUs and payment amounts for these services, generally on an individual basis following review of documentation such as an operative report

M = multiple surgery adjustment applies

Me = multiple endoscopy rules may apply

M+ = multiple therapy rules apply

Mtc = multiple diagnostic imaging rules apply

T = team surgeons permitted

T+ = team surgeons payable if medical necessity established with documentation

§ = indicates code is not covered by Medicare

GS = procedure must be performed under the general supervision of a physician

DS = procedure must be performed under the direct supervision of a physician

PS = procedure must be performed under the personal supervision of a physician

DRA = procedure subject to DRA limitation

Relative Value Units

CPT Code and Modifier	Description	Work RVU	Nonfacility Practice Expense RVU	Facility Practice Expense RVU	PLI RVU	Total Non-facility RVUs	Medicare Payment Nonfacility	Total Facility RVUs	Medicare Payment Facility	Global Period	Payment Policy Indicators
26665	Treat thumb fracture	7.94	NA	9.35	1.29	NA	NA	18.58	$642.98	090	A B C+ M
26670	Treat hand dislocation	3.83	5.93	4.81	0.77	10.53	$364.40	9.41	$325.64	090	A+ M
26675	Treat hand dislocation	4.83	8.08	6.86	1.00	13.91	$481.37	12.69	$439.15	090	A+ M
26676	Pin hand dislocation	5.74	NA	8.42	1.07	NA	NA	15.23	$527.05	090	A M
26685	Treat hand dislocation	7.07	NA	8.77	1.34	NA	NA	17.18	$594.53	090	A C+ M
26686	Treat hand dislocation	8.17	NA	8.77	1.68	NA	NA	18.62	$644.37	090	M
26700	Treat knuckle dislocation	3.83	5.60	4.78	0.76	10.19	$352.64	9.37	$324.26	090	A M
26705	Treat knuckle dislocation	4.38	7.58	6.39	0.79	12.75	$441.23	11.56	$400.05	090	A+ M
26706	Pin knuckle dislocation	5.31	NA	7.06	1.00	NA	NA	13.37	$462.68	090	A M
26715	Treat knuckle dislocation	7.03	NA	8.73	1.33	NA	NA	17.09	$591.42	090	A+ M
26720	Treat finger fracture each	1.76	3.92	3.56	0.34	6.02	$208.33	5.66	$195.87	090	A M
26725	Treat finger fracture each	3.48	6.15	5.01	0.67	10.30	$356.44	9.16	$316.99	090	A M
26727	Treat finger fracture each	5.42	NA	7.76	1.01	NA	NA	14.19	$491.06	090	A M
26735	Treat finger fracture each	7.42	NA	8.90	1.40	NA	NA	17.72	$613.22	090	A M
26740	Treat finger fracture each	2.07	4.54	4.17	0.39	7.00	$242.24	6.63	$229.44	090	A M
26742	Treat finger fracture each	3.99	6.52	5.36	0.76	11.27	$390.01	10.11	$349.87	090	A M
26746	Treat finger fracture each	9.80	NA	10.47	1.82	NA	NA	22.09	$764.45	090	A M
26750	Treat finger fracture each	1.80	3.49	3.53	0.34	5.63	$194.83	5.67	$196.22	090	A M
26755	Treat finger fracture each	3.23	5.77	4.40	0.64	9.64	$333.60	8.27	$286.19	090	A M
26756	Pin finger fracture each	4.58	NA	7.28	0.87	NA	NA	12.73	$440.54	090	A+ M
26765	Treat finger fracture each	5.86	NA	8.03	1.09	NA	NA	14.98	$518.40	090	A M
26770	Treat finger dislocation	3.15	4.84	4.06	0.61	8.60	$297.61	7.82	$270.62	090	A M
26775	Treat finger dislocation	3.90	7.19	5.97	0.73	11.82	$409.05	10.60	$366.83	090	A M
26776	Pin finger dislocation	4.99	NA	7.55	0.95	NA	NA	13.49	$466.84	090	A M
26785	Treat finger dislocation	6.60	NA	8.45	1.24	NA	NA	16.29	$563.73	090	A M
26820	Thumb fusion with graft	8.45	NA	14.98	1.73	NA	NA	25.16	$870.69	090	B C+ M
26841	Fusion of thumb	7.35	NA	14.66	1.40	NA	NA	23.41	$810.13	090	A+ B C+ M
26842	Thumb fusion with graft	8.49	NA	15.00	1.73	NA	NA	25.22	$872.77	090	B C+ M
26843	Fusion of hand joint	7.78	NA	14.38	1.61	NA	NA	23.77	$822.59	090	C+ M
26844	Fusion/graft of hand joint	8.98	NA	15.25	1.84	NA	NA	26.07	$902.18	090	C+ M
26850	Fusion of knuckle	7.14	NA	13.79	1.33	NA	NA	22.26	$770.33	090	A+ M
26852	Fusion of knuckle with graft	8.71	NA	14.86	1.59	NA	NA	25.16	$870.69	090	C+ M
26860	Fusion of finger joint	4.88	NA	12.80	0.90	NA	NA	18.58	$642.98	090	A M

26861		Fusion of finger jnt add-on	1.74	NA	0.94	0.32	NA	NA	3.00	$103.82	ZZZ	A
26862		Fusion/graft of finger joint	7.56	NA	14.25	1.38	NA	NA	23.19	$802.52	090	C+ M
26863		Fuse/graft added joint	3.89	NA	2.10	0.70	NA	NA	6.69	$231.52	ZZZ	
26910		Amputate metacarpal bone	7.79	NA	13.78	1.49	NA	NA	23.06	$798.02	090	A M
26951		Amputation of finger/thumb	6.04	NA	13.96	1.17	NA	NA	21.17	$732.61	090	A M
26952		Amputation of finger/thumb	6.48	NA	13.03	1.21	NA	NA	20.72	$717.04	090	A M
26989	CP	Hand/finger surgery	0.00	0.00	0.00	0.00	0.00	$0.00	0.00	$0.00	YYY	A C+ M T+
26990		Drainage of pelvis lesion	7.95	NA	10.81	1.68	NA	NA	20.44	$707.35	090	A M
26991		Drainage of pelvis bursa	7.06	12.73	7.13	1.41	21.20	$733.65	15.60	$539.86	090	A+ M
26992		Drainage of bone lesion	13.48	NA	13.80	2.79	NA	NA	30.07	$1040.61	090	A+ M
27000		Incision of hip tendon	5.74	NA	5.57	0.65	NA	NA	11.96	$413.89	090	A B C+ M
27001		Incision of hip tendon	7.14	NA	7.51	1.47	NA	NA	16.12	$557.85	090	B C+ M
27003		Incision of hip tendon	7.81	NA	8.46	1.61	NA	NA	17.88	$618.76	090	B C+ M
27005		Incision of hip tendon	10.07	NA	9.44	2.01	NA	NA	21.52	$744.73	090	B C+ M
27006		Incision of hip tendons	10.11	NA	9.57	1.61	NA	NA	21.29	$736.77	090	B C+ M
27025		Incision of hip/thigh fascia	12.89	NA	11.87	2.66	NA	NA	27.42	$948.90	090	A+ B C+ M
27027		Buttock fasciotomy	13.04	NA	10.65	2.60	NA	NA	26.29	$909.80	090	A+ B M
27030		Drainage of hip joint	13.65	NA	11.38	2.80	NA	NA	27.83	$963.09	090	B C+ M
27033		Exploration of hip joint	14.11	NA	11.87	2.88	NA	NA	28.86	$998.73	090	B C+ M
27035		Denervation of hip joint	17.37	NA	15.64	0.89	NA	NA	33.90	$1173.15	090	B C+ M
27036		Excision of hip joint/muscle	14.38	NA	12.90	2.96	NA	NA	30.24	$1046.49	090	B C+ M
27040		Biopsy of soft tissues	2.92	6.85	2.50	0.42	10.19	$352.64	5.84	$202.10	010	A B M
27041		Biopsy of soft tissues	10.18	NA	8.86	2.04	NA	NA	21.08	$729.50	090	A B M
27043		Exc hip pelvis les sc 3 cm/>	6.88	NA	5.49	1.62	NA	NA	13.99	$484.14	090	A B M
27045		Exc hip/pelv tum deep 5 cm/>	11.13	NA	8.34	2.38	NA	NA	21.85	$756.15	090	B C+ M
27047		Exc hip/pelvis les sc < 3 cm	4.94	8.93	4.74	1.07	14.94	$517.02	10.75	$372.02	090	A B M
27048		Exc hip/pelv tum deep < 5 cm	8.85	NA	7.34	1.96	NA	NA	18.15	$628.10	090	B C+ M
27049		Resect hip/pelv tum < 5 cm	21.55	NA	13.40	5.04	NA	NA	39.99	$1383.90	090	B C+ M

*Please note that these calculations are based on the Medicare 2022 Conversion Factor of $34.6062 and the DRA RVU cap rates at time of publication.

A = assistant-at-surgery restriction
A+ = assistant-at-surgery restriction unless medical necessity established with documentation
B = bilateral surgery adjustment applies
C = cosurgeons payable
C+ = cosurgeons payable if medical necessity established with documentation
CP = carriers may establish RVUs and payment amounts for these services, generally on an individual basis following review of documentation such as an operative report
M = multiple surgery adjustment applies
Me = multiple endoscopy rules may apply
M+ = multiple therapy rules apply
Mtc = multiple diagnostic imaging rules apply
T = team surgeons permitted
T+ = team surgeons payable if medical necessity established with documentation
§ = indicates code is not covered by Medicare
GS = procedure must be performed under the general supervision of a physician
DS = procedure must be performed under the direct supervision of a physician
PS = procedure must be performed under the personal supervision of a physician
DRA = procedure subject to DRA limitation

Relative Value Units

CPT Code and Modifier	Description	Work RVU	Nonfacility Practice Expense RVU	Facility Practice Expense RVU	PLI RVU	Total Non-facility RVUs	Medicare Payment Nonfacility	Total Facility RVUs	Medicare Payment Facility	Global Period	Payment Policy Indicators
27050	Biopsy of sacroiliac joint	4.74	NA	6.39	0.98	NA	NA	12.11	$419.08	090	A+ B C+ M
27052	Biopsy of hip joint	7.42	NA	8.29	1.52	NA	NA	17.23	$596.26	090	B C+ M
27054	Removal of hip joint lining	9.21	NA	9.41	1.86	NA	NA	20.48	$708.73	090	B C+ M
27057	Buttock fasciotomy w/dbrdmt	14.91	NA	12.00	3.06	NA	NA	29.97	$1037.15	090	A+ B M
27059	Resect hip/pelv tum 5 cm/>	29.35	NA	18.17	6.12	NA	NA	53.64	$1856.28	090	B C+ M
27060	Removal of ischial bursa	5.87	NA	6.83	1.20	NA	NA	13.90	$481.03	090	A B M
27062	Remove femur lesion/bursa	5.75	NA	6.68	1.16	NA	NA	13.59	$470.30	090	A B C+ M
27065	Remove hip bone les super	6.55	NA	7.81	1.33	NA	NA	15.69	$542.97	090	B C+ M
27066	Remove hip bone les deep	11.20	NA	10.76	2.29	NA	NA	24.25	$839.20	090	B C+ M
27067	Remove/graft hip bone lesion	14.72	NA	13.01	3.02	NA	NA	30.75	$1064.14	090	B M
27070	Part remove hip bone super	11.56	NA	12.75	2.23	NA	NA	26.54	$918.45	090	B C+ M
27071	Part removal hip bone deep	12.39	NA	14.16	2.55	NA	NA	29.10	$1007.04	090	B C+ M
27075	Resect hip tumor	32.71	NA	22.12	6.74	NA	NA	61.57	$2130.70	090	C+ M
27076	Resect hip tum incl acetabul	40.21	NA	25.91	8.29	NA	NA	74.41	$2575.05	090	C+ M
27077	Resect hip tum w/innom bone	45.21	NA	28.45	9.33	NA	NA	82.99	$2871.97	090	C+ M
27078	Rsect hip tum incl femur	32.21	NA	21.86	6.64	NA	NA	60.71	$2100.94	090	B C+ M
27080	Removal of tail bone	6.89	NA	6.73	1.64	NA	NA	15.26	$528.09	090	C+ M
27086	Remove hip foreign body	1.92	7.06	2.68	0.40	9.38	$324.61	5.00	$173.03	010	A+ B M
27087	Remove hip foreign body	8.83	NA	7.47	2.01	NA	NA	18.31	$633.64	090	B C+ M
27090	Removal of hip prosthesis	11.69	NA	10.63	2.38	NA	NA	24.70	$854.77	090	B C+ M
27091	Removal of hip prosthesis	24.35	NA	17.79	5.01	NA	NA	47.15	$1631.68	090	B C+ M
27093	Injection for hip x-ray	1.30	5.81	0.56	0.12	7.23	$250.20	1.98	$68.52	000	A B M
27095	Injection for hip x-ray	1.50	8.01	0.70	0.24	9.75	$337.41	2.44	$84.44	000	A B M
27096	Inject sacroiliac joint	1.48	3.25	0.81	0.12	4.85	$167.84	2.41	$83.40	000	A B M
27097	Revision of hip tendon	9.27	NA	9.19	1.93	NA	NA	20.39	$705.62	090	B M
27098	Transfer tendon to pelvis	9.32	NA	9.48	1.94	NA	NA	20.74	$717.73	090	B M
27100	Transfer of abdominal muscle	11.35	NA	11.03	2.33	NA	NA	24.71	$855.12	090	B C+ M
27105	Transfer of spinal muscle	12.04	NA	11.38	2.49	NA	NA	25.91	$896.65	090	B M
27110	Transfer of iliopsoas muscle	13.77	NA	12.25	2.85	NA	NA	28.87	$999.08	090	B C+ M
27111	Transfer of iliopsoas muscle	12.60	NA	11.67	2.61	NA	NA	26.88	$930.21	090	B C+ M
27120	Reconstruction of hip socket	19.25	NA	15.28	3.97	NA	NA	38.50	$1332.34	090	B C+ M
27122	Reconstruction of hip socket	16.09	NA	13.36	3.31	NA	NA	32.76	$1133.70	090	B C+ M
27125	Partial hip replacement	16.64	NA	13.49	3.41	NA	NA	33.54	$1160.69	090	B C+ M

27130		Total hip arthroplasty	19.60	NA	14.41	4.01	NA	NA	38.02	$1315.73	090	B C+ M
27132		Total hip arthroplasty	25.69	NA	18.46	5.28	NA	NA	49.43	$1710.58	090	B C+ M
27134		Revise hip joint replacement	30.28	NA	19.82	6.22	NA	NA	56.32	$1949.02	090	B C+ M
27137		Revise hip joint replacement	22.70	NA	15.99	4.67	NA	NA	43.36	$1500.52	090	B C+ M
27138		Revise hip joint replacement	23.70	NA	16.49	4.88	NA	NA	45.07	$1559.70	090	B C+ M
27140		Transplant femur ridge	12.78	NA	11.16	2.62	NA	NA	26.56	$919.14	090	B C+ M
27146		Incision of hip bone	18.92	NA	15.09	3.94	NA	NA	37.95	$1313.31	090	B C+ M
27147		Revision of hip bone	22.07	NA	16.68	4.56	NA	NA	43.31	$1498.79	090	B C+ M
27151		Incision of hip bones	24.12	NA	17.71	4.97	NA	NA	46.80	$1619.57	090	B C+ M
27156		Revision of hip bones	26.23	NA	18.78	5.41	NA	NA	50.42	$1744.84	090	B C+ M
27158		Revision of pelvis	21.04	NA	16.09	4.33	NA	NA	41.46	$1434.77	090	M
27161		Incision of neck of femur	17.89	NA	14.61	3.70	NA	NA	36.20	$1252.74	090	B C+ M
27165		Incision/fixation of femur	20.29	NA	16.38	4.19	NA	NA	40.86	$1414.01	090	B C+ M
27170		Repair/graft femur head/neck	17.61	NA	13.35	3.60	NA	NA	34.56	$1195.99	090	B C+ M
27175		Treat slipped epiphysis	9.38	NA	8.51	1.94	NA	NA	19.83	$686.24	090	A+ B M
27176		Treat slipped epiphysis	12.92	NA	11.83	2.67	NA	NA	27.42	$948.90	090	B C+ M
27177		Treat slipped epiphysis	16.09	NA	13.70	3.32	NA	NA	33.11	$1145.81	090	B C+ M
27178		Treat slipped epiphysis	12.92	NA	11.83	2.67	NA	NA	27.42	$948.90	090	B C+ M
27179		Revise head/neck of femur	13.97	NA	12.24	2.89	NA	NA	29.10	$1007.04	090	B M
27181		Treat slipped epiphysis	16.18	NA	13.69	3.34	NA	NA	33.21	$1149.27	090	B M
27185		Revision of femur epiphysis	9.79	NA	9.60	2.01	NA	NA	21.40	$740.57	090	A B C+ M
27187		Reinforce hip bones	14.23	NA	12.45	2.94	NA	NA	29.62	$1025.04	090	B C+ M
27197		Clsd tx pelvic ring fx	1.53	NA	2.15	0.31	NA	NA	3.99	$138.08	000	A M
27198		Clsd tx pelvic ring fx	4.75	NA	3.84	0.87	NA	NA	9.46	$327.37	000	A+ C M
27200		Treat tail bone fracture	1.92	3.35	3.37	0.37	5.64	$195.18	5.66	$195.87	090	A M
27202		Treat tail bone fracture	7.31	NA	6.90	1.50	NA	NA	15.71	$543.66	090	M
27215	§	Treat pelvic fracture(s)	10.45	NA	6.46	0.87	NA	NA	17.78	$615.30	090	
27216	§	Treat pelvic ring fracture	15.73	NA	9.26	1.29	NA	NA	26.28	$909.45	090	

*Please note that these calculations are based on the Medicare 2022 Conversion Factor of $34.6062 and the DRA RVU cap rates at time of publication.

A = assistant-at-surgery restriction
A+ = assistant-at-surgery restriction unless medical necessity established with documentation
B = bilateral surgery adjustment applies
C = cosurgeons payable
C+ = cosurgeons payable if medical necessity established with documentation
CP = carriers may establish RVUs and payment amounts for these services, generally on an individual basis following review of documentation such as an operative report
M = multiple surgery adjustment applies
Me = multiple endoscopy rules may apply
M+ = multiple therapy rules apply
Mtc = multiple diagnostic imaging rules apply
T = team surgeons permitted
T+ = team surgeons payable if medical necessity established with documentation
§ = indicates code is not covered by Medicare
GS = procedure must be performed under the general supervision of a physician
DS = procedure must be performed under the direct supervision of a physician
PS = procedure must be performed under the personal supervision of a physician
DRA = procedure subject to DRA limitation

Relative Value Units

CPT Code and Modifier		Description	Work RVU	Nonfacility Practice Expense RVU	Facility Practice Expense RVU	PLI RVU	Total Non-facility RVUs	Medicare Payment Nonfacility	Total Facility RVUs	Medicare Payment Facility	Global Period	Payment Policy Indicators
27217	§	Treat pelvic ring fracture	14.65	NA	8.85	1.20	NA	NA	24.70	$854.77	090	
27218	§	Treat pelvic ring fracture	20.93	NA	11.26	1.71	NA	NA	33.90	$1173.15	090	
27220		Treat hip socket fracture	5.50	5.90	5.71	1.11	12.51	$432.92	12.32	$426.35	090	A B M
27222		Treat hip socket fracture	14.11	NA	12.23	2.91	NA	NA	29.25	$1012.23	090	A B M
27226		Treat hip wall fracture	15.57	NA	12.54	3.20	NA	NA	31.31	$1083.52	090	B C M
27227		Treat hip fracture(s)	25.41	NA	18.22	5.20	NA	NA	48.83	$1689.82	090	B C M
27228		Treat hip fracture(s)	29.33	NA	20.13	6.04	NA	NA	55.50	$1920.64	090	B C M
27230		Treat thigh fracture	5.81	7.58	7.29	1.18	14.57	$504.21	14.28	$494.18	090	A B M
27232		Treat thigh fracture	11.72	NA	7.79	2.44	NA	NA	21.95	$759.61	090	A B M
27235		Treat thigh fracture	13.00	NA	11.30	2.66	NA	NA	26.96	$932.98	090	A B C+ M
27236		Treat thigh fracture	17.61	NA	14.16	3.60	NA	NA	35.37	$1224.02	090	B C+ M
27238		Treat thigh fracture	5.75	NA	7.06	1.17	NA	NA	13.98	$483.79	090	A B M
27240		Treat thigh fracture	13.81	NA	11.86	2.83	NA	NA	28.50	$986.28	090	A B M
27244		Treat thigh fracture	18.18	NA	14.47	3.73	NA	NA	36.38	$1258.97	090	B C+ M
27245		Treat thigh fracture	18.18	NA	14.46	3.71	NA	NA	36.35	$1257.94	090	B C M
27246		Treat thigh fracture	4.83	5.90	5.75	0.98	11.71	$405.24	11.56	$400.05	090	A B M
27248		Treat thigh fracture	10.78	NA	9.22	2.20	NA	NA	22.20	$768.26	090	B C+ M
27250		Treat hip dislocation	3.82	NA	0.73	0.78	NA	NA	5.33	$184.45	000	A B M
27252		Treat hip dislocation	11.03	NA	9.22	2.23	NA	NA	22.48	$777.95	090	A B M
27253		Treat hip dislocation	13.58	NA	11.58	2.79	NA	NA	27.95	$967.24	090	B C+ M
27254		Treat hip dislocation	18.94	NA	14.87	3.90	NA	NA	37.71	$1305.00	090	B C+ M
27256		Treat hip dislocation	4.28	3.97	1.89	0.90	9.15	$316.65	7.07	$244.67	010	A+ B M
27257		Treat hip dislocation	5.38	NA	4.21	1.10	NA	NA	10.69	$369.94	010	A+ B M
27258		Treat hip dislocation	16.18	NA	13.48	3.34	NA	NA	33.00	$1142.00	090	B C+ M
27259		Treat hip dislocation	23.26	NA	17.62	4.79	NA	NA	45.67	$1580.47	090	B M
27265		Treat hip dislocation	5.24	NA	5.97	1.07	NA	NA	12.28	$424.96	090	A B M
27266		Treat hip dislocation	7.78	NA	8.09	1.59	NA	NA	17.46	$604.22	090	A B M
27267		Cltx thigh fx	5.50	NA	6.59	1.09	NA	NA	13.18	$456.11	090	B C+ M
27268		Cltx thigh fx w/mnpj	7.12	NA	7.66	1.47	NA	NA	16.25	$562.35	090	B C+ M
27269		Optx thigh fx	18.89	NA	13.96	3.89	NA	NA	36.74	$1271.43	090	B C+ M
27275		Manipulation of hip joint	2.32	NA	2.69	0.43	NA	NA	5.44	$188.26	010	A M
27279		Arthrodesis sacroiliac joint	12.13	NA	9.89	2.84	NA	NA	24.86	$860.31	090	B C+ M
27280		Fusion of sacroiliac joint	20.00	NA	14.71	5.72	NA	NA	40.43	$1399.13	090	B C+ M

27282		Fusion of pubic bones	11.85	NA	11.29	2.45	NA	NA	25.59	$885.57	090	C+ M
27284		Fusion of hip joint	25.06	NA	17.23	5.17	NA	NA	47.46	$1642.41	090	B C+ M
27286		Fusion of hip joint	25.17	NA	18.24	5.19	NA	NA	48.60	$1681.86	090	B C+ M
27290		Amputation of leg at hip	24.55	NA	18.51	5.06	NA	NA	48.12	$1665.25	090	C+ M
27295		Amputation of leg at hip	19.66	NA	13.59	4.20	NA	NA	37.45	$1296.00	090	B C+ M
27299	CP	Pelvis/hip joint surgery	0.00	0.00	0.00	0.00	0.00	$0.00	0.00	$0.00	YYY	B C+ M T+
27301		Drain thigh/knee lesion	6.78	11.98	6.89	1.43	20.19	$698.70	15.10	$522.55	090	A B M
27303		Drainage of bone lesion	8.63	NA	8.56	1.84	NA	NA	19.03	$658.56	090	B C+ M
27305		Incise thigh tendon & fascia	6.18	NA	6.99	1.26	NA	NA	14.43	$499.37	090	B C+ M
27306		Incision of thigh tendon	4.74	NA	4.88	0.44	NA	NA	10.06	$348.14	090	B M
27307		Incision of thigh tendons	6.06	NA	5.71	0.65	NA	NA	12.42	$429.81	090	A+ B C+ M
27310		Exploration of knee joint	10.00	NA	9.77	2.03	NA	NA	21.80	$754.42	090	B C+ M
27323		Biopsy thigh soft tissues	2.33	5.52	2.46	0.34	8.19	$283.42	5.13	$177.53	010	A B M
27324		Biopsy thigh soft tissues	5.04	NA	5.98	1.11	NA	NA	12.13	$419.77	090	A B M
27325		Neurectomy hamstring	7.20	NA	8.19	1.48	NA	NA	16.87	$583.81	090	B M
27326		Neurectomy popliteal	6.47	NA	7.82	1.33	NA	NA	15.62	$540.55	090	B C+ M
27327		Exc thigh/knee les sc < 3 cm	3.96	10.40	4.55	0.87	15.23	$527.05	9.38	$324.61	090	A B M
27328		Exc thigh/knee tum deep <5cm	8.85	NA	7.75	1.94	NA	NA	18.54	$641.60	090	A B M
27329		Resect thigh/knee tum < 5 cm	15.72	NA	11.65	3.55	NA	NA	30.92	$1070.02	090	B C+ M
27330		Biopsy knee joint lining	5.11	NA	6.46	1.05	NA	NA	12.62	$436.73	090	A B C+ M
27331		Explore/treat knee joint	6.02	NA	6.99	1.21	NA	NA	14.22	$492.10	090	B C+ M
27332		Removal of knee cartilage	8.46	NA	9.06	1.73	NA	NA	19.25	$666.17	090	B C+ M
27333		Removal of knee cartilage	7.55	NA	8.48	1.55	NA	NA	17.58	$608.38	090	B C+ M
27334		Remove knee joint lining	9.19	NA	9.39	1.86	NA	NA	20.44	$707.35	090	B C+ M
27335		Remove knee joint lining	10.55	NA	10.09	2.17	NA	NA	22.81	$789.37	090	B C+ M
27337		Exc thigh/knee les sc 3 cm/>	5.91	NA	5.24	1.37	NA	NA	12.52	$433.27	090	B M
27339		Exc thigh/knee tum dep 5cm/>	11.13	NA	8.85	2.50	NA	NA	22.48	$777.95	090	B M
27340		Removal of kneecap bursa	4.32	NA	6.00	0.89	NA	NA	11.21	$387.94	090	A B M

*Please note that these calculations are based on the Medicare 2022 Conversion Factor of $34.6062 and the DRA RVU cap rates at time of publication.

A = assistant-at-surgery restriction
A+ = assistant-at-surgery restriction unless medical necessity established with documentation
B = bilateral surgery adjustment applies
C = cosurgeons payable
C+ = cosurgeons payable if medical necessity established with documentation
CP = carriers may establish RVUs and payment amounts for these services, generally on an individual basis following review of documentation such as an operative report
M = multiple surgery adjustment applies
Me = multiple endoscopy rules may apply
M+ = multiple therapy rules apply
Mtc = multiple diagnostic imaging rules apply
T = team surgeons permitted
T+ = team surgeons payable if medical necessity established with documentation
§ = indicates code is not covered by Medicare
GS = procedure must be performed under the general supervision of a physician
DS = procedure must be performed under the direct supervision of a physician
PS = procedure must be performed under the personal supervision of a physician
DRA = procedure subject to DRA limitation

Relative Value Units

CPT Code and Modifier	Description	Work RVU	Nonfacility Practice Expense RVU	Facility Practice Expense RVU	PLI RVU	Total Non-facility RVUs	Medicare Payment Nonfacility	Total Facility RVUs	Medicare Payment Facility	Global Period	Payment Policy Indicators
27345	Removal of knee cyst	6.09	NA	7.18	1.24	NA	NA	14.51	$502.14	090	B C+ M
27347	Remove knee cyst	6.73	NA	7.60	1.37	NA	NA	15.70	$543.32	090	B C+ M
27350	Removal of kneecap	8.66	NA	9.10	1.76	NA	NA	19.52	$675.51	090	B C+ M
27355	Remove femur lesion	8.00	NA	8.52	1.64	NA	NA	18.16	$628.45	090	B C+ M
27356	Remove femur lesion/graft	10.09	NA	9.88	2.07	NA	NA	22.04	$762.72	090	B C+ M
27357	Remove femur lesion/graft	11.16	NA	10.94	2.31	NA	NA	24.41	$844.74	090	B C+ M
27358	Remove femur lesion/fixation	4.73	NA	2.40	0.98	NA	NA	8.11	$280.66	ZZZ	
27360	Partial removal leg bone(s)	11.46	NA	13.25	2.34	NA	NA	27.05	$936.10	090	B C+ M
27364	Resect thigh/knee tum 5 cm/>	24.49	NA	16.42	5.41	NA	NA	46.32	$1602.96	090	B C+ M
27365	Resect femur/knee tumor	32.21	NA	21.81	6.65	NA	NA	60.67	$2099.56	090	B C+ M
27369	Njx cntrst kne arthg/ct/mri	0.77	4.44	0.30	0.10	5.31	$183.76	1.17	$40.49	000	A B M
27372	Removal of foreign body	5.21	11.57	5.70	1.07	17.85	$617.72	11.98	$414.58	090	A+ B M
27380	Repair of kneecap tendon	7.45	NA	9.74	1.50	NA	NA	18.69	$646.79	090	B C+ M
27381	Repair/graft kneecap tendon	10.76	NA	11.64	2.17	NA	NA	24.57	$850.27	090	B C+ M
27385	Repair of thigh muscle	6.93	NA	9.89	1.39	NA	NA	18.21	$630.18	090	B C+ M
27386	Repair/graft of thigh muscle	11.13	NA	12.30	2.23	NA	NA	25.66	$888.00	090	B C+ M
27390	Incision of thigh tendon	5.53	NA	6.77	1.12	NA	NA	13.42	$464.42	090	B M
27391	Incision of thigh tendons	7.49	NA	7.70	1.41	NA	NA	16.60	$574.46	090	A+ C+ M
27392	Incision of thigh tendons	9.63	NA	9.63	1.99	NA	NA	21.25	$735.38	090	C+ M
27393	Lengthening of thigh tendon	6.59	NA	7.10	1.30	NA	NA	14.99	$518.75	090	B C+ M
27394	Lengthening of thigh tendons	8.79	NA	8.93	1.81	NA	NA	19.53	$675.86	090	M
27395	Lengthening of thigh tendons	12.24	NA	11.48	2.51	NA	NA	26.23	$907.72	090	C+ M
27396	Transplant of thigh tendon	8.15	NA	8.62	1.68	NA	NA	18.45	$638.48	090	B C+ M
27397	Transplants of thigh tendons	12.66	NA	11.91	2.62	NA	NA	27.19	$940.94	090	B M
27400	Revise thigh muscles/tendons	9.33	NA	9.48	1.94	NA	NA	20.75	$718.08	090	B C+ M
27403	Repair of knee cartilage	8.62	NA	8.86	1.75	NA	NA	19.23	$665.48	090	B C+ M
27405	Repair of knee ligament	9.08	NA	9.27	1.83	NA	NA	20.18	$698.35	090	B C+ M
27407	Repair of knee ligament	10.85	NA	10.66	2.23	NA	NA	23.74	$821.55	090	B C+ M
27409	Repair of knee ligaments	13.71	NA	12.22	2.83	NA	NA	28.76	$995.27	090	B C+ M
27412	Autochondrocyte implant knee	24.74	NA	18.94	5.10	NA	NA	48.78	$1688.09	090	B C+ M
27415	Osteochondral knee allograft	20.00	NA	16.54	4.12	NA	NA	40.66	$1407.09	090	B C+ M
27416	Osteochondral knee autograft	14.16	NA	12.03	2.93	NA	NA	29.12	$1007.73	090	A+ B M
27418	Repair degenerated kneecap	11.60	NA	10.83	2.31	NA	NA	24.74	$856.16	090	B C+ M

27420	Revision of unstable kneecap	10.26	NA	9.81	2.04	NA	NA	22.11	$765.14	090	B C+ M
27422	Revision of unstable kneecap	10.21	NA	9.87	2.04	NA	NA	22.12	$765.49	090	B C+ M
27424	Revision/removal of kneecap	10.24	NA	9.94	2.13	NA	NA	22.31	$772.06	090	B C+ M
27425	Lat retinacular release open	5.39	NA	7.07	1.09	NA	NA	13.55	$468.91	090	A B C+ M
27427	Reconstruction knee	9.79	NA	9.44	1.94	NA	NA	21.17	$732.61	090	B C+ M
27428	Reconstruction knee	15.58	NA	14.36	3.23	NA	NA	33.17	$1147.89	090	B C+ M
27429	Reconstruction knee	17.54	NA	16.18	3.61	NA	NA	37.33	$1291.85	090	B C+ M
27430	Revision of thigh muscles	10.16	NA	9.88	2.08	NA	NA	22.12	$765.49	090	B C+ M
27435	Incision of knee joint	10.88	NA	10.90	2.17	NA	NA	23.95	$828.82	090	B C+ M
27437	Revise kneecap	8.93	NA	8.94	1.81	NA	NA	19.68	$681.05	090	A B C+ M
27438	Revise kneecap with implant	11.89	NA	10.70	2.39	NA	NA	24.98	$864.46	090	B C+ M
27440	Revision of knee joint	11.09	NA	10.37	2.28	NA	NA	23.74	$821.55	090	B C+ M
27441	Revision of knee joint	11.54	NA	10.60	2.37	NA	NA	24.51	$848.20	090	B C+ M
27442	Revision of knee joint	12.37	NA	10.98	2.54	NA	NA	25.89	$895.95	090	B C+ M
27443	Revision of knee joint	11.41	NA	10.53	2.34	NA	NA	24.28	$840.24	090	B C+ M
27445	Revision of knee joint	18.66	NA	14.70	3.82	NA	NA	37.18	$1286.66	090	B C+ M
27446	Revision of knee joint	17.48	NA	13.13	3.57	NA	NA	34.18	$1182.84	090	B C+ M
27447	Total knee arthroplasty	19.60	NA	14.38	4.00	NA	NA	37.98	$1314.34	090	B C+ M
27448	Incision of thigh	11.60	NA	10.14	2.34	NA	NA	24.08	$833.32	090	B C+ M
27450	Incision of thigh	14.61	NA	12.49	2.96	NA	NA	30.06	$1040.26	090	B C+ M
27454	Realignment of thigh bone	19.17	NA	15.20	3.95	NA	NA	38.32	$1326.11	090	B C+ M
27455	Realignment of knee	13.36	NA	12.51	2.76	NA	NA	28.63	$990.78	090	B C+ M
27457	Realignment of knee	14.03	NA	11.62	2.90	NA	NA	28.55	$988.01	090	B C+ M
27465	Shortening of thigh bone	18.60	NA	14.55	3.84	NA	NA	36.99	$1280.08	090	B C+ M
27466	Lengthening of thigh bone	17.28	NA	14.30	3.56	NA	NA	35.14	$1216.06	090	B C+ M
27468	Shorten/lengthen thighs	19.97	NA	15.66	4.12	NA	NA	39.75	$1375.60	090	B C+ M
27470	Repair of thigh	17.14	NA	14.32	3.52	NA	NA	34.98	$1210.52	090	B C+ M
27472	Repair/graft of thigh	18.72	NA	14.90	3.84	NA	NA	37.46	$1296.35	090	B C+ M

*Please note that these calculations are based on the Medicare 2022 Conversion Factor of $34.6062 and the DRA RVU cap rates at time of publication.

A = assistant-at-surgery restriction
A+ = assistant-at-surgery restriction unless medical necessity established with documentation
B = bilateral surgery adjustment applies
C = cosurgeons payable
C+ = cosurgeons payable if medical necessity established with documentation
CP = carriers may establish RVUs and payment amounts for these services, generally on an individual basis following review of documentation such as an operative report
M = multiple surgery adjustment applies
Me = multiple endoscopy rules may apply
M+ = multiple therapy rules apply
Mtc = multiple diagnostic imaging rules apply
T = team surgeons permitted
T+ = team surgeons payable if medical necessity established with documentation
§ = indicates code is not covered by Medicare
GS = procedure must be performed under the general supervision of a physician
DS = procedure must be performed under the direct supervision of a physician
PS = procedure must be performed under the personal supervision of a physician
DRA = procedure subject to DRA limitation

Relative Value Units

CPT Code and Modifier	Description	Work RVU	Nonfacility Practice Expense RVU	Facility Practice Expense RVU	PLI RVU	Total Non-facility RVUs	Medicare Payment Nonfacility	Total Facility RVUs	Medicare Payment Facility	Global Period	Payment Policy Indicators
27475	Surgery to stop leg growth	8.93	NA	9.02	1.84	NA	NA	19.79	$684.86	090	A B C+ M
27477	Surgery to stop leg growth	10.14	NA	9.63	2.09	NA	NA	21.86	$756.49	090	A B C+ M
27479	Surgery to stop leg growth	13.16	NA	11.43	2.71	NA	NA	27.30	$944.75	090	B M
27485	Surgery to stop leg growth	9.13	NA	9.03	1.87	NA	NA	20.03	$693.16	090	A B M
27486	Revise/replace knee joint	21.12	NA	16.12	4.32	NA	NA	41.56	$1438.23	090	B C+ M
27487	Revise/replace knee joint	27.11	NA	19.18	5.56	NA	NA	51.85	$1794.33	090	B C+ M
27488	Removal of knee prosthesis	17.60	NA	14.35	3.61	NA	NA	35.56	$1230.60	090	B C+ M
27495	Reinforce thigh	16.54	NA	13.60	3.39	NA	NA	33.53	$1160.35	090	B C+ M
27496	Decompression of thigh/knee	6.78	NA	8.19	1.40	NA	NA	16.37	$566.50	090	A B M
27497	Decompression of thigh/knee	7.79	NA	7.92	1.61	NA	NA	17.32	$599.38	090	A+ B C M
27498	Decompression of thigh/knee	8.66	NA	9.15	1.78	NA	NA	19.59	$677.94	090	B C M
27499	Decompression of thigh/knee	9.43	NA	9.53	1.94	NA	NA	20.90	$723.27	090	B C M
27500	Treatment of thigh fracture	6.30	8.04	6.78	1.27	15.61	$540.20	14.35	$496.60	090	A B M
27501	Treatment of thigh fracture	6.45	7.40	7.11	1.32	15.17	$524.98	14.88	$514.94	090	A+ B M
27502	Treatment of thigh fracture	11.36	NA	8.91	2.33	NA	NA	22.60	$782.10	090	A B M
27503	Treatment of thigh fracture	11.27	NA	10.22	2.29	NA	NA	23.78	$822.94	090	A+ B M
27506	Treatment of thigh fracture	19.65	NA	15.97	4.00	NA	NA	39.62	$1371.10	090	B C+ M
27507	Treatment of thigh fracture	14.48	NA	11.27	2.97	NA	NA	28.72	$993.89	090	B C M
27508	Treatment of thigh fracture	6.20	8.30	7.48	1.25	15.75	$545.05	14.93	$516.67	090	A B M
27509	Treatment of thigh fracture	8.14	NA	10.49	1.65	NA	NA	20.28	$701.81	090	A+ B M
27510	Treatment of thigh fracture	9.80	NA	8.43	1.99	NA	NA	20.22	$699.74	090	A B M
27511	Treatment of thigh fracture	15.11	NA	11.37	3.06	NA	NA	29.54	$1022.27	090	B C M
27513	Treatment of thigh fracture	19.25	NA	13.46	3.94	NA	NA	36.65	$1268.32	090	B C M
27514	Treatment of thigh fracture	14.60	NA	11.11	2.97	NA	NA	28.68	$992.51	090	B C+ M
27516	Treat thigh fx growth plate	5.59	8.79	7.77	1.16	15.54	$537.78	14.52	$502.48	090	A B M
27517	Treat thigh fx growth plate	9.12	NA	9.56	1.86	NA	NA	20.54	$710.81	090	A+ B M
27519	Treat thigh fx growth plate	13.25	NA	10.49	2.72	NA	NA	26.46	$915.68	090	B C+ M
27520	Treat kneecap fracture	3.04	6.16	5.42	0.60	9.80	$339.14	9.06	$313.53	090	A B M
27524	Treat kneecap fracture	10.37	NA	9.95	2.11	NA	NA	22.43	$776.22	090	B C+ M
27530	Treat knee fracture	2.65	6.09	5.53	0.54	9.28	$321.15	8.72	$301.77	090	A B M
27532	Treat knee fracture	7.55	9.47	8.22	1.54	18.56	$642.29	17.31	$599.03	090	A B M
27535	Treat knee fracture	13.41	NA	10.50	2.72	NA	NA	26.63	$921.56	090	B C M
27536	Treat knee fracture	17.39	NA	14.23	3.56	NA	NA	35.18	$1217.45	090	B C+ M

27538		Treat knee fracture(s)	5.09	8.49	7.45	1.04	14.62	$505.94	13.58	$469.95	090	A+ B M
27540		Treat knee fracture	11.30	NA	10.60	2.31	NA	NA	24.21	$837.82	090	B C+ M
27550		Treat knee dislocation	5.98	8.24	6.98	1.24	15.46	$535.01	14.20	$491.41	090	A+ B M
27552		Treat knee dislocation	8.18	NA	9.09	1.66	NA	NA	18.93	$655.10	090	A+ B M
27556		Treat knee dislocation	13.00	NA	10.36	2.68	NA	NA	26.04	$901.15	090	B C+ M
27557		Treat knee dislocation	15.90	NA	11.84	3.29	NA	NA	31.03	$1073.83	090	B C+ M
27558		Treat knee dislocation	18.39	NA	13.09	3.79	NA	NA	35.27	$1220.56	090	B C M
27560		Treat kneecap dislocation	3.99	6.32	5.34	0.79	11.10	$384.13	10.12	$350.21	090	A B M
27562		Treat kneecap dislocation	5.98	NA	7.45	1.24	NA	NA	14.67	$507.67	090	A+ B M
27566		Treat kneecap dislocation	12.71	NA	11.21	2.62	NA	NA	26.54	$918.45	090	B C+ M
27570		Fixation of knee joint	1.79	NA	2.38	0.37	NA	NA	4.54	$157.11	010	A B M
27580		Fusion of knee	21.10	NA	18.44	4.32	NA	NA	43.86	$1517.83	090	B C+ M
27590		Amputate leg at thigh	13.47	NA	6.65	3.26	NA	NA	23.38	$809.09	090	B C+ M
27591		Amputate leg at thigh	13.94	NA	11.83	2.88	NA	NA	28.65	$991.47	090	B C+ M
27592		Amputate leg at thigh	10.98	NA	6.31	2.62	NA	NA	19.91	$689.01	090	B C+ M
27594		Amputation follow-up surgery	7.29	NA	6.14	1.68	NA	NA	15.11	$522.90	090	A B M
27596		Amputation follow-up surgery	11.29	NA	7.28	2.66	NA	NA	21.23	$734.69	090	A B C+ M
27598		Amputate lower leg at knee	11.22	NA	6.98	2.62	NA	NA	20.82	$720.50	090	B C+ M
27599	CP	Leg surgery procedure	0.00	0.00	0.00	0.00	0.00	$0.00	0.00	$0.00	YYY	B C+ M T+
27600		Decompression of lower leg	6.03	NA	4.74	1.25	NA	NA	12.02	$415.97	090	A B C+ M
27601		Decompression of lower leg	6.05	NA	6.07	1.20	NA	NA	13.32	$460.95	090	A B M
27602		Decompression of lower leg	7.82	NA	4.60	1.84	NA	NA	14.26	$493.48	090	B C+ M
27603		Drain lower leg lesion	5.23	9.69	5.43	1.02	15.94	$551.62	11.68	$404.20	090	A B M
27604		Drain lower leg bursa	4.59	8.15	4.27	0.65	13.39	$463.38	9.51	$329.10	090	A+ B M
27605		Incision of achilles tendon	2.92	6.70	2.19	0.27	9.89	$342.26	5.38	$186.18	010	A+ B M
27606		Incision of achilles tendon	4.18	NA	3.25	0.65	NA	NA	8.08	$279.62	010	A B C+ M
27607		Treat lower leg bone lesion	8.62	NA	7.66	1.43	NA	NA	17.71	$612.88	090	A B M
27610		Explore/treat ankle joint	9.13	NA	8.49	1.63	NA	NA	19.25	$666.17	090	A B M

*Please note that these calculations are based on the Medicare 2022 Conversion Factor of $34.6062 and the DRA RVU cap rates at time of publication.

A = assistant-at-surgery restriction

A+ = assistant-at-surgery restriction unless medical necessity established with documentation

B = bilateral surgery adjustment applies

C = cosurgeons payable

C+ = cosurgeons payable if medical necessity established with documentation

CP = carriers may establish RVUs and payment amounts for these services, generally on an individual basis following review of documentation such as an operative report

M = multiple surgery adjustment applies

Me = multiple endoscopy rules may apply

M+ = multiple therapy rules apply

Mtc = multiple diagnostic imaging rules apply

T = team surgeons permitted

T+ = team surgeons payable if medical necessity established with documentation

§ = indicates code is not covered by Medicare

GS = procedure must be performed under the general supervision of a physician

DS = procedure must be performed under the direct supervision of a physician

PS = procedure must be performed under the personal supervision of a physician

DRA = procedure subject to DRA limitation

Relative Value Units

CPT Code and Modifier	Description	Work RVU	Nonfacility Practice Expense RVU	Facility Practice Expense RVU	PLI RVU	Total Non-facility RVUs	Medicare Payment Nonfacility	Total Facility RVUs	Medicare Payment Facility	Global Period	Payment Policy Indicators
27612	Exploration of ankle joint	8.15	NA	7.24	1.18	NA	NA	16.57	$573.42	090	B C+ M
27613	Biopsy lower leg soft tissue	2.22	5.04	2.22	0.29	7.55	$261.28	4.73	$163.69	010	A B M
27614	Biopsy lower leg soft tissue	5.80	10.60	5.43	1.01	17.41	$602.49	12.24	$423.58	090	A B M
27615	Resect leg/ankle tum < 5 cm	15.72	NA	11.41	3.22	NA	NA	30.35	$1050.30	090	A+ B C+ M
27616	Resect leg/ankle tum 5 cm/>	19.63	NA	13.69	4.31	NA	NA	37.63	$1302.23	090	A+ B C+ M
27618	Exc leg/ankle tum < 3 cm	3.96	10.03	4.37	0.77	14.76	$510.79	9.10	$314.92	090	A B M
27619	Exc leg/ankle tum deep <5 cm	6.91	NA	5.66	1.12	NA	NA	13.69	$473.76	090	A B M
27620	Explore/treat ankle joint	6.15	NA	6.25	0.98	NA	NA	13.38	$463.03	090	B C+ M
27625	Remove ankle joint lining	8.49	NA	7.23	1.32	NA	NA	17.04	$589.69	090	B C+ M
27626	Remove ankle joint lining	9.10	NA	7.43	1.33	NA	NA	17.86	$618.07	090	B M
27630	Removal of tendon lesion	4.94	10.51	4.97	0.73	16.18	$559.93	10.64	$368.21	090	A B M
27632	Exc leg/ankle les sc 3 cm/>	5.91	NA	5.08	1.29	NA	NA	12.28	$424.96	090	B M
27634	Exc leg/ankle tum dep 5 cm/>	10.13	NA	7.93	2.01	NA	NA	20.07	$694.55	090	B M
27635	Remove lower leg bone lesion	8.03	NA	7.78	1.41	NA	NA	17.22	$595.92	090	A B C+ M
27637	Remove/graft leg bone lesion	10.31	NA	9.63	1.90	NA	NA	21.84	$755.80	090	B C+ M
27638	Remove/graft leg bone lesion	10.99	NA	9.36	1.94	NA	NA	22.29	$771.37	090	B C+ M
27640	Partial removal of tibia	12.24	NA	10.24	2.22	NA	NA	24.70	$854.77	090	A B C+ M
27641	Partial removal of fibula	9.84	NA	7.91	1.60	NA	NA	19.35	$669.63	090	A B C+ M
27645	Resect tibia tumor	27.21	NA	19.44	5.60	NA	NA	52.25	$1808.17	090	B C+ M
27646	Resect fibula tumor	23.21	NA	17.42	4.78	NA	NA	45.41	$1571.47	090	B C+ M
27647	Resect talus/calcaneus tum	20.26	NA	7.38	1.63	NA	NA	29.27	$1012.92	090	B M
27648	Injection for ankle x-ray	0.96	5.55	0.42	0.12	6.63	$229.44	1.50	$51.91	000	A+ B M
27650	Repair achilles tendon	9.21	NA	8.90	1.44	NA	NA	19.55	$676.55	090	B C+ M
27652	Repair/graft achilles tendon	10.78	NA	7.43	1.30	NA	NA	19.51	$675.17	090	A B C+ M
27654	Repair of achilles tendon	10.53	NA	9.03	1.57	NA	NA	21.13	$731.23	090	B C+ M
27656	Repair leg fascia defect	4.71	10.97	5.03	0.72	16.40	$567.54	10.46	$361.98	090	B M
27658	Repair of leg tendon each	5.12	NA	5.08	0.73	NA	NA	10.93	$378.25	090	C+ M
27659	Repair of leg tendon each	7.10	NA	5.87	0.96	NA	NA	13.93	$482.06	090	C+ M
27664	Repair of leg tendon each	4.73	NA	5.34	0.77	NA	NA	10.84	$375.13	090	A+ M
27665	Repair of leg tendon each	5.57	NA	6.04	0.93	NA	NA	12.54	$433.96	090	C+ M
27675	Repair lower leg tendons	7.35	NA	6.22	1.01	NA	NA	14.58	$504.56	090	B C+ M
27676	Repair lower leg tendons	8.73	NA	7.85	1.47	NA	NA	18.05	$624.64	090	B M
27680	Release of lower leg tendon	5.88	NA	5.63	0.89	NA	NA	12.40	$429.12	090	A C+ M

27681	Release of lower leg tendons	7.05	NA	6.87	1.18	NA	NA	15.10	$522.55	090	A B C+ M
27685	Revision of lower leg tendon	6.69	11.90	6.13	0.93	19.52	$675.51	13.75	$475.84	090	B C+ M
27686	Revise lower leg tendons	7.75	NA	6.84	1.20	NA	NA	15.79	$546.43	090	A B C+ M
27687	Revision of calf tendon	6.41	NA	6.09	0.95	NA	NA	13.45	$465.45	090	B C+ M
27690	Revise lower leg tendon	9.17	NA	8.46	1.37	NA	NA	19.00	$657.52	090	B C+ M
27691	Revise lower leg tendon	10.49	NA	9.81	1.78	NA	NA	22.08	$764.10	090	B C+ M
27692	Revise additional leg tendon	1.87	NA	0.79	0.31	NA	NA	2.97	$102.78	ZZZ	C+
27695	Repair of ankle ligament	6.70	NA	6.53	1.00	NA	NA	14.23	$492.45	090	A B C+ M
27696	Repair of ankle ligaments	8.58	NA	6.52	1.16	NA	NA	16.26	$562.70	090	A B C+ M
27698	Repair of ankle ligament	9.61	NA	7.79	1.49	NA	NA	18.89	$653.71	090	B C+ M
27700	Revision of ankle joint	9.66	NA	7.24	1.25	NA	NA	18.15	$628.10	090	B C+ M
27702	Reconstruct ankle joint	14.42	NA	11.50	2.63	NA	NA	28.55	$988.01	090	B C+ M
27703	Reconstruction ankle joint	16.94	NA	12.81	3.09	NA	NA	32.84	$1136.47	090	B M
27704	Removal of ankle implant	7.81	NA	7.75	1.40	NA	NA	16.96	$586.92	090	A B C+ M
27705	Incision of tibia	10.86	NA	9.63	2.06	NA	NA	22.55	$780.37	090	B C+ M
27707	Incision of fibula	4.78	NA	6.37	0.87	NA	NA	12.02	$415.97	090	A B C+ M
27709	Incision of tibia & fibula	17.48	NA	13.10	3.30	NA	NA	33.88	$1172.46	090	B C+ M
27712	Realignment of lower leg	15.87	NA	13.54	3.28	NA	NA	32.69	$1131.28	090	B C+ M
27715	Revision of lower leg	15.50	NA	13.14	3.22	NA	NA	31.86	$1102.55	090	B C+ M
27720	Repair of tibia	12.36	NA	11.17	2.46	NA	NA	25.99	$899.42	090	B C+ M
27722	Repair/graft of tibia	12.45	NA	11.60	2.56	NA	NA	26.61	$920.87	090	B C+ M
27724	Repair/graft of tibia	19.31	NA	13.93	3.92	NA	NA	37.16	$1285.97	090	B C+ M
27725	Repair of lower leg	17.41	NA	15.01	3.60	NA	NA	36.02	$1246.52	090	B C+ M
27726	Repair fibula nonunion	14.34	NA	11.33	2.79	NA	NA	28.46	$984.89	090	A B C+ M
27727	Repair of lower leg	14.84	NA	12.95	3.05	NA	NA	30.84	$1067.26	090	B C+ M
27730	Repair of tibia epiphysis	7.70	NA	8.28	1.59	NA	NA	17.57	$608.03	090	A B C+ M
27732	Repair of fibula epiphysis	5.46	NA	6.97	1.11	NA	NA	13.54	$468.57	090	A B M
27734	Repair lower leg epiphyses	8.83	NA	8.98	1.81	NA	NA	19.62	$678.97	090	A B M

*Please note that these calculations are based on the Medicare 2022 Conversion Factor of $34.6062 and the DRA RVU cap rates at time of publication.

A = assistant-at-surgery restriction
A+ = assistant-at-surgery restriction unless medical necessity established with documentation
B = bilateral surgery adjustment applies
C = cosurgeons payable
C+ = cosurgeons payable if medical necessity established with documentation
CP = carriers may establish RVUs and payment amounts for these services, generally on an individual basis following review of documentation such as an operative report
M = multiple surgery adjustment applies
Me = multiple endoscopy rules may apply
M+ = multiple therapy rules apply
Mtc = multiple diagnostic imaging rules apply
T = team surgeons permitted
T+ = team surgeons payable if medical necessity established with documentation
§ = indicates code is not covered by Medicare
GS = procedure must be performed under the general supervision of a physician
DS = procedure must be performed under the direct supervision of a physician
PS = procedure must be performed under the personal supervision of a physician
DRA = procedure subject to DRA limitation

Relative Value Units

CPT Code and Modifier	Description	Work RVU	Nonfacility Practice Expense RVU	Facility Practice Expense RVU	PLI RVU	Total Non-facility RVUs	Medicare Payment Nonfacility	Total Facility RVUs	Medicare Payment Facility	Global Period	Payment Policy Indicators
27740	Repair of leg epiphyses	9.61	NA	9.50	1.99	NA	NA	21.10	$730.19	090	B M
27742	Repair of leg epiphyses	10.63	NA	10.31	2.18	NA	NA	23.12	$800.10	090	B C+ M
27745	Reinforce tibia	10.49	NA	9.91	2.13	NA	NA	22.53	$779.68	090	B C+ M
27750	Treatment of tibia fracture	3.37	6.42	5.67	0.66	10.45	$361.63	9.70	$335.68	090	A B M
27752	Treatment of tibia fracture	6.27	8.51	7.15	1.28	16.06	$555.78	14.70	$508.71	090	A B M
27756	Treatment of tibia fracture	7.45	NA	8.36	1.48	NA	NA	17.29	$598.34	090	B C+ M
27758	Treatment of tibia fracture	12.54	NA	11.56	2.55	NA	NA	26.65	$922.26	090	B C+ M
27759	Treatment of tibia fracture	14.45	NA	12.20	2.96	NA	NA	29.61	$1024.69	090	B C M
27760	Cltx medial ankle fx	3.21	6.22	5.46	0.57	10.00	$346.06	9.24	$319.76	090	A B M
27762	Cltx med ankle fx w/mnpj	5.47	7.93	6.56	1.09	14.49	$501.44	13.12	$454.03	090	A B M
27766	Optx medial ankle fx	7.89	NA	8.63	1.49	NA	NA	18.01	$623.26	090	A B C+ M
27767	Cltx post ankle fx	2.64	5.65	5.57	0.50	8.79	$304.19	8.71	$301.42	090	A B M
27768	Cltx post ankle fx w/mnpj	5.14	NA	7.21	1.05	NA	NA	13.40	$463.72	090	A B M
27769	Optx post ankle fx	10.14	NA	9.55	1.99	NA	NA	21.68	$750.26	090	A B M
27780	Treatment of fibula fracture	2.83	5.94	5.20	0.56	9.33	$322.88	8.59	$297.27	090	A B M
27781	Treatment of fibula fracture	4.59	7.58	6.54	0.93	13.10	$453.34	12.06	$417.35	090	A B M
27784	Treatment of fibula fracture	9.67	NA	9.54	1.84	NA	NA	21.05	$728.46	090	A B C+ M
27786	Treatment of ankle fracture	3.02	5.88	5.10	0.56	9.46	$327.37	8.68	$300.38	090	A B M
27788	Treatment of ankle fracture	4.64	7.23	6.02	0.90	12.77	$441.92	11.56	$400.05	090	A B M
27792	Treatment of ankle fracture	8.75	NA	8.83	1.63	NA	NA	19.21	$664.79	090	A B C+ M
27808	Treatment of ankle fracture	3.03	6.50	5.61	0.57	10.10	$349.52	9.21	$318.72	090	A B M
27810	Treatment of ankle fracture	5.32	7.79	6.39	1.06	14.17	$490.37	12.77	$441.92	090	A B M
27814	Treatment of ankle fracture	10.62	NA	10.07	2.05	NA	NA	22.74	$786.94	090	B C+ M
27816	Treatment of ankle fracture	3.07	6.29	5.18	0.60	9.96	$344.68	8.85	$306.26	090	A B M
27818	Treatment of ankle fracture	5.69	7.87	6.30	1.12	14.68	$508.02	13.11	$453.69	090	A B M
27822	Treatment of ankle fracture	11.21	NA	12.79	2.17	NA	NA	26.17	$905.64	090	B C+ M
27823	Treatment of ankle fracture	13.16	NA	13.69	2.54	NA	NA	29.39	$1017.08	090	B C+ M
27824	Treat lower leg fracture	3.31	5.63	5.23	0.61	9.55	$330.49	9.15	$316.65	090	A B M
27825	Treat lower leg fracture	6.69	8.24	6.66	1.33	16.26	$562.70	14.68	$508.02	090	A+ B M
27826	Treat lower leg fracture	11.10	NA	12.42	2.01	NA	NA	25.53	$883.50	090	B C M
27827	Treat lower leg fracture	14.79	NA	15.69	2.93	NA	NA	33.41	$1156.19	090	B C M
27828	Treat lower leg fracture	18.43	NA	17.51	3.67	NA	NA	39.61	$1370.75	090	B C M
27829	Treat lower leg joint	8.80	NA	10.71	1.65	NA	NA	21.16	$732.27	090	B C M

27830		Treat lower leg dislocation	3.96	6.97	6.05	0.83	11.76	$406.97	10.84	$375.13	090	A+ B M
27831		Treat lower leg dislocation	4.73	NA	6.56	0.98	NA	NA	12.27	$424.62	090	A+ B M
27832		Treat lower leg dislocation	10.17	NA	10.28	2.09	NA	NA	22.54	$780.02	090	B C+ M
27840		Treat ankle dislocation	4.77	NA	5.74	0.95	NA	NA	11.46	$396.59	090	A B M
27842		Treat ankle dislocation	6.46	NA	7.13	1.25	NA	NA	14.84	$513.56	090	A B M
27846		Treat ankle dislocation	10.28	NA	9.29	1.94	NA	NA	21.51	$744.38	090	B C+ M
27848		Treat ankle dislocation	11.68	NA	9.66	2.16	NA	NA	23.50	$813.25	090	B C+ M
27860		Fixation of ankle joint	2.39	NA	2.17	0.35	NA	NA	4.91	$169.92	010	A+ B M
27870		Fusion of ankle joint open	15.41	NA	11.86	2.71	NA	NA	29.98	$1037.49	090	B C+ M
27871		Fusion of tibiofibular joint	9.54	NA	9.15	1.83	NA	NA	20.52	$710.12	090	B C+ M
27880		Amputation of lower leg	15.37	NA	7.69	3.66	NA	NA	26.72	$924.68	090	B C+ M
27881		Amputation of lower leg	13.47	NA	8.81	3.09	NA	NA	25.37	$877.96	090	B C+ M
27882		Amputation of lower leg	9.79	NA	5.43	2.37	NA	NA	17.59	$608.72	090	A+ B C+ M
27884		Amputation follow-up surgery	8.76	NA	6.38	2.03	NA	NA	17.17	$594.19	090	A B M
27886		Amputation follow-up surgery	10.02	NA	6.97	2.33	NA	NA	19.32	$668.59	090	A B C+ M
27888		Amputation of foot at ankle	10.37	NA	6.95	1.94	NA	NA	19.26	$666.52	090	B C+ M
27889		Amputation of foot at ankle	10.86	NA	5.63	2.40	NA	NA	18.89	$653.71	090	A B C+ M
27892		Decompression of leg	7.94	NA	6.41	1.59	NA	NA	15.94	$551.62	090	A+ B M
27893		Decompression of leg	7.90	NA	8.76	1.63	NA	NA	18.29	$632.95	090	A+ B M
27894		Decompression of leg	12.67	NA	9.03	2.62	NA	NA	24.32	$841.62	090	B M
27899	CP	Leg/ankle surgery procedure	0.00	0.00	0.00	0.00	0.00	$0.00	0.00	$0.00	YYY	A+ B C+ M T+
28001		Drainage of bursa of foot	2.00	2.98	0.66	0.19	5.17	$178.91	2.85	$98.63	000	A M
28002		Treatment of foot infection	2.79	4.37	1.10	0.27	7.43	$257.12	4.16	$143.96	000	A M
28003		Treatment of foot infection	5.28	5.46	1.80	0.64	11.38	$393.82	7.72	$267.16	000	A M
28005		Treat foot bone lesion	9.44	NA	6.53	0.90	NA	NA	16.87	$583.81	090	A M
28008		Incision of foot fascia	4.59	7.67	3.65	0.41	12.67	$438.46	8.65	$299.34	090	A B M
28010		Incision of toe tendon	2.97	3.63	2.86	0.25	6.85	$237.05	6.08	$210.41	090	A M
28011		Incision of toe tendons	4.28	4.57	3.53	0.40	9.25	$320.11	8.21	$284.12	090	A M

*Please note that these calculations are based on the Medicare 2022 Conversion Factor of $34.6062 and the DRA RVU cap rates at time of publication.

A = assistant-at-surgery restriction
A+ = assistant-at-surgery restriction unless medical necessity established with documentation
B = bilateral surgery adjustment applies
C = cosurgeons payable
C+ = cosurgeons payable if medical necessity established with documentation
CP = carriers may establish RVUs and payment amounts for these services, generally on an individual basis following review of documentation such as an operative report
M = multiple surgery adjustment applies
Me = multiple endoscopy rules may apply
M+ = multiple therapy rules apply
Mtc = multiple diagnostic imaging rules apply
T = team surgeons permitted
T+ = team surgeons payable if medical necessity established with documentation
§ = indicates code is not covered by Medicare
GS = procedure must be performed under the general supervision of a physician
DS = procedure must be performed under the direct supervision of a physician
PS = procedure must be performed under the personal supervision of a physician
DRA = procedure subject to DRA limitation

Relative Value Units

CPT Code and Modifier	Description	Work RVU	Nonfacility Practice Expense RVU	Facility Practice Expense RVU	PLI RVU	Total Non-facility RVUs	Medicare Payment Nonfacility	Total Facility RVUs	Medicare Payment Facility	Global Period	Payment Policy Indicators
28020	Exploration of foot joint	5.15	10.47	5.05	0.73	16.35	$565.81	10.93	$378.25	090	A C+ M
28022	Exploration of foot joint	4.81	9.05	4.25	0.55	14.41	$498.68	9.61	$332.57	090	A M
28024	Exploration of toe joint	4.52	8.52	3.98	0.43	13.47	$466.15	8.93	$309.03	090	A M
28035	Decompression of tibia nerve	5.23	9.65	4.60	0.64	15.52	$537.09	10.47	$362.33	090	A B C+ M
28039	Exc foot/toe tum sc 1.5 cm/>	5.42	8.34	4.04	0.78	14.54	$503.17	10.24	$354.37	090	B M
28041	Exc foot/toe tum dep 1.5cm/>	7.13	NA	5.27	0.85	NA	NA	13.25	$458.53	090	A+ B M
28043	Exc foot/toe tum sc < 1.5 cm	3.96	6.99	3.28	0.39	11.34	$392.43	7.63	$264.05	090	A B M
28045	Exc foot/toe tum deep <1.5cm	5.45	8.15	4.17	0.52	14.12	$488.64	10.14	$350.91	090	A+ B M
28046	Resect foot/toe tumor < 3 cm	12.38	NA	7.17	1.41	NA	NA	20.96	$725.35	090	A B C+ M
28047	Resect foot/toe tumor 3 cm/>	17.45	NA	10.39	2.60	NA	NA	30.44	$1053.41	090	B C+ M
28050	Biopsy of foot joint lining	4.39	7.54	3.42	0.34	12.27	$424.62	8.15	$282.04	090	A B C+ M
28052	Biopsy of foot joint lining	4.06	7.13	3.10	0.33	11.52	$398.66	7.49	$259.20	090	A B C+ M
28054	Biopsy of toe joint lining	3.57	6.98	3.00	0.28	10.83	$374.79	6.85	$237.05	090	A+ B M
28055	Neurectomy foot	6.29	NA	4.34	0.60	NA	NA	11.23	$388.63	090	A+ B M
28060	Partial removal foot fascia	5.40	9.40	4.63	0.60	15.40	$532.94	10.63	$367.86	090	A B M
28062	Removal of foot fascia	6.69	9.52	4.48	0.60	16.81	$581.73	11.77	$407.31	090	A B C+ M
28070	Removal of foot joint lining	5.24	9.41	4.39	0.60	15.25	$527.74	10.23	$354.02	090	A M
28072	Removal of foot joint lining	4.72	9.26	4.29	0.55	14.53	$502.83	9.56	$330.84	090	A M
28080	Removal of foot lesion	4.86	10.33	5.67	0.54	15.73	$544.36	11.07	$383.09	090	A+ M
28086	Excise foot tendon sheath	4.92	10.33	4.92	0.67	15.92	$550.93	10.51	$363.71	090	B C+ M
28088	Excise foot tendon sheath	3.98	9.07	4.05	0.44	13.49	$466.84	8.47	$293.11	090	A+ B M
28090	Removal of foot lesion	4.55	8.71	4.01	0.47	13.73	$475.14	9.03	$312.49	090	A B M
28092	Removal of toe lesions	3.78	8.20	3.74	0.39	12.37	$428.08	7.91	$273.74	090	A M
28100	Removal of ankle/heel lesion	5.83	11.56	5.73	0.85	18.24	$631.22	12.41	$429.46	090	B C+ M
28102	Remove/graft foot lesion	7.92	NA	8.66	1.64	NA	NA	18.22	$630.52	090	B M
28103	Remove/graft foot lesion	6.67	NA	4.17	0.55	NA	NA	11.39	$394.16	090	B M
28104	Removal of foot lesion	5.26	9.64	4.52	0.60	15.50	$536.40	10.38	$359.21	090	C+ M
28106	Remove/graft foot lesion	7.35	NA	4.56	0.60	NA	NA	12.51	$432.92	090	C+ M
28107	Remove/graft foot lesion	5.73	8.71	3.97	0.44	14.88	$514.94	10.14	$350.91	090	M
28108	Removal of toe lesions	4.30	8.13	3.75	0.40	12.83	$444.00	8.45	$292.42	090	A M
28110	Part removal of metatarsal	4.22	8.95	3.90	0.42	13.59	$470.30	8.54	$295.54	090	A B C+ M
28111	Part removal of metatarsal	5.15	8.52	3.75	0.56	14.23	$492.45	9.46	$327.37	090	A B C+ M
28112	Part removal of metatarsal	4.63	9.15	4.05	0.52	14.30	$494.87	9.20	$318.38	090	A B C+ M

28113	Part removal of metatarsal	6.11	10.53	5.76	0.61	17.25	$596.96	12.48	$431.89	090	A+ B M
28114	Removal of metatarsal heads	12.00	17.86	11.00	1.68	31.54	$1091.48	24.68	$854.08	090	B C+ M
28116	Revision of foot	9.14	12.55	6.92	1.16	22.85	$790.75	17.22	$595.92	090	A B M
28118	Removal of heel bone	6.13	10.90	5.46	0.83	17.86	$618.07	12.42	$429.81	090	B C+ M
28119	Removal of heel spur	5.56	9.42	4.57	0.57	15.55	$538.13	10.70	$370.29	090	A B C+ M
28120	Part removal of ankle/heel	7.31	11.66	6.38	0.98	19.95	$690.39	14.67	$507.67	090	A B C+ M
28122	Partial removal of foot bone	6.76	9.96	5.38	0.73	17.45	$603.88	12.87	$445.38	090	B C+ M
28124	Partial removal of toe	5.00	8.61	4.33	0.44	14.05	$486.22	9.77	$338.10	090	A B M
28126	Partial removal of toe	3.64	7.49	3.26	0.37	11.50	$397.97	7.27	$251.59	090	A M
28130	Removal of ankle bone	9.50	NA	7.39	1.21	NA	NA	18.10	$626.37	090	B C+ M
28140	Removal of metatarsal	7.14	8.97	4.59	0.95	17.06	$590.38	12.68	$438.81	090	A C+ M
28150	Removal of toe	4.23	7.69	3.52	0.40	12.32	$426.35	8.15	$282.04	090	A M
28153	Partial removal of toe	3.80	7.87	3.60	0.37	12.04	$416.66	7.77	$268.89	090	A M
28160	Partial removal of toe	3.88	7.89	3.59	0.39	12.16	$420.81	7.86	$272.00	090	A M
28171	Resect tarsal tumor	16.41	NA	13.00	3.39	NA	NA	32.80	$1135.08	090	M
28173	Resect metatarsal tumor	14.16	NA	5.99	1.12	NA	NA	21.27	$736.07	090	A C+ M
28175	Resect phalanx of toe tumor	8.29	NA	4.79	0.66	NA	NA	13.74	$475.49	090	A C+ M
28190	Removal of foot foreign body	2.01	5.02	1.68	0.20	7.23	$250.20	3.89	$134.62	010	A B M
28192	Removal of foot foreign body	4.78	8.39	3.90	0.44	13.61	$470.99	9.12	$315.61	090	A B M
28193	Removal of foot foreign body	5.90	9.00	4.33	0.52	15.42	$533.63	10.75	$372.02	090	A B M
28200	Repair of foot tendon	4.74	9.40	4.35	0.56	14.70	$508.71	9.65	$333.95	090	A C+ M
28202	Repair/graft of foot tendon	7.07	9.83	4.82	0.68	17.58	$608.38	12.57	$435.00	090	C+ M
28208	Repair of foot tendon	4.51	9.23	4.34	0.56	14.30	$494.87	9.41	$325.64	090	A C+ M
28210	Repair/graft of foot tendon	6.52	10.07	5.07	0.73	17.32	$599.38	12.32	$426.35	090	M
28220	Release of foot tendon	4.67	8.20	3.84	0.43	13.30	$460.26	8.94	$309.38	090	A B M
28222	Release of foot tendons	5.76	9.03	4.23	0.60	15.39	$532.59	10.59	$366.48	090	A B M
28225	Release of foot tendon	3.78	8.08	3.58	0.41	12.27	$424.62	7.77	$268.89	090	A B C+ M
28226	Release of foot tendons	4.67	12.81	6.22	0.96	18.44	$638.14	11.85	$410.08	090	A B M

*Please note that these calculations are based on the Medicare 2022 Conversion Factor of $34.6062 and the DRA RVU cap rates at time of publication.

A = assistant-at-surgery restriction

A+ = assistant-at-surgery restriction unless medical necessity established with documentation

B = bilateral surgery adjustment applies

C = cosurgeons payable

C+ = cosurgeons payable if medical necessity established with documentation

CP = carriers may establish RVUs and payment amounts for these services, generally on an individual basis following review of documentation such as an operative report

M = multiple surgery adjustment applies

Me = multiple endoscopy rules may apply

M+ = multiple therapy rules apply

Mtc = multiple diagnostic imaging rules apply

T = team surgeons permitted

T+ = team surgeons payable if medical necessity established with documentation

§ = indicates code is not covered by Medicare

GS = procedure must be performed under the general supervision of a physician

DS = procedure must be performed under the direct supervision of a physician

PS = procedure must be performed under the personal supervision of a physician

DRA = procedure subject to DRA limitation

Relative Value Units

CPT Code and Modifier	Description	Work RVU	Nonfacility Practice Expense RVU	Facility Practice Expense RVU	PLI RVU	Total Non-facility RVUs	Medicare Payment Nonfacility	Total Facility RVUs	Medicare Payment Facility	Global Period	Payment Policy Indicators
28230	Incision of foot tendon(s)	4.36	8.01	3.56	0.41	12.78	$442.27	8.33	$288.27	090	A B M
28232	Incision of toe tendon	3.51	7.36	3.23	0.32	11.19	$387.24	7.06	$244.32	090	A M
28234	Incision of foot tendon	3.54	8.18	3.96	0.34	12.06	$417.35	7.84	$271.31	090	A M
28238	Revision of foot tendon	7.96	10.98	5.55	0.90	19.84	$686.59	14.41	$498.68	090	B C+ M
28240	Release of big toe	4.48	8.25	3.72	0.42	13.15	$455.07	8.62	$298.31	090	A B M
28250	Revision of foot fascia	6.06	10.34	5.12	0.77	17.17	$594.19	11.95	$413.54	090	B C+ M
28260	Release of midfoot joint	8.19	11.71	6.25	1.11	21.01	$727.08	15.55	$538.13	090	B C+ M
28261	Revision of foot tendon	13.11	19.92	12.02	2.70	35.73	$1236.48	27.83	$963.09	090	A+ B M
28262	Revision of foot and ankle	17.21	21.08	12.98	3.16	41.45	$1434.43	33.35	$1154.12	090	B C+ M
28264	Release of midfoot joint	10.65	14.50	8.21	1.65	26.80	$927.45	20.51	$709.77	090	B M
28270	Release of foot contracture	4.93	8.95	4.37	0.50	14.38	$497.64	9.80	$339.14	090	A B M
28272	Release of toe joint each	3.92	7.09	3.11	0.32	11.33	$392.09	7.35	$254.36	090	A B M
28280	Fusion of toes	5.33	9.21	4.33	0.57	15.11	$522.90	10.23	$354.02	090	A+ B M
28285	Repair of hammertoe	5.62	9.64	5.06	0.60	15.86	$548.85	11.28	$390.36	090	A B C+ M
28286	Repair of hammertoe	4.70	7.95	3.61	0.40	13.05	$451.61	8.71	$301.42	090	A B M
28288	Partial removal of foot bone	6.02	11.18	6.08	0.67	17.87	$618.41	12.77	$441.92	090	A M
28289	Corrj halux rigdus w/o implt	6.90	12.65	5.80	0.79	20.34	$703.89	13.49	$466.84	090	B C+ M
28291	Corrj halux rigdus w/implt	8.01	12.13	5.61	0.79	20.93	$724.31	14.41	$498.68	090	B C+ M
28292	Correction hallux valgus	7.44	12.34	5.96	0.73	20.51	$709.77	14.13	$488.99	090	B C+ M
28295	Correction hallux valgus	8.57	22.61	8.32	1.32	32.50	$1124.70	18.21	$630.18	090	B C+ M
28296	Correction hallux valgus	8.25	17.36	6.02	0.77	26.38	$912.91	15.04	$520.48	090	B C+ M
28297	Correction hallux valgus	9.29	20.37	7.35	1.16	30.82	$1066.56	17.80	$615.99	090	B C+ M
28298	Correction hallux valgus	7.75	16.03	6.13	0.90	24.68	$854.08	14.78	$511.48	090	B C+ M
28299	Correction hallux valgus	9.29	19.57	6.99	1.02	29.88	$1034.03	17.30	$598.69	090	B C+ M
28300	Incision of heel bone	9.73	NA	7.95	1.55	NA	NA	19.23	$665.48	090	B C+ M
28302	Incision of ankle bone	9.74	NA	9.57	2.01	NA	NA	21.32	$737.80	090	B C+ M
28304	Incision of midfoot bones	9.41	13.72	7.29	1.36	24.49	$847.51	18.06	$624.99	090	B C+ M
28305	Incise/graft midfoot bones	10.77	NA	7.79	1.49	NA	NA	20.05	$693.85	090	B C+ M
28306	Incision of metatarsal	6.00	11.14	5.10	0.78	17.92	$620.14	11.88	$411.12	090	B C+ M
28307	Incision of metatarsal	6.50	15.60	7.55	1.33	23.43	$810.82	15.38	$532.24	090	A+ B M
28308	Incision of metatarsal	5.48	10.73	5.21	0.65	16.86	$583.46	11.34	$392.43	090	B C+ M
28309	Incision of metatarsals	14.16	NA	10.02	2.17	NA	NA	26.35	$911.87	090	A+ B M
28310	Revision of big toe	5.57	9.92	4.44	0.62	16.11	$557.51	10.63	$367.86	090	A B C+ M

28312	Revision of toe	4.69	10.08	4.42	0.56	15.33	$530.51	9.67	$334.64	090	A C+ M
28313	Repair deformity of toe	5.15	9.80	4.77	0.66	15.61	$540.20	10.58	$366.13	090	A M
28315	Removal of sesamoid bone	5.00	8.67	4.08	0.54	14.21	$491.75	9.62	$332.91	090	A B C+ M
28320	Repair of foot bones	9.37	NA	7.29	1.38	NA	NA	18.04	$624.30	090	B C+ M
28322	Repair of metatarsals	8.53	13.43	7.22	1.29	23.25	$804.59	17.04	$589.69	090	C+ M
28340	Resect enlarged toe tissue	7.15	8.98	4.27	0.57	16.70	$577.92	11.99	$414.93	090	A M
28341	Resect enlarged toe	8.72	9.93	4.86	0.70	19.35	$669.63	14.28	$494.18	090	A M
28344	Repair extra toe(s)	4.40	7.61	3.42	0.34	12.35	$427.39	8.16	$282.39	090	A B C+ M
28345	Repair webbed toe(s)	6.09	8.53	4.04	0.50	15.12	$523.25	10.63	$367.86	090	A+ M
28360	Reconstruct cleft foot	14.92	NA	14.66	3.06	NA	NA	32.64	$1129.55	090	B M
28400	Treatment of heel fracture	2.31	4.71	4.17	0.37	7.39	$255.74	6.85	$237.05	090	A B M
28405	Treatment of heel fracture	4.74	6.21	5.06	0.67	11.62	$402.12	10.47	$362.33	090	A+ B M
28406	Treatment of heel fracture	6.56	NA	9.09	1.20	NA	NA	16.85	$583.11	090	A+ B M
28415	Treat heel fracture	16.19	NA	14.55	2.71	NA	NA	33.45	$1157.58	090	B C+ M
28420	Treat/graft heel fracture	17.52	NA	17.52	3.61	NA	NA	38.65	$1337.53	090	B C+ M
28430	Treatment of ankle fracture	2.22	4.62	3.73	0.35	7.19	$248.82	6.30	$218.02	090	A B M
28435	Treatment of ankle fracture	3.54	6.81	5.55	0.73	11.08	$383.44	9.82	$339.83	090	A+ B M
28436	Treatment of ankle fracture	4.90	NA	8.99	1.00	NA	NA	14.89	$515.29	090	A B M
28445	Treat ankle fracture	15.76	NA	12.02	2.50	NA	NA	30.28	$1047.88	090	B C+ M
28446	Osteochondral talus autogrft	17.71	NA	14.95	3.66	NA	NA	36.32	$1256.90	090	B C+ M
28450	Treat midfoot fracture each	2.03	4.00	3.39	0.28	6.31	$218.37	5.70	$197.26	090	A M
28455	Treat midfoot fracture each	3.24	5.03	4.08	0.39	8.66	$299.69	7.71	$266.81	090	A+ M
28456	Treat midfoot fracture	2.86	NA	7.69	0.60	NA	NA	11.15	$385.86	090	A M
28465	Treat midfoot fracture each	8.80	NA	8.82	1.27	NA	NA	18.89	$653.71	090	A M
28470	Treat metatarsal fracture	2.03	4.19	3.80	0.29	6.51	$225.29	6.12	$211.79	090	A M
28475	Treat metatarsal fracture	3.01	4.25	3.34	0.34	7.60	$263.01	6.69	$231.52	090	A M
28476	Treat metatarsal fracture	3.60	NA	7.45	0.57	NA	NA	11.62	$402.12	090	A+ M
28485	Treat metatarsal fracture	7.44	NA	8.25	0.96	NA	NA	16.65	$576.19	090	A C+ M

*Please note that these calculations are based on the Medicare 2022 Conversion Factor of $34.6062 and the DRA RVU cap rates at time of publication.

A = assistant-at-surgery restriction
A+ = assistant-at-surgery restriction unless medical necessity established with documentation
B = bilateral surgery adjustment applies
C = cosurgeons payable
C+ = cosurgeons payable if medical necessity established with documentation
CP = carriers may establish RVUs and payment amounts for these services, generally on an individual basis following review of documentation such as an operative report
M = multiple surgery adjustment applies
Me = multiple endoscopy rules may apply
M+ = multiple therapy rules apply
Mtc = multiple diagnostic imaging rules apply
T = team surgeons permitted
T+ = team surgeons payable if medical necessity established with documentation
§ = indicates code is not covered by Medicare
GS = procedure must be performed under the general supervision of a physician
DS = procedure must be performed under the direct supervision of a physician
PS = procedure must be performed under the personal supervision of a physician
DRA = procedure subject to DRA limitation

Relative Value Units

CPT Code and Modifier	Description	Work RVU	Nonfacility Practice Expense RVU	Facility Practice Expense RVU	PLI RVU	Total Non-facility RVUs	Medicare Payment Nonfacility	Total Facility RVUs	Medicare Payment Facility	Global Period	Payment Policy Indicators
28490	Treat big toe fracture	1.17	2.86	2.35	0.17	4.20	$145.35	3.69	$127.70	090	A B M
28495	Treat big toe fracture	1.68	3.43	2.53	0.20	5.31	$183.76	4.41	$152.61	090	A B M
28496	Treat big toe fracture	2.48	10.52	4.37	0.40	13.40	$463.72	7.25	$250.89	090	A B M
28505	Treat big toe fracture	7.44	11.17	6.34	0.94	19.55	$676.55	14.72	$509.40	090	A B M
28510	Treatment of toe fracture	1.17	2.27	2.23	0.12	3.56	$123.20	3.52	$121.81	090	A M
28515	Treatment of toe fracture	1.56	3.11	2.48	0.18	4.85	$167.84	4.22	$146.04	090	A M
28525	Treat toe fracture	5.62	10.54	5.64	0.70	16.86	$583.46	11.96	$413.89	090	A+ M
28530	Treat sesamoid bone fracture	1.11	2.15	1.70	0.10	3.36	$116.28	2.91	$100.70	090	A+ B M
28531	Treat sesamoid bone fracture	2.57	6.98	2.52	0.21	9.76	$337.76	5.30	$183.41	090	A B C M
28540	Treat foot dislocation	2.19	3.40	2.80	0.19	5.78	$200.02	5.18	$179.26	090	A+ B M
28545	Treat foot dislocation	2.60	6.11	4.95	0.55	9.26	$320.45	8.10	$280.31	090	A+ B M
28546	Treat foot dislocation	3.40	13.48	6.36	0.70	17.58	$608.38	10.46	$361.98	090	A+ B M
28555	Repair foot dislocation	9.65	14.34	8.30	1.53	25.52	$883.15	19.48	$674.13	090	B C+ M
28570	Treat foot dislocation	1.76	4.90	3.75	0.35	7.01	$242.59	5.86	$202.79	090	A+ B M
28575	Treat foot dislocation	3.49	7.11	5.93	0.73	11.33	$392.09	10.15	$351.25	090	A+ B M
28576	Treat foot dislocation	4.60	NA	5.91	0.95	NA	NA	11.46	$396.59	090	A+ B M
28585	Repair foot dislocation	11.13	13.70	8.09	1.36	26.19	$906.34	20.58	$712.20	090	B C+ M
28600	Treat foot dislocation	2.02	4.16	3.21	0.25	6.43	$222.52	5.48	$189.64	090	A+ M
28605	Treat foot dislocation	2.89	6.74	5.62	0.60	10.23	$354.02	9.11	$315.26	090	A+ M
28606	Treat foot dislocation	5.09	NA	5.34	0.86	NA	NA	11.29	$390.70	090	A M
28615	Repair foot dislocation	10.70	NA	12.07	1.78	NA	NA	24.55	$849.58	090	C+ M
28630	Treat toe dislocation	1.75	2.55	1.26	0.25	4.55	$157.46	3.26	$112.82	010	A+ M
28635	Treat toe dislocation	1.96	2.96	1.72	0.23	5.15	$178.22	3.91	$135.31	010	A+ M
28636	Treat toe dislocation	2.77	6.14	2.71	0.41	9.32	$322.53	5.89	$203.83	010	A C M
28645	Repair toe dislocation	7.44	10.93	5.98	0.87	19.24	$665.82	14.29	$494.52	090	A C+ M
28660	Treat toe dislocation	1.28	2.14	1.24	0.23	3.65	$126.31	2.75	$95.17	010	A M
28665	Treat toe dislocation	1.97	2.28	1.55	0.20	4.45	$154.00	3.72	$128.74	010	A+ M
28666	Treat toe dislocation	2.66	NA	2.39	0.21	NA	NA	5.26	$182.03	010	A C M
28675	Repair of toe dislocation	5.62	10.74	5.79	0.73	17.09	$591.42	12.14	$420.12	090	A M
28705	Fusion of foot bones	20.33	NA	12.63	3.20	NA	NA	36.16	$1251.36	090	B C+ M
28715	Fusion of foot bones	13.42	NA	12.11	2.31	NA	NA	27.84	$963.44	090	B C+ M
28725	Fusion of foot bones	11.22	NA	9.95	1.84	NA	NA	23.01	$796.29	090	B C+ M
28730	Fusion of foot bones	10.70	NA	9.31	1.65	NA	NA	21.66	$749.57	090	B C+ M

28735		Fusion of foot bones	12.23	NA	9.10	1.81	NA	NA	23.14	$800.79	090	B C+ M
28737		Revision of foot bones	11.03	NA	7.84	1.41	NA	NA	20.28	$701.81	090	B C+ M
28740		Fusion of foot bones	9.29	13.95	7.65	1.30	24.54	$849.24	18.24	$631.22	090	B C+ M
28750		Fusion of big toe joint	8.57	13.51	7.35	1.18	23.26	$804.94	17.10	$591.77	090	A+ B M
28755		Fusion of big toe joint	4.88	9.57	4.41	0.57	15.02	$519.79	9.86	$341.22	090	A B C+ M
28760		Fusion of big toe joint	9.14	12.41	6.57	1.00	22.55	$780.37	16.71	$578.27	090	B C+ M
28800		Amputation of midfoot	8.79	NA	5.76	1.06	NA	NA	15.61	$540.20	090	B C+ M
28805		Amputation thru metatarsal	12.71	NA	6.56	1.68	NA	NA	20.95	$725.00	090	A+ B M
28810		Amputation toe & metatarsal	6.64	NA	4.85	1.05	NA	NA	12.54	$433.96	090	A+ M
28820		Amputation of toe	3.51	4.99	1.32	0.42	8.92	$308.69	5.25	$181.68	000	A M
28825		Partial amputation of toe	3.41	4.94	1.29	0.40	8.75	$302.80	5.10	$176.49	000	A M
28890		Hi enrgy eswt plantar fascia	3.45	5.38	2.71	0.28	9.11	$315.26	6.44	$222.86	090	A B C+ M
28899	CP	Foot/toes surgery procedure	0.00	0.00	0.00	0.00	0.00	$0.00	0.00	$0.00	YYY	A+ C+ M T+
29000		Application of body cast	2.25	7.20	2.67	0.87	10.32	$357.14	5.79	$200.37	000	A+ M
29010		Application of body cast	2.06	5.47	2.20	0.42	7.95	$275.12	4.68	$161.96	000	A+ M
29015		Application of body cast	2.41	5.65	2.37	0.50	8.56	$296.23	5.28	$182.72	000	A+ M
29035		Application of body cast	1.77	5.33	2.05	0.37	7.47	$258.51	4.19	$145.00	000	A+ M
29040		Application of body cast	2.22	5.86	2.38	0.44	8.52	$294.84	5.04	$174.42	000	A+ M
29044		Application of body cast	2.12	5.81	2.33	0.42	8.35	$288.96	4.87	$168.53	000	A+ M
29046		Application of body cast	2.41	6.26	2.58	0.50	9.17	$317.34	5.49	$189.99	000	A+ M
29049		Application of figure eight	0.89	1.83	0.97	0.19	2.91	$100.70	2.05	$70.94	000	A+ M
29055		Application of shoulder cast	1.78	4.35	1.87	0.37	6.50	$224.94	4.02	$139.12	000	A+ M
29058		Application of shoulder cast	1.31	2.05	1.18	0.25	3.61	$124.93	2.74	$94.82	000	A+ M
29065		Application of long arm cast	0.87	1.78	0.96	0.18	2.83	$97.94	2.01	$69.56	000	A B M
29075		Application of forearm cast	0.77	1.63	0.90	0.14	2.54	$87.90	1.81	$62.64	000	A B M
29085		Apply hand/wrist cast	0.87	1.76	0.94	0.17	2.80	$96.90	1.98	$68.52	000	A B M
29086		Apply finger cast	0.62	1.53	0.74	0.08	2.23	$77.17	1.44	$49.83	000	A B M
29105		Apply long arm splint	0.80	1.45	0.28	0.14	2.39	$82.71	1.22	$42.22	000	A B M

*Please note that these calculations are based on the Medicare 2022 Conversion Factor of $34.6062 and the DRA RVU cap rates at time of publication.

A = assistant-at-surgery restriction
A+ = assistant-at-surgery restriction unless medical necessity established with documentation
B = bilateral surgery adjustment applies
C = cosurgeons payable
C+ = cosurgeons payable if medical necessity established with documentation
CP = carriers may establish RVUs and payment amounts for these services, generally on an individual basis following review of documentation such as an operative report
M = multiple surgery adjustment applies
Me = multiple endoscopy rules may apply
M+ = multiple therapy rules apply
Mtc = multiple diagnostic imaging rules apply
T = team surgeons permitted
T+ = team surgeons payable if medical necessity established with documentation
§ = indicates code is not covered by Medicare
GS = procedure must be performed under the general supervision of a physician
DS = procedure must be performed under the direct supervision of a physician
PS = procedure must be performed under the personal supervision of a physician
DRA = procedure subject to DRA limitation

Relative Value Units

CPT Code and Modifier	Description	Work RVU	Nonfacility Practice Expense RVU	Facility Practice Expense RVU	PLI RVU	Total Non-facility RVUs	Medicare Payment Nonfacility	Total Facility RVUs	Medicare Payment Facility	Global Period	Payment Policy Indicators
29125	Apply forearm splint	0.50	1.33	0.58	0.09	1.92	$66.44	1.17	$40.49	000	A B M
29126	Apply forearm splint	0.68	1.48	0.66	0.10	2.26	$78.21	1.44	$49.83	000	A B M
29130	Application of finger splint	0.50	0.62	0.27	0.09	1.21	$41.87	0.86	$29.76	000	A B M
29131	Application of finger splint	0.55	0.91	0.37	0.09	1.55	$53.64	1.01	$34.95	000	A B M
29200	Strapping of chest	0.39	0.57	0.14	0.02	0.98	$33.91	0.55	$19.03	000	A M
29240	Strapping of shoulder	0.39	0.48	0.13	0.02	0.89	$30.80	0.54	$18.69	000	A B M
29260	Strapping of elbow or wrist	0.39	0.45	0.14	0.04	0.88	$30.45	0.57	$19.73	000	A B M
29280	Strapping of hand or finger	0.39	0.44	0.15	0.04	0.87	$30.11	0.58	$20.07	000	A B M
29305	Application of hip cast	2.03	4.77	2.18	0.41	7.21	$249.51	4.62	$159.88	000	A+ M
29325	Application of hip casts	2.32	5.18	2.39	0.47	7.97	$275.81	5.18	$179.26	000	A+ M
29345	Application of long leg cast	1.40	2.30	1.25	0.27	3.97	$137.39	2.92	$101.05	000	A B M
29355	Application of long leg cast	1.53	2.34	1.30	0.29	4.16	$143.96	3.12	$107.97	000	A B M
29358	Apply long leg cast brace	1.43	2.96	1.30	0.29	4.68	$161.96	3.02	$104.51	000	A B M
29365	Application of long leg cast	1.18	2.18	1.14	0.24	3.60	$124.58	2.56	$88.59	000	A B M
29405	Apply short leg cast	0.80	1.41	0.78	0.12	2.33	$80.63	1.70	$58.83	000	A B M
29425	Apply short leg cast	0.80	1.30	0.68	0.10	2.20	$76.13	1.58	$54.68	000	A B M
29435	Apply short leg cast	1.18	1.91	0.96	0.20	3.29	$113.85	2.34	$80.98	000	A B M
29440	Addition of walker to cast	0.57	0.62	0.20	0.05	1.24	$42.91	0.82	$28.38	000	A B M
29445	Apply rigid leg cast	1.78	1.79	0.93	0.20	3.77	$130.47	2.91	$100.70	000	A B M
29450	Application of leg cast	2.08	1.95	1.02	0.25	4.28	$148.11	3.35	$115.93	000	A B M
29505	Application long leg splint	0.69	1.75	0.70	0.11	2.55	$88.25	1.50	$51.91	000	A B M
29515	Application lower leg splint	0.73	1.24	0.60	0.11	2.08	$71.98	1.44	$49.83	000	A B M
29520	Strapping of hip	0.39	0.63	0.13	0.02	1.04	$35.99	0.54	$18.69	000	A+ B M
29530	Strapping of knee	0.39	0.48	0.12	0.02	0.89	$30.80	0.53	$18.34	000	A B M
29540	Strapping of ankle and/or ft	0.39	0.39	0.09	0.04	0.82	$28.38	0.52	$18.00	000	A B M
29550	Strapping of toes	0.25	0.29	0.06	0.02	0.56	$19.38	0.33	$11.42	000	A B M
29580	Application of paste boot	0.55	1.27	0.16	0.08	1.90	$65.75	0.79	$27.34	000	A B M
29581	Apply multlay comprs lwr leg	0.60	2.04	0.18	0.02	2.66	$92.05	0.80	$27.68	000	A+ B M
29584	Appl multlay comprs arm/hand	0.35	2.10	0.10	0.01	2.46	$85.13	0.46	$15.92	000	A+ B M
29700	Removal/revision of cast	0.57	1.14	0.30	0.10	1.81	$62.64	0.97	$33.57	000	A M
29705	Removal/revision of cast	0.76	0.98	0.44	0.11	1.85	$64.02	1.31	$45.33	000	A B M
29710	Removal/revision of cast	1.34	1.96	0.82	0.27	3.57	$123.54	2.43	$84.09	000	A+ B M
29720	Repair of body cast	0.68	1.67	0.46	0.12	2.47	$85.48	1.26	$43.60	000	A M

29730		Windowing of cast	0.75	1.00	0.43	0.12	1.87	$64.71	1.30	$44.99	000	A M
29740		Wedging of cast	1.12	1.55	0.69	0.23	2.90	$100.36	2.04	$70.60	000	A M
29750		Wedging of clubfoot cast	1.26	1.62	0.76	0.25	3.13	$108.32	2.27	$78.56	000	A+ B M
29799	CP	Casting/strapping procedure	0.00	0.00	0.00	0.00	0.00	$0.00	0.00	$0.00	YYY	A+ C+ M T+
29800		Jaw arthroscopy/surgery	6.84	NA	7.55	1.40	NA	NA	15.79	$546.43	090	A+ B M
29804		Jaw arthroscopy/surgery	8.87	NA	8.02	0.87	NA	NA	17.76	$614.61	090	B C+ M
29805		Sho arthrs dx +- synovial bx	6.03	NA	6.75	1.18	NA	NA	13.96	$483.10	090	A B C+ M
29806		Sho arthrs srg capsulorraphy	15.14	NA	13.28	3.02	NA	NA	31.44	$1088.02	090	A B C+ Me
29807		Sho arthrs srg rpr slap les	14.67	NA	13.08	2.92	NA	NA	30.67	$1061.37	090	A B C+ Me
29819		Sho arthrs srg rmvl loose/fb	7.79	NA	8.15	1.54	NA	NA	17.48	$604.92	090	A B C+ Me
29820		Sho arthrs srg prtl synvct	7.21	NA	7.37	1.40	NA	NA	15.98	$553.01	090	B C+ Me
29821		Sho arthrs srg compl synvct	7.89	NA	8.25	1.57	NA	NA	17.71	$612.88	090	B C+ Me
29822		Sho arthrs srg lmtd dbrdmt	7.03	NA	7.69	1.40	NA	NA	16.12	$557.85	090	B Me
29823		Sho arthrs srg xtnsv dbrdmt	7.98	NA	8.09	1.57	NA	NA	17.64	$610.45	090	B C+ Me
29824		Sho arthrs srg dstl claviclc	8.98	NA	9.39	1.78	NA	NA	20.15	$697.31	090	B C+ Me
29825		Sho arthrs srg lss&rescj ads	7.79	NA	8.16	1.53	NA	NA	17.48	$604.92	090	B C+ Me
29826		Sho arthrs srg decompression	3.00	NA	1.50	0.60	NA	NA	5.10	$176.49	ZZZ	B C+
29827		Sho arthrs srg rt8tr cuf rpr	15.59	NA	13.06	3.06	NA	NA	31.71	$1097.36	090	B C+ Me
29828		Sho arthrs srg bicp tenodsis	13.16	NA	11.45	2.61	NA	NA	27.22	$941.98	090	B C+ Me
29830		Elbow arthroscopy	5.88	NA	6.62	1.04	NA	NA	13.54	$468.57	090	A B M
29834		Elbow arthroscopy/surgery	6.42	NA	7.00	1.24	NA	NA	14.66	$507.33	090	B C+ Me
29835		Elbow arthroscopy/surgery	6.62	NA	7.20	1.37	NA	NA	15.19	$525.67	090	B C+ Me
29836		Elbow arthroscopy/surgery	7.72	NA	8.20	1.51	NA	NA	17.43	$603.19	090	B C+ Me
29837		Elbow arthroscopy/surgery	7.01	NA	7.40	1.36	NA	NA	15.77	$545.74	090	B C+ Me
29838		Elbow arthroscopy/surgery	7.88	NA	8.27	1.52	NA	NA	17.67	$611.49	090	A+ B Me
29840		Wrist arthroscopy	5.68	NA	6.72	1.02	NA	NA	13.42	$464.42	090	A+ B M
29843		Wrist arthroscopy/surgery	6.15	NA	7.08	1.27	NA	NA	14.50	$501.79	090	B C+ Me
29844		Wrist arthroscopy/surgery	6.51	NA	7.17	1.18	NA	NA	14.86	$514.25	090	B Me

*Please note that these calculations are based on the Medicare 2022 Conversion Factor of $34.6062 and the DRA RVU cap rates at time of publication.

A = assistant-at-surgery restriction
A+ = assistant-at-surgery restriction unless medical necessity established with documentation
B = bilateral surgery adjustment applies
C = cosurgeons payable
C+ = cosurgeons payable if medical necessity established with documentation
CP = carriers may establish RVUs and payment amounts for these services, generally on an individual basis following review of documentation such as an operative report
M = multiple surgery adjustment applies
Me = multiple endoscopy rules may apply
M+ = multiple therapy rules apply
Mtc = multiple diagnostic imaging rules apply
T = team surgeons permitted
T+ = team surgeons payable if medical necessity established with documentation
§ = indicates code is not covered by Medicare
GS = procedure must be performed under the general supervision of a physician
DS = procedure must be performed under the direct supervision of a physician
PS = procedure must be performed under the personal supervision of a physician
DRA = procedure subject to DRA limitation

Relative Value Units

CPT Code and Modifier	Description	Work RVU	Nonfacility Practice Expense RVU	Facility Practice Expense RVU	PLI RVU	Total Non-facility RVUs	Medicare Payment Nonfacility	Total Facility RVUs	Medicare Payment Facility	Global Period	Payment Policy Indicators
29845	Wrist arthroscopy/surgery	7.69	NA	8.29	1.44	NA	NA	17.42	$602.84	090	B C+ Me
29846	Wrist arthroscopy/surgery	6.89	NA	7.37	1.28	NA	NA	15.54	$537.78	090	A+ B Me
29847	Wrist arthroscopy/surgery	7.22	NA	7.51	1.48	NA	NA	16.21	$560.97	090	B Me
29848	Wrist endoscopy/surgery	6.39	NA	7.61	1.20	NA	NA	15.20	$526.01	090	A B M
29850	Knee arthroscopy/surgery	8.27	NA	8.59	1.70	NA	NA	18.56	$642.29	090	A+ B C M
29851	Knee arthroscopy/surgery	13.26	NA	11.60	2.72	NA	NA	27.58	$954.44	090	B C M
29855	Tibial arthroscopy/surgery	10.76	NA	10.29	2.17	NA	NA	23.22	$803.56	090	B C M
29856	Tibial arthroscopy/surgery	14.28	NA	12.23	2.95	NA	NA	29.46	$1019.50	090	B C M
29860	Hip arthroscopy dx	9.00	NA	8.45	1.66	NA	NA	19.11	$661.32	090	B C+ M
29861	Hip arthro w/fb removal	10.10	NA	9.26	1.98	NA	NA	21.34	$738.50	090	B C+ Me
29862	Hip arthr0 w/debridement	11.17	NA	10.82	2.22	NA	NA	24.21	$837.82	090	B C+ Me
29863	Hip arthr0 w/synovectomy	11.17	NA	10.73	2.22	NA	NA	24.12	$834.70	090	B C+ Me
29866	Autgrft implnt knee w/scope	14.67	NA	13.54	3.02	NA	NA	31.23	$1080.75	090	A+ B M
29867	Allgrft implnt knee w/scope	18.39	NA	15.72	3.79	NA	NA	37.90	$1311.57	090	A+ B M
29868	Meniscal trnspl knee w/scpe	25.10	NA	19.12	5.18	NA	NA	49.40	$1709.55	090	A+ B M
29870	Knee arthroscopy dx	5.19	10.33	5.94	0.99	16.51	$571.35	12.12	$419.43	090	A B C+ M
29871	Knee arthroscopy/drainage	6.69	NA	7.29	1.34	NA	NA	15.32	$530.17	090	A B Me
29873	Knee arthroscopy/surgery	6.24	NA	8.51	1.27	NA	NA	16.02	$554.39	090	A B C+ Me
29874	Knee arthroscopy/surgery	7.19	NA	7.35	1.42	NA	NA	15.96	$552.31	090	A+ B Me
29875	Knee arthroscopy/surgery	6.45	NA	7.04	1.29	NA	NA	14.78	$511.48	090	A+ B Me
29876	Knee arthroscopy/surgery	8.87	NA	8.78	1.78	NA	NA	19.43	$672.40	090	A B Me
29877	Knee arthroscopy/surgery	8.30	NA	8.51	1.68	NA	NA	18.49	$639.87	090	A+ B Me
29879	Knee arthroscopy/surgery	8.99	NA	8.86	1.82	NA	NA	19.67	$680.70	090	A+ B Me
29880	Knee arthroscopy/surgery	7.39	NA	7.86	1.48	NA	NA	16.73	$578.96	090	A+ B C+ Me
29881	Knee arthroscopy/surgery	7.03	NA	7.68	1.41	NA	NA	16.12	$557.85	090	A+ B Me
29882	Knee arthroscopy/surgery	9.60	NA	9.00	1.87	NA	NA	20.47	$708.39	090	A B Me
29883	Knee arthroscopy/surgery	11.77	NA	10.82	2.38	NA	NA	24.97	$864.12	090	A+ B Me
29884	Knee arthroscopy/surgery	8.28	NA	8.46	1.65	NA	NA	18.39	$636.41	090	B C+ Me
29885	Knee arthroscopy/surgery	10.21	NA	10.17	2.11	NA	NA	22.49	$778.29	090	B C+ Me
29886	Knee arthroscopy/surgery	8.49	NA	8.70	1.73	NA	NA	18.92	$654.75	090	A B Me
29887	Knee arthroscopy/surgery	10.16	NA	10.14	2.09	NA	NA	22.39	$774.83	090	B C+ Me
29888	Knee arthroscopy/surgery	14.30	NA	11.89	2.80	NA	NA	28.99	$1003.23	090	B C+ M
29889	Knee arthroscopy/surgery	17.41	NA	15.30	3.60	NA	NA	36.31	$1256.55	090	B C+ M

29891		Ankle arthroscopy/surgery	9.67	NA	8.65	1.55	NA	NA	19.87	$687.63	090	B M
29892		Ankle arthroscopy/surgery	10.27	NA	7.31	1.24	NA	NA	18.82	$651.29	090	B M
29893		Scope plantar fasciotomy	6.32	12.85	5.88	0.55	19.72	$682.43	12.75	$441.23	090	A B C+ M
29894		Ankle arthroscopy/surgery	7.35	NA	6.43	1.18	NA	NA	14.96	$517.71	090	B C+ M
29895		Ankle arthroscopy/surgery	7.13	NA	5.72	1.02	NA	NA	13.87	$479.99	090	B C+ M
29897		Ankle arthroscopy/surgery	7.32	NA	6.16	1.11	NA	NA	14.59	$504.90	090	B M
29898		Ankle arthroscopy/surgery	8.49	NA	6.88	1.26	NA	NA	16.63	$575.50	090	B C+ M
29899		Ankle arthroscopy/surgery	15.41	NA	11.91	2.79	NA	NA	30.11	$1041.99	090	B C+ M
29900		Mcp joint arthroscopy dx	5.88	NA	7.91	1.21	NA	NA	15.00	$519.09	090	A+ B M
29901		Mcp joint arthroscopy surg	6.59	NA	8.15	1.36	NA	NA	16.10	$557.16	090	A+ B M
29902		Mcp joint arthroscopy surg	7.16	NA	8.44	1.47	NA	NA	17.07	$590.73	090	A+ B M
29904		Subtalar arthro w/fb rmvl	8.65	NA	8.57	1.78	NA	NA	19.00	$657.52	090	B M
29905		Subtalar arthro w/exc	9.18	NA	5.17	0.73	NA	NA	15.08	$521.86	090	B M
29906		Subtalar arthro w/deb	9.65	NA	8.17	1.53	NA	NA	19.35	$669.63	090	B M
29907		Subtalar arthro w/fusion	12.18	NA	11.37	2.50	NA	NA	26.05	$901.49	090	B M
29914		Hip arthro w/femoroplasty	14.67	NA	12.09	2.85	NA	NA	29.61	$1024.69	090	B C+ Me
29915		Hip arthro acetabuloplasty	15.00	NA	12.45	3.02	NA	NA	30.47	$1054.45	090	B C+ Me
29916		Hip arthro w/labral repair	15.00	NA	12.30	2.97	NA	NA	30.27	$1047.53	090	B C+ Me
29999	CP	Arthroscopy of joint	0.00	0.00	0.00	0.00	0.00	$0.00	0.00	$0.00	YYY	A+ B C+ M T+
30000		Drainage of nose lesion	1.48	6.44	1.87	0.21	8.13	$281.35	3.56	$123.20	010	A+ M
30020		Drainage of nose lesion	1.48	6.51	1.90	0.22	8.21	$284.12	3.60	$124.58	010	A M
30100		Intranasal biopsy	0.94	3.21	0.92	0.12	4.27	$147.77	1.98	$68.52	000	A M
30110		Removal of nose polyp(s)	1.68	5.57	1.98	0.24	7.49	$259.20	3.90	$134.96	010	A B M
30115		Removal of nose polyp(s)	4.44	NA	9.04	0.62	NA	NA	14.10	$487.95	090	A B M
30117		Removal of intranasal lesion	3.26	25.92	6.18	0.44	29.62	$1025.04	9.88	$341.91	090	A M
30118		Removal of intranasal lesion	9.92	NA	12.52	1.40	NA	NA	23.84	$825.01	090	A C+ M
30120		Revision of nose	5.39	8.99	6.26	0.77	15.15	$524.28	12.42	$429.81	090	A M
30124		Removal of nose lesion	3.20	NA	5.45	0.44	NA	NA	9.09	$314.57	090	A M

*Please note that these calculations are based on the Medicare 2022 Conversion Factor of $34.6062 and the DRA RVU cap rates at time of publication.

A = assistant-at-surgery restriction
A+ = assistant-at-surgery restriction unless medical necessity established with documentation
B = bilateral surgery adjustment applies
C = cosurgeons payable
C+ = cosurgeons payable if medical necessity established with documentation
CP = carriers may establish RVUs and payment amounts for these services, generally on an individual basis following review of documentation such as an operative report
M = multiple surgery adjustment applies
Me = multiple endoscopy rules may apply
M+ = multiple therapy rules apply
Mtc = multiple diagnostic imaging rules apply
T = team surgeons permitted
T+ = team surgeons payable if medical necessity established with documentation
§ = indicates code is not covered by Medicare
GS = procedure must be performed under the general supervision of a physician
DS = procedure must be performed under the direct supervision of a physician
PS = procedure must be performed under the personal supervision of a physician
DRA = procedure subject to DRA limitation

Relative Value Units

CPT Code and Modifier	Description	Work RVU	Nonfacility Practice Expense RVU	Facility Practice Expense RVU	PLI RVU	Total Non-facility RVUs	Medicare Payment Nonfacility	Total Facility RVUs	Medicare Payment Facility	Global Period	Payment Policy Indicators
30125	Removal of nose lesion	7.30	NA	11.39	1.04	NA	NA	19.73	$682.78	090	M
30130	Excise inferior turbinate	3.47	NA	8.67	0.47	NA	NA	12.61	$436.38	090	A B M
30140	Resect inferior turbinate	3.00	5.46	1.81	0.42	8.88	$307.30	5.23	$180.99	000	A B M
30150	Partial removal of nose	9.55	NA	13.18	1.44	NA	NA	24.17	$836.43	090	A C+ M
30160	Removal of nose	9.99	NA	13.11	1.41	NA	NA	24.51	$848.20	090	C+ M
30200	Injection treatment of nose	0.78	2.43	0.84	0.11	3.32	$114.89	1.73	$59.87	000	A M
30210	Nasal sinus therapy	1.13	3.23	1.74	0.17	4.53	$156.77	3.04	$105.20	010	A M
30220	Insert nasal septal button	1.59	7.45	1.95	0.23	9.27	$320.80	3.77	$130.47	010	A M
30300	Remove nasal foreign body	1.09	5.11	2.47	0.14	6.34	$219.40	3.70	$128.04	010	A M
30310	Remove nasal foreign body	2.01	NA	3.98	0.28	NA	NA	6.27	$216.98	010	A+ M
30320	Remove nasal foreign body	4.64	NA	9.44	0.65	NA	NA	14.73	$509.75	090	A+ M
30400	Reconstruction of nose	10.86	NA	24.37	1.99	NA	NA	37.22	$1288.04	090	A+ M
30410	Reconstruction of nose	14.00	NA	26.18	2.56	NA	NA	42.74	$1479.07	090	M
30420	Reconstruction of nose	16.90	NA	24.41	2.47	NA	NA	43.78	$1515.06	090	A M
30430	Revision of nose	8.24	NA	22.86	1.50	NA	NA	32.60	$1128.16	090	M
30435	Revision of nose	12.73	NA	25.46	2.33	NA	NA	40.52	$1402.24	090	M
30450	Revision of nose	19.66	NA	29.46	3.61	NA	NA	52.73	$1824.78	090	M
30460	Revision of nose	10.32	NA	12.66	1.87	NA	NA	24.85	$859.96	090	C M
30462	Revision of nose	20.28	NA	23.89	3.73	NA	NA	47.90	$1657.64	090	C M
30465	Repair nasal stenosis	12.36	NA	16.77	1.78	NA	NA	30.91	$1069.68	090	A+ M
30468	Rpr nsl vlv collapse w/implt	2.80	76.30	1.74	0.40	79.50	$2751.19	4.94	$170.95	000	A B M
30520	Repair of nasal septum	7.01	NA	12.30	1.00	NA	NA	20.31	$702.85	090	A M
30540	Repair nasal defect	7.92	NA	13.26	1.11	NA	NA	22.29	$771.37	090	M
30545	Repair nasal defect	11.62	NA	16.99	1.64	NA	NA	30.25	$1046.84	090	M
30560	Release of nasal adhesions	1.31	8.37	3.01	0.20	9.88	$341.91	4.52	$156.42	010	A M
30580	Repair upper jaw fistula	6.88	10.70	6.04	0.67	18.25	$631.56	13.59	$470.30	090	A M
30600	Repair mouth/nose fistula	6.16	8.65	4.56	0.56	15.37	$531.90	11.28	$390.36	090	A+ M
30620	Intranasal reconstruction	6.16	NA	13.41	0.89	NA	NA	20.46	$708.04	090	A M
30630	Repair nasal septum defect	7.29	NA	11.87	1.04	NA	NA	20.20	$699.05	090	A+ M
30801	Ablate inf turbinate superf	1.14	5.32	3.30	0.17	6.63	$229.44	4.61	$159.53	010	A M
30802	Ablate inf turbinate submuc	2.08	6.02	3.74	0.29	8.39	$290.35	6.11	$211.44	010	A M
30901	Control of nosebleed	1.10	3.47	0.38	0.19	4.76	$164.73	1.67	$57.79	000	A B M
30903	Control of nosebleed	1.54	5.66	0.48	0.25	7.45	$257.82	2.27	$78.56	000	A B M

30905		Control of nosebleed	1.97	8.35	0.80	0.34	10.66	$368.90	3.11	$107.63	000	A M
30906		Repeat control of nosebleed	2.45	8.35	1.16	0.39	11.19	$387.24	4.00	$138.42	000	A M
30915		Ligation nasal sinus artery	7.44	NA	9.60	1.05	NA	NA	18.09	$626.03	090	A M
30920		Ligation upper jaw artery	11.14	NA	13.50	1.59	NA	NA	26.23	$907.72	090	A M
30930		Ther fx nasal inf turbinate	1.31	NA	1.98	0.19	NA	NA	3.48	$120.43	010	A M
30999	CP	Nasal surgery procedure	0.00	0.00	0.00	0.00	0.00	$0.00	0.00	$0.00	YYY	A+ C+ M T+
31000		Irrigation maxillary sinus	1.20	4.14	1.85	0.18	5.52	$191.03	3.23	$111.78	010	A B M
31002		Irrigation sphenoid sinus	1.96	NA	3.62	0.24	NA	NA	5.82	$201.41	010	A+ B M
31020		Exploration maxillary sinus	3.07	10.33	7.67	0.39	13.79	$477.22	11.13	$385.17	090	A B M
31030		Exploration maxillary sinus	6.01	12.42	8.62	0.66	19.09	$660.63	15.29	$529.13	090	A B M
31032		Explore sinus remove polyps	6.69	NA	10.25	0.85	NA	NA	17.79	$615.64	090	A B M
31040		Exploration behind upper jaw	9.77	NA	13.05	1.39	NA	NA	24.21	$837.82	090	A B C+ M
31050		Exploration sphenoid sinus	5.37	NA	9.47	0.76	NA	NA	15.60	$539.86	090	A B M
31051		Sphenoid sinus surgery	7.25	NA	12.69	1.02	NA	NA	20.96	$725.35	090	A B M
31070		Exploration of frontal sinus	4.40	NA	9.35	0.62	NA	NA	14.37	$497.29	090	A B M
31075		Exploration of frontal sinus	9.51	NA	14.10	1.34	NA	NA	24.95	$863.42	090	B C+ M
31080		Removal of frontal sinus	12.74	NA	18.27	1.81	NA	NA	32.82	$1135.78	090	B M
31081		Removal of frontal sinus	14.19	NA	18.93	2.01	NA	NA	35.13	$1215.72	090	B C+ M
31084		Removal of frontal sinus	14.95	NA	19.28	2.14	NA	NA	36.37	$1258.63	090	B C+ M
31085		Removal of frontal sinus	15.64	NA	19.60	2.22	NA	NA	37.46	$1296.35	090	B C+ M
31086		Removal of frontal sinus	14.36	NA	19.01	2.03	NA	NA	35.40	$1225.06	090	B M
31087		Removal of frontal sinus	14.57	NA	16.98	2.06	NA	NA	33.61	$1163.11	090	B C+ M
31090		Exploration of sinuses	11.17	NA	20.88	1.50	NA	NA	33.55	$1161.04	090	A B M
31200		Removal of ethmoid sinus	5.14	NA	13.15	0.44	NA	NA	18.73	$648.17	090	A B M
31201		Removal of ethmoid sinus	8.60	NA	14.15	1.30	NA	NA	24.05	$832.28	090	A B M
31205		Removal of ethmoid sinus	10.58	NA	16.51	0.90	NA	NA	27.99	$968.63	090	B C+ M
31225		Removal of upper jaw	26.70	NA	23.22	3.74	NA	NA	53.66	$1856.97	090	B C+ M
31230		Removal of upper jaw	30.82	NA	24.54	4.38	NA	NA	59.74	$2067.37	090	B C+ M

*Please note that these calculations are based on the Medicare 2022 Conversion Factor of $34.6062 and the DRA RVU cap rates at time of publication.

A = assistant-at-surgery restriction

A+ = assistant-at-surgery restriction unless medical necessity established with documentation

B = bilateral surgery adjustment applies

C = cosurgeons payable

C+ = cosurgeons payable if medical necessity established with documentation

CP = carriers may establish RVUs and payment amounts for these services, generally on an individual basis following review of documentation such as an operative report

M = multiple surgery adjustment applies

Me = multiple endoscopy rules may apply

M+ = multiple therapy rules apply

Mtc = multiple diagnostic imaging rules apply

T = team surgeons permitted

T+ = team surgeons payable if medical necessity established with documentation

§ = indicates code is not covered by Medicare

GS = procedure must be performed under the general supervision of a physician

DS = procedure must be performed under the direct supervision of a physician

PS = procedure must be performed under the personal supervision of a physician

DRA = procedure subject to DRA limitation

Relative Value Units

CPT Code and Modifier		Description	Work RVU	Nonfacility Practice Expense RVU	Facility Practice Expense RVU	PLI RVU	Total Non-facility RVUs	Medicare Payment Nonfacility	Total Facility RVUs	Medicare Payment Facility	Global Period	Payment Policy Indicators
31231		Nasal endoscopy dx	1.10	4.42	0.63	0.14	5.66	$195.87	1.87	$64.71	000	A M
31233		Nsl/sins ndsc dx max sinusc	2.18	5.75	1.47	0.31	8.24	$285.16	3.96	$137.04	000	A+ B Me
31235		Nsl/sins ndsc dx sphn sinusc	2.64	6.38	1.68	0.33	9.35	$323.57	4.65	$160.92	000	A+ B Me
31237		Nasal/sinus endoscopy surg	2.60	4.66	1.71	0.37	7.63	$264.05	4.68	$161.96	000	A B Me
31238		Nasal/sinus endoscopy surg	2.74	4.32	1.77	0.39	7.45	$257.82	4.90	$169.57	000	A+ B Me
31239		Nasal/sinus endoscopy surg	9.04	NA	7.90	0.95	NA	NA	17.89	$619.10	010	A+ B Me
31240		Nasal/sinus endoscopy surg	2.61	NA	1.67	0.37	NA	NA	4.65	$160.92	000	A+ B Me
31241		Nsl/sins ndsc w/artery lig	8.00	NA	3.93	1.12	NA	NA	13.05	$451.61	000	A+ B Me
31253		Nsl/sins ndsc total	9.00	NA	4.42	1.29	NA	NA	14.71	$509.06	000	A B Me
31254		Nsl/sins ndsc w/prtl ethmdct	4.27	8.31	2.27	0.60	13.18	$456.11	7.14	$247.09	000	A B Me
31255		Nsl/sins ndsc w/tot ethmdct	5.75	NA	2.95	0.83	NA	NA	9.53	$329.80	000	A B Me
31256		Exploration maxillary sinus	3.11	NA	1.74	0.42	NA	NA	5.27	$182.37	000	A B Me
31257		Nsl/sins ndsc tot w/sphendt	8.00	NA	3.98	1.11	NA	NA	13.09	$453.00	000	A B Me
31259		Nsl/sins ndsc sphn tiss rmvl	8.48	NA	4.18	1.20	NA	NA	13.86	$479.64	000	A B Me
31267		Endoscopy maxillary sinus	4.68	NA	2.45	0.66	NA	NA	7.79	$269.58	000	A B Me
31276		Nsl/sins ndsc frnt tiss rmvl	6.75	NA	3.40	0.95	NA	NA	11.10	$384.13	000	A B Me
31287		Nasal/sinus endoscopy surg	3.50	NA	1.92	0.50	NA	NA	5.92	$204.87	000	A+ B Me
31288		Nasal/sinus endoscopy surg	4.10	NA	2.19	0.60	NA	NA	6.89	$238.44	000	A+ B Me
31290		Nasal/sinus endoscopy surg	18.61	NA	12.56	2.80	NA	NA	33.97	$1175.57	010	A+ B Me
31291		Nasal/sinus endoscopy surg	19.56	NA	13.12	3.05	NA	NA	35.73	$1236.48	010	A+ B Me
31292		Nsl/sins ndsc med/inf dcmprn	15.90	NA	11.30	2.34	NA	NA	29.54	$1022.27	010	A+ B Me
31293		Nsl/sins ndsc med&inf dcmprn	17.47	NA	11.95	2.49	NA	NA	31.91	$1104.28	010	A+ B Me
31294		Nsl/sins ndsc surg on dcmprn	20.31	NA	13.24	2.89	NA	NA	36.44	$1261.05	010	A+ B Me
31295		Nsl/sins ndsc surg max sins	2.70	48.76	1.55	0.39	51.85	$1794.33	4.64	$160.57	000	B Me
31296		Nsl/sins ndsc surg frnt sins	3.10	49.06	1.73	0.42	52.58	$1819.59	5.25	$181.68	000	B Me
31297		Nsl/sins ndsc surg sphn sins	2.44	48.64	1.43	0.34	51.42	$1779.45	4.21	$145.69	000	A+ B Me
31298		Nsl/sins ndsc surg frnt&sphn	4.50	92.54	2.37	0.64	97.68	$3380.33	7.51	$259.89	000	A+ B Me
31299	CP	Sinus surgery procedure	0.00	0.00	0.00	0.00	0.00	$0.00	0.00	$0.00	YYY	A+ C+ M T+
31300		Removal of larynx lesion	15.91	NA	19.18	2.26	NA	NA	37.35	$1292.54	090	C+ M
31360		Removal of larynx	29.91	NA	26.87	4.32	NA	NA	61.10	$2114.44	090	C+ M
31365		Removal of larynx	38.81	NA	30.89	5.59	NA	NA	75.29	$2605.50	090	C+ M
31367		Partial removal of larynx	30.57	NA	29.85	4.33	NA	NA	64.75	$2240.75	090	C+ M
31368		Partial removal of larynx	34.19	NA	32.58	4.87	NA	NA	71.64	$2479.19	090	C+ M

31370	Partial removal of larynx	27.57	NA	29.37	3.92	NA	NA	60.86	$2106.13	090	C+ M
31375	Partial removal of larynx	26.07	NA	28.06	3.71	NA	NA	57.84	$2001.62	090	C+ M
31380	Partial removal of larynx	25.57	NA	27.83	3.63	NA	NA	57.03	$1973.59	090	C+ M
31382	Partial removal of larynx	28.57	NA	29.83	4.06	NA	NA	62.46	$2161.50	090	C+ M
31390	Removal of larynx & pharynx	42.51	NA	34.65	6.04	NA	NA	83.20	$2879.24	090	C+ M
31395	Reconstruct larynx & pharynx	43.80	NA	37.40	6.23	NA	NA	87.43	$3025.62	090	C+ M
31400	Revision of larynx	11.60	NA	17.00	1.64	NA	NA	30.24	$1046.49	090	M
31420	Removal of epiglottis	11.43	NA	11.71	1.63	NA	NA	24.77	$857.20	090	C+ M
31500	Insert emergency airway	3.00	NA	0.73	0.42	NA	NA	4.15	$143.62	000	A
31502	Change of windpipe airway	0.65	NA	0.29	0.09	NA	NA	1.03	$35.64	000	A M
31505	Diagnostic laryngoscopy	0.61	2.03	0.74	0.09	2.73	$94.47	1.44	$49.83	000	A M
31510	Laryngoscopy with biopsy	1.92	4.24	1.35	0.25	6.41	$221.83	3.52	$121.81	000	A+ Me
31511	Remove foreign body larynx	2.16	3.85	1.39	0.33	6.34	$219.40	3.88	$134.27	000	A Me
31512	Removal of larynx lesion	2.07	4.09	1.42	0.28	6.44	$222.86	3.77	$130.47	000	A+ Me
31513	Injection into vocal cord	2.10	NA	1.43	0.29	NA	NA	3.82	$132.20	000	A+ Me
31515	Laryngoscopy for aspiration	1.80	4.36	1.22	0.25	6.41	$221.83	3.27	$113.16	000	A M
31520	Dx laryngoscopy newborn	2.56	NA	1.64	0.35	NA	NA	4.55	$157.46	000	A+ M
31525	Dx laryngoscopy excl nb	2.63	4.45	1.67	0.39	7.47	$258.51	4.69	$162.30	000	A M
31526	Dx laryngoscopy w/oper scope	2.57	NA	1.65	0.37	NA	NA	4.59	$158.84	000	A M
31527	Laryngoscopy for treatment	3.27	NA	1.97	0.45	NA	NA	5.69	$196.91	000	A+ Me
31528	Laryngoscopy and dilation	2.37	NA	1.50	0.33	NA	NA	4.20	$145.35	000	A+ Me
31529	Laryngoscopy and dilation	2.68	NA	1.65	0.39	NA	NA	4.72	$163.34	000	A+ Me
31530	Laryngoscopy w/fb removal	3.38	NA	1.95	0.51	NA	NA	5.84	$202.10	000	A Me
31531	Laryngoscopy w/fb & op scope	3.58	NA	2.09	0.51	NA	NA	6.18	$213.87	000	A+ Me
31535	Laryngoscopy w/biopsy	3.16	NA	1.92	0.44	NA	NA	5.52	$191.03	000	A Me
31536	Laryngoscopy w/bx & op scope	3.55	NA	2.10	0.51	NA	NA	6.16	$213.17	000	A Me
31540	Laryngoscopy w/exc of tumor	4.12	NA	2.36	0.60	NA	NA	7.08	$245.01	000	A Me
31541	Larynscop w/tumr exc + scope	4.52	NA	2.54	0.64	NA	NA	7.70	$266.47	000	A Me

*Please note that these calculations are based on the Medicare 2022 Conversion Factor of $34.6062 and the DRA RVU cap rates at time of publication.

A = assistant-at-surgery restriction
A+ = assistant-at-surgery restriction unless medical necessity established with documentation
B = bilateral surgery adjustment applies
C = cosurgeons payable
C+ = cosurgeons payable if medical necessity established with documentation
CP = carriers may establish RVUs and payment amounts for these services, generally on an individual basis following review of documentation such as an operative report
M = multiple surgery adjustment applies
Me = multiple endoscopy rules may apply
M+ = multiple therapy rules apply
Mtc = multiple diagnostic imaging rules apply
T = team surgeons permitted
T+ = team surgeons payable if medical necessity established with documentation
§ = indicates code is not covered by Medicare
GS = procedure must be performed under the general supervision of a physician
DS = procedure must be performed under the direct supervision of a physician
PS = procedure must be performed under the personal supervision of a physician
DRA = procedure subject to DRA limitation

Relative Value Units

CPT Code and Modifier		Description	Work RVU	Nonfacility Practice Expense RVU	Facility Practice Expense RVU	PLI RVU	Total Non-facility RVUs	Medicare Payment Nonfacility	Total Facility RVUs	Medicare Payment Facility	Global Period	Payment Policy Indicators
31545		Remove vc lesion w/scope	6.30	NA	3.39	0.90	NA	NA	10.59	$366.48	000	A B Me
31546		Remove vc lesion scope/graft	9.73	NA	4.95	1.39	NA	NA	16.07	$556.12	000	A B Me
31551		Laryngoplasty laryngeal sten	21.50	NA	21.37	3.04	NA	NA	45.91	$1588.77	090	A+ C+ M
31552		Laryngoplasty laryngeal sten	20.50	NA	20.94	2.92	NA	NA	44.36	$1535.13	090	A+ C+ M
31553		Laryngoplasty laryngeal sten	22.00	NA	25.13	3.13	NA	NA	50.26	$1739.31	090	A+ C+ M
31554		Laryngoplasty laryngeal sten	22.00	NA	25.16	3.13	NA	NA	50.29	$1740.35	090	A+ C+ M
31560		Laryngoscop w/arytenoidectom	5.45	NA	2.92	0.77	NA	NA	9.14	$316.30	000	A+ Me
31561		Larynscop remve cart + scop	5.99	NA	3.16	0.86	NA	NA	10.01	$346.41	000	A+ Me
31570		Laryngoscope w/vc inj	3.86	5.75	2.26	0.60	10.21	$353.33	6.72	$232.55	000	A Me
31571		Laryngoscop w/vc inj + scope	4.26	NA	2.42	0.60	NA	NA	7.28	$251.93	000	A Me
31572		Largsc w/laser dstrj les	3.01	12.56	1.85	0.42	15.99	$553.35	5.28	$182.72	000	A+ B Me
31573		Largsc w/ther injection	2.43	5.81	1.57	0.34	8.58	$296.92	4.34	$150.19	000	A+ B Me
31574		Largsc w/njx augmentation	2.43	26.39	1.58	0.34	29.16	$1009.12	4.35	$150.54	000	A+ B Me
31575		Diagnostic laryngoscopy	0.94	2.79	0.91	0.12	3.85	$133.23	1.97	$68.17	000	A M
31576		Laryngoscopy with biopsy	1.89	5.90	1.33	0.25	8.04	$278.23	3.47	$120.08	000	A Me
31577		Largsc w/rmvl foreign bdy(s)	2.19	5.74	1.47	0.31	8.24	$285.16	3.97	$137.39	000	A+ Me
31578		Largsc w/removal lesion	2.43	6.39	1.58	0.34	9.16	$316.99	4.35	$150.54	000	A+ Me
31579		Laryngoscopy telescopic	1.88	3.78	1.36	0.25	5.91	$204.52	3.49	$120.78	000	A Me
31580		Laryngoplasty laryngeal web	14.60	NA	21.79	2.07	NA	NA	38.46	$1330.95	090	A+ C+ M
31584		Laryngoplasty fx rdctj fixj	17.58	NA	22.27	2.49	NA	NA	42.34	$1465.23	090	A+ C+ M
31587		Laryngoplasty cricoid split	15.27	NA	18.56	2.17	NA	NA	36.00	$1245.82	090	A+ C+ M
31590		Reinnervate larynx	7.85	NA	18.72	1.11	NA	NA	27.68	$957.90	090	C+ M
31591		Laryngoplasty medialization	13.56	NA	17.33	1.94	NA	NA	32.83	$1136.12	090	A+ B C+ M
31592		Cricotracheal resection	25.00	NA	22.99	3.55	NA	NA	51.54	$1783.60	090	A+ C+ M
31599	CP	Larynx surgery procedure	0.00	0.00	0.00	0.00	0.00	$0.00	0.00	$0.00	YYY	A+ C+ M T+
31600		Incision of windpipe	5.56	NA	2.41	1.05	NA	NA	9.02	$312.15	000	A M
31601		Incision of windpipe	8.00	NA	4.08	1.12	NA	NA	13.20	$456.80	000	C+ M
31603		Incision of windpipe	6.00	NA	2.37	1.09	NA	NA	9.46	$327.37	000	A M
31605		Incision of windpipe	6.45	NA	2.07	1.30	NA	NA	9.82	$339.83	000	A M
31610		Incision of windpipe	12.00	NA	14.85	1.82	NA	NA	28.67	$992.16	090	A M
31611		Surgery/speech prosthesis	6.00	NA	9.16	0.89	NA	NA	16.05	$555.43	090	C+ M
31612		Puncture/clear windpipe	0.91	1.76	0.38	0.12	2.79	$96.55	1.41	$48.79	000	A+ M
31613		Repair windpipe opening	4.71	NA	7.31	0.77	NA	NA	12.79	$442.61	090	A M

31614	Repair windpipe opening	8.63	NA	11.39	1.28	NA	NA	21.30	$737.11	090	A M
31615	Visualization of windpipe	1.84	3.07	1.29	0.25	5.16	$178.57	3.38	$116.97	000	A M
31622	Dx bronchoscope/wash	2.53	4.60	1.04	0.28	7.41	$256.43	3.85	$133.23	000	A M
31623	Dx bronchoscope/brush	2.63	5.48	1.02	0.22	8.33	$288.27	3.87	$133.93	000	A Me
31624	Dx bronchoscope/lavage	2.63	4.82	1.05	0.23	7.68	$265.78	3.91	$135.31	000	A Me
31625	Bronchoscopy w/biopsy(s)	3.11	7.26	1.18	0.28	10.65	$368.56	4.57	$158.15	000	A Me
31626	Bronchoscopy w/markers	3.91	20.18	1.41	0.42	24.51	$848.20	5.74	$198.64	000	A+ M
31627	Navigational bronchoscopy	2.00	32.15	0.62	0.20	34.35	$1188.72	2.82	$97.59	ZZZ	A+
31628	Bronchoscopy/lung bx each	3.55	7.48	1.30	0.28	11.31	$391.40	5.13	$177.53	000	A Me
31629	Bronchoscopy/needle bx each	3.75	9.80	1.36	0.33	13.88	$480.33	5.44	$188.26	000	A Me
31630	Bronchoscopy dilate/fx repr	3.81	NA	1.55	0.43	NA	NA	5.79	$200.37	000	A Me
31631	Bronchoscopy dilate w/stent	4.36	NA	1.73	0.52	NA	NA	6.61	$228.75	000	A Me
31632	Bronchoscopy/lung bx addl	1.03	0.80	0.32	0.09	1.92	$66.44	1.44	$49.83	ZZZ	A
31633	Bronchoscopy/needle bx addl	1.32	0.95	0.41	0.11	2.38	$82.36	1.84	$63.68	ZZZ	A
31634	Bronch w/balloon occlusion	3.75	44.36	1.45	0.39	48.50	$1678.40	5.59	$193.45	000	Me
31635	Bronchoscopy w/fb removal	3.42	5.03	1.35	0.35	8.80	$304.53	5.12	$177.18	000	A Me
31636	Bronchoscopy bronch stents	4.30	NA	1.62	0.43	NA	NA	6.35	$219.75	000	A Me
31637	Bronchoscopy stent add-on	1.58	NA	0.53	0.14	NA	NA	2.25	$77.86	ZZZ	A
31638	Bronchoscopy revise stent	4.88	NA	1.82	0.52	NA	NA	7.22	$249.86	000	A Me
31640	Bronchoscopy w/tumor excise	4.93	NA	1.84	0.50	NA	NA	7.27	$251.59	000	A Me
31641	Bronchoscopy treat blockage	5.02	NA	1.91	0.54	NA	NA	7.47	$258.51	000	A Me
31643	Diag bronchoscope/catheter	3.49	NA	1.34	0.29	NA	NA	5.12	$177.18	000	A M
31645	Brnchsc w/ther aspir 1st	2.88	5.07	1.15	0.25	8.20	$283.77	4.28	$148.11	000	A Me
31646	Brnchsc w/ther aspir sbsq	2.78	NA	1.11	0.25	NA	NA	4.14	$143.27	000	A M
31647	Bronchial valve init insert	4.15	NA	1.49	0.39	NA	NA	6.03	$208.68	000	A Me
31648	Bronchial valve remov init	3.95	NA	1.44	0.39	NA	NA	5.78	$200.02	000	A Me
31649	Bronchial valve remov addl	1.44	0.41	0.41	0.11	1.96	$67.83	1.96	$67.83	ZZZ	A
31651	Bronchial valve addl insert	1.58	0.50	0.50	0.14	2.22	$76.83	2.22	$76.83	ZZZ	A

*Please note that these calculations are based on the Medicare 2022 Conversion Factor of $34.6062 and the DRA RVU cap rates at time of publication.

A = assistant-at-surgery restriction
A+ = assistant-at-surgery restriction unless medical necessity established with documentation
B = bilateral surgery adjustment applies
C = cosurgeons payable
C+ = cosurgeons payable if medical necessity established with documentation
CP = carriers may establish RVUs and payment amounts for these services, generally on an individual basis following review of documentation such as an operative report
M = multiple surgery adjustment applies
Me = multiple endoscopy rules may apply
M+ = multiple therapy rules apply
Mtc = multiple diagnostic imaging rules apply
T = team surgeons permitted
T+ = team surgeons payable if medical necessity established with documentation
§ = indicates code is not covered by Medicare
GS = procedure must be performed under the general supervision of a physician
DS = procedure must be performed under the direct supervision of a physician
PS = procedure must be performed under the personal supervision of a physician
DRA = procedure subject to DRA limitation

Relative Value Units

CPT Code and Modifier		Description	Work RVU	Nonfacility Practice Expense RVU	Facility Practice Expense RVU	PLI RVU	Total Non-facility RVUs	Medicare Payment Nonfacility	Total Facility RVUs	Medicare Payment Facility	Global Period	Payment Policy Indicators
31652		Bronch ebus samplng 1/2 node	4.46	34.63	1.59	0.41	39.50	$1366.94	6.46	$223.56	000	A M
31653		Bronch ebus samplng 3/> node	4.96	35.59	1.75	0.45	41.00	$1418.85	7.16	$247.78	000	A M
31654		Bronch ebus ivntj perph les	1.40	2.12	0.44	0.11	3.63	$125.62	1.95	$67.48	ZZZ	A
31660		Bronch thermoplsty 1 lobe	4.00	NA	1.40	0.34	NA	NA	5.74	$198.64	000	A Me
31661		Bronch thermoplsty 2/> lobes	4.25	NA	1.44	0.33	NA	NA	6.02	$208.33	000	A Me
31717		Bronchial brush biopsy	2.12	6.56	0.83	0.17	8.85	$306.26	3.12	$107.97	000	A M
31720		Clearance of airways	1.06	NA	0.58	0.10	NA	NA	1.74	$60.21	000	A M
31725		Clearance of airways	1.71	NA	0.49	0.12	NA	NA	2.32	$80.29	000	A M
31730		Intro windpipe wire/tube	2.85	30.34	0.97	0.60	33.79	$1169.34	4.42	$152.96	000	A M
31750		Repair of windpipe	15.39	NA	22.93	2.38	NA	NA	40.70	$1408.47	090	C+ M
31755		Repair of windpipe	17.54	NA	31.90	2.49	NA	NA	51.93	$1797.10	090	C+ M
31760		Repair of windpipe	23.48	NA	11.42	5.56	NA	NA	40.46	$1400.17	090	C+ M
31766		Reconstruction of windpipe	31.67	NA	12.99	7.50	NA	NA	52.16	$1805.06	090	C+ M
31770		Repair/graft of bronchus	23.54	NA	9.91	5.57	NA	NA	39.02	$1350.33	090	C+ M
31775		Reconstruct bronchus	24.59	NA	10.69	5.83	NA	NA	41.11	$1422.66	090	M
31780		Reconstruct windpipe	19.84	NA	11.69	3.38	NA	NA	34.91	$1208.10	090	C+ M
31781		Reconstruct windpipe	24.85	NA	14.09	3.54	NA	NA	42.48	$1470.07	090	C+ M
31785		Remove windpipe lesion	18.35	NA	10.49	2.96	NA	NA	31.80	$1100.48	090	C+ M
31786		Remove windpipe lesion	25.42	NA	10.93	6.03	NA	NA	42.38	$1466.61	090	C+ M
31800		Repair of windpipe injury	8.18	NA	11.94	1.16	NA	NA	21.28	$736.42	090	A+ M
31805		Repair of windpipe injury	13.42	NA	7.51	3.20	NA	NA	24.13	$835.05	090	C+ M
31820		Closure of windpipe lesion	4.64	7.99	4.49	0.72	13.35	$461.99	9.85	$340.87	090	A+ M
31825		Repair of windpipe defect	7.07	10.18	6.26	1.04	18.29	$632.95	14.37	$497.29	090	A+ M
31830		Revise windpipe scar	4.62	9.51	5.50	0.77	14.90	$515.63	10.89	$376.86	090	A+ M
31899	CP	Airways surgical procedure	0.00	0.00	0.00	0.00	0.00	$0.00	0.00	$0.00	YYY	A+ C+ M T+
32035		Thoracostomy w/rib resection	11.29	NA	7.75	2.68	NA	NA	21.72	$751.65	090	B C+ M
32036		Thoracostomy w/flap drainage	12.30	NA	8.19	2.90	NA	NA	23.39	$809.44	090	B C+ M
32096		Open wedge/bx lung infiltr	13.75	NA	6.54	3.23	NA	NA	23.52	$813.94	090	C+ M
32097		Open wedge/bx lung nodule	13.75	NA	6.58	3.24	NA	NA	23.57	$815.67	090	C+ M
32098		Open biopsy of lung pleura	12.91	NA	6.39	3.03	NA	NA	22.33	$772.76	090	C+ M
32100		Exploration of chest	13.75	NA	6.85	3.24	NA	NA	23.84	$825.01	090	C+ M
32110		Explore/repair chest	25.28	NA	12.19	5.92	NA	NA	43.39	$1501.56	090	C+ M
32120		Re-exploration of chest	14.39	NA	7.92	3.39	NA	NA	25.70	$889.38	090	C+ M

32124	Explore chest free adhesions	15.45	NA	8.18	3.63	NA	NA	27.26	$943.37	090	C+ M
32140	Removal of lung lesion(s)	16.66	NA	8.53	3.95	NA	NA	29.14	$1008.42	090	C+ M
32141	Remove/treat lung lesions	27.18	NA	11.08	6.45	NA	NA	44.71	$1547.24	090	C+ M
32150	Removal of lung lesion(s)	16.82	NA	9.01	3.93	NA	NA	29.76	$1029.88	090	C+ M
32151	Remove lung foreign body	16.94	NA	8.61	4.01	NA	NA	29.56	$1022.96	090	C+ M
32160	Open chest heart massage	13.10	NA	7.30	3.06	NA	NA	23.46	$811.86	090	C+ M
32200	Drain open lung lesion	18.68	NA	10.42	4.44	NA	NA	33.54	$1160.69	090	C+ M
32215	Treat chest lining	13.05	NA	7.39	3.09	NA	NA	23.53	$814.28	090	B C+ M
32220	Release of lung	26.65	NA	14.02	6.32	NA	NA	46.99	$1626.15	090	B C+ M
32225	Partial release of lung	16.75	NA	8.65	3.99	NA	NA	29.39	$1017.08	090	B C+ M
32310	Removal of chest lining	15.28	NA	8.19	3.61	NA	NA	27.08	$937.14	090	C+ M
32320	Free/remove chest lining	27.25	NA	13.50	6.47	NA	NA	47.22	$1634.10	090	C+ M
32400	Needle biopsy chest lining	1.76	3.05	0.55	0.17	4.98	$172.34	2.48	$85.82	000	A M
32408	Core ndl bx lng/med perq	3.18	23.07	1.00	0.27	26.52	$917.76	4.45	$154.00	000	A M
32440	Remove lung pneumonectomy	27.28	NA	12.44	6.47	NA	NA	46.19	$1598.46	090	C+ M
32442	Sleeve pneumonectomy	56.47	NA	19.69	13.41	NA	NA	89.57	$3099.68	090	C+ M
32445	Removal of lung extrapleural	63.84	NA	24.55	15.12	NA	NA	103.51	$3582.09	090	C+ M
32480	Partial removal of lung	25.82	NA	11.61	6.12	NA	NA	43.55	$1507.10	090	C+ M
32482	Bilobectomy	27.44	NA	12.65	6.51	NA	NA	46.60	$1612.65	090	C+ M
32484	Segmentectomy	25.38	NA	10.77	6.03	NA	NA	42.18	$1459.69	090	C+ M
32486	Sleeve lobectomy	42.88	NA	15.62	10.17	NA	NA	68.67	$2376.41	090	C+ M
32488	Completion pneumonectomy	42.99	NA	16.98	10.20	NA	NA	70.17	$2428.32	090	C+ M
32491	Lung volume reduction	25.24	NA	12.07	5.98	NA	NA	43.29	$1498.10	090	B C+ M
32501	Repair bronchus add-on	4.68	NA	1.32	1.10	NA	NA	7.10	$245.70	ZZZ	C+
32503	Resect apical lung tumor	31.74	NA	13.45	7.51	NA	NA	52.70	$1823.75	090	C+ M
32504	Resect apical lung tum/chest	36.54	NA	14.82	8.66	NA	NA	60.02	$2077.06	090	C+ M
32505	Wedge resect of lung initial	15.75	NA	7.93	3.73	NA	NA	27.41	$948.56	090	C+ M
32506	Wedge resect of lung add-on	3.00	NA	0.87	0.72	NA	NA	4.59	$158.84	ZZZ	C+

*Please note that these calculations are based on the Medicare 2022 Conversion Factor of $34.6062 and the DRA RVU cap rates at time of publication.

A = assistant-at-surgery restriction
A+ = assistant-at-surgery restriction unless medical necessity established with documentation
B = bilateral surgery adjustment applies
C = cosurgeons payable
C+ = cosurgeons payable if medical necessity established with documentation
CP = carriers may establish RVUs and payment amounts for these services, generally on an individual basis following review of documentation such as an operative report
M = multiple surgery adjustment applies
Me = multiple endoscopy rules may apply
M+ = multiple therapy rules apply
Mtc = multiple diagnostic imaging rules apply
T = team surgeons permitted
T+ = team surgeons payable if medical necessity established with documentation
§ = indicates code is not covered by Medicare
GS = procedure must be performed under the general supervision of a physician
DS = procedure must be performed under the direct supervision of a physician
PS = procedure must be performed under the personal supervision of a physician
DRA = procedure subject to DRA limitation

Relative Value Units

CPT Code and Modifier	Description	Work RVU	Nonfacility Practice Expense RVU	Facility Practice Expense RVU	PLI RVU	Total Non-facility RVUs	Medicare Payment Nonfacility	Total Facility RVUs	Medicare Payment Facility	Global Period	Payment Policy Indicators
32507	Wedge resect of lung diag	3.00	NA	0.87	0.72	NA	NA	4.59	$158.84	ZZZ	C+
32540	Removal of lung lesion	30.35	NA	13.24	7.20	NA	NA	50.79	$1757.65	090	C+ M
32550	Insert pleural cath	3.92	20.18	1.53	0.54	24.64	$852.70	5.99	$207.29	000	A
32551	Insertion of chest tube	3.04	NA	1.02	0.55	NA	NA	4.61	$159.53	000	A B M
32552	Remove lung catheter	2.53	2.54	1.74	0.35	5.42	$187.57	4.62	$159.88	010	A+ M
32553	Ins mark thor for rt perq	3.55	11.71	1.25	0.33	15.59	$539.51	5.13	$177.53	000	M
32554	Aspirate pleura w/o imaging	1.82	5.19	0.60	0.20	7.21	$249.51	2.62	$90.67	000	A B M
32555	Aspirate pleura w/ imaging	2.27	7.19	0.74	0.20	9.66	$334.30	3.21	$111.09	000	A B M
32556	Insert cath pleura w/o image	2.50	20.19	0.81	0.32	23.01	$796.29	3.63	$125.62	000	A B M
32557	Insert cath pleura w/ image	3.12	17.11	0.97	0.27	20.50	$709.43	4.36	$150.88	000	A B M
32560	Treat pleurodesis w/agent	1.54	6.14	0.48	0.24	7.92	$274.08	2.26	$78.21	000	A M
32561	Lyse chest fibrin init day	1.39	1.25	0.44	0.17	2.81	$97.24	2.00	$69.21	000	M
32562	Lyse chest fibrin subq day	1.24	1.13	0.39	0.12	2.49	$86.17	1.75	$60.56	000	M
32601	Thoracoscopy diagnostic	5.50	NA	2.24	1.29	NA	NA	9.03	$312.49	000	A+ M
32604	Thoracoscopy wbx sac	8.77	NA	3.19	2.07	NA	NA	14.03	$485.52	000	A+ M
32606	Thoracoscopy w/bx med space	8.39	NA	3.16	1.99	NA	NA	13.54	$468.57	000	A+ M
32607	Thoracoscopy w/bx infiltrate	5.50	NA	2.23	1.29	NA	NA	9.02	$312.15	000	A+ M
32608	Thoracoscopy w/bx nodule	6.84	NA	2.63	1.63	NA	NA	11.10	$384.13	000	A+ M
32609	Thoracoscopy w/bx pleura	4.58	NA	1.96	0.96	NA	NA	7.50	$259.55	000	A+ M
32650	Thoracoscopy w/pleurodesis	10.83	NA	6.33	2.50	NA	NA	19.66	$680.36	090	B C+ M
32651	Thoracoscopy remove cortex	18.78	NA	8.98	4.45	NA	NA	32.21	$1114.67	090	B C+ M
32652	Thoracoscopy rem totl cortex	29.13	NA	12.81	6.89	NA	NA	48.83	$1689.82	090	B C+ M
32653	Thoracoscopy remov fb/fibrin	18.17	NA	8.78	4.22	NA	NA	31.17	$1078.68	090	C+ M
32654	Thoracoscopy contrl bleeding	20.52	NA	9.44	4.27	NA	NA	34.23	$1184.57	090	B C+ M
32655	Thoracoscopy resect bullae	16.17	NA	8.12	3.84	NA	NA	28.13	$973.47	090	B C+ M
32656	Thoracoscopy w/pleurectomy	13.26	NA	7.26	3.16	NA	NA	23.68	$819.47	090	B C+ M
32658	Thoracoscopy w/sac fb remove	11.71	NA	6.55	2.78	NA	NA	21.04	$728.11	090	C+ M
32659	Thoracoscopy w/sac drainage	11.94	NA	6.77	2.84	NA	NA	21.55	$745.76	090	C+ M
32661	Thoracoscopy w/pericard exc	13.33	NA	7.01	3.17	NA	NA	23.51	$813.59	090	C+ M
32662	Thoracoscopy w/mediast exc	14.99	NA	7.73	3.56	NA	NA	26.28	$909.45	090	C+ M
32663	Thoracoscopy w/lobectomy	24.64	NA	10.60	5.85	NA	NA	41.09	$1421.97	090	C+ M
32664	Thoracoscopy w/ th nrv exc	14.28	NA	7.28	3.39	NA	NA	24.95	$863.42	090	B C+ M
32665	Thoracoscop w/esoph musc exc	21.53	NA	9.54	5.10	NA	NA	36.17	$1251.71	090	C+ M

32666		Thoracoscopy w/wedge resect	14.50	NA	7.64	3.46	NA	NA	25.60	$885.92	090	B C+ M
32667		Thoracoscopy w/w resect addl	3.00	NA	0.88	0.72	NA	NA	4.60	$159.19	ZZZ	C+
32668		Thoracoscopy w/w resect diag	3.00	NA	0.88	0.73	NA	NA	4.61	$159.53	ZZZ	C+
32669		Thoracoscopy remove segment	23.53	NA	10.31	5.59	NA	NA	39.43	$1364.52	090	C+ M
32670		Thoracoscopy bilobectomy	28.52	NA	11.82	6.77	NA	NA	47.11	$1630.30	090	C+ M
32671		Thoracoscopy pneumonectomy	31.92	NA	12.53	7.55	NA	NA	52.00	$1799.52	090	C+ M
32672		Thoracoscopy for lvrs	27.00	NA	11.21	6.40	NA	NA	44.61	$1543.78	090	C+ M
32673		Thoracoscopy w/thymus resect	21.13	NA	9.56	5.01	NA	NA	35.70	$1235.44	090	C+ M
32674		Thoracoscopy lymph node exc	4.12	NA	1.20	0.98	NA	NA	6.30	$218.02	ZZZ	C+
32701		Thorax stereo rad targetw/tx	4.18	NA	1.23	0.84	NA	NA	6.25	$216.29	XXX	A+ C+
32800		Repair lung hernia	15.71	NA	8.37	3.73	NA	NA	27.81	$962.40	090	C+ M
32810		Close chest after drainage	14.95	NA	8.02	3.55	NA	NA	26.52	$917.76	090	M
32815		Close bronchial fistula	50.03	NA	20.45	11.78	NA	NA	82.26	$2846.71	090	C+ M
32820		Reconstruct injured chest	22.51	NA	11.32	5.33	NA	NA	39.16	$1355.18	090	C+ M
32851		Lung transplant single	59.64	NA	22.23	14.09	NA	NA	95.96	$3320.81	090	C+ M T
32852		Lung transplant with bypass	65.50	NA	23.19	15.33	NA	NA	104.02	$3599.74	090	C+ M T
32853		Lung transplant double	84.48	NA	29.86	19.68	NA	NA	134.02	$4637.92	090	C+ M T
32854		Lung transplant with bypass	90.00	NA	30.85	21.22	NA	NA	142.07	$4916.50	090	C+ M T
32855	CP	Prepare donor lung single	0.00	0.00	0.00	0.00	0.00	$0.00	0.00	$0.00	XXX	C+ M
32856	CP	Prepare donor lung double	0.00	0.00	0.00	0.00	0.00	$0.00	0.00	$0.00	XXX	C+ M
32900		Removal of rib(s)	23.81	NA	12.28	5.54	NA	NA	41.63	$1440.66	090	C+ M
32905		Revise & repair chest wall	23.29	NA	10.40	5.51	NA	NA	39.20	$1356.56	090	C+ M
32906		Revise & repair chest wall	29.30	NA	12.11	6.95	NA	NA	48.36	$1673.56	090	C+ M
32940		Revision of lung	21.34	NA	9.84	5.06	NA	NA	36.24	$1254.13	090	C+ M
32960		Therapeutic pneumothorax	1.84	1.77	0.69	0.12	3.73	$129.08	2.65	$91.71	000	A M
32994		Ablate pulm tumor perq crybl	9.03	143.66	2.84	0.85	153.54	$5313.44	12.72	$440.19	000	B M
32997		Total lung lavage	7.31	NA	2.08	0.56	NA	NA	9.95	$344.33	000	A B M
32998		Ablate pulm tumor perq rf	9.03	87.10	2.81	0.86	96.99	$3356.46	12.70	$439.50	000	B M

*Please note that these calculations are based on the Medicare 2022 Conversion Factor of $34.6062 and the DRA RVU cap rates at time of publication.

A = assistant-at-surgery restriction
A+ = assistant-at-surgery restriction unless medical necessity established with documentation
B = bilateral surgery adjustment applies
C = cosurgeons payable
C+ = cosurgeons payable if medical necessity established with documentation
CP = carriers may establish RVUs and payment amounts for these services, generally on an individual basis following review of documentation such as an operative report
M = multiple surgery adjustment applies
Me = multiple endoscopy rules may apply
M+ = multiple therapy rules apply
Mtc = multiple diagnostic imaging rules apply
T = team surgeons permitted
T+ = team surgeons payable if medical necessity established with documentation
§ = indicates code is not covered by Medicare
GS = procedure must be performed under the general supervision of a physician
DS = procedure must be performed under the direct supervision of a physician
PS = procedure must be performed under the personal supervision of a physician
DRA = procedure subject to DRA limitation

Relative Value Units

CPT Code and Modifier		Description	Work RVU	Nonfacility Practice Expense RVU	Facility Practice Expense RVU	PLI RVU	Total Non-facility RVUs	Medicare Payment Nonfacility	Total Facility RVUs	Medicare Payment Facility	Global Period	Payment Policy Indicators
32999	CP	Chest surgery procedure	0.00	0.00	0.00	0.00	0.00	$0.00	0.00	$0.00	YYY	A C+ M T+
33016		Pericardiocentesis w/imaging	4.40	NA	1.54	0.96	NA	NA	6.90	$238.78	000	A M
33017		Prcrd drg 6yr+ w/o cgen car	4.62	NA	1.61	0.99	NA	NA	7.22	$249.86	000	A M
33018		Prcrd drg 0-5yr or w/anomly	5.40	NA	1.86	1.27	NA	NA	8.53	$295.19	000	A M
33019		Perq prcrd drg insj cath ct	4.29	NA	1.42	0.60	NA	NA	6.31	$218.37	000	A M
33020		Incision of heart sac	14.31	NA	6.69	3.38	NA	NA	24.38	$843.70	090	C+ M
33025		Incision of heart sac	13.20	NA	6.33	3.09	NA	NA	22.62	$782.79	090	C+ M
33030		Partial removal of heart sac	36.00	NA	14.25	8.50	NA	NA	58.75	$2033.11	090	C+ M
33031		Partial removal of heart sac	45.00	NA	16.97	10.64	NA	NA	72.61	$2512.76	090	C+ M
33050		Resect heart sac lesion	16.97	NA	8.60	4.01	NA	NA	29.58	$1023.65	090	C+ M
33120		Removal of heart lesion	38.45	NA	13.88	9.05	NA	NA	61.38	$2124.13	090	C+ M
33130		Removal of heart lesion	24.17	NA	10.34	5.65	NA	NA	40.16	$1389.78	090	C+ M
33140		Heart revascularize (tmr)	28.34	NA	10.75	6.64	NA	NA	45.73	$1582.54	090	M
33141		Heart tmr w/other procedure	2.54	NA	0.72	0.60	NA	NA	3.86	$133.58	ZZZ	C+
33202		Insert epicard eltrd open	13.20	NA	6.36	3.12	NA	NA	22.68	$784.87	090	A M
33203		Insert epicard eltrd endo	13.97	NA	6.47	3.32	NA	NA	23.76	$822.24	090	A M
33206		Insert heart pm atrial	7.14	NA	4.72	1.64	NA	NA	13.50	$467.18	090	A C M
33207		Insert heart pm ventricular	7.80	NA	4.57	1.80	NA	NA	14.17	$490.37	090	A C M
33208		Insrt heart pm atrial & vent	8.52	NA	4.89	1.96	NA	NA	15.37	$531.90	090	A C M
33210		Insert electrd/pm cath sngl	3.05	NA	1.07	0.64	NA	NA	4.76	$164.73	000	A M
33211		Insert card electrodes dual	3.14	NA	1.17	0.67	NA	NA	4.98	$172.34	000	A M
33212		Insert pulse gen sngl lead	5.01	NA	3.39	1.16	NA	NA	9.56	$330.84	090	A M
33213		Insert pulse gen dual leads	5.28	NA	3.49	1.20	NA	NA	9.97	$345.02	090	A M
33214		Upgrade of pacemaker system	7.59	NA	4.88	1.72	NA	NA	14.19	$491.06	090	A+ C M
33215		Reposition pacing-defib lead	4.92	NA	3.13	1.12	NA	NA	9.17	$317.34	090	A M
33216		Insert 1 electrode pm-defib	5.62	NA	4.12	1.29	NA	NA	11.03	$381.71	090	A M
33217		Insert 2 electrode pm-defib	5.59	NA	4.06	1.28	NA	NA	10.93	$378.25	090	A M
33218		Repair lead pace-defib one	5.82	NA	4.39	1.33	NA	NA	11.54	$399.36	090	A M
33220		Repair lead pace-defib dual	5.90	NA	3.90	1.38	NA	NA	11.18	$386.90	090	A M
33221		Insert pulse gen mult leads	5.55	NA	3.88	1.27	NA	NA	10.70	$370.29	090	A M
33222		Relocation pocket pacemaker	4.85	NA	4.21	1.10	NA	NA	10.16	$351.60	090	A M
33223		Relocate pocket for defib	6.30	NA	4.41	1.44	NA	NA	12.15	$420.47	090	A+ M
33224		Insert pacing lead & connect	9.04	NA	4.06	2.07	NA	NA	15.17	$524.98	000	A M

33225	L ventric pacing lead add-on	8.33	NA	3.51	1.94	NA	NA	13.78	$476.87	ZZZ	A
33226	Reposition l ventric lead	8.68	NA	3.85	2.01	NA	NA	14.54	$503.17	000	A M
33227	Remove&replace pm gen singl	5.25	NA	3.61	1.20	NA	NA	10.06	$348.14	090	A M
33228	Remv&replc pm gen dual lead	5.52	NA	3.73	1.28	NA	NA	10.53	$364.40	090	A M
33229	Remv&replc pm gen mult leads	5.79	NA	4.00	1.33	NA	NA	11.12	$384.82	090	A M
33230	Insrt pulse gen w/dual leads	6.07	NA	3.93	1.39	NA	NA	11.39	$394.16	090	A M
33231	Insrt pulse gen w/mult leads	6.34	NA	4.06	1.43	NA	NA	11.83	$409.39	090	A M
33233	Removal of pm generator	3.14	NA	3.06	0.73	NA	NA	6.93	$239.82	090	A M
33234	Removal of pacemaker system	7.66	NA	4.96	1.75	NA	NA	14.37	$497.29	090	A M
33235	Removal pacemaker electrode	9.90	NA	6.70	2.29	NA	NA	18.89	$653.71	090	A M
33236	Remove electrode/thoracotomy	12.73	NA	7.39	2.98	NA	NA	23.10	$799.40	090	A+ C M
33237	Remove electrode/thoracotomy	13.84	NA	7.70	3.24	NA	NA	24.78	$857.54	090	A+ C M
33238	Remove electrode/thoracotomy	15.40	NA	8.92	3.63	NA	NA	27.95	$967.24	090	A+ C M
33240	Insrt pulse gen w/singl lead	5.80	NA	3.71	1.36	NA	NA	10.87	$376.17	090	A M
33241	Remove pulse generator	3.04	NA	2.63	0.72	NA	NA	6.39	$221.13	090	A M
33243	Remove eltrd/thoracotomy	23.57	NA	11.30	5.54	NA	NA	40.41	$1398.44	090	C+ M
33244	Remove elctrd transvenously	13.74	NA	8.74	3.20	NA	NA	25.68	$888.69	090	A C+ M
33249	Insj/rplcmt defib w/lead(s)	14.92	NA	8.76	3.46	NA	NA	27.14	$939.21	090	A C+ M
33250	Ablate heart dysrhythm focus	25.90	NA	10.82	6.06	NA	NA	42.78	$1480.45	090	C+ M
33251	Ablate heart dysrhythm focus	28.92	NA	12.01	6.84	NA	NA	47.77	$1653.14	090	C+ M
33254	Ablate atria lmtd	23.71	NA	10.72	5.59	NA	NA	40.02	$1384.94	090	C+ M
33255	Ablate atria w/o bypass ext	29.04	NA	11.93	6.80	NA	NA	47.77	$1653.14	090	C+ M
33256	Ablate atria w/bypass exten	34.90	NA	13.54	8.16	NA	NA	56.60	$1958.71	090	C+ M
33257	Ablate atria lmtd add-on	9.63	NA	5.21	2.26	NA	NA	17.10	$591.77	ZZZ	
33258	Ablate atria x10sv add-on	11.00	NA	5.53	2.57	NA	NA	19.10	$660.98	ZZZ	
33259	Ablate atria w/bypass add-on	14.14	NA	7.43	3.29	NA	NA	24.86	$860.31	ZZZ	
33261	Ablate heart dysrhythm focus	28.92	NA	11.65	6.77	NA	NA	47.34	$1638.26	090	C+ M
33262	Rmvl& replc pulse gen 1 lead	5.81	NA	3.94	1.33	NA	NA	11.08	$383.44	090	A M

*Please note that these calculations are based on the Medicare 2022 Conversion Factor of $34.6062 and the DRA RVU cap rates at time of publication.

A = assistant-at-surgery restriction
A+ = assistant-at-surgery restriction unless medical necessity established with documentation
B = bilateral surgery adjustment applies
C = cosurgeons payable
C+ = cosurgeons payable if medical necessity established with documentation
CP = carriers may establish RVUs and payment amounts for these services, generally on an individual basis following review of documentation such as an operative report
M = multiple surgery adjustment applies
Me = multiple endoscopy rules may apply
M+ = multiple therapy rules apply
Mtc = multiple diagnostic imaging rules apply
T = team surgeons permitted
T+ = team surgeons payable if medical necessity established with documentation
§ = indicates code is not covered by Medicare
GS = procedure must be performed under the general supervision of a physician
DS = procedure must be performed under the direct supervision of a physician
PS = procedure must be performed under the personal supervision of a physician
DRA = procedure subject to DRA limitation

Relative Value Units

CPT Code and Modifier	Description	Work RVU	Nonfacility Practice Expense RVU	Facility Practice Expense RVU	PLI RVU	Total Non-facility RVUs	Medicare Payment Nonfacility	Total Facility RVUs	Medicare Payment Facility	Global Period	Payment Policy Indicators
33263	Rmvl & rplcmt dfb gen 2 lead	6.08	NA	4.04	1.40	NA	NA	11.52	$398.66	090	A M
33264	Rmvl & rplcmt dfb gen mlt ld	6.35	NA	4.18	1.47	NA	NA	12.00	$415.27	090	A M
33265	Ablate atria lmtd endo	23.71	NA	10.69	5.58	NA	NA	39.98	$1383.56	090	C+ M
33266	Ablate atria x10sv endo	33.04	NA	13.23	7.77	NA	NA	54.04	$1870.12	090	C+ M
33267	Excl laa open any method	18.50	NA	8.01	4.26	NA	NA	30.77	$1064.83	090	C+ M
33268	Excl laa opn oth px any meth	2.50	NA	0.77	0.57	NA	NA	3.84	$132.89	ZZZ	
33269	Excl laa thrscp any method	14.31	NA	6.72	3.31	NA	NA	24.34	$842.31	090	C+ M
33270	Ins/rep subq defibrillator	9.10	NA	5.50	2.08	NA	NA	16.68	$577.23	090	A M
33271	Insj subq impltbl dfb elctrd	7.50	NA	4.13	1.75	NA	NA	13.38	$463.03	090	A M
33272	Rmvl of subq defibrillator	5.42	NA	3.62	1.25	NA	NA	10.29	$356.10	090	A M
33273	Repos prev impltbl subq dfb	6.50	NA	3.79	1.51	NA	NA	11.80	$408.35	090	A M
33274	Tcat insj/rpl perm ldls pm	7.80	NA	4.66	1.80	NA	NA	14.26	$493.48	090	A C M
33275	Tcat rmvl perm ldls pm w/img	8.59	NA	4.25	2.01	NA	NA	14.85	$513.90	090	A M
33285	Insj subq car rhythm mntr	1.53	135.25	0.71	0.34	137.12	$4745.20	2.58	$89.28	000	A M
33286	Rmvl subq car rhythm mntr	1.50	2.15	0.71	0.34	3.99	$138.08	2.55	$88.25	000	A M
33289	Tcat impl wrls p-art prs snr	6.00	NA	2.45	1.38	NA	NA	9.83	$340.18	000	A+ M
33300	Repair of heart wound	44.97	NA	16.10	10.60	NA	NA	71.67	$2480.23	090	C+ M
33305	Repair of heart wound	76.93	NA	24.79	18.10	NA	NA	119.82	$4146.51	090	C+ M
33310	Exploratory heart surgery	20.34	NA	9.29	4.76	NA	NA	34.39	$1190.11	090	C+ M
33315	Exploratory heart surgery	35.00	NA	13.04	8.25	NA	NA	56.29	$1947.98	090	C+ M
33320	Repair major blood vessel(s)	18.54	NA	8.21	4.26	NA	NA	31.01	$1073.14	090	C+ M
33321	Repair major vessel	20.81	NA	9.26	4.88	NA	NA	34.95	$1209.49	090	C+ M
33322	Repair major blood vessel(s)	24.42	NA	10.70	5.72	NA	NA	40.84	$1413.32	090	C+ M
33330	Insert major vessel graft	25.29	NA	10.65	5.92	NA	NA	41.86	$1448.62	090	C+ M
33335	Insert major vessel graft	33.91	NA	13.02	7.94	NA	NA	54.87	$1898.84	090	C+ M
33340	Perq clsr tcat l atr apndge	14.00	NA	5.90	3.23	NA	NA	23.13	$800.44	000	A+ C M T+
33361	Replace aortic valve perq	22.47	NA	7.80	5.23	NA	NA	35.50	$1228.52	000	A+ C M T+
33362	Replace aortic valve open	24.54	NA	8.42	5.74	NA	NA	38.70	$1339.26	000	A+ C M T+
33363	Replace aortic valve open	25.47	NA	8.69	5.96	NA	NA	40.12	$1388.40	000	A+ C M T+
33364	Replace aortic valve open	25.97	NA	8.04	6.07	NA	NA	40.08	$1387.02	000	A+ C M T+
33365	Replace aortic valve open	26.59	NA	9.10	6.17	NA	NA	41.86	$1448.62	000	A+ C M T+
33366	Trcath replace aortic valve	29.35	NA	9.95	6.83	NA	NA	46.13	$1596.38	000	A+ C M T+
33367	Replace aortic valve w/byp	11.88	NA	3.27	2.79	NA	NA	17.94	$620.84	ZZZ	A+ T+

33368	Replace aortic valve w/byp	14.39	NA	3.97	3.38	NA	NA	21.74	$752.34	ZZZ	A+ T+
33369	Replace aortic valve w/byp	19.00	NA	5.23	4.45	NA	NA	28.68	$992.51	ZZZ	A+ T+
33370	Tcat plmt&rmvl cepd perq	2.50	NA	0.90	0.50	NA	NA	3.90	$134.96	ZZZ	A+
33390	Valvuloplasty aortic valve	35.00	NA	13.33	8.25	NA	NA	56.58	$1958.02	090	C+ M
33391	Valvuloplasty aortic valve	41.50	NA	15.93	9.84	NA	NA	67.27	$2327.96	090	C+ M
33404	Prepare heart-aorta conduit	31.37	NA	12.64	7.35	NA	NA	51.36	$1777.37	090	C+ M
33405	Replacement aortic valve opn	41.32	NA	15.56	9.73	NA	NA	66.61	$2305.12	090	C+ M
33406	Replacement aortic valve opn	52.68	NA	19.19	12.44	NA	NA	84.31	$2917.65	090	C+ M
33410	Replacement aortic valve opn	46.41	NA	17.12	10.98	NA	NA	74.51	$2578.51	090	C+ M
33411	Replacement of aortic valve	62.07	NA	21.68	14.60	NA	NA	98.35	$3403.52	090	M
33412	Replacement of aortic valve	59.00	NA	19.50	13.80	NA	NA	92.30	$3194.15	090	C+ M
33413	Replacement of aortic valve	59.87	NA	20.68	14.02	NA	NA	94.57	$3272.71	090	C+ M
33414	Repair of aortic valve	39.37	NA	14.24	9.34	NA	NA	62.95	$2178.46	090	C+ M
33415	Revision subvalvular tissue	37.27	NA	13.45	8.78	NA	NA	59.50	$2059.07	090	C+ M
33416	Revise ventricle muscle	36.56	NA	14.23	8.56	NA	NA	59.35	$2053.88	090	C+ M
33417	Repair of aortic valve	29.33	NA	12.69	6.95	NA	NA	48.97	$1694.67	090	C+ M
33418	Repair tcat mitral valve	32.25	NA	13.17	7.41	NA	NA	52.83	$1828.25	090	C+ M
33419	Repair tcat mitral valve	7.93	NA	2.69	1.82	NA	NA	12.44	$430.50	ZZZ	C+
33420	Revision of mitral valve	25.79	NA	10.80	6.04	NA	NA	42.63	$1475.26	090	A C+ M
33422	Revision of mitral valve	29.73	NA	12.19	6.95	NA	NA	48.87	$1691.20	090	C+ M
33425	Repair of mitral valve	49.96	NA	18.38	11.76	NA	NA	80.10	$2771.96	090	C+ M
33426	Repair of mitral valve	43.28	NA	16.42	10.15	NA	NA	69.85	$2417.24	090	C+ M
33427	Repair of mitral valve	44.83	NA	16.43	10.23	NA	NA	71.49	$2474.00	090	C+ M
33430	Replacement of mitral valve	50.93	NA	19.28	11.98	NA	NA	82.19	$2844.28	090	C+ M
33440	Rplcmt a-valve tlcj autol pv	64.00	NA	20.88	14.99	NA	NA	99.87	$3456.12	090	C+ M
33460	Revision of tricuspid valve	44.70	NA	15.25	10.45	NA	NA	70.40	$2436.28	090	C+ M
33463	Valvuloplasty tricuspid	57.08	NA	20.69	12.27	NA	NA	90.04	$3115.94	090	C+ M
33464	Valvuloplasty tricuspid	44.62	NA	16.57	10.29	NA	NA	71.48	$2473.65	090	C+ M

*Please note that these calculations are based on the Medicare 2022 Conversion Factor of $34.6062 and the DRA RVU cap rates at time of publication.

A = assistant-at-surgery restriction
A+ = assistant-at-surgery restriction unless medical necessity established with documentation
B = bilateral surgery adjustment applies
C = cosurgeons payable
C+ = cosurgeons payable if medical necessity established with documentation
CP = carriers may establish RVUs and payment amounts for these services, generally on an individual basis following review of documentation such as an operative report
M = multiple surgery adjustment applies
Me = multiple endoscopy rules may apply
M+ = multiple therapy rules apply
Mtc = multiple diagnostic imaging rules apply
T = team surgeons permitted
T+ = team surgeons payable if medical necessity established with documentation
§ = indicates code is not covered by Medicare
GS = procedure must be performed under the general supervision of a physician
DS = procedure must be performed under the direct supervision of a physician
PS = procedure must be performed under the personal supervision of a physician
DRA = procedure subject to DRA limitation

Relative Value Units

CPT Code and Modifier	Description	Work RVU	Nonfacility Practice Expense RVU	Facility Practice Expense RVU	PLI RVU	Total Non-facility RVUs	Medicare Payment Nonfacility	Total Facility RVUs	Medicare Payment Facility	Global Period	Payment Policy Indicators
33465	Replace tricuspid valve	50.72	NA	18.18	11.82	NA	NA	80.72	$2793.41	090	C+ M
33468	Revision of tricuspid valve	45.13	NA	15.98	10.69	NA	NA	71.80	$2484.73	090	C+ M
33471	Vlvt pv clsd hrt via p-art	22.96	NA	10.52	5.43	NA	NA	38.91	$1346.53	090	C+ M
33474	Revision of pulmonary valve	39.40	NA	15.17	9.35	NA	NA	63.92	$2212.03	090	C+ M
33475	Replacement pulmonary valve	42.40	NA	15.91	9.78	NA	NA	68.09	$2356.34	090	C+ M
33476	Revision of heart chamber	26.57	NA	11.88	6.29	NA	NA	44.74	$1548.28	090	C+ M
33477	Implant tcat pulm vlv perq	25.00	NA	8.94	5.84	NA	NA	39.78	$1376.63	000	A+ C+ M T+
33478	Revision of heart chamber	27.54	NA	12.15	6.52	NA	NA	46.21	$1599.15	090	C+ M
33496	Repair prosth valve clot	29.84	NA	12.09	6.99	NA	NA	48.92	$1692.94	090	C+ M
33500	Repair heart vessel fistula	27.94	NA	11.38	6.54	NA	NA	45.86	$1587.04	090	C+ M
33501	Repair heart vessel fistula	19.51	NA	8.75	4.57	NA	NA	32.83	$1136.12	090	C M
33502	Coronary artery correction	21.85	NA	10.54	5.18	NA	NA	37.57	$1300.15	090	C+ M
33503	Coronary artery graft	22.51	NA	11.18	5.33	NA	NA	39.02	$1350.33	090	A+ C+ M
33504	Coronary artery graft	25.46	NA	11.60	6.04	NA	NA	43.10	$1491.53	090	C+ M
33505	Repair artery w/tunnel	38.40	NA	12.88	9.09	NA	NA	60.37	$2089.18	090	C+ M
33506	Repair artery translocation	37.85	NA	13.32	8.97	NA	NA	60.14	$2081.22	090	C+ M
33507	Repair art intramural	31.40	NA	11.62	7.44	NA	NA	50.46	$1746.23	090	C+ M
33508	Endoscopic vein harvest	0.31	NA	0.09	0.08	NA	NA	0.48	$16.61	ZZZ	C+
33509	Ndsc hrv uxtr art 1 sgm cab	3.34	NA	0.95	0.78	NA	NA	5.07	$175.45	ZZZ	C+
33510	Cabg vein single	34.98	NA	13.57	8.23	NA	NA	56.78	$1964.94	090	M
33511	Cabg vein two	38.45	NA	14.82	9.06	NA	NA	62.33	$2157.00	090	M
33512	Cabg vein three	43.98	NA	16.76	10.33	NA	NA	71.07	$2459.46	090	M
33513	Cabg vein four	45.37	NA	16.74	10.66	NA	NA	72.77	$2518.29	090	M
33514	Cabg vein five	48.08	NA	17.25	11.24	NA	NA	76.57	$2649.80	090	M
33516	Cabg vein six or more	49.76	NA	17.88	11.65	NA	NA	79.29	$2743.93	090	M
33517	Cabg artery-vein single	3.61	NA	1.03	0.86	NA	NA	5.50	$190.33	ZZZ	
33518	Cabg artery-vein two	7.93	NA	2.25	1.85	NA	NA	12.03	$416.31	ZZZ	
33519	Cabg artery-vein three	10.49	NA	2.97	2.48	NA	NA	15.94	$551.62	ZZZ	
33521	Cabg artery-vein four	12.59	NA	3.55	2.97	NA	NA	19.11	$661.32	ZZZ	
33522	Cabg artery-vein five	14.14	NA	3.98	3.33	NA	NA	21.45	$742.30	ZZZ	
33523	Cabg art-vein six or more	16.08	NA	4.42	3.77	NA	NA	24.27	$839.89	ZZZ	
33530	Coronary artery bypass/reop	10.13	NA	2.87	2.37	NA	NA	15.37	$531.90	ZZZ	
33533	Cabg arterial single	33.75	NA	13.24	7.95	NA	NA	54.94	$1901.26	090	M

33534	Cabg arterial two	39.88	NA	15.22	9.39	NA	NA	64.49	$2231.75	090	M
33535	Cabg arterial three	44.75	NA	16.55	10.49	NA	NA	71.79	$2484.38	090	M
33536	Cabg arterial four or more	48.43	NA	17.60	11.29	NA	NA	77.32	$2675.75	090	M
33542	Removal of heart lesion	48.21	NA	17.33	11.21	NA	NA	76.75	$2656.03	090	C+ M
33545	Repair of heart damage	57.06	NA	19.59	13.36	NA	NA	90.01	$3114.90	090	C+ M
33548	Restore/remodel ventricle	54.14	NA	20.24	12.78	NA	NA	87.16	$3016.28	090	C+ M
33572	Open coronary endarterectomy	4.44	NA	1.26	1.04	NA	NA	6.74	$233.25	ZZZ	
33600	Closure of valve	30.31	NA	12.98	7.17	NA	NA	50.46	$1746.23	090	C+ M
33602	Closure of valve	29.34	NA	12.70	6.95	NA	NA	48.99	$1695.36	090	C+ M
33606	Anastomosis/artery-aorta	31.53	NA	13.20	7.47	NA	NA	52.20	$1806.44	090	C+ M
33608	Repair anomaly w/conduit	31.88	NA	13.42	7.55	NA	NA	52.85	$1828.94	090	C+ M
33610	Repair by enlargement	31.40	NA	13.29	7.44	NA	NA	52.13	$1804.02	090	C+ M
33611	Repair double ventricle	35.57	NA	13.16	8.44	NA	NA	57.17	$1978.44	090	C+ M
33612	Repair double ventricle	36.57	NA	13.44	8.67	NA	NA	58.68	$2030.69	090	C+ M
33615	Repair modified fontan	35.89	NA	14.21	8.52	NA	NA	58.62	$2028.62	090	C+ M
33617	Repair single ventricle	39.09	NA	15.11	9.26	NA	NA	63.46	$2196.11	090	C+ M
33619	Repair single ventricle	48.76	NA	20.30	11.56	NA	NA	80.62	$2789.95	090	C+ M
33620	Apply r&l pulm art bands	30.00	NA	11.22	7.11	NA	NA	48.33	$1672.52	090	C+ M
33621	Transthor cath for stent	16.18	NA	7.28	3.84	NA	NA	27.30	$944.75	090	C+ M
33622	Redo compl cardiac anomaly	64.00	NA	21.27	15.18	NA	NA	100.45	$3476.19	090	C+ M
33641	Repair heart septum defect	29.58	NA	11.46	7.02	NA	NA	48.06	$1663.17	090	C+ M
33645	Revision of heart veins	31.30	NA	12.05	7.43	NA	NA	50.78	$1757.30	090	C+ M
33647	Repair heart septum defects	33.00	NA	12.42	7.84	NA	NA	53.26	$1843.13	090	C+ M
33660	Repair of heart defects	31.83	NA	12.10	7.54	NA	NA	51.47	$1781.18	090	C+ M
33665	Repair of heart defects	34.85	NA	12.95	8.27	NA	NA	56.07	$1940.37	090	C+ M
33670	Repair of heart chambers	36.63	NA	12.46	8.69	NA	NA	57.78	$1999.55	090	C+ M
33675	Close mult vsd	35.95	NA	13.28	8.53	NA	NA	57.76	$1998.85	090	C+ M
33676	Close mult vsd w/resection	36.95	NA	13.57	8.77	NA	NA	59.29	$2051.80	090	C+ M

*Please note that these calculations are based on the Medicare 2022 Conversion Factor of $34.6062 and the DRA RVU cap rates at time of publication.

A = assistant-at-surgery restriction
A+ = assistant-at-surgery restriction unless medical necessity established with documentation
B = bilateral surgery adjustment applies
C = cosurgeons payable
C+ = cosurgeons payable if medical necessity established with documentation
CP = carriers may establish RVUs and payment amounts for these services, generally on an individual basis following review of documentation such as an operative report
M = multiple surgery adjustment applies
Me = multiple endoscopy rules may apply
M+ = multiple therapy rules apply
Mtc = multiple diagnostic imaging rules apply
T = team surgeons permitted
T+ = team surgeons payable if medical necessity established with documentation
§ = indicates code is not covered by Medicare
GS = procedure must be performed under the general supervision of a physician
DS = procedure must be performed under the direct supervision of a physician
PS = procedure must be performed under the personal supervision of a physician
DRA = procedure subject to DRA limitation

Relative Value Units

CPT Code and Modifier	Description	Work RVU	Nonfacility Practice Expense RVU	Facility Practice Expense RVU	PLI RVU	Total Non-facility RVUs	Medicare Payment Nonfacility	Total Facility RVUs	Medicare Payment Facility	Global Period	Payment Policy Indicators
33677	Cl mult vsd w/rem pul band	38.45	NA	14.00	9.12	NA	NA	61.57	$2130.70	090	C+ M
33681	Repair heart septum defect	32.34	NA	14.15	7.66	NA	NA	54.15	$1873.93	090	C+ M
33684	Repair heart septum defect	34.37	NA	12.81	8.16	NA	NA	55.34	$1915.11	090	C+ M
33688	Repair heart septum defect	34.75	NA	12.19	8.25	NA	NA	55.19	$1909.92	090	C+ M
33690	Reinforce pulmonary artery	20.36	NA	10.14	4.83	NA	NA	35.33	$1222.64	090	C+ M
33692	Repair of heart defects	36.15	NA	12.59	8.57	NA	NA	57.31	$1983.28	090	C+ M
33694	Repair of heart defects	35.57	NA	13.16	8.44	NA	NA	57.17	$1978.44	090	C+ M
33697	Repair of heart defects	37.57	NA	13.73	8.91	NA	NA	60.21	$2083.64	090	C+ M
33702	Repair of heart defects	27.24	NA	11.74	6.46	NA	NA	45.44	$1572.51	090	C+ M
33710	Repair of heart defects	37.50	NA	13.71	8.91	NA	NA	60.12	$2080.52	090	M
33720	Repair of heart defect	27.26	NA	11.75	6.47	NA	NA	45.48	$1573.89	090	C+ M
33724	Repair venous anomaly	27.63	NA	10.91	6.56	NA	NA	45.10	$1560.74	090	C+ M
33726	Repair pul venous stenosis	37.12	NA	13.62	8.80	NA	NA	59.54	$2060.45	090	C+ M
33730	Repair heart-vein defect(s)	36.14	NA	14.15	8.57	NA	NA	58.86	$2036.92	090	C+ M
33732	Repair heart-vein defect	28.96	NA	12.59	6.86	NA	NA	48.41	$1675.29	090	C+ M
33735	Revision of heart chamber	22.20	NA	10.67	5.27	NA	NA	38.14	$1319.88	090	M
33736	Revision of heart chamber	24.32	NA	11.27	5.79	NA	NA	41.38	$1432.00	090	C+ M
33737	Revision of heart chamber	22.47	NA	10.38	5.32	NA	NA	38.17	$1320.92	090	C+ M
33741	Tas congenital car anomal	14.00	NA	4.83	3.28	NA	NA	22.11	$765.14	000	M
33745	Tis cgen car anomal 1st shnt	20.00	NA	6.90	4.67	NA	NA	31.57	$1092.52	000	M
33746	Tis cgen car anomal ea addl	8.00	NA	2.76	1.86	NA	NA	12.62	$436.73	ZZZ	
33750	Major vessel shunt	22.22	NA	9.63	5.28	NA	NA	37.13	$1284.93	090	C+ M
33755	Major vessel shunt	22.60	NA	10.78	5.36	NA	NA	38.74	$1340.64	090	C+ M
33762	Major vessel shunt	22.60	NA	9.73	5.36	NA	NA	37.69	$1304.31	090	C+ M
33764	Major vessel shunt & graft	22.60	NA	10.78	5.36	NA	NA	38.74	$1340.64	090	C+ M
33766	Major vessel shunt	23.57	NA	10.01	5.58	NA	NA	39.16	$1355.18	090	C+ M
33767	Major vessel shunt	25.30	NA	10.51	6.00	NA	NA	41.81	$1446.89	090	C+ M
33768	Cavopulmonary shunting	8.00	NA	2.28	1.90	NA	NA	12.18	$421.50	ZZZ	C
33770	Repair great vessels defect	39.07	NA	13.67	9.25	NA	NA	61.99	$2145.24	090	C+ M
33771	Repair great vessels defect	40.63	NA	13.51	9.63	NA	NA	63.77	$2206.84	090	C+ M
33774	Repair great vessels defect	31.73	NA	13.60	7.51	NA	NA	52.84	$1828.59	090	C+ M
33775	Repair great vessels defect	32.99	NA	13.61	7.84	NA	NA	54.44	$1883.96	090	M
33776	Repair great vessels defect	34.75	NA	14.55	8.25	NA	NA	57.55	$1991.59	090	C+ M

33777	Repair great vessels defect	34.17	NA	13.25	8.11	NA	NA	55.53	$1921.68	090	M
33778	Repair great vessels defect	42.75	NA	16.03	10.14	NA	NA	68.92	$2385.06	090	C+ M
33779	Repair great vessels defect	43.23	NA	14.61	10.24	NA	NA	68.08	$2355.99	090	C+ M
33780	Repair great vessels defect	43.90	NA	15.04	10.41	NA	NA	69.35	$2399.94	090	C+ M
33781	Repair great vessels defect	43.21	NA	14.25	10.24	NA	NA	67.70	$2342.84	090	M
33782	Nikaidoh proc	60.08	NA	20.16	14.26	NA	NA	94.50	$3270.29	090	C+ M
33783	Nikaidoh proc w/ostia implt	65.08	NA	21.58	15.43	NA	NA	102.09	$3532.95	090	C+ M
33786	Repair arterial trunk	41.87	NA	14.96	9.93	NA	NA	66.76	$2310.31	090	C+ M
33788	Revision of pulmonary artery	27.42	NA	11.11	6.50	NA	NA	45.03	$1558.32	090	C+ M
33800	Aortic suspension	17.28	NA	7.58	4.10	NA	NA	28.96	$1002.20	090	C M
33802	Repair vessel defect	18.37	NA	9.22	4.34	NA	NA	31.93	$1104.98	090	C+ M
33803	Repair vessel defect	20.31	NA	8.73	4.83	NA	NA	33.87	$1172.11	090	C+ M
33813	Repair septal defect	21.36	NA	10.06	5.06	NA	NA	36.48	$1262.43	090	C+ M
33814	Repair septal defect	26.57	NA	11.92	6.29	NA	NA	44.78	$1549.67	090	C+ M
33820	Revise major vessel	16.69	NA	7.78	3.96	NA	NA	28.43	$983.85	090	M
33822	Revise major vessel	17.71	NA	8.07	4.22	NA	NA	30.00	$1038.19	090	C+ M
33824	Revise major vessel	20.23	NA	9.71	4.79	NA	NA	34.73	$1201.87	090	C+ M
33840	Remove aorta constriction	21.34	NA	10.06	5.06	NA	NA	36.46	$1261.74	090	C+ M
33845	Remove aorta constriction	22.93	NA	10.88	5.43	NA	NA	39.24	$1357.95	090	C+ M
33851	Remove aorta constriction	21.98	NA	10.24	5.21	NA	NA	37.43	$1295.31	090	C+ M
33852	Repair septal defect	24.41	NA	10.93	5.81	NA	NA	41.15	$1424.05	090	M
33853	Repair septal defect	32.51	NA	13.60	7.71	NA	NA	53.82	$1862.51	090	C+ M
33858	As-aort grf f/aortic dsj	63.40	NA	21.19	14.90	NA	NA	99.49	$3442.97	090	C+ M
33859	As-aort grf f/ds oth/thn dsj	45.13	NA	15.73	10.64	NA	NA	71.50	$2474.34	090	C+ M
33863	Ascending aortic graft	58.79	NA	19.58	13.84	NA	NA	92.21	$3191.04	090	C+ M
33864	Ascending aortic graft	60.08	NA	20.05	14.22	NA	NA	94.35	$3265.09	090	C+ M
33866	Aortic hemiarch graft	17.75	NA	5.05	4.19	NA	NA	26.99	$934.02	ZZZ	A+ T+
33871	Transvrs a-arch grf hypthrm	60.88	NA	20.22	14.39	NA	NA	95.49	$3304.55	090	C+ M

*Please note that these calculations are based on the Medicare 2022 Conversion Factor of $34.6062 and the DRA RVU cap rates at time of publication.

A = assistant-at-surgery restriction
A+ = assistant-at-surgery restriction unless medical necessity established with documentation
B = bilateral surgery adjustment applies
C = cosurgeons payable
C+ = cosurgeons payable if medical necessity established with documentation
CP = carriers may establish RVUs and payment amounts for these services, generally on an individual basis following review of documentation such as an operative report
M = multiple surgery adjustment applies
Me = multiple endoscopy rules may apply
M+ = multiple therapy rules apply
Mtc = multiple diagnostic imaging rules apply
T = team surgeons permitted
T+ = team surgeons payable if medical necessity established with documentation
§ = indicates code is not covered by Medicare
GS = procedure must be performed under the general supervision of a physician
DS = procedure must be performed under the direct supervision of a physician
PS = procedure must be performed under the personal supervision of a physician
DRA = procedure subject to DRA limitation

Relative Value Units

CPT Code and Modifier		Description	Work RVU	Nonfacility Practice Expense RVU	Facility Practice Expense RVU	PLI RVU	Total Non-facility RVUs	Medicare Payment Nonfacility	Total Facility RVUs	Medicare Payment Facility	Global Period	Payment Policy Indicators
33875		Thoracic aortic graft	50.72	NA	17.12	12.04	NA	NA	79.88	$2764.34	090	C M
33877		Thoracoabdominal graft	69.03	NA	20.21	16.67	NA	NA	105.91	$3665.14	090	C M
33880		Endovasc taa repr incl subcl	34.58	NA	9.64	8.23	NA	NA	52.45	$1815.10	090	C M
33881		Endovasc taa repr w/o subcl	29.58	NA	8.36	7.02	NA	NA	44.96	$1555.89	090	C M
33883		Insert endovasc prosth taa	21.09	NA	6.55	4.94	NA	NA	32.58	$1127.47	090	C M
33884		Endovasc prosth taa add-on	8.20	NA	1.31	2.04	NA	NA	11.55	$399.70	ZZZ	C
33886		Endovasc prosth delayed	18.09	NA	5.75	4.39	NA	NA	28.23	$976.93	090	C M
33889		Artery transpose/endovas taa	15.92	NA	3.45	3.88	NA	NA	23.25	$804.59	000	B C M
33891		Car-car bp grft/endovas taa	20.00	NA	3.18	5.00	NA	NA	28.18	$975.20	000	B C M
33894		Evasc st rpr thrc/aa acrs br	18.27	NA	6.58	3.63	NA	NA	28.48	$985.58	000	A+ M
33895		Evasc st rpr thrc/aa x crsg	14.54	NA	5.23	2.89	NA	NA	22.66	$784.18	000	A+ M
33897		Perq trluml angp nt/recr coa	10.81	NA	3.89	2.17	NA	NA	16.87	$583.81	000	A+ M
33910		Remove lung artery emboli	48.21	NA	17.55	11.40	NA	NA	77.16	$2670.21	090	C+ M
33915		Remove lung artery emboli	24.95	NA	9.68	5.83	NA	NA	40.46	$1400.17	090	C+ M
33916		Surgery of great vessel	78.00	NA	26.04	18.30	NA	NA	122.34	$4233.72	090	C+ M
33917		Repair pulmonary artery	25.30	NA	11.55	6.00	NA	NA	42.85	$1482.88	090	C+ M
33920		Repair pulmonary atresia	32.74	NA	12.62	7.77	NA	NA	53.13	$1838.63	090	C+ M
33922		Transect pulmonary artery	24.22	NA	10.88	5.74	NA	NA	40.84	$1413.32	090	C+ M
33924		Remove pulmonary shunt	5.49	NA	1.56	1.29	NA	NA	8.34	$288.62	ZZZ	C+
33925		Rpr pul art unifocal w/o cpb	31.30	NA	11.59	7.43	NA	NA	50.32	$1741.38	090	C+ M
33926		Repr pul art unifocal w/cpb	44.73	NA	15.41	10.61	NA	NA	70.75	$2448.39	090	C+ M
33927		Impltj tot rplcmt hrt sys	49.00	NA	13.96	11.62	NA	NA	74.58	$2580.93	XXX	M
33928	CP	Rmvl & rplcmt tot hrt sys	0.00	0.00	0.00	0.00	0.00	$0.00	0.00	$0.00	XXX	M
33929	CP	Rmvl rplcmt hrt sys f/trnspl	0.00	0.00	0.00	0.00	0.00	$0.00	0.00	$0.00	ZZZ	
33933	CP	Prepare donor heart/lung	0.00	0.00	0.00	0.00	0.00	$0.00	0.00	$0.00	XXX	C+ M
33935		Transplantation heart/lung	91.78	NA	31.36	21.47	NA	NA	144.61	$5004.40	090	C+ M T
33944	CP	Prepare donor heart	0.00	0.00	0.00	0.00	0.00	$0.00	0.00	$0.00	XXX	C+ M
33945		Transplantation of heart	89.50	NA	31.93	21.06	NA	NA	142.49	$4931.04	090	C+ M T
33946		Ecmo/ecls initiation venous	6.00	NA	1.83	1.25	NA	NA	9.08	$314.22	XXX	A
33947		Ecmo/ecls initiation artery	6.63	NA	2.00	1.41	NA	NA	10.04	$347.45	XXX	A
33948		Ecmo/ecls daily mgmt-venous	4.73	NA	1.48	0.77	NA	NA	6.98	$241.55	XXX	A
33949		Ecmo/ecls daily mgmt artery	4.60	NA	1.40	0.77	NA	NA	6.77	$234.28	XXX	A
33951		Ecmo/ecls insj prph cannula	8.15	NA	2.35	1.91	NA	NA	12.41	$429.46	000	A+ M

33952	Ecmo/ecls insj prph cannula	8.15	NA	2.57	1.81	NA	NA	12.53	$433.62	000	A+ M
33953	Ecmo/ecls insj prph cannula	9.11	NA	2.61	2.16	NA	NA	13.88	$480.33	000	A+ M
33954	Ecmo/ecls insj prph cannula	9.11	NA	2.74	2.14	NA	NA	13.99	$484.14	000	A+ M
33955	Ecmo/ecls insj ctr cannula	16.00	NA	4.50	3.75	NA	NA	24.25	$839.20	000	A+ C+ M T+
33956	Ecmo/ecls insj ctr cannula	16.00	NA	4.70	3.74	NA	NA	24.44	$845.78	000	A+ C+ M T+
33957	Ecmo/ecls repos perph cnula	3.51	NA	1.07	0.83	NA	NA	5.41	$187.22	000	A+ M
33958	Ecmo/ecls repos perph cnula	3.51	NA	1.07	0.83	NA	NA	5.41	$187.22	000	A+ M
33959	Ecmo/ecls repos perph cnula	4.47	NA	1.34	1.04	NA	NA	6.85	$237.05	000	A+ M
33962	Ecmo/ecls repos perph cnula	4.47	NA	1.34	1.04	NA	NA	6.85	$237.05	000	A+ M
33963	Ecmo/ecls repos perph cnula	9.00	NA	2.58	2.11	NA	NA	13.69	$473.76	000	A+ C+ M T+
33964	Ecmo/ecls repos perph cnula	9.50	NA	2.72	2.22	NA	NA	14.44	$499.71	000	A+ C+ M T+
33965	Ecmo/ecls rmvl perph cannula	3.51	NA	1.07	0.83	NA	NA	5.41	$187.22	000	A+ M
33966	Ecmo/ecls rmvl prph cannula	4.50	NA	1.43	0.99	NA	NA	6.92	$239.47	000	A+ M
33967	Insert i-aort percut device	4.84	NA	1.65	1.10	NA	NA	7.59	$262.66	000	A+ M
33968	Remove aortic assist device	0.64	NA	0.21	0.12	NA	NA	0.97	$33.57	000	A
33969	Ecmo/ecls rmvl perph cannula	5.22	NA	1.54	1.21	NA	NA	7.97	$275.81	000	A+ M
33970	Aortic circulation assist	6.74	NA	2.10	1.54	NA	NA	10.38	$359.21	000	C+ M
33971	Aortic circulation assist	11.99	NA	6.02	2.82	NA	NA	20.83	$720.85	090	A M
33973	Insert balloon device	9.75	NA	2.68	2.28	NA	NA	14.71	$509.06	000	C+ M
33974	Remove intra-aortic balloon	15.03	NA	7.66	3.52	NA	NA	26.21	$907.03	090	A M
33975	Implant ventricular device	25.00	NA	7.30	5.81	NA	NA	38.11	$1318.84	XXX	M
33976	Implant ventricular device	30.75	NA	8.47	7.18	NA	NA	46.40	$1605.73	XXX	M
33977	Remove ventricular device	20.86	NA	7.17	4.76	NA	NA	32.79	$1134.74	XXX	M
33978	Remove ventricular device	25.00	NA	8.12	5.84	NA	NA	38.96	$1348.26	XXX	M
33979	Insert intracorporeal device	37.50	NA	10.58	8.83	NA	NA	56.91	$1969.44	XXX	M
33980	Remove intracorporeal device	33.50	NA	10.71	7.85	NA	NA	52.06	$1801.60	XXX	M
33981	Replace vad pump ext	16.11	NA	4.43	3.78	NA	NA	24.32	$841.62	XXX	M
33982	Replace vad intra w/o bp	37.86	NA	10.42	8.87	NA	NA	57.15	$1977.74	XXX	M

*Please note that these calculations are based on the Medicare 2022 Conversion Factor of $34.6062 and the DRA RVU cap rates at time of publication.

A = assistant-at-surgery restriction

A+ = assistant-at-surgery restriction unless medical necessity established with documentation

B = bilateral surgery adjustment applies

C = cosurgeons payable

C+ = cosurgeons payable if medical necessity established with documentation

CP = carriers may establish RVUs and payment amounts for these services, generally on an individual basis following review of documentation such as an operative report

M = multiple surgery adjustment applies

Me = multiple endoscopy rules may apply

M+ = multiple therapy rules apply

Mtc = multiple diagnostic imaging rules apply

T = team surgeons permitted

T+ = team surgeons payable if medical necessity established with documentation

§ = indicates code is not covered by Medicare

GS = procedure must be performed under the general supervision of a physician

DS = procedure must be performed under the direct supervision of a physician

PS = procedure must be performed under the personal supervision of a physician

DRA = procedure subject to DRA limitation

Relative Value Units

CPT Code and Modifier		Description	Work RVU	Nonfacility Practice Expense RVU	Facility Practice Expense RVU	PLI RVU	Total Non-facility RVUs	Medicare Payment Nonfacility	Total Facility RVUs	Medicare Payment Facility	Global Period	Payment Policy Indicators
33983		Replace vad intra w/bp	44.54	NA	12.50	10.49	NA	NA	67.53	$2336.96	XXX	M
33984		Ecmo/ecls rmvl prph cannula	5.46	NA	1.56	1.29	NA	NA	8.31	$287.58	000	A+ M
33985		Ecmo/ecls rmvl ctr cannula	9.89	NA	2.83	2.31	NA	NA	15.03	$520.13	000	A+ C+ M T+
33986		Ecmo/ecls rmvl ctr cannula	10.00	NA	2.99	2.33	NA	NA	15.32	$530.17	000	A+ C+ M T+
33987		Artery expos/graft artery	4.04	NA	1.12	0.95	NA	NA	6.11	$211.44	ZZZ	A+ C+ T+
33988		Insertion of left heart vent	15.00	NA	4.23	3.52	NA	NA	22.75	$787.29	000	A+ C+ M T+
33989		Removal of left heart vent	9.50	NA	2.72	2.22	NA	NA	14.44	$499.71	000	A+ C+ M T+
33990		Insj perq vad l hrt arterial	6.75	NA	2.31	1.54	NA	NA	10.60	$366.83	000	M
33991		Insj perq vad l hrt artl&ven	8.84	NA	3.04	2.01	NA	NA	13.89	$480.68	000	M
33992		Rmvl perq left heart vad	3.55	NA	1.16	0.83	NA	NA	5.54	$191.72	000	M
33993		Reposg perq r/l hrt vad	3.10	NA	1.11	0.66	NA	NA	4.87	$168.53	000	M
33995		Insj perq vad r hrt venous	6.75	NA	2.43	1.41	NA	NA	10.59	$366.48	000	M
33997		Rmvl perq right heart vad	3.00	NA	1.09	0.62	NA	NA	4.71	$163.00	000	M
33999	CP	Cardiac surgery procedure	0.00	0.00	0.00	0.00	0.00	$0.00	0.00	$0.00	YYY	C+ M T+
34001		Removal of artery clot	17.88	NA	4.46	4.47	NA	NA	26.81	$927.79	090	B C+ M
34051		Removal of artery clot	16.99	NA	8.29	3.97	NA	NA	29.25	$1012.23	090	B C+ M
34101		Removal of artery clot	10.93	NA	3.91	2.70	NA	NA	17.54	$606.99	090	B C+ M
34111		Removal of arm artery clot	10.93	NA	4.01	2.69	NA	NA	17.63	$610.11	090	B C+ M
34151		Removal of artery clot	26.52	NA	7.92	6.37	NA	NA	40.81	$1412.28	090	B C+ M
34201		Removal of artery clot	19.48	NA	5.69	4.83	NA	NA	30.00	$1038.19	090	B C+ M
34203		Removal of leg artery clot	17.86	NA	5.54	4.44	NA	NA	27.84	$963.44	090	B C+ M
34401		Removal of vein clot	26.52	NA	10.94	6.10	NA	NA	43.56	$1507.45	090	B C+ M
34421		Removal of vein clot	13.37	NA	3.67	3.35	NA	NA	20.39	$705.62	090	B C+ M
34451		Removal of vein clot	28.52	NA	6.43	7.12	NA	NA	42.07	$1455.88	090	B C+ M
34471		Removal of vein clot	21.11	NA	5.25	5.28	NA	NA	31.64	$1094.94	090	A B C+ M
34490		Removal of vein clot	10.91	NA	5.53	2.71	NA	NA	19.15	$662.71	090	A B M
34501		Repair valve femoral vein	16.85	NA	5.14	4.22	NA	NA	26.21	$907.03	090	B C+ M
34502		Reconstruct vena cava	28.07	NA	10.90	6.28	NA	NA	45.25	$1565.93	090	M
34510		Transposition of vein valve	19.91	NA	5.06	4.97	NA	NA	29.94	$1036.11	090	B C+ M
34520		Cross-over vein graft	19.18	NA	5.04	4.78	NA	NA	29.00	$1003.58	090	B C+ M
34530		Leg vein fusion	17.93	NA	5.20	4.50	NA	NA	27.63	$956.17	090	B C+ M
34701		Evasc rpr a-ao ndgft	23.71	NA	6.99	5.65	NA	NA	36.35	$1257.94	090	C M
34702		Evasc rpr a-ao ndgft rpt	36.00	NA	9.41	8.74	NA	NA	54.15	$1873.93	090	C M

34703		Evasc rpr a-unilac ndgft	26.52	NA	7.36	6.39	NA	NA	40.27	$1393.59	090	C M
34704		Evasc rpr a-unilac ndgft rpt	45.00	NA	10.84	11.06	NA	NA	66.90	$2315.15	090	C M
34705		Evac rpr a-biiliac ndgft	29.58	NA	8.06	7.10	NA	NA	44.74	$1548.28	090	C M
34706		Evasc rpr a-biiliac rpt	45.00	NA	10.84	10.97	NA	NA	66.81	$2312.04	090	C M
34707		Evasc rpr ilio-iliac ndgft	22.28	NA	6.34	5.28	NA	NA	33.90	$1173.15	090	B C M
34708		Evasc rpr ilio-iliac rpt	36.50	NA	9.06	8.55	NA	NA	54.11	$1872.54	090	B C M
34709		Plmt xtn prosth evasc rpr	6.50	NA	1.38	1.55	NA	NA	9.43	$326.34	ZZZ	C
34710		Dlyd plmt xtn prosth 1st vsl	15.00	NA	4.70	3.60	NA	NA	23.30	$806.32	090	C M
34711		Dlyd plmt xtn prosth ea addl	6.00	NA	1.19	1.43	NA	NA	8.62	$298.31	ZZZ	C
34712		Tcat dlvr enhncd fixj dev	12.00	NA	4.34	2.84	NA	NA	19.18	$663.75	090	C M
34713		Perq access & clsr fem art	2.50	NA	0.51	0.60	NA	NA	3.61	$124.93	ZZZ	B C
34714		Opn fem art expos cndt crtj	5.25	NA	1.37	1.26	NA	NA	7.88	$272.70	ZZZ	B C
34715		Opn ax/subcla art expos	6.00	NA	1.29	1.47	NA	NA	8.76	$303.15	ZZZ	B C
34716		Opn ax/subcla art expos cndt	7.19	NA	1.99	1.68	NA	NA	10.86	$375.82	ZZZ	B C
34717		Evasc rpr a-iliac ndgft	9.00	NA	1.85	2.17	NA	NA	13.02	$450.57	ZZZ	C
34718		Evasc rpr n/a a-iliac ndgft	24.00	NA	6.46	5.73	NA	NA	36.19	$1252.40	090	C M
34808		Endovas iliac a device addon	4.12	NA	0.67	1.02	NA	NA	5.81	$201.06	ZZZ	C
34812		Opn fem art expos	4.13	NA	0.90	1.00	NA	NA	6.03	$208.68	ZZZ	B C
34813		Femoral endovas graft add-on	4.79	NA	0.94	1.18	NA	NA	6.91	$239.13	ZZZ	C
34820		Opn iliac art expos	7.00	NA	1.12	1.73	NA	NA	9.85	$340.87	ZZZ	B C
34830		Open aortic tube prosth repr	35.23	NA	7.58	8.80	NA	NA	51.61	$1786.03	090	C M
34831		Open aortoiliac prosth repr	37.98	NA	9.01	9.40	NA	NA	56.39	$1951.44	090	C M
34832		Open aortofemor prosth repr	37.98	NA	8.02	9.49	NA	NA	55.49	$1920.30	090	C M
34833		Opn ilac art expos cndt crtj	8.16	NA	1.30	2.03	NA	NA	11.49	$397.63	ZZZ	B C
34834		Opn brach art expos	2.65	NA	0.48	0.65	NA	NA	3.78	$130.81	ZZZ	B C
34841	CP	Endovasc visc aorta 1 graft	0.00	0.00	0.00	0.00	0.00	$0.00	0.00	$0.00	YYY	C M
34842	CP	Endovasc visc aorta 2 graft	0.00	0.00	0.00	0.00	0.00	$0.00	0.00	$0.00	YYY	C M
34843	CP	Endovasc visc aorta 3 graft	0.00	0.00	0.00	0.00	0.00	$0.00	0.00	$0.00	YYY	C M

*Please note that these calculations are based on the Medicare 2022 Conversion Factor of $34.6062 and the DRA RVU cap rates at time of publication.

A = assistant-at-surgery restriction
A+ = assistant-at-surgery restriction unless medical necessity established with documentation
B = bilateral surgery adjustment applies
C = cosurgeons payable
C+ = cosurgeons payable if medical necessity established with documentation
CP = carriers may establish RVUs and payment amounts for these services, generally on an individual basis following review of documentation such as an operative report
M = multiple surgery adjustment applies
Me = multiple endoscopy rules may apply
M+ = multiple therapy rules apply
Mtc = multiple diagnostic imaging rules apply
T = team surgeons permitted
T+ = team surgeons payable if medical necessity established with documentation
§ = indicates code is not covered by Medicare
GS = procedure must be performed under the general supervision of a physician
DS = procedure must be performed under the direct supervision of a physician
PS = procedure must be performed under the personal supervision of a physician
DRA = procedure subject to DRA limitation

Relative Value Units

CPT Code and Modifier		Description	Work RVU	Nonfacility Practice Expense RVU	Facility Practice Expense RVU	PLI RVU	Total Non-facility RVUs	Medicare Payment Nonfacility	Total Facility RVUs	Medicare Payment Facility	Global Period	Payment Policy Indicators
34844	CP	Endovasc visc aorta 4 graft	0.00	0.00	0.00	0.00	0.00	$0.00	0.00	$0.00	YYY	C M
34845	CP	Visc & infraren abd 1 prosth	0.00	0.00	0.00	0.00	0.00	$0.00	0.00	$0.00	YYY	C M
34846	CP	Visc & infraren abd 2 prosth	0.00	0.00	0.00	0.00	0.00	$0.00	0.00	$0.00	YYY	C M
34847	CP	Visc & infraren abd 3 prosth	0.00	0.00	0.00	0.00	0.00	$0.00	0.00	$0.00	YYY	C M
34848	CP	Visc & infraren abd 4+ prost	0.00	0.00	0.00	0.00	0.00	$0.00	0.00	$0.00	YYY	C M
35001		Repair defect of artery	20.81	NA	7.14	5.10	NA	NA	33.05	$1143.73	090	B C+ M
35002		Repair artery rupture neck	22.23	NA	5.58	5.54	NA	NA	33.35	$1154.12	090	B C+ M
35005		Repair defect of artery	19.29	NA	5.11	4.83	NA	NA	29.23	$1011.54	090	B C+ M
35011		Repair defect of artery	18.58	NA	6.46	4.62	NA	NA	29.66	$1026.42	090	B C+ M
35013		Repair artery rupture arm	23.23	NA	8.05	5.79	NA	NA	37.07	$1282.85	090	B C+ M
35021		Repair defect of artery	22.17	NA	9.71	5.19	NA	NA	37.07	$1282.85	090	B C+ M
35022		Repair artery rupture chest	25.70	NA	10.69	6.02	NA	NA	42.41	$1467.65	090	B C+ M
35045		Repair defect of arm artery	18.01	NA	6.24	4.36	NA	NA	28.61	$990.08	090	B C+ M
35081		Repair defect of artery	33.53	NA	8.88	8.28	NA	NA	50.69	$1754.19	090	C+ M
35082		Repair artery rupture aorta	42.09	NA	11.08	10.38	NA	NA	63.55	$2199.22	090	C+ M
35091		Repair defect of artery	35.35	NA	8.32	8.74	NA	NA	52.41	$1813.71	090	B C+ M
35092		Repair artery rupture aorta	50.97	NA	12.77	12.61	NA	NA	76.35	$2642.18	090	B C+ M
35102		Repair defect of artery	36.53	NA	9.39	9.06	NA	NA	54.98	$1902.65	090	B C+ M
35103		Repair artery rupture aorta	43.62	NA	10.57	10.78	NA	NA	64.97	$2248.36	090	B C+ M
35111		Repair defect of artery	26.28	NA	6.08	6.57	NA	NA	38.93	$1347.22	090	C+ M
35112		Repair artery rupture spleen	32.57	NA	7.15	8.12	NA	NA	47.84	$1655.56	090	B C+ M
35121		Repair defect of artery	31.52	NA	6.90	7.87	NA	NA	46.29	$1601.92	090	B M
35122		Repair artery rupture belly	37.89	NA	8.00	9.46	NA	NA	55.35	$1915.45	090	B C+ M
35131		Repair defect of artery	26.40	NA	7.15	6.56	NA	NA	40.11	$1388.05	090	B C+ M
35132		Repair artery rupture groin	32.57	NA	7.15	8.12	NA	NA	47.84	$1655.56	090	B C+ M
35141		Repair defect of artery	20.91	NA	6.09	5.17	NA	NA	32.17	$1113.28	090	B C+ M
35142		Repair artery rupture thigh	25.16	NA	7.42	6.21	NA	NA	38.79	$1342.37	090	B C+ M
35151		Repair defect of artery	23.72	NA	6.65	5.90	NA	NA	36.27	$1255.17	090	B C+ M
35152		Repair ruptd popliteal art	27.66	NA	6.38	6.89	NA	NA	40.93	$1416.43	090	B C+ M
35180		Repair blood vessel lesion	15.10	NA	4.15	3.78	NA	NA	23.03	$796.98	090	C+ M
35182		Repair blood vessel lesion	31.71	NA	13.39	7.51	NA	NA	52.61	$1820.63	090	C+ M
35184		Repair blood vessel lesion	18.82	NA	4.76	4.71	NA	NA	28.29	$979.01	090	C+ M
35188		Repair blood vessel lesion	18.00	NA	13.21	6.89	NA	NA	38.10	$1318.50	090	C+ M

35189	Repair blood vessel lesion	29.98	NA	6.74	7.47	NA	NA	44.19	$1529.25	090	C+ M
35190	Repair blood vessel lesion	13.42	NA	5.82	3.31	NA	NA	22.55	$780.37	090	C+ M
35201	Repair blood vessel lesion	16.93	NA	6.75	4.00	NA	NA	27.68	$957.90	090	B C+ M
35206	Repair blood vessel lesion	13.84	NA	5.95	3.27	NA	NA	23.06	$798.02	090	B C+ M
35207	Repair blood vessel lesion	10.94	NA	9.37	2.04	NA	NA	22.35	$773.45	090	A B C+ M
35211	Repair blood vessel lesion	24.58	NA	10.68	5.78	NA	NA	41.04	$1420.24	090	B C+ M
35216	Repair blood vessel lesion	36.61	NA	16.30	8.48	NA	NA	61.39	$2124.47	090	B C+ M
35221	Repair blood vessel lesion	26.62	NA	10.36	6.46	NA	NA	43.44	$1503.29	090	B C+ M
35226	Repair blood vessel lesion	15.30	NA	5.43	3.73	NA	NA	24.46	$846.47	090	B C+ M
35231	Repair blood vessel lesion	21.16	NA	11.52	3.96	NA	NA	36.64	$1267.97	090	B C+ M
35236	Repair blood vessel lesion	18.02	NA	7.16	4.23	NA	NA	29.41	$1017.77	090	B C+ M
35241	Repair blood vessel lesion	25.58	NA	10.66	5.98	NA	NA	42.22	$1461.07	090	B C+ M
35246	Repair blood vessel lesion	28.23	NA	11.11	6.60	NA	NA	45.94	$1589.81	090	B C+ M
35251	Repair blood vessel lesion	31.91	NA	11.37	7.77	NA	NA	51.05	$1766.65	090	B C+ M
35256	Repair blood vessel lesion	19.06	NA	6.15	4.65	NA	NA	29.86	$1033.34	090	B C+ M
35261	Repair blood vessel lesion	18.96	NA	5.02	4.75	NA	NA	28.73	$994.24	090	B C+ M
35266	Repair blood vessel lesion	15.83	NA	5.70	3.84	NA	NA	25.37	$877.96	090	B C+ M
35271	Repair blood vessel lesion	24.58	NA	10.27	5.79	NA	NA	40.64	$1406.40	090	B C+ M
35276	Repair blood vessel lesion	25.83	NA	11.00	6.05	NA	NA	42.88	$1483.91	090	B C+ M
35281	Repair blood vessel lesion	30.06	NA	10.26	7.29	NA	NA	47.61	$1647.60	090	B C+ M
35286	Repair blood vessel lesion	17.19	NA	5.99	4.22	NA	NA	27.40	$948.21	090	B C+ M
35301	Rechanneling of artery	21.16	NA	6.70	5.29	NA	NA	33.15	$1147.20	090	B C+ M
35302	Rechanneling of artery	21.35	NA	6.25	5.28	NA	NA	32.88	$1137.85	090	B C+ M
35303	Rechanneling of artery	23.60	NA	6.74	5.83	NA	NA	36.17	$1251.71	090	B C+ M
35304	Rechanneling of artery	24.60	NA	6.66	6.11	NA	NA	37.37	$1293.23	090	B C+ M
35305	Rechanneling of artery	23.60	NA	6.55	5.80	NA	NA	35.95	$1244.09	090	B C+ M
35306	Rechanneling of artery	9.25	NA	1.47	2.31	NA	NA	13.03	$450.92	ZZZ	C+
35311	Rechanneling of artery	28.60	NA	10.42	6.68	NA	NA	45.70	$1581.50	090	B C+ M

*Please note that these calculations are based on the Medicare 2022 Conversion Factor of $34.6062 and the DRA RVU cap rates at time of publication.

A = assistant-at-surgery restriction
A+ = assistant-at-surgery restriction unless medical necessity established with documentation
B = bilateral surgery adjustment applies
C = cosurgeons payable
C+ = cosurgeons payable if medical necessity established with documentation
CP = carriers may establish RVUs and payment amounts for these services, generally on an individual basis following review of documentation such as an operative report
M = multiple surgery adjustment applies
Me = multiple endoscopy rules may apply
M+ = multiple therapy rules apply
Mtc = multiple diagnostic imaging rules apply
T = team surgeons permitted
T+ = team surgeons payable if medical necessity established with documentation
§ = indicates code is not covered by Medicare
GS = procedure must be performed under the general supervision of a physician
DS = procedure must be performed under the direct supervision of a physician
PS = procedure must be performed under the personal supervision of a physician
DRA = procedure subject to DRA limitation

Relative Value Units

CPT Code and Modifier	Description	Work RVU	Nonfacility Practice Expense RVU	Facility Practice Expense RVU	PLI RVU	Total Non-facility RVUs	Medicare Payment Nonfacility	Total Facility RVUs	Medicare Payment Facility	Global Period	Payment Policy Indicators
35321	Rechanneling of artery	16.59	NA	5.49	4.13	NA	NA	26.21	$907.03	090	B C+ M
35331	Rechanneling of artery	27.72	NA	7.95	6.86	NA	NA	42.53	$1471.80	090	B C+ M
35341	Rechanneling of artery	26.21	NA	7.99	6.40	NA	NA	40.60	$1405.01	090	B C+ M
35351	Rechanneling of artery	24.61	NA	7.04	6.11	NA	NA	37.76	$1306.73	090	B C+ M
35355	Rechanneling of artery	19.86	NA	5.39	4.93	NA	NA	30.18	$1044.42	090	B C+ M
35361	Rechanneling of artery	30.24	NA	6.78	7.55	NA	NA	44.57	$1542.40	090	B C+ M
35363	Rechanneling of artery	32.35	NA	7.12	8.09	NA	NA	47.56	$1645.87	090	B C+ M
35371	Rechanneling of artery	15.31	NA	4.82	3.79	NA	NA	23.92	$827.78	090	B C+ M
35372	Rechanneling of artery	18.58	NA	5.38	4.60	NA	NA	28.56	$988.35	090	B C+ M
35390	Reoperation carotid add-on	3.19	NA	0.68	0.77	NA	NA	4.64	$160.57	ZZZ	C+
35400	Angioscopy	3.00	NA	0.58	0.75	NA	NA	4.33	$149.84	ZZZ	A+ C+
35500	Harvest vein for bypass	6.44	NA	1.28	1.59	NA	NA	9.31	$322.18	ZZZ	C+
35501	Art byp grft ipsilat carotid	29.09	NA	6.37	7.26	NA	NA	42.72	$1478.38	090	B C+ M
35506	Art byp grft subclav-carotid	25.33	NA	5.65	6.33	NA	NA	37.31	$1291.16	090	B C+ M
35508	Art byp grft carotid-vertbrl	26.09	NA	6.27	6.51	NA	NA	38.87	$1345.14	090	B C+ M
35509	Art byp grft contral carotid	28.09	NA	6.24	7.02	NA	NA	41.35	$1430.97	090	B C+ M
35510	Art byp grft carotid-brchial	24.39	NA	5.52	6.10	NA	NA	36.01	$1246.17	090	B C+ M
35511	Art byp grft subclav-subclav	22.20	NA	5.07	5.54	NA	NA	32.81	$1135.43	090	B C+ M
35512	Art byp grft subclav-brchial	23.89	NA	5.44	5.96	NA	NA	35.29	$1221.25	090	B C+ M
35515	Art byp grft subclav-vertbrl	26.09	NA	6.27	6.51	NA	NA	38.87	$1345.14	090	B C+ M
35516	Art byp grft subclav-axilary	24.21	NA	5.47	6.05	NA	NA	35.73	$1236.48	090	B C+ M
35518	Art byp grft axillary-axilry	22.65	NA	5.14	5.65	NA	NA	33.44	$1157.23	090	B C+ M
35521	Art byp grft axill-femoral	24.13	NA	5.82	6.03	NA	NA	35.98	$1245.13	090	B C+ M
35522	Art byp grft axill-brachial	23.15	NA	5.32	5.80	NA	NA	34.27	$1185.95	090	B C+ M
35523	Art byp grft brchl-ulnr-rdl	24.13	NA	7.58	5.88	NA	NA	37.59	$1300.85	090	B C+ M
35525	Art byp grft brachial-brchl	21.69	NA	6.16	5.39	NA	NA	33.24	$1150.31	090	B C+ M
35526	Art byp grft aor/carot/innom	31.55	NA	11.89	7.39	NA	NA	50.83	$1759.03	090	B C+ M
35531	Art byp grft aorcel/aormesen	39.11	NA	8.20	9.78	NA	NA	57.09	$1975.67	090	B C+ M
35533	Art byp grft axill/fem/fem	29.92	NA	6.74	7.47	NA	NA	44.13	$1527.17	090	B C+ M
35535	Art byp grft hepatorenal	38.13	NA	8.06	9.52	NA	NA	55.71	$1927.91	090	B C+ M
35536	Art byp grft splenorenal	33.73	NA	7.34	8.43	NA	NA	49.50	$1713.01	090	B C+ M
35537	Art byp grft aortoiliac	41.88	NA	8.67	10.45	NA	NA	61.00	$2110.98	090	C+ M
35538	Art byp grft aortobi-iliac	47.03	NA	9.59	11.73	NA	NA	68.35	$2365.33	090	C+ M

35539	Art byp grft aortofemoral	44.11	NA	9.03	11.01	NA	NA	64.15	$2219.99	090	B C+ M
35540	Art byp grft aortbifemoral	49.33	NA	9.85	12.32	NA	NA	71.50	$2474.34	090	A B C+ M
35556	Art byp grft fem-popliteal	26.75	NA	7.58	6.62	NA	NA	40.95	$1417.12	090	B C+ M
35558	Art byp grft fem-femoral	23.13	NA	7.25	5.74	NA	NA	36.12	$1249.98	090	B C+ M
35560	Art byp grft aortorenal	34.03	NA	7.39	8.51	NA	NA	49.93	$1727.89	090	B C+ M
35563	Art byp grft ilioiliac	26.12	NA	6.13	6.52	NA	NA	38.77	$1341.68	090	B C+ M
35565	Art byp grft iliofemoral	25.13	NA	7.07	6.22	NA	NA	38.42	$1329.57	090	B C+ M
35566	Art byp fem-ant-post tib/prl	32.35	NA	8.45	8.04	NA	NA	48.84	$1690.17	090	B C+ M
35570	Art byp tibial-tib/peroneal	29.15	NA	6.72	7.29	NA	NA	43.16	$1493.60	090	B C+ M
35571	Art byp pop-tibl-prl-other	25.52	NA	6.99	6.34	NA	NA	38.85	$1344.45	090	B C+ M
35572	Harvest femoropopliteal vein	6.81	NA	1.60	1.65	NA	NA	10.06	$348.14	ZZZ	
35583	Vein byp grft fem-popliteal	27.75	NA	7.54	6.90	NA	NA	42.19	$1460.04	090	B C+ M
35585	Vein byp fem-tibial peroneal	32.35	NA	8.53	8.06	NA	NA	48.94	$1693.63	090	B C+ M
35587	Vein byp pop-tibl peroneal	26.21	NA	6.91	6.56	NA	NA	39.68	$1373.17	090	B C+ M
35600	Open hrv uxtr art 1 sgm cab	3.59	NA	1.02	0.86	NA	NA	5.47	$189.30	ZZZ	C+
35601	Art byp common ipsi carotid	27.09	NA	7.24	6.78	NA	NA	41.11	$1422.66	090	B C+ M
35606	Art byp carotid-subclavian	22.46	NA	6.37	5.51	NA	NA	34.34	$1188.38	090	B C+ M
35612	Art byp subclav-subclavian	20.35	NA	5.20	5.08	NA	NA	30.63	$1059.99	090	B C+ M
35616	Art byp subclav-axillary	21.82	NA	5.00	5.43	NA	NA	32.25	$1116.05	090	B C+ M
35621	Art byp axillary-femoral	21.03	NA	5.94	5.21	NA	NA	32.18	$1113.63	090	B C+ M
35623	Art byp axillary-pop-tibial	25.92	NA	6.10	6.49	NA	NA	38.51	$1332.68	090	B C+ M
35626	Art byp aorsubcl/carot/innom	29.14	NA	10.79	6.95	NA	NA	46.88	$1622.34	090	B C+ M
35631	Art byp aor-celiac-msn-renal	36.03	NA	9.15	8.93	NA	NA	54.11	$1872.54	090	B C+ M
35632	Art byp ilio-celiac	36.13	NA	7.74	9.03	NA	NA	52.90	$1830.67	090	B C+ M
35633	Art byp ilio-mesenteric	39.11	NA	9.22	9.69	NA	NA	58.02	$2007.85	090	B C+ M
35634	Art byp iliorenal	35.33	NA	7.61	8.83	NA	NA	51.77	$1791.56	090	B C+ M
35636	Art byp spenorenal	31.75	NA	7.02	7.94	NA	NA	46.71	$1616.46	090	B C+ M
35637	Art byp aortoiliac	33.05	NA	7.26	8.25	NA	NA	48.56	$1680.48	090	C+ M

*Please note that these calculations are based on the Medicare 2022 Conversion Factor of $34.6062 and the DRA RVU cap rates at time of publication.

A = assistant-at-surgery restriction
A+ = assistant-at-surgery restriction unless medical necessity established with documentation
B = bilateral surgery adjustment applies
C = cosurgeons payable
C+ = cosurgeons payable if medical necessity established with documentation
CP = carriers may establish RVUs and payment amounts for these services, generally on an individual basis following review of documentation such as an operative report
M = multiple surgery adjustment applies
Me = multiple endoscopy rules may apply
M+ = multiple therapy rules apply
Mtc = multiple diagnostic imaging rules apply
T = team surgeons permitted
T+ = team surgeons payable if medical necessity established with documentation
§ = indicates code is not covered by Medicare
GS = procedure must be performed under the general supervision of a physician
DS = procedure must be performed under the direct supervision of a physician
PS = procedure must be performed under the personal supervision of a physician
DRA = procedure subject to DRA limitation

Relative Value Units

CPT Code and Modifier	Description	Work RVU	Nonfacility Practice Expense RVU	Facility Practice Expense RVU	PLI RVU	Total Non-facility RVUs	Medicare Payment Nonfacility	Total Facility RVUs	Medicare Payment Facility	Global Period	Payment Policy Indicators
35638	Art byp aortobi-iliac	33.60	NA	8.93	8.30	NA	NA	50.83	$1759.03	090	C+ M
35642	Art byp carotid-vertebral	18.94	NA	5.28	4.75	NA	NA	28.97	$1002.54	090	B C+ M
35645	Art byp subclav-vertebrl	18.43	NA	4.74	4.60	NA	NA	27.77	$961.01	090	B C+ M
35646	Art byp aortobifemoral	32.98	NA	8.88	8.16	NA	NA	50.02	$1731.00	090	C+ M
35647	Art byp aortofemoral	29.73	NA	8.33	7.35	NA	NA	45.41	$1571.47	090	B C+ M
35650	Art byp axillary-axillary	20.16	NA	4.74	5.04	NA	NA	29.94	$1036.11	090	B C+ M
35654	Art byp axill-fem-femoral	26.28	NA	7.24	6.52	NA	NA	40.04	$1385.63	090	C+ M
35656	Art byp femoral-popliteal	20.47	NA	6.02	5.06	NA	NA	31.55	$1091.83	090	B C+ M
35661	Art byp femoral-femoral	20.35	NA	6.41	5.03	NA	NA	31.79	$1100.13	090	B C+ M
35663	Art byp ilioiliac	23.93	NA	5.79	5.97	NA	NA	35.69	$1235.10	090	B C+ M
35665	Art byp iliofemoral	22.35	NA	6.54	5.45	NA	NA	34.34	$1188.38	090	B C+ M
35666	Art byp fem-ant-post tib/prl	23.66	NA	8.31	5.87	NA	NA	37.84	$1309.50	090	B C+ M
35671	Art byp pop-tibl-prl-other	20.77	NA	7.43	5.17	NA	NA	33.37	$1154.81	090	B C+ M
35681	Composite byp grft pros&vein	1.60	NA	0.34	0.39	NA	NA	2.33	$80.63	ZZZ	C+
35682	Composite byp grft 2 veins	7.19	NA	1.37	1.78	NA	NA	10.34	$357.83	ZZZ	A+ C+
35683	Composite byp grft 3/> segmt	8.49	NA	1.35	2.14	NA	NA	11.98	$414.58	ZZZ	A+ C+
35685	Bypass graft patency/patch	4.04	NA	0.75	1.00	NA	NA	5.79	$200.37	ZZZ	C+
35686	Bypass graft/av fist patency	3.34	NA	0.53	0.85	NA	NA	4.72	$163.34	ZZZ	C+
35691	Art trnsposj vertbrl carotid	18.41	NA	4.74	4.60	NA	NA	27.75	$960.32	090	B C+ M
35693	Art trnsposj subclavian	15.73	NA	4.84	3.93	NA	NA	24.50	$847.85	090	B C+ M
35694	Art trnsposj subclav carotid	19.28	NA	4.87	4.83	NA	NA	28.98	$1002.89	090	B C+ M
35695	Art trnsposj carotid subclav	20.06	NA	5.00	5.01	NA	NA	30.07	$1040.61	090	B C+ M
35697	Reimplant artery each	3.00	NA	0.56	0.73	NA	NA	4.29	$148.46	ZZZ	C
35700	Reoperation bypass graft	3.08	NA	0.60	0.76	NA	NA	4.44	$153.65	ZZZ	C+
35701	Expl n/flwd surg neck art	7.50	NA	4.09	1.29	NA	NA	12.88	$445.73	090	B C+ M
35702	Expl n/flwd surg uxtr art	7.12	NA	3.20	1.66	NA	NA	11.98	$414.58	090	B C+ M
35703	Expl n/flwd surg lxtr art	7.50	NA	3.04	1.78	NA	NA	12.32	$426.35	090	B C+ M
35800	Explore neck vessels	12.00	NA	7.13	2.38	NA	NA	21.51	$744.38	090	C+ M
35820	Explore chest vessels	36.89	NA	13.51	8.64	NA	NA	59.04	$2043.15	090	C+ M
35840	Explore abdominal vessels	20.75	NA	10.07	4.93	NA	NA	35.75	$1237.17	090	C+ M
35860	Explore limb vessels	15.25	NA	5.68	3.74	NA	NA	24.67	$853.73	090	C+ M
35870	Repair vessel graft defect	24.50	NA	5.95	6.12	NA	NA	36.57	$1265.55	090	C+ M
35875	Removal of clot in graft	10.72	NA	4.06	2.66	NA	NA	17.44	$603.53	090	A C+ M

35876		Removal of clot in graft	17.82	NA	5.53	4.34	NA	NA	27.69	$958.25	090	C+ M
35879		Revise graft w/vein	17.41	NA	5.33	4.31	NA	NA	27.05	$936.10	090	B C+ M
35881		Revise graft w/vein	19.35	NA	5.79	4.83	NA	NA	29.97	$1037.15	090	B C+ M
35883		Revise graft w/nonauto graft	23.15	NA	6.33	5.76	NA	NA	35.24	$1219.52	090	B C+ M
35884		Revise graft w/vein	24.65	NA	5.49	6.16	NA	NA	36.30	$1256.21	090	B C+ M
35901		Excision graft neck	8.38	NA	3.51	2.09	NA	NA	13.98	$483.79	090	C+ M
35903		Excision graft extremity	9.53	NA	4.79	2.36	NA	NA	16.68	$577.23	090	C+ M
35905		Excision graft thorax	33.52	NA	7.31	8.40	NA	NA	49.23	$1703.66	090	C+ M
35907		Excision graft abdomen	37.27	NA	9.39	9.23	NA	NA	55.89	$1934.14	090	C+ M
36000	§	Place needle in vein	0.18	0.70	0.07	0.01	0.89	$30.80	0.26	$9.00	XXX	
36002		Pseudoaneurysm injection trt	1.96	2.21	0.78	0.29	4.46	$154.34	3.03	$104.86	000	A B M
36005		Injection ext venography	0.95	6.85	0.30	0.14	7.94	$274.77	1.39	$48.10	000	A+ B M
36010		Place catheter in vein	2.18	14.32	0.61	0.39	16.89	$584.50	3.18	$110.05	XXX	A B M
36011		Place catheter in vein	3.14	21.59	0.92	0.52	25.25	$873.81	4.58	$158.50	XXX	A B M
36012		Place catheter in vein	3.51	21.75	0.98	0.57	25.83	$893.88	5.06	$175.11	XXX	A B M
36013		Place catheter in artery	2.52	21.32	0.77	0.33	24.17	$836.43	3.62	$125.27	XXX	A M
36014		Place catheter in artery	3.02	21.02	0.93	0.45	24.49	$847.51	4.40	$152.27	XXX	A B M
36015		Place catheter in artery	3.51	22.54	1.05	0.40	26.45	$915.33	4.96	$171.65	XXX	A B M
36100		Establish access to artery	3.02	13.03	0.75	0.73	16.78	$580.69	4.50	$155.73	XXX	A B M
36140		Intro ndl icath upr/lxtr art	1.76	13.78	0.50	0.35	15.89	$549.89	2.61	$90.32	XXX	A M
36160		Establish access to aorta	2.52	14.36	0.76	0.34	17.22	$595.92	3.62	$125.27	XXX	A M
36200		Place catheter in aorta	2.77	15.06	0.70	0.60	18.43	$637.79	4.07	$140.85	000	A B M
36215		Place catheter in artery	4.17	27.20	1.46	0.57	31.94	$1105.32	6.20	$214.56	000	A M
36216		Place catheter in artery	5.27	26.59	1.63	0.98	32.84	$1136.47	7.88	$272.70	000	A M
36217		Place catheter in artery	6.29	46.84	1.99	1.26	54.39	$1882.23	9.54	$330.14	000	A M
36218		Place catheter in artery	1.01	4.97	0.31	0.18	6.16	$213.17	1.50	$51.91	ZZZ	A
36221		Place cath thoracic aorta	3.92	25.89	1.09	0.89	30.70	$1062.41	5.90	$204.18	000	A M
36222		Place cath carotid/inom art	5.28	30.52	1.79	1.26	37.06	$1282.51	8.33	$288.27	000	A B M

*Please note that these calculations are based on the Medicare 2022 Conversion Factor of $34.6062 and the DRA RVU cap rates at time of publication.

A = assistant-at-surgery restriction
A+ = assistant-at-surgery restriction unless medical necessity established with documentation
B = bilateral surgery adjustment applies
C = cosurgeons payable
C+ = cosurgeons payable if medical necessity established with documentation
CP = carriers may establish RVUs and payment amounts for these services, generally on an individual basis following review of documentation such as an operative report
M = multiple surgery adjustment applies
Me = multiple endoscopy rules may apply
M+ = multiple therapy rules apply
Mtc = multiple diagnostic imaging rules apply
T = team surgeons permitted
T+ = team surgeons payable if medical necessity established with documentation
§ = indicates code is not covered by Medicare
GS = procedure must be performed under the general supervision of a physician
DS = procedure must be performed under the direct supervision of a physician
PS = procedure must be performed under the personal supervision of a physician
DRA = procedure subject to DRA limitation

Relative Value Units

CPT Code and Modifier		Description	Work RVU	Nonfacility Practice Expense RVU	Facility Practice Expense RVU	PLI RVU	Total Non-facility RVUs	Medicare Payment Nonfacility	Total Facility RVUs	Medicare Payment Facility	Global Period	Payment Policy Indicators
36223		Place cath carotid/inom art	5.75	41.86	2.25	1.44	49.05	$1697.43	9.44	$326.68	000	A B M
36224		Place cath carotd art	6.25	53.61	2.70	1.68	61.54	$2129.67	10.63	$367.86	000	A B M
36225		Place cath subclavian art	5.75	39.34	2.17	1.47	46.56	$1611.26	9.39	$324.95	000	A B M
36226		Place cath vertebral art	6.25	51.43	2.65	1.66	59.34	$2053.53	10.56	$365.44	000	A B M
36227		Place cath xtrnl carotid	2.09	4.40	0.84	0.56	7.05	$243.97	3.49	$120.78	ZZZ	A B
36228		Place cath intracranial art	4.25	32.82	1.71	1.18	38.25	$1323.69	7.14	$247.09	ZZZ	A B
36245		Ins cath abd/l-ext art 1st	4.65	33.01	1.42	0.79	38.45	$1330.61	6.86	$237.40	XXX	A B M
36246		Ins cath abd/l-ext art 2nd	5.02	19.75	1.34	1.01	25.78	$892.15	7.37	$255.05	000	A B M
36247		Ins cath abd/l-ext art 3rd	6.04	37.03	1.63	1.02	44.09	$1525.79	8.69	$300.73	000	A B M
36248		Ins cath abd/l-ext art addl	1.01	2.43	0.28	0.11	3.55	$122.85	1.40	$48.45	ZZZ	A
36251		Ins cath ren art 1st unilat	5.10	33.88	1.49	0.89	39.87	$1379.75	7.48	$258.85	000	A M
36252		Ins cath ren art 1st bilat	6.74	34.76	2.25	1.48	42.98	$1487.37	10.47	$362.33	000	A M
36253		Ins cath ren art 2nd+ unilat	7.30	54.16	2.15	0.85	62.31	$2156.31	10.30	$356.44	000	A M
36254		Ins cath ren art 2nd+ bilat	7.90	52.13	2.50	1.61	61.64	$2133.13	12.01	$415.62	000	A M
36260		Insertion of infusion pump	9.91	NA	7.19	2.50	NA	NA	19.60	$678.28	090	A M
36261		Revision of infusion pump	5.63	NA	5.25	1.41	NA	NA	12.29	$425.31	090	M
36262		Removal of infusion pump	4.11	NA	4.23	1.04	NA	NA	9.38	$324.61	090	A M
36299	CP	Vessel injection procedure	0.00	0.00	0.00	0.00	0.00	$0.00	0.00	$0.00	YYY	A+ C+ M T+
36400		Bl draw < 3 yrs fem/jugular	0.38	0.39	0.14	0.04	0.81	$28.03	0.56	$19.38	XXX	A M
36405		Bl draw <3 yrs scalp vein	0.31	0.37	0.11	0.02	0.70	$24.22	0.44	$15.23	XXX	A M
36406		Bl draw <3 yrs other vein	0.18	0.32	0.07	0.01	0.51	$17.65	0.26	$9.00	XXX	A M
36410		Non-routine bl draw 3/> yrs	0.18	0.32	0.07	0.02	0.52	$18.00	0.27	$9.34	XXX	A M
36420		Vein access cutdown < 1 yr	1.01	NA	0.17	0.21	NA	NA	1.39	$48.10	XXX	A+ M
36425		Vein access cutdown > 1 yr	0.76	NA	0.32	0.10	NA	NA	1.18	$40.84	XXX	A M
36430		Blood transfusion service	0.00	1.11	NA	0.02	1.13	$39.11	NA	NA	XXX	A
36440		Bl push transfuse 2 yr/<	1.03	NA	0.38	0.08	NA	NA	1.49	$51.56	XXX	A+ M
36450		Bl exchange/transfuse nb	3.50	NA	1.30	0.23	NA	NA	5.03	$174.07	XXX	A+ M
36455		Bl exchange/transfuse non-nb	2.43	NA	0.69	0.57	NA	NA	3.69	$127.70	XXX	A M
36456		Prtl exchange transfuse nb	2.00	NA	0.74	0.12	NA	NA	2.86	$98.97	XXX	A+ M
36460		Transfusion service fetal	6.58	NA	2.49	1.07	NA	NA	10.14	$350.91	XXX	M
36465		Njx noncmpnd sclrsnt 1 vein	2.35	37.92	0.68	0.43	40.70	$1408.47	3.46	$119.74	000	A B M
36466		Njx noncmpnd sclrsnt mlt vn	3.00	41.43	0.94	0.56	44.99	$1556.93	4.50	$155.73	000	A B M
36468		Njx sclrsnt spider veins	0.00	0.00	0.00	0.00	0.00	$0.00	0.00	$0.00	000	A+ M

36470	Njx sclrsnt 1 incmptnt vein	0.75	2.55	0.22	0.14	3.44	$119.05	1.11	$38.41	000	A B M
36471	Njx sclrsnt mlt incmptnt vn	1.50	4.20	0.43	0.28	5.98	$206.95	2.21	$76.48	000	A B M
36473	Endovenous mchnchem 1st vein	3.50	33.78	1.07	0.67	37.95	$1313.31	5.24	$181.34	000	A B M
36474	Endovenous mchnchem add-on	1.75	5.76	0.52	0.34	7.85	$271.66	2.61	$90.32	ZZZ	A B
36475	Endovenous rf 1st vein	5.30	26.97	1.72	1.11	33.38	$1155.15	8.13	$281.35	000	A B M
36476	Endovenous rf vein add-on	2.65	5.47	0.72	0.57	8.69	$300.73	3.94	$136.35	ZZZ	A B
36478	Endovenous laser 1st vein	5.30	24.09	1.76	1.05	30.44	$1053.41	8.11	$280.66	000	A B M
36479	Endovenous laser vein addon	2.65	5.91	0.78	0.55	9.11	$315.26	3.98	$137.73	ZZZ	A B
36481	Insertion of catheter vein	6.73	46.31	2.01	0.64	53.68	$1857.66	9.38	$324.61	000	A M
36482	Endoven ther chem adhes 1st	3.50	47.62	1.04	0.72	51.84	$1793.99	5.26	$182.03	000	A B M
36483	Endoven ther chem adhes sbsq	1.75	1.94	0.48	0.39	4.08	$141.19	2.62	$90.67	ZZZ	A B
36500	Insertion of catheter vein	3.51	NA	1.16	0.64	NA	NA	5.31	$183.76	000	A M
36510	Insertion of catheter vein	1.09	1.36	0.40	0.08	2.53	$87.55	1.57	$54.33	000	A+ M
36511	Apheresis wbc	2.00	NA	1.07	0.12	NA	NA	3.19	$110.39	000	A M
36512	Apheresis rbc	2.00	NA	1.00	0.12	NA	NA	3.12	$107.97	000	A M
36513	Apheresis platelets	2.00	NA	0.90	0.21	NA	NA	3.11	$107.63	000	A M
36514	Apheresis plasma	1.81	15.21	0.79	0.14	17.16	$593.84	2.74	$94.82	000	A M
36516	Apheresis immunoads slctv	1.56	52.81	0.65	0.28	54.65	$1891.23	2.49	$86.17	000	A M
36522	Photopheresis	1.75	39.97	0.97	0.11	41.83	$1447.58	2.83	$97.94	000	A M
36555	Insert non-tunnel cv cath	1.93	3.64	0.38	0.17	5.74	$198.64	2.48	$85.82	000	A
36556	Insert non-tunnel cv cath	1.75	4.53	0.50	0.22	6.50	$224.94	2.47	$85.48	000	A
36557	Insert tunneled cv cath	4.89	30.20	3.40	1.24	36.33	$1257.24	9.53	$329.80	010	A+ B M
36558	Insert tunneled cv cath	4.59	20.62	2.39	0.61	25.82	$893.53	7.59	$262.66	010	A+ B M
36560	Insert tunneled cv cath	6.04	31.10	3.83	1.52	38.66	$1337.88	11.39	$394.16	010	A+ B M
36561	Insert tunneled cv cath	5.79	23.91	3.07	0.95	30.65	$1060.68	9.81	$339.49	010	A+ B M
36563	Insert tunneled cv cath	5.99	27.50	3.41	1.40	34.89	$1207.41	10.80	$373.75	010	A+ M
36565	Insert tunneled cv cath	5.79	18.47	2.86	1.27	25.53	$883.50	9.92	$343.29	010	A+ B M
36566	Insert tunneled cv cath	6.29	126.19	3.09	1.20	133.68	$4626.16	10.58	$366.13	010	A+ B M

*Please note that these calculations are based on the Medicare 2022 Conversion Factor of $34.6062 and the DRA RVU cap rates at time of publication.

A = assistant-at-surgery restriction
A+ = assistant-at-surgery restriction unless medical necessity established with documentation
B = bilateral surgery adjustment applies
C = cosurgeons payable
C+ = cosurgeons payable if medical necessity established with documentation
CP = carriers may establish RVUs and payment amounts for these services, generally on an individual basis following review of documentation such as an operative report
M = multiple surgery adjustment applies
Me = multiple endoscopy rules may apply
M+ = multiple therapy rules apply
Mtc = multiple diagnostic imaging rules apply
T = team surgeons permitted
T+ = team surgeons payable if medical necessity established with documentation
§ = indicates code is not covered by Medicare
GS = procedure must be performed under the general supervision of a physician
DS = procedure must be performed under the direct supervision of a physician
PS = procedure must be performed under the personal supervision of a physician
DRA = procedure subject to DRA limitation

Relative Value Units

CPT Code and Modifier	Description	Work RVU	Nonfacility Practice Expense RVU	Facility Practice Expense RVU	PLI RVU	Total Non-facility RVUs	Medicare Payment Nonfacility	Total Facility RVUs	Medicare Payment Facility	Global Period	Payment Policy Indicators
36568	Insj picc <5 yr w/o imaging	2.11	NA	0.35	0.21	NA	NA	2.67	$92.40	000	A
36569	Insj picc 5 yr+ w/o imaging	1.90	NA	0.60	0.24	NA	NA	2.74	$94.82	000	A
36570	Insert picvad cath	5.11	39.39	3.48	1.29	45.79	$1584.62	9.88	$341.91	010	A+ B M
36571	Insert picvad cath	5.09	33.75	3.16	1.01	39.85	$1379.06	9.26	$320.45	010	A+ B M
36572	Insj picc rs&i <5 yr	1.82	9.46	0.33	0.20	11.48	$397.28	2.35	$81.32	000	A
36573	Insj picc rs&i 5 yr+	1.70	9.96	0.56	0.20	11.86	$410.43	2.46	$85.13	000	A
36575	Repair tunneled cv cath	0.67	3.80	0.24	0.08	4.55	$157.46	0.99	$34.26	000	A+ M
36576	Repair tunneled cv cath	2.99	7.06	1.88	0.57	10.62	$367.52	5.44	$188.26	010	A+ M
36578	Replace tunneled cv cath	3.29	9.52	2.08	0.61	13.42	$464.42	5.98	$206.95	010	A+ M
36580	Replace cvad cath	1.31	4.34	0.44	0.17	5.82	$201.41	1.92	$66.44	000	A
36581	Replace tunneled cv cath	3.23	20.65	1.73	0.40	24.28	$840.24	5.36	$185.49	010	A+ M
36582	Replace tunneled cv cath	4.99	21.61	2.62	0.86	27.46	$950.29	8.47	$293.11	010	A+ M
36583	Replace tunneled cv cath	5.04	29.71	3.46	1.28	36.03	$1246.86	9.78	$338.45	010	A+ M
36584	Compl rplcmt picc rs&i	1.20	8.86	0.40	0.11	10.17	$351.95	1.71	$59.18	000	A
36585	Replace picvad cath	4.59	30.87	2.94	0.79	36.25	$1254.47	8.32	$287.92	010	A+ M
36589	Removal tunneled cv cath	2.28	2.34	1.42	0.33	4.95	$171.30	4.03	$139.46	010	A+ M
36590	Removal tunneled cv cath	3.10	3.06	1.96	0.55	6.71	$232.21	5.61	$194.14	010	A+ M
36591	Draw blood off venous device	0.00	0.78	NA	0.01	0.79	$27.34	NA	NA	XXX	A+
36592	Collect blood from picc	0.00	0.87	NA	0.01	0.88	$30.45	NA	NA	XXX	A+
36593	Declot vascular device	0.00	0.95	NA	0.02	0.97	$33.57	NA	NA	XXX	A+
36595	Mech remov tunneled cv cath	3.59	14.39	1.30	0.40	18.38	$636.06	5.29	$183.07	000	A M
36596	Mech remov tunneled cv cath	0.75	2.56	0.44	0.10	3.41	$118.01	1.29	$44.64	000	A M
36597	Reposition venous catheter	1.21	1.99	0.41	0.12	3.32	$114.89	1.74	$60.21	000	A M
36598	Inj w/fluor eval cv device	0.74	2.87	0.24	0.08	3.69	$127.70	1.06	$36.68	000	A+ B M
36600	Withdrawal of arterial blood	0.32	0.49	0.10	0.04	0.85	$29.42	0.46	$15.92	XXX	A M
36620	Insertion catheter artery	1.00	NA	0.20	0.09	NA	NA	1.29	$44.64	000	A
36625	Insertion catheter artery	2.11	NA	0.65	0.34	NA	NA	3.10	$107.28	000	A
36640	Insertion catheter artery	2.10	NA	1.14	0.14	NA	NA	3.38	$116.97	000	A M
36660	Insertion catheter artery	1.40	NA	0.52	0.09	NA	NA	2.01	$69.56	000	A+ M
36680	Insert needle bone cavity	1.20	NA	0.32	0.22	NA	NA	1.74	$60.21	000	A+ M
36800	Insertion of cannula	2.43	NA	0.85	0.29	NA	NA	3.57	$123.54	000	A M
36810	Insertion of cannula	3.96	NA	1.79	0.43	NA	NA	6.18	$213.87	000	A M
36815	Insertion of cannula	2.62	NA	0.69	0.65	NA	NA	3.96	$137.04	000	A M

36818	Av fuse uppr arm cephalic	12.39	NA	4.83	3.04	NA	NA	20.26	$701.12	090	C+ M
36819	Av fuse uppr arm basilic	13.29	NA	4.90	3.29	NA	NA	21.48	$743.34	090	C+ M
36820	Av fusion/forearm vein	13.07	NA	4.88	3.18	NA	NA	21.13	$731.23	090	B C+ M
36821	Av fusion direct any site	11.90	NA	4.63	2.94	NA	NA	19.47	$673.78	090	C+ M
36823	Insertion of cannula(s)	22.98	NA	13.05	5.81	NA	NA	41.84	$1447.92	090	A M
36825	Artery-vein autograft	14.17	NA	5.64	3.53	NA	NA	23.34	$807.71	090	C+ M
36830	Artery-vein nonautograft	12.03	NA	4.60	2.97	NA	NA	19.60	$678.28	090	C+ M
36831	Open thrombect av fistula	11.00	NA	4.37	2.71	NA	NA	18.08	$625.68	090	C+ M
36832	Av fistula revision open	13.50	NA	5.39	3.33	NA	NA	22.22	$768.95	090	C+ M
36833	Av fistula revision	14.50	NA	5.66	3.60	NA	NA	23.76	$822.24	090	C+ M
36835	Artery to vein shunt	7.51	NA	5.01	1.78	NA	NA	14.30	$494.87	090	A M
36838	Dist revas ligation hemo	21.69	NA	6.45	5.39	NA	NA	33.53	$1160.35	090	B C+ M
36860	External cannula declotting	2.01	4.50	0.75	0.51	7.02	$242.94	3.27	$113.16	000	A M
36861	Cannula declotting	2.52	NA	0.94	0.64	NA	NA	4.10	$141.89	000	A M
36901	Intro cath dialysis circuit	3.36	17.91	1.05	0.50	21.77	$753.38	4.91	$169.92	000	A M
36902	Intro cath dialysis circuit	4.83	31.90	1.47	0.68	37.41	$1294.62	6.98	$241.55	000	A M
36903	Intro cath dialysis circuit	6.39	127.30	1.82	0.99	134.68	$4660.76	9.20	$318.38	000	A M
36904	Thrmbc/nfs dialysis circuit	7.50	47.32	2.15	1.04	55.86	$1933.10	10.69	$369.94	000	A C+ M
36905	Thrmbc/nfs dialysis circuit	9.00	60.63	2.72	1.20	70.83	$2451.16	12.92	$447.11	000	A C+ M
36906	Thrmbc/nfs dialysis circuit	10.42	158.47	3.01	1.42	170.31	$5893.78	14.85	$513.90	000	A C+ M
36907	Balo angiop ctr dialysis seg	3.00	14.83	0.83	0.42	18.25	$631.56	4.25	$147.08	ZZZ	A
36908	Stent plmt ctr dialysis seg	4.25	39.30	1.11	0.67	44.22	$1530.29	6.03	$208.68	ZZZ	A
36909	Dialysis circuit embolj	4.12	55.62	1.11	0.64	60.38	$2089.52	5.87	$203.14	ZZZ	A
37140	Revision of circulation	40.00	NA	18.99	10.12	NA	NA	69.11	$2391.63	090	A C+ M
37145	Revision of circulation	37.00	NA	17.76	9.36	NA	NA	64.12	$2218.95	090	M
37160	Revision of circulation	38.00	NA	18.24	9.60	NA	NA	65.84	$2278.47	090	C+ M
37180	Revision of circulation	36.50	NA	17.53	9.23	NA	NA	63.26	$2189.19	090	C+ M
37181	Splice spleen/kidney veins	40.00	NA	18.99	10.12	NA	NA	69.11	$2391.63	090	C+ M

*Please note that these calculations are based on the Medicare 2022 Conversion Factor of $34.6062 and the DRA RVU cap rates at time of publication.

A = assistant-at-surgery restriction
A+ = assistant-at-surgery restriction unless medical necessity established with documentation
B = bilateral surgery adjustment applies
C = cosurgeons payable
C+ = cosurgeons payable if medical necessity established with documentation
CP = carriers may establish RVUs and payment amounts for these services, generally on an individual basis following review of documentation such as an operative report
M = multiple surgery adjustment applies
Me = multiple endoscopy rules may apply
M+ = multiple therapy rules apply
Mtc = multiple diagnostic imaging rules apply
T = team surgeons permitted
T+ = team surgeons payable if medical necessity established with documentation
§ = indicates code is not covered by Medicare
GS = procedure must be performed under the general supervision of a physician
DS = procedure must be performed under the direct supervision of a physician
PS = procedure must be performed under the personal supervision of a physician
DRA = procedure subject to DRA limitation

Relative Value Units

CPT Code and Modifier		Description	Work RVU	Nonfacility Practice Expense RVU	Facility Practice Expense RVU	PLI RVU	Total Non-facility RVUs	Medicare Payment Nonfacility	Total Facility RVUs	Medicare Payment Facility	Global Period	Payment Policy Indicators
37182		Insert hepatic shunt (tips)	16.97	NA	5.07	1.54	NA	NA	23.58	$816.01	000	A+ M
37183		Remove hepatic shunt (tips)	7.74	174.69	2.35	0.72	183.15	$6338.13	10.81	$374.09	000	A+ M
37184		Prim art m-thrmbc 1st vsl	8.41	43.25	2.51	1.64	53.30	$1844.51	12.56	$434.65	000	A B C M
37185		Prim art m-thrmbc sbsq vsl	3.28	10.62	0.80	0.66	14.56	$503.87	4.74	$164.03	ZZZ	A C
37186		Sec art thrombectomy add-on	4.92	31.08	1.21	0.98	36.98	$1279.74	7.11	$246.05	ZZZ	A C
37187		Venous mech thrombectomy	7.78	44.42	2.45	1.20	53.40	$1847.97	11.43	$395.55	000	A B C M
37188		Ven mechnl thrmbc repeat tx	5.46	39.29	1.76	0.87	45.62	$1578.73	8.09	$279.96	000	A B C
37191		Ins endovas vena cava filtr	4.46	58.48	1.36	0.61	63.55	$2199.22	6.43	$222.52	000	A M
37192		Redo endovas vena cava filtr	7.10	30.64	1.21	1.78	39.52	$1367.64	10.09	$349.18	000	A M
37193		Rem endovas vena cava filter	7.10	38.17	1.99	0.99	46.26	$1600.88	10.08	$348.83	000	A M
37195	CP	Thrombolytic therapy stroke	0.00	0.00	0.00	0.00	0.00	$0.00	0.00	$0.00	XXX	A+
37197		Remove intrvas foreign body	6.04	41.40	1.73	0.95	48.39	$1674.59	8.72	$301.77	000	A M
37200		Transcatheter biopsy	4.55	NA	1.25	0.41	NA	NA	6.21	$214.90	000	A M
37211		Thrombolytic art therapy	7.75	NA	2.10	1.40	NA	NA	11.25	$389.32	000	A B M
37212		Thrombolytic venous therapy	6.81	NA	1.89	1.11	NA	NA	9.81	$339.49	000	A B M
37213		Thromblytic art/ven therapy	4.75	NA	1.22	0.78	NA	NA	6.75	$233.59	000	A M
37214		Cessj therapy cath removal	2.49	NA	0.64	0.41	NA	NA	3.54	$122.51	000	A M
37215		Transcath stent cca w/eps	17.75	NA	6.97	4.43	NA	NA	29.15	$1008.77	090	A+ B M
37216	§	Transcath stent cca w/o eps	17.98	NA	9.14	1.48	NA	NA	28.60	$989.74	090	
37217		Stent placemt retro carotid	20.38	NA	6.32	4.97	NA	NA	31.67	$1095.98	090	A+ B M
37218		Stent placemt ante carotid	14.75	NA	5.85	3.35	NA	NA	23.95	$828.82	090	A+ B M
37220		Iliac revasc	7.90	68.59	2.02	1.78	78.27	$2708.63	11.70	$404.89	000	A B M
37221		Iliac revasc w/stent	9.75	84.63	2.47	2.20	96.58	$3342.27	14.42	$499.02	000	A+ B M
37222		Iliac revasc add-on	3.73	14.34	0.85	0.85	18.92	$654.75	5.43	$187.91	ZZZ	A+ B
37223		Iliac revasc w/stent add-on	4.25	34.68	0.98	0.98	39.91	$1381.13	6.21	$214.90	ZZZ	A+ B
37224		Fem/popl revas w/tla	8.75	80.87	2.27	1.95	91.57	$3168.89	12.97	$448.84	000	A+ B M
37225		Fem/popl revas w/ather	11.75	261.72	3.21	2.56	276.03	$9552.35	17.52	$606.30	000	A+ B M
37226		Fem/popl revasc w/stent	10.24	244.93	2.60	2.33	257.50	$8911.10	15.17	$524.98	000	A+ B M
37227		Fem/popl revasc stnt & ather	14.25	336.35	3.65	3.09	353.69	$12239.87	20.99	$726.38	000	A+ B M
37228		Tib/per revasc w/tla	10.75	117.11	2.69	2.36	130.22	$4506.42	15.80	$546.78	000	A+ B M
37229		Tib/per revasc w/ather	13.80	262.74	3.66	2.85	279.39	$9668.63	20.31	$702.85	000	A+ B M
37230		Tib/per revasc w/stent	13.55	264.62	3.78	3.00	281.17	$9730.23	20.33	$703.54	000	A+ B M
37231		Tib/per revasc stent & ather	14.75	349.39	4.00	2.73	366.87	$12695.98	21.48	$743.34	000	A+ B M

37232		Tib/per revasc add-on	4.00	20.61	1.01	0.79	25.40	$879.00	5.80	$200.72	ZZZ	A+ B
37233		Tibper revasc w/ather add-on	6.50	24.00	1.62	1.33	31.83	$1101.52	9.45	$327.03	ZZZ	A+ B
37234		Revsc opn/prq tib/pero stent	5.50	106.58	1.56	1.20	113.28	$3920.19	8.26	$285.85	ZZZ	A+ B
37235		Tib/per revasc stnt & ather	7.80	112.18	2.12	1.26	121.24	$4195.66	11.18	$386.90	ZZZ	A+ B
37236		Open/perq place stent 1st	8.75	75.20	2.28	1.87	85.82	$2969.90	12.90	$446.42	000	A+ B M
37237		Open/perq place stent ea add	4.25	34.98	0.97	0.95	40.18	$1390.48	6.17	$213.52	ZZZ	A+ B
37238		Open/perq place stent same	6.04	100.31	1.71	1.18	107.53	$3721.20	8.93	$309.03	000	A+ B M
37239		Open/perq place stent ea add	2.97	49.57	0.82	0.61	53.15	$1839.32	4.40	$152.27	ZZZ	A+ B
37241		Vasc embolize/occlude venous	8.75	136.01	2.47	1.29	146.05	$5054.24	12.51	$432.92	000	A M
37242		Vasc embolize/occlude artery	9.80	212.05	2.55	1.44	223.29	$7727.22	13.79	$477.22	000	A M
37243		Vasc embolize/occlude organ	11.74	256.53	3.33	1.09	269.36	$9321.53	16.16	$559.24	000	A M
37244		Vasc embolize/occlude bleed	13.75	190.53	4.05	1.33	205.61	$7115.38	19.13	$662.02	000	A M
37246		Trluml balo angiop 1st art	7.00	48.61	1.89	1.24	56.85	$1967.36	10.13	$350.56	000	A B M
37247		Trluml balo angiop addl art	3.50	12.64	0.73	0.73	16.87	$583.81	4.96	$171.65	ZZZ	A B
37248		Trluml balo angiop 1st vein	6.00	35.48	1.79	0.86	42.34	$1465.23	8.65	$299.34	000	A B M
37249		Trluml balo angiop addl vein	2.97	10.13	0.76	0.50	13.60	$470.64	4.23	$146.38	ZZZ	A B
37252		Intrvasc us noncoronary 1st	1.80	27.51	0.45	0.34	29.65	$1026.07	2.59	$89.63	ZZZ	A+ C+
37253		Intrvasc us noncoronary addl	1.44	3.38	0.36	0.25	5.07	$175.45	2.05	$70.94	ZZZ	A+ C+
37500		Endoscopy ligate perf veins	11.67	NA	3.94	2.92	NA	NA	18.53	$641.25	090	A B C+ M
37501	CP	Vascular endoscopy procedure	0.00	0.00	0.00	0.00	0.00	$0.00	0.00	$0.00	YYY	A B C+ M T+
37565		Ligation of neck vein	12.05	NA	6.98	2.50	NA	NA	21.53	$745.07	090	A+ B C+ M
37600		Ligation of neck artery	12.42	NA	7.13	2.18	NA	NA	21.73	$751.99	090	C+ M
37605		Ligation of neck artery	14.28	NA	3.81	3.56	NA	NA	21.65	$749.22	090	C+ M
37606		Ligation of neck artery	8.81	NA	9.49	3.38	NA	NA	21.68	$750.26	090	M
37607		Ligation of a-v fistula	6.25	NA	3.29	1.48	NA	NA	11.02	$381.36	090	A C+ M
37609		Temporal artery procedure	3.05	5.74	2.36	0.64	9.43	$326.34	6.05	$209.37	010	A B M
37615		Ligation of neck artery	7.80	NA	6.17	1.96	NA	NA	15.93	$551.28	090	C+ M
37616		Ligation of chest artery	18.97	NA	9.10	4.45	NA	NA	32.52	$1125.39	090	C+ M

*Please note that these calculations are based on the Medicare 2022 Conversion Factor of $34.6062 and the DRA RVU cap rates at time of publication.

A = assistant-at-surgery restriction

A+ = assistant-at-surgery restriction unless medical necessity established with documentation

B = bilateral surgery adjustment applies

C = cosurgeons payable

C+ = cosurgeons payable if medical necessity established with documentation

CP = carriers may establish RVUs and payment amounts for these services, generally on an individual basis following review of documentation such as an operative report

M = multiple surgery adjustment applies

Me = multiple endoscopy rules may apply

M+ = multiple therapy rules apply

Mtc = multiple diagnostic imaging rules apply

T = team surgeons permitted

T+ = team surgeons payable if medical necessity established with documentation

§ = indicates code is not covered by Medicare

GS = procedure must be performed under the general supervision of a physician

DS = procedure must be performed under the direct supervision of a physician

PS = procedure must be performed under the personal supervision of a physician

DRA = procedure subject to DRA limitation

Relative Value Units

CPT Code and Modifier		Description	Work RVU	Nonfacility Practice Expense RVU	Facility Practice Expense RVU	PLI RVU	Total Non-facility RVUs	Medicare Payment Nonfacility	Total Facility RVUs	Medicare Payment Facility	Global Period	Payment Policy Indicators
37617		Ligation of abdomen artery	23.79	NA	9.68	5.39	NA	NA	38.86	$1344.80	090	C+ M
37618		Ligation of extremity artery	6.03	NA	4.10	1.41	NA	NA	11.54	$399.36	090	C+ M
37619		Ligation of inf vena cava	30.00	NA	13.84	7.57	NA	NA	51.41	$1779.10	090	M
37650		Revision of major vein	8.49	NA	2.89	2.14	NA	NA	13.52	$467.88	090	A B C+ M
37660		Revision of major vein	22.28	NA	11.27	5.61	NA	NA	39.16	$1355.18	090	B C+ M
37700		Revise leg vein	3.82	NA	2.47	0.95	NA	NA	7.24	$250.55	090	A B M
37718		Ligate/strip short leg vein	7.13	NA	2.65	1.78	NA	NA	11.56	$400.05	090	A B C+ M
37722		Ligate/strip long leg vein	8.16	NA	3.62	2.01	NA	NA	13.79	$477.22	090	A B C+ M
37735		Removal of leg veins/lesion	10.90	NA	3.49	2.71	NA	NA	17.10	$591.77	090	A B C+ M
37760		Ligate leg veins radical	10.78	NA	3.47	2.69	NA	NA	16.94	$586.23	090	A B C+ M
37761		Ligate leg veins open	9.13	NA	4.46	2.20	NA	NA	15.79	$546.43	090	B C+ M
37765		Stab phleb veins xtr 10-20	4.80	7.04	2.12	1.05	12.89	$446.07	7.97	$275.81	010	A B C+ M
37766		Phleb veins - extrem 20+	6.00	7.69	2.44	1.32	15.01	$519.44	9.76	$337.76	010	A B C+ M
37780		Revision of leg vein	3.93	NA	2.02	0.98	NA	NA	6.93	$239.82	090	A B C+ M
37785		Ligate/divide/excise vein	3.93	5.77	2.69	0.95	10.65	$368.56	7.57	$261.97	090	A B M
37788		Revascularization penis	23.33	NA	10.77	2.78	NA	NA	36.88	$1276.28	090	C+ M
37790		Penile venous occlusion	8.43	NA	4.77	1.00	NA	NA	14.20	$491.41	090	A+ M
37799	CP	Vascular surgery procedure	0.00	0.00	0.00	0.00	0.00	$0.00	0.00	$0.00	YYY	A+ C+ M T+
38100		Removal of spleen total	19.55	NA	10.05	4.65	NA	NA	34.25	$1185.26	090	C+ M
38101		Removal of spleen partial	19.55	NA	10.25	4.94	NA	NA	34.74	$1202.22	090	C+ M
38102		Removal of spleen total	4.79	NA	1.86	1.07	NA	NA	7.72	$267.16	ZZZ	C+
38115		Repair of ruptured spleen	21.88	NA	11.12	5.53	NA	NA	38.53	$1333.38	090	C+ M
38120		Laparoscopy splenectomy	17.07	NA	10.22	4.22	NA	NA	31.51	$1090.44	090	C+ M
38129	CP	Laparoscope proc spleen	0.00	0.00	0.00	0.00	0.00	$0.00	0.00	$0.00	YYY	C+ M T+
38200		Injection for spleen x-ray	2.64	NA	0.96	0.22	NA	NA	3.82	$132.20	000	A+ M
38204	§	Bl donor search management	2.00	NA	0.77	0.18	NA	NA	2.95	$102.09	XXX	
38205		Harvest allogeneic stem cell	1.50	NA	0.91	0.10	NA	NA	2.51	$86.86	000	A+ M
38206		Harvest auto stem cells	1.50	NA	0.88	0.10	NA	NA	2.48	$85.82	000	A+ M
38207	§	Cryopreserve stem cells	0.89	NA	0.34	0.08	NA	NA	1.31	$45.33	XXX	
38208	§	Thaw preserved stem cells	0.56	NA	0.22	0.05	NA	NA	0.83	$28.72	XXX	
38209	§	Wash harvest stem cells	0.24	NA	0.09	0.02	NA	NA	0.35	$12.11	XXX	
38210	§	T-cell depletion of harvest	1.57	NA	0.61	0.12	NA	NA	2.30	$79.59	XXX	
38211	§	Tumor cell deplete of harvst	1.42	NA	0.55	0.11	NA	NA	2.08	$71.98	XXX	

38212	§	Rbc depletion of harvest	0.94	NA	0.36	0.09	NA	NA	1.39	$48.10	XXX	
38213	§	Platelet deplete of harvest	0.24	NA	0.09	0.02	NA	NA	0.35	$12.11	XXX	
38214	§	Volume deplete of harvest	0.81	NA	0.31	0.08	NA	NA	1.20	$41.53	XXX	
38215	§	Harvest stem cell concentrte	0.94	NA	0.36	0.09	NA	NA	1.39	$48.10	XXX	
38220		Dx bone marrow aspirations	1.20	3.35	0.70	0.09	4.64	$160.57	1.99	$68.87	XXX	A+ B M
38221		Dx bone marrow biopsies	1.28	3.46	0.70	0.09	4.83	$167.15	2.07	$71.63	XXX	A+ B M
38222		Dx bone marrow bx & aspir	1.44	3.68	0.68	0.11	5.23	$180.99	2.23	$77.17	XXX	A+ B M
38230		Bone marrow harvest allogen	3.50	NA	1.77	0.73	NA	NA	6.00	$207.64	000	A+ M
38232		Bone marrow harvest autolog	3.50	NA	1.71	0.60	NA	NA	5.81	$201.06	000	A+ M
38240		Transplt allo hct/donor	4.00	NA	2.84	0.27	NA	NA	7.11	$246.05	XXX	A+ M
38241		Transplt autol hct/donor	3.00	NA	2.03	0.21	NA	NA	5.24	$181.34	XXX	A+ M
38242		Transplt allo lymphocytes	2.11	NA	1.47	0.12	NA	NA	3.70	$128.04	000	A+ M
38243		Transplj hematopoietic boost	2.13	NA	1.35	0.12	NA	NA	3.60	$124.58	000	A+ M
38300		Drainage lymph node lesion	2.36	7.35	3.30	0.60	10.31	$356.79	6.26	$216.63	010	A M
38305		Drainage lymph node lesion	6.68	NA	6.41	1.68	NA	NA	14.77	$511.13	090	A M
38308		Incision of lymph channels	6.81	NA	5.41	1.57	NA	NA	13.79	$477.22	090	C+ M
38380		Thoracic duct procedure	8.46	NA	7.02	1.40	NA	NA	16.88	$584.15	090	C+ M
38381		Thoracic duct procedure	13.38	NA	7.11	3.17	NA	NA	23.66	$818.78	090	C+ M
38382		Thoracic duct procedure	10.65	NA	7.11	2.51	NA	NA	20.27	$701.47	090	C+ M
38500		Biopsy/removal lymph nodes	3.79	5.45	2.93	0.89	10.13	$350.56	7.61	$263.35	010	A B M
38505		Needle biopsy lymph nodes	1.59	3.60	0.77	0.14	5.33	$184.45	2.50	$86.52	000	A B M
38510		Biopsy/removal lymph nodes	6.74	7.80	4.39	1.29	15.83	$547.82	12.42	$429.81	010	A B M
38520		Biopsy/removal lymph nodes	7.03	NA	5.36	1.47	NA	NA	13.86	$479.64	090	A B M
38525		Biopsy/removal lymph nodes	6.43	NA	5.13	1.59	NA	NA	13.15	$455.07	090	A B M
38530		Biopsy/removal lymph nodes	8.34	NA	6.63	1.72	NA	NA	16.69	$577.58	090	B C+ M
38531		Open bx/exc inguinofem nodes	6.74	NA	5.00	1.55	NA	NA	13.29	$459.92	090	A+ B M
38542		Explore deep node(s) neck	7.95	NA	6.19	1.37	NA	NA	15.51	$536.74	090	B C+ M
38550		Removal neck/armpit lesion	7.11	NA	6.74	1.80	NA	NA	15.65	$541.59	090	A+ M

*Please note that these calculations are based on the Medicare 2022 Conversion Factor of $34.6062 and the DRA RVU cap rates at time of publication.

A = assistant-at-surgery restriction

A+ = assistant-at-surgery restriction unless medical necessity established with documentation

B = bilateral surgery adjustment applies

C = cosurgeons payable

C+ = cosurgeons payable if medical necessity established with documentation

CP = carriers may establish RVUs and payment amounts for these services, generally on an individual basis following review of documentation such as an operative report

M = multiple surgery adjustment applies

Me = multiple endoscopy rules may apply

M+ = multiple therapy rules apply

Mtc = multiple diagnostic imaging rules apply

T = team surgeons permitted

T+ = team surgeons payable if medical necessity established with documentation

§ = indicates code is not covered by Medicare

GS = procedure must be performed under the general supervision of a physician

DS = procedure must be performed under the direct supervision of a physician

PS = procedure must be performed under the personal supervision of a physician

DRA = procedure subject to DRA limitation

Relative Value Units

CPT Code and Modifier		Description	Work RVU	Nonfacility Practice Expense RVU	Facility Practice Expense RVU	PLI RVU	Total Non-facility RVUs	Medicare Payment Nonfacility	Total Facility RVUs	Medicare Payment Facility	Global Period	Payment Policy Indicators
38555		Removal neck/armpit lesion	15.59	NA	11.14	3.94	NA	NA	30.67	$1061.37	090	C+ M
38562		Removal pelvic lymph nodes	11.06	NA	7.91	1.94	NA	NA	20.91	$723.62	090	C+ M
38564		Removal abdomen lymph nodes	11.38	NA	7.10	2.50	NA	NA	20.98	$726.04	090	C+ M
38570		Laparoscopy lymph node biop	8.49	NA	5.28	1.47	NA	NA	15.24	$527.40	010	C Me
38571		Laparoscopy lymphadenectomy	12.00	NA	5.89	1.53	NA	NA	19.42	$672.05	010	C Me
38572		Laparoscopy lymphadenectomy	15.60	NA	8.72	2.46	NA	NA	26.78	$926.75	010	C Me
38573		Laps pelvic lymphadec	20.00	NA	11.30	3.31	NA	NA	34.61	$1197.72	010	C Me
38589	CP	Laparoscope proc lymphatic	0.00	0.00	0.00	0.00	0.00	$0.00	0.00	$0.00	YYY	B C+ M T+
38700		Removal of lymph nodes neck	12.81	NA	9.15	1.94	NA	NA	23.90	$827.09	090	B C+ M
38720		Removal of lymph nodes neck	21.95	NA	14.06	3.67	NA	NA	39.68	$1373.17	090	B C+ M
38724		Removal of lymph nodes neck	23.95	NA	15.30	3.63	NA	NA	42.88	$1483.91	090	B C+ M
38740		Remove armpit lymph nodes	10.70	NA	7.59	2.62	NA	NA	20.91	$723.62	090	B C+ M
38745		Remove armpit lymph nodes	13.87	NA	9.00	3.41	NA	NA	26.28	$909.45	090	B C+ M
38746		Remove thoracic lymph nodes	4.12	NA	1.20	0.98	NA	NA	6.30	$218.02	ZZZ	C+
38747		Remove abdominal lymph nodes	4.88	NA	1.84	1.17	NA	NA	7.89	$273.04	ZZZ	C+
38760		Remove groin lymph nodes	13.62	NA	8.35	2.85	NA	NA	24.82	$858.93	090	B C+ M
38765		Remove groin lymph nodes	21.91	NA	12.46	4.45	NA	NA	38.82	$1343.41	090	B C+ M
38770		Remove pelvis lymph nodes	14.06	NA	7.53	2.07	NA	NA	23.66	$818.78	090	B C+ M
38780		Remove abdomen lymph nodes	17.70	NA	9.95	3.03	NA	NA	30.68	$1061.72	090	C+ M
38790		Inject for lymphatic x-ray	1.29	NA	0.89	0.20	NA	NA	2.38	$82.36	000	A B M
38792		Ra tracer id of sentinl node	0.65	1.72	0.23	0.09	2.46	$85.13	0.97	$33.57	000	A B M
38794		Access thoracic lymph duct	4.62	NA	3.58	0.39	NA	NA	8.59	$297.27	090	A+ M
38900		Io map of sent lymph node	2.50	0.98	0.98	0.60	4.08	$141.19	4.08	$141.19	ZZZ	B C+
38999	CP	Blood/lymph system procedure	0.00	0.00	0.00	0.00	0.00	$0.00	0.00	$0.00	YYY	A+ C+ M T+
39000		Exploration of chest	7.57	NA	5.56	1.64	NA	NA	14.77	$511.13	090	C+ M
39010		Exploration of chest	13.19	NA	6.98	3.06	NA	NA	23.23	$803.90	090	C+ M
39200		Resect mediastinal cyst	15.09	NA	6.94	3.58	NA	NA	25.61	$886.26	090	C+ M
39220		Resect mediastinal tumor	19.55	NA	9.54	4.28	NA	NA	33.37	$1154.81	090	C+ M
39401		Mediastinoscpy w/medstnl bx	5.44	NA	2.32	1.29	NA	NA	9.05	$313.19	000	A M
39402		Mediastinoscpy w/lmph nod bx	7.25	NA	2.87	1.70	NA	NA	11.82	$409.05	000	A M
39499	CP	Chest procedure	0.00	0.00	0.00	0.00	0.00	$0.00	0.00	$0.00	YYY	C+ M T+
39501		Repair diaphragm laceration	13.98	NA	8.10	3.29	NA	NA	25.37	$877.96	090	C+ M
39503		Repair of diaphragm hernia	108.91	NA	36.01	25.82	NA	NA	170.74	$5908.66	090	C+ M

39540		Repair of diaphragm hernia	14.57	NA	7.57	3.49	NA	NA	25.63	$886.96	090	C+ M
39541		Repair of diaphragm hernia	15.75	NA	8.38	3.79	NA	NA	27.92	$966.21	090	C+ M
39545		Revision of diaphragm	14.67	NA	8.34	3.46	NA	NA	26.47	$916.03	090	C+ M
39560		Resect diaphragm simple	13.06	NA	7.80	2.85	NA	NA	23.71	$820.51	090	C+ M
39561		Resect diaphragm complex	19.99	NA	12.21	4.66	NA	NA	36.86	$1275.58	090	C+ M
39599	CP	Diaphragm surgery procedure	0.00	0.00	0.00	0.00	0.00	$0.00	0.00	$0.00	YYY	C+ M T+
40490		Biopsy of lip	1.22	2.32	0.68	0.11	3.65	$126.31	2.01	$69.56	000	A M
40500		Partial excision of lip	4.47	10.61	5.80	0.60	15.68	$542.63	10.87	$376.17	090	A M
40510		Partial excision of lip	4.82	9.20	4.85	0.65	14.67	$507.67	10.32	$357.14	090	A M
40520		Partial excision of lip	4.79	9.56	5.05	0.70	15.05	$520.82	10.54	$364.75	090	A M
40525		Reconstruct lip with flap	7.72	NA	7.43	1.18	NA	NA	16.33	$565.12	090	A M
40527		Reconstruct lip with flap	9.32	NA	7.92	1.33	NA	NA	18.57	$642.64	090	A+ M
40530		Partial removal of lip	5.54	10.33	5.64	0.86	16.73	$578.96	12.04	$416.66	090	A M
40650		Repair lip	3.78	9.90	4.74	0.73	14.41	$498.68	9.25	$320.11	090	A+ M
40652		Repair lip	4.43	10.25	5.41	0.76	15.44	$534.32	10.60	$366.83	090	A+ M
40654		Repair lip	5.48	11.09	6.24	0.83	17.40	$602.15	12.55	$434.31	090	A M
40700		Repair cleft lip/nasal	14.17	NA	13.00	2.61	NA	NA	29.78	$1030.57	090	A+ M
40701		Repair cleft lip/nasal	17.23	NA	14.78	3.16	NA	NA	35.17	$1217.10	090	M
40702		Repair cleft lip/nasal	14.27	NA	12.64	2.62	NA	NA	29.53	$1021.92	090	M
40720		Repair cleft lip/nasal	14.72	NA	12.90	2.69	NA	NA	30.31	$1048.91	090	A+ B M
40761		Repair cleft lip/nasal	15.84	NA	13.14	2.91	NA	NA	31.89	$1103.59	090	A M
40799	CP	Lip surgery procedure	0.00	0.00	0.00	0.00	0.00	$0.00	0.00	$0.00	YYY	C+ M T+
40800		Drainage of mouth lesion	1.23	4.76	2.15	0.12	6.11	$211.44	3.50	$121.12	010	A M
40801		Drainage of mouth lesion	2.63	5.75	2.91	0.25	8.63	$298.65	5.79	$200.37	010	A M
40804		Removal foreign body mouth	1.30	4.17	1.86	0.14	5.61	$194.14	3.30	$114.20	010	A+ M
40805		Removal foreign body mouth	2.79	5.44	2.76	0.25	8.48	$293.46	5.80	$200.72	010	A+ M
40806		Incision of lip fold	0.31	2.63	0.48	0.04	2.98	$103.13	0.83	$28.72	000	A+ M
40808		Biopsy of mouth lesion	1.05	3.89	1.40	0.11	5.05	$174.76	2.56	$88.59	010	A M

*Please note that these calculations are based on the Medicare 2022 Conversion Factor of $34.6062 and the DRA RVU cap rates at time of publication.

A = assistant-at-surgery restriction

A+ = assistant-at-surgery restriction unless medical necessity established with documentation

B = bilateral surgery adjustment applies

C = cosurgeons payable

C+ = cosurgeons payable if medical necessity established with documentation

CP = carriers may establish RVUs and payment amounts for these services, generally on an individual basis following review of documentation such as an operative report

M = multiple surgery adjustment applies

Me = multiple endoscopy rules may apply

M+ = multiple therapy rules apply

Mtc = multiple diagnostic imaging rules apply

T = team surgeons permitted

T+ = team surgeons payable if medical necessity established with documentation

§ = indicates code is not covered by Medicare

GS = procedure must be performed under the general supervision of a physician

DS = procedure must be performed under the direct supervision of a physician

PS = procedure must be performed under the personal supervision of a physician

DRA = procedure subject to DRA limitation

Relative Value Units

CPT Code and Modifier		Description	Work RVU	Nonfacility Practice Expense RVU	Facility Practice Expense RVU	PLI RVU	Total Non-facility RVUs	Medicare Payment Nonfacility	Total Facility RVUs	Medicare Payment Facility	Global Period	Payment Policy Indicators
40810		Excision of mouth lesion	1.36	4.97	2.08	0.17	6.50	$224.94	3.61	$124.93	010	A M
40812		Excise/repair mouth lesion	2.37	5.94	2.85	0.25	8.56	$296.23	5.47	$189.30	010	A M
40814		Excise/repair mouth lesion	3.52	7.26	4.48	0.37	11.15	$385.86	8.37	$289.65	090	A M
40816		Excision of mouth lesion	3.77	7.77	4.73	0.42	11.96	$413.89	8.92	$308.69	090	A M
40818		Excise oral mucosa for graft	2.83	7.84	4.74	0.31	10.98	$379.98	7.88	$272.70	090	A+ M
40819		Excise lip or cheek fold	2.51	5.30	3.11	0.22	8.03	$277.89	5.84	$202.10	090	A+ M
40820		Treatment of mouth lesion	1.34	6.44	3.54	0.12	7.90	$273.39	5.00	$173.03	010	A M
40830		Repair mouth laceration	1.82	4.99	2.32	0.25	7.06	$244.32	4.39	$151.92	010	A+ M
40831		Repair mouth laceration	2.57	6.42	3.25	0.33	9.32	$322.53	6.15	$212.83	010	A+ M
40840		Reconstruction of mouth	9.15	15.33	8.23	1.37	25.85	$894.57	18.75	$648.87	090	M
40842		Reconstruction of mouth	9.15	16.96	9.22	1.68	27.79	$961.71	20.05	$693.85	090	A+ M
40843		Reconstruction of mouth	12.79	20.66	10.65	2.33	35.78	$1238.21	25.77	$891.80	090	M
40844		Reconstruction of mouth	16.80	24.93	14.94	3.06	44.79	$1550.01	34.80	$1204.30	090	M
40845		Reconstruction of mouth	19.36	22.19	13.73	2.71	44.26	$1531.67	35.80	$1238.90	090	A+ M
40899	CP	Mouth surgery procedure	0.00	0.00	0.00	0.00	0.00	$0.00	0.00	$0.00	YYY	A+ C+ M T+
41000		Drainage of mouth lesion	1.35	3.01	1.62	0.17	4.53	$156.77	3.14	$108.66	010	A M
41005		Drainage of mouth lesion	1.31	5.03	1.78	0.11	6.45	$223.21	3.20	$110.74	010	A+ M
41006		Drainage of mouth lesion	3.34	7.13	3.38	0.34	10.81	$374.09	7.06	$244.32	090	A+ M
41007		Drainage of mouth lesion	3.20	6.31	2.97	0.27	9.78	$338.45	6.44	$222.86	090	A+ M
41008		Drainage of mouth lesion	3.46	7.77	3.65	0.40	11.63	$402.47	7.51	$259.89	090	A+ M
41009		Drainage of mouth lesion	3.71	8.48	4.21	0.39	12.58	$435.35	8.31	$287.58	090	A+ M
41010		Incision of tongue fold	1.11	5.31	1.98	0.17	6.59	$228.05	3.26	$112.82	010	A+ M
41015		Drainage of mouth lesion	4.08	7.45	4.35	0.35	11.88	$411.12	8.78	$303.84	090	A+ M
41016		Drainage of mouth lesion	4.19	9.48	5.64	0.43	14.10	$487.95	10.26	$355.06	090	A+ M
41017		Drainage of mouth lesion	4.19	9.29	5.49	0.42	13.90	$481.03	10.10	$349.52	090	A+ M
41018		Drainage of mouth lesion	5.22	9.79	5.97	0.56	15.57	$538.82	11.75	$406.62	090	A+ M
41019		Place needles h&n for rt	8.84	NA	4.71	0.65	NA	NA	14.20	$491.41	000	A+ C+ M T+
41100		Biopsy of tongue	1.42	4.02	1.56	0.19	5.63	$194.83	3.17	$109.70	010	A M
41105		Biopsy of tongue	1.47	3.96	1.58	0.19	5.62	$194.49	3.24	$112.12	010	A M
41108		Biopsy of floor of mouth	1.10	3.79	1.42	0.14	5.03	$174.07	2.66	$92.05	010	A M
41110		Excision of tongue lesion	1.56	5.14	2.07	0.21	6.91	$239.13	3.84	$132.89	010	A M
41112		Excision of tongue lesion	2.83	6.97	4.01	0.34	10.14	$350.91	7.18	$248.47	090	A M
41113		Excision of tongue lesion	3.29	7.23	4.17	0.39	10.91	$377.55	7.85	$271.66	090	A M

41114		Excision of tongue lesion	8.82	NA	8.18	1.12	NA	NA	18.12	$627.06	090	A+ M
41115		Excision of tongue fold	1.79	5.86	2.29	0.25	7.90	$273.39	4.33	$149.84	010	A+ M
41116		Excision of mouth lesion	2.52	7.21	3.52	0.32	10.05	$347.79	6.36	$220.10	090	A M
41120		Partial removal of tongue	11.14	NA	19.04	1.60	NA	NA	31.78	$1099.79	090	C+ M
41130		Partial removal of tongue	15.74	NA	21.10	2.26	NA	NA	39.10	$1353.10	090	C+ M
41135		Tongue and neck surgery	30.14	NA	29.74	4.25	NA	NA	64.13	$2219.30	090	C+ M
41140		Removal of tongue	29.15	NA	31.55	4.14	NA	NA	64.84	$2243.87	090	C+ M
41145		Tongue removal neck surgery	37.93	NA	38.40	5.39	NA	NA	81.72	$2828.02	090	C+ M
41150		Tongue mouth jaw surgery	29.86	NA	31.08	4.26	NA	NA	65.20	$2256.32	090	C+ M
41153		Tongue mouth neck surgery	33.59	NA	32.56	4.77	NA	NA	70.92	$2454.27	090	C+ M
41155		Tongue jaw & neck surgery	44.30	NA	38.19	6.17	NA	NA	88.66	$3068.19	090	C+ M
41250		Repair tongue laceration	1.96	6.20	2.19	0.37	8.53	$295.19	4.52	$156.42	010	A+ M
41251		Repair tongue laceration	2.32	6.57	2.53	0.50	9.39	$324.95	5.35	$185.14	010	A+ M
41252		Repair tongue laceration	3.02	6.34	2.64	0.50	9.86	$341.22	6.16	$213.17	010	A+ M
41510		Tongue to lip surgery	3.51	NA	9.62	0.50	NA	NA	13.63	$471.68	090	A+ M
41512		Tongue suspension	6.86	NA	12.15	0.98	NA	NA	19.99	$691.78	090	A+ M
41520		Reconstruction tongue fold	2.83	7.75	4.19	0.40	10.98	$379.98	7.42	$256.78	090	A+ M
41530		Tongue base vol reduction	3.50	24.36	7.41	0.50	28.36	$981.43	11.41	$394.86	000	A+ M
41599	CP	Tongue and mouth surgery	0.00	0.00	0.00	0.00	0.00	$0.00	0.00	$0.00	YYY	A+ C+ M T+
41800		Drainage of gum lesion	1.27	7.30	3.07	0.20	8.77	$303.50	4.54	$157.11	010	A M
41805		Removal foreign body gum	1.34	7.98	4.44	0.12	9.44	$326.68	5.90	$204.18	010	A+ M
41806		Removal foreign body jawbone	2.79	9.37	5.28	0.25	12.41	$429.46	8.32	$287.92	010	A+ M
41820		Excision gum each quadrant	0.00	0.00	0.00	0.00	0.00	$0.00	0.00	$0.00	000	A+ M
41821		Excision of gum flap	0.00	0.00	0.00	0.00	0.00	$0.00	0.00	$0.00	000	A+ M
41822		Excision of gum lesion	2.41	7.77	3.08	0.42	10.60	$366.83	5.91	$204.52	010	A+ M
41823		Excision of gum lesion	3.77	11.34	6.31	0.68	15.79	$546.43	10.76	$372.36	090	A+ M
41825		Excision of gum lesion	1.41	5.04	1.97	0.14	6.59	$228.05	3.52	$121.81	010	A M
41826		Excision of gum lesion	2.41	6.48	3.21	0.24	9.13	$315.95	5.86	$202.79	010	A M

*Please note that these calculations are based on the Medicare 2022 Conversion Factor of $34.6062 and the DRA RVU cap rates at time of publication.

A = assistant-at-surgery restriction
A+ = assistant-at-surgery restriction unless medical necessity established with documentation
B = bilateral surgery adjustment applies
C = cosurgeons payable
C+ = cosurgeons payable if medical necessity established with documentation
CP = carriers may establish RVUs and payment amounts for these services, generally on an individual basis following review of documentation such as an operative report
M = multiple surgery adjustment applies
Me = multiple endoscopy rules may apply
M+ = multiple therapy rules apply
Mtc = multiple diagnostic imaging rules apply
T = team surgeons permitted
T+ = team surgeons payable if medical necessity established with documentation
§ = indicates code is not covered by Medicare
GS = procedure must be performed under the general supervision of a physician
DS = procedure must be performed under the direct supervision of a physician
PS = procedure must be performed under the personal supervision of a physician
DRA = procedure subject to DRA limitation

Relative Value Units

CPT Code and Modifier		Description	Work RVU	Nonfacility Practice Expense RVU	Facility Practice Expense RVU	PLI RVU	Total Non-facility RVUs	Medicare Payment Nonfacility	Total Facility RVUs	Medicare Payment Facility	Global Period	Payment Policy Indicators
41827		Excision of gum lesion	3.83	8.78	4.26	0.40	13.01	$450.23	8.49	$293.81	090	A M
41828		Excision of gum lesion	3.14	6.82	2.85	0.57	10.53	$364.40	6.56	$227.02	010	A+ M
41830		Removal of gum tissue	3.45	9.97	5.25	0.62	14.04	$485.87	9.32	$322.53	010	A+ M
41850		Treatment of gum lesion	0.00	0.00	0.00	0.00	0.00	$0.00	0.00	$0.00	000	A+ M
41870		Gum graft	0.00	0.00	0.00	0.00	0.00	$0.00	0.00	$0.00	000	A+ M
41872		Repair gum	3.01	10.47	5.35	0.56	14.04	$485.87	8.92	$308.69	090	A+ M
41874		Repair tooth socket	3.19	8.05	3.67	0.32	11.56	$400.05	7.18	$248.47	090	A+ M
41899	CP	Dental surgery procedure	0.00	0.00	0.00	0.00	0.00	$0.00	0.00	$0.00	YYY	A+ C+ M T+
42000		Drainage mouth roof lesion	1.28	3.36	1.71	0.19	4.83	$167.15	3.18	$110.05	010	A+ M
42100		Biopsy roof of mouth	1.36	2.86	1.69	0.18	4.40	$152.27	3.23	$111.78	010	A M
42104		Excision lesion mouth roof	1.69	4.58	2.06	0.22	6.49	$224.59	3.97	$137.39	010	A M
42106		Excision lesion mouth roof	2.15	5.34	2.44	0.24	7.73	$267.51	4.83	$167.15	010	A M
42107		Excision lesion mouth roof	4.56	8.63	4.70	0.55	13.74	$475.49	9.81	$339.49	090	A M
42120		Remove palate/lesion	11.86	NA	16.46	1.70	NA	NA	30.02	$1038.88	090	C+ M
42140		Excision of uvula	1.70	7.45	2.81	0.24	9.39	$324.95	4.75	$164.38	090	A M
42145		Repair palate pharynx/uvula	9.78	NA	9.25	1.39	NA	NA	20.42	$706.66	090	A M
42160		Treatment mouth roof lesion	1.85	4.90	2.13	0.24	6.99	$241.90	4.22	$146.04	010	A+ M
42180		Repair palate	2.55	4.77	2.61	0.35	7.67	$265.43	5.51	$190.68	010	A+ M
42182		Repair palate	3.87	5.49	3.21	0.56	9.92	$343.29	7.64	$264.39	010	A+ M
42200		Reconstruct cleft palate	12.53	NA	12.68	2.29	NA	NA	27.50	$951.67	090	M
42205		Reconstruct cleft palate	13.66	NA	12.46	2.50	NA	NA	28.62	$990.43	090	M
42210		Reconstruct cleft palate	15.03	NA	14.17	2.76	NA	NA	31.96	$1106.01	090	M
42215		Reconstruct cleft palate	8.99	NA	10.22	1.64	NA	NA	20.85	$721.54	090	M
42220		Reconstruct cleft palate	7.16	NA	8.71	1.30	NA	NA	17.17	$594.19	090	M
42225		Reconstruct cleft palate	9.77	NA	17.85	1.78	NA	NA	29.40	$1017.42	090	M
42226		Lengthening of palate	10.35	NA	15.20	1.47	NA	NA	27.02	$935.06	090	M
42227		Lengthening of palate	9.90	NA	13.88	1.40	NA	NA	25.18	$871.38	090	M
42235		Repair palate	8.01	NA	13.02	1.12	NA	NA	22.15	$766.53	090	M
42260		Repair nose to lip fistula	10.22	13.99	8.15	1.44	25.65	$887.65	19.81	$685.55	090	M
42280		Preparation palate mold	1.59	3.58	1.48	0.14	5.31	$183.76	3.21	$111.09	010	A+ M
42281		Insertion palate prosthesis	1.98	4.57	2.57	0.20	6.75	$233.59	4.75	$164.38	010	A+ M
42299	CP	Palate/uvula surgery	0.00	0.00	0.00	0.00	0.00	$0.00	0.00	$0.00	YYY	C+ M T+
42300		Drainage of salivary gland	1.98	4.20	2.34	0.27	6.45	$223.21	4.59	$158.84	010	A M

42305		Drainage of salivary gland	6.31	NA	5.42	0.89	NA	NA	12.62	$436.73	090	A+ M
42310		Drainage of salivary gland	1.61	3.35	2.19	0.17	5.13	$177.53	3.97	$137.39	010	A+ M
42320		Drainage of salivary gland	2.40	5.11	2.54	0.34	7.85	$271.66	5.28	$182.72	010	A+ M
42330		Removal of salivary stone	2.26	4.40	2.31	0.31	6.97	$241.21	4.88	$168.88	010	A M
42335		Removal of salivary stone	3.41	9.13	3.85	0.45	12.99	$449.53	7.71	$266.81	090	A M
42340		Removal of salivary stone	4.72	10.62	4.78	0.66	16.00	$553.70	10.16	$351.60	090	A+ B M
42400		Biopsy of salivary gland	0.78	2.08	0.68	0.09	2.95	$102.09	1.55	$53.64	000	A M
42405		Biopsy of salivary gland	3.34	5.26	2.91	0.44	9.04	$312.84	6.69	$231.52	010	A M
42408		Excision of salivary cyst	4.66	11.26	5.17	0.43	16.35	$565.81	10.26	$355.06	090	A+ M
42409		Drainage of salivary cyst	2.91	8.60	3.49	0.40	11.91	$412.16	6.80	$235.32	090	M
42410		Excise parotid gland/lesion	9.57	NA	7.60	1.49	NA	NA	18.66	$645.75	090	B C+ M
42415		Excise parotid gland/lesion	17.16	NA	11.64	2.50	NA	NA	31.30	$1083.17	090	B C+ M
42420		Excise parotid gland/lesion	19.53	NA	12.70	2.85	NA	NA	35.08	$1213.99	090	B C+ M
42425		Excise parotid gland/lesion	13.42	NA	9.44	1.95	NA	NA	24.81	$858.58	090	B C+ M
42426		Excise parotid gland/lesion	22.66	NA	13.84	3.41	NA	NA	39.91	$1381.13	090	B C+ M
42440		Excise submaxillary gland	6.14	NA	5.27	0.89	NA	NA	12.30	$425.66	090	B C+ M
42450		Excise sublingual gland	4.74	8.71	5.41	0.67	14.12	$488.64	10.82	$374.44	090	A+ M
42500		Repair salivary duct	4.42	8.43	5.24	0.60	13.45	$465.45	10.26	$355.06	090	A+ M
42505		Repair salivary duct	6.32	9.95	6.42	0.89	17.16	$593.84	13.63	$471.68	090	A M
42507		Parotid duct diversion	6.25	NA	7.59	0.89	NA	NA	14.73	$509.75	090	M
42509		Parotid duct diversion	11.76	NA	10.91	1.66	NA	NA	24.33	$841.97	090	A+ M
42510		Parotid duct diversion	8.35	NA	8.55	1.18	NA	NA	18.08	$625.68	090	C+ M
42550		Injection for salivary x-ray	1.25	3.42	0.45	0.10	4.77	$165.07	1.80	$62.29	000	A M
42600		Closure of salivary fistula	4.94	10.74	4.88	0.70	16.38	$566.85	10.52	$364.06	090	A+ M
42650		Dilation of salivary duct	0.77	1.35	0.83	0.11	2.23	$77.17	1.71	$59.18	000	A M
42660		Dilation of salivary duct	1.13	2.06	1.17	0.28	3.47	$120.08	2.58	$89.28	000	A+ M
42665		Ligation of salivary duct	2.63	8.33	3.36	0.37	11.33	$392.09	6.36	$220.10	090	A+ M
42699	CP	Salivary surgery procedure	0.00	0.00	0.00	0.00	0.00	$0.00	0.00	$0.00	YYY	C+ M T+

*Please note that these calculations are based on the Medicare 2022 Conversion Factor of $34.6062 and the DRA RVU cap rates at time of publication.

A = assistant-at-surgery restriction
A+ = assistant-at-surgery restriction unless medical necessity established with documentation
B = bilateral surgery adjustment applies
C = cosurgeons payable
C+ = cosurgeons payable if medical necessity established with documentation
CP = carriers may establish RVUs and payment amounts for these services, generally on an individual basis following review of documentation such as an operative report
M = multiple surgery adjustment applies
Me = multiple endoscopy rules may apply
M+ = multiple therapy rules apply
Mtc = multiple diagnostic imaging rules apply
T = team surgeons permitted
T+ = team surgeons payable if medical necessity established with documentation
§ = indicates code is not covered by Medicare
GS = procedure must be performed under the general supervision of a physician
DS = procedure must be performed under the direct supervision of a physician
PS = procedure must be performed under the personal supervision of a physician
DRA = procedure subject to DRA limitation

Relative Value Units

CPT Code and Modifier	Description	Work RVU	Nonfacility Practice Expense RVU	Facility Practice Expense RVU	PLI RVU	Total Non-facility RVUs	Medicare Payment Nonfacility	Total Facility RVUs	Medicare Payment Facility	Global Period	Payment Policy Indicators
42700	Drainage of tonsil abscess	1.67	3.84	2.08	0.25	5.76	$199.33	4.00	$138.42	010	A M
42720	Drainage of throat abscess	6.31	6.16	4.22	0.89	13.36	$462.34	11.42	$395.20	010	A+ M
42725	Drainage of throat abscess	12.41	NA	9.42	1.81	NA	NA	23.64	$818.09	090	C+ M
42800	Biopsy of throat	1.44	3.09	1.78	0.20	4.73	$163.69	3.42	$118.35	010	A M
42804	Biopsy of upper nose/throat	1.29	4.99	2.14	0.20	6.48	$224.25	3.63	$125.62	010	A M
42806	Biopsy of upper nose/throat	1.63	5.34	2.30	0.23	7.20	$249.16	4.16	$143.96	010	A M
42808	Excise pharynx lesion	2.35	4.23	2.21	0.33	6.91	$239.13	4.89	$169.22	010	A M
42809	Remove pharynx foreign body	1.86	3.93	1.59	0.29	6.08	$210.41	3.74	$129.43	010	A M
42810	Excision of neck cyst	3.38	7.78	4.49	0.47	11.63	$402.47	8.34	$288.62	090	B M
42815	Excision of neck cyst	7.31	NA	7.68	1.06	NA	NA	16.05	$555.43	090	B C+ M
42820	Remove tonsils and adenoids	4.22	NA	3.79	0.60	NA	NA	8.61	$297.96	090	A+ M
42821	Remove tonsils and adenoids	4.36	NA	4.02	0.61	NA	NA	8.99	$311.11	090	A+ M
42825	Removal of tonsils	3.51	NA	3.93	0.50	NA	NA	7.94	$274.77	090	A+ M
42826	Removal of tonsils	3.45	NA	3.61	0.50	NA	NA	7.56	$261.62	090	A M
42830	Removal of adenoids	2.65	NA	3.24	0.39	NA	NA	6.28	$217.33	090	A+ M
42831	Removal of adenoids	2.81	NA	3.61	0.40	NA	NA	6.82	$236.01	090	A+ M
42835	Removal of adenoids	2.38	NA	3.12	0.34	NA	NA	5.84	$202.10	090	A+ M
42836	Removal of adenoids	3.26	NA	3.52	0.44	NA	NA	7.22	$249.86	090	A+ M
42842	Extensive surgery of throat	12.23	NA	16.13	1.80	NA	NA	30.16	$1043.72	090	A+ M
42844	Extensive surgery of throat	17.78	NA	20.68	2.45	NA	NA	40.91	$1415.74	090	C+ M
42845	Extensive surgery of throat	32.56	NA	28.32	4.62	NA	NA	65.50	$2266.71	090	C+ M
42860	Excision of tonsil tags	2.30	NA	3.08	0.33	NA	NA	5.71	$197.60	090	A+ M
42870	Excision of lingual tonsil	5.52	NA	11.38	0.78	NA	NA	17.68	$611.84	090	A+ M
42890	Partial removal of pharynx	19.13	NA	20.30	2.79	NA	NA	42.22	$1461.07	090	C+ M
42892	Revision of pharyngeal walls	26.03	NA	25.84	3.79	NA	NA	55.66	$1926.18	090	C+ M
42894	Revision of pharyngeal walls	33.92	NA	31.48	4.83	NA	NA	70.23	$2430.39	090	C+ M
42900	Repair throat wound	5.29	NA	3.76	0.75	NA	NA	9.80	$339.14	010	A+ M
42950	Reconstruction of throat	8.27	NA	14.42	1.20	NA	NA	23.89	$826.74	090	C+ M
42953	Repair throat esophagus	9.45	NA	17.75	1.41	NA	NA	28.61	$990.08	090	M
42955	Surgical opening of throat	8.01	NA	13.57	1.12	NA	NA	22.70	$785.56	090	M
42960	Control throat bleeding	2.38	NA	2.07	0.33	NA	NA	4.78	$165.42	010	A+ M
42961	Control throat bleeding	5.77	NA	5.83	0.83	NA	NA	12.43	$430.16	090	M
42962	Control throat bleeding	7.40	NA	6.83	1.04	NA	NA	15.27	$528.44	090	A M

42970		Control nose/throat bleeding	5.82	NA	5.55	0.84	NA	NA	12.21	$422.54	090	A M
42971		Control nose/throat bleeding	6.60	NA	5.90	0.95	NA	NA	13.45	$465.45	090	M
42972		Control nose/throat bleeding	7.59	NA	6.36	1.07	NA	NA	15.02	$519.79	090	M
42975		Dise eval slp do brth flx dx	1.90	NA	1.17	0.25	NA	NA	3.32	$114.89	000	A Me
42999	CP	Throat surgery procedure	0.00	0.00	0.00	0.00	0.00	$0.00	0.00	$0.00	YYY	A+ C+ M T+
43020		Incision of esophagus	8.23	NA	6.62	2.07	NA	NA	16.92	$585.54	090	C+ M
43030		Throat muscle surgery	7.99	NA	6.31	1.20	NA	NA	15.50	$536.40	090	C+ M
43045		Incision of esophagus	21.88	NA	11.39	5.19	NA	NA	38.46	$1330.95	090	C+ M
43100		Excision of esophagus lesion	9.66	NA	7.78	1.38	NA	NA	18.82	$651.29	090	C+ M
43101		Excision of esophagus lesion	17.07	NA	8.59	4.06	NA	NA	29.72	$1028.50	090	C+ M
43107		Removal of esophagus	52.05	NA	23.13	12.42	NA	NA	87.60	$3031.50	090	C+ M
43108		Removal of esophagus	82.87	NA	28.01	19.65	NA	NA	130.53	$4517.15	090	C+ M
43112		Esphg tot w/thrcm	62.00	NA	25.22	14.87	NA	NA	102.09	$3532.95	090	C M
43113		Removal of esophagus	80.06	NA	28.51	18.98	NA	NA	127.55	$4414.02	090	C M
43116		Partial removal of esophagus	92.99	NA	30.89	22.06	NA	NA	145.94	$5050.43	090	C+ M
43117		Partial removal of esophagus	57.50	NA	24.47	13.79	NA	NA	95.76	$3313.89	090	C M
43118		Partial removal of esophagus	67.07	NA	23.50	15.91	NA	NA	106.48	$3684.87	090	C M
43121		Partial removal of esophagus	51.43	NA	20.33	12.19	NA	NA	83.95	$2905.19	090	C M
43122		Partial removal of esophagus	44.18	NA	20.72	10.60	NA	NA	75.50	$2612.77	090	C+ M
43123		Partial removal of esophagus	83.12	NA	29.39	19.72	NA	NA	132.23	$4575.98	090	C+ M
43124		Removal of esophagus	69.09	NA	26.35	16.38	NA	NA	111.82	$3869.67	090	C+ M
43130		Removal of esophagus pouch	12.53	NA	8.78	2.22	NA	NA	23.53	$814.28	090	C+ M
43135		Removal of esophagus pouch	26.17	NA	10.89	6.21	NA	NA	43.27	$1497.41	090	C+ M
43180		Esophagoscopy rigid trnso	9.03	NA	5.81	1.33	NA	NA	16.17	$559.58	090	A M
43191		Esophagoscopy rigid trnso dx	2.49	NA	1.69	0.37	NA	NA	4.55	$157.46	000	A M
43192		Esophagoscp rig trnso inject	2.79	NA	1.79	0.40	NA	NA	4.98	$172.34	000	A Me
43193		Esophagoscp rig trnso biopsy	2.79	NA	1.78	0.40	NA	NA	4.97	$171.99	000	A Me
43194		Esophagoscp rig trnso rem fb	3.51	NA	1.60	0.57	NA	NA	5.68	$196.56	000	A Me

*Please note that these calculations are based on the Medicare 2022 Conversion Factor of $34.6062 and the DRA RVU cap rates at time of publication.

A = assistant-at-surgery restriction
A+ = assistant-at-surgery restriction unless medical necessity established with documentation
B = bilateral surgery adjustment applies
C = cosurgeons payable
C+ = cosurgeons payable if medical necessity established with documentation
CP = carriers may establish RVUs and payment amounts for these services, generally on an individual basis following review of documentation such as an operative report
M = multiple surgery adjustment applies
Me = multiple endoscopy rules may apply
M+ = multiple therapy rules apply
Mtc = multiple diagnostic imaging rules apply
T = team surgeons permitted
T+ = team surgeons payable if medical necessity established with documentation
§ = indicates code is not covered by Medicare
GS = procedure must be performed under the general supervision of a physician
DS = procedure must be performed under the direct supervision of a physician
PS = procedure must be performed under the personal supervision of a physician
DRA = procedure subject to DRA limitation

Relative Value Units

CPT Code and Modifier	Description	Work RVU	Nonfacility Practice Expense RVU	Facility Practice Expense RVU	PLI RVU	Total Non-facility RVUs	Medicare Payment Nonfacility	Total Facility RVUs	Medicare Payment Facility	Global Period	Payment Policy Indicators
43195	Esophagoscopy rigid balloon	3.07	NA	1.91	0.43	NA	NA	5.41	$187.22	000	A Me
43196	Esophagoscp guide wire dilat	3.31	NA	2.00	0.42	NA	NA	5.73	$198.29	000	A Me
43197	Esophagoscopy flex dx brush	1.52	4.04	0.67	0.24	5.80	$200.72	2.43	$84.09	000	A M
43198	Esophagosc flex trnsn biopsy	1.82	4.33	0.82	0.25	6.40	$221.48	2.89	$100.01	000	A Me
43200	Esophagoscopy flexible brush	1.42	6.43	0.94	0.21	8.06	$278.93	2.57	$88.94	000	A M
43201	Esoph scope w/submucous inj	1.72	5.98	1.06	0.25	7.95	$275.12	3.03	$104.86	000	A Me
43202	Esophagoscopy flex biopsy	1.72	9.12	1.07	0.23	11.07	$383.09	3.02	$104.51	000	A Me
43204	Esoph scope w/sclerosis inj	2.33	NA	1.36	0.25	NA	NA	3.94	$136.35	000	A Me
43205	Esophagus endoscopy/ligation	2.44	NA	1.41	0.25	NA	NA	4.10	$141.89	000	A Me
43206	Esoph optical endomicroscopy	2.29	6.70	1.35	0.25	9.24	$319.76	3.89	$134.62	000	A Me
43210	Egd esophagogastrc fndoplsty	7.75	NA	3.60	1.33	NA	NA	12.68	$438.81	000	A Me
43211	Esophagoscop mucosal resect	4.20	NA	2.20	0.45	NA	NA	6.85	$237.05	000	A Me
43212	Esophagoscop stent placement	3.40	NA	1.58	0.57	NA	NA	5.55	$192.06	000	A Me
43213	Esophagoscopy retro balloon	4.63	33.29	2.26	0.72	38.64	$1337.18	7.61	$263.35	000	A Me
43214	Esophagosc dilate balloon 30	3.40	NA	1.81	0.44	NA	NA	5.65	$195.53	000	A Me
43215	Esophagoscopy flex remove fb	2.44	9.33	1.34	0.37	12.14	$420.12	4.15	$143.62	000	A Me
43216	Esophagoscopy lesion removal	2.30	10.15	1.35	0.25	12.70	$439.50	3.90	$134.96	000	A Me
43217	Esophagoscopy snare les remv	2.80	9.85	1.57	0.31	12.96	$448.50	4.68	$161.96	000	A Me
43220	Esophagoscopy balloon <30mm	2.00	26.03	1.20	0.25	28.28	$978.66	3.45	$119.39	000	A Me
43226	Esoph endoscopy dilation	2.24	9.29	1.25	0.33	11.86	$410.43	3.82	$132.20	000	A Me
43227	Esophagoscopy control bleed	2.89	15.26	1.59	0.34	18.49	$639.87	4.82	$166.80	000	A Me
43229	Esophagoscopy lesion ablate	3.49	18.25	1.85	0.41	22.15	$766.53	5.75	$198.99	000	A Me
43231	Esophagoscop ultrasound exam	2.80	NA	1.55	0.29	NA	NA	4.64	$160.57	000	A C Me
43232	Esophagoscopy w/us needle bx	3.59	NA	1.85	0.39	NA	NA	5.83	$201.75	000	A C Me
43233	Egd balloon dil esoph30 mm/>	4.07	NA	2.06	0.60	NA	NA	6.73	$232.90	000	A Me
43235	Egd diagnostic brush wash	2.09	6.75	1.25	0.25	9.09	$314.57	3.59	$124.24	000	A M
43236	Uppr gi scope w/submuc inj	2.39	9.76	1.38	0.25	12.40	$429.12	4.02	$139.12	000	A Me
43237	Endoscopic us exam esoph	3.47	NA	1.87	0.39	NA	NA	5.73	$198.29	000	A Me
43238	Egd us fine needle bx/aspir	4.16	NA	2.18	0.44	NA	NA	6.78	$234.63	000	A Me
43239	Egd biopsy single/multiple	2.39	8.97	1.38	0.27	11.63	$402.47	4.04	$139.81	000	A Me
43240	Egd w/transmural drain cyst	7.15	NA	3.51	0.79	NA	NA	11.45	$396.24	000	A Me
43241	Egd tube/cath insertion	2.49	NA	1.37	0.31	NA	NA	4.17	$144.31	000	A Me
43242	Egd us fine needle bx/aspir	4.73	NA	2.44	0.52	NA	NA	7.69	$266.12	000	A Me

43243	Egd injection varices	4.27	NA	2.16	0.50	NA	NA	6.93	$239.82	000	A Me
43244	Egd varices ligation	4.40	NA	2.29	0.47	NA	NA	7.16	$247.78	000	A Me
43245	Egd dilate stricture	3.08	15.01	1.65	0.41	18.50	$640.21	5.14	$177.88	000	A Me
43246	Egd place gastrostomy tube	3.56	NA	1.79	0.52	NA	NA	5.87	$203.14	000	A+ C Me
43247	Egd remove foreign body	3.11	8.25	1.68	0.39	11.75	$406.62	5.18	$179.26	000	A Me
43248	Egd guide wire insertion	2.91	9.47	1.61	0.33	12.71	$439.84	4.85	$167.84	000	A Me
43249	Esoph egd dilation <30 mm	2.67	31.12	1.50	0.32	34.11	$1180.42	4.49	$155.38	000	A Me
43250	Egd cautery tumor polyp	2.97	10.58	1.59	0.42	13.97	$483.45	4.98	$172.34	000	A Me
43251	Egd remove lesion snare	3.47	11.44	1.86	0.40	15.31	$529.82	5.73	$198.29	000	A Me
43252	Egd optical endomicroscopy	2.96	7.03	1.62	0.34	10.33	$357.48	4.92	$170.26	000	A Me
43253	Egd us transmural injxn/mark	4.73	NA	2.43	0.52	NA	NA	7.68	$265.78	000	A Me
43254	Egd endo mucosal resection	4.87	NA	2.49	0.56	NA	NA	7.92	$274.08	000	A Me
43255	Egd control bleeding any	3.56	15.52	1.91	0.40	19.48	$674.13	5.87	$203.14	000	A Me
43257	Egd w/thrml txmnt gerd	4.15	NA	2.13	0.56	NA	NA	6.84	$236.71	000	A Me
43259	Egd us exam duodenum/jejunum	4.04	NA	2.13	0.42	NA	NA	6.59	$228.05	000	A Me
43260	Ercp w/specimen collection	5.85	NA	2.93	0.65	NA	NA	9.43	$326.34	000	A M
43261	Endo cholangiopancreatograph	6.15	NA	3.07	0.67	NA	NA	9.89	$342.26	000	A Me
43262	Endo cholangiopancreatograph	6.50	NA	3.23	0.73	NA	NA	10.46	$361.98	000	A Me
43263	Ercp sphincter pressure meas	6.50	NA	3.23	0.73	NA	NA	10.46	$361.98	000	A Me
43264	Ercp remove duct calculi	6.63	NA	3.28	0.73	NA	NA	10.64	$368.21	000	A Me
43265	Ercp lithotripsy calculi	7.93	NA	3.87	0.89	NA	NA	12.69	$439.15	000	A Me
43266	Egd endoscopic stent place	3.92	NA	1.96	0.50	NA	NA	6.38	$220.79	000	A Me
43270	Egd lesion ablation	4.01	18.26	2.11	0.43	22.70	$785.56	6.55	$226.67	000	A Me
43273	Endoscopic pancreatoscopy	2.24	NA	1.00	0.25	NA	NA	3.49	$120.78	ZZZ	A+
43274	Ercp duct stent placement	8.48	NA	4.10	0.95	NA	NA	13.53	$468.22	000	A Me
43275	Ercp remove forgn body duct	6.86	NA	3.38	0.76	NA	NA	11.00	$380.67	000	A Me
43276	Ercp stent exchange w/dilate	8.84	NA	4.27	0.98	NA	NA	14.09	$487.60	000	A Me
43277	Ercp ea duct/ampulla dilate	6.90	NA	3.41	0.76	NA	NA	11.07	$383.09	000	A Me

*Please note that these calculations are based on the Medicare 2022 Conversion Factor of $34.6062 and the DRA RVU cap rates at time of publication.

A = assistant-at-surgery restriction
A+ = assistant-at-surgery restriction unless medical necessity established with documentation
B = bilateral surgery adjustment applies
C = cosurgeons payable
C+ = cosurgeons payable if medical necessity established with documentation
CP = carriers may establish RVUs and payment amounts for these services, generally on an individual basis following review of documentation such as an operative report
M = multiple surgery adjustment applies
Me = multiple endoscopy rules may apply
M+ = multiple therapy rules apply
Mtc = multiple diagnostic imaging rules apply
T = team surgeons permitted
T+ = team surgeons payable if medical necessity established with documentation
§ = indicates code is not covered by Medicare
GS = procedure must be performed under the general supervision of a physician
DS = procedure must be performed under the direct supervision of a physician
PS = procedure must be performed under the personal supervision of a physician
DRA = procedure subject to DRA limitation

Relative Value Units

CPT Code and Modifier		Description	Work RVU	Nonfacility Practice Expense RVU	Facility Practice Expense RVU	PLI RVU	Total Non-facility RVUs	Medicare Payment Nonfacility	Total Facility RVUs	Medicare Payment Facility	Global Period	Payment Policy Indicators
43278		Ercp lesion ablate w/dilate	7.92	NA	3.86	0.89	NA	NA	12.67	$438.46	000	A Me
43279		Lap myotomy heller	22.10	NA	10.73	5.39	NA	NA	38.22	$1322.65	090	C+ M
43280		Laparoscopy fundoplasty	18.10	NA	9.59	4.46	NA	NA	32.15	$1112.59	090	C+ M
43281		Lap paraesophag hern repair	26.60	NA	12.64	6.58	NA	NA	45.82	$1585.66	090	C+ M
43282		Lap paraesoph her rpr w/mesh	30.10	NA	13.97	7.44	NA	NA	51.51	$1782.57	090	C+ M
43283		Lap esoph lengthening	2.95	NA	1.00	0.73	NA	NA	4.68	$161.96	ZZZ	C+
43284		Laps esophgl sphnctr agmntj	10.13	NA	6.81	2.55	NA	NA	19.49	$674.47	090	C+ M
43285		Rmvl esophgl sphnctr dev	10.47	NA	6.94	2.66	NA	NA	20.07	$694.55	090	C+ M
43286		Esphg tot w/laps moblj	55.00	NA	25.46	13.36	NA	NA	93.82	$3246.75	090	C+ M
43287		Esphg dstl 2/3 w/laps moblj	63.00	NA	26.38	15.22	NA	NA	104.60	$3619.81	090	C M
43288		Esphg thrsc moblj	66.42	NA	28.14	15.65	NA	NA	110.21	$3813.95	090	C M
43289	CP	Laparoscope proc esoph	0.00	0.00	0.00	0.00	0.00	$0.00	0.00	$0.00	YYY	B C+ M T+
43300		Repair of esophagus	9.33	NA	7.86	1.33	NA	NA	18.52	$640.91	090	C+ M
43305		Repair esophagus and fistula	18.10	NA	11.70	2.57	NA	NA	32.37	$1120.20	090	C+ M
43310		Repair of esophagus	26.26	NA	11.17	6.23	NA	NA	43.66	$1510.91	090	C+ M
43312		Repair esophagus and fistula	29.25	NA	10.50	6.94	NA	NA	46.69	$1615.76	090	C+ M
43313		Esophagoplasty congenital	48.45	NA	25.65	12.26	NA	NA	86.36	$2988.59	090	C+ M
43314		Tracheo-esophagoplasty cong	53.43	NA	25.76	13.50	NA	NA	92.69	$3207.65	090	C+ M
43320		Fuse esophagus & stomach	23.31	NA	12.53	5.88	NA	NA	41.72	$1443.77	090	C+ M
43325		Revise esophagus & stomach	22.60	NA	12.27	5.72	NA	NA	40.59	$1404.67	090	C+ M
43327		Esoph fundoplasty lap	13.35	NA	7.78	3.31	NA	NA	24.44	$845.78	090	C+ M
43328		Esoph fundoplasty thor	19.91	NA	8.47	4.74	NA	NA	33.12	$1146.16	090	C+ M
43330		Esophagomyotomy abdominal	22.19	NA	12.13	5.60	NA	NA	39.92	$1381.48	090	C+ M
43331		Esophagomyotomy thoracic	23.06	NA	10.96	5.46	NA	NA	39.48	$1366.25	090	C+ M
43332		Transab esoph hiat hern rpr	19.62	NA	9.83	4.78	NA	NA	34.23	$1184.57	090	C+ M
43333		Transab esoph hiat hern rpr	21.46	NA	10.66	5.26	NA	NA	37.38	$1293.58	090	C+ M
43334		Transthor diaphrag hern rpr	22.12	NA	9.31	5.28	NA	NA	36.71	$1270.39	090	C+ M
43335		Transthor diaphrag hern rpr	23.97	NA	9.62	5.69	NA	NA	39.28	$1359.33	090	C+ M
43336		Thorabd diaphr hern repair	25.81	NA	10.76	6.12	NA	NA	42.69	$1477.34	090	C+ M
43337		Thorabd diaphr hern repair	27.65	NA	11.28	6.56	NA	NA	45.49	$1574.24	090	C+ M
43338		Esoph lengthening	2.21	NA	0.63	0.54	NA	NA	3.38	$116.97	ZZZ	C+
43340		Fuse esophagus & intestine	22.99	NA	12.41	5.81	NA	NA	41.21	$1426.12	090	C+ M
43341		Fuse esophagus & intestine	24.23	NA	11.29	5.76	NA	NA	41.28	$1428.54	090	C+ M

43351		Surgical opening esophagus	22.05	NA	11.63	5.23	NA	NA	38.91	$1346.53	090	C+ M
43352		Surgical opening esophagus	17.81	NA	9.46	4.22	NA	NA	31.49	$1089.75	090	C+ M
43360		Gastrointestinal repair	40.11	NA	16.55	9.51	NA	NA	66.17	$2289.89	090	C+ M
43361		Gastrointestinal repair	45.68	NA	23.10	11.53	NA	NA	80.31	$2779.22	090	C+ M
43400		Ligate esophagus veins	25.60	NA	13.39	6.47	NA	NA	45.46	$1573.20	090	C+ M
43405		Ligate/staple esophagus	24.73	NA	12.39	5.87	NA	NA	42.99	$1487.72	090	C+ M
43410		Repair esophagus wound	16.41	NA	11.71	2.33	NA	NA	30.45	$1053.76	090	C+ M
43415		Repair esophagus wound	44.88	NA	19.99	10.50	NA	NA	75.37	$2608.27	090	C+ M
43420		Repair esophagus opening	16.78	NA	10.91	2.38	NA	NA	30.07	$1040.61	090	A+ C+ M
43425		Repair esophagus opening	25.04	NA	11.52	5.94	NA	NA	42.50	$1470.76	090	C+ M
43450		Dilate esophagus 1/mult pass	1.28	4.29	0.90	0.14	5.71	$197.60	2.32	$80.29	000	A M
43453		Dilate esophagus	1.41	23.63	0.94	0.18	25.22	$872.77	2.53	$87.55	000	A M
43460		Pressure treatment esophagus	3.79	NA	2.00	0.41	NA	NA	6.20	$214.56	000	A M
43496	CP	Free jejunum flap microvasc	0.00	0.00	0.00	0.00	0.00	$0.00	0.00	$0.00	090	C+ M
43497		Transorl lwr esophgl myotomy	13.29	NA	8.17	1.94	NA	NA	23.40	$809.79	090	A Me
43499	CP	Esophagus surgery procedure	0.00	0.00	0.00	0.00	0.00	$0.00	0.00	$0.00	YYY	A C+ M T+
43500		Surgical opening of stomach	12.79	NA	7.57	3.13	NA	NA	23.49	$812.90	090	C+ M
43501		Surgical repair of stomach	22.60	NA	12.07	5.62	NA	NA	40.29	$1394.28	090	C+ M
43502		Surgical repair of stomach	25.69	NA	13.39	6.49	NA	NA	45.57	$1577.00	090	C+ M
43510		Surgical opening of stomach	15.14	NA	9.45	3.82	NA	NA	28.41	$983.16	090	C+ M
43520		Incision of pyloric muscle	11.29	NA	6.76	2.60	NA	NA	20.65	$714.62	090	C+ M
43605		Biopsy of stomach	13.72	NA	7.95	3.34	NA	NA	25.01	$865.50	090	C+ M
43610		Excision of stomach lesion	16.34	NA	8.93	3.95	NA	NA	29.22	$1011.19	090	C+ M
43611		Excision of stomach lesion	20.38	NA	11.13	4.90	NA	NA	36.41	$1260.01	090	C+ M
43620		Removal of stomach	34.04	NA	16.50	8.61	NA	NA	59.15	$2046.96	090	C+ M
43621		Removal of stomach	39.53	NA	18.33	9.74	NA	NA	67.60	$2339.38	090	C+ M
43622		Removal of stomach	40.03	NA	18.73	10.12	NA	NA	68.88	$2383.68	090	C+ M
43631		Removal of stomach partial	24.51	NA	12.72	5.98	NA	NA	43.21	$1495.33	090	C+ M

*Please note that these calculations are based on the Medicare 2022 Conversion Factor of $34.6062 and the DRA RVU cap rates at time of publication.

A = assistant-at-surgery restriction
A+ = assistant-at-surgery restriction unless medical necessity established with documentation
B = bilateral surgery adjustment applies
C = cosurgeons payable
C+ = cosurgeons payable if medical necessity established with documentation
CP = carriers may establish RVUs and payment amounts for these services, generally on an individual basis following review of documentation such as an operative report
M = multiple surgery adjustment applies
Me = multiple endoscopy rules may apply
M+ = multiple therapy rules apply
Mtc = multiple diagnostic imaging rules apply
T = team surgeons permitted
T+ = team surgeons payable if medical necessity established with documentation
§ = indicates code is not covered by Medicare
GS = procedure must be performed under the general supervision of a physician
DS = procedure must be performed under the direct supervision of a physician
PS = procedure must be performed under the personal supervision of a physician
DRA = procedure subject to DRA limitation

Relative Value Units

CPT Code and Modifier		Description	Work RVU	Nonfacility Practice Expense RVU	Facility Practice Expense RVU	PLI RVU	Total Non-facility RVUs	Medicare Payment Nonfacility	Total Facility RVUs	Medicare Payment Facility	Global Period	Payment Policy Indicators
43632		Removal of stomach partial	35.14	NA	16.74	8.64	NA	NA	60.52	$2094.37	090	C+ M
43633		Removal of stomach partial	33.14	NA	15.96	8.12	NA	NA	57.22	$1980.17	090	C+ M
43634		Removal of stomach partial	36.64	NA	17.47	9.25	NA	NA	63.36	$2192.65	090	C+ M
43635		Removal of stomach partial	2.06	NA	0.77	0.50	NA	NA	3.33	$115.24	ZZZ	C+
43640		Vagotomy & pylorus repair	19.56	NA	11.11	4.94	NA	NA	35.61	$1232.33	090	C+ M
43641		Vagotomy & pylorus repair	19.81	NA	11.20	5.01	NA	NA	36.02	$1246.52	090	C+ M
43644		Lap gastric bypass/roux-en-y	29.40	NA	15.03	7.37	NA	NA	51.80	$1792.60	090	C+ M
43645		Lap gastr bypass incl smll i	31.53	NA	15.55	7.71	NA	NA	54.79	$1896.07	090	C+ M
43647	CP	Lap impl electrode antrum	0.00	0.00	0.00	0.00	0.00	$0.00	0.00	$0.00	YYY	C+ M
43648	CP	Lap revise/remv eltrd antrum	0.00	0.00	0.00	0.00	0.00	$0.00	0.00	$0.00	YYY	C+ M
43651		Laparoscopy vagus nerve	10.13	NA	6.97	2.55	NA	NA	19.65	$680.01	090	C+ M
43652		Laparoscopy vagus nerve	12.13	NA	7.72	3.05	NA	NA	22.90	$792.48	090	C+ M
43653		Laparoscopy gastrostomy	8.48	NA	6.74	2.09	NA	NA	17.31	$599.03	090	C+ M
43659	CP	Laparoscope proc stom	0.00	0.00	0.00	0.00	0.00	$0.00	0.00	$0.00	YYY	B C+ M T+
43752		Nasal/orogastric w/tube plmt	0.81	NA	0.28	0.09	NA	NA	1.18	$40.84	000	A
43753		Tx gastro intub w/asp	0.45	NA	0.11	0.09	NA	NA	0.65	$22.49	000	
43754		Dx gastr intub w/asp spec	0.45	6.40	0.51	0.10	6.95	$240.51	1.06	$36.68	000	
43755		Dx gastr intub w/asp specs	0.94	5.19	0.70	0.10	6.23	$215.60	1.74	$60.21	000	
43756		Dx duod intub w/asp spec	0.77	7.81	0.63	0.09	8.67	$300.04	1.49	$51.56	000	
43757		Dx duod intub w/asp specs	1.26	10.21	0.85	0.12	11.59	$401.09	2.23	$77.17	000	
43761		Reposition gastrostomy tube	2.01	1.36	0.73	0.32	3.69	$127.70	3.06	$105.89	000	A M
43762		Rplc gtube no revj trc	0.75	6.14	0.22	0.12	7.01	$242.59	1.09	$37.72	000	A M
43763		Rplc gtube revj gstrst trc	1.41	8.92	0.84	0.25	10.58	$366.13	2.50	$86.52	000	A M
43770		Lap place gastr adj device	18.00	NA	11.17	4.56	NA	NA	33.73	$1167.27	090	C+ M
43771		Lap revise gastr adj device	20.79	NA	12.20	5.26	NA	NA	38.25	$1323.69	090	C+ M
43772		Lap rmvl gastr adj device	15.70	NA	8.78	3.91	NA	NA	28.39	$982.47	090	C+ M
43773		Lap replace gastr adj device	20.79	NA	12.20	5.26	NA	NA	38.25	$1323.69	090	C+ M
43774		Lap rmvl gastr adj all parts	15.76	NA	9.00	3.95	NA	NA	28.71	$993.54	090	C+ M
43775		Lap sleeve gastrectomy	20.38	NA	7.55	5.10	NA	NA	33.03	$1143.04	090	C+ M
43800		Reconstruction of pylorus	15.43	NA	8.55	3.82	NA	NA	27.80	$962.05	090	C+ M
43810		Fusion of stomach and bowel	16.88	NA	9.26	4.25	NA	NA	30.39	$1051.68	090	C+ M
43820		Fusion of stomach and bowel	22.53	NA	12.05	5.50	NA	NA	40.08	$1387.02	090	C+ M
43825		Fusion of stomach and bowel	21.76	NA	11.93	5.50	NA	NA	39.19	$1356.22	090	C+ M

43830		Place gastrostomy tube	10.85	NA	7.56	2.62	NA	NA	21.03	$727.77	090	C+ M
43831		Place gastrostomy tube	8.49	NA	7.68	2.17	NA	NA	18.34	$634.68	090	C+ M
43832		Place gastrostomy tube	17.34	NA	9.58	4.25	NA	NA	31.17	$1078.68	090	C+ M
43840		Repair of stomach lesion	22.83	NA	12.16	5.56	NA	NA	40.55	$1403.28	090	C+ M
43842	§	V-band gastroplasty	21.03	NA	11.07	1.72	NA	NA	33.82	$1170.38	090	
43843		Gastroplasty w/o v-band	21.21	NA	11.83	5.36	NA	NA	38.40	$1328.88	090	C M
43845		Gastroplasty duodenal switch	33.30	NA	16.78	8.21	NA	NA	58.29	$2017.20	090	C+ M
43846		Gastric bypass for obesity	27.41	NA	15.02	6.92	NA	NA	49.35	$1707.82	090	C+ M
43847		Gastric bypass incl small i	30.28	NA	16.09	7.65	NA	NA	54.02	$1869.43	090	C+ M
43848		Revision gastroplasty	32.75	NA	16.75	8.05	NA	NA	57.55	$1991.59	090	C+ M
43860		Revise stomach-bowel fusion	27.89	NA	14.18	6.71	NA	NA	48.78	$1688.09	090	C+ M
43865		Revise stomach-bowel fusion	29.05	NA	14.64	7.35	NA	NA	51.04	$1766.30	090	C+ M
43870		Repair stomach opening	11.44	NA	7.09	2.68	NA	NA	21.21	$734.00	090	C+ M
43880		Repair stomach-bowel fistula	27.18	NA	13.99	6.52	NA	NA	47.69	$1650.37	090	C+ M
43881	CP	Impl/redo electrd antrum	0.00	0.00	0.00	0.00	0.00	$0.00	0.00	$0.00	YYY	C+ M
43882	CP	Revise/remove electrd antrum	0.00	0.00	0.00	0.00	0.00	$0.00	0.00	$0.00	YYY	C+ M
43886		Revise gastric port open	4.64	NA	5.23	1.17	NA	NA	11.04	$382.05	090	C+ M
43887		Remove gastric port open	4.32	NA	4.52	1.09	NA	NA	9.93	$343.64	090	C+ M
43888		Change gastric port open	6.44	NA	5.90	1.63	NA	NA	13.97	$483.45	090	C+ M
43999	CP	Stomach surgery procedure	0.00	0.00	0.00	0.00	0.00	$0.00	0.00	$0.00	YYY	A+ C+ M T+
44005		Freeing of bowel adhesion	18.46	NA	9.67	4.42	NA	NA	32.55	$1126.43	090	C+ M
44010		Incision of small bowel	14.26	NA	8.57	2.62	NA	NA	25.45	$880.73	090	C+ M
44015		Insert needle cath bowel	2.62	NA	0.94	0.64	NA	NA	4.20	$145.35	ZZZ	C+
44020		Explore small intestine	16.22	NA	8.94	3.94	NA	NA	29.10	$1007.04	090	C+ M
44021		Decompress small bowel	16.31	NA	8.77	3.87	NA	NA	28.95	$1001.85	090	C+ M
44025		Incision of large bowel	16.51	NA	9.04	3.68	NA	NA	29.23	$1011.54	090	C+ M
44050		Reduce bowel obstruction	15.52	NA	8.65	3.75	NA	NA	27.92	$966.21	090	C+ M
44055		Correct malrotation of bowel	25.63	NA	12.48	6.20	NA	NA	44.31	$1533.40	090	C+ M

*Please note that these calculations are based on the Medicare 2022 Conversion Factor of $34.6062 and the DRA RVU cap rates at time of publication.

A = assistant-at-surgery restriction
A+ = assistant-at-surgery restriction unless medical necessity established with documentation
B = bilateral surgery adjustment applies
C = cosurgeons payable
C+ = cosurgeons payable if medical necessity established with documentation
CP = carriers may establish RVUs and payment amounts for these services, generally on an individual basis following review of documentation such as an operative report
M = multiple surgery adjustment applies
Me = multiple endoscopy rules may apply
M+ = multiple therapy rules apply
Mtc = multiple diagnostic imaging rules apply
T = team surgeons permitted
T+ = team surgeons payable if medical necessity established with documentation
§ = indicates code is not covered by Medicare
GS = procedure must be performed under the general supervision of a physician
DS = procedure must be performed under the direct supervision of a physician
PS = procedure must be performed under the personal supervision of a physician
DRA = procedure subject to DRA limitation

Relative Value Units

CPT Code and Modifier		Description	Work RVU	Nonfacility Practice Expense RVU	Facility Practice Expense RVU	PLI RVU	Total Non-facility RVUs	Medicare Payment Nonfacility	Total Facility RVUs	Medicare Payment Facility	Global Period	Payment Policy Indicators
44100		Biopsy of bowel	2.01	NA	0.90	0.22	NA	NA	3.13	$108.32	000	A M
44110		Excise intestine lesion(s)	14.04	NA	8.23	2.91	NA	NA	25.18	$871.38	090	C+ M
44111		Excision of bowel lesion(s)	16.52	NA	9.02	3.58	NA	NA	29.12	$1007.73	090	C+ M
44120		Removal of small intestine	20.82	NA	10.59	4.95	NA	NA	36.36	$1258.28	090	C+ M
44121		Removal of small intestine	4.44	NA	1.66	1.02	NA	NA	7.12	$246.40	ZZZ	C+
44125		Removal of small intestine	20.03	NA	10.41	4.55	NA	NA	34.99	$1210.87	090	C+ M
44126		Enterectomy w/o taper cong	42.23	NA	20.71	10.67	NA	NA	73.61	$2547.36	090	C+ M
44127		Enterectomy w/taper cong	49.30	NA	23.24	12.46	NA	NA	85.00	$2941.53	090	C+ M
44128		Enterectomy cong add-on	4.44	NA	1.65	1.11	NA	NA	7.20	$249.16	ZZZ	C+
44130		Bowel to bowel fusion	22.11	NA	11.87	5.18	NA	NA	39.16	$1355.18	090	C+ M
44132		Enterectomy cadaver donor	0.00	0.00	0.00	0.00	0.00	$0.00	0.00	$0.00	XXX	A+
44133		Enterectomy live donor	0.00	0.00	0.00	0.00	0.00	$0.00	0.00	$0.00	XXX	A+
44135		Intestine transplnt cadaver	0.00	0.00	0.00	0.00	0.00	$0.00	0.00	$0.00	XXX	A+
44136		Intestine transplant live	0.00	0.00	0.00	0.00	0.00	$0.00	0.00	$0.00	XXX	A+
44137	CP	Remove intestinal allograft	0.00	0.00	0.00	0.00	0.00	$0.00	0.00	$0.00	XXX	C+ M
44139		Mobilization of colon	2.23	NA	0.84	0.50	NA	NA	3.57	$123.54	ZZZ	C+
44140		Partial removal of colon	22.59	NA	12.06	5.28	NA	NA	39.93	$1381.83	090	C+ M
44141		Partial removal of colon	29.91	NA	17.14	6.99	NA	NA	54.04	$1870.12	090	C+ M
44143		Partial removal of colon	27.79	NA	15.00	6.46	NA	NA	49.25	$1704.36	090	C+ M
44144		Partial removal of colon	29.91	NA	15.63	6.84	NA	NA	52.38	$1812.67	090	C+ M
44145		Partial removal of colon	28.58	NA	14.25	6.06	NA	NA	48.89	$1691.90	090	C+ M
44146		Partial removal of colon	35.30	NA	19.45	7.51	NA	NA	62.26	$2154.58	090	C+ M
44147		Partial removal of colon	33.69	NA	16.03	7.57	NA	NA	57.29	$1982.59	090	C+ M
44150		Removal of colon	30.18	NA	18.27	6.59	NA	NA	55.04	$1904.73	090	C+ M
44151		Removal of colon/ileostomy	34.92	NA	20.50	8.83	NA	NA	64.25	$2223.45	090	C+ M
44155		Removal of colon/ileostomy	34.42	NA	19.89	6.95	NA	NA	61.26	$2119.98	090	C+ M
44156		Removal of colon/ileostomy	37.42	NA	21.86	9.44	NA	NA	68.72	$2378.14	090	C+ M
44157		Colectomy w/ileoanal anast	35.70	NA	20.52	9.03	NA	NA	65.25	$2258.05	090	C+ M
44158		Colectomy w/neo-rectum pouch	36.70	NA	20.90	9.26	NA	NA	66.86	$2313.77	090	C+ M
44160		Removal of colon	20.89	NA	11.25	4.77	NA	NA	36.91	$1277.31	090	C+ M
44180		Lap enterolysis	15.27	NA	8.48	3.68	NA	NA	27.43	$949.25	090	C+ M
44186		Lap jejunostomy	10.38	NA	6.54	2.55	NA	NA	19.47	$673.78	090	C+ M
44187		Lap ileo/jejuno-stomy	17.40	NA	11.63	3.38	NA	NA	32.41	$1121.59	090	C+ M

44188		Lap colostomy	19.35	NA	12.61	4.17	NA	NA	36.13	$1250.32	090	C+ M
44202		Lap enterectomy	23.39	NA	12.36	5.50	NA	NA	41.25	$1427.51	090	C+ M
44203		Lap resect s/intestine addl	4.44	NA	1.63	1.04	NA	NA	7.11	$246.05	ZZZ	C+
44204		Laparo partial colectomy	26.42	NA	13.44	5.69	NA	NA	45.55	$1576.31	090	C+ M
44205		Lap colectomy part w/ileum	22.95	NA	11.81	4.79	NA	NA	39.55	$1368.68	090	C+ M
44206		Lap part colectomy w/stoma	29.79	NA	15.43	6.43	NA	NA	51.65	$1787.41	090	C+ M
44207		L colectomy/coloproctostomy	31.92	NA	15.29	6.34	NA	NA	53.55	$1853.16	090	C+ M
44208		L colectomy/coloproctostomy	33.99	NA	17.64	6.65	NA	NA	58.28	$2016.85	090	C+ M
44210		Laparo total proctocolectomy	30.09	NA	16.65	5.49	NA	NA	52.23	$1807.48	090	C+ M
44211		Lap colectomy w/proctectomy	37.08	NA	20.05	4.90	NA	NA	62.03	$2146.62	090	C+ M
44212		Laparo total proctocolectomy	34.58	NA	19.31	5.87	NA	NA	59.76	$2068.07	090	C+ M
44213		Lap mobil splenic fl add-on	3.50	NA	1.30	0.72	NA	NA	5.52	$191.03	ZZZ	C+
44227		Lap close enterostomy	28.62	NA	14.35	6.26	NA	NA	49.23	$1703.66	090	C+ M
44238	CP	Laparoscope proc intestine	0.00	0.00	0.00	0.00	0.00	$0.00	0.00	$0.00	YYY	B C+ M T+
44300		Open bowel to skin	13.75	NA	8.01	3.35	NA	NA	25.11	$868.96	090	C+ M
44310		Ileostomy/jejunostomy	17.59	NA	9.51	3.76	NA	NA	30.86	$1067.95	090	C+ M
44312		Revision of ileostomy	9.43	NA	6.41	1.94	NA	NA	17.78	$615.30	090	A+ M
44314		Revision of ileostomy	16.74	NA	9.72	3.36	NA	NA	29.82	$1031.96	090	C+ M
44316		Devise bowel pouch	23.59	NA	12.70	5.96	NA	NA	42.25	$1462.11	090	C+ M
44320		Colostomy	19.91	NA	11.31	4.45	NA	NA	35.67	$1234.40	090	C+ M
44322		Colostomy with biopsies	13.32	NA	13.53	3.38	NA	NA	30.23	$1046.15	090	C+ M
44340		Revision of colostomy	9.28	NA	7.34	2.03	NA	NA	18.65	$645.41	090	A C+ M
44345		Revision of colostomy	17.22	NA	10.29	3.66	NA	NA	31.17	$1078.68	090	C+ M
44346		Revision of colostomy	19.63	NA	11.20	4.26	NA	NA	35.09	$1214.33	090	C+ M
44360		Small bowel endoscopy	2.49	NA	1.43	0.27	NA	NA	4.19	$145.00	000	A M
44361		Small bowel endoscopy/biopsy	2.77	NA	1.56	0.31	NA	NA	4.64	$160.57	000	A Me
44363		Small bowel endoscopy	3.39	NA	1.83	0.39	NA	NA	5.61	$194.14	000	A+ Me
44364		Small bowel endoscopy	3.63	NA	1.94	0.40	NA	NA	5.97	$206.60	000	A+ Me

*Please note that these calculations are based on the Medicare 2022 Conversion Factor of $34.6062 and the DRA RVU cap rates at time of publication.

A = assistant-at-surgery restriction

A+ = assistant-at-surgery restriction unless medical necessity established with documentation

B = bilateral surgery adjustment applies

C = cosurgeons payable

C+ = cosurgeons payable if medical necessity established with documentation

CP = carriers may establish RVUs and payment amounts for these services, generally on an individual basis following review of documentation such as an operative report

M = multiple surgery adjustment applies

Me = multiple endoscopy rules may apply

M+ = multiple therapy rules apply

Mtc = multiple diagnostic imaging rules apply

T = team surgeons permitted

T+ = team surgeons payable if medical necessity established with documentation

§ = indicates code is not covered by Medicare

GS = procedure must be performed under the general supervision of a physician

DS = procedure must be performed under the direct supervision of a physician

PS = procedure must be performed under the personal supervision of a physician

DRA = procedure subject to DRA limitation

Relative Value Units

CPT Code and Modifier	Description	Work RVU	Nonfacility Practice Expense RVU	Facility Practice Expense RVU	PLI RVU	Total Non-facility RVUs	Medicare Payment Nonfacility	Total Facility RVUs	Medicare Payment Facility	Global Period	Payment Policy Indicators
44365	Small bowel endoscopy	3.21	NA	1.76	0.34	NA	NA	5.31	$183.76	000	A+ Me
44366	Small bowel endoscopy	4.30	NA	2.24	0.45	NA	NA	6.99	$241.90	000	A Me
44369	Small bowel endoscopy	4.41	NA	2.29	0.47	NA	NA	7.17	$248.13	000	A+ Me
44370	Small bowel endoscopy/stent	4.69	NA	2.58	0.52	NA	NA	7.79	$269.58	000	A+ Me
44372	Small bowel endoscopy	4.30	NA	2.16	0.55	NA	NA	7.01	$242.59	000	A Me
44373	Small bowel endoscopy	3.39	NA	1.80	0.42	NA	NA	5.61	$194.14	000	A Me
44376	Small bowel endoscopy	5.15	NA	2.60	0.56	NA	NA	8.31	$287.58	000	A+ M
44377	Small bowel endoscopy/biopsy	5.42	NA	2.72	0.60	NA	NA	8.74	$302.46	000	A+ Me
44378	Small bowel endoscopy	7.02	NA	3.46	0.77	NA	NA	11.25	$389.32	000	A+ Me
44379	S bowel endoscope w/stent	7.36	NA	3.78	0.83	NA	NA	11.97	$414.24	000	A+ Me
44380	Small bowel endoscopy br/wa	0.87	5.01	0.68	0.10	5.98	$206.95	1.65	$57.10	000	A M
44381	Small bowel endoscopy br/wa	1.38	28.87	0.90	0.18	30.43	$1053.07	2.46	$85.13	000	A Me
44382	Small bowel endoscopy	1.17	7.95	0.84	0.12	9.24	$319.76	2.13	$73.71	000	A Me
44384	Small bowel endoscopy	2.85	NA	1.32	0.35	NA	NA	4.52	$156.42	000	A Me
44385	Endoscopy of bowel pouch	1.20	5.18	0.76	0.17	6.55	$226.67	2.13	$73.71	000	A M
44386	Endoscopy bowel pouch/biop	1.50	7.92	0.92	0.20	9.62	$332.91	2.62	$90.67	000	A M
44388	Colonoscopy thru stoma spx	2.72	6.49	1.46	0.40	9.61	$332.57	4.58	$158.50	000	A M
44388-53	Colonoscopy thru stoma spx	1.36	3.24	0.73	0.20	4.80	$166.11	2.29	$79.25	000	A M
44389	Colonoscopy with biopsy	3.02	9.22	1.62	0.39	12.63	$437.08	5.03	$174.07	000	A Me
44390	Colonoscopy for foreign body	3.74	8.16	1.99	0.40	12.30	$425.66	6.13	$212.14	000	A Me
44391	Colonoscopy for bleeding	4.12	15.15	2.13	0.50	19.77	$684.16	6.75	$233.59	000	A Me
44392	Colonoscopy & polypectomy	3.53	7.67	1.77	0.54	11.74	$406.28	5.84	$202.10	000	A Me
44394	Colonoscopy w/snare	4.03	8.82	2.05	0.54	13.39	$463.38	6.62	$229.09	000	A Me
44401	Colonoscopy with ablation	4.34	70.35	2.26	0.47	75.16	$2601.00	7.07	$244.67	000	A Me
44402	Colonoscopy w/stent plcmt	4.70	NA	2.43	0.52	NA	NA	7.65	$264.74	000	A Me
44403	Colonoscopy w/resection	5.50	NA	2.78	0.60	NA	NA	8.88	$307.30	000	A Me
44404	Colonoscopy w/injection	3.02	9.55	1.62	0.40	12.97	$448.84	5.04	$174.42	000	A Me
44405	Colonoscopy w/dilation	3.23	13.62	1.77	0.35	17.20	$595.23	5.35	$185.14	000	A Me
44406	Colonoscopy w/ultrasound	4.10	NA	2.16	0.43	NA	NA	6.69	$231.52	000	A Me
44407	Colonoscopy w/ndl aspir/bx	4.96	NA	2.54	0.56	NA	NA	8.06	$278.93	000	A Me
44408	Colonoscopy w/decompression	4.14	NA	2.17	0.44	NA	NA	6.75	$233.59	000	A Me
44500	Intro gastrointestinal tube	0.39	NA	0.14	0.04	NA	NA	0.57	$19.73	000	A+
44602	Suture small intestine	24.72	NA	11.31	5.82	NA	NA	41.85	$1448.27	090	C+ M

44603		Suture small intestine	28.16	NA	13.46	6.34	NA	NA	47.96	$1659.71	090	C+ M
44604		Suture large intestine	18.16	NA	9.05	4.11	NA	NA	31.32	$1083.87	090	C+ M
44605		Repair of bowel lesion	22.08	NA	11.52	5.03	NA	NA	38.63	$1336.84	090	C+ M
44615		Intestinal stricturoplasty	18.16	NA	9.69	4.03	NA	NA	31.88	$1103.25	090	C+ M
44620		Repair bowel opening	14.43	NA	8.17	3.05	NA	NA	25.65	$887.65	090	C+ M
44625		Repair bowel opening	17.28	NA	9.20	3.45	NA	NA	29.93	$1035.76	090	C+ M
44626		Repair bowel opening	27.90	NA	13.18	6.23	NA	NA	47.31	$1637.22	090	C+ M
44640		Repair bowel-skin fistula	24.20	NA	11.86	5.41	NA	NA	41.47	$1435.12	090	C+ M
44650		Repair bowel fistula	25.12	NA	12.16	5.51	NA	NA	42.79	$1480.80	090	C+ M
44660		Repair bowel-bladder fistula	23.91	NA	11.08	4.32	NA	NA	39.31	$1360.37	090	C+ M
44661		Repair bowel-bladder fistula	27.35	NA	12.71	5.68	NA	NA	45.74	$1582.89	090	C+ M
44680		Surgical revision intestine	17.96	NA	9.67	4.55	NA	NA	32.18	$1113.63	090	C+ M
44700		Suspend bowel w/prosthesis	17.48	NA	9.04	2.98	NA	NA	29.50	$1020.88	090	C+ M
44701		Intraop colon lavage add-on	3.10	NA	1.16	0.77	NA	NA	5.03	$174.07	ZZZ	C+
44705	§	Prepare fecal microbiota	1.42	1.73	0.55	0.11	3.26	$112.82	2.08	$71.98	XXX	
44715	CP	Prepare donor intestine	0.00	0.00	0.00	0.00	0.00	$0.00	0.00	$0.00	XXX	C+ M
44720		Prep donor intestine/venous	5.00	NA	1.86	1.27	NA	NA	8.13	$281.35	XXX	C+ M
44721		Prep donor intestine/artery	7.00	NA	2.61	1.76	NA	NA	11.37	$393.47	XXX	C+ M
44799	CP	Unlisted px small intestine	0.00	0.00	0.00	0.00	0.00	$0.00	0.00	$0.00	YYY	A C+ M T+
44800		Excision of bowel pouch	12.05	NA	8.21	2.73	NA	NA	22.99	$795.60	090	C+ M
44820		Excision of mesentery lesion	13.73	NA	8.26	3.48	NA	NA	25.47	$881.42	090	C+ M
44850		Repair of mesentery	12.11	NA	7.44	2.85	NA	NA	22.40	$775.18	090	C+ M
44899	CP	Bowel surgery procedure	0.00	0.00	0.00	0.00	0.00	$0.00	0.00	$0.00	YYY	C+ M T+
44900		Drain appendix abscess open	12.57	NA	7.74	3.18	NA	NA	23.49	$812.90	090	C+ M
44950		Appendectomy	10.60	NA	6.01	2.57	NA	NA	19.18	$663.75	090	C+ M
44955		Appendectomy add-on	1.53	NA	0.60	0.33	NA	NA	2.46	$85.13	ZZZ	C+
44960		Appendectomy	14.50	NA	8.17	3.57	NA	NA	26.24	$908.07	090	C+ M
44970		Laparoscopy appendectomy	9.45	NA	6.25	2.31	NA	NA	18.01	$623.26	090	C M

*Please note that these calculations are based on the Medicare 2022 Conversion Factor of $34.6062 and the DRA RVU cap rates at time of publication.

A = assistant-at-surgery restriction
A+ = assistant-at-surgery restriction unless medical necessity established with documentation
B = bilateral surgery adjustment applies
C = cosurgeons payable
C+ = cosurgeons payable if medical necessity established with documentation
CP = carriers may establish RVUs and payment amounts for these services, generally on an individual basis following review of documentation such as an operative report
M = multiple surgery adjustment applies
Me = multiple endoscopy rules may apply
M+ = multiple therapy rules apply
Mtc = multiple diagnostic imaging rules apply
T = team surgeons permitted
T+ = team surgeons payable if medical necessity established with documentation
§ = indicates code is not covered by Medicare
GS = procedure must be performed under the general supervision of a physician
DS = procedure must be performed under the direct supervision of a physician
PS = procedure must be performed under the personal supervision of a physician
DRA = procedure subject to DRA limitation

Relative Value Units

CPT Code and Modifier		Description	Work RVU	Nonfacility Practice Expense RVU	Facility Practice Expense RVU	PLI RVU	Total Non-facility RVUs	Medicare Payment Nonfacility	Total Facility RVUs	Medicare Payment Facility	Global Period	Payment Policy Indicators
44979	CP	Laparoscope proc app	0.00	0.00	0.00	0.00	0.00	$0.00	0.00	$0.00	YYY	B C+ M T+
45000		Drainage of pelvic abscess	6.30	NA	5.26	1.18	NA	NA	12.74	$440.88	090	A M
45005		Drainage of rectal abscess	2.02	7.23	2.50	0.51	9.76	$337.76	5.03	$174.07	010	A M
45020		Drainage of rectal abscess	8.56	NA	6.80	1.73	NA	NA	17.09	$591.42	090	A M
45100		Biopsy of rectum	4.04	NA	4.18	0.75	NA	NA	8.97	$310.42	090	A M
45108		Removal of anorectal lesion	5.12	NA	4.78	1.29	NA	NA	11.19	$387.24	090	A C+ M
45110		Removal of rectum	30.76	NA	17.49	5.61	NA	NA	53.86	$1863.89	090	C+ M
45111		Partial removal of rectum	18.01	NA	10.67	3.57	NA	NA	32.25	$1116.05	090	C+ M
45112		Removal of rectum	33.18	NA	15.83	5.51	NA	NA	54.52	$1886.73	090	C+ M
45113		Partial proctectomy	33.22	NA	17.21	4.38	NA	NA	54.81	$1896.77	090	C+ M
45114		Partial removal of rectum	30.79	NA	15.62	7.80	NA	NA	54.21	$1876.00	090	C+ M
45116		Partial removal of rectum	27.72	NA	13.94	3.66	NA	NA	45.32	$1568.35	090	C+ M
45119		Remove rectum w/reservoir	33.48	NA	17.31	4.42	NA	NA	55.21	$1910.61	090	C+ M
45120		Removal of rectum	26.40	NA	14.73	6.65	NA	NA	47.78	$1653.48	090	C+ M
45121		Removal of rectum and colon	29.08	NA	15.73	7.35	NA	NA	52.16	$1805.06	090	C+ M
45123		Partial proctectomy	18.86	NA	10.77	3.33	NA	NA	32.96	$1140.62	090	C+ M
45126		Pelvic exenteration	49.10	NA	23.58	8.10	NA	NA	80.78	$2795.49	090	C+ M
45130		Excision of rectal prolapse	18.50	NA	10.39	3.06	NA	NA	31.95	$1105.67	090	C+ M
45135		Excision of rectal prolapse	22.36	NA	12.75	2.95	NA	NA	38.06	$1317.11	090	C+ M
45136		Excise ileoanal reservior	30.82	NA	17.58	4.06	NA	NA	52.46	$1815.44	090	C+ M
45150		Excision of rectal stricture	5.85	NA	5.36	1.47	NA	NA	12.68	$438.81	090	A+ M
45160		Excision of rectal lesion	16.33	NA	10.22	4.12	NA	NA	30.67	$1061.37	090	C+ M
45171		Exc rect tum transanal part	8.13	NA	8.81	1.52	NA	NA	18.46	$638.83	090	C+ M
45172		Exc rect tum transanal full	12.13	NA	10.29	2.14	NA	NA	24.56	$849.93	090	C+ M
45190		Destruction rectal tumor	10.42	NA	9.00	1.64	NA	NA	21.06	$728.81	090	A C+ M
45300		Proctosigmoidoscopy dx	0.80	2.98	0.49	0.11	3.89	$134.62	1.40	$48.45	000	A M
45303		Proctosigmoidoscopy dilate	1.40	28.09	0.87	0.22	29.71	$1028.15	2.49	$86.17	000	A Me
45305		Proctosigmoidoscopy w/bx	1.15	4.18	0.79	0.20	5.53	$191.37	2.14	$74.06	000	A Me
45307		Proctosigmoidoscopy fb	1.60	4.58	0.98	0.40	6.58	$227.71	2.98	$103.13	000	A+ Me
45308		Proctosigmoidoscopy removal	1.30	4.66	0.87	0.33	6.29	$217.67	2.50	$86.52	000	A Me
45309		Proctosigmoidoscopy removal	1.40	4.74	0.90	0.34	6.48	$224.25	2.64	$91.36	000	A Me
45315		Proctosigmoidoscopy removal	1.70	4.88	1.02	0.42	7.00	$242.24	3.14	$108.66	000	A Me
45317		Proctosigmoidoscopy bleed	1.90	4.53	1.07	0.27	6.70	$231.86	3.24	$112.12	000	A Me

45320	Proctosigmoidoscopy ablate	1.68	4.78	1.01	0.42	6.88	$238.09	3.11	$107.63	000	A Me
45321	Proctosigmoidoscopy volvul	1.65	NA	1.00	0.41	NA	NA	3.06	$105.89	000	A Me
45327	Proctosigmoidoscopy w/stent	1.90	NA	1.09	0.47	NA	NA	3.46	$119.74	000	A Me
45330	Diagnostic sigmoidoscopy	0.84	4.72	0.69	0.11	5.67	$196.22	1.64	$56.75	000	A M
45331	Sigmoidoscopy and biopsy	1.14	7.58	0.83	0.12	8.84	$305.92	2.09	$72.33	000	A Me
45332	Sigmoidoscopy w/fb removal	1.76	6.51	1.09	0.23	8.50	$294.15	3.08	$106.59	000	A Me
45333	Sigmoidoscopy & polypectomy	1.55	8.40	0.98	0.22	10.17	$351.95	2.75	$95.17	000	A Me
45334	Sigmoidoscopy for bleeding	2.00	13.14	1.21	0.23	15.37	$531.90	3.44	$119.05	000	A Me
45335	Sigmoidoscopy w/submuc inj	1.04	7.84	0.77	0.12	9.00	$311.46	1.93	$66.79	000	A Me
45337	Sigmoidoscopy & decompress	2.10	NA	1.01	0.25	NA	NA	3.36	$116.28	000	A Me
45338	Sigmoidoscopy w/tumr remove	2.05	6.87	1.22	0.25	9.17	$317.34	3.52	$121.81	000	A Me
45340	Sig w/tndsc balloon dilation	1.25	12.88	0.86	0.18	14.31	$495.21	2.29	$79.25	000	A Me
45341	Sigmoidoscopy w/ultrasound	2.12	NA	1.27	0.24	NA	NA	3.63	$125.62	000	A Me
45342	Sigmoidoscopy w/us guide bx	2.98	NA	1.65	0.33	NA	NA	4.96	$171.65	000	A Me
45346	Sigmoidoscopy w/ablation	2.81	69.68	1.55	0.33	72.82	$2520.02	4.69	$162.30	000	A Me
45347	Sigmoidoscopy w/plcmt stent	2.72	NA	1.48	0.31	NA	NA	4.51	$156.07	000	A Me
45349	Sigmoidoscopy w/resection	3.52	NA	1.88	0.40	NA	NA	5.80	$200.72	000	A Me
45350	Sgmdsc w/band ligation	1.68	19.15	1.06	0.21	21.04	$728.11	2.95	$102.09	000	A Me
45378	Diagnostic colonoscopy	3.26	6.66	1.74	0.40	10.32	$357.14	5.40	$186.87	000	A M
45378-53	Diagnostic colonoscopy	1.63	3.33	0.87	0.20	5.16	$178.57	2.70	$93.44	000	A M
45379	Colonoscopy w/fb removal	4.28	8.45	2.20	0.52	13.25	$458.53	7.00	$242.24	000	A Me
45380	Colonoscopy and biopsy	3.56	9.33	1.89	0.41	13.30	$460.26	5.86	$202.79	000	A Me
45381	Colonoscopy submucous njx	3.56	9.60	1.89	0.41	13.57	$469.61	5.86	$202.79	000	A Me
45382	Colonoscopy w/control bleed	4.66	15.39	2.39	0.54	20.59	$712.54	7.59	$262.66	000	A Me
45384	Colonoscopy w/lesion removal	4.07	10.30	2.03	0.60	14.97	$518.05	6.70	$231.86	000	A Me
45385	Colonoscopy w/lesion removal	4.57	8.72	2.34	0.54	13.83	$478.60	7.45	$257.82	000	A Me
45386	Colonoscopy w/balloon dilat	3.77	14.69	1.97	0.44	18.90	$654.06	6.18	$213.87	000	A Me
45388	Colonoscopy w/ablation	4.88	72.13	2.43	0.60	77.61	$2685.79	7.91	$273.74	000	A Me

*Please note that these calculations are based on the Medicare 2022 Conversion Factor of $34.6062 and the DRA RVU cap rates at time of publication.

A = assistant-at-surgery restriction
A+ = assistant-at-surgery restriction unless medical necessity established with documentation
B = bilateral surgery adjustment applies
C = cosurgeons payable
C+ = cosurgeons payable if medical necessity established with documentation
CP = carriers may establish RVUs and payment amounts for these services, generally on an individual basis following review of documentation such as an operative report
M = multiple surgery adjustment applies
Me = multiple endoscopy rules may apply
M+ = multiple therapy rules apply
Mtc = multiple diagnostic imaging rules apply
T = team surgeons permitted
T+ = team surgeons payable if medical necessity established with documentation
§ = indicates code is not covered by Medicare
GS = procedure must be performed under the general supervision of a physician
DS = procedure must be performed under the direct supervision of a physician
PS = procedure must be performed under the personal supervision of a physician
DRA = procedure subject to DRA limitation

Relative Value Units

CPT Code and Modifier		Description	Work RVU	Nonfacility Practice Expense RVU	Facility Practice Expense RVU	PLI RVU	Total Non-facility RVUs	Medicare Payment Nonfacility	Total Facility RVUs	Medicare Payment Facility	Global Period	Payment Policy Indicators
45389		Colonoscopy w/stent plcmt	5.24	NA	2.64	0.60	NA	NA	8.48	$293.46	000	A Me
45390		Colonoscopy w/resection	6.04	NA	3.01	0.66	NA	NA	9.71	$336.03	000	A Me
45391		Colonoscopy w/endoscope us	4.64	NA	2.39	0.51	NA	NA	7.54	$260.93	000	A Me
45392		Colonoscopy w/endoscopic fnb	5.50	NA	2.77	0.61	NA	NA	8.88	$307.30	000	A Me
45393		Colonoscopy w/decompression	4.68	NA	2.12	0.60	NA	NA	7.40	$256.09	000	A Me
45395		Lap removal of rectum	33.00	NA	18.88	5.81	NA	NA	57.69	$1996.43	090	C+ M
45397		Lap remove rectum w/pouch	36.50	NA	20.16	6.01	NA	NA	62.67	$2168.77	090	C+ M
45398		Colonoscopy w/band ligation	4.20	20.94	2.09	0.60	25.74	$890.76	6.89	$238.44	000	A Me
45399	CP	Unlisted procedure colon	0.00	0.00	0.00	0.00	0.00	$0.00	0.00	$0.00	YYY	A C+ M T+
45400		Laparoscopic proc	19.44	NA	10.73	3.26	NA	NA	33.43	$1156.89	090	C+ M
45402		Lap proctopexy w/sig resect	26.51	NA	13.40	4.77	NA	NA	44.68	$1546.21	090	C+ M
45499	CP	Laparoscope proc rectum	0.00	0.00	0.00	0.00	0.00	$0.00	0.00	$0.00	YYY	C+ M T+
45500		Repair of rectum	7.73	NA	7.45	1.95	NA	NA	17.13	$592.80	090	A+ M
45505		Repair of rectum	8.36	NA	8.11	1.48	NA	NA	17.95	$621.18	090	A M
45520		Treatment of rectal prolapse	0.55	4.29	0.55	0.08	4.92	$170.26	1.18	$40.84	000	A M
45540		Correct rectal prolapse	18.12	NA	10.00	3.06	NA	NA	31.18	$1079.02	090	C+ M
45541		Correct rectal prolapse	14.85	NA	10.33	2.88	NA	NA	28.06	$971.05	090	C+ M
45550		Repair rectum/remove sigmoid	24.80	NA	13.96	4.36	NA	NA	43.12	$1492.22	090	C+ M
45560		Repair of rectocele	11.50	NA	7.17	1.81	NA	NA	20.48	$708.73	090	C+ M
45562		Exploration/repair of rectum	17.98	NA	12.10	3.84	NA	NA	33.92	$1173.84	090	C+ M
45563		Exploration/repair of rectum	26.38	NA	16.61	6.65	NA	NA	49.64	$1717.85	090	C+ M
45800		Repair rect/bladder fistula	20.31	NA	12.62	5.13	NA	NA	38.06	$1317.11	090	C+ M
45805		Repair fistula w/colostomy	23.32	NA	14.78	5.88	NA	NA	43.98	$1521.98	090	C+ M
45820		Repair rectourethral fistula	20.37	NA	12.64	5.15	NA	NA	38.16	$1320.57	090	C+ M
45825		Repair fistula w/colostomy	24.17	NA	15.78	6.12	NA	NA	46.07	$1594.31	090	C+ M
45900		Reduction of rectal prolapse	2.99	NA	2.61	0.76	NA	NA	6.36	$220.10	010	A+ M
45905		Dilation of anal sphincter	2.35	NA	2.26	0.41	NA	NA	5.02	$173.72	010	A M
45910		Dilation of rectal narrowing	2.85	NA	2.39	0.50	NA	NA	5.74	$198.64	010	A M
45915		Remove rectal obstruction	3.19	6.92	3.09	0.57	10.68	$369.59	6.85	$237.05	010	A M
45990		Surg dx exam anorectal	1.80	NA	0.99	0.31	NA	NA	3.10	$107.28	000	A+ C+ M T+
45999	CP	Rectum surgery procedure	0.00	0.00	0.00	0.00	0.00	$0.00	0.00	$0.00	YYY	A+ C+ M T+
46020		Placement of seton	1.86	NA	1.22	0.34	NA	NA	3.42	$118.35	000	A M
46030		Removal of rectal marker	1.48	6.09	0.84	0.25	7.82	$270.62	2.57	$88.94	000	A+ M

46040	Incision of rectal abscess	5.37	10.26	6.20	1.16	16.79	$581.04	12.73	$440.54	090	A M
46045	Incision of rectal abscess	5.87	NA	6.13	1.16	NA	NA	13.16	$455.42	090	A M
46050	Incision of anal abscess	1.24	5.71	1.50	0.24	7.19	$248.82	2.98	$103.13	010	A M
46060	Incision of rectal abscess	6.37	NA	6.99	1.16	NA	NA	14.52	$502.48	090	A M
46070	Incision of anal septum	2.79	NA	4.69	0.72	NA	NA	8.20	$283.77	090	A+ M
46080	Incision of anal sphincter	2.52	5.71	1.67	0.50	8.73	$302.11	4.69	$162.30	010	A M
46083	Incise external hemorrhoid	1.45	4.64	1.55	0.27	6.36	$220.10	3.27	$113.16	010	A M
46200	Removal of anal fissure	3.59	10.13	5.85	0.62	14.34	$496.25	10.06	$348.14	090	A M
46220	Excise anal ext tag/papilla	1.61	5.72	1.69	0.29	7.62	$263.70	3.59	$124.24	010	A M
46221	Ligation of hemorrhoid(s)	2.36	5.91	3.08	0.34	8.61	$297.96	5.78	$200.02	010	A M
46230	Removal of anal tags	2.62	6.38	2.07	0.42	9.42	$325.99	5.11	$176.84	010	A M
46250	Remove ext hem groups 2+	4.25	9.48	4.52	0.77	14.50	$501.79	9.54	$330.14	090	A M
46255	Remove int/ext hem 1 group	4.96	9.89	4.77	0.93	15.78	$546.09	10.66	$368.90	090	A M
46257	Remove in/ex hem grp & fiss	5.76	NA	5.86	0.76	NA	NA	12.38	$428.42	090	A M
46258	Remove in/ex hem grp w/fistu	6.41	NA	6.41	1.62	NA	NA	14.44	$499.71	090	A+ M
46260	Remove in/ex hem groups 2+	6.73	NA	6.39	1.32	NA	NA	14.44	$499.71	090	A M
46261	Remove in/ex hem grps & fiss	7.76	NA	6.64	1.38	NA	NA	15.78	$546.09	090	A M
46262	Remove in/ex hem grps w/fist	7.91	NA	7.74	1.99	NA	NA	17.64	$610.45	090	A M
46270	Remove anal fist subq	4.92	10.31	6.09	0.96	16.19	$560.27	11.97	$414.24	090	A M
46275	Remove anal fist inter	5.42	10.67	6.23	0.96	17.05	$590.04	12.61	$436.38	090	A M
46280	Remove anal fist complex	6.39	NA	6.85	1.11	NA	NA	14.35	$496.60	090	A M
46285	Remove anal fist 2 stage	5.42	10.60	6.23	0.94	16.96	$586.92	12.59	$435.69	090	A M
46288	Repair anal fistula	7.81	NA	7.51	1.30	NA	NA	16.62	$575.16	090	A M
46320	Removal of hemorrhoid clot	1.64	4.54	1.44	0.28	6.46	$223.56	3.36	$116.28	010	A M
46500	Injection into hemorrhoid(s)	1.74	7.59	3.56	0.25	9.58	$331.53	5.55	$192.06	010	A M
46505	Chemodenervation anal musc	3.18	5.76	3.78	0.56	9.50	$328.76	7.52	$260.24	010	A B M
46600	Diagnostic anoscopy spx	0.55	3.02	0.56	0.09	3.66	$126.66	1.20	$41.53	000	A M
46601	Diagnostic anoscopy	1.60	2.73	0.97	0.23	4.56	$157.80	2.80	$96.90	000	A Me

*Please note that these calculations are based on the Medicare 2022 Conversion Factor of $34.6062 and the DRA RVU cap rates at time of publication.

A = assistant-at-surgery restriction
A+ = assistant-at-surgery restriction unless medical necessity established with documentation
B = bilateral surgery adjustment applies
C = cosurgeons payable
C+ = cosurgeons payable if medical necessity established with documentation
CP = carriers may establish RVUs and payment amounts for these services, generally on an individual basis following review of documentation such as an operative report
M = multiple surgery adjustment applies
Me = multiple endoscopy rules may apply
M+ = multiple therapy rules apply
Mtc = multiple diagnostic imaging rules apply
T = team surgeons permitted
T+ = team surgeons payable if medical necessity established with documentation
§ = indicates code is not covered by Medicare
GS = procedure must be performed under the general supervision of a physician
DS = procedure must be performed under the direct supervision of a physician
PS = procedure must be performed under the personal supervision of a physician
DRA = procedure subject to DRA limitation

Relative Value Units

CPT Code and Modifier	Description	Work RVU	Nonfacility Practice Expense RVU	Facility Practice Expense RVU	PLI RVU	Total Non-facility RVUs	Medicare Payment Nonfacility	Total Facility RVUs	Medicare Payment Facility	Global Period	Payment Policy Indicators
46604	Anoscopy and dilation	1.03	19.72	0.74	0.19	20.94	$724.65	1.96	$67.83	000	A Me
46606	Anoscopy and biopsy	1.20	7.27	0.81	0.21	8.68	$300.38	2.22	$76.83	000	A Me
46607	Diagnostic anoscopy & biopsy	2.20	3.85	1.23	0.31	6.36	$220.10	3.74	$129.43	000	A Me
46608	Anoscopy remove for body	1.30	7.46	0.87	0.33	9.09	$314.57	2.50	$86.52	000	A Me
46610	Anoscopy remove lesion	1.28	7.04	0.84	0.25	8.57	$296.58	2.37	$82.02	000	A Me
46611	Anoscopy	1.30	5.44	0.87	0.20	6.94	$240.17	2.37	$82.02	000	A Me
46612	Anoscopy remove lesions	1.50	8.56	0.94	0.39	10.45	$361.63	2.83	$97.94	000	A Me
46614	Anoscopy control bleeding	1.00	3.99	0.72	0.14	5.13	$177.53	1.86	$64.37	000	A Me
46615	Anoscopy	1.50	3.81	0.99	0.20	5.51	$190.68	2.69	$93.09	000	A Me
46700	Repair of anal stricture	9.81	NA	8.16	1.55	NA	NA	19.52	$675.51	090	A M
46705	Repair of anal stricture	7.43	NA	7.90	1.86	NA	NA	17.19	$594.88	090	C+ M
46706	Repr of anal fistula w/glue	2.44	NA	2.30	0.61	NA	NA	5.35	$185.14	010	A M
46707	Repair anorectal fist w/plug	6.39	NA	7.17	1.62	NA	NA	15.18	$525.32	090	A+ M
46710	Repr per/vag pouch sngl proc	17.14	NA	11.83	4.32	NA	NA	33.29	$1152.04	090	C+ M
46712	Repr per/vag pouch dbl proc	36.45	NA	20.69	9.21	NA	NA	66.35	$2296.12	090	C+ M
46715	Rep perf anoper fistu	7.62	NA	7.18	1.94	NA	NA	16.74	$579.31	090	M
46716	Rep perf anoper/vestib fistu	17.54	NA	14.96	4.44	NA	NA	36.94	$1278.35	090	C+ M
46730	Construction of absent anus	30.65	NA	21.00	7.74	NA	NA	59.39	$2055.26	090	C+ M
46735	Construction of absent anus	36.14	NA	23.05	9.13	NA	NA	68.32	$2364.30	090	C+ M
46740	Construction of absent anus	33.90	NA	22.32	8.56	NA	NA	64.78	$2241.79	090	C+ M
46742	Repair of imperforated anus	40.14	NA	24.54	10.14	NA	NA	74.82	$2589.24	090	C+ M
46744	Repair of cloacal anomaly	58.94	NA	31.64	14.89	NA	NA	105.47	$3649.92	090	C+ M
46746	Repair of cloacal anomaly	65.44	NA	34.21	16.53	NA	NA	116.18	$4020.55	090	C+ M
46748	Repair of cloacal anomaly	71.42	NA	36.43	18.03	NA	NA	125.88	$4356.23	090	C+ M
46750	Repair of anal sphincter	12.15	NA	8.19	1.94	NA	NA	22.28	$771.03	090	C+ M
46751	Repair of anal sphincter	9.30	NA	8.50	2.33	NA	NA	20.13	$696.62	090	C+ M
46753	Reconstruction of anus	8.89	NA	7.52	2.23	NA	NA	18.64	$645.06	090	A M
46754	Removal of suture from anus	3.01	6.97	3.69	0.40	10.38	$359.21	7.10	$245.70	010	A+ M
46760	Repair of anal sphincter	17.45	NA	12.79	2.29	NA	NA	32.53	$1125.74	090	C+ M
46761	Repair of anal sphincter	15.29	NA	9.37	2.50	NA	NA	27.16	$939.90	090	C+ M
46900	Destruction anal lesion(s)	1.91	4.98	1.87	0.25	7.14	$247.09	4.03	$139.46	010	A M
46910	Destruction anal lesion(s)	1.91	5.78	1.78	0.31	8.00	$276.85	4.00	$138.42	010	A M
46916	Cryosurgery anal lesion(s)	1.91	5.71	2.04	0.20	7.82	$270.62	4.15	$143.62	010	A M

46917		Laser surgery anal lesions	1.91	11.02	1.56	0.29	13.22	$457.49	3.76	$130.12	010	A M
46922		Excision of anal lesion(s)	1.91	7.30	1.82	0.34	9.55	$330.49	4.07	$140.85	010	A M
46924		Destruction anal lesion(s)	2.81	13.46	2.08	0.42	16.69	$577.58	5.31	$183.76	010	A M
46930		Destroy internal hemorrhoids	1.61	4.73	2.72	0.22	6.56	$227.02	4.55	$157.46	090	A+ M
46940		Treatment of anal fissure	2.35	5.32	1.58	0.33	8.00	$276.85	4.26	$147.42	010	A M
46942		Treatment of anal fissure	2.07	5.27	1.47	0.28	7.62	$263.70	3.82	$132.20	010	A+ M
46945		Int hrhc lig 1 hroid w/o img	3.69	NA	5.87	0.60	NA	NA	10.16	$351.60	090	A M
46946		Int hrhc lig 2+hroid w/o img	4.50	NA	6.22	0.73	NA	NA	11.45	$396.24	090	A M
46947		Hemorrhoidopexy by stapling	5.57	NA	4.83	1.20	NA	NA	11.60	$401.43	090	A M
46948		Int hrhc tranal dartlzj 2+	5.57	NA	6.69	1.11	NA	NA	13.37	$462.68	090	A M
46999	CP	Anus surgery procedure	0.00	0.00	0.00	0.00	0.00	$0.00	0.00	$0.00	YYY	A+ C+ M T+
47000		Needle biopsy of liver	1.65	7.40	0.76	0.14	9.19	$318.03	2.55	$88.25	000	A M
47001		Needle biopsy liver add-on	1.90	NA	0.71	0.45	NA	NA	3.06	$105.89	ZZZ	A C+
47010		Open drainage liver lesion	19.40	NA	12.08	4.78	NA	NA	36.26	$1254.82	090	C+ M
47015		Inject/aspirate liver cyst	18.50	NA	11.72	4.67	NA	NA	34.89	$1207.41	090	C+ M
47100		Wedge biopsy of liver	12.91	NA	9.32	3.16	NA	NA	25.39	$878.65	090	C+ M
47120		Partial removal of liver	39.01	NA	20.96	9.49	NA	NA	69.46	$2403.75	090	C+ M
47122		Extensive removal of liver	59.48	NA	28.05	14.57	NA	NA	102.10	$3533.29	090	C+ M
47125		Partial removal of liver	53.04	NA	25.30	13.14	NA	NA	91.48	$3165.78	090	C+ M
47130		Partial removal of liver	57.19	NA	26.95	14.00	NA	NA	98.14	$3396.25	090	C+ M
47135		Transplantation of liver	90.00	NA	47.67	22.31	NA	NA	159.98	$5536.30	090	C+ M T
47140		Partial removal donor liver	59.40	NA	31.79	15.01	NA	NA	106.20	$3675.18	090	C+ M T
47141		Partial removal donor liver	71.50	NA	37.39	18.06	NA	NA	126.95	$4393.26	090	C+ M T
47142		Partial removal donor liver	79.44	NA	40.25	19.82	NA	NA	139.51	$4827.91	090	C+ M
47143	CP	Prep donor liver whole	0.00	0.00	0.00	0.00	0.00	$0.00	0.00	$0.00	XXX	C+ M
47144	CP	Prep donor liver 3-segment	0.00	0.00	0.00	0.00	0.00	$0.00	0.00	$0.00	090	C+ M
47145	CP	Prep donor liver lobe split	0.00	0.00	0.00	0.00	0.00	$0.00	0.00	$0.00	XXX	C+ M
47146		Prep donor liver/venous	6.00	NA	2.23	1.49	NA	NA	9.72	$336.37	XXX	C+ M

*Please note that these calculations are based on the Medicare 2022 Conversion Factor of $34.6062 and the DRA RVU cap rates at time of publication.

A = assistant-at-surgery restriction
A+ = assistant-at-surgery restriction unless medical necessity established with documentation
B = bilateral surgery adjustment applies
C = cosurgeons payable
C+ = cosurgeons payable if medical necessity established with documentation
CP = carriers may establish RVUs and payment amounts for these services, generally on an individual basis following review of documentation such as an operative report
M = multiple surgery adjustment applies
Me = multiple endoscopy rules may apply
M+ = multiple therapy rules apply
Mtc = multiple diagnostic imaging rules apply
T = team surgeons permitted
T+ = team surgeons payable if medical necessity established with documentation
§ = indicates code is not covered by Medicare
GS = procedure must be performed under the general supervision of a physician
DS = procedure must be performed under the direct supervision of a physician
PS = procedure must be performed under the personal supervision of a physician
DRA = procedure subject to DRA limitation

Relative Value Units

CPT Code and Modifier		Description	Work RVU	Nonfacility Practice Expense RVU	Facility Practice Expense RVU	PLI RVU	Total Non-facility RVUs	Medicare Payment Nonfacility	Total Facility RVUs	Medicare Payment Facility	Global Period	Payment Policy Indicators
47147		Prep donor liver/arterial	7.00	NA	2.59	1.70	NA	NA	11.29	$390.70	XXX	C+ M
47300		Surgery for liver lesion	18.14	NA	11.27	4.44	NA	NA	33.85	$1171.42	090	C+ M
47350		Repair liver wound	22.49	NA	12.99	5.33	NA	NA	40.81	$1412.28	090	C+ M
47360		Repair liver wound	31.31	NA	16.81	7.90	NA	NA	56.02	$1938.64	090	C+ M
47361		Repair liver wound	52.60	NA	24.50	12.58	NA	NA	89.68	$3103.48	090	C+ M
47362		Repair liver wound	23.54	NA	13.70	5.32	NA	NA	42.56	$1472.84	090	C+ M
47370		Laparo ablate liver tumor rf	20.80	NA	11.41	5.10	NA	NA	37.31	$1291.16	090	C+ M
47371		Laparo ablate liver cryosurg	20.80	NA	11.56	5.27	NA	NA	37.63	$1302.23	090	C+ M
47379	CP	Laparoscope procedure liver	0.00	0.00	0.00	0.00	0.00	$0.00	0.00	$0.00	YYY	C+ M T+
47380		Open ablate liver tumor rf	24.56	NA	12.63	5.89	NA	NA	43.08	$1490.84	090	C+ M
47381		Open ablate liver tumor cryo	24.88	NA	13.08	6.28	NA	NA	44.24	$1530.98	090	C+ M
47382		Percut ablate liver rf	14.97	97.90	5.00	1.39	114.26	$3954.10	21.36	$739.19	010	A M
47383		Perq abltj lvr cryoablation	8.88	175.79	3.25	0.84	185.51	$6419.80	12.97	$448.84	010	A M
47399	CP	Liver surgery procedure	0.00	0.00	0.00	0.00	0.00	$0.00	0.00	$0.00	YYY	A C+ M T+
47400		Incision of liver duct	36.36	NA	18.69	9.18	NA	NA	64.23	$2222.76	090	C+ M
47420		Incision of bile duct	22.03	NA	12.36	5.43	NA	NA	39.82	$1378.02	090	C+ M
47425		Incision of bile duct	22.31	NA	12.98	5.62	NA	NA	40.91	$1415.74	090	C+ M
47460		Incise bile duct sphincter	20.52	NA	12.31	5.19	NA	NA	38.02	$1315.73	090	C+ M
47480		Incision of gallbladder	13.25	NA	9.78	3.12	NA	NA	26.15	$904.95	090	C+ M
47490		Incision of gallbladder	4.76	NA	4.57	0.42	NA	NA	9.75	$337.41	010	A M
47531		Injection for cholangiogram	1.30	11.78	0.62	0.11	13.19	$456.46	2.03	$70.25	000	A M
47532		Injection for cholangiogram	4.25	21.33	1.46	0.41	25.99	$899.42	6.12	$211.79	000	A M
47533		Plmt biliary drainage cath	5.38	30.26	1.78	0.50	36.14	$1250.67	7.66	$265.08	000	A M
47534		Plmt biliary drainage cath	7.60	31.09	2.39	0.68	39.37	$1362.45	10.67	$369.25	000	A M
47535		Conversion ext bil drg cath	3.95	23.20	1.36	0.35	27.50	$951.67	5.66	$195.87	000	A M
47536		Exchange biliary drg cath	2.61	16.89	0.95	0.24	19.74	$683.13	3.80	$131.50	000	A M
47537		Removal biliary drg cath	1.84	13.28	0.77	0.18	15.30	$529.47	2.79	$96.55	000	A M
47538		Perq plmt bile duct stent	4.75	113.39	1.60	0.42	118.56	$4102.91	6.77	$234.28	000	A M
47539		Perq plmt bile duct stent	8.75	121.81	2.60	0.86	131.42	$4547.95	12.21	$422.54	000	A M
47540		Perq plmt bile duct stent	9.03	123.24	2.83	0.84	133.11	$4606.43	12.70	$439.50	000	A M
47541		Plmt access bil tree sm bwl	6.75	28.35	2.26	0.65	35.75	$1237.17	9.66	$334.30	000	A M
47542		Dilate biliary duct/ampulla	2.85	12.27	0.81	0.25	15.37	$531.90	3.91	$135.31	ZZZ	A
47543		Endoluminal bx biliary tree	3.00	8.76	0.88	0.25	12.01	$415.62	4.13	$142.92	ZZZ	A

47544		Removal duct glbldr calculi	3.28	22.48	0.91	0.31	26.07	$902.18	4.50	$155.73	ZZZ	A
47550		Bile duct endoscopy add-on	3.02	NA	1.13	0.73	NA	NA	4.88	$168.88	ZZZ	C+
47552		Biliary endo perq dx w/speci	6.03	NA	1.34	0.60	NA	NA	7.97	$275.81	000	A C+ M
47553		Biliary endoscopy thru skin	6.34	NA	1.04	0.65	NA	NA	8.03	$277.89	000	A Me
47554		Biliary endoscopy thru skin	9.05	NA	3.94	2.28	NA	NA	15.27	$528.44	000	A C+ Me
47555		Biliary endoscopy thru skin	7.55	NA	1.23	0.77	NA	NA	9.55	$330.49	000	A Me
47556		Biliary endoscopy thru skin	8.55	NA	1.39	0.89	NA	NA	10.83	$374.79	000	A Me
47562		Laparoscopic cholecystectomy	10.47	NA	6.68	2.61	NA	NA	19.76	$683.82	090	C+ M
47563		Laparo cholecystectomy/graph	11.47	NA	7.18	2.85	NA	NA	21.50	$744.03	090	C+ M
47564		Laparo cholecystectomy/explr	18.00	NA	10.91	4.45	NA	NA	33.36	$1154.46	090	C+ M
47570		Laparo cholecystoenterostomy	12.56	NA	7.49	3.18	NA	NA	23.23	$803.90	090	C+ M
47579	CP	Laparoscope proc biliary	0.00	0.00	0.00	0.00	0.00	$0.00	0.00	$0.00	YYY	B C+ M T+
47600		Removal of gallbladder	17.48	NA	10.19	4.26	NA	NA	31.93	$1104.98	090	C+ M
47605		Removal of gallbladder	18.48	NA	10.65	4.57	NA	NA	33.70	$1166.23	090	C+ M
47610		Removal of gallbladder	20.92	NA	11.38	5.18	NA	NA	37.48	$1297.04	090	C+ M
47612		Removal of gallbladder	21.21	NA	11.53	5.36	NA	NA	38.10	$1318.50	090	C+ M
47620		Removal of gallbladder	23.07	NA	12.22	5.83	NA	NA	41.12	$1423.01	090	C+ M
47700		Exploration of bile ducts	16.50	NA	11.11	4.18	NA	NA	31.79	$1100.13	090	C+ M
47701		Bile duct revision	28.73	NA	15.98	7.25	NA	NA	51.96	$1798.14	090	A+ M
47711		Excision of bile duct tumor	25.90	NA	14.21	6.34	NA	NA	46.45	$1607.46	090	C+ M
47712		Excision of bile duct tumor	33.72	NA	17.39	8.53	NA	NA	59.64	$2063.91	090	C+ M
47715		Excision of bile duct cyst	21.55	NA	12.85	5.43	NA	NA	39.83	$1378.36	090	C+ M
47720		Fuse gallbladder & bowel	18.34	NA	11.66	4.62	NA	NA	34.62	$1198.07	090	C+ M
47721		Fuse upper gi structures	21.99	NA	13.02	5.55	NA	NA	40.56	$1403.63	090	C+ M
47740		Fuse gallbladder & bowel	21.23	NA	12.73	5.38	NA	NA	39.34	$1361.41	090	C+ M
47741		Fuse gallbladder & bowel	24.21	NA	13.85	6.12	NA	NA	44.18	$1528.90	090	C+ M
47760		Fuse bile ducts and bowel	38.32	NA	19.26	9.44	NA	NA	67.02	$2319.31	090	C+ M
47765		Fuse liver ducts & bowel	52.19	NA	25.05	13.17	NA	NA	90.41	$3128.75	090	C+ M

*Please note that these calculations are based on the Medicare 2022 Conversion Factor of $34.6062 and the DRA RVU cap rates at time of publication.

A = assistant-at-surgery restriction
A+ = assistant-at-surgery restriction unless medical necessity established with documentation
B = bilateral surgery adjustment applies
C = cosurgeons payable
C+ = cosurgeons payable if medical necessity established with documentation
CP = carriers may establish RVUs and payment amounts for these services, generally on an individual basis following review of documentation such as an operative report
M = multiple surgery adjustment applies
Me = multiple endoscopy rules may apply
M+ = multiple therapy rules apply
Mtc = multiple diagnostic imaging rules apply
T = team surgeons permitted
T+ = team surgeons payable if medical necessity established with documentation
§ = indicates code is not covered by Medicare
GS = procedure must be performed under the general supervision of a physician
DS = procedure must be performed under the direct supervision of a physician
PS = procedure must be performed under the personal supervision of a physician
DRA = procedure subject to DRA limitation

Relative Value Units

CPT Code and Modifier		Description	Work RVU	Nonfacility Practice Expense RVU	Facility Practice Expense RVU	PLI RVU	Total Non-facility RVUs	Medicare Payment Nonfacility	Total Facility RVUs	Medicare Payment Facility	Global Period	Payment Policy Indicators
47780		Fuse bile ducts and bowel	42.32	NA	20.81	10.45	NA	NA	73.58	$2546.32	090	C+ M
47785		Fuse bile ducts and bowel	56.19	NA	26.21	13.51	NA	NA	95.91	$3319.08	090	C+ M
47800		Reconstruction of bile ducts	26.17	NA	14.08	5.58	NA	NA	45.83	$1586.00	090	C+ M
47801		Placement bile duct support	17.60	NA	11.39	4.45	NA	NA	33.44	$1157.23	090	C+ M
47802		Fuse liver duct & intestine	24.93	NA	14.43	6.29	NA	NA	45.65	$1579.77	090	C+ M
47900		Suture bile duct injury	22.44	NA	12.79	5.54	NA	NA	40.77	$1410.89	090	C+ M
47999	CP	Bile tract surgery procedure	0.00	0.00	0.00	0.00	0.00	$0.00	0.00	$0.00	YYY	A C+ M T+
48000		Drainage of abdomen	31.95	NA	16.18	8.08	NA	NA	56.21	$1945.21	090	C+ M
48001		Placement of drain pancreas	39.69	NA	19.07	10.04	NA	NA	68.80	$2380.91	090	C+ M
48020		Removal of pancreatic stone	19.09	NA	11.39	4.83	NA	NA	35.31	$1221.94	090	C+ M
48100		Biopsy of pancreas open	14.46	NA	8.43	3.33	NA	NA	26.22	$907.37	090	C+ M
48102		Needle biopsy pancreas	4.70	10.59	1.74	0.41	15.70	$543.32	6.85	$237.05	010	A M
48105		Resect/debride pancreas	49.26	NA	24.00	11.22	NA	NA	84.48	$2923.53	090	C+ M
48120		Removal of pancreas lesion	18.41	NA	10.06	4.45	NA	NA	32.92	$1139.24	090	C+ M
48140		Partial removal of pancreas	26.32	NA	13.83	6.42	NA	NA	46.57	$1611.61	090	C+ M
48145		Partial removal of pancreas	27.39	NA	14.49	6.90	NA	NA	48.78	$1688.09	090	C+ M
48146		Pancreatectomy	30.60	NA	18.08	7.73	NA	NA	56.41	$1952.14	090	C+ M
48148		Removal of pancreatic duct	20.39	NA	11.88	5.15	NA	NA	37.42	$1294.96	090	C+ M
48150		Partial removal of pancreas	52.84	NA	26.84	12.95	NA	NA	92.63	$3205.57	090	C+ M
48152		Pancreatectomy	48.65	NA	25.31	12.29	NA	NA	86.25	$2984.78	090	C+ M
48153		Pancreatectomy	52.79	NA	26.55	13.12	NA	NA	92.46	$3199.69	090	C+ M
48154		Pancreatectomy	48.88	NA	25.40	12.35	NA	NA	86.63	$2997.94	090	C+ M
48155		Removal of pancreas	29.45	NA	17.67	7.18	NA	NA	54.30	$1879.12	090	C+ M
48400		Injection intraop add-on	1.95	NA	0.73	0.50	NA	NA	3.18	$110.05	ZZZ	A+
48500		Surgery of pancreatic cyst	18.16	NA	11.71	4.60	NA	NA	34.47	$1192.88	090	C+ M
48510		Drain pancreatic pseudocyst	17.19	NA	11.35	4.33	NA	NA	32.87	$1137.51	090	C+ M
48520		Fuse pancreas cyst and bowel	18.15	NA	10.19	4.60	NA	NA	32.94	$1139.93	090	C+ M
48540		Fuse pancreas cyst and bowel	21.94	NA	11.61	5.54	NA	NA	39.09	$1352.76	090	C+ M
48545		Pancreatorrhaphy	22.23	NA	12.41	5.61	NA	NA	40.25	$1392.90	090	C+ M
48547		Duodenal exclusion	30.38	NA	15.45	7.67	NA	NA	53.50	$1851.43	090	C+ M
48548		Fuse pancreas and bowel	28.09	NA	14.75	7.10	NA	NA	49.94	$1728.23	090	C+ M
48551	CP	Prep donor pancreas	0.00	0.00	0.00	0.00	0.00	$0.00	0.00	$0.00	XXX	C+ M
48552		Prep donor pancreas/venous	4.30	NA	1.60	1.09	NA	NA	6.99	$241.90	XXX	C+ M

48554		Transpl allograft pancreas	37.80	NA	30.34	9.39	NA	NA	77.53	$2683.02	090	C M T
48556		Removal allograft pancreas	19.47	NA	13.97	4.93	NA	NA	38.37	$1327.84	090	C M T
48999	CP	Pancreas surgery procedure	0.00	0.00	0.00	0.00	0.00	$0.00	0.00	$0.00	YYY	C+ M T+
49000		Exploration of abdomen	12.54	NA	7.45	2.93	NA	NA	22.92	$793.17	090	C+ M
49002		Reopening of abdomen	17.63	NA	9.27	4.16	NA	NA	31.06	$1074.87	090	C+ M
49010		Exploration behind abdomen	16.06	NA	7.69	3.71	NA	NA	27.46	$950.29	090	C+ M
49013		Prpertl pel pack hemrrg trma	8.35	NA	3.11	2.11	NA	NA	13.57	$469.61	000	A M
49014		Reexploration pelvic wound	6.73	NA	2.85	1.69	NA	NA	11.27	$390.01	000	A M
49020		Drainage abdom abscess open	26.67	NA	14.60	6.18	NA	NA	47.45	$1642.06	090	M
49040		Drain open abdom abscess	16.52	NA	9.57	3.95	NA	NA	30.04	$1039.57	090	C+ M
49060		Drain open retroperi abscess	18.53	NA	9.98	4.18	NA	NA	32.69	$1131.28	090	A C+ M
49062		Drain to peritoneal cavity	12.22	NA	7.68	3.06	NA	NA	22.96	$794.56	090	C+ M
49082		Abd paracentesis	1.24	5.05	0.73	0.19	6.48	$224.25	2.16	$74.75	000	A M
49083		Abd paracentesis w/imaging	2.00	6.78	0.91	0.19	8.97	$310.42	3.10	$107.28	000	A M
49084		Peritoneal lavage	2.00	NA	0.74	0.42	NA	NA	3.16	$109.36	000	A M
49180		Biopsy abdominal mass	1.73	3.35	0.54	0.14	5.22	$180.64	2.41	$83.40	000	A M
49185		Sclerotx fluid collection	2.35	37.00	0.87	0.23	39.58	$1369.71	3.45	$119.39	000	A
49203		Exc abd tum 5 cm or less	20.13	NA	10.97	4.43	NA	NA	35.53	$1229.56	090	C+ M
49204		Exc abd tum over 5 cm	26.13	NA	13.42	5.58	NA	NA	45.13	$1561.78	090	C+ M
49205		Exc abd tum over 10 cm	30.13	NA	15.11	6.50	NA	NA	51.74	$1790.52	090	C+ M
49215		Excise sacral spine tumor	37.81	NA	19.95	7.94	NA	NA	65.70	$2273.63	090	C+ M
49250		Excision of umbilicus	9.01	NA	6.61	2.08	NA	NA	17.70	$612.53	090	A C+ M
49255		Removal of omentum	12.56	NA	8.29	2.68	NA	NA	23.53	$814.28	090	C+ M
49320		Diag laparo separate proc	5.14	NA	3.47	1.18	NA	NA	9.79	$338.79	010	M
49321		Laparoscopy biopsy	5.44	NA	3.62	1.20	NA	NA	10.26	$355.06	010	C Me
49322		Laparoscopy aspiration	6.01	NA	3.80	1.37	NA	NA	11.18	$386.90	010	C Me
49323		Laparo drain lymphocele	10.23	NA	6.40	2.25	NA	NA	18.88	$653.37	090	C Me
49324		Lap insert tunnel ip cath	6.32	NA	3.70	1.55	NA	NA	11.57	$400.39	010	C Me

*Please note that these calculations are based on the Medicare 2022 Conversion Factor of $34.6062 and the DRA RVU cap rates at time of publication.

A = assistant-at-surgery restriction
A+ = assistant-at-surgery restriction unless medical necessity established with documentation
B = bilateral surgery adjustment applies
C = cosurgeons payable
C+ = cosurgeons payable if medical necessity established with documentation
CP = carriers may establish RVUs and payment amounts for these services, generally on an individual basis following review of documentation such as an operative report
M = multiple surgery adjustment applies
Me = multiple endoscopy rules may apply
M+ = multiple therapy rules apply
Mtc = multiple diagnostic imaging rules apply
T = team surgeons permitted
T+ = team surgeons payable if medical necessity established with documentation
§ = indicates code is not covered by Medicare
GS = procedure must be performed under the general supervision of a physician
DS = procedure must be performed under the direct supervision of a physician
PS = procedure must be performed under the personal supervision of a physician
DRA = procedure subject to DRA limitation

Relative Value Units

CPT Code and Modifier		Description	Work RVU	Nonfacility Practice Expense RVU	Facility Practice Expense RVU	PLI RVU	Total Non-facility RVUs	Medicare Payment Nonfacility	Total Facility RVUs	Medicare Payment Facility	Global Period	Payment Policy Indicators
49325		Lap revision perm ip cath	6.82	NA	3.85	1.69	NA	NA	12.36	$427.73	010	C Me
49326		Lap w/omentopexy add-on	3.50	NA	1.22	0.89	NA	NA	5.61	$194.14	ZZZ	C+
49327		Lap ins device for rt	2.38	NA	0.89	0.60	NA	NA	3.87	$133.93	ZZZ	C+
49329	CP	Laparo proc abdm/per/oment	0.00	0.00	0.00	0.00	0.00	$0.00	0.00	$0.00	YYY	B C+ M T+
49400		Air injection into abdomen	1.88	2.46	0.57	0.20	4.54	$157.11	2.65	$91.71	000	A M
49402		Remove foreign body adbomen	14.09	NA	8.01	3.34	NA	NA	25.44	$880.38	090	A C+ M
49405		Image cath fluid colxn visc	4.00	23.06	1.31	0.35	27.41	$948.56	5.66	$195.87	000	A M
49406		Image cath fluid peri/retro	4.00	23.05	1.30	0.35	27.40	$948.21	5.65	$195.53	000	A M
49407		Image cath fluid trns/vgnl	4.25	18.40	1.33	0.41	23.06	$798.02	5.99	$207.29	000	A M
49411		Ins mark abd/pel for rt perq	3.57	10.70	1.45	0.31	14.58	$504.56	5.33	$184.45	000	A+ M
49412		Ins device for rt guide open	1.50	NA	0.56	0.39	NA	NA	2.45	$84.79	ZZZ	A+ C+
49418		Insert tun ip cath perc	3.96	26.16	1.49	0.40	30.52	$1056.18	5.85	$202.45	000	A+ M
49419		Insert tun ip cath w/port	7.08	NA	4.14	1.41	NA	NA	12.63	$437.08	090	A M
49421		Ins tun ip cath for dial opn	4.21	NA	1.52	0.99	NA	NA	6.72	$232.55	000	A M
49422		Remove tunneled ip cath	4.00	NA	1.63	0.94	NA	NA	6.57	$227.36	000	A M
49423		Exchange drainage catheter	1.46	16.88	0.45	0.12	18.46	$638.83	2.03	$70.25	000	A+ M
49424		Assess cyst contrast inject	0.76	4.82	0.26	0.08	5.66	$195.87	1.10	$38.07	000	A+ M
49425		Insert abdomen-venous drain	12.22	NA	6.51	1.94	NA	NA	20.67	$715.31	090	C+ M
49426		Revise abdomen-venous shunt	10.41	NA	7.04	2.63	NA	NA	20.08	$694.89	090	A M
49427		Injection abdominal shunt	0.89	NA	0.15	0.09	NA	NA	1.13	$39.11	000	A+ M
49428		Ligation of shunt	6.87	NA	4.28	1.72	NA	NA	12.87	$445.38	010	A M
49429		Removal of shunt	7.44	NA	4.37	1.86	NA	NA	13.67	$473.07	010	A M
49435		Insert subq exten to ip cath	2.25	NA	0.72	0.56	NA	NA	3.53	$122.16	ZZZ	C+
49436		Embedded ip cath exit-site	2.72	NA	2.23	0.67	NA	NA	5.62	$194.49	010	C+ M
49440		Place gastrostomy tube perc	3.93	21.43	1.58	0.39	25.75	$891.11	5.90	$204.18	010	A+ M
49441		Place duod/jej tube perc	4.52	24.03	1.86	0.57	29.12	$1007.73	6.95	$240.51	010	A+ M
49442		Place cecostomy tube perc	3.75	20.52	1.93	0.31	24.58	$850.62	5.99	$207.29	010	A+ M
49446		Change g-tube to g-j perc	3.06	21.39	0.91	0.28	24.73	$855.81	4.25	$147.08	000	A+ M
49450		Replace g/c tube perc	1.36	17.06	0.41	0.12	18.54	$641.60	1.89	$65.41	000	A+ M
49451		Replace duod/jej tube perc	1.84	17.89	0.56	0.19	19.92	$689.36	2.59	$89.63	000	A+ M
49452		Replace g-j tube perc	2.86	20.99	0.85	0.25	24.10	$834.01	3.96	$137.04	000	A+ M
49460		Fix g/colon tube w/device	0.96	19.73	0.35	0.11	20.80	$719.81	1.42	$49.14	000	A+ M
49465		Fluoro exam of g/colon tube	0.62	3.43	0.21	0.05	4.10	$141.89	0.88	$30.45	000	A+ M

49491	Rpr hern preemie reduc	12.53	NA	8.22	3.17	NA	NA	23.92	$827.78	090	B C+ M
49492	Rpr ing hern premie blocked	15.43	NA	9.41	3.90	NA	NA	28.74	$994.58	090	B C+ M
49495	Rpr ing hernia baby reduc	6.20	NA	4.48	1.55	NA	NA	12.23	$423.23	090	B C+ M
49496	Rpr ing hernia baby blocked	9.42	NA	6.65	2.38	NA	NA	18.45	$638.48	090	B C+ M
49500	Rpr ing hernia init reduce	5.84	NA	5.14	1.47	NA	NA	12.45	$430.85	090	B C+ M
49501	Rpr ing hernia init blocked	9.36	NA	6.46	2.36	NA	NA	18.18	$629.14	090	B C+ M
49505	Prp i/hern init reduc >5 yr	7.96	NA	5.72	1.98	NA	NA	15.66	$541.93	090	B C+ M
49507	Prp i/hern init block >5 yr	9.09	NA	6.26	2.23	NA	NA	17.58	$608.38	090	B C+ M
49520	Rerepair ing hernia reduce	9.99	NA	6.49	2.49	NA	NA	18.97	$656.48	090	B C+ M
49521	Rerepair ing hernia blocked	11.48	NA	7.11	2.84	NA	NA	21.43	$741.61	090	B C+ M
49525	Repair ing hernia sliding	8.93	NA	6.05	2.20	NA	NA	17.18	$594.53	090	B C+ M
49540	Repair lumbar hernia	10.74	NA	6.93	2.57	NA	NA	20.24	$700.43	090	B C+ M
49550	Rpr rem hernia init reduce	8.99	NA	6.07	2.20	NA	NA	17.26	$597.30	090	B C+ M
49553	Rpr fem hernia init blocked	9.92	NA	6.58	2.45	NA	NA	18.95	$655.79	090	B C+ M
49555	Rerepair fem hernia reduce	9.39	NA	6.37	2.37	NA	NA	18.13	$627.41	090	B C+ M
49557	Rerepair fem hernia blocked	11.62	NA	7.17	2.89	NA	NA	21.68	$750.26	090	B C+ M
49560	Rpr ventral hern init reduc	11.92	NA	7.23	2.90	NA	NA	22.05	$763.07	090	B C+ M
49561	Rpr ventral hern init block	15.38	NA	8.59	3.77	NA	NA	27.74	$959.98	090	B C+ M
49565	Rerepair ventrl hern reduce	12.37	NA	7.58	3.00	NA	NA	22.95	$794.21	090	B C+ M
49566	Rerepair ventrl hern block	15.53	NA	8.66	3.79	NA	NA	27.98	$968.28	090	B C+ M
49568	Hernia repair w/mesh	4.88	NA	1.83	1.18	NA	NA	7.89	$273.04	ZZZ	C+
49570	Rpr epigastric hern reduce	6.05	NA	5.03	1.49	NA	NA	12.57	$435.00	090	B C+ M
49572	Rpr epigastric hern blocked	7.87	NA	5.73	1.96	NA	NA	15.56	$538.47	090	B C+ M
49580	Rpr umbil hern reduc < 5 yr	4.47	NA	4.53	1.11	NA	NA	10.11	$349.87	090	C+ M
49582	Rpr umbil hern block < 5 yr	7.13	NA	5.63	1.81	NA	NA	14.57	$504.21	090	C+ M
49585	Rpr umbil hern reduc > 5 yr	6.59	NA	5.20	1.62	NA	NA	13.41	$464.07	090	C+ M
49587	Rpr umbil hern block > 5 yr	7.08	NA	5.51	1.73	NA	NA	14.32	$495.56	090	C+ M
49590	Repair spigelian hernia	8.90	NA	6.09	2.18	NA	NA	17.17	$594.19	090	B C+ M

*Please note that these calculations are based on the Medicare 2022 Conversion Factor of $34.6062 and the DRA RVU cap rates at time of publication.

A = assistant-at-surgery restriction

A+ = assistant-at-surgery restriction unless medical necessity established with documentation

B = bilateral surgery adjustment applies

C = cosurgeons payable

C+ = cosurgeons payable if medical necessity established with documentation

CP = carriers may establish RVUs and payment amounts for these services, generally on an individual basis following review of documentation such as an operative report

M = multiple surgery adjustment applies

Me = multiple endoscopy rules may apply

M+ = multiple therapy rules apply

Mtc = multiple diagnostic imaging rules apply

T = team surgeons permitted

T+ = team surgeons payable if medical necessity established with documentation

§ = indicates code is not covered by Medicare

GS = procedure must be performed under the general supervision of a physician

DS = procedure must be performed under the direct supervision of a physician

PS = procedure must be performed under the personal supervision of a physician

DRA = procedure subject to DRA limitation

Relative Value Units

CPT Code and Modifier		Description	Work RVU	Nonfacility Practice Expense RVU	Facility Practice Expense RVU	PLI RVU	Total Non-facility RVUs	Medicare Payment Nonfacility	Total Facility RVUs	Medicare Payment Facility	Global Period	Payment Policy Indicators
49600		Repair umbilical lesion	11.55	NA	7.57	2.92	NA	NA	22.04	$762.72	090	C+ M
49605		Repair umbilical lesion	87.09	NA	37.33	21.99	NA	NA	146.41	$5066.69	090	C+ M
49606		Repair umbilical lesion	19.00	NA	10.15	4.79	NA	NA	33.94	$1174.53	090	C+ M
49610		Repair umbilical lesion	10.91	NA	7.14	2.76	NA	NA	20.81	$720.16	090	C+ M
49611		Repair umbilical lesion	9.34	NA	6.65	2.34	NA	NA	18.33	$634.33	090	C+ M
49650		Lap ing hernia repair init	6.36	NA	5.02	1.57	NA	NA	12.95	$448.15	090	B C+ M
49651		Lap ing hernia repair recur	8.38	NA	6.45	2.08	NA	NA	16.91	$585.19	090	B C+ M
49652		Lap vent/abd hernia repair	11.92	NA	7.37	2.95	NA	NA	22.24	$769.64	090	B C+ M
49653		Lap vent/abd hern proc comp	14.94	NA	9.19	3.73	NA	NA	27.86	$964.13	090	B C+ M
49654		Lap inc hernia repair	13.76	NA	8.08	3.39	NA	NA	25.23	$873.11	090	B C+ M
49655		Lap inc hern repair comp	16.84	NA	9.90	4.18	NA	NA	30.92	$1070.02	090	B C+ M
49656		Lap inc hernia repair recur	15.08	NA	8.59	3.74	NA	NA	27.41	$948.56	090	B C+ M
49657		Lap inc hern recur comp	22.11	NA	11.79	5.45	NA	NA	39.35	$1361.75	090	B C+ M
49659	CP	Laparo proc hernia repair	0.00	0.00	0.00	0.00	0.00	$0.00	0.00	$0.00	YYY	B C+ M T+
49900		Repair of abdominal wall	12.41	NA	9.18	2.91	NA	NA	24.50	$847.85	090	C+ M
49904		Omental flap extra-abdom	22.35	NA	14.03	4.82	NA	NA	41.20	$1425.78	090	A C+ M T+
49905		Omental flap intra-abdom	6.54	NA	2.41	1.47	NA	NA	10.42	$360.60	ZZZ	C
49906	CP	Free omental flap microvasc	0.00	0.00	0.00	0.00	0.00	$0.00	0.00	$0.00	090	A C+ M
49999	CP	Abdomen surgery procedure	0.00	0.00	0.00	0.00	0.00	$0.00	0.00	$0.00	YYY	A C+ M T+
50010		Exploration of kidney	12.28	NA	6.88	1.47	NA	NA	20.63	$713.93	090	B C+ M
50020		Renal abscess open drain	18.08	NA	9.43	2.17	NA	NA	29.68	$1027.11	090	A C+ M
50040		Drainage of kidney	16.68	NA	8.37	1.99	NA	NA	27.04	$935.75	090	A B C+ M
50045		Exploration of kidney	16.82	NA	8.42	2.01	NA	NA	27.25	$943.02	090	B C+ M
50060		Removal of kidney stone	20.95	NA	9.81	2.49	NA	NA	33.25	$1150.66	090	B C+ M
50065		Incision of kidney	22.32	NA	10.27	2.66	NA	NA	35.25	$1219.87	090	B M
50070		Incision of kidney	21.85	NA	10.11	2.62	NA	NA	34.58	$1196.68	090	B C+ M
50075		Removal of kidney stone	27.09	NA	12.17	3.23	NA	NA	42.49	$1470.42	090	B C+ M
50080		Removal of kidney stone	15.74	NA	7.76	1.86	NA	NA	25.36	$877.61	090	A B M
50081		Removal of kidney stone	23.50	NA	10.98	2.82	NA	NA	37.30	$1290.81	090	B C+ M
50100		Revise kidney blood vessels	17.45	NA	10.48	4.42	NA	NA	32.35	$1119.51	090	B C+ M
50120		Exploration of kidney	17.21	NA	8.48	2.04	NA	NA	27.73	$959.63	090	B C+ M
50125		Explore and drain kidney	17.82	NA	8.76	2.14	NA	NA	28.72	$993.89	090	B C+ M
50130		Removal of kidney stone	18.82	NA	9.10	2.23	NA	NA	30.15	$1043.38	090	B C+ M

50135		Exploration of kidney	20.59	NA	9.69	2.46	NA	NA	32.74	$1133.01	090	B C+ M
50200		Renal biopsy perq	2.38	13.33	1.10	0.22	15.93	$551.28	3.70	$128.04	000	A B M
50205		Renal biopsy open	12.29	NA	7.29	2.85	NA	NA	22.43	$776.22	090	B C+ M
50220		Remove kidney open	18.68	NA	9.40	2.85	NA	NA	30.93	$1070.37	090	B C+ M
50225		Removal kidney open complex	21.88	NA	10.25	3.06	NA	NA	35.19	$1217.79	090	B C+ M
50230		Removal kidney open radical	23.81	NA	10.47	3.12	NA	NA	37.40	$1294.27	090	B C M
50234		Removal of kidney & ureter	24.05	NA	10.96	3.12	NA	NA	38.13	$1319.53	090	B C+ M
50236		Removal of kidney & ureter	26.94	NA	12.57	3.27	NA	NA	42.78	$1480.45	090	B C+ M
50240		Partial removal of kidney	24.21	NA	11.56	2.98	NA	NA	38.75	$1340.99	090	B C+ M
50250		Cryoablate renal mass open	22.22	NA	10.65	2.66	NA	NA	35.53	$1229.56	090	C+ M
50280		Removal of kidney lesion	17.09	NA	8.67	2.37	NA	NA	28.13	$973.47	090	B C+ M
50290		Removal of kidney lesion	16.15	NA	8.19	1.94	NA	NA	26.28	$909.45	090	C+ M
50320		Remove kidney living donor	22.43	NA	17.16	5.65	NA	NA	45.24	$1565.58	090	B C+ M
50323	CP	Prep cadaver renal allograft	0.00	0.00	0.00	0.00	0.00	$0.00	0.00	$0.00	XXX	C+ M
50325	CP	Prep donor renal graft	0.00	0.00	0.00	0.00	0.00	$0.00	0.00	$0.00	XXX	C+ M
50327		Prep renal graft/venous	4.00	NA	1.46	0.95	NA	NA	6.41	$221.83	XXX	C+ M
50328		Prep renal graft/arterial	3.50	NA	1.29	0.83	NA	NA	5.62	$194.49	XXX	C+ M
50329		Prep renal graft/ureteral	3.34	NA	1.23	0.75	NA	NA	5.32	$184.10	XXX	C+ M
50340		Removal of kidney	14.04	NA	10.99	3.55	NA	NA	28.58	$989.05	090	B C+ M
50360		Transplantation of kidney	39.88	NA	22.73	9.60	NA	NA	72.21	$2498.91	090	C M T
50365		Transplantation of kidney	46.13	NA	29.03	10.97	NA	NA	86.13	$2980.63	090	B C M T
50370		Remove transplanted kidney	18.88	NA	12.81	4.46	NA	NA	36.15	$1251.01	090	C+ M
50380		Reimplantation of kidney	30.11	NA	22.96	7.61	NA	NA	60.68	$2099.90	090	C+ M
50382		Change ureter stent percut	5.25	25.41	1.57	0.50	31.16	$1078.33	7.32	$253.32	000	A B M
50384		Remove ureter stent percut	4.75	21.44	1.37	0.44	26.63	$921.56	6.56	$227.02	000	A B M
50385		Change stent via transureth	4.19	26.65	1.65	0.44	31.28	$1082.48	6.28	$217.33	000	A+ B M
50386		Remove stent via transureth	3.05	19.70	1.30	0.34	23.09	$799.06	4.69	$162.30	000	A+ B M
50387		Change nephroureteral cath	1.75	15.44	0.50	0.17	17.36	$600.76	2.42	$83.75	000	A+ B M

*Please note that these calculations are based on the Medicare 2022 Conversion Factor of $34.6062 and the DRA RVU cap rates at time of publication.

A = assistant-at-surgery restriction
A+ = assistant-at-surgery restriction unless medical necessity established with documentation
B = bilateral surgery adjustment applies
C = cosurgeons payable
C+ = cosurgeons payable if medical necessity established with documentation
CP = carriers may establish RVUs and payment amounts for these services, generally on an individual basis following review of documentation such as an operative report
M = multiple surgery adjustment applies
Me = multiple endoscopy rules may apply
M+ = multiple therapy rules apply
Mtc = multiple diagnostic imaging rules apply
T = team surgeons permitted
T+ = team surgeons payable if medical necessity established with documentation
§ = indicates code is not covered by Medicare
GS = procedure must be performed under the general supervision of a physician
DS = procedure must be performed under the direct supervision of a physician
PS = procedure must be performed under the personal supervision of a physician
DRA = procedure subject to DRA limitation

Relative Value Units

CPT Code and Modifier		Description	Work RVU	Nonfacility Practice Expense RVU	Facility Practice Expense RVU	PLI RVU	Total Non-facility RVUs	Medicare Payment Nonfacility	Total Facility RVUs	Medicare Payment Facility	Global Period	Payment Policy Indicators
50389		Remove renal tube w/fluoro	1.10	11.78	0.34	0.10	12.98	$449.19	1.54	$53.29	000	A B M
50390		Drainage of kidney lesion	1.96	NA	0.62	0.19	NA	NA	2.77	$95.86	000	A B M
50391		Instll rx agnt into rnal tub	1.96	1.50	0.66	0.23	3.69	$127.70	2.85	$98.63	000	A B M
50396		Measure kidney pressure	2.09	NA	1.11	0.18	NA	NA	3.38	$116.97	000	A+ B M
50400		Revision of kidney/ureter	21.27	NA	9.92	2.54	NA	NA	33.73	$1167.27	090	B C+ M
50405		Revision of kidney/ureter	25.86	NA	11.76	3.06	NA	NA	40.68	$1407.78	090	B C+ M
50430		Njx px nfrosgrm &/urtrgrm	2.90	16.23	1.27	0.28	19.41	$671.71	4.45	$154.00	000	A+ B M
50431		Njx px nfrosgrm &/urtrgrm	1.10	8.78	0.69	0.10	9.98	$345.37	1.89	$65.41	000	A B M
50432		Plmt nephrostomy catheter	4.00	23.66	1.56	0.35	28.01	$969.32	5.91	$204.52	000	A B M
50433		Plmt nephroureteral catheter	5.05	29.40	1.83	0.45	34.90	$1207.76	7.33	$253.66	000	A B M
50434		Convert nephrostomy catheter	3.75	23.98	1.42	0.34	28.07	$971.40	5.51	$190.68	000	A B M
50435		Exchange nephrostomy cath	1.82	16.69	0.89	0.18	18.69	$646.79	2.89	$100.01	000	A B M
50436		Dilat xst trc ndurlgc px	2.78	NA	1.31	0.27	NA	NA	4.36	$150.88	000	A B M
50437		Dilat xst trc new access rcs	4.85	NA	1.92	0.43	NA	NA	7.20	$249.16	000	A B M
50500		Repair of kidney wound	21.22	NA	11.17	4.68	NA	NA	37.07	$1282.85	090	C+ M
50520		Close kidney-skin fistula	18.88	NA	11.01	4.77	NA	NA	34.66	$1199.45	090	C+ M
50525		Close nephrovisceral fistula	24.39	NA	13.39	6.17	NA	NA	43.95	$1520.94	090	C+ M
50526		Close nephrovisceral fistula	26.31	NA	14.10	6.64	NA	NA	47.05	$1628.22	090	M
50540		Revision of horseshoe kidney	21.10	NA	9.86	2.50	NA	NA	33.46	$1157.92	090	C+ M
50541		Laparo ablate renal cyst	16.86	NA	7.87	2.05	NA	NA	26.78	$926.75	090	B C+ M
50542		Laparo ablate renal mass	21.36	NA	10.11	2.61	NA	NA	34.08	$1179.38	090	B C+ M
50543		Laparo partial nephrectomy	27.41	NA	12.77	3.31	NA	NA	43.49	$1505.02	090	B C+ M
50544		Laparoscopy pyeloplasty	23.37	NA	10.05	2.82	NA	NA	36.24	$1254.13	090	B C+ M
50545		Laparo radical nephrectomy	25.06	NA	10.85	3.03	NA	NA	38.94	$1347.57	090	B C+ M
50546		Laparoscopic nephrectomy	21.87	NA	10.46	2.85	NA	NA	35.18	$1217.45	090	B C+ M
50547		Laparo removal donor kidney	26.34	NA	15.71	5.94	NA	NA	47.99	$1660.75	090	B C+ M
50548		Laparo remove w/ureter	25.36	NA	10.74	3.06	NA	NA	39.16	$1355.18	090	B C+ M
50549	CP	Laparoscope proc renal	0.00	0.00	0.00	0.00	0.00	$0.00	0.00	$0.00	YYY	B C+ M T+
50551		Kidney endoscopy	5.59	4.35	2.28	0.66	10.60	$366.83	8.53	$295.19	000	A+ B M
50553		Kidney endoscopy	5.98	4.66	2.41	0.72	11.36	$393.13	9.11	$315.26	000	A B M
50555		Kidney endoscopy & biopsy	6.52	4.80	2.59	0.77	12.09	$418.39	9.88	$341.91	000	A+ B Me
50557		Kidney endoscopy & treatment	6.61	4.91	2.62	0.78	12.30	$425.66	10.01	$346.41	000	A+ B Me
50561		Kidney endoscopy & treatment	7.58	5.46	2.95	0.90	13.94	$482.41	11.43	$395.55	000	A+ B Me

50562	Renal scope w/tumor resect	10.90	NA	4.59	1.29	NA	NA	16.78	$580.69	090	C+ M
50570	Kidney endoscopy	9.53	NA	3.57	1.12	NA	NA	14.22	$492.10	000	A+ B M
50572	Kidney endoscopy	10.33	NA	3.84	1.22	NA	NA	15.39	$532.59	000	A+ B Me
50574	Kidney endoscopy & biopsy	11.00	NA	4.06	1.30	NA	NA	16.36	$566.16	000	A+ B Me
50575	Kidney endoscopy	13.96	NA	5.06	1.66	NA	NA	20.68	$715.66	000	A B Me
50576	Kidney endoscopy & treatment	10.97	NA	4.05	1.30	NA	NA	16.32	$564.77	000	A+ B Me
50580	Kidney endoscopy & treatment	11.84	NA	4.34	1.40	NA	NA	17.58	$608.38	000	A+ B Me
50590	Fragmenting of kidney stone	9.77	11.05	5.78	1.17	21.99	$760.99	16.72	$578.62	090	A B M
50592	Perc rf ablate renal tumor	6.55	81.32	2.80	0.60	88.47	$3061.61	9.95	$344.33	010	A B M
50593	Perc cryo ablate renal tum	8.88	108.61	3.56	0.79	118.28	$4093.22	13.23	$457.84	010	B M
50600	Exploration of ureter	17.17	NA	8.17	2.04	NA	NA	27.38	$947.52	090	B C+ M
50605	Insert ureteral support	16.79	NA	9.26	3.75	NA	NA	29.80	$1031.26	090	B C+ M
50606	Endoluminal bx urtr rnl plvs	3.16	11.31	0.52	0.32	14.79	$511.83	4.00	$138.42	ZZZ	A B
50610	Removal of ureter stone	17.25	NA	8.27	2.05	NA	NA	27.57	$954.09	090	B C+ M
50620	Removal of ureter stone	16.43	NA	7.99	1.95	NA	NA	26.37	$912.57	090	B C+ M
50630	Removal of ureter stone	16.21	NA	7.92	1.94	NA	NA	26.07	$902.18	090	B C+ M
50650	Removal of ureter	18.82	NA	9.19	2.36	NA	NA	30.37	$1050.99	090	B C+ M
50660	Removal of ureter	21.02	NA	9.83	2.50	NA	NA	33.35	$1154.12	090	C+ M
50684	Injection for ureter x-ray	0.76	2.99	0.61	0.09	3.84	$132.89	1.46	$50.53	000	A B M
50686	Measure ureter pressure	1.51	2.54	0.87	0.19	4.24	$146.73	2.57	$88.94	000	A+ M
50688	Change of ureter tube/stent	1.20	NA	0.93	0.11	NA	NA	2.24	$77.52	010	A M
50690	Injection for ureter x-ray	1.16	2.30	0.75	0.11	3.57	$123.54	2.02	$69.90	000	A M
50693	Plmt ureteral stent prq	3.96	26.44	1.56	0.35	30.75	$1064.14	5.87	$203.14	000	A B M
50694	Plmt ureteral stent prq	5.25	28.70	1.97	0.45	34.40	$1190.45	7.67	$265.43	000	A B M
50695	Plmt ureteral stent prq	6.80	33.93	2.48	0.60	41.33	$1430.27	9.88	$341.91	000	A B M
50700	Revision of ureter	16.69	NA	8.38	1.99	NA	NA	27.06	$936.44	090	B C+ M
50705	Ureteral embolization/occl	4.03	52.88	0.66	0.40	57.31	$1983.28	5.09	$176.15	ZZZ	A B
50706	Balloon dilate urtrl strix	3.80	21.82	1.09	0.34	25.96	$898.38	5.23	$180.99	ZZZ	A B

*Please note that these calculations are based on the Medicare 2022 Conversion Factor of $34.6062 and the DRA RVU cap rates at time of publication.

A = assistant-at-surgery restriction
A+ = assistant-at-surgery restriction unless medical necessity established with documentation
B = bilateral surgery adjustment applies
C = cosurgeons payable
C+ = cosurgeons payable if medical necessity established with documentation
CP = carriers may establish RVUs and payment amounts for these services, generally on an individual basis following review of documentation such as an operative report
M = multiple surgery adjustment applies
Me = multiple endoscopy rules may apply
M+ = multiple therapy rules apply
Mtc = multiple diagnostic imaging rules apply
T = team surgeons permitted
T+ = team surgeons payable if medical necessity established with documentation
§ = indicates code is not covered by Medicare
GS = procedure must be performed under the general supervision of a physician
DS = procedure must be performed under the direct supervision of a physician
PS = procedure must be performed under the personal supervision of a physician
DRA = procedure subject to DRA limitation

Relative Value Units

CPT Code and Modifier		Description	Work RVU	Nonfacility Practice Expense RVU	Facility Practice Expense RVU	PLI RVU	Total Non-facility RVUs	Medicare Payment Nonfacility	Total Facility RVUs	Medicare Payment Facility	Global Period	Payment Policy Indicators
50715		Release of ureter	20.64	NA	11.34	3.48	NA	NA	35.46	$1227.14	090	B C+ M
50722		Release of ureter	17.95	NA	9.32	2.94	NA	NA	30.21	$1045.45	090	C+ M
50725		Release/revise ureter	20.20	NA	9.55	2.39	NA	NA	32.14	$1112.24	090	C+ M
50727		Revise ureter	8.28	NA	5.66	1.10	NA	NA	15.04	$520.48	090	C M
50728		Revise ureter	12.18	NA	7.39	1.99	NA	NA	21.56	$746.11	090	C M
50740		Fusion of ureter & kidney	20.07	NA	11.46	5.06	NA	NA	36.59	$1266.24	090	B C+ M
50750		Fusion of ureter & kidney	21.22	NA	9.90	2.51	NA	NA	33.63	$1163.81	090	B M
50760		Fusion of ureters	20.07	NA	10.04	3.29	NA	NA	33.40	$1155.85	090	B C+ M
50770		Splicing of ureters	21.22	NA	9.90	2.51	NA	NA	33.63	$1163.81	090	C+ M
50780		Reimplant ureter in bladder	19.95	NA	9.75	2.82	NA	NA	32.52	$1125.39	090	B C+ M
50782		Reimplant ureter in bladder	19.66	NA	9.38	2.33	NA	NA	31.37	$1085.60	090	B C M
50783		Reimplant ureter in bladder	20.70	NA	9.72	2.47	NA	NA	32.89	$1138.20	090	B C M
50785		Reimplant ureter in bladder	22.23	NA	10.40	2.82	NA	NA	35.45	$1226.79	090	B C+ M
50800		Implant ureter in bowel	16.41	NA	8.60	2.01	NA	NA	27.02	$935.06	090	B C+ M
50810		Fusion of ureter & bowel	22.61	NA	13.68	5.72	NA	NA	42.01	$1453.81	090	C+ M
50815		Urine shunt to intestine	22.26	NA	10.84	2.66	NA	NA	35.76	$1237.52	090	B C+ M
50820		Construct bowel bladder	24.07	NA	11.25	3.00	NA	NA	38.32	$1326.11	090	B C+ M
50825		Construct bowel bladder	30.68	NA	13.68	3.66	NA	NA	48.02	$1661.79	090	C+ M
50830		Revise urine flow	33.77	NA	14.72	4.01	NA	NA	52.50	$1816.83	090	C+ M
50840		Replace ureter by bowel	22.39	NA	10.88	2.67	NA	NA	35.94	$1243.75	090	B C+ M
50845		Appendico-vesicostomy	22.46	NA	11.50	2.68	NA	NA	36.64	$1267.97	090	C+ M
50860		Transplant ureter to skin	17.08	NA	8.51	2.03	NA	NA	27.62	$955.82	090	B C+ M
50900		Repair of ureter	15.04	NA	7.82	1.80	NA	NA	24.66	$853.39	090	B C+ M
50920		Closure ureter/skin fistula	15.81	NA	8.08	1.87	NA	NA	25.76	$891.46	090	C+ M
50930		Closure ureter/bowel fistula	20.19	NA	9.55	2.39	NA	NA	32.13	$1111.90	090	C+ M
50940		Release of ureter	15.93	NA	8.12	1.90	NA	NA	25.95	$898.03	090	B C+ M
50945		Laparoscopy ureterolithotomy	17.97	NA	8.22	2.17	NA	NA	28.36	$981.43	090	B C+ M
50947		Laparo new ureter/bladder	25.78	NA	11.50	3.13	NA	NA	40.41	$1398.44	090	B C+ M
50948		Laparo new ureter/bladder	23.82	NA	10.44	2.94	NA	NA	37.20	$1287.35	090	B C+ M
50949	CP	Laparoscope proc ureter	0.00	0.00	0.00	0.00	0.00	$0.00	0.00	$0.00	YYY	B C+ M T+
50951		Endoscopy of ureter	5.83	4.60	2.37	0.68	11.11	$384.47	8.88	$307.30	000	A+ B M
50953		Endoscopy of ureter	6.23	4.79	2.49	0.73	11.75	$406.62	9.45	$327.03	000	A+ B Me
50955		Ureter endoscopy & biopsy	6.74	4.99	2.66	0.79	12.52	$433.27	10.19	$352.64	000	A+ B Me

50957	Ureter endoscopy & treatment	6.78	5.06	2.68	0.79	12.63	$437.08	10.25	$354.71	000	A+ B Me
50961	Ureter endoscopy & treatment	6.04	4.66	2.43	0.73	11.43	$395.55	9.20	$318.38	000	A+ B Me
50970	Ureter endoscopy	7.13	NA	2.76	0.86	NA	NA	10.75	$372.02	000	A+ B M
50972	Ureter endoscopy & catheter	6.88	NA	2.68	0.83	NA	NA	10.39	$359.56	000	A+ B M
50974	Ureter endoscopy & biopsy	9.16	NA	3.45	1.09	NA	NA	13.70	$474.10	000	A+ B Me
50976	Ureter endoscopy & treatment	9.03	NA	3.40	1.07	NA	NA	13.50	$467.18	000	A+ B Me
50980	Ureter endoscopy & treatment	6.84	NA	2.66	0.83	NA	NA	10.33	$357.48	000	A+ B M
51020	Incise & treat bladder	7.69	NA	5.18	0.93	NA	NA	13.80	$477.57	090	C+ M
51030	Incise & treat bladder	7.81	NA	5.15	0.94	NA	NA	13.90	$481.03	090	A+ M
51040	Incise & drain bladder	4.49	NA	3.51	0.55	NA	NA	8.55	$295.88	090	C+ M
51045	Incise bladder/drain ureter	7.81	NA	5.75	1.39	NA	NA	14.95	$517.36	090	M
51050	Removal of bladder stone	7.97	NA	4.90	0.95	NA	NA	13.82	$478.26	090	C+ M
51060	Removal of ureter stone	9.95	NA	5.95	1.18	NA	NA	17.08	$591.07	090	C+ M
51065	Remove ureter calculus	9.95	NA	5.88	1.18	NA	NA	17.01	$588.65	090	A+ M
51080	Drainage of bladder abscess	6.71	NA	4.48	0.79	NA	NA	11.98	$414.58	090	C+ M
51100	Drain bladder by needle	0.78	1.32	0.26	0.09	2.19	$75.79	1.13	$39.11	000	A M
51101	Drain bladder by trocar/cath	1.02	3.57	0.35	0.11	4.70	$162.65	1.48	$51.22	000	A M
51102	Drain bl w/cath insertion	2.70	4.24	1.22	0.29	7.23	$250.20	4.21	$145.69	000	A M
51500	Removal of bladder cyst	11.05	NA	6.31	1.32	NA	NA	18.68	$646.44	090	C+ M
51520	Removal of bladder lesion	10.21	NA	6.04	1.21	NA	NA	17.46	$604.22	090	C+ M
51525	Removal of bladder lesion	15.42	NA	7.84	1.87	NA	NA	25.13	$869.65	090	C+ M
51530	Removal of bladder lesion	13.71	NA	7.20	1.64	NA	NA	22.55	$780.37	090	C+ M
51535	Repair of ureter lesion	13.90	NA	7.26	1.65	NA	NA	22.81	$789.37	090	B C+ M
51550	Partial removal of bladder	17.23	NA	8.65	2.33	NA	NA	28.21	$976.24	090	C+ M
51555	Partial removal of bladder	23.18	NA	10.73	2.98	NA	NA	36.89	$1276.62	090	C+ M
51565	Revise bladder & ureter(s)	23.68	NA	11.12	2.83	NA	NA	37.63	$1302.23	090	C+ M
51570	Removal of bladder	27.46	NA	12.11	3.34	NA	NA	42.91	$1484.95	090	C+ M
51575	Removal of bladder & nodes	34.18	NA	14.73	4.20	NA	NA	53.11	$1837.94	090	C+ M

*Please note that these calculations are based on the Medicare 2022 Conversion Factor of $34.6062 and the DRA RVU cap rates at time of publication.

A = assistant-at-surgery restriction
A+ = assistant-at-surgery restriction unless medical necessity established with documentation
B = bilateral surgery adjustment applies
C = cosurgeons payable
C+ = cosurgeons payable if medical necessity established with documentation
CP = carriers may establish RVUs and payment amounts for these services, generally on an individual basis following review of documentation such as an operative report
M = multiple surgery adjustment applies
Me = multiple endoscopy rules may apply
M+ = multiple therapy rules apply
Mtc = multiple diagnostic imaging rules apply
T = team surgeons permitted
T+ = team surgeons payable if medical necessity established with documentation
§ = indicates code is not covered by Medicare
GS = procedure must be performed under the general supervision of a physician
DS = procedure must be performed under the direct supervision of a physician
PS = procedure must be performed under the personal supervision of a physician
DRA = procedure subject to DRA limitation

Relative Value Units

CPT Code and Modifier	Description	Work RVU	Nonfacility Practice Expense RVU	Facility Practice Expense RVU	PLI RVU	Total Non-facility RVUs	Medicare Payment Nonfacility	Total Facility RVUs	Medicare Payment Facility	Global Period	Payment Policy Indicators
51580	Remove bladder/revise tract	35.37	NA	15.69	4.22	NA	NA	55.28	$1913.03	090	C+ M
51585	Removal of bladder & nodes	39.64	NA	17.13	4.74	NA	NA	61.51	$2128.63	090	C+ M
51590	Remove bladder/revise tract	36.33	NA	15.50	4.50	NA	NA	56.33	$1949.37	090	C+ M
51595	Remove bladder/revise tract	41.32	NA	17.38	5.00	NA	NA	63.70	$2204.41	090	C+ M
51596	Remove bladder/create pouch	44.26	NA	18.97	5.39	NA	NA	68.62	$2374.68	090	C+ M
51597	Removal of pelvic structures	42.86	NA	18.74	5.43	NA	NA	67.03	$2319.65	090	C+ M
51600	Injection for bladder x-ray	0.88	5.56	0.31	0.09	6.53	$225.98	1.28	$44.30	000	A M
51605	Preparation for bladder xray	0.64	NA	0.40	0.09	NA	NA	1.13	$39.11	000	A M
51610	Injection for bladder x-ray	1.05	2.73	0.70	0.11	3.89	$134.62	1.86	$64.37	000	A M
51700	Irrigation of bladder	0.60	1.60	0.21	0.09	2.29	$79.25	0.90	$31.15	000	A M
51701	Insert bladder catheter	0.50	0.75	0.18	0.08	1.33	$46.03	0.76	$26.30	000	A M
51702	Insert temp bladder cath	0.50	1.28	0.18	0.07	1.85	$64.02	0.75	$25.95	000	A M
51703	Insert bladder cath complex	1.47	2.84	0.58	0.19	4.50	$155.73	2.24	$77.52	000	A M
51705	Change of bladder tube	0.90	1.87	0.49	0.11	2.88	$99.67	1.50	$51.91	000	A M
51710	Change of bladder tube	1.35	2.54	0.80	0.17	4.06	$140.50	2.32	$80.29	000	A M
51715	Endoscopic injection/implant	3.73	6.99	1.59	0.50	11.22	$388.28	5.82	$201.41	000	A+ M
51720	Treatment of bladder lesion	0.87	1.62	0.30	0.10	2.59	$89.63	1.27	$43.95	000	A M
51725	Simple cystometrogram	1.51	5.22	NA	0.16	6.89	$238.44	NA	NA	000	A+ M
51725-26	Simple cystometrogram	1.51	0.55	0.55	0.14	2.20	$76.13	2.20	$76.13	000	A+ M
51725-TC	Simple cystometrogram	0.00	4.67	NA	0.02	4.69	$162.30	NA	NA	000	A+ M DS
51726	Complex cystometrogram	1.71	7.24	NA	0.16	9.11	$315.26	NA	NA	000	A M
51726-26	Complex cystometrogram	1.71	0.60	0.60	0.14	2.45	$84.79	2.45	$84.79	000	A M
51726-TC	Complex cystometrogram	0.00	6.64	NA	0.02	6.66	$230.48	NA	NA	000	A M DS
51727	Cystometrogram w/up	2.11	8.66	NA	0.23	11.00	$380.67	NA	NA	000	A+ M
51727-26	Cystometrogram w/up	2.11	0.76	0.76	0.21	3.08	$106.59	3.08	$106.59	000	A+ M
51727-TC	Cystometrogram w/up	0.00	7.90	NA	0.02	7.92	$274.08	NA	NA	000	A+ M DS
51728	Cystometrogram w/vp	2.11	8.76	NA	0.21	11.08	$383.44	NA	NA	000	A+ M
51728-26	Cystometrogram w/vp	2.11	0.72	0.72	0.19	3.02	$104.51	3.02	$104.51	000	A+ M
51728-TC	Cystometrogram w/vp	0.00	8.04	NA	0.02	8.06	$278.93	NA	NA	000	A+ M DS
51729	Cystometrogram w/vp&up	2.51	8.93	NA	0.27	11.71	$405.24	NA	NA	000	A+ M
51729-26	Cystometrogram w/vp&up	2.51	0.90	0.90	0.25	3.66	$126.66	3.66	$126.66	000	A+ M
51729-TC	Cystometrogram w/vp&up	0.00	8.03	NA	0.02	8.05	$278.58	NA	NA	000	A+ M DS
51736	Urine flow measurement	0.17	0.20	NA	0.02	0.39	$13.50	NA	NA	XXX	A+ M

51736-26	Urine flow measurement	0.17	0.06	0.06	0.01	0.24	$8.31	0.24	$8.31	XXX	A+ M
51736-TC	Urine flow measurement	0.00	0.14	NA	0.01	0.15	$5.19	NA	NA	XXX	A+ M DS
51741	Electro-uroflowmetry first	0.17	0.21	NA	0.03	0.41	$14.19	NA	NA	XXX	A M
51741-26	Electro-uroflowmetry first	0.17	0.06	0.06	0.02	0.25	$8.65	0.25	$8.65	XXX	A M
51741-TC	Electro-uroflowmetry first	0.00	0.15	NA	0.01	0.16	$5.54	NA	NA	XXX	A M DS
51784	Anal/urinary muscle study	0.75	1.06	NA	0.09	1.90	$65.75	NA	NA	XXX	A M
51784-26	Anal/urinary muscle study	0.75	0.26	0.26	0.08	1.09	$37.72	1.09	$37.72	XXX	A M
51784-TC	Anal/urinary muscle study	0.00	0.80	NA	0.01	0.81	$28.03	NA	NA	XXX	A M DS
51785	Anal/urinary muscle study	1.53	11.43	NA	0.49	13.45	$465.45	NA	NA	XXX	A+ M
51785-26	Anal/urinary muscle study	1.53	0.73	0.73	0.47	2.73	$94.47	2.73	$94.47	XXX	A+ M
51785-TC	Anal/urinary muscle study	0.00	10.70	NA	0.02	10.72	$370.98	NA	NA	XXX	A+ M PS
51792	Urinary reflex study	1.10	6.98	NA	0.13	8.21	$284.12	NA	NA	000	A+ M
51792-26	Urinary reflex study	1.10	0.38	0.38	0.09	1.57	$54.33	1.57	$54.33	000	A+ M
51792-TC	Urinary reflex study	0.00	6.60	NA	0.04	6.64	$229.79	NA	NA	000	A+ M DS
51797	Intraabdominal pressure test	0.80	5.04	NA	0.08	5.92	$204.87	NA	NA	ZZZ	A+
51797-26	Intraabdominal pressure test	0.80	0.28	0.28	0.08	1.16	$40.14	1.16	$40.14	ZZZ	A+
51797-TC	Intraabdominal pressure test	0.00	4.76	NA	0.00	4.76	$164.73	NA	NA	ZZZ	A+ DS
51798	Us urine capacity measure	0.00	0.30	NA	0.01	0.31	$10.73	NA	NA	XXX	A+
51800	Revision of bladder/urethra	18.89	NA	9.19	2.23	NA	NA	30.31	$1048.91	090	C+ M
51820	Revision of urinary tract	19.59	NA	9.78	2.33	NA	NA	31.70	$1097.02	090	C+ M
51840	Attach bladder/urethra	11.36	NA	7.73	1.48	NA	NA	20.57	$711.85	090	C+ M
51841	Attach bladder/urethra	13.68	NA	8.43	1.63	NA	NA	23.74	$821.55	090	C+ M
51845	Repair bladder neck	10.15	NA	5.73	1.20	NA	NA	17.08	$591.07	090	C+ M
51860	Repair of bladder wound	12.60	NA	7.44	1.93	NA	NA	21.97	$760.30	090	C+ M
51865	Repair of bladder wound	15.80	NA	8.38	2.17	NA	NA	26.35	$911.87	090	C+ M
51880	Repair of bladder opening	7.87	NA	4.76	1.04	NA	NA	13.67	$473.07	090	C+ M
51900	Repair bladder/vagina lesion	14.63	NA	7.74	1.73	NA	NA	24.10	$834.01	090	C+ M
51920	Close bladder-uterus fistula	13.41	NA	7.33	1.60	NA	NA	22.34	$773.10	090	C+ M

*Please note that these calculations are based on the Medicare 2022 Conversion Factor of $34.6062 and the DRA RVU cap rates at time of publication.

A = assistant-at-surgery restriction

A+ = assistant-at-surgery restriction unless medical necessity established with documentation

B = bilateral surgery adjustment applies

C = cosurgeons payable

C+ = cosurgeons payable if medical necessity established with documentation

CP = carriers may establish RVUs and payment amounts for these services, generally on an individual basis following review of documentation such as an operative report

M = multiple surgery adjustment applies

Me = multiple endoscopy rules may apply

M+ = multiple therapy rules apply

Mtc = multiple diagnostic imaging rules apply

T = team surgeons permitted

T+ = team surgeons payable if medical necessity established with documentation

§ = indicates code is not covered by Medicare

GS = procedure must be performed under the general supervision of a physician

DS = procedure must be performed under the direct supervision of a physician

PS = procedure must be performed under the personal supervision of a physician

DRA = procedure subject to DRA limitation

Relative Value Units

CPT Code and Modifier		Description	Work RVU	Nonfacility Practice Expense RVU	Facility Practice Expense RVU	PLI RVU	Total Non-facility RVUs	Medicare Payment Nonfacility	Total Facility RVUs	Medicare Payment Facility	Global Period	Payment Policy Indicators
51925		Hysterectomy/bladder repair	17.53	NA	11.75	2.88	NA	NA	32.16	$1112.94	090	C+ M
51940		Correction of bladder defect	30.66	NA	13.54	3.66	NA	NA	47.86	$1656.25	090	C+ M
51960		Revision of bladder & bowel	25.40	NA	11.99	3.02	NA	NA	40.41	$1398.44	090	C+ M
51980		Construct bladder opening	12.57	NA	6.83	1.49	NA	NA	20.89	$722.92	090	C+ M
51990		Laparo urethral suspension	13.36	NA	6.83	1.64	NA	NA	21.83	$755.45	090	C+ M
51992		Laparo sling operation	14.87	NA	7.55	2.23	NA	NA	24.65	$853.04	090	C+ M
51999	CP	Laparoscope proc bla	0.00	0.00	0.00	0.00	0.00	$0.00	0.00	$0.00	YYY	A+ C+ T+
52000		Cystoscopy	1.53	5.59	0.63	0.19	7.31	$252.97	2.35	$81.32	000	A M
52001		Cystoscopy removal of clots	5.44	7.08	2.23	0.65	13.17	$455.76	8.32	$287.92	000	A Me
52005		Cystoscopy & ureter catheter	2.37	6.56	1.20	0.28	9.21	$318.72	3.85	$133.23	000	A Me
52007		Cystoscopy and biopsy	3.02	10.37	1.41	0.37	13.76	$476.18	4.80	$166.11	000	A B Me
52010		Cystoscopy & duct catheter	3.02	8.21	1.41	0.35	11.58	$400.74	4.78	$165.42	000	A Me
52204		Cystoscopy w/biopsy(s)	2.59	8.63	1.20	0.31	11.53	$399.01	4.10	$141.89	000	A Me
52214		Cystoscopy and treatment	3.50	19.10	1.19	0.41	23.01	$796.29	5.10	$176.49	000	A Me
52224		Cystoscopy and treatment	4.05	19.48	1.36	0.50	24.03	$831.59	5.91	$204.52	000	A Me
52234		Cystoscopy and treatment	4.62	NA	1.95	0.56	NA	NA	7.13	$246.74	000	A Me
52235		Cystoscopy and treatment	5.44	NA	2.26	0.65	NA	NA	8.35	$288.96	000	A Me
52240		Cystoscopy and treatment	7.50	NA	2.96	0.90	NA	NA	11.36	$393.13	000	A Me
52250		Cystoscopy and radiotracer	4.49	NA	1.90	0.55	NA	NA	6.94	$240.17	000	A Me
52260		Cystoscopy and treatment	3.91	NA	1.71	0.50	NA	NA	6.12	$211.79	000	A Me
52265		Cystoscopy and treatment	2.94	8.06	1.39	0.39	11.39	$394.16	4.72	$163.34	000	A Me
52270		Cystoscopy & revise urethra	3.36	9.04	1.50	0.40	12.80	$442.96	5.26	$182.03	000	A Me
52275		Cystoscopy & revise urethra	4.69	11.17	1.95	0.56	16.42	$568.23	7.20	$249.16	000	A Me
52276		Cystoscopy and treatment	4.99	NA	2.07	0.60	NA	NA	7.66	$265.08	000	A Me
52277		Cystoscopy and treatment	6.16	NA	2.47	0.73	NA	NA	9.36	$323.91	000	A+ Me
52281		Cystoscopy and treatment	2.75	6.81	1.33	0.33	9.89	$342.26	4.41	$152.61	000	A Me
52282		Cystoscopy implant stent	6.39	NA	2.58	0.76	NA	NA	9.73	$336.72	000	A Me
52283		Cystoscopy and treatment	3.73	6.50	1.66	0.43	10.66	$368.90	5.82	$201.41	000	A Me
52285		Cystoscopy and treatment	3.60	6.52	1.63	0.43	10.55	$365.10	5.66	$195.87	000	A Me
52287		Cystoscopy chemodenervation	3.20	8.19	1.32	0.40	11.79	$408.01	4.92	$170.26	000	A Me
52290		Cystoscopy and treatment	4.58	NA	1.93	0.56	NA	NA	7.07	$244.67	000	A Me
52300		Cystoscopy and treatment	5.30	NA	2.18	0.62	NA	NA	8.10	$280.31	000	A+ Me
52301		Cystoscopy and treatment	5.50	NA	2.24	0.65	NA	NA	8.39	$290.35	000	A+ Me

52305	Cystoscopy and treatment	5.30	NA	2.13	0.62	NA	NA	8.05	$278.58	000	A Me
52310	Cystoscopy and treatment	2.81	6.45	1.24	0.34	9.60	$332.22	4.39	$151.92	000	A Me
52315	Cystoscopy and treatment	5.20	8.28	2.13	0.62	14.10	$487.95	7.95	$275.12	000	A Me
52317	Remove bladder stone	6.71	19.51	2.55	0.79	27.01	$934.71	10.05	$347.79	000	A Me
52318	Remove bladder stone	9.18	NA	3.44	1.09	NA	NA	13.71	$474.45	000	A Me
52320	Cystoscopy and treatment	4.69	NA	1.89	0.56	NA	NA	7.14	$247.09	000	A B Me
52325	Cystoscopy stone removal	6.15	NA	2.39	0.73	NA	NA	9.27	$320.80	000	A B Me
52327	Cystoscopy inject material	5.18	NA	1.79	0.67	NA	NA	7.64	$264.39	000	A B Me
52330	Cystoscopy and treatment	5.03	12.71	2.00	0.60	18.34	$634.68	7.63	$264.05	000	A B Me
52332	Cystoscopy and treatment	2.82	9.07	1.35	0.34	12.23	$423.23	4.51	$156.07	000	A B Me
52334	Create passage to kidney	3.37	NA	1.52	0.40	NA	NA	5.29	$183.07	000	A Me
52341	Cysto w/ureter stricture tx	5.35	NA	2.23	0.64	NA	NA	8.22	$284.46	000	A B Me
52342	Cysto w/up stricture tx	5.85	NA	2.40	0.70	NA	NA	8.95	$309.73	000	A B Me
52343	Cysto w/renal stricture tx	6.55	NA	2.64	0.77	NA	NA	9.96	$344.68	000	A B Me
52344	Cysto/uretero stricture tx	7.05	NA	2.81	0.85	NA	NA	10.71	$370.63	000	A B Me
52345	Cysto/uretero w/up stricture	7.55	NA	2.97	0.90	NA	NA	11.42	$395.20	000	A+ B Me
52346	Cystouretero w/renal strict	8.58	NA	3.34	1.00	NA	NA	12.92	$447.11	000	A+ B Me
52351	Cystouretero & or pyeloscope	5.75	NA	2.33	0.68	NA	NA	8.76	$303.15	000	A M
52352	Cystouretero w/stone remove	6.75	NA	2.71	0.79	NA	NA	10.25	$354.71	000	A B Me
52353	Cystouretero w/lithotripsy	7.50	NA	2.96	0.90	NA	NA	11.36	$393.13	000	A B Me
52354	Cystouretero w/biopsy	8.00	NA	3.13	0.95	NA	NA	12.08	$418.04	000	A B Me
52355	Cystouretero w/excise tumor	9.00	NA	3.46	1.06	NA	NA	13.52	$467.88	000	A B Me
52356	Cysto/uretero w/lithotripsy	8.00	NA	3.09	0.95	NA	NA	12.04	$416.66	000	A B Me
52400	Cystouretero w/congen repr	8.69	NA	4.20	1.04	NA	NA	13.93	$482.06	090	A Me
52402	Cystourethro cut ejacul duct	5.27	NA	1.82	0.62	NA	NA	7.71	$266.81	000	A Me
52441	Cystourethro w/implant	4.00	34.78	1.61	0.47	39.25	$1358.29	6.08	$210.41	000	A Me
52442	Cystourethro w/addl implant	1.01	25.86	0.34	0.11	26.98	$933.68	1.46	$50.53	ZZZ	A
52450	Incision of prostate	7.78	NA	5.17	0.94	NA	NA	13.89	$480.68	090	A M

*Please note that these calculations are based on the Medicare 2022 Conversion Factor of $34.6062 and the DRA RVU cap rates at time of publication.

A = assistant-at-surgery restriction
A+ = assistant-at-surgery restriction unless medical necessity established with documentation
B = bilateral surgery adjustment applies
C = cosurgeons payable
C+ = cosurgeons payable if medical necessity established with documentation
CP = carriers may establish RVUs and payment amounts for these services, generally on an individual basis following review of documentation such as an operative report
M = multiple surgery adjustment applies
Me = multiple endoscopy rules may apply
M+ = multiple therapy rules apply
Mtc = multiple diagnostic imaging rules apply
T = team surgeons permitted
T+ = team surgeons payable if medical necessity established with documentation
§ = indicates code is not covered by Medicare
GS = procedure must be performed under the general supervision of a physician
DS = procedure must be performed under the direct supervision of a physician
PS = procedure must be performed under the personal supervision of a physician
DRA = procedure subject to DRA limitation

Relative Value Units

CPT Code and Modifier	Description	Work RVU	Nonfacility Practice Expense RVU	Facility Practice Expense RVU	PLI RVU	Total Non-facility RVUs	Medicare Payment Nonfacility	Total Facility RVUs	Medicare Payment Facility	Global Period	Payment Policy Indicators
52500	Revision of bladder neck	8.14	NA	5.29	0.96	NA	NA	14.39	$497.98	090	A M
52601	Prostatectomy (turp)	13.16	NA	6.58	1.55	NA	NA	21.29	$736.77	090	A M
52630	Remove prostate regrowth	6.55	NA	4.54	0.77	NA	NA	11.86	$410.43	090	A M
52640	Relieve bladder contracture	4.79	NA	4.05	0.57	NA	NA	9.41	$325.64	090	A M
52647	Laser surgery of prostate	11.30	34.95	6.36	1.33	47.58	$1646.56	18.99	$657.17	090	A M
52648	Laser surgery of prostate	12.15	35.48	6.66	1.43	49.06	$1697.78	20.24	$700.43	090	A M
52649	Prostate laser enucleation	14.56	NA	7.87	1.72	NA	NA	24.15	$835.74	090	A+ M
52700	Drainage of prostate abscess	7.49	NA	4.56	0.90	NA	NA	12.95	$448.15	090	A+ M
53000	Incision of urethra	2.33	NA	1.74	0.27	NA	NA	4.34	$150.19	010	A M
53010	Incision of urethra	4.45	NA	3.71	0.54	NA	NA	8.70	$301.07	090	A M
53020	Incision of urethra	1.77	NA	0.83	0.21	NA	NA	2.81	$97.24	000	A M
53025	Incision of urethra	1.13	NA	0.72	0.12	NA	NA	1.97	$68.17	000	A+ M
53040	Drainage of urethra abscess	6.55	NA	4.17	0.77	NA	NA	11.49	$397.63	090	A+ M
53060	Drainage of urethra abscess	2.68	2.49	1.78	0.42	5.59	$193.45	4.88	$168.88	010	A M
53080	Drainage of urinary leakage	6.92	NA	4.58	0.84	NA	NA	12.34	$427.04	090	A M
53085	Drainage of urinary leakage	11.18	NA	6.51	1.33	NA	NA	19.02	$658.21	090	C+ M
53200	Biopsy of urethra	2.59	1.72	1.21	0.33	4.64	$160.57	4.13	$142.92	000	A M
53210	Removal of urethra	13.72	NA	7.33	1.68	NA	NA	22.73	$786.60	090	C+ M
53215	Removal of urethra	16.85	NA	8.24	2.03	NA	NA	27.12	$938.52	090	C+ M
53220	Treatment of urethra lesion	7.63	NA	4.70	0.90	NA	NA	13.23	$457.84	090	A+ M
53230	Removal of urethra lesion	10.44	NA	6.13	1.34	NA	NA	17.91	$619.80	090	C+ M
53235	Removal of urethra lesion	10.99	NA	6.28	1.30	NA	NA	18.57	$642.64	090	C+ M
53240	Surgery for urethra pouch	7.08	NA	4.53	0.86	NA	NA	12.47	$431.54	090	A M
53250	Removal of urethra gland	6.52	NA	4.32	0.77	NA	NA	11.61	$401.78	090	A M
53260	Treatment of urethra lesion	3.03	2.68	1.89	0.40	6.11	$211.44	5.32	$184.10	010	A M
53265	Treatment of urethra lesion	3.17	3.18	1.94	0.42	6.77	$234.28	5.53	$191.37	010	A M
53270	Removal of urethra gland	3.14	2.72	1.90	0.37	6.23	$215.60	5.41	$187.22	010	A M
53275	Repair of urethra defect	4.57	NA	2.56	0.60	NA	NA	7.73	$267.51	010	A M
53400	Revise urethra stage 1	14.13	NA	7.57	1.70	NA	NA	23.40	$809.79	090	C+ M
53405	Revise urethra stage 2	15.66	NA	8.01	1.85	NA	NA	25.52	$883.15	090	C+ M
53410	Reconstruction of urethra	17.68	NA	8.84	2.14	NA	NA	28.66	$991.81	090	C+ M
53415	Reconstruction of urethra	20.70	NA	9.83	2.48	NA	NA	33.01	$1142.35	090	C+ M
53420	Reconstruct urethra stage 1	15.17	NA	7.62	1.81	NA	NA	24.60	$851.31	090	A C+ M

53425		Reconstruct urethra stage 2	17.07	NA	8.27	2.03	NA	NA	27.37	$947.17	090	C+ M
53430		Reconstruction of urethra	17.43	NA	8.73	2.37	NA	NA	28.53	$987.31	090	C+ M
53431		Reconstruct urethra/bladder	21.18	NA	9.95	2.51	NA	NA	33.64	$1164.15	090	C+ M
53440		Male sling procedure	13.36	NA	7.08	1.59	NA	NA	22.03	$762.37	090	C+ M
53442		Remove/revise male sling	13.49	NA	7.89	1.61	NA	NA	22.99	$795.60	090	M
53444		Insert tandem cuff	14.19	NA	7.34	1.68	NA	NA	23.21	$803.21	090	C+ M
53445		Insert uro/ves nck sphincter	13.00	NA	7.60	1.54	NA	NA	22.14	$766.18	090	C+ M
53446		Remove uro sphincter	11.02	NA	6.50	1.32	NA	NA	18.84	$651.98	090	C+ M
53447		Remove/replace ur sphincter	14.28	NA	7.63	1.70	NA	NA	23.61	$817.05	090	C+ M
53448		Remov/replc ur sphinctr comp	23.44	NA	11.03	2.80	NA	NA	37.27	$1289.77	090	C+ M
53449		Repair uro sphincter	10.56	NA	6.14	1.27	NA	NA	17.97	$621.87	090	C+ M
53450		Revision of urethra	6.77	NA	4.44	0.79	NA	NA	12.00	$415.27	090	A M
53451	CP	Tprnl balo cntnc dev bi	0.00	0.00	0.00	0.00	0.00	$0.00	0.00	$0.00	010	A+
53452	CP	Tprnl balo cntnc dev uni	0.00	0.00	0.00	0.00	0.00	$0.00	0.00	$0.00	010	A+
53453	CP	Tprnl balo cntnc dev rmvl ea	0.00	0.00	0.00	0.00	0.00	$0.00	0.00	$0.00	000	A+
53454	CP	Tprnl balo cntnc dev adjmt	0.00	0.00	0.00	0.00	0.00	$0.00	0.00	$0.00	000	A+
53460		Revision of urethra	7.75	NA	4.74	0.94	NA	NA	13.43	$464.76	090	A+ M
53500		Urethrlys transvag w/ scope	13.00	NA	7.18	1.82	NA	NA	22.00	$761.34	090	C+ M
53502		Repair of urethra injury	8.26	NA	5.00	0.99	NA	NA	14.25	$493.14	090	A M
53505		Repair of urethra injury	8.26	NA	4.99	0.99	NA	NA	14.24	$492.79	090	M
53510		Repair of urethra injury	10.96	NA	6.27	1.30	NA	NA	18.53	$641.25	090	C+ M
53515		Repair of urethra injury	14.22	NA	7.36	1.69	NA	NA	23.27	$805.29	090	C+ M
53520		Repair of urethra defect	9.48	NA	5.77	1.11	NA	NA	16.36	$566.16	090	A M
53600		Dilate urethra stricture	1.21	1.26	0.49	0.14	2.61	$90.32	1.84	$63.68	000	A M
53601		Dilate urethra stricture	0.98	1.41	0.45	0.11	2.50	$86.52	1.54	$53.29	000	A M
53605		Dilate urethra stricture	1.28	NA	0.43	0.14	NA	NA	1.85	$64.02	000	A M
53620		Dilate urethra stricture	1.62	3.34	0.72	0.20	5.16	$178.57	2.54	$87.90	000	A M
53621		Dilate urethra stricture	1.35	3.40	0.58	0.17	4.92	$170.26	2.10	$72.67	000	A M

*Please note that these calculations are based on the Medicare 2022 Conversion Factor of $34.6062 and the DRA RVU cap rates at time of publication.

A = assistant-at-surgery restriction
A+ = assistant-at-surgery restriction unless medical necessity established with documentation
B = bilateral surgery adjustment applies
C = cosurgeons payable
C+ = cosurgeons payable if medical necessity established with documentation
CP = carriers may establish RVUs and payment amounts for these services, generally on an individual basis following review of documentation such as an operative report
M = multiple surgery adjustment applies
Me = multiple endoscopy rules may apply
M+ = multiple therapy rules apply
Mtc = multiple diagnostic imaging rules apply
T = team surgeons permitted
T+ = team surgeons payable if medical necessity established with documentation
§ = indicates code is not covered by Medicare
GS = procedure must be performed under the general supervision of a physician
DS = procedure must be performed under the direct supervision of a physician
PS = procedure must be performed under the personal supervision of a physician
DRA = procedure subject to DRA limitation

Relative Value Units

CPT Code and Modifier		Description	Work RVU	Nonfacility Practice Expense RVU	Facility Practice Expense RVU	PLI RVU	Total Non-facility RVUs	Medicare Payment Nonfacility	Total Facility RVUs	Medicare Payment Facility	Global Period	Payment Policy Indicators
53660		Dilation of urethra	0.71	1.43	0.41	0.09	2.23	$77.17	1.21	$41.87	000	A M
53661		Dilation of urethra	0.72	1.38	0.36	0.09	2.19	$75.79	1.17	$40.49	000	A M
53665		Dilation of urethra	0.76	NA	0.26	0.10	NA	NA	1.12	$38.76	000	A M
53850		Prostatic microwave thermotx	5.42	37.52	4.31	0.65	43.59	$1508.48	10.38	$359.21	090	A M
53852		Prostatic rf thermotx	5.93	35.87	4.48	0.72	42.52	$1471.46	11.13	$385.17	090	A M
53854		Trurl dstrj prst8 tiss rf wv	5.93	44.92	4.49	0.72	51.57	$1784.64	11.14	$385.51	090	A M
53855		Insert prost urethral stent	1.64	18.47	0.56	0.20	20.31	$702.85	2.40	$83.05	000	A+ M
53860		Transurethral rf treatment	3.97	69.78	2.05	0.45	74.20	$2567.78	6.47	$223.90	090	A+ M
53899	CP	Urology surgery procedure	0.00	0.00	0.00	0.00	0.00	$0.00	0.00	$0.00	YYY	A+ C+ M T+
54000		Slitting of prepuce	1.59	3.06	1.45	0.20	4.85	$167.84	3.24	$112.12	010	A+ M
54001		Slitting of prepuce	2.24	3.38	1.60	0.25	5.87	$203.14	4.09	$141.54	010	A M
54015		Drain penis lesion	5.36	NA	2.92	0.64	NA	NA	8.92	$308.69	010	A+ M
54050		Destruction penis lesion(s)	1.29	2.78	1.66	0.12	4.19	$145.00	3.07	$106.24	010	A M
54055		Destruction penis lesion(s)	1.25	2.64	1.38	0.12	4.01	$138.77	2.75	$95.17	010	A M
54056		Cryosurgery penis lesion(s)	1.29	2.80	1.80	0.12	4.21	$145.69	3.21	$111.09	010	A M
54057		Laser surg penis lesion(s)	1.29	2.75	1.40	0.14	4.18	$144.65	2.83	$97.94	010	A M
54060		Excision of penis lesion(s)	1.98	3.59	1.62	0.24	5.81	$201.06	3.84	$132.89	010	A M
54065		Destruction penis lesion(s)	2.47	3.83	2.27	0.25	6.55	$226.67	4.99	$172.68	010	A M
54100		Biopsy of penis	1.90	3.92	1.41	0.20	6.02	$208.33	3.51	$121.47	000	A M
54105		Biopsy of penis	3.54	4.21	2.26	0.41	8.16	$282.39	6.21	$214.90	010	A M
54110		Treatment of penis lesion	10.92	NA	6.14	1.32	NA	NA	18.38	$636.06	090	M
54111		Treat penis lesion graft	14.42	NA	7.24	1.70	NA	NA	23.36	$808.40	090	C+ M
54112		Treat penis lesion graft	16.98	NA	8.40	2.01	NA	NA	27.39	$947.86	090	C+ M
54115		Treatment of penis lesion	6.95	5.65	4.72	0.84	13.44	$465.11	12.51	$432.92	090	M
54120		Partial removal of penis	11.01	NA	6.19	1.33	NA	NA	18.53	$641.25	090	C+ M
54125		Removal of penis	14.56	NA	7.64	1.83	NA	NA	24.03	$831.59	090	C+ M
54130		Remove penis & nodes	21.84	NA	10.40	2.62	NA	NA	34.86	$1206.37	090	C+ M
54135		Remove penis & nodes	28.17	NA	12.54	3.36	NA	NA	44.07	$1525.10	090	M
54150		Circumcision w/regionl block	1.90	2.27	0.69	0.25	4.42	$152.96	2.84	$98.28	000	A+ M
54160		Circumcision neonate	2.53	3.71	1.43	0.29	6.53	$225.98	4.25	$147.08	010	A M
54161		Circum 28 days or older	3.32	NA	2.06	0.40	NA	NA	5.78	$200.02	010	A M
54162		Lysis penil circumic lesion	3.32	3.92	2.15	0.40	7.64	$264.39	5.87	$203.14	010	A M
54163		Repair of circumcision	3.32	NA	2.67	0.40	NA	NA	6.39	$221.13	010	A M

54164	Frenulotomy of penis	2.82	NA	2.52	0.34	NA	NA	5.68	$196.56	010	A M
54200	Treatment of penis lesion	1.11	2.17	1.28	0.12	3.40	$117.66	2.51	$86.86	010	A M
54205	Treatment of penis lesion	8.97	NA	5.57	1.06	NA	NA	15.60	$539.86	090	M
54220	Treatment of penis lesion	2.42	3.73	1.11	0.37	6.52	$225.63	3.90	$134.96	000	A M
54230	Prepare penis study	1.34	1.61	0.81	0.17	3.12	$107.97	2.32	$80.29	000	A M
54231	Dynamic cavernosometry	2.04	1.90	1.08	0.24	4.18	$144.65	3.36	$116.28	000	A M
54235	Penile injection	1.19	1.27	0.80	0.12	2.58	$89.28	2.11	$73.02	000	A M
54240	Penis study	1.31	1.62	NA	0.18	3.11	$107.63	NA	NA	000	A+
54240-26	Penis study	1.31	0.44	0.44	0.17	1.92	$66.44	1.92	$66.44	000	A+
54240-TC	Penis study	0.00	1.18	NA	0.01	1.19	$41.18	NA	NA	000	A+ DS
54250	Penis study	2.22	1.16	NA	0.20	3.58	$123.89	NA	NA	000	A+
54250-26	Penis study	2.22	0.75	0.75	0.19	3.16	$109.36	3.16	$109.36	000	A+
54250-TC	Penis study	0.00	0.41	NA	0.01	0.42	$14.53	NA	NA	000	A+ GS
54300	Revision of penis	11.20	NA	6.40	1.36	NA	NA	18.96	$656.13	090	C+ M
54304	Revision of penis	13.28	NA	7.03	1.59	NA	NA	21.90	$757.88	090	M
54308	Reconstruction of urethra	12.62	NA	6.85	1.50	NA	NA	20.97	$725.69	090	C+ M
54312	Reconstruction of urethra	14.51	NA	7.71	1.71	NA	NA	23.93	$828.13	090	C+ M
54316	Reconstruction of urethra	18.05	NA	8.87	2.17	NA	NA	29.09	$1006.69	090	C+ M
54318	Reconstruction of urethra	12.43	NA	6.93	1.47	NA	NA	20.83	$720.85	090	C+ M
54322	Reconstruction of urethra	13.98	NA	7.22	1.66	NA	NA	22.86	$791.10	090	M
54324	Reconstruction of urethra	17.55	NA	8.67	2.08	NA	NA	28.30	$979.36	090	C+ M
54326	Reconstruction of urethra	17.02	NA	8.51	2.01	NA	NA	27.54	$953.05	090	C+ M
54328	Revise penis/urethra	16.89	NA	8.48	2.01	NA	NA	27.38	$947.52	090	C+ M
54332	Revise penis/urethra	18.37	NA	8.98	2.18	NA	NA	29.53	$1021.92	090	C+ M
54336	Revise penis/urethra	21.62	NA	10.52	2.57	NA	NA	34.71	$1201.18	090	C+ M
54340	Rpr hypspad comp simple	9.71	NA	5.83	1.16	NA	NA	16.70	$577.92	090	C+ M
54344	Rrp hypspad comp moblj&urtp	17.06	NA	8.53	2.03	NA	NA	27.62	$955.82	090	C+ M
54348	Rpr hypspad comp dsj & urtp	18.32	NA	9.03	2.18	NA	NA	29.53	$1021.92	090	C+ M

*Please note that these calculations are based on the Medicare 2022 Conversion Factor of $34.6062 and the DRA RVU cap rates at time of publication.

A = assistant-at-surgery restriction
A+ = assistant-at-surgery restriction unless medical necessity established with documentation
B = bilateral surgery adjustment applies
C = cosurgeons payable
C+ = cosurgeons payable if medical necessity established with documentation
CP = carriers may establish RVUs and payment amounts for these services, generally on an individual basis following review of documentation such as an operative report
M = multiple surgery adjustment applies
Me = multiple endoscopy rules may apply
M+ = multiple therapy rules apply
Mtc = multiple diagnostic imaging rules apply
T = team surgeons permitted
T+ = team surgeons payable if medical necessity established with documentation
§ = indicates code is not covered by Medicare
GS = procedure must be performed under the general supervision of a physician
DS = procedure must be performed under the direct supervision of a physician
PS = procedure must be performed under the personal supervision of a physician
DRA = procedure subject to DRA limitation

Relative Value Units

CPT Code and Modifier		Description	Work RVU	Nonfacility Practice Expense RVU	Facility Practice Expense RVU	PLI RVU	Total Non-facility RVUs	Medicare Payment Nonfacility	Total Facility RVUs	Medicare Payment Facility	Global Period	Payment Policy Indicators
54352		Revj prior hypspad repair	26.13	NA	12.04	3.12	NA	NA	41.29	$1428.89	090	C+ M
54360		Penis plastic surgery	12.78	NA	6.81	1.52	NA	NA	21.11	$730.54	090	C+ M
54380		Repair penis	14.18	NA	7.53	1.68	NA	NA	23.39	$809.44	090	C+ M
54385		Repair penis	16.56	NA	8.70	1.98	NA	NA	27.24	$942.67	090	C+ M
54390		Repair penis and bladder	22.77	NA	10.79	2.71	NA	NA	36.27	$1255.17	090	C+ M
54400		Insert semi-rigid prosthesis	9.17	NA	5.35	1.09	NA	NA	15.61	$540.20	090	A C+ M
54401		Insert self-contd prosthesis	10.44	NA	7.75	1.25	NA	NA	19.44	$672.74	090	A C+ M
54405		Insert multi-comp penis pros	14.52	NA	7.41	1.72	NA	NA	23.65	$818.44	090	C+ M
54406		Remove muti-comp penis pros	12.89	NA	6.98	1.54	NA	NA	21.41	$740.92	090	C+ M
54408		Repair multi-comp penis pros	13.91	NA	7.58	1.66	NA	NA	23.15	$801.13	090	C+ M
54410		Remove/replace penis prosth	15.18	NA	8.27	1.81	NA	NA	25.26	$874.15	090	C+ M
54411		Remov/replc penis pros comp	18.35	NA	9.57	2.17	NA	NA	30.09	$1041.30	090	C+ M
54415		Remove self-contd penis pros	8.88	NA	5.64	1.06	NA	NA	15.58	$539.16	090	C+ M
54416		Remv/repl penis contain pros	12.08	NA	7.45	1.47	NA	NA	21.00	$726.73	090	C+ M
54417		Remv/replc penis pros compl	16.10	NA	8.27	1.93	NA	NA	26.30	$910.14	090	C+ M
54420		Revision of penis	12.39	NA	6.72	1.47	NA	NA	20.58	$712.20	090	M
54430		Revision of penis	11.06	NA	6.34	1.32	NA	NA	18.72	$647.83	090	M
54435		Revision of penis	6.81	NA	4.53	0.79	NA	NA	12.13	$419.77	090	A M
54437		Repair corporeal tear	11.50	NA	6.98	1.37	NA	NA	19.85	$686.93	090	C+ M
54438		Replantation of penis	24.50	NA	11.62	2.92	NA	NA	39.04	$1351.03	090	C+ M
54440	CP	Repair of penis	0.00	0.00	0.00	0.00	0.00	$0.00	0.00	$0.00	090	C+ M
54450		Preputial stretching	1.12	0.75	0.41	0.12	1.99	$68.87	1.65	$57.10	000	A M
54500		Biopsy of testis	1.31	NA	0.69	0.17	NA	NA	2.17	$75.10	000	A+ B M
54505		Biopsy of testis	3.50	NA	2.22	0.41	NA	NA	6.13	$212.14	010	A+ B M
54512		Excise lesion testis	9.33	NA	5.29	1.12	NA	NA	15.74	$544.70	090	A B C+ M
54520		Removal of testis	5.30	NA	3.64	0.70	NA	NA	9.64	$333.60	090	A B M
54522		Orchiectomy partial	10.25	NA	5.76	1.21	NA	NA	17.22	$595.92	090	B C+ M
54530		Removal of testis	8.46	NA	5.41	1.04	NA	NA	14.91	$515.98	090	B C+ M
54535		Extensive testis surgery	13.19	NA	7.03	1.55	NA	NA	21.77	$753.38	090	B M
54550		Exploration for testis	8.41	NA	5.00	1.00	NA	NA	14.41	$498.68	090	B M
54560		Exploration for testis	12.10	NA	6.60	1.42	NA	NA	20.12	$696.28	090	B C+ M
54600		Reduce testis torsion	7.64	NA	4.73	0.90	NA	NA	13.27	$459.22	090	A B M
54620		Suspension of testis	5.21	NA	2.91	0.61	NA	NA	8.73	$302.11	010	A B M

54640		Orchiopexy ingun/scrot appr	7.73	NA	3.95	1.00	NA	NA	12.68	$438.81	090	A+ B M
54650		Orchiopexy (fowler-stephens)	12.39	NA	6.99	1.47	NA	NA	20.85	$721.54	090	B M
54660		Revision of testis	5.74	NA	4.09	0.68	NA	NA	10.51	$363.71	090	A+ B M
54670		Repair testis injury	6.65	NA	4.57	0.78	NA	NA	12.00	$415.27	090	A+ B M
54680		Relocation of testis(es)	14.04	NA	7.34	1.68	NA	NA	23.06	$798.02	090	B C+ M
54690		Laparoscopy orchiectomy	11.70	NA	6.10	1.40	NA	NA	19.20	$664.44	090	B C+ M
54692		Laparoscopy orchiopexy	13.74	NA	6.74	1.64	NA	NA	22.12	$765.49	090	A B M
54699	CP	Laparoscope proc testis	0.00	0.00	0.00	0.00	0.00	$0.00	0.00	$0.00	YYY	B C+ M T+
54700		Drainage of scrotum	3.47	NA	2.33	0.45	NA	NA	6.25	$216.29	010	A B M
54800		Biopsy of epididymis	2.33	NA	1.04	0.27	NA	NA	3.64	$125.97	000	A+ B M
54830		Remove epididymis lesion	6.01	NA	4.20	0.73	NA	NA	10.94	$378.59	090	A+ B M
54840		Remove epididymis lesion	5.27	NA	3.57	0.62	NA	NA	9.46	$327.37	090	A B M
54860		Removal of epididymis	6.95	NA	4.51	0.84	NA	NA	12.30	$425.66	090	A M
54861		Removal of epididymis	9.70	NA	5.81	1.16	NA	NA	16.67	$576.89	090	A+ M
54865		Explore epididymis	5.77	NA	4.10	0.68	NA	NA	10.55	$365.10	090	A+ M
54900		Fusion of spermatic ducts	14.20	NA	7.54	1.69	NA	NA	23.43	$810.82	090	A+ M
54901		Fusion of spermatic ducts	19.10	NA	9.57	2.27	NA	NA	30.94	$1070.72	090	A+ M
55000		Drainage of hydrocele	1.43	1.96	0.85	0.19	3.58	$123.89	2.47	$85.48	000	A B M
55040		Removal of hydrocele	5.45	NA	3.82	0.68	NA	NA	9.95	$344.33	090	A M
55041		Removal of hydroceles	8.54	NA	5.45	1.04	NA	NA	15.03	$520.13	090	A M
55060		Repair of hydrocele	6.15	NA	4.25	0.76	NA	NA	11.16	$386.21	090	A+ B M
55100		Drainage of scrotum abscess	2.45	4.07	2.12	0.35	6.87	$237.74	4.92	$170.26	010	A M
55110		Explore scrotum	6.33	NA	4.27	0.83	NA	NA	11.43	$395.55	090	A M
55120		Removal of scrotum lesion	5.72	NA	4.02	0.67	NA	NA	10.41	$360.25	090	A+ M
55150		Removal of scrotum	8.14	NA	5.35	1.05	NA	NA	14.54	$503.17	090	C+ M
55175		Revision of scrotum	5.87	NA	4.12	0.73	NA	NA	10.72	$370.98	090	A+ M
55180		Revision of scrotum	11.78	NA	6.99	1.54	NA	NA	20.31	$702.85	090	A+ M
55200		Incision of sperm duct	4.55	6.36	3.04	0.55	11.46	$396.59	8.14	$281.69	090	A+ M

*Please note that these calculations are based on the Medicare 2022 Conversion Factor of $34.6062 and the DRA RVU cap rates at time of publication.

A = assistant-at-surgery restriction
A+ = assistant-at-surgery restriction unless medical necessity established with documentation
B = bilateral surgery adjustment applies
C = cosurgeons payable
C+ = cosurgeons payable if medical necessity established with documentation
CP = carriers may establish RVUs and payment amounts for these services, generally on an individual basis following review of documentation such as an operative report
M = multiple surgery adjustment applies
Me = multiple endoscopy rules may apply
M+ = multiple therapy rules apply
Mtc = multiple diagnostic imaging rules apply
T = team surgeons permitted
T+ = team surgeons payable if medical necessity established with documentation
§ = indicates code is not covered by Medicare
GS = procedure must be performed under the general supervision of a physician
DS = procedure must be performed under the direct supervision of a physician
PS = procedure must be performed under the personal supervision of a physician
DRA = procedure subject to DRA limitation

Relative Value Units

CPT Code and Modifier		Description	Work RVU	Nonfacility Practice Expense RVU	Facility Practice Expense RVU	PLI RVU	Total Non-facility RVUs	Medicare Payment Nonfacility	Total Facility RVUs	Medicare Payment Facility	Global Period	Payment Policy Indicators
55250		Removal of sperm duct(s)	3.37	6.24	2.93	0.40	10.01	$346.41	6.70	$231.86	090	A M
55300		Prepare sperm duct x-ray	3.50	NA	1.50	0.41	NA	NA	5.41	$187.22	000	A+ M
55400		Repair of sperm duct	8.61	NA	5.01	1.02	NA	NA	14.64	$506.63	090	B C+ M
55500		Removal of hydrocele	6.22	NA	4.45	0.93	NA	NA	11.60	$401.43	090	A+ B M
55520		Removal of sperm cord lesion	6.66	NA	5.43	1.61	NA	NA	13.70	$474.10	090	B C+ M
55530		Revise spermatic cord veins	5.75	NA	3.90	0.73	NA	NA	10.38	$359.21	090	A B C+ M
55535		Revise spermatic cord veins	7.19	NA	4.58	0.87	NA	NA	12.64	$437.42	090	B C+ M
55540		Revise hernia & sperm veins	8.30	NA	6.22	2.09	NA	NA	16.61	$574.81	090	A B C+ M
55550		Laparo ligate spermatic vein	7.20	NA	4.54	0.87	NA	NA	12.61	$436.38	090	B C+ M
55559	CP	Laparo proc spermatic cord	0.00	0.00	0.00	0.00	0.00	$0.00	0.00	$0.00	YYY	B C+ M T+
55600		Incise sperm duct pouch	7.01	NA	4.53	0.85	NA	NA	12.39	$428.77	090	A+ B M
55605		Incise sperm duct pouch	8.76	NA	5.56	1.04	NA	NA	15.36	$531.55	090	A+ B M
55650		Remove sperm duct pouch	12.65	NA	6.89	1.51	NA	NA	21.05	$728.46	090	B C+ M
55680		Remove sperm pouch lesion	5.67	NA	3.85	0.67	NA	NA	10.19	$352.64	090	A+ B M
55700		Biopsy of prostate	2.50	4.43	0.99	0.29	7.22	$249.86	3.78	$130.81	000	A M
55705		Biopsy of prostate	4.61	NA	2.60	0.56	NA	NA	7.77	$268.89	010	A C+ M
55706		Prostate saturation sampling	6.28	NA	4.00	0.73	NA	NA	11.01	$381.01	010	C+ M
55720		Drainage of prostate abscess	7.73	NA	4.61	0.93	NA	NA	13.27	$459.22	090	C+ M
55725		Drainage of prostate abscess	10.05	NA	6.20	1.20	NA	NA	17.45	$603.88	090	C+ M
55801		Removal of prostate	19.80	NA	9.85	2.34	NA	NA	31.99	$1107.05	090	C+ M
55810		Extensive prostate surgery	24.29	NA	10.97	2.90	NA	NA	38.16	$1320.57	090	C+ M
55812		Extensive prostate surgery	29.89	NA	13.45	3.56	NA	NA	46.90	$1623.03	090	C+ M
55815		Extensive prostate surgery	32.95	NA	14.48	3.92	NA	NA	51.35	$1777.03	090	C+ M
55821		Removal of prostate	15.76	NA	7.89	1.86	NA	NA	25.51	$882.80	090	C+ M
55831		Removal of prostate	17.19	NA	8.38	2.07	NA	NA	27.64	$956.52	090	C+ M
55840		Extensive prostate surgery	21.36	NA	10.22	2.56	NA	NA	34.14	$1181.46	090	C+ M
55842		Extensive prostate surgery	21.36	NA	10.23	2.56	NA	NA	34.15	$1181.80	090	C+ M
55845		Extensive prostate surgery	25.18	NA	11.51	3.02	NA	NA	39.71	$1374.21	090	C+ M
55860		Surgical exposure prostate	15.84	NA	7.86	1.87	NA	NA	25.57	$884.88	090	A C+ M
55862		Extensive prostate surgery	20.04	NA	9.57	2.38	NA	NA	31.99	$1107.05	090	C+ M
55865		Extensive prostate surgery	24.57	NA	11.48	2.93	NA	NA	38.98	$1348.95	090	C+ M
55866		Laparo radical prostatectomy	26.80	NA	12.02	3.22	NA	NA	42.04	$1454.84	090	C+ M
55870		Electroejaculation	2.58	2.27	1.23	0.31	5.16	$178.57	4.12	$142.58	000	A C+ M

55873		Cryoablate prostate	13.60	162.77	7.14	1.62	177.99	$6159.56	22.36	$773.79	090	A M
55874		Tprnl plmt biodegrdabl matrl	3.03	85.56	1.47	0.29	88.88	$3075.80	4.79	$165.76	000	A C+ M T+
55875		Transperi needle place pros	13.46	NA	7.83	1.40	NA	NA	22.69	$785.21	090	A+ M
55876		Place rt device/marker pros	1.73	2.56	1.04	0.19	4.48	$155.04	2.96	$102.43	000	A C+ M T+
55880		Abltj mal prst8 tiss hifu	17.73	NA	8.78	2.16	NA	NA	28.67	$992.16	090	A M
55899	CP	Genital surgery procedure	0.00	0.00	0.00	0.00	0.00	$0.00	0.00	$0.00	YYY	A+ C+ M T+
55920		Place needles pelvic for rt	8.31	NA	4.42	0.65	NA	NA	13.38	$463.03	000	A+ M
55970	CP	Sex transformation m to f	0.00	0.00	0.00	0.00	0.00	$0.00	0.00	$0.00	YYY	
55980	CP	Sex transformation f to m	0.00	0.00	0.00	0.00	0.00	$0.00	0.00	$0.00	YYY	
56405		I & d of vulva/perineum	1.49	2.73	2.06	0.25	4.47	$154.69	3.80	$131.50	010	A C M
56420		Drainage of gland abscess	1.44	3.95	1.64	0.25	5.64	$195.18	3.33	$115.24	010	A M
56440		Surgery for vulva lesion	2.89	NA	2.01	0.45	NA	NA	5.35	$185.14	010	A M
56441		Lysis of labial lesion(s)	2.02	3.21	2.28	0.31	5.54	$191.72	4.61	$159.53	010	A+ M
56442		Hymenotomy	0.68	NA	0.59	0.11	NA	NA	1.38	$47.76	000	A+ M
56501		Destroy vulva lesions sim	1.58	4.01	2.15	0.24	5.83	$201.75	3.97	$137.39	010	A M
56515		Destroy vulva lesion/s compl	3.08	4.79	2.76	0.50	8.37	$289.65	6.34	$219.40	010	A M
56605		Biopsy of vulva/perineum	1.10	1.62	0.47	0.18	2.90	$100.36	1.75	$60.56	000	A C M
56606		Biopsy of vulva/perineum	0.55	0.50	0.22	0.09	1.14	$39.45	0.86	$29.76	ZZZ	A C
56620		Partial removal of vulva	7.53	NA	8.74	1.24	NA	NA	17.51	$605.95	090	C+ M
56625		Complete removal of vulva	9.68	NA	8.64	1.60	NA	NA	19.92	$689.36	090	C+ M
56630		Extensive vulva surgery	14.80	NA	11.39	2.40	NA	NA	28.59	$989.39	090	C+ M
56631		Extensive vulva surgery	18.99	NA	13.09	3.12	NA	NA	35.20	$1218.14	090	C M
56632		Extensive vulva surgery	21.86	NA	17.23	3.57	NA	NA	42.66	$1476.30	090	C M
56633		Extensive vulva surgery	19.62	NA	13.71	3.22	NA	NA	36.55	$1264.86	090	C M
56634		Extensive vulva surgery	20.66	NA	14.36	3.39	NA	NA	38.41	$1329.22	090	C M
56637		Extensive vulva surgery	24.75	NA	16.17	4.06	NA	NA	44.98	$1556.59	090	C M
56640		Extensive vulva surgery	24.78	NA	16.47	4.06	NA	NA	45.31	$1568.01	090	B C+ M
56700		Partial removal of hymen	2.84	NA	2.78	0.45	NA	NA	6.07	$210.06	010	C+ M

*Please note that these calculations are based on the Medicare 2022 Conversion Factor of $34.6062 and the DRA RVU cap rates at time of publication.

A = assistant-at-surgery restriction

A+ = assistant-at-surgery restriction unless medical necessity established with documentation

B = bilateral surgery adjustment applies

C = cosurgeons payable

C+ = cosurgeons payable if medical necessity established with documentation

CP = carriers may establish RVUs and payment amounts for these services, generally on an individual basis following review of documentation such as an operative report

M = multiple surgery adjustment applies

Me = multiple endoscopy rules may apply

M+ = multiple therapy rules apply

Mtc = multiple diagnostic imaging rules apply

T = team surgeons permitted

T+ = team surgeons payable if medical necessity established with documentation

§ = indicates code is not covered by Medicare

GS = procedure must be performed under the general supervision of a physician

DS = procedure must be performed under the direct supervision of a physician

PS = procedure must be performed under the personal supervision of a physician

DRA = procedure subject to DRA limitation

Relative Value Units

CPT Code and Modifier	Description	Work RVU	Nonfacility Practice Expense RVU	Facility Practice Expense RVU	PLI RVU	Total Non-facility RVUs	Medicare Payment Nonfacility	Total Facility RVUs	Medicare Payment Facility	Global Period	Payment Policy Indicators
56740	Remove vagina gland lesion	4.88	NA	3.72	0.84	NA	NA	9.44	$326.68	010	A B M
56800	Repair of vagina	3.93	NA	2.98	0.62	NA	NA	7.53	$260.58	010	C+ M
56805	Repair clitoris	19.88	NA	11.63	3.26	NA	NA	34.77	$1203.26	090	C+ M
56810	Repair of perineum	4.29	NA	3.13	0.68	NA	NA	8.10	$280.31	010	C M
56820	Exam of vulva w/scope	1.50	1.99	0.74	0.25	3.74	$129.43	2.49	$86.17	000	A M
56821	Exam/biopsy of vulva w/scope	2.05	2.62	0.96	0.34	5.01	$173.38	3.35	$115.93	000	A M
57000	Exploration of vagina	3.02	NA	2.52	0.50	NA	NA	6.04	$209.02	010	A+ M
57010	Drainage of pelvic abscess	6.84	NA	5.72	1.11	NA	NA	13.67	$473.07	090	A+ M
57020	Drainage of pelvic fluid	1.50	2.07	0.60	0.25	3.82	$132.20	2.35	$81.32	000	A+ M
57022	I & d vaginal hematoma pp	2.73	NA	2.26	0.43	NA	NA	5.42	$187.57	010	A+ M
57023	I & d vag hematoma non-ob	5.18	NA	3.51	0.86	NA	NA	9.55	$330.49	010	A+ M
57061	Destroy vag lesions simple	1.30	3.57	1.92	0.21	5.08	$175.80	3.43	$118.70	010	A M
57065	Destroy vag lesions complex	2.66	4.38	2.46	0.42	7.46	$258.16	5.54	$191.72	010	A M
57100	Biopsy of vagina	1.20	1.70	0.54	0.20	3.10	$107.28	1.94	$67.14	000	A M
57105	Biopsy of vagina	1.74	3.33	2.36	0.27	5.34	$184.80	4.37	$151.23	010	A M
57106	Remove vagina wall partial	7.50	NA	7.37	1.20	NA	NA	16.07	$556.12	090	C+ M
57107	Remove vagina tissue part	24.56	NA	14.84	3.88	NA	NA	43.28	$1497.76	090	C+ M
57109	Vaginectomy partial w/nodes	28.40	NA	18.27	4.65	NA	NA	51.32	$1775.99	090	C+ M
57110	Remove vagina wall complete	15.48	NA	8.98	2.47	NA	NA	26.93	$931.94	090	C+ M
57111	Remove vagina tissue compl	28.40	NA	18.27	4.65	NA	NA	51.32	$1775.99	090	C+ M
57120	Closure of vagina	8.28	NA	6.27	1.29	NA	NA	15.84	$548.16	090	C+ M
57130	Remove vagina lesion	2.46	4.12	2.31	0.40	6.98	$241.55	5.17	$178.91	010	C+ M
57135	Remove vagina lesion	2.70	4.34	2.47	0.42	7.46	$258.16	5.59	$193.45	010	A M
57150	Treat vagina infection	0.50	1.20	0.19	0.09	1.79	$61.95	0.78	$26.99	000	A M
57155	Insert uteri tandem/ovoids	5.15	6.05	2.72	0.42	11.62	$402.12	8.29	$286.89	000	A C M
57156	Ins vag brachytx device	2.69	3.84	1.51	0.20	6.73	$232.90	4.40	$152.27	000	A+ M
57160	Insert pessary/other device	0.89	1.21	0.33	0.12	2.22	$76.83	1.34	$46.37	000	A M
57170	Fitting of diaphragm/cap	0.91	1.29	0.35	0.14	2.34	$80.98	1.40	$48.45	000	A+ M
57180	Treat vaginal bleeding	1.63	4.17	1.75	0.25	6.05	$209.37	3.63	$125.62	010	A M
57200	Repair of vagina	4.42	NA	4.80	0.73	NA	NA	9.95	$344.33	090	C+ M
57210	Repair vagina/perineum	5.71	NA	5.15	0.93	NA	NA	11.79	$408.01	090	C+ M
57220	Revision of urethra	4.85	NA	4.76	0.77	NA	NA	10.38	$359.21	090	C+ M
57230	Repair of urethral lesion	6.30	NA	5.21	1.02	NA	NA	12.53	$433.62	090	C+ M

57240	Anterior colporrhaphy	10.08	NA	6.66	1.51	NA	NA	18.25	$631.56	090	C+ M
57250	Repair rectum & vagina	10.08	NA	6.70	1.59	NA	NA	18.37	$635.72	090	C+ M
57260	Cmbn ant pst colprhy	13.25	NA	7.86	2.08	NA	NA	23.19	$802.52	090	C+ M
57265	Cmbn ap colprhy w/ntrcl rpr	15.00	NA	8.57	2.39	NA	NA	25.96	$898.38	090	C+ M
57267	Insert mesh/pelvic flr addon	4.88	NA	1.78	0.73	NA	NA	7.39	$255.74	ZZZ	C+
57268	Repair of bowel bulge	7.57	NA	6.38	1.18	NA	NA	15.13	$523.59	090	C+ M
57270	Repair of bowel pouch	13.67	NA	8.38	2.18	NA	NA	24.23	$838.51	090	C+ M
57280	Suspension of vagina	16.72	NA	9.45	2.56	NA	NA	28.73	$994.24	090	C+ M
57282	Colpopexy extraperitoneal	11.63	NA	7.25	1.78	NA	NA	20.66	$714.96	090	C+ M
57283	Colpopexy intraperitoneal	11.66	NA	7.31	1.84	NA	NA	20.81	$720.16	090	C+ M
57284	Repair paravag defect open	14.33	NA	8.28	2.17	NA	NA	24.78	$857.54	090	C M
57285	Repair paravag defect vag	11.60	NA	7.28	1.76	NA	NA	20.64	$714.27	090	C M
57287	Revise/remove sling repair	11.15	NA	9.37	1.62	NA	NA	22.14	$766.18	090	C+ M
57288	Repair bladder defect	12.13	NA	8.17	1.78	NA	NA	22.08	$764.10	090	C+ M
57289	Repair bladder & vagina	12.80	NA	8.83	2.09	NA	NA	23.72	$820.86	090	C+ M
57291	Construction of vagina	8.64	NA	6.37	1.41	NA	NA	16.42	$568.23	090	M
57292	Construct vagina with graft	14.01	NA	8.40	2.29	NA	NA	24.70	$854.77	090	C+ M
57295	Revise vag graft via vagina	7.82	NA	5.96	1.18	NA	NA	14.96	$517.71	090	C+ M
57296	Revise vag graft open abd	16.56	NA	9.28	2.71	NA	NA	28.55	$988.01	090	C+ M
57300	Repair rectum-vagina fistula	8.71	NA	8.12	1.52	NA	NA	18.35	$635.02	090	C+ M
57305	Repair rectum-vagina fistula	15.35	NA	11.18	2.98	NA	NA	29.51	$1021.23	090	C+ M
57307	Fistula repair & colostomy	17.17	NA	12.74	2.26	NA	NA	32.17	$1113.28	090	C+ M
57308	Fistula repair transperine	10.59	NA	7.66	1.40	NA	NA	19.65	$680.01	090	C+ M
57310	Repair urethrovaginal lesion	7.65	NA	6.04	0.90	NA	NA	14.59	$504.90	090	C+ M
57311	Repair urethrovaginal lesion	8.91	NA	6.47	1.05	NA	NA	16.43	$568.58	090	C+ M
57320	Repair bladder-vagina lesion	8.88	NA	6.55	1.44	NA	NA	16.87	$583.81	090	C+ M
57330	Repair bladder-vagina lesion	13.21	NA	7.85	1.57	NA	NA	22.63	$783.14	090	C+ M
57335	Repair vagina	20.02	NA	11.81	3.28	NA	NA	35.11	$1215.02	090	C+ M

*Please note that these calculations are based on the Medicare 2022 Conversion Factor of $34.6062 and the DRA RVU cap rates at time of publication.

A = assistant-at-surgery restriction

A+ = assistant-at-surgery restriction unless medical necessity established with documentation

B = bilateral surgery adjustment applies

C = cosurgeons payable

C+ = cosurgeons payable if medical necessity established with documentation

CP = carriers may establish RVUs and payment amounts for these services, generally on an individual basis following review of documentation such as an operative report

M = multiple surgery adjustment applies

Me = multiple endoscopy rules may apply

M+ = multiple therapy rules apply

Mtc = multiple diagnostic imaging rules apply

T = team surgeons permitted

T+ = team surgeons payable if medical necessity established with documentation

§ = indicates code is not covered by Medicare

GS = procedure must be performed under the general supervision of a physician

DS = procedure must be performed under the direct supervision of a physician

PS = procedure must be performed under the personal supervision of a physician

DRA = procedure subject to DRA limitation

Relative Value Units

CPT Code and Modifier	Description	Work RVU	Nonfacility Practice Expense RVU	Facility Practice Expense RVU	PLI RVU	Total Non-facility RVUs	Medicare Payment Nonfacility	Total Facility RVUs	Medicare Payment Facility	Global Period	Payment Policy Indicators
57400	Dilation of vagina	2.27	NA	1.24	0.35	NA	NA	3.86	$133.58	000	A+ M
57410	Pelvic examination	1.75	NA	1.09	0.27	NA	NA	3.11	$107.63	000	A M
57415	Remove vaginal foreign body	2.49	NA	2.36	0.39	NA	NA	5.24	$181.34	010	A+ M
57420	Exam of vagina w/scope	1.60	2.09	0.78	0.25	3.94	$136.35	2.63	$91.01	000	A M
57421	Exam/biopsy of vag w/scope	2.20	2.75	1.03	0.35	5.30	$183.41	3.58	$123.89	000	A M
57423	Repair paravag defect lap	16.08	NA	9.04	2.50	NA	NA	27.62	$955.82	090	C M
57425	Laparoscopy surg colpopexy	17.03	NA	9.29	2.60	NA	NA	28.92	$1000.81	090	C+ M
57426	Revise prosth vag graft lap	14.30	NA	9.49	2.16	NA	NA	25.95	$898.03	090	C+ M
57452	Exam of cervix w/scope	1.50	2.05	0.93	0.24	3.79	$131.16	2.67	$92.40	000	A M
57454	Bx/curett of cervix w/scope	2.33	2.35	1.23	0.39	5.07	$175.45	3.95	$136.69	000	A Me
57455	Biopsy of cervix w/scope	1.99	2.53	0.90	0.32	4.84	$167.49	3.21	$111.09	000	A Me
57456	Endocerv curettage w/scope	1.85	2.40	0.84	0.29	4.54	$157.11	2.98	$103.13	000	A Me
57460	Bx of cervix w/scope leep	2.83	6.30	1.41	0.44	9.57	$331.18	4.68	$161.96	000	A Me
57461	Conz of cervix w/scope leep	3.43	6.69	1.44	0.56	10.68	$369.59	5.43	$187.91	000	A Me
57465	Cam cervix uteri drg colp	0.81	0.67	0.31	0.12	1.60	$55.37	1.24	$42.91	ZZZ	A+
57500	Biopsy of cervix	1.20	3.30	0.81	0.20	4.70	$162.65	2.21	$76.48	000	A M
57505	Endocervical curettage	1.19	3.32	1.88	0.20	4.71	$163.00	3.27	$113.16	010	A M
57510	Cauterization of cervix	1.90	2.86	1.12	0.31	5.07	$175.45	3.33	$115.24	010	A M
57511	Cryocautery of cervix	1.95	3.79	2.13	0.32	6.06	$209.71	4.40	$152.27	010	A M
57513	Laser surgery of cervix	1.95	3.99	2.12	0.32	6.26	$216.63	4.39	$151.92	010	A M
57520	Conization of cervix	4.11	5.84	4.05	0.66	10.61	$367.17	8.82	$305.23	090	A M
57522	Conization of cervix	3.67	4.85	3.33	0.60	9.12	$315.61	7.60	$263.01	090	A M
57530	Removal of cervix	5.27	NA	5.04	0.86	NA	NA	11.17	$386.55	090	C+ M
57531	Removal of cervix radical	29.95	NA	15.74	8.61	NA	NA	54.30	$1879.12	090	C+ M
57540	Removal of residual cervix	13.29	NA	8.15	2.17	NA	NA	23.61	$817.05	090	C+ M
57545	Remove cervix/repair pelvis	14.10	NA	8.46	2.31	NA	NA	24.87	$860.66	090	C+ M
57550	Removal of residual cervix	6.34	NA	5.53	1.04	NA	NA	12.91	$446.77	090	C+ M
57555	Remove cervix/repair vagina	9.94	NA	6.92	1.63	NA	NA	18.49	$639.87	090	C+ M
57556	Remove cervix repair bowel	9.36	NA	6.67	1.53	NA	NA	17.56	$607.68	090	C+ M
57558	D&c of cervical stump	1.72	2.77	1.86	0.27	4.76	$164.73	3.85	$133.23	010	A M
57700	Revision of cervix	4.35	NA	5.64	0.72	NA	NA	10.71	$370.63	090	A+ M
57720	Revision of cervix	4.61	NA	4.66	0.76	NA	NA	10.03	$347.10	090	M
57800	Dilation of cervical canal	0.77	1.44	0.51	0.12	2.33	$80.63	1.40	$48.45	000	A M

58100		Biopsy of uterus lining	1.21	1.66	0.47	0.20	3.07	$106.24	1.88	$65.06	000	A M
58110		Bx done w/colposcopy add-on	0.77	0.59	0.30	0.12	1.48	$51.22	1.19	$41.18	ZZZ	A+
58120		Dilation and curettage	3.59	4.77	2.78	0.60	8.96	$310.07	6.97	$241.21	010	A M
58140		Myomectomy abdom method	15.79	NA	9.32	2.72	NA	NA	27.83	$963.09	090	C+ M
58145		Myomectomy vag method	8.91	NA	6.63	1.44	NA	NA	16.98	$587.61	090	C+ M
58146		Myomectomy abdom complex	20.34	NA	10.72	3.34	NA	NA	34.40	$1190.45	090	C+ M
58150		Total hysterectomy	17.31	NA	9.90	2.85	NA	NA	30.06	$1040.26	090	C+ M
58152		Total hysterectomy	21.86	NA	11.39	3.58	NA	NA	36.83	$1274.55	090	C+ M
58180		Partial hysterectomy	16.60	NA	9.19	2.72	NA	NA	28.51	$986.62	090	C+ M
58200		Extensive hysterectomy	23.10	NA	13.04	3.78	NA	NA	39.92	$1381.48	090	C+ M
58210		Extensive hysterectomy	30.91	NA	18.00	5.10	NA	NA	54.01	$1869.08	090	C+ M
58240		Removal of pelvis contents	49.33	NA	29.72	8.16	NA	NA	87.21	$3018.01	090	C+ M
58260		Vaginal hysterectomy	14.15	NA	8.56	2.29	NA	NA	25.00	$865.16	090	C+ M
58262		Vag hyst including t/o	15.94	NA	9.10	2.57	NA	NA	27.61	$955.48	090	C M
58263		Vag hyst w/t/o & vag repair	17.23	NA	9.58	2.78	NA	NA	29.59	$1024.00	090	C M
58267		Vag hyst w/urinary repair	18.36	NA	10.53	3.00	NA	NA	31.89	$1103.59	090	C+ M
58270		Vag hyst w/enterocele repair	15.30	NA	8.90	2.49	NA	NA	26.69	$923.64	090	C+ M
58275		Hysterectomy/revise vagina	17.03	NA	9.74	2.69	NA	NA	29.46	$1019.50	090	C+ M
58280		Hysterectomy/revise vagina	18.33	NA	10.25	3.00	NA	NA	31.58	$1092.86	090	C+ M
58285		Extensive hysterectomy	23.38	NA	14.96	3.82	NA	NA	42.16	$1459.00	090	C+ M
58290		Vag hyst complex	20.27	NA	10.69	3.32	NA	NA	34.28	$1186.30	090	C+ M
58291		Vag hyst incl t/o complex	22.06	NA	11.37	3.61	NA	NA	37.04	$1281.81	090	C M
58292		Vag hyst t/o & repair compl	23.35	NA	11.86	3.82	NA	NA	39.03	$1350.68	090	C M
58294		Vag hyst w/enterocele compl	21.55	NA	11.18	3.53	NA	NA	36.26	$1254.82	090	C+ M
58300	§	Insert intrauterine device	1.01	2.25	0.39	0.09	3.35	$115.93	1.49	$51.56	XXX	
58301		Remove intrauterine device	1.27	1.85	0.49	0.20	3.32	$114.89	1.96	$67.83	000	A+ M
58321		Artificial insemination	0.92	1.36	0.35	0.14	2.42	$83.75	1.41	$48.79	000	A+ M
58322		Artificial insemination	1.10	1.43	0.42	0.19	2.72	$94.13	1.71	$59.18	000	A+ M

*Please note that these calculations are based on the Medicare 2022 Conversion Factor of $34.6062 and the DRA RVU cap rates at time of publication.

A = assistant-at-surgery restriction
A+ = assistant-at-surgery restriction unless medical necessity established with documentation
B = bilateral surgery adjustment applies
C = cosurgeons payable
C+ = cosurgeons payable if medical necessity established with documentation
CP = carriers may establish RVUs and payment amounts for these services, generally on an individual basis following review of documentation such as an operative report
M = multiple surgery adjustment applies
Me = multiple endoscopy rules may apply
M+ = multiple therapy rules apply
Mtc = multiple diagnostic imaging rules apply
T = team surgeons permitted
T+ = team surgeons payable if medical necessity established with documentation
§ = indicates code is not covered by Medicare
GS = procedure must be performed under the general supervision of a physician
DS = procedure must be performed under the direct supervision of a physician
PS = procedure must be performed under the personal supervision of a physician
DRA = procedure subject to DRA limitation

Relative Value Units

CPT Code and Modifier	Description	Work RVU	Nonfacility Practice Expense RVU	Facility Practice Expense RVU	PLI RVU	Total Non-facility RVUs	Medicare Payment Nonfacility	Total Facility RVUs	Medicare Payment Facility	Global Period	Payment Policy Indicators
58323	Sperm washing	0.23	0.17	0.09	0.04	0.44	$15.23	0.36	$12.46	000	A+ M
58340	Catheter for hysterography	0.88	6.57	0.66	0.12	7.57	$261.97	1.66	$57.45	000	A M
58345	Reopen fallopian tube	4.70	NA	3.16	0.77	NA	NA	8.63	$298.65	010	B C M
58346	Insert heyman uteri capsule	7.56	NA	6.44	0.56	NA	NA	14.56	$503.87	090	A M
58350	Reopen fallopian tube	1.06	3.45	1.62	0.18	4.69	$162.30	2.86	$98.97	010	A B M
58353	Endometr ablate thermal	3.60	24.84	2.71	0.60	29.04	$1004.96	6.91	$239.13	010	A C M
58356	Endometrial cryoablation	6.41	44.71	3.12	1.04	52.16	$1805.06	10.57	$365.79	010	C M
58400	Suspension of uterus	7.14	NA	5.66	1.04	NA	NA	13.84	$478.95	090	C+ M
58410	Suspension of uterus	13.80	NA	8.28	2.25	NA	NA	24.33	$841.97	090	C+ M
58520	Repair of ruptured uterus	13.48	NA	8.16	2.20	NA	NA	23.84	$825.01	090	C+ M
58540	Revision of uterus	15.71	NA	9.07	2.57	NA	NA	27.35	$946.48	090	M
58541	Lsh uterus 250 g or less	12.29	NA	7.58	1.85	NA	NA	21.72	$751.65	090	C Me
58542	Lsh w/t/o ut 250 g or less	14.16	NA	8.34	2.25	NA	NA	24.75	$856.50	090	C M
58543	Lsh uterus above 250 g	14.39	NA	8.39	2.34	NA	NA	25.12	$869.31	090	C M
58544	Lsh w/t/o uterus above 250 g	15.60	NA	8.83	2.54	NA	NA	26.97	$933.33	090	C M
58545	Laparoscopic myomectomy	15.55	NA	8.63	2.62	NA	NA	26.80	$927.45	090	C M
58546	Laparo-myomectomy complex	19.94	NA	9.91	3.27	NA	NA	33.12	$1146.16	090	C M
58548	Lap radical hyst	31.63	NA	18.99	5.17	NA	NA	55.79	$1930.68	090	C M
58550	Laparo-asst vag hysterectomy	15.10	NA	8.65	2.47	NA	NA	26.22	$907.37	090	C Me
58552	Laparo-vag hyst incl t/o	16.91	NA	9.46	2.76	NA	NA	29.13	$1008.08	090	C M
58553	Laparo-vag hyst complex	20.06	NA	9.95	3.29	NA	NA	33.30	$1152.39	090	C M
58554	Laparo-vag hyst w/t/o compl	23.11	NA	11.86	3.78	NA	NA	38.75	$1340.99	090	C M
58555	Hysteroscopy dx sep proc	2.65	8.03	1.37	0.42	11.10	$384.13	4.44	$153.65	000	A+ C M
58558	Hysteroscopy biopsy	4.17	36.73	1.96	0.67	41.57	$1438.58	6.80	$235.32	000	A C Me
58559	Hysteroscopy lysis	5.20	NA	2.34	0.86	NA	NA	8.40	$290.69	000	A C Me
58560	Hysteroscopy resect septum	5.75	NA	2.53	0.95	NA	NA	9.23	$319.42	000	C Me
58561	Hysteroscopy remove myoma	6.60	NA	2.88	1.07	NA	NA	10.55	$365.10	000	A+ C Me
58562	Hysteroscopy remove fb	4.00	8.54	1.88	0.65	13.19	$456.46	6.53	$225.98	000	A C Me
58563	Hysteroscopy ablation	4.47	61.14	2.05	0.73	66.34	$2295.78	7.25	$250.89	000	A+ C Me
58565	Hysteroscopy sterilization	7.12	43.58	5.38	1.17	51.87	$1795.02	13.67	$473.07	090	A C Me
58570	Tlh uterus 250 g or less	13.36	NA	8.43	2.17	NA	NA	23.96	$829.16	090	C M
58571	Tlh w/t/o 250 g or less	15.00	NA	9.53	2.46	NA	NA	26.99	$934.02	090	C M
58572	Tlh uterus over 250 g	17.71	NA	10.24	2.85	NA	NA	30.80	$1065.87	090	C M

58573		Tlh w/t/o uterus over 250 g	20.79	NA	11.97	3.39	NA	NA	36.15	$1251.01	090	C M
58575		Laps tot hyst resj mal	32.60	NA	19.44	5.33	NA	NA	57.37	$1985.36	090	C M
58578	CP	Laparo proc uterus	0.00	0.00	0.00	0.00	0.00	$0.00	0.00	$0.00	YYY	B C+ M T+
58579	CP	Hysteroscope procedure	0.00	0.00	0.00	0.00	0.00	$0.00	0.00	$0.00	YYY	B C+ M T+
58600		Division of fallopian tube	5.91	NA	4.18	0.96	NA	NA	11.05	$382.40	090	C+ M
58605		Division of fallopian tube	5.28	NA	3.91	0.89	NA	NA	10.08	$348.83	090	M
58611		Ligate oviduct(s) add-on	1.45	NA	0.55	0.24	NA	NA	2.24	$77.52	ZZZ	
58615		Occlude fallopian tube(s)	3.94	NA	3.00	0.65	NA	NA	7.59	$262.66	010	M
58660		Laparoscopy lysis	11.59	NA	6.57	2.14	NA	NA	20.30	$702.51	090	C Me
58661		Laparoscopy remove adnexa	11.35	NA	6.17	1.86	NA	NA	19.38	$670.67	010	B C Me
58662		Laparoscopy excise lesions	12.15	NA	6.99	2.01	NA	NA	21.15	$731.92	090	C Me
58670		Laparoscopy tubal cautery	5.91	NA	4.22	0.96	NA	NA	11.09	$383.78	090	A C Me
58671		Laparoscopy tubal block	5.91	NA	4.20	0.96	NA	NA	11.07	$383.09	090	A C Me
58672		Laparoscopy fimbrioplasty	12.91	NA	6.74	2.13	NA	NA	21.78	$753.72	090	B Me
58673		Laparoscopy salpingostomy	14.04	NA	7.27	2.29	NA	NA	23.60	$816.71	090	B Me
58674		Laps abltj uterine fibroids	14.08	NA	7.82	2.31	NA	NA	24.21	$837.82	090	C M
58679	CP	Laparo proc oviduct-ovary	0.00	0.00	0.00	0.00	0.00	$0.00	0.00	$0.00	YYY	B C+ M T+
58700		Removal of fallopian tube	12.95	NA	8.59	2.33	NA	NA	23.87	$826.05	090	C+ M
58720		Removal of ovary/tube(s)	12.16	NA	8.32	2.09	NA	NA	22.57	$781.06	090	C+ M
58740		Adhesiolysis tube ovary	14.90	NA	9.26	2.68	NA	NA	26.84	$928.83	090	C+ M
58750		Repair oviduct	15.64	NA	8.94	2.56	NA	NA	27.14	$939.21	090	B C+ M
58752		Revise ovarian tube(s)	15.64	NA	8.87	2.56	NA	NA	27.07	$936.79	090	B M
58760		Fimbrioplasty	13.93	NA	8.29	2.27	NA	NA	24.49	$847.51	090	B C+ M
58770		Create new tubal opening	14.77	NA	8.54	2.40	NA	NA	25.71	$889.73	090	B M
58800		Drainage of ovarian cyst(s)	4.62	5.55	4.07	0.76	10.93	$378.25	9.45	$327.03	090	A M
58805		Drainage of ovarian cyst(s)	6.42	NA	5.34	1.04	NA	NA	12.80	$442.96	090	C+ M
58820		Drain ovary abscess open	4.70	NA	4.69	0.77	NA	NA	10.16	$351.60	090	B M
58822		Drain ovary abscess percut	11.81	NA	7.59	1.94	NA	NA	21.34	$738.50	090	B C+ M

*Please note that these calculations are based on the Medicare 2022 Conversion Factor of $34.6062 and the DRA RVU cap rates at time of publication.

A = assistant-at-surgery restriction
A+ = assistant-at-surgery restriction unless medical necessity established with documentation
B = bilateral surgery adjustment applies
C = cosurgeons payable
C+ = cosurgeons payable if medical necessity established with documentation
CP = carriers may establish RVUs and payment amounts for these services, generally on an individual basis following review of documentation such as an operative report
M = multiple surgery adjustment applies
Me = multiple endoscopy rules may apply
M+ = multiple therapy rules apply
Mtc = multiple diagnostic imaging rules apply
T = team surgeons permitted
T+ = team surgeons payable if medical necessity established with documentation
§ = indicates code is not covered by Medicare
GS = procedure must be performed under the general supervision of a physician
DS = procedure must be performed under the direct supervision of a physician
PS = procedure must be performed under the personal supervision of a physician
DRA = procedure subject to DRA limitation

Relative Value Units

CPT Code and Modifier		Description	Work RVU	Nonfacility Practice Expense RVU	Facility Practice Expense RVU	PLI RVU	Total Non-facility RVUs	Medicare Payment Nonfacility	Total Facility RVUs	Medicare Payment Facility	Global Period	Payment Policy Indicators
58825		Transposition ovary(s)	11.78	NA	7.47	1.94	NA	NA	21.19	$733.31	090	C+ M
58900		Biopsy of ovary(s)	6.59	NA	5.41	1.07	NA	NA	13.07	$452.30	090	C+ M
58920		Partial removal of ovary(s)	11.95	NA	7.43	1.95	NA	NA	21.33	$738.15	090	C+ M
58925		Removal of ovarian cyst(s)	12.43	NA	8.26	2.20	NA	NA	22.89	$792.14	090	C+ M
58940		Removal of ovary(s)	8.22	NA	6.86	1.53	NA	NA	16.61	$574.81	090	C+ M
58943		Removal of ovary(s)	19.52	NA	11.98	3.22	NA	NA	34.72	$1201.53	090	C+ M
58950		Resect ovarian malignancy	18.37	NA	12.88	3.01	NA	NA	34.26	$1185.61	090	C+ M
58951		Resect ovarian malignancy	24.26	NA	14.52	3.99	NA	NA	42.77	$1480.11	090	C+ M
58952		Resect ovarian malignancy	27.29	NA	17.03	4.52	NA	NA	48.84	$1690.17	090	C+ M
58953		Tah rad dissect for debulk	34.13	NA	19.53	5.61	NA	NA	59.27	$2051.11	090	C+ M
58954		Tah rad debulk/lymph remove	37.13	NA	20.88	6.12	NA	NA	64.13	$2219.30	090	C+ M
58956		Bso omentectomy w/tah	22.80	NA	13.69	3.78	NA	NA	40.27	$1393.59	090	C+ M
58957		Resect recurrent gyn mal	26.22	NA	16.63	4.42	NA	NA	47.27	$1635.84	090	C+ M
58958		Resect recur gyn mal w/lym	29.22	NA	15.33	4.77	NA	NA	49.32	$1706.78	090	C+ M
58960		Exploration of abdomen	15.79	NA	11.16	2.60	NA	NA	29.55	$1022.61	090	C+ M
58970		Retrieval of oocyte	3.52	3.10	1.69	0.57	7.19	$248.82	5.78	$200.02	000	A+ M
58974	CP	Transfer of embryo	0.00	0.00	0.00	0.00	0.00	$0.00	0.00	$0.00	000	C+ M
58976		Transfer of embryo	3.82	3.25	1.80	0.62	7.69	$266.12	6.24	$215.94	000	C+ M
58999	CP	Genital surgery procedure	0.00	0.00	0.00	0.00	0.00	$0.00	0.00	$0.00	YYY	A C+ M T+
59000		Amniocentesis diagnostic	1.30	1.79	0.69	0.37	3.46	$119.74	2.36	$81.67	000	A M
59001		Amniocentesis therapeutic	3.00	NA	1.38	0.87	NA	NA	5.25	$181.68	000	A M
59012		Fetal cord puncture prenatal	3.44	NA	1.49	0.99	NA	NA	5.92	$204.87	000	A+ M
59015		Chorion biopsy	2.20	1.80	1.03	0.62	4.62	$159.88	3.85	$133.23	000	A+ M
59020		Fetal contract stress test	0.66	1.23	NA	0.19	2.08	$71.98	NA	NA	000	A+
59020-26		Fetal contract stress test	0.66	0.25	0.25	0.18	1.09	$37.72	1.09	$37.72	000	A+
59020-TC		Fetal contract stress test	0.00	0.98	NA	0.01	0.99	$34.26	NA	NA	000	A+ DS
59025		Fetal non-stress test	0.53	0.77	NA	0.12	1.42	$49.14	NA	NA	000	A+
59025-26		Fetal non-stress test	0.53	0.20	0.20	0.11	0.84	$29.07	0.84	$29.07	000	A+
59025-TC		Fetal non-stress test	0.00	0.57	NA	0.01	0.58	$20.07	NA	NA	000	A+ GS
59030		Fetal scalp blood sample	1.99	NA	0.75	0.57	NA	NA	3.31	$114.55	000	A+ M
59050		Fetal monitor w/report	0.89	NA	0.34	0.25	NA	NA	1.48	$51.22	XXX	A+
59051		Fetal monitor/interpret only	0.74	NA	0.28	0.21	NA	NA	1.23	$42.57	XXX	A+
59070		Transabdom amnioinfus w/us	5.24	5.10	2.34	1.50	11.84	$409.74	9.08	$314.22	000	M

59072	Umbilical cord occlud w/us	8.99	NA	3.76	2.60	NA	NA	15.35	$531.21	000	A M
59074	Fetal fluid drainage w/us	5.24	4.61	2.34	1.50	11.35	$392.78	9.08	$314.22	000	M
59076	Fetal shunt placement w/us	8.99	NA	3.76	2.60	NA	NA	15.35	$531.21	000	M
59100	Remove uterus lesion	13.37	NA	8.28	3.84	NA	NA	25.49	$882.11	090	C+ M
59120	Treat ectopic pregnancy	12.67	NA	8.01	3.65	NA	NA	24.33	$841.97	090	C+ M
59121	Treat ectopic pregnancy	12.74	NA	7.94	3.67	NA	NA	24.35	$842.66	090	C+ M
59130	Treat ectopic pregnancy	15.08	NA	8.83	4.32	NA	NA	28.23	$976.93	090	A+ M
59136	Treat ectopic pregnancy	14.25	NA	8.45	4.10	NA	NA	26.80	$927.45	090	M
59140	Treat ectopic pregnancy	5.94	NA	4.84	1.70	NA	NA	12.48	$431.89	090	M
59150	Treat ectopic pregnancy	12.29	NA	7.79	3.54	NA	NA	23.62	$817.40	090	M
59151	Treat ectopic pregnancy	12.11	NA	7.53	3.46	NA	NA	23.10	$799.40	090	M
59160	D & c after delivery	2.76	4.76	2.09	0.78	8.30	$287.23	5.63	$194.83	010	A+ M
59200	Insert cervical dilator	0.79	2.19	0.30	0.22	3.20	$110.74	1.31	$45.33	000	A M
59300	Episiotomy or vaginal repair	2.41	3.87	1.24	0.68	6.96	$240.86	4.33	$149.84	000	A+ M
59320	Revision of cervix	2.48	NA	1.27	0.72	NA	NA	4.47	$154.69	000	A+ M
59325	Revision of cervix	4.06	NA	1.86	1.17	NA	NA	7.09	$245.36	000	A+ M
59350	Repair of uterus	4.94	NA	1.86	1.41	NA	NA	8.21	$284.12	000	M
59400	Obstetrical care	36.58	NA	24.98	9.53	NA	NA	71.09	$2460.15	MMM	A M
59409	Obstetrical care	14.37	NA	5.63	3.73	NA	NA	23.73	$821.21	MMM	A+ M
59410	Obstetrical care	18.34	NA	8.29	4.75	NA	NA	31.38	$1085.94	MMM	A M
59412	Antepartum manipulation	1.71	NA	0.82	0.50	NA	NA	3.03	$104.86	MMM	A+
59414	Deliver placenta	1.61	NA	0.61	0.44	NA	NA	2.66	$92.05	MMM	A+ M
59425	Antepartum care only	7.80	6.81	3.02	2.01	16.62	$575.16	12.83	$444.00	MMM	A+
59426	Antepartum care only	14.30	12.43	5.57	3.63	30.36	$1050.64	23.50	$813.25	MMM	A+
59430	Care after delivery	3.22	3.84	1.25	0.85	7.91	$273.74	5.32	$184.10	MMM	A M
59510	Cesarean delivery	40.39	NA	26.62	11.49	NA	NA	78.50	$2716.59	MMM	A M
59514	Cesarean delivery only	16.13	NA	6.19	4.51	NA	NA	26.83	$928.48	MMM	C+ M
59515	Cesarean delivery	22.13	NA	10.21	6.32	NA	NA	38.66	$1337.88	MMM	A M

*Please note that these calculations are based on the Medicare 2022 Conversion Factor of $34.6062 and the DRA RVU cap rates at time of publication.

A = assistant-at-surgery restriction
A+ = assistant-at-surgery restriction unless medical necessity established with documentation
B = bilateral surgery adjustment applies
C = cosurgeons payable
C+ = cosurgeons payable if medical necessity established with documentation
CP = carriers may establish RVUs and payment amounts for these services, generally on an individual basis following review of documentation such as an operative report
M = multiple surgery adjustment applies
Me = multiple endoscopy rules may apply
M+ = multiple therapy rules apply
Mtc = multiple diagnostic imaging rules apply
T = team surgeons permitted
T+ = team surgeons payable if medical necessity established with documentation
§ = indicates code is not covered by Medicare
GS = procedure must be performed under the general supervision of a physician
DS = procedure must be performed under the direct supervision of a physician
PS = procedure must be performed under the personal supervision of a physician
DRA = procedure subject to DRA limitation

Relative Value Units

CPT Code and Modifier		Description	Work RVU	Nonfacility Practice Expense RVU	Facility Practice Expense RVU	PLI RVU	Total Non-facility RVUs	Medicare Payment Nonfacility	Total Facility RVUs	Medicare Payment Facility	Global Period	Payment Policy Indicators
59525		Remove uterus after cesarean	8.53	NA	3.23	2.46	NA	NA	14.22	$492.10	ZZZ	C+
59610		Vbac delivery	38.29	NA	25.05	11.00	NA	NA	74.34	$2572.62	MMM	A+ M
59612		Vbac delivery only	16.09	NA	6.08	4.62	NA	NA	26.79	$927.10	MMM	A+ M
59614		Vbac care after delivery	20.06	NA	8.04	5.79	NA	NA	33.89	$1172.80	MMM	A+ M
59618		Attempted vbac delivery	40.91	NA	26.67	11.75	NA	NA	79.33	$2745.31	MMM	A+ M
59620		Attempted vbac delivery only	16.66	NA	6.30	4.78	NA	NA	27.74	$959.98	MMM	M
59622		Attempted vbac after care	22.66	NA	10.94	6.50	NA	NA	40.10	$1387.71	MMM	A+ M
59812		Treatment of miscarriage	4.44	5.20	3.47	1.27	10.91	$377.55	9.18	$317.68	090	A M
59820		Care of miscarriage	4.84	6.97	5.28	1.38	13.19	$456.46	11.50	$397.97	090	A M
59821		Treatment of miscarriage	5.09	6.44	4.69	1.47	13.00	$449.88	11.25	$389.32	090	A+ M
59830		Treat uterus infection	6.59	NA	5.38	1.90	NA	NA	13.87	$479.99	090	A+ M
59840		Abortion	3.01	3.62	2.75	0.89	7.52	$260.24	6.65	$230.13	010	A+ M
59841		Abortion	5.65	5.53	3.83	1.63	12.81	$443.31	11.11	$384.47	010	A+ M
59850		Abortion	5.90	NA	4.06	1.69	NA	NA	11.65	$403.16	090	A+ M
59851		Abortion	5.92	NA	5.17	1.69	NA	NA	12.78	$442.27	090	A+ M
59852		Abortion	8.23	NA	7.03	2.36	NA	NA	17.62	$609.76	090	A+ M
59855		Abortion	6.43	NA	4.38	1.84	NA	NA	12.65	$437.77	090	A+ M
59856		Abortion	7.79	NA	4.78	2.23	NA	NA	14.80	$512.17	090	A+ M
59857		Abortion	9.33	NA	5.26	2.68	NA	NA	17.27	$597.65	090	A+ M
59866		Abortion (mpr)	3.99	NA	1.87	1.16	NA	NA	7.02	$242.94	000	C+ M
59870		Evacuate mole of uterus	6.57	NA	7.61	1.87	NA	NA	16.05	$555.43	090	M
59871		Remove cerclage suture	2.13	NA	1.17	0.60	NA	NA	3.90	$134.96	000	A+ M
59897	CP	Fetal invas px w/us	0.00	0.00	0.00	0.00	0.00	$0.00	0.00	$0.00	YYY	A M
59898	CP	Laparo proc ob care/deliver	0.00	0.00	0.00	0.00	0.00	$0.00	0.00	$0.00	YYY	B C+ M T+
59899	CP	Maternity care procedure	0.00	0.00	0.00	0.00	0.00	$0.00	0.00	$0.00	YYY	C+ M T+
60000		Drain thyroid/tongue cyst	1.81	3.43	2.55	0.25	5.49	$189.99	4.61	$159.53	010	A+ M
60100		Biopsy of thyroid	1.56	1.54	0.54	0.14	3.24	$112.12	2.24	$77.52	000	A M
60200		Remove thyroid lesion	10.02	NA	7.89	1.95	NA	NA	19.86	$687.28	090	C+ M
60210		Partial thyroid excision	11.23	NA	7.57	2.23	NA	NA	21.03	$727.77	090	C+ M
60212		Partial thyroid excision	16.43	NA	10.13	4.16	NA	NA	30.72	$1063.10	090	C+ M
60220		Partial removal of thyroid	11.19	NA	7.70	2.11	NA	NA	21.00	$726.73	090	C+ M
60225		Partial removal of thyroid	14.79	NA	10.34	2.72	NA	NA	27.85	$963.78	090	C+ M
60240		Removal of thyroid	15.04	NA	9.23	3.00	NA	NA	27.27	$943.71	090	C+ M

60252		Removal of thyroid	22.01	NA	12.85	4.38	NA	NA	39.24	$1357.95	090	C+ M
60254		Extensive thyroid surgery	28.42	NA	15.62	5.43	NA	NA	49.47	$1711.97	090	C+ M
60260		Repeat thyroid surgery	18.26	NA	10.61	3.44	NA	NA	32.31	$1118.13	090	B C+ M
60270		Removal of thyroid	23.20	NA	12.64	4.56	NA	NA	40.40	$1398.09	090	C+ M
60271		Removal of thyroid	17.62	NA	10.33	3.36	NA	NA	31.31	$1083.52	090	C+ M
60280		Remove thyroid duct lesion	6.16	NA	6.38	0.95	NA	NA	13.49	$466.84	090	C+ M
60281		Remove thyroid duct lesion	8.82	NA	7.58	1.26	NA	NA	17.66	$611.15	090	C+ M
60300		Aspir/inj thyroid cyst	0.97	2.15	0.36	0.10	3.22	$111.43	1.43	$49.49	000	A M
60500		Explore parathyroid glands	15.60	NA	9.90	3.34	NA	NA	28.84	$998.04	090	C+ M
60502		Re-explore parathyroids	21.15	NA	12.89	4.63	NA	NA	38.67	$1338.22	090	C+ M
60505		Explore parathyroid glands	23.06	NA	13.95	4.62	NA	NA	41.63	$1440.66	090	C+ M
60512		Autotransplant parathyroid	4.44	NA	1.79	0.90	NA	NA	7.13	$246.74	ZZZ	C+
60520		Removal of thymus gland	17.16	NA	10.09	4.01	NA	NA	31.26	$1081.79	090	C+ M
60521		Removal of thymus gland	19.18	NA	9.35	4.55	NA	NA	33.08	$1144.77	090	C+ M
60522		Removal of thymus gland	23.48	NA	11.28	5.51	NA	NA	40.27	$1393.59	090	C+ M
60540		Explore adrenal gland	18.02	NA	10.16	3.65	NA	NA	31.83	$1101.52	090	B C+ M
60545		Explore adrenal gland	20.93	NA	11.45	4.55	NA	NA	36.93	$1278.01	090	B C+ M
60600		Remove carotid body lesion	25.09	NA	9.43	5.60	NA	NA	40.12	$1388.40	090	C+ M
60605		Remove carotid body lesion	31.96	NA	8.55	7.99	NA	NA	48.50	$1678.40	090	C+ M
60650		Laparoscopy adrenalectomy	20.73	NA	10.19	4.30	NA	NA	35.22	$1218.83	090	B C+ M
60659	CP	Laparo proc endocrine	0.00	0.00	0.00	0.00	0.00	$0.00	0.00	$0.00	YYY	B M
60699	CP	Endocrine surgery procedure	0.00	0.00	0.00	0.00	0.00	$0.00	0.00	$0.00	YYY	C+ M T+
61000		Remove cranial cavity fluid	1.58	NA	1.16	0.60	NA	NA	3.34	$115.58	000	A M
61001		Remove cranial cavity fluid	1.49	NA	1.12	0.57	NA	NA	3.18	$110.05	000	A M
61020		Remove brain cavity fluid	1.51	NA	1.11	0.51	NA	NA	3.13	$108.32	000	A M
61026		Injection into brain canal	1.69	NA	1.07	0.39	NA	NA	3.15	$109.01	000	A M
61050		Remove brain canal fluid	1.51	NA	0.72	0.12	NA	NA	2.35	$81.32	000	A+ M
61055		Injection into brain canal	2.10	NA	1.03	0.32	NA	NA	3.45	$119.39	000	A

*Please note that these calculations are based on the Medicare 2022 Conversion Factor of $34.6062 and the DRA RVU cap rates at time of publication.

A = assistant-at-surgery restriction
A+ = assistant-at-surgery restriction unless medical necessity established with documentation
B = bilateral surgery adjustment applies
C = cosurgeons payable
C+ = cosurgeons payable if medical necessity established with documentation
CP = carriers may establish RVUs and payment amounts for these services, generally on an individual basis following review of documentation such as an operative report
M = multiple surgery adjustment applies
Me = multiple endoscopy rules may apply
M+ = multiple therapy rules apply
Mtc = multiple diagnostic imaging rules apply
T = team surgeons permitted
T+ = team surgeons payable if medical necessity established with documentation
§ = indicates code is not covered by Medicare
GS = procedure must be performed under the general supervision of a physician
DS = procedure must be performed under the direct supervision of a physician
PS = procedure must be performed under the personal supervision of a physician
DRA = procedure subject to DRA limitation

Relative Value Units

CPT Code and Modifier	Description	Work RVU	Nonfacility Practice Expense RVU	Facility Practice Expense RVU	PLI RVU	Total Non-facility RVUs	Medicare Payment Nonfacility	Total Facility RVUs	Medicare Payment Facility	Global Period	Payment Policy Indicators
61070	Brain canal shunt procedure	0.89	NA	0.61	0.17	NA	NA	1.67	$57.79	000	A M
61105	Twist drill hole	5.45	NA	6.28	2.08	NA	NA	13.81	$477.91	090	A+ M
61107	Drill skull for implantation	4.99	NA	2.37	1.86	NA	NA	9.22	$319.07	000	A
61108	Drill skull for drainage	11.64	NA	11.04	4.26	NA	NA	26.94	$932.29	090	A M
61120	Burr hole for puncture	9.60	NA	9.09	3.69	NA	NA	22.38	$774.49	090	A+ M
61140	Pierce skull for biopsy	17.23	NA	14.03	6.58	NA	NA	37.84	$1309.50	090	M
61150	Pierce skull for drainage	18.90	NA	14.04	7.24	NA	NA	40.18	$1390.48	090	A C+ M
61151	Pierce skull for drainage	13.49	NA	10.95	5.17	NA	NA	29.61	$1024.69	090	A M
61154	Pierce skull & remove clot	17.07	NA	14.46	6.51	NA	NA	38.04	$1316.42	090	B C+ M
61156	Pierce skull for drainage	17.45	NA	12.84	6.67	NA	NA	36.96	$1279.05	090	C+ M
61210	Pierce skull implant device	5.83	NA	2.78	2.20	NA	NA	10.81	$374.09	000	A M
61215	Insert brain-fluid device	5.85	NA	7.26	2.23	NA	NA	15.34	$530.86	090	A C+ M
61250	Pierce skull & explore	11.49	NA	9.99	4.42	NA	NA	25.90	$896.30	090	B C+ M
61253	Pierce skull & explore	13.49	NA	10.95	5.17	NA	NA	29.61	$1024.69	090	M
61304	Open skull for exploration	23.41	NA	16.57	8.84	NA	NA	48.82	$1689.47	090	C+ M
61305	Open skull for exploration	28.64	NA	20.00	10.99	NA	NA	59.63	$2063.57	090	C+ M
61312	Open skull for drainage	30.17	NA	19.83	11.49	NA	NA	61.49	$2127.94	090	C+ M
61313	Open skull for drainage	28.09	NA	20.17	10.69	NA	NA	58.95	$2040.04	090	C+ M
61314	Open skull for drainage	25.90	NA	18.68	9.84	NA	NA	54.42	$1883.27	090	C+ M
61315	Open skull for drainage	29.65	NA	20.39	11.29	NA	NA	61.33	$2122.40	090	C+ M
61316	Implt cran bone flap to abdo	1.39	NA	0.67	0.54	NA	NA	2.60	$89.98	ZZZ	A
61320	Open skull for drainage	27.42	NA	18.48	10.35	NA	NA	56.25	$1946.60	090	C+ M
61321	Open skull for drainage	30.53	NA	20.90	11.71	NA	NA	63.14	$2185.04	090	C+ M
61322	Decompressive craniotomy	34.26	NA	23.42	13.06	NA	NA	70.74	$2448.04	090	C+ M
61323	Decompressive lobectomy	35.06	NA	22.44	13.36	NA	NA	70.86	$2452.20	090	C+ M
61330	Decompress eye socket	25.30	NA	18.34	9.71	NA	NA	53.35	$1846.24	090	B C+ M
61333	Explore orbit/remove lesion	29.27	NA	19.41	11.21	NA	NA	59.89	$2072.57	090	B C+ M
61340	Subtemporal decompression	20.11	NA	15.02	7.71	NA	NA	42.84	$1482.53	090	B C+ M
61343	Incise skull (press relief)	31.86	NA	21.39	12.00	NA	NA	65.25	$2258.05	090	C+ M
61345	Relieve cranial pressure	29.23	NA	20.28	11.20	NA	NA	60.71	$2100.94	090	C+ M
61450	Incise skull for surgery	27.69	NA	18.73	10.63	NA	NA	57.05	$1974.28	090	C+ M
61458	Incise skull for brain wound	28.84	NA	20.04	10.99	NA	NA	59.87	$2071.87	090	C+ M
61460	Incise skull for surgery	30.24	NA	20.77	11.60	NA	NA	62.61	$2166.69	090	C M

61500	Removal of skull lesion	19.18	NA	14.02	5.51	NA	NA	38.71	$1339.61	090	C+ M
61501	Remove infected skull bone	16.35	NA	12.77	4.43	NA	NA	33.55	$1161.04	090	C+ M
61510	Removal of brain lesion	30.83	NA	22.81	11.76	NA	NA	65.40	$2263.25	090	C+ M
61512	Remove brain lining lesion	37.14	NA	24.51	14.17	NA	NA	75.82	$2623.84	090	C+ M
61514	Removal of brain abscess	27.23	NA	19.32	10.37	NA	NA	56.92	$1969.78	090	C+ M
61516	Removal of brain lesion	26.58	NA	18.96	10.05	NA	NA	55.59	$1923.76	090	C+ M
61517	Implt brain chemotx add-on	1.38	NA	0.66	0.54	NA	NA	2.58	$89.28	ZZZ	A
61518	Removal of brain lesion	39.89	NA	27.14	15.20	NA	NA	82.23	$2845.67	090	C+ M
61519	Remove brain lining lesion	43.43	NA	27.37	16.35	NA	NA	87.15	$3015.93	090	C+ M
61520	Removal of brain lesion	57.09	NA	34.13	19.63	NA	NA	110.85	$3836.10	090	C M
61521	Removal of brain lesion	46.99	NA	29.24	17.82	NA	NA	94.05	$3254.71	090	C+ M
61522	Removal of brain abscess	31.54	NA	21.39	12.10	NA	NA	65.03	$2250.44	090	C+ M
61524	Removal of brain lesion	29.89	NA	20.60	11.46	NA	NA	61.95	$2143.85	090	C+ M
61526	Removal of brain lesion	54.08	NA	30.47	14.77	NA	NA	99.32	$3437.09	090	A C M
61530	Removal of brain lesion	45.56	NA	28.10	17.46	NA	NA	91.12	$3153.32	090	A C M
61531	Implant brain electrodes	16.41	NA	13.81	6.28	NA	NA	36.50	$1263.13	090	C M
61533	Implant brain electrodes	21.46	NA	15.75	8.23	NA	NA	45.44	$1572.51	090	C+ M
61534	Removal of brain lesion	23.01	NA	17.32	8.83	NA	NA	49.16	$1701.24	090	C+ M
61535	Remove brain electrodes	13.15	NA	11.78	5.04	NA	NA	29.97	$1037.15	090	C+ M
61536	Removal of brain lesion	37.72	NA	24.35	14.45	NA	NA	76.52	$2648.07	090	C+ M
61537	Removal of brain tissue	36.45	NA	22.52	13.97	NA	NA	72.94	$2524.18	090	C+ M
61538	Removal of brain tissue	39.45	NA	24.35	15.12	NA	NA	78.92	$2731.12	090	C+ M
61539	Removal of brain tissue	34.28	NA	22.71	13.14	NA	NA	70.13	$2426.93	090	C+ M
61540	Removal of brain tissue	31.43	NA	21.20	12.04	NA	NA	64.67	$2237.98	090	C+ M
61541	Incision of brain tissue	30.94	NA	21.10	11.85	NA	NA	63.89	$2210.99	090	C+ M
61543	Removal of brain tissue	31.31	NA	21.28	12.00	NA	NA	64.59	$2235.21	090	C+ M
61544	Remove & treat brain lesion	27.36	NA	18.57	10.48	NA	NA	56.41	$1952.14	090	M
61545	Excision of brain tumor	46.43	NA	30.33	17.80	NA	NA	94.56	$3272.36	090	C+ M

*Please note that these calculations are based on the Medicare 2022 Conversion Factor of $34.6062 and the DRA RVU cap rates at time of publication.

A = assistant-at-surgery restriction
A+ = assistant-at-surgery restriction unless medical necessity established with documentation
B = bilateral surgery adjustment applies
C = cosurgeons payable
C+ = cosurgeons payable if medical necessity established with documentation
CP = carriers may establish RVUs and payment amounts for these services, generally on an individual basis following review of documentation such as an operative report
M = multiple surgery adjustment applies
Me = multiple endoscopy rules may apply
M+ = multiple therapy rules apply
Mtc = multiple diagnostic imaging rules apply
T = team surgeons permitted
T+ = team surgeons payable if medical necessity established with documentation
§ = indicates code is not covered by Medicare
GS = procedure must be performed under the general supervision of a physician
DS = procedure must be performed under the direct supervision of a physician
PS = procedure must be performed under the personal supervision of a physician
DRA = procedure subject to DRA limitation

Relative Value Units

CPT Code and Modifier	Description	Work RVU	Nonfacility Practice Expense RVU	Facility Practice Expense RVU	PLI RVU	Total Non-facility RVUs	Medicare Payment Nonfacility	Total Facility RVUs	Medicare Payment Facility	Global Period	Payment Policy Indicators
61546	Removal of pituitary gland	33.44	NA	22.30	12.81	NA	NA	68.55	$2372.26	090	C+ M
61548	Removal of pituitary gland	23.37	NA	15.58	7.71	NA	NA	46.66	$1614.73	090	C M
61550	Release of skull seams	15.59	NA	14.10	5.97	NA	NA	35.66	$1234.06	090	C+ M
61552	Release of skull seams	20.40	NA	16.07	7.84	NA	NA	44.31	$1533.40	090	C+ M
61556	Incise skull/sutures	24.09	NA	17.52	9.23	NA	NA	50.84	$1759.38	090	C+ M
61557	Incise skull/sutures	23.31	NA	17.95	8.93	NA	NA	50.19	$1736.89	090	C+ M
61558	Excision of skull/sutures	26.50	NA	19.32	10.16	NA	NA	55.98	$1937.26	090	C+ M
61559	Excision of skull/sutures	34.02	NA	24.23	13.05	NA	NA	71.30	$2467.42	090	C+ M
61563	Excision of skull tumor	28.44	NA	19.61	10.90	NA	NA	58.95	$2040.04	090	C+ M
61564	Excision of skull tumor	34.74	NA	23.42	13.34	NA	NA	71.50	$2474.34	090	B C+ M
61566	Removal of brain tissue	32.45	NA	21.69	12.44	NA	NA	66.58	$2304.08	090	C+ M
61567	Incision of brain tissue	37.00	NA	24.62	14.19	NA	NA	75.81	$2623.50	090	C+ M
61570	Remove foreign body brain	26.51	NA	18.99	10.16	NA	NA	55.66	$1926.18	090	C+ M
61571	Incise skull for brain wound	28.42	NA	19.90	10.90	NA	NA	59.22	$2049.38	090	C+ M
61575	Skull base/brainstem surgery	36.56	NA	23.79	14.02	NA	NA	74.37	$2573.66	090	C+ M
61576	Skull base/brainstem surgery	55.31	NA	47.93	21.20	NA	NA	124.44	$4306.40	090	C+ M
61580	Craniofacial approach skull	34.51	NA	32.98	7.08	NA	NA	74.57	$2580.58	090	A B C+ M T
61581	Craniofacial approach skull	39.13	NA	38.79	6.95	NA	NA	84.87	$2937.03	090	A B C M T
61582	Craniofacial approach skull	35.14	NA	43.13	12.12	NA	NA	90.39	$3128.05	090	C+ M T
61583	Craniofacial approach skull	38.50	NA	35.05	13.63	NA	NA	87.18	$3016.97	090	C+ M T
61584	Orbitocranial approach/skull	37.70	NA	35.17	13.29	NA	NA	86.16	$2981.67	090	B C+ M T
61585	Orbitocranial approach/skull	42.57	NA	39.45	16.32	NA	NA	98.34	$3403.17	090	B C+ M T
61586	Resect nasopharynx skull	27.48	NA	38.39	10.53	NA	NA	76.40	$2643.91	090	C+ M T
61590	Infratemporal approach/skull	47.04	NA	34.33	9.15	NA	NA	90.52	$3132.55	090	B C+ M T
61591	Infratemporal approach/skull	47.02	NA	34.36	9.57	NA	NA	90.95	$3147.43	090	B C+ M T
61592	Orbitocranial approach/skull	43.08	NA	36.38	15.17	NA	NA	94.63	$3274.78	090	B C+ M T
61595	Transtemporal approach/skull	33.74	NA	29.61	8.22	NA	NA	71.57	$2476.77	090	A B C+ M T
61596	Transcochlear approach/skull	39.43	NA	27.47	5.59	NA	NA	72.49	$2508.60	090	B C+ M T
61597	Transcondylar approach/skull	40.82	NA	33.10	14.95	NA	NA	88.87	$3075.45	090	B C+ M T
61598	Transpetrosal approach/skull	36.53	NA	34.99	14.01	NA	NA	85.53	$2959.87	090	C+ M T
61600	Resect/excise cranial lesion	30.01	NA	27.30	6.42	NA	NA	63.73	$2205.45	090	C+ M T
61601	Resect/excise cranial lesion	31.14	NA	30.56	11.11	NA	NA	72.81	$2519.68	090	C+ M T
61605	Resect/excise cranial lesion	32.57	NA	26.82	5.22	NA	NA	64.61	$2235.91	090	C+ M T

61606		Resect/excise cranial lesion	42.05	NA	31.71	13.16	NA	NA	86.92	$3007.97	090	C+ M T
61607		Resect/excise cranial lesion	40.93	NA	28.60	9.78	NA	NA	79.31	$2744.62	090	C+ M T
61608		Resect/excise cranial lesion	45.54	NA	35.25	16.81	NA	NA	97.60	$3377.57	090	C+ M T
61611		Transect artery sinus	7.41	NA	3.55	2.85	NA	NA	13.81	$477.91	ZZZ	C+ T
61613		Remove aneurysm sinus	45.03	NA	35.89	17.27	NA	NA	98.19	$3397.98	090	B C+ M T
61615		Resect/excise lesion skull	35.77	NA	34.91	13.72	NA	NA	84.40	$2920.76	090	C+ M T
61616		Resect/excise lesion skull	46.74	NA	37.08	15.71	NA	NA	99.53	$3444.36	090	C+ M T
61618		Repair dura	18.69	NA	13.72	5.88	NA	NA	38.29	$1325.07	090	C+ M T
61619		Repair dura	22.10	NA	14.48	5.55	NA	NA	42.13	$1457.96	090	C+ M T
61623		Endovasc tempory vessel occl	9.95	NA	4.24	2.76	NA	NA	16.95	$586.58	000	A M
61624		Transcath occlusion cns	20.12	NA	8.27	5.55	NA	NA	33.94	$1174.53	000	A M
61626		Transcath occlusion non-cns	16.60	NA	6.14	3.48	NA	NA	26.22	$907.37	000	A M
61630		Intracranial angioplasty	22.07	NA	11.99	6.20	NA	NA	40.26	$1393.25	XXX	C+ M
61635		Intracran angioplsty w/stent	24.28	NA	12.52	6.06	NA	NA	42.86	$1483.22	XXX	C+ M
61640	§	Dilate ic vasospasm init	12.32	0.00	0.00	1.69	14.01	$484.83	14.01	$484.83	000	
61641	§	Dilat ic vspsm ea vsl sm ter	4.33	0.00	0.00	0.59	4.92	$170.26	4.92	$170.26	ZZZ	
61642	§	Dilat ic vspsm ea diff ter	8.66	0.00	0.00	1.18	9.84	$340.53	9.84	$340.53	ZZZ	
61645		Perq art m-thrombect &/nfs	15.00	NA	5.94	3.73	NA	NA	24.67	$853.73	000	A+ B
61650		Evasc prlng admn rx agnt 1st	10.00	NA	4.11	2.79	NA	NA	16.90	$584.84	000	A M
61651		Evasc prlng admn rx agnt add	4.25	NA	1.75	1.12	NA	NA	7.12	$246.40	ZZZ	A
61680		Intracranial vessel surgery	32.55	NA	22.25	12.37	NA	NA	67.17	$2324.50	090	C+ M
61682		Intracranial vessel surgery	63.41	NA	35.62	24.12	NA	NA	123.15	$4261.75	090	C+ M
61684		Intracranial vessel surgery	41.64	NA	26.72	15.97	NA	NA	84.33	$2918.34	090	C+ M
61686		Intracranial vessel surgery	67.50	NA	39.55	25.87	NA	NA	132.92	$4599.86	090	C+ M
61690		Intracranial vessel surgery	31.34	NA	21.41	12.01	NA	NA	64.76	$2241.10	090	C+ M
61692		Intracranial vessel surgery	54.59	NA	32.53	20.92	NA	NA	108.04	$3738.85	090	C+ M
61697		Brain aneurysm repr complx	63.40	NA	37.47	24.14	NA	NA	125.01	$4326.12	090	C+ M
61698		Brain aneurysm repr complx	69.63	NA	40.57	26.69	NA	NA	136.89	$4737.24	090	C+ M

*Please note that these calculations are based on the Medicare 2022 Conversion Factor of $34.6062 and the DRA RVU cap rates at time of publication.

A = assistant-at-surgery restriction
A+ = assistant-at-surgery restriction unless medical necessity established with documentation
B = bilateral surgery adjustment applies
C = cosurgeons payable
C+ = cosurgeons payable if medical necessity established with documentation
CP = carriers may establish RVUs and payment amounts for these services, generally on an individual basis following review of documentation such as an operative report
M = multiple surgery adjustment applies
Me = multiple endoscopy rules may apply
M+ = multiple therapy rules apply
Mtc = multiple diagnostic imaging rules apply
T = team surgeons permitted
T+ = team surgeons payable if medical necessity established with documentation
§ = indicates code is not covered by Medicare
GS = procedure must be performed under the general supervision of a physician
DS = procedure must be performed under the direct supervision of a physician
PS = procedure must be performed under the personal supervision of a physician
DRA = procedure subject to DRA limitation

Relative Value Units

CPT Code and Modifier	Description	Work RVU	Nonfacility Practice Expense RVU	Facility Practice Expense RVU	PLI RVU	Total Non-facility RVUs	Medicare Payment Nonfacility	Total Facility RVUs	Medicare Payment Facility	Global Period	Payment Policy Indicators
61700	Brain aneurysm repr simple	50.62	NA	31.18	18.99	NA	NA	100.79	$3487.96	090	C+ M
61702	Inner skull vessel surgery	60.04	NA	35.99	23.02	NA	NA	119.05	$4119.87	090	C+ M
61703	Clamp neck artery	18.80	NA	14.48	7.20	NA	NA	40.48	$1400.86	090	C+ M
61705	Revise circulation to head	38.10	NA	24.53	14.63	NA	NA	77.26	$2673.68	090	C+ M
61708	Revise circulation to head	37.20	NA	24.10	14.27	NA	NA	75.57	$2615.19	090	M
61710	Revise circulation to head	31.29	NA	20.45	11.99	NA	NA	63.73	$2205.45	090	A+ M
61711	Fusion of skull arteries	38.23	NA	24.13	13.89	NA	NA	76.25	$2638.72	090	C+ M
61720	Incise skull/brain surgery	17.62	NA	13.51	6.76	NA	NA	37.89	$1311.23	090	A M
61735	Incise skull/brain surgery	22.35	NA	16.60	8.57	NA	NA	47.52	$1644.49	090	A C+ M
61736	Litt icr 1 traj 1 smpl les	19.06	NA	5.49	2.17	NA	NA	26.72	$924.68	000	A
61737	Litt icr mlt trj mlt/cplx ls	22.67	NA	6.45	2.71	NA	NA	31.83	$1101.52	000	A+ B
61750	Incise skull/brain biopsy	19.83	NA	14.56	7.56	NA	NA	41.95	$1451.73	090	A C+ M
61751	Brain biopsy w/ct/mr guide	18.79	NA	15.32	7.17	NA	NA	41.28	$1428.54	090	A C+ M
61760	Implant brain electrodes	22.39	NA	16.26	8.59	NA	NA	47.24	$1634.80	090	A C M
61770	Incise skull for treatment	23.19	NA	16.17	8.91	NA	NA	48.27	$1670.44	090	A C+ M
61781	Scan proc cranial intra	3.75	NA	1.78	1.41	NA	NA	6.94	$240.17	ZZZ	A+
61782	Scan proc cranial extra	3.18	NA	1.45	0.45	NA	NA	5.08	$175.80	ZZZ	A+
61783	Scan proc spinal	3.75	NA	1.82	1.28	NA	NA	6.85	$237.05	ZZZ	A+
61790	Treat trigeminal nerve	11.60	NA	10.39	4.38	NA	NA	26.37	$912.57	090	A B M
61791	Treat trigeminal tract	15.41	NA	12.29	5.90	NA	NA	33.60	$1162.77	090	A+ B M
61796	Srs cranial lesion simple	13.93	NA	11.07	5.30	NA	NA	30.30	$1048.57	090	
61797	Srs cran les simple addl	3.48	NA	1.66	1.33	NA	NA	6.47	$223.90	ZZZ	
61798	Srs cranial lesion complex	19.85	NA	13.75	7.44	NA	NA	41.04	$1420.24	090	
61799	Srs cran les complex addl	4.81	NA	2.29	1.83	NA	NA	8.93	$309.03	ZZZ	
61800	Apply srs headframe add-on	2.25	NA	1.36	0.87	NA	NA	4.48	$155.04	ZZZ	
61850	Implant neuroelectrodes	13.34	NA	10.97	5.10	NA	NA	29.41	$1017.77	090	M
61860	Implant neuroelectrodes	22.26	NA	15.73	8.55	NA	NA	46.54	$1610.57	090	M
61863	Implant neuroelectrode	20.71	NA	16.15	7.94	NA	NA	44.80	$1550.36	090	B C+ M
61864	Implant neuroelectrde addl	4.49	NA	2.14	1.70	NA	NA	8.33	$288.27	ZZZ	C+
61867	Implant neuroelectrode	33.03	NA	22.01	12.64	NA	NA	67.68	$2342.15	090	B C+ M
61868	Implant neuroelectrde addl	7.91	NA	3.78	3.02	NA	NA	14.71	$509.06	ZZZ	C+
61880	Revise/remove neuroelectrode	6.95	NA	7.89	2.66	NA	NA	17.50	$605.61	090	B C+ M
61885	Insrt/redo neurostim 1 array	6.05	NA	7.43	2.20	NA	NA	15.68	$542.63	090	A+ B M

61886	Implant neurostim arrays	9.93	NA	12.38	3.78	NA	NA	26.09	$902.88	090	A+ M
61888	Revise/remove neuroreceiver	5.23	NA	4.73	1.94	NA	NA	11.90	$411.81	010	A B M
62000	Treat skull fracture	13.93	NA	11.59	5.33	NA	NA	30.85	$1067.60	090	A M
62005	Treat skull fracture	17.63	NA	13.52	6.76	NA	NA	37.91	$1311.92	090	C+ M
62010	Treatment of head injury	21.43	NA	16.16	8.23	NA	NA	45.82	$1585.66	090	C+ M
62100	Repair brain fluid leakage	23.53	NA	15.86	7.47	NA	NA	46.86	$1621.65	090	C+ M
62115	Reduction of skull defect	22.91	NA	18.52	8.77	NA	NA	50.20	$1737.23	090	C+ M
62117	Reduction of skull defect	28.35	NA	19.22	10.87	NA	NA	58.44	$2022.39	090	C+ M
62120	Repair skull cavity lesion	24.59	NA	28.25	9.42	NA	NA	62.26	$2154.58	090	C+ M
62121	Incise skull repair	23.03	NA	17.96	5.71	NA	NA	46.70	$1616.11	090	C+ M
62140	Repair of skull defect	14.55	NA	11.11	4.66	NA	NA	30.32	$1049.26	090	C+ M
62141	Repair of skull defect	16.07	NA	12.34	5.53	NA	NA	33.94	$1174.53	090	C+ M
62142	Remove skull plate/flap	11.83	NA	10.46	4.31	NA	NA	26.60	$920.52	090	M
62143	Replace skull plate/flap	14.15	NA	11.72	5.28	NA	NA	31.15	$1077.98	090	C+ M
62145	Repair of skull & brain	20.09	NA	14.42	7.25	NA	NA	41.76	$1445.15	090	C+ M
62146	Repair of skull with graft	17.28	NA	13.35	6.62	NA	NA	37.25	$1289.08	090	C+ M
62147	Repair of skull with graft	20.67	NA	14.58	7.15	NA	NA	42.40	$1467.30	090	C+ M
62148	Retr bone flap to fix skull	2.00	NA	0.96	0.77	NA	NA	3.73	$129.08	ZZZ	A
62160	Neuroendoscopy add-on	3.00	NA	1.43	1.16	NA	NA	5.59	$193.45	ZZZ	A
62161	Dissect brain w/scope	21.23	NA	15.91	8.04	NA	NA	45.18	$1563.51	090	C+ M
62162	Remove colloid cyst w/scope	26.80	NA	19.10	10.28	NA	NA	56.18	$1944.18	090	C+ M
62164	Remove brain tumor w/scope	29.43	NA	21.57	11.29	NA	NA	62.29	$2155.62	090	C+ M
62165	Remove pituit tumor w/scope	23.23	NA	15.45	6.32	NA	NA	45.00	$1557.28	090	A+ C+ M
62180	Establish brain cavity shunt	22.58	NA	16.35	8.65	NA	NA	47.58	$1646.56	090	M
62190	Establish brain cavity shunt	12.17	NA	10.91	4.67	NA	NA	27.75	$960.32	090	A C+ M
62192	Establish brain cavity shunt	13.35	NA	11.16	4.91	NA	NA	29.42	$1018.11	090	C+ M
62194	Replace/irrigate catheter	5.78	NA	6.76	2.20	NA	NA	14.74	$510.10	010	A+ M
62200	Establish brain cavity shunt	19.29	NA	14.31	7.40	NA	NA	41.00	$1418.85	090	C+ M

*Please note that these calculations are based on the Medicare 2022 Conversion Factor of $34.6062 and the DRA RVU cap rates at time of publication.

A = assistant-at-surgery restriction

A+ = assistant-at-surgery restriction unless medical necessity established with documentation

B = bilateral surgery adjustment applies

C = cosurgeons payable

C+ = cosurgeons payable if medical necessity established with documentation

CP = carriers may establish RVUs and payment amounts for these services, generally on an individual basis following review of documentation such as an operative report

M = multiple surgery adjustment applies

Me = multiple endoscopy rules may apply

M+ = multiple therapy rules apply

Mtc = multiple diagnostic imaging rules apply

T = team surgeons permitted

T+ = team surgeons payable if medical necessity established with documentation

§ = indicates code is not covered by Medicare

GS = procedure must be performed under the general supervision of a physician

DS = procedure must be performed under the direct supervision of a physician

PS = procedure must be performed under the personal supervision of a physician

DRA = procedure subject to DRA limitation

Relative Value Units

CPT Code and Modifier	Description	Work RVU	Nonfacility Practice Expense RVU	Facility Practice Expense RVU	PLI RVU	Total Non-facility RVUs	Medicare Payment Nonfacility	Total Facility RVUs	Medicare Payment Facility	Global Period	Payment Policy Indicators
62201	Brain cavity shunt w/scope	16.04	NA	13.96	6.10	NA	NA	36.10	$1249.28	090	A M
62220	Establish brain cavity shunt	14.10	NA	10.04	4.94	NA	NA	29.08	$1006.35	090	C+ M
62223	Establish brain cavity shunt	14.05	NA	12.02	4.93	NA	NA	31.00	$1072.79	090	C+ M
62225	Replace/irrigate catheter	6.19	NA	7.41	2.33	NA	NA	15.93	$551.28	090	A M
62230	Replace/revise brain shunt	11.43	NA	9.52	4.16	NA	NA	25.11	$868.96	090	C+ M
62252	Csf shunt reprogram	0.74	1.44	NA	0.26	2.44	$84.44	NA	NA	XXX	A+
62252-26	Csf shunt reprogram	0.74	0.36	0.36	0.25	1.35	$46.72	1.35	$46.72	XXX	A+
62252-TC	Csf shunt reprogram	0.00	1.08	NA	0.01	1.09	$37.72	NA	NA	XXX	A+ PS
62256	Remove brain cavity shunt	7.38	NA	8.02	2.79	NA	NA	18.19	$629.49	090	M
62258	Replace brain cavity shunt	15.64	NA	11.91	5.64	NA	NA	33.19	$1148.58	090	C+ M
62263	Epidural lysis mult sessions	5.00	13.50	3.70	0.50	19.00	$657.52	9.20	$318.38	010	A M
62264	Epidural lysis on single day	4.42	8.42	2.29	0.44	13.28	$459.57	7.15	$247.43	010	A M
62267	Interdiscal perq aspir dx	3.00	4.80	1.25	0.25	8.05	$278.58	4.50	$155.73	000	A+ M
62268	Drain spinal cord cyst	4.73	NA	2.27	0.50	NA	NA	7.50	$259.55	000	A M
62269	Needle biopsy spinal cord	5.01	NA	2.19	0.41	NA	NA	7.61	$263.35	000	A+ M
62270	Dx lmbr spi pnxr	1.22	2.35	0.40	0.20	3.77	$130.47	1.82	$62.98	000	A M
62272	Ther spi pnxr drg csf	1.58	3.17	0.66	0.39	5.14	$177.88	2.63	$91.01	000	A M
62273	Inject epidural patch	2.15	2.65	0.95	0.21	5.01	$173.38	3.31	$114.55	000	A M
62280	Treat spinal cord lesion	2.63	6.94	1.74	0.28	9.85	$340.87	4.65	$160.92	010	A M
62281	Treat spinal cord lesion	2.66	4.20	1.73	0.25	7.11	$246.05	4.64	$160.57	010	A M
62282	Treat spinal canal lesion	2.33	7.16	1.67	0.20	9.69	$335.33	4.20	$145.35	010	A M
62284	Injection for myelogram	1.54	4.11	0.76	0.18	5.83	$201.75	2.48	$85.82	000	A M
62287	Dcmprn px perq 1/mlt lumbar	9.03	NA	6.98	0.95	NA	NA	16.96	$586.92	090	A M
62290	Njx px discography lumbar	3.00	7.56	1.42	0.27	10.83	$374.79	4.69	$162.30	000	A M
62291	Njx px discography crv/thrc	2.91	6.66	1.18	0.25	9.82	$339.83	4.34	$150.19	000	A M
62292	Njx chemonucleolysis lmbr	9.24	NA	6.71	1.01	NA	NA	16.96	$586.92	090	A+ M
62294	Injection into spinal artery	12.87	NA	10.56	4.93	NA	NA	28.36	$981.43	090	A M
62302	Myelography lumbar injection	2.29	5.35	1.00	0.20	7.84	$271.31	3.49	$120.78	000	A M
62303	Myelography lumbar injection	2.29	5.49	1.01	0.20	7.98	$276.16	3.50	$121.12	000	A M
62304	Myelography lumbar injection	2.25	5.30	0.99	0.20	7.75	$268.20	3.44	$119.05	000	A M
62305	Myelography lumbar injection	2.35	5.89	1.03	0.21	8.45	$292.42	3.59	$124.24	000	A M
62320	Njx interlaminar crv/thrc	1.80	2.87	0.89	0.24	4.91	$169.92	2.93	$101.40	000	A M
62321	Njx interlaminar crv/thrc	1.95	5.77	0.99	0.20	7.92	$274.08	3.14	$108.66	000	A M

62322		Njx interlaminar lmbr/sac	1.55	2.43	0.64	0.19	4.17	$144.31	2.38	$82.36	000	A M
62323		Njx interlaminar lmbr/sac	1.80	5.82	0.92	0.19	7.81	$270.27	2.91	$100.70	000	A M
62324		Njx interlaminar crv/thrc	1.89	2.06	0.56	0.17	4.12	$142.58	2.62	$90.67	000	A M
62325		Njx interlaminar crv/thrc	2.20	5.26	0.85	0.21	7.67	$265.43	3.26	$112.82	000	A M
62326		Njx interlaminar lmbr/sac	1.78	2.22	0.57	0.17	4.17	$144.31	2.52	$87.21	000	A M
62327		Njx interlaminar lmbr/sac	1.90	5.89	0.97	0.20	7.99	$276.50	3.07	$106.24	000	A M
62328		Dx lmbr spi pnxr w/fluor/ct	1.73	5.32	0.62	0.22	7.27	$251.59	2.57	$88.94	000	A M
62329		Ther spi pnxr csf fluor/ct	2.03	6.76	0.82	0.42	9.21	$318.72	3.27	$113.16	000	A M
62350		Implant spinal canal cath	6.05	NA	4.54	1.18	NA	NA	11.77	$407.31	010	A C+ M
62351		Implant spinal canal cath	11.66	NA	11.46	3.96	NA	NA	27.08	$937.14	090	C M
62355		Remove spinal canal catheter	3.55	NA	3.75	0.77	NA	NA	8.07	$279.27	010	A+ M
62360		Insert spine infusion device	4.33	NA	4.23	1.05	NA	NA	9.61	$332.57	010	A+ C+ M
62361		Implant spine infusion pump	5.00	NA	6.00	1.93	NA	NA	12.93	$447.46	010	A+ C+ M
62362		Implant spine infusion pump	5.60	NA	4.53	1.26	NA	NA	11.39	$394.16	010	A+ C+ M
62365		Remove spine infusion device	3.93	NA	3.89	0.95	NA	NA	8.77	$303.50	010	A+ M
62367		Analyze spine infus pump	0.48	0.39	0.19	0.07	0.94	$32.53	0.74	$25.61	XXX	A
62368		Analyze sp inf pump w/reprog	0.67	0.55	0.27	0.09	1.31	$45.33	1.03	$35.64	XXX	A
62369		Anal sp inf pmp w/reprg&fill	0.67	2.00	0.28	0.09	2.76	$95.51	1.04	$35.99	XXX	A
62370		Anl sp inf pmp w/mdreprg&fil	0.90	1.78	0.35	0.10	2.78	$96.21	1.35	$46.72	XXX	A
62380	CP	Ndsc dcmprn 1 ntrspc lumbar	0.00	0.00	0.00	0.00	0.00	$0.00	0.00	$0.00	090	B C M
63001		Remove spine lamina 1/2 crvl	17.61	NA	13.02	6.06	NA	NA	36.69	$1269.70	090	C M
63003		Remove spine lamina 1/2 thrc	17.74	NA	12.99	5.95	NA	NA	36.68	$1269.36	090	C M
63005		Remove spine lamina 1/2 lmbr	16.43	NA	13.61	5.57	NA	NA	35.61	$1232.33	090	C M
63011		Remove spine lamina 1/2 scrl	15.91	NA	12.44	4.20	NA	NA	32.55	$1126.43	090	C M
63012		Remove lamina/facets lumbar	16.85	NA	13.26	5.42	NA	NA	35.53	$1229.56	090	C M
63015		Remove spine lamina >2 crvcl	20.85	NA	15.85	7.27	NA	NA	43.97	$1521.63	090	C M
63016		Remove spine lamina >2 thrc	22.03	NA	15.81	7.48	NA	NA	45.32	$1568.35	090	C M
63017		Remove spine lamina >2 lmbr	17.33	NA	14.16	6.06	NA	NA	37.55	$1299.46	090	C M

*Please note that these calculations are based on the Medicare 2022 Conversion Factor of $34.6062 and the DRA RVU cap rates at time of publication.

A = assistant-at-surgery restriction

A+ = assistant-at-surgery restriction unless medical necessity established with documentation

B = bilateral surgery adjustment applies

C = cosurgeons payable

C+ = cosurgeons payable if medical necessity established with documentation

CP = carriers may establish RVUs and payment amounts for these services, generally on an individual basis following review of documentation such as an operative report

M = multiple surgery adjustment applies

Me = multiple endoscopy rules may apply

M+ = multiple therapy rules apply

Mtc = multiple diagnostic imaging rules apply

T = team surgeons permitted

T+ = team surgeons payable if medical necessity established with documentation

§ = indicates code is not covered by Medicare

GS = procedure must be performed under the general supervision of a physician

DS = procedure must be performed under the direct supervision of a physician

PS = procedure must be performed under the personal supervision of a physician

DRA = procedure subject to DRA limitation

Relative Value Units

CPT Code and Modifier		Description	Work RVU	Nonfacility Practice Expense RVU	Facility Practice Expense RVU	PLI RVU	Total Non-facility RVUs	Medicare Payment Nonfacility	Total Facility RVUs	Medicare Payment Facility	Global Period	Payment Policy Indicators
63020		Neck spine disk surgery	16.20	NA	13.26	4.99	NA	NA	34.45	$1192.18	090	B C M
63030		Low back disk surgery	13.18	NA	11.76	4.06	NA	NA	29.00	$1003.58	090	B C M
63035		Spinal disk surgery add-on	3.15	NA	1.54	0.95	NA	NA	5.64	$195.18	ZZZ	B C
63040		Laminotomy single cervical	20.31	NA	14.69	6.04	NA	NA	41.04	$1420.24	090	B C M
63042		Laminotomy single lumbar	18.76	NA	14.36	5.32	NA	NA	38.44	$1330.26	090	B C M
63043	CP	Laminotomy addl cervical	0.00	0.00	0.00	0.00	0.00	$0.00	0.00	$0.00	ZZZ	B C
63044	CP	Laminotomy addl lumbar	0.00	0.00	0.00	0.00	0.00	$0.00	0.00	$0.00	ZZZ	B C
63045		Lam facetec & foramot crv	17.95	NA	14.31	6.02	NA	NA	38.28	$1324.73	090	C M
63046		Lam facetec & foramot thrc	17.25	NA	13.80	5.43	NA	NA	36.48	$1262.43	090	C M
63047		Lam facetec & foramot lumbar	15.37	NA	12.81	4.66	NA	NA	32.84	$1136.47	090	C M
63048		Lam facetec &foramot ea addl	3.47	NA	1.70	1.04	NA	NA	6.21	$214.90	ZZZ	C
63050		Cervical laminoplsty 2/> seg	22.01	NA	15.85	6.13	NA	NA	43.99	$1522.33	090	C M
63051		C-laminoplasty w/graft/plate	25.51	NA	17.54	7.30	NA	NA	50.35	$1742.42	090	C M
63052		Lam facetc/frmt arthrd lum 1	4.25	NA	2.08	1.29	NA	NA	7.62	$263.70	ZZZ	C
63053		Lam factc/frmt arthrd lum ea	3.19	NA	1.56	0.95	NA	NA	5.70	$197.26	ZZZ	C
63055		Decompress spinal cord thrc	23.55	NA	16.63	8.08	NA	NA	48.26	$1670.10	090	C+ M
63056		Decompress spinal cord lmbr	21.86	NA	15.60	6.86	NA	NA	44.32	$1533.75	090	C+ M
63057		Decompress spine cord add-on	5.25	NA	2.57	1.65	NA	NA	9.47	$327.72	ZZZ	C+
63064		Decompress spinal cord thrc	26.22	NA	17.83	8.77	NA	NA	52.82	$1827.90	090	C+ M
63066		Decompress spine cord add-on	3.26	NA	1.55	1.25	NA	NA	6.06	$209.71	ZZZ	C+
63075		Neck spine disk surgery	19.60	NA	14.70	6.07	NA	NA	40.37	$1397.05	090	C M
63076		Neck spine disk surgery	4.04	NA	1.98	1.16	NA	NA	7.18	$248.47	ZZZ	C
63077		Spine disk surgery thorax	22.88	NA	15.06	6.64	NA	NA	44.58	$1542.74	090	C M
63078		Spine disk surgery thorax	3.28	NA	1.56	1.26	NA	NA	6.10	$211.10	ZZZ	C
63081		Remove vert body dcmprn crvl	26.10	NA	17.99	8.08	NA	NA	52.17	$1805.41	090	C+ M T
63082		Remove vertebral body add-on	4.36	NA	2.13	1.32	NA	NA	7.81	$270.27	ZZZ	C+ T
63085		Remove vert body dcmprn thrc	29.47	NA	18.78	8.92	NA	NA	57.17	$1978.44	090	C M T
63086		Remove vertebral body add-on	3.19	NA	1.50	0.93	NA	NA	5.62	$194.49	ZZZ	C T
63087		Remov vertbr dcmprn thrclmbr	37.53	NA	22.77	10.99	NA	NA	71.29	$2467.08	090	C M T
63088		Remove vertebral body add-on	4.32	NA	2.02	1.22	NA	NA	7.56	$261.62	ZZZ	C T
63090		Remove vert body dcmprn lmbr	30.93	NA	18.90	8.23	NA	NA	58.06	$2009.24	090	C M T
63091		Remove vertebral body add-on	3.03	NA	1.41	0.79	NA	NA	5.23	$180.99	ZZZ	C T
63101		Remove vert body dcmprn thrc	34.10	NA	23.45	11.44	NA	NA	68.99	$2387.48	090	C+ M

63102	Remove vert body dcmprn lmbr	34.10	NA	22.91	10.21	NA	NA	67.22	$2326.23	090	C+ M
63103	Remove vertebral body add-on	4.82	NA	2.34	1.50	NA	NA	8.66	$299.69	ZZZ	C+
63170	Incise spinal cord tract(s)	22.21	NA	16.72	8.52	NA	NA	47.45	$1642.06	090	C+ M
63172	Drainage of spinal cyst	19.76	NA	14.73	7.56	NA	NA	42.05	$1455.19	090	C+ M
63173	Drainage of spinal cyst	24.31	NA	17.72	9.33	NA	NA	51.36	$1777.37	090	C+ M
63185	Incise spine nrv half segmnt	16.49	NA	12.86	4.39	NA	NA	33.74	$1167.61	090	C+ M
63190	Incise spine nrv >2 segmnts	18.89	NA	13.99	3.89	NA	NA	36.77	$1272.47	090	C+ M
63191	Incise spine accessory nerve	18.92	NA	14.98	7.25	NA	NA	41.15	$1424.05	090	B C+ M
63197	Lam w/cordotomy 1stg thrc	24.08	NA	17.61	9.23	NA	NA	50.92	$1762.15	090	C+ M
63200	Release spinal cord lumbar	21.44	NA	16.31	7.35	NA	NA	45.10	$1560.74	090	M
63250	Revise spinal cord vsls crvl	43.86	NA	27.28	16.82	NA	NA	87.96	$3043.96	090	C+ M
63251	Revise spinal cord vsls thrc	44.64	NA	28.16	17.12	NA	NA	89.92	$3111.79	090	C+ M
63252	Revise spine cord vsl thrlmb	44.63	NA	28.15	17.12	NA	NA	89.90	$3111.10	090	C+ M
63265	Excise intraspinl lesion crv	23.82	NA	17.39	8.41	NA	NA	49.62	$1717.16	090	C+ M
63266	Excise intrspinl lesion thrc	24.68	NA	17.80	8.69	NA	NA	51.17	$1770.80	090	C+ M
63267	Excise intrspinl lesion lmbr	19.45	NA	15.03	6.34	NA	NA	40.82	$1412.63	090	C+ M
63268	Excise intrspinl lesion scrl	20.02	NA	15.48	6.71	NA	NA	42.21	$1460.73	090	C+ M
63270	Excise intrspinl lesion crvl	29.80	NA	20.56	11.44	NA	NA	61.80	$2138.66	090	C+ M
63271	Excise intrspinl lesion thrc	29.92	NA	20.48	11.17	NA	NA	61.57	$2130.70	090	C+ M
63272	Excise intrspinl lesion lmbr	27.50	NA	19.01	9.16	NA	NA	55.67	$1926.53	090	C+ M
63273	Excise intrspinl lesion scrl	26.47	NA	18.97	10.15	NA	NA	55.59	$1923.76	090	M
63275	Bx/exc xdrl spine lesn crvl	25.86	NA	18.46	9.46	NA	NA	53.78	$1861.12	090	C+ M
63276	Bx/exc xdrl spine lesn thrc	25.69	NA	18.31	9.18	NA	NA	53.18	$1840.36	090	C+ M
63277	Bx/exc xdrl spine lesn lmbr	22.39	NA	16.52	7.47	NA	NA	46.38	$1605.04	090	C+ M
63278	Bx/exc xdrl spine lesn scrl	22.12	NA	16.89	8.49	NA	NA	47.50	$1643.79	090	C+ M
63280	Bx/exc idrl spine lesn crvl	30.29	NA	21.25	11.46	NA	NA	63.00	$2180.19	090	C+ M
63281	Bx/exc idrl spine lesn thrc	29.99	NA	21.07	11.29	NA	NA	62.35	$2157.70	090	C+ M
63282	Bx/exc idrl spine lesn lmbr	28.15	NA	20.13	10.58	NA	NA	58.86	$2036.92	090	C+ M

*Please note that these calculations are based on the Medicare 2022 Conversion Factor of $34.6062 and the DRA RVU cap rates at time of publication.

A = assistant-at-surgery restriction
A+ = assistant-at-surgery restriction unless medical necessity established with documentation
B = bilateral surgery adjustment applies
C = cosurgeons payable
C+ = cosurgeons payable if medical necessity established with documentation
CP = carriers may establish RVUs and payment amounts for these services, generally on an individual basis following review of documentation such as an operative report
M = multiple surgery adjustment applies
Me = multiple endoscopy rules may apply
M+ = multiple therapy rules apply
Mtc = multiple diagnostic imaging rules apply
T = team surgeons permitted
T+ = team surgeons payable if medical necessity established with documentation
§ = indicates code is not covered by Medicare
GS = procedure must be performed under the general supervision of a physician
DS = procedure must be performed under the direct supervision of a physician
PS = procedure must be performed under the personal supervision of a physician
DRA = procedure subject to DRA limitation

Relative Value Units

CPT Code and Modifier	Description	Work RVU	Nonfacility Practice Expense RVU	Facility Practice Expense RVU	PLI RVU	Total Non-facility RVUs	Medicare Payment Nonfacility	Total Facility RVUs	Medicare Payment Facility	Global Period	Payment Policy Indicators
63283	Bx/exc idrl spine lesn scrl	26.76	NA	19.61	10.26	NA	NA	56.63	$1959.75	090	C+ M
63285	Bx/exc idrl imed lesn cervl	38.05	NA	25.00	14.60	NA	NA	77.65	$2687.17	090	C+ M
63286	Bx/exc idrl imed lesn thrc	37.62	NA	24.76	14.19	NA	NA	76.57	$2649.80	090	C+ M
63287	Bx/exc idrl imed lesn thrlmb	40.08	NA	25.97	15.37	NA	NA	81.42	$2817.64	090	C+ M
63290	Bx/exc xdrl/idrl lsn any lvl	40.82	NA	26.32	15.65	NA	NA	82.79	$2865.05	090	C+ M
63295	Repair laminectomy defect	5.25	NA	2.52	1.91	NA	NA	9.68	$334.99	ZZZ	C
63300	Remove vert xdrl body crvcl	26.80	NA	18.43	8.64	NA	NA	53.87	$1864.24	090	C+ M
63301	Remove vert xdrl body thrc	31.57	NA	21.90	12.11	NA	NA	65.58	$2269.47	090	C+ M
63302	Remove vert xdrl body thrlmb	31.15	NA	21.70	11.95	NA	NA	64.80	$2242.48	090	C+ M
63303	Remov vert xdrl bdy lmbr/sac	33.55	NA	22.36	12.87	NA	NA	68.78	$2380.21	090	C+ M
63304	Remove vert idrl body crvcl	33.85	NA	22.99	12.98	NA	NA	69.82	$2416.20	090	C+ M
63305	Remove vert idrl body thrc	36.24	NA	24.13	13.90	NA	NA	74.27	$2570.20	090	C+ M
63306	Remov vert idrl bdy thrclmbr	35.55	NA	23.80	13.63	NA	NA	72.98	$2525.56	090	C+ M
63307	Remov vert idrl bdy lmbr/sac	34.96	NA	23.12	13.42	NA	NA	71.50	$2474.34	090	C+ M
63308	Remove vertebral body add-on	5.24	NA	2.50	1.65	NA	NA	9.39	$324.95	ZZZ	C+
63600	Remove spinal cord lesion	15.12	NA	11.64	5.81	NA	NA	32.57	$1127.12	090	A+ M
63610	Stimulation of spinal cord	8.72	NA	5.05	3.35	NA	NA	17.12	$592.46	000	A+ M
63620	Srs spinal lesion	15.60	NA	11.88	5.96	NA	NA	33.44	$1157.23	090	
63621	Srs spinal lesion addl	4.00	NA	1.91	1.53	NA	NA	7.44	$257.47	ZZZ	
63650	Implant neuroelectrodes	7.15	62.84	4.23	0.79	70.78	$2449.43	12.17	$421.16	010	A M
63655	Implant neuroelectrodes	10.92	NA	10.41	3.58	NA	NA	24.91	$862.04	090	C+ M
63661	Remove spine eltrd perq aray	5.08	14.57	3.66	0.95	20.60	$712.89	9.69	$335.33	010	C+ M
63662	Remove spine eltrd plate	11.00	NA	10.58	3.65	NA	NA	25.23	$873.11	090	C+ M
63663	Revise spine eltrd perq aray	7.75	18.26	4.45	1.06	27.07	$936.79	13.26	$458.88	010	C+ M
63664	Revise spine eltrd plate	11.52	NA	10.88	3.85	NA	NA	26.25	$908.41	090	C+ M
63685	Insrt/redo spine n generator	5.19	NA	4.43	1.09	NA	NA	10.71	$370.63	010	C+ M
63688	Revise/remove neuroreceiver	5.30	NA	4.57	1.16	NA	NA	11.03	$381.71	010	A M
63700	Repair of spinal herniation	17.47	NA	14.97	6.68	NA	NA	39.12	$1353.79	090	C+ M
63702	Repair of spinal herniation	19.41	NA	15.90	7.44	NA	NA	42.75	$1479.42	090	C+ M
63704	Repair of spinal herniation	22.43	NA	18.66	8.61	NA	NA	49.70	$1719.93	090	C+ M
63706	Repair of spinal herniation	25.35	NA	20.06	9.73	NA	NA	55.14	$1908.19	090	C+ M
63707	Repair spinal fluid leakage	12.65	NA	11.23	4.01	NA	NA	27.89	$965.17	090	C+ M
63709	Repair spinal fluid leakage	15.65	NA	12.73	4.83	NA	NA	33.21	$1149.27	090	C+ M

63710	Graft repair of spine defect	15.40	NA	12.46	4.39	NA	NA	32.25	$1116.05	090	C+ M
63740	Install spinal shunt	12.63	NA	11.95	4.84	NA	NA	29.42	$1018.11	090	C+ M
63741	Install spinal shunt	9.12	NA	8.06	3.02	NA	NA	20.20	$699.05	090	C+ M
63744	Revision of spinal shunt	8.94	NA	8.41	3.26	NA	NA	20.61	$713.23	090	C+ M
63746	Removal of spinal shunt	7.33	NA	8.10	2.82	NA	NA	18.25	$631.56	090	A+ M
64400	Njx aa&/strd trigeminal nrv	0.75	2.44	0.54	0.20	3.39	$117.32	1.49	$51.56	000	A B M
64405	Njx aa&/strd gr ocpl nrv	0.94	1.09	0.41	0.21	2.24	$77.52	1.56	$53.99	000	A B M
64408	Njx aa&/strd vagus nrv	0.75	1.58	0.46	0.11	2.44	$84.44	1.32	$45.68	000	A+ B M
64415	Njx aa&/strd brach plexus	1.35	1.89	0.38	0.11	3.35	$115.93	1.84	$63.68	000	A B M
64416	Njx aa&/strd brach plex nfs	1.48	NA	0.27	0.11	NA	NA	1.86	$64.37	000	A B M
64417	Njx aa&/strd axillary nrv	1.27	2.80	0.40	0.11	4.18	$144.65	1.78	$61.60	000	A B M
64418	Njx aa&/strd sprscap nrv	1.10	1.40	0.43	0.12	2.62	$90.67	1.65	$57.10	000	A B M
64420	Njx aa&/strd ntrcost nrv 1	1.08	1.71	0.54	0.11	2.90	$100.36	1.73	$59.87	000	A B M
64421	Njx aa&/strd ntrcost nrv ea	0.50	0.43	0.18	0.05	0.98	$33.91	0.73	$25.26	ZZZ	A B
64425	Njx aa&/strd ii ih nerves	1.00	2.23	0.51	0.10	3.33	$115.24	1.61	$55.72	000	A B M
64430	Njx aa&/strd pudendal nerve	1.00	1.83	0.48	0.11	2.94	$101.74	1.59	$55.02	000	A B M
64435	Njx aa&/strd paracrv nrv	0.75	1.56	0.41	0.11	2.42	$83.75	1.27	$43.95	000	A B M
64445	Njx aa&/strd sciatic nerve	1.00	2.66	0.47	0.10	3.76	$130.12	1.57	$54.33	000	A B M
64446	Njx aa&/strd sciatic nrv nfs	1.36	NA	0.25	0.11	NA	NA	1.72	$59.52	000	A B M
64447	Njx aa&/strd femoral nerve	1.10	1.44	0.35	0.09	2.63	$91.01	1.54	$53.29	000	A B M
64448	Njx aa&/strd fem nerve nfs	1.41	NA	0.25	0.11	NA	NA	1.77	$61.25	000	A B M
64449	Njx aa&/strd lmbr plex nfs	1.27	NA	0.42	0.11	NA	NA	1.80	$62.29	000	A B M
64450	Njx aa&/strd other pn/branch	0.75	1.42	0.40	0.09	2.26	$78.21	1.24	$42.91	000	A B M
64451	Njx aa&/strd nrv nrvtg si jt	1.52	5.27	0.73	0.14	6.93	$239.82	2.39	$82.71	000	A B M
64454	Njx aa&/strd gnclr nrv brnch	1.52	5.05	0.74	0.17	6.74	$233.25	2.43	$84.09	000	A B M
64455	Njx aa&/strd pltr com dg nrv	0.75	0.65	0.17	0.07	1.47	$50.87	0.99	$34.26	000	A+ B M
64461	Pvb thoracic single inj site	1.75	2.14	0.38	0.17	4.06	$140.50	2.30	$79.59	000	A B M
64462	Pvb thoracic 2nd+ inj site	1.10	0.97	0.24	0.09	2.16	$74.75	1.43	$49.49	ZZZ	A B

*Please note that these calculations are based on the Medicare 2022 Conversion Factor of $34.6062 and the DRA RVU cap rates at time of publication.

A = assistant-at-surgery restriction
A+ = assistant-at-surgery restriction unless medical necessity established with documentation
B = bilateral surgery adjustment applies
C = cosurgeons payable
C+ = cosurgeons payable if medical necessity established with documentation
CP = carriers may establish RVUs and payment amounts for these services, generally on an individual basis following review of documentation such as an operative report
M = multiple surgery adjustment applies
Me = multiple endoscopy rules may apply
M+ = multiple therapy rules apply
Mtc = multiple diagnostic imaging rules apply
T = team surgeons permitted
T+ = team surgeons payable if medical necessity established with documentation
§ = indicates code is not covered by Medicare
GS = procedure must be performed under the general supervision of a physician
DS = procedure must be performed under the direct supervision of a physician
PS = procedure must be performed under the personal supervision of a physician
DRA = procedure subject to DRA limitation

Relative Value Units

CPT Code and Modifier	Description	Work RVU	Nonfacility Practice Expense RVU	Facility Practice Expense RVU	PLI RVU	Total Non-facility RVUs	Medicare Payment Nonfacility	Total Facility RVUs	Medicare Payment Facility	Global Period	Payment Policy Indicators
64463	Pvb thoracic cont infusion	1.90	5.02	0.35	0.17	7.09	$245.36	2.42	$83.75	000	A B M
64479	Njx aa&/strd tfrm epi c/t 1	2.29	5.49	1.33	0.22	8.00	$276.85	3.84	$132.89	000	A B M
64480	Njx aa&/strd tfrm epi c/t ea	1.20	2.75	0.48	0.11	4.06	$140.50	1.79	$61.95	ZZZ	A B
64483	Njx aa&/strd tfrm epi l/s 1	1.90	5.35	1.17	0.19	7.44	$257.47	3.26	$112.82	000	A B M
64484	Njx aa&/strd tfrm epi l/s ea	1.00	2.27	0.41	0.10	3.37	$116.62	1.51	$52.26	ZZZ	A B
64486	Tap block unil by injection	1.27	1.98	0.25	0.11	3.36	$116.28	1.63	$56.41	000	A B M
64487	Tap block uni by infusion	1.48	5.01	0.27	0.11	6.60	$228.40	1.86	$64.37	000	A B M
64488	Tap block bi injection	1.60	2.44	0.29	0.12	4.16	$143.96	2.01	$69.56	000	A M
64489	Tap block bi by infusion	1.80	8.88	0.32	0.14	10.82	$374.44	2.26	$78.21	000	A M
64490	Inj paravert f jnt c/t 1 lev	1.82	3.68	1.08	0.20	5.70	$197.26	3.10	$107.28	000	B M
64491	Inj paravert f jnt c/t 2 lev	1.16	1.60	0.47	0.11	2.87	$99.32	1.74	$60.21	ZZZ	B
64492	Inj paravert f jnt c/t 3 lev	1.16	1.61	0.49	0.11	2.88	$99.67	1.76	$60.91	ZZZ	B
64493	Inj paravert f jnt l/s 1 lev	1.52	3.56	0.97	0.14	5.22	$180.64	2.63	$91.01	000	B M
64494	Inj paravert f jnt l/s 2 lev	1.00	1.60	0.40	0.10	2.70	$93.44	1.50	$51.91	ZZZ	B
64495	Inj paravert f jnt l/s 3 lev	1.00	1.59	0.42	0.10	2.69	$93.09	1.52	$52.60	ZZZ	B
64505	N block spenopalatine gangl	1.36	2.55	1.36	0.34	4.25	$147.08	3.06	$105.89	000	A B M
64510	N block stellate ganglion	1.22	3.07	0.92	0.11	4.40	$152.27	2.25	$77.86	000	A B M
64517	N block inj hypogas plxs	2.20	3.36	1.30	0.20	5.76	$199.33	3.70	$128.04	000	A M
64520	N block lumbar/thoracic	1.35	5.48	1.00	0.12	6.95	$240.51	2.47	$85.48	000	A B M
64530	N block inj celiac pelus	1.58	5.29	1.04	0.14	7.01	$242.59	2.76	$95.51	000	A M
64553	Implant neuroelectrodes	6.13	69.85	4.32	0.70	76.68	$2653.60	11.15	$385.86	010	A+ M
64555	Implant neuroelectrodes	5.76	60.81	3.21	0.64	67.21	$2325.88	9.61	$332.57	010	A M
64561	Implant neuroelectrodes	5.44	16.41	2.75	0.72	22.57	$781.06	8.91	$308.34	010	A B M
64566	Neuroeltrd stim post tibial	0.60	2.89	0.21	0.09	3.58	$123.89	0.90	$31.15	000	A+ M
64568	Opn impltj crnl nrv nea&pg	9.00	NA	7.06	2.08	NA	NA	18.14	$627.76	090	A+ B M
64569	Revise/repl vagus n eltrd	11.00	NA	8.45	3.41	NA	NA	22.86	$791.10	090	A+ B C+ M T+
64570	Remove vagus n eltrd	9.10	NA	9.32	3.49	NA	NA	21.91	$758.22	090	A+ B C+ M T+
64575	Opn impltj nea perph nerve	4.42	NA	4.22	0.87	NA	NA	9.51	$329.10	090	A M
64580	Opn impltj nea neuromuscular	4.19	NA	4.16	1.05	NA	NA	9.40	$325.30	090	M
64581	Opn impltj nea sacral nerve	12.20	NA	5.49	1.63	NA	NA	19.32	$668.59	090	A M
64582	Opn mpltj hpglsl nstm ary pg	14.00	NA	8.80	2.85	NA	NA	25.65	$887.65	090	A+ B M
64583	Rev/rplct hpglsl nstm ary pg	14.50	NA	7.63	1.20	NA	NA	23.33	$807.36	090	A+ B C+ M T+
64584	Rmvl hpglsl nstim ary pg	12.00	NA	6.67	0.99	NA	NA	19.66	$680.36	090	A+ B C+ M T+

64585	Revise/remove neuroelectrode	2.11	4.94	1.83	0.28	7.33	$253.66	4.22	$146.04	010	A M
64590	Insrt/redo pn/gastr stimul	2.45	5.11	1.94	0.34	7.90	$273.39	4.73	$163.69	010	A C+ M
64595	Revise/rmv pn/gastr stimul	1.78	4.93	1.70	0.25	6.96	$240.86	3.73	$129.08	010	A M
64600	Injection treatment of nerve	3.49	9.77	2.60	0.67	13.93	$482.06	6.76	$233.94	010	A M
64605	Injection treatment of nerve	5.65	12.59	3.65	0.99	19.23	$665.48	10.29	$356.10	010	A+ B M
64610	Injection treatment of nerve	7.20	14.49	4.86	2.33	24.02	$831.24	14.39	$497.98	010	A B M
64611	Chemodenerv saliv glands	1.03	2.44	1.89	0.37	3.84	$132.89	3.29	$113.85	010	A+ M
64612	Destroy nerve face muscle	1.41	2.34	1.79	0.28	4.03	$139.46	3.48	$120.43	010	A B M
64615	Chemodenerv musc migraine	1.85	2.14	1.19	0.60	4.59	$158.84	3.64	$125.97	010	A M
64616	Chemodenerv musc neck dyston	1.53	2.07	1.20	0.50	4.10	$141.89	3.23	$111.78	010	A B M
64617	Chemodener muscle larynx emg	1.90	2.69	1.02	0.25	4.84	$167.49	3.17	$109.70	010	A B M
64620	Injection treatment of nerve	2.89	2.98	1.98	0.33	6.20	$214.56	5.20	$179.95	010	A M
64624	Dstrj nulyt agt gnclr nrv	2.50	9.08	1.55	0.24	11.82	$409.05	4.29	$148.46	010	A+ B M
64625	Rf abltj nrv nrvtg si jt	3.39	10.60	2.00	0.33	14.32	$495.56	5.72	$197.95	010	A B M
64628	Trml dstrj ios bvn 1st 2 l/s	7.15	NA	4.79	1.64	NA	NA	13.58	$469.95	010	A M
64629	Trml dstrj ios bvn ea addl	3.77	NA	1.70	0.89	NA	NA	6.36	$220.10	ZZZ	A
64630	Injection treatment of nerve	3.05	4.17	2.13	0.54	7.76	$268.54	5.72	$197.95	010	A+ M
64632	N block inj common digit	1.23	1.33	0.62	0.10	2.66	$92.05	1.95	$67.48	010	A+ B M
64633	Destroy cerv/thor facet jnt	3.32	9.61	1.97	0.33	13.26	$458.88	5.62	$194.49	010	A B M
64634	Destroy c/th facet jnt addl	1.32	6.41	0.52	0.12	7.85	$271.66	1.96	$67.83	ZZZ	A B
64635	Destroy lumb/sac facet jnt	3.32	9.74	1.98	0.32	13.38	$463.03	5.62	$194.49	010	A B M
64636	Destroy l/s facet jnt addl	1.16	6.14	0.46	0.11	7.41	$256.43	1.73	$59.87	ZZZ	A B
64640	Injection treatment of nerve	1.98	5.25	1.30	0.20	7.43	$257.12	3.48	$120.43	010	A B M
64642	Chemodenerv 1 extremity 1-4	1.65	2.48	1.14	0.39	4.52	$156.42	3.18	$110.05	000	A M
64643	Chemodenerv 1 extrem 1-4 ea	1.22	1.32	0.63	0.24	2.78	$96.21	2.09	$72.33	ZZZ	A
64644	Chemodenerv 1 extrem 5/> mus	1.82	3.09	1.24	0.40	5.31	$183.76	3.46	$119.74	000	A M
64645	Chemodenerv 1 extrem 5/> ea	1.39	1.90	0.72	0.32	3.61	$124.93	2.43	$84.09	ZZZ	A
64646	Chemodenerv trunk musc 1-5	1.80	2.48	1.17	0.43	4.71	$163.00	3.40	$117.66	000	A M

*Please note that these calculations are based on the Medicare 2022 Conversion Factor of $34.6062 and the DRA RVU cap rates at time of publication.

A = assistant-at-surgery restriction
A+ = assistant-at-surgery restriction unless medical necessity established with documentation
B = bilateral surgery adjustment applies
C = cosurgeons payable
C+ = cosurgeons payable if medical necessity established with documentation
CP = carriers may establish RVUs and payment amounts for these services, generally on an individual basis following review of documentation such as an operative report
M = multiple surgery adjustment applies
Me = multiple endoscopy rules may apply
M+ = multiple therapy rules apply
Mtc = multiple diagnostic imaging rules apply
T = team surgeons permitted
T+ = team surgeons payable if medical necessity established with documentation
§ = indicates code is not covered by Medicare
GS = procedure must be performed under the general supervision of a physician
DS = procedure must be performed under the direct supervision of a physician
PS = procedure must be performed under the personal supervision of a physician
DRA = procedure subject to DRA limitation

Relative Value Units

CPT Code and Modifier	Description	Work RVU	Nonfacility Practice Expense RVU	Facility Practice Expense RVU	PLI RVU	Total Non-facility RVUs	Medicare Payment Nonfacility	Total Facility RVUs	Medicare Payment Facility	Global Period	Payment Policy Indicators
64647	Chemodenerv trunk musc 6/>	2.11	2.72	1.28	0.57	5.40	$186.87	3.96	$137.04	000	A M
64650	Chemodenerv eccrine glands	0.70	1.83	0.38	0.11	2.64	$91.36	1.19	$41.18	000	A+ M
64653	Chemodenerv eccrine glands	0.88	2.09	0.47	0.19	3.16	$109.36	1.54	$53.29	000	A+ M
64680	Injection treatment of nerve	2.67	7.64	1.80	0.25	10.56	$365.44	4.72	$163.34	010	A M
64681	Injection treatment of nerve	3.78	10.06	2.46	0.35	14.19	$491.06	6.59	$228.05	010	A M
64702	Revise finger/toe nerve	6.26	NA	7.79	1.09	NA	NA	15.14	$523.94	090	A M
64704	Revise hand/foot nerve	4.69	NA	4.33	0.56	NA	NA	9.58	$331.53	090	C+ M
64708	Revise arm/leg nerve	6.36	NA	7.41	1.16	NA	NA	14.93	$516.67	090	C+ M
64712	Revision of sciatic nerve	8.07	NA	7.96	1.66	NA	NA	17.69	$612.18	090	B C+ M
64713	Revision of arm nerve(s)	11.40	NA	9.52	2.55	NA	NA	23.47	$812.21	090	B C+ M
64714	Revise low back nerve(s)	10.55	NA	9.62	2.29	NA	NA	22.46	$777.26	090	B C+ M
64716	Revision of cranial nerve	6.99	NA	7.08	1.12	NA	NA	15.19	$525.67	090	C+ M
64718	Revise ulnar nerve at elbow	7.26	NA	9.16	1.44	NA	NA	17.86	$618.07	090	A+ B M
64719	Revise ulnar nerve at wrist	4.97	NA	6.20	0.95	NA	NA	12.12	$419.43	090	A B M
64721	Carpal tunnel surgery	4.97	7.26	7.01	0.99	13.22	$457.49	12.97	$448.84	090	A B M
64722	Relieve pressure on nerve(s)	4.82	NA	4.89	0.99	NA	NA	10.70	$370.29	090	C+ M
64726	Release foot/toe nerve	4.27	NA	3.26	0.40	NA	NA	7.93	$274.43	090	A M
64727	Internal nerve revision	3.10	NA	1.66	0.54	NA	NA	5.30	$183.41	ZZZ	A
64732	Incision of brow nerve	4.89	NA	6.76	1.86	NA	NA	13.51	$467.53	090	B M
64734	Incision of cheek nerve	5.55	NA	7.58	2.14	NA	NA	15.27	$528.44	090	A+ B M
64736	Incision of chin nerve	5.23	NA	4.03	0.44	NA	NA	9.70	$335.68	090	B M
64738	Incision of jaw nerve	6.36	NA	6.31	0.60	NA	NA	13.27	$459.22	090	B M
64740	Incision of tongue nerve	6.22	NA	6.78	0.60	NA	NA	13.60	$470.64	090	B M
64742	Incision of facial nerve	6.85	NA	7.00	0.54	NA	NA	14.39	$497.98	090	B M
64744	Incise nerve back of head	5.72	NA	7.16	2.18	NA	NA	15.06	$521.17	090	A+ B M
64746	Incise diaphragm nerve	6.56	NA	4.73	1.55	NA	NA	12.84	$444.34	090	B C+ M
64755	Incision of stomach nerves	15.05	NA	8.71	3.80	NA	NA	27.56	$953.75	090	C+ M
64760	Incision of vagus nerve	7.59	NA	6.09	1.93	NA	NA	15.61	$540.20	090	C+ M
64763	Incise hip/thigh nerve	7.56	NA	5.97	1.91	NA	NA	15.44	$534.32	090	B C+ M
64766	Incise hip/thigh nerve	9.47	NA	7.20	2.38	NA	NA	19.05	$659.25	090	B M
64771	Sever cranial nerve	8.15	NA	7.62	1.39	NA	NA	17.16	$593.84	090	M
64772	Incision of spinal nerve	7.84	NA	7.32	1.51	NA	NA	16.67	$576.89	090	C+ M
64774	Remove skin nerve lesion	5.80	NA	5.55	1.04	NA	NA	12.39	$428.77	090	A M

64776	Remove digit nerve lesion	5.60	NA	5.19	0.87	NA	NA	11.66	$403.51	090	A+ M
64778	Digit nerve surgery add-on	3.11	NA	1.57	0.64	NA	NA	5.32	$184.10	ZZZ	A
64782	Remove limb nerve lesion	6.86	NA	5.67	0.96	NA	NA	13.49	$466.84	090	A C+ M
64783	Limb nerve surgery add-on	3.71	NA	1.88	0.77	NA	NA	6.36	$220.10	ZZZ	A
64784	Remove nerve lesion	10.62	NA	8.95	2.01	NA	NA	21.58	$746.80	090	A+ M
64786	Remove sciatic nerve lesion	16.25	NA	9.73	4.10	NA	NA	30.08	$1040.95	090	B M
64787	Implant nerve end	4.29	NA	1.99	0.73	NA	NA	7.01	$242.59	ZZZ	A+
64788	Remove skin nerve lesion	5.24	NA	5.71	1.09	NA	NA	12.04	$416.66	090	A M
64790	Removal of nerve lesion	12.10	NA	9.94	2.84	NA	NA	24.88	$861.00	090	A+ C+ M
64792	Removal of nerve lesion	15.86	NA	12.01	3.78	NA	NA	31.65	$1095.29	090	C+ M
64795	Biopsy of nerve	3.01	NA	1.87	0.75	NA	NA	5.63	$194.83	000	A M
64802	Sympathectomy cervical	10.37	NA	10.87	3.97	NA	NA	25.21	$872.42	090	B C+ M
64804	Remove sympathetic nerves	15.91	NA	13.52	6.11	NA	NA	35.54	$1229.90	090	B C+ M
64809	Remove sympathetic nerves	14.71	NA	12.13	5.62	NA	NA	32.46	$1123.32	090	B C+ M
64818	Remove sympathetic nerves	11.34	NA	9.43	2.33	NA	NA	23.10	$799.40	090	B C+ M
64820	Sympathectomy digital artery	10.74	NA	9.05	1.78	NA	NA	21.57	$746.46	090	A M
64821	Remove sympathetic nerves	9.33	NA	9.46	1.70	NA	NA	20.49	$709.08	090	A B M
64822	Remove sympathetic nerves	9.33	NA	9.51	1.94	NA	NA	20.78	$719.12	090	A B M
64823	Sympathectomy supfc palmar	10.94	NA	10.33	2.25	NA	NA	23.52	$813.94	090	A B M
64831	Repair of digit nerve	9.16	NA	9.71	1.69	NA	NA	20.56	$711.50	090	A B M
64832	Repair nerve add-on	5.65	NA	3.08	1.04	NA	NA	9.77	$338.10	ZZZ	A+
64834	Repair of hand or foot nerve	10.81	NA	9.15	1.99	NA	NA	21.95	$759.61	090	A+ B M
64835	Repair of hand or foot nerve	11.73	NA	10.10	2.40	NA	NA	24.23	$838.51	090	B M
64836	Repair of hand or foot nerve	11.73	NA	10.10	2.40	NA	NA	24.23	$838.51	090	B M
64837	Repair nerve add-on	6.25	NA	3.17	1.29	NA	NA	10.71	$370.63	ZZZ	
64840	Repair of leg nerve	14.02	NA	11.63	2.90	NA	NA	28.55	$988.01	090	B M
64856	Repair/transpose nerve	15.07	NA	11.87	2.99	NA	NA	29.93	$1035.76	090	A C+ M
64857	Repair arm/leg nerve	15.82	NA	12.30	3.11	NA	NA	31.23	$1080.75	090	C+ M

*Please note that these calculations are based on the Medicare 2022 Conversion Factor of $34.6062 and the DRA RVU cap rates at time of publication.

A = assistant-at-surgery restriction
A+ = assistant-at-surgery restriction unless medical necessity established with documentation
B = bilateral surgery adjustment applies
C = cosurgeons payable
C+ = cosurgeons payable if medical necessity established with documentation
CP = carriers may establish RVUs and payment amounts for these services, generally on an individual basis following review of documentation such as an operative report
M = multiple surgery adjustment applies
Me = multiple endoscopy rules may apply
M+ = multiple therapy rules apply
Mtc = multiple diagnostic imaging rules apply
T = team surgeons permitted
T+ = team surgeons payable if medical necessity established with documentation
§ = indicates code is not covered by Medicare
GS = procedure must be performed under the general supervision of a physician
DS = procedure must be performed under the direct supervision of a physician
PS = procedure must be performed under the personal supervision of a physician
DRA = procedure subject to DRA limitation

Relative Value Units

CPT Code and Modifier	Description	Work RVU	Nonfacility Practice Expense RVU	Facility Practice Expense RVU	PLI RVU	Total Non-facility RVUs	Medicare Payment Nonfacility	Total Facility RVUs	Medicare Payment Facility	Global Period	Payment Policy Indicators
64858	Repair sciatic nerve	17.82	NA	13.31	3.68	NA	NA	34.81	$1204.64	090	B C+ M
64859	Nerve surgery	4.25	NA	2.15	0.89	NA	NA	7.29	$252.28	ZZZ	C+
64861	Repair of arm nerves	20.89	NA	16.39	8.01	NA	NA	45.29	$1567.31	090	B C+ M
64862	Repair of low back nerves	21.09	NA	15.20	4.34	NA	NA	40.63	$1406.05	090	B M
64864	Repair of facial nerve	13.41	NA	9.81	2.07	NA	NA	25.29	$875.19	090	C+ M
64865	Repair of facial nerve	16.09	NA	13.88	2.28	NA	NA	32.25	$1116.05	090	C+ M
64866	Fusion of facial/other nerve	16.83	NA	17.11	3.06	NA	NA	37.00	$1280.43	090	C+ M
64868	Fusion of facial/other nerve	14.90	NA	12.57	2.13	NA	NA	29.60	$1024.34	090	C+ M
64872	Subsequent repair of nerve	1.99	NA	1.01	0.40	NA	NA	3.40	$117.66	ZZZ	C+
64874	Repair & revise nerve add-on	2.98	NA	1.51	0.61	NA	NA	5.10	$176.49	ZZZ	C+
64876	Repair nerve/shorten bone	3.37	NA	1.70	0.70	NA	NA	5.77	$199.68	ZZZ	C+
64885	Nerve graft head/neck </4 cm	17.60	NA	12.31	2.67	NA	NA	32.58	$1127.47	090	C+ M
64886	Nerve graft head/neck >4 cm	20.82	NA	14.03	3.06	NA	NA	37.91	$1311.92	090	C+ M
64890	Nerve graft hand/foot </4 cm	16.24	NA	12.39	3.36	NA	NA	31.99	$1107.05	090	M
64891	Nerve graft hand/foot >4 cm	17.35	NA	13.07	3.58	NA	NA	34.00	$1176.61	090	M
64892	Nerve graft arm/leg <4 cm	15.74	NA	12.13	3.24	NA	NA	31.11	$1076.60	090	C+ M
64893	Nerve graft arm/leg >4 cm	16.87	NA	12.82	3.48	NA	NA	33.17	$1147.89	090	M
64895	Nerve graft hand/foot </4 cm	20.39	NA	14.62	4.22	NA	NA	39.23	$1357.60	090	C+ M
64896	Nerve graft hand/foot >4 cm	21.96	NA	15.76	4.54	NA	NA	42.26	$1462.46	090	C+ M
64897	Nerve graft arm/leg </4 cm	19.38	NA	14.10	3.99	NA	NA	37.47	$1296.69	090	C+ M
64898	Nerve graft arm/leg >4 cm	20.97	NA	15.26	4.31	NA	NA	40.54	$1402.94	090	C+ M
64901	Nerve graft add-on	10.20	NA	5.17	2.11	NA	NA	17.48	$604.92	ZZZ	C+
64902	Nerve graft add-on	11.81	NA	5.99	2.44	NA	NA	20.24	$700.43	ZZZ	C+
64905	Nerve pedicle transfer	15.11	NA	11.83	2.84	NA	NA	29.78	$1030.57	090	C+ M
64907	Nerve pedicle transfer	20.03	NA	14.31	4.13	NA	NA	38.47	$1331.30	090	C+ M
64910	Nerve repair w/allograft	10.52	NA	10.50	1.80	NA	NA	22.82	$789.71	090	C+ M
64911	Neurorraphy w/vein autograft	14.00	NA	13.47	2.89	NA	NA	30.36	$1050.64	090	C+ M
64912	Nrv rpr w/nrv algrft 1st	12.00	NA	12.14	2.17	NA	NA	26.31	$910.49	090	C+ M
64913	Nrv rpr w/nrv algrft ea addl	3.00	NA	1.61	0.55	NA	NA	5.16	$178.57	ZZZ	C+
64999 CP	Nervous system surgery	0.00	0.00	0.00	0.00	0.00	$0.00	0.00	$0.00	YYY	A+ C+ M T+
65091	Revise eye	7.26	NA	14.34	0.56	NA	NA	22.16	$766.87	090	A+ B C+ M
65093	Revise eye with implant	7.04	NA	14.38	0.56	NA	NA	21.98	$760.64	090	A B C+ M
65101	Removal of eye	8.30	NA	16.33	0.64	NA	NA	25.27	$874.50	090	A B M

65103	Remove eye/insert implant	8.84	NA	16.53	0.67	NA	NA	26.04	$901.15	090	A B C+ M
65105	Remove eye/attach implant	9.93	NA	17.60	0.77	NA	NA	28.30	$979.36	090	B C+ M
65110	Removal of eye	15.70	NA	22.00	1.20	NA	NA	38.90	$1346.18	090	B C+ M
65112	Remove eye/revise socket	18.51	NA	24.56	1.41	NA	NA	44.48	$1539.28	090	B C+ M
65114	Remove eye/revise socket	19.65	NA	25.27	1.51	NA	NA	46.43	$1606.77	090	B C+ M
65125	Revise ocular implant	3.27	9.98	4.97	0.25	13.50	$467.18	8.49	$293.81	090	A B C+ M
65130	Insert ocular implant	8.42	NA	16.28	0.65	NA	NA	25.35	$877.27	090	A B C+ M
65135	Insert ocular implant	8.60	NA	16.39	0.65	NA	NA	25.64	$887.30	090	A B M
65140	Attach ocular implant	9.46	NA	17.34	0.73	NA	NA	27.53	$952.71	090	A B M
65150	Revise ocular implant	6.43	NA	14.01	0.50	NA	NA	20.94	$724.65	090	A+ B M
65155	Reinsert ocular implant	10.10	NA	17.72	0.77	NA	NA	28.59	$989.39	090	A B M
65175	Removal of ocular implant	7.40	NA	15.22	0.57	NA	NA	23.19	$802.52	090	A B C+ M
65205	Remove foreign body from eye	0.49	0.32	0.32	0.04	0.85	$29.42	0.85	$29.42	000	A B M
65210	Remove foreign body from eye	0.61	0.49	0.40	0.04	1.14	$39.45	1.05	$36.34	000	A B M
65220	Remove foreign body from eye	0.71	0.97	0.40	0.09	1.77	$61.25	1.20	$41.53	000	A B M
65222	Remove foreign body from eye	0.84	1.09	0.57	0.05	1.98	$68.52	1.46	$50.53	000	A B M
65235	Remove foreign body from eye	9.01	NA	11.54	0.70	NA	NA	21.25	$735.38	090	A+ B M
65260	Remove foreign body from eye	12.54	NA	15.08	0.96	NA	NA	28.58	$989.05	090	B M
65265	Remove foreign body from eye	14.34	NA	16.73	1.10	NA	NA	32.17	$1113.28	090	B C+ M
65270	Repair of eye wound	1.95	6.40	1.98	0.14	8.49	$293.81	4.07	$140.85	010	A+ B M
65272	Repair of eye wound	4.62	10.65	5.28	0.35	15.62	$540.55	10.25	$354.71	090	A B M
65273	Repair of eye wound	5.16	NA	5.46	0.40	NA	NA	11.02	$381.36	090	A B C+ M
65275	Repair of eye wound	6.29	10.49	6.60	0.50	17.28	$598.00	13.39	$463.38	090	A+ B M
65280	Repair of eye wound	9.10	NA	9.63	0.70	NA	NA	19.43	$672.40	090	A+ B M
65285	Repair of eye wound	15.36	NA	15.47	1.20	NA	NA	32.03	$1108.44	090	A B M
65286	Repair of eye wound	6.63	13.47	7.23	0.51	20.61	$713.23	14.37	$497.29	090	A B M
65290	Repair of eye socket wound	6.53	NA	7.17	0.50	NA	NA	14.20	$491.41	090	A B C+ M
65400	Removal of eye lesion	7.50	12.15	9.37	0.57	20.22	$699.74	17.44	$603.53	090	A B M

*Please note that these calculations are based on the Medicare 2022 Conversion Factor of $34.6062 and the DRA RVU cap rates at time of publication.

A = assistant-at-surgery restriction
A+ = assistant-at-surgery restriction unless medical necessity established with documentation
B = bilateral surgery adjustment applies
C = cosurgeons payable
C+ = cosurgeons payable if medical necessity established with documentation
CP = carriers may establish RVUs and payment amounts for these services, generally on an individual basis following review of documentation such as an operative report
M = multiple surgery adjustment applies
Me = multiple endoscopy rules may apply
M+ = multiple therapy rules apply
Mtc = multiple diagnostic imaging rules apply
T = team surgeons permitted
T+ = team surgeons payable if medical necessity established with documentation
§ = indicates code is not covered by Medicare
GS = procedure must be performed under the general supervision of a physician
DS = procedure must be performed under the direct supervision of a physician
PS = procedure must be performed under the personal supervision of a physician
DRA = procedure subject to DRA limitation

Relative Value Units

CPT Code and Modifier		Description	Work RVU	Nonfacility Practice Expense RVU	Facility Practice Expense RVU	PLI RVU	Total Non-facility RVUs	Medicare Payment Nonfacility	Total Facility RVUs	Medicare Payment Facility	Global Period	Payment Policy Indicators
65410		Biopsy of cornea	1.47	2.60	1.36	0.11	4.18	$144.65	2.94	$101.74	000	A+ B M
65420		Removal of eye lesion	4.36	11.24	6.28	0.34	15.94	$551.62	10.98	$379.98	090	A B M
65426		Removal of eye lesion	6.05	13.27	7.32	0.45	19.77	$684.16	13.82	$478.26	090	A B M
65430		Corneal smear	1.47	1.77	1.35	0.11	3.35	$115.93	2.93	$101.40	000	A B M
65435		Curette/treat cornea	0.92	1.40	1.00	0.08	2.40	$83.05	2.00	$69.21	000	A B M
65436		Curette/treat cornea	4.82	6.06	5.49	0.37	11.25	$389.32	10.68	$369.59	090	A B M
65450		Treatment of corneal lesion	3.47	5.81	5.58	0.25	9.53	$329.80	9.30	$321.84	090	A B M
65600		Revision of cornea	4.20	8.35	5.30	0.32	12.87	$445.38	9.82	$339.83	090	A B M
65710		Corneal transplant	14.45	NA	17.67	1.10	NA	NA	33.22	$1149.62	090	B C+ M
65730		Corneal transplant	16.35	NA	18.80	1.26	NA	NA	36.41	$1260.01	090	B C+ M
65750		Corneal transplant	16.90	NA	18.51	1.29	NA	NA	36.70	$1270.05	090	B C+ M
65755		Corneal transplant	16.79	NA	18.45	1.29	NA	NA	36.53	$1264.16	090	B C+ M
65756		Corneal trnspl endothelial	16.84	NA	15.93	1.29	NA	NA	34.06	$1178.69	090	B C+ M
65757	CP	Prep corneal endo allograft	0.00	0.00	0.00	0.00	0.00	$0.00	0.00	$0.00	ZZZ	A+
65770		Revise cornea with implant	19.74	NA	19.55	1.52	NA	NA	40.81	$1412.28	090	B M
65772		Correction of astigmatism	5.09	7.84	6.22	0.39	13.32	$460.95	11.70	$404.89	090	A B M
65775		Correction of astigmatism	6.91	NA	9.26	0.54	NA	NA	16.71	$578.27	090	A B M
65778		Cover eye w/membrane	1.00	39.77	0.50	0.05	40.82	$1412.63	1.55	$53.64	000	A+ B M
65779		Cover eye w/membrane suture	2.50	32.68	1.60	0.20	35.38	$1224.37	4.30	$148.81	000	A+ B M
65780		Ocular reconst transplant	7.81	NA	10.96	0.60	NA	NA	19.37	$670.32	090	A B C+ M
65781		Ocular reconst transplant	18.14	NA	18.84	1.40	NA	NA	38.38	$1328.19	090	B C+ M
65782		Ocular reconst transplant	15.43	NA	16.53	1.18	NA	NA	33.14	$1146.85	090	A B C+ M
65785		Impltj ntrstrml crnl rng seg	5.39	59.95	7.01	0.41	65.75	$2275.36	12.81	$443.31	090	A B C+ M
65800		Drainage of eye	1.53	1.83	0.94	0.11	3.47	$120.08	2.58	$89.28	000	A B M
65810		Drainage of eye	5.82	NA	7.17	0.43	NA	NA	13.42	$464.42	090	A B M
65815		Drainage of eye	6.00	12.49	7.33	0.44	18.93	$655.10	13.77	$476.53	090	A B M
65820		Relieve inner eye pressure	8.91	NA	14.63	0.68	NA	NA	24.22	$838.16	090	A+ B M
65850		Incision of eye	11.39	NA	12.22	0.89	NA	NA	24.50	$847.85	090	A B C+ M
65855		Trabeculoplasty laser surg	3.00	3.95	2.71	0.23	7.18	$248.47	5.94	$205.56	010	A B C+ M T+
65860		Incise inner eye adhesions	3.59	5.11	3.31	0.27	8.97	$310.42	7.17	$248.13	090	A+ B M
65865		Incise inner eye adhesions	5.77	NA	7.69	0.43	NA	NA	13.89	$480.68	090	A B C+ M
65870		Incise inner eye adhesions	7.39	NA	9.32	0.57	NA	NA	17.28	$598.00	090	A B C+ M
65875		Incise inner eye adhesions	7.81	NA	10.01	0.60	NA	NA	18.42	$637.45	090	A B C+ M

65880	Incise inner eye adhesions	8.36	NA	10.35	0.65	NA	NA	19.36	$669.98	090	A B M
65900	Remove eye lesion	12.51	NA	15.41	0.96	NA	NA	28.88	$999.43	090	B M
65920	Remove implant of eye	9.99	NA	12.22	0.77	NA	NA	22.98	$795.25	090	A B C+ M
65930	Remove blood clot from eye	8.39	NA	9.61	0.65	NA	NA	18.65	$645.41	090	A B C+ M
66020	Injection treatment of eye	1.64	4.05	2.02	0.12	5.81	$201.06	3.78	$130.81	010	A B M
66030	Injection treatment of eye	1.30	3.85	1.81	0.10	5.25	$181.68	3.21	$111.09	010	A B M
66130	Remove eye lesion	7.83	12.33	7.91	0.60	20.76	$718.42	16.34	$565.47	090	A+ B M
66150	Glaucoma surgery	10.53	NA	14.11	0.79	NA	NA	25.43	$880.04	090	A B C+ M
66155	Glaucoma surgery	10.52	NA	14.11	0.79	NA	NA	25.42	$879.69	090	A B M
66160	Glaucoma surgery	12.39	NA	15.25	0.95	NA	NA	28.59	$989.39	090	A B C+ M
66170	Glaucoma surgery	13.94	NA	16.66	1.07	NA	NA	31.67	$1095.98	090	B C+ M
66172	Incision of eye	14.84	NA	18.58	1.16	NA	NA	34.58	$1196.68	090	B C+ M
66174	Translum dil eye canal	7.62	NA	13.77	0.60	NA	NA	21.99	$760.99	090	B C+ M
66175	Trnslum dil eye canal w/stnt	9.34	NA	13.02	0.73	NA	NA	23.09	$799.06	090	B C+ M
66179	Aqueous shunt eye w/o graft	14.00	NA	16.23	1.07	NA	NA	31.30	$1083.17	090	B M
66180	Aqueous shunt eye w/graft	15.00	NA	16.83	1.16	NA	NA	32.99	$1141.66	090	B M
66183	Insert ant drainage device	13.20	NA	15.60	1.01	NA	NA	29.81	$1031.61	090	B M
66184	Revision of aqueous shunt	9.58	NA	12.62	0.73	NA	NA	22.93	$793.52	090	B M
66185	Revise aqueous shunt eye	10.58	NA	13.24	0.83	NA	NA	24.65	$853.04	090	B M
66225	Repair/graft eye lesion	12.63	NA	13.51	0.98	NA	NA	27.12	$938.52	090	A B C+ M
66250	Follow-up surgery of eye	7.10	14.54	8.44	0.56	22.20	$768.26	16.10	$557.16	090	A B M
66500	Incision of iris	3.83	NA	7.49	0.29	NA	NA	11.61	$401.78	090	A B C+ M
66505	Incision of iris	4.22	NA	8.07	0.33	NA	NA	12.62	$436.73	090	A B M
66600	Remove iris and lesion	10.12	NA	15.71	0.77	NA	NA	26.60	$920.52	090	A B M
66605	Removal of iris	14.22	NA	16.46	1.09	NA	NA	31.77	$1099.44	090	A B M
66625	Removal of iris	5.30	NA	6.71	0.40	NA	NA	12.41	$429.46	090	A B M
66630	Removal of iris	7.28	NA	8.56	0.56	NA	NA	16.40	$567.54	090	A B M
66635	Removal of iris	7.37	NA	8.62	0.57	NA	NA	16.56	$573.08	090	A B M

*Please note that these calculations are based on the Medicare 2022 Conversion Factor of $34.6062 and the DRA RVU cap rates at time of publication.

A = assistant-at-surgery restriction
A+ = assistant-at-surgery restriction unless medical necessity established with documentation
B = bilateral surgery adjustment applies
C = cosurgeons payable
C+ = cosurgeons payable if medical necessity established with documentation
CP = carriers may establish RVUs and payment amounts for these services, generally on an individual basis following review of documentation such as an operative report
M = multiple surgery adjustment applies
Me = multiple endoscopy rules may apply
M+ = multiple therapy rules apply
Mtc = multiple diagnostic imaging rules apply
T = team surgeons permitted
T+ = team surgeons payable if medical necessity established with documentation
§ = indicates code is not covered by Medicare
GS = procedure must be performed under the general supervision of a physician
DS = procedure must be performed under the direct supervision of a physician
PS = procedure must be performed under the personal supervision of a physician
DRA = procedure subject to DRA limitation

Relative Value Units

CPT Code and Modifier		Description	Work RVU	Nonfacility Practice Expense RVU	Facility Practice Expense RVU	PLI RVU	Total Non-facility RVUs	Medicare Payment Nonfacility	Total Facility RVUs	Medicare Payment Facility	Global Period	Payment Policy Indicators
66680		Repair iris & ciliary body	6.39	NA	8.26	0.50	NA	NA	15.15	$524.28	090	A B C+ M
66682		Repair iris & ciliary body	7.33	NA	13.11	0.57	NA	NA	21.01	$727.08	090	A B M
66700		Destruction ciliary body	5.14	7.64	5.79	0.40	13.18	$456.11	11.33	$392.09	090	A+ B M
66710		Ciliary transsleral therapy	5.14	7.38	5.79	0.40	12.92	$447.11	11.33	$392.09	090	A B M
66711		Ecp ciliary body destruction	5.62	NA	8.60	0.42	NA	NA	14.64	$506.63	090	A B Me
66720		Destruction ciliary body	4.75	8.48	6.74	0.37	13.60	$470.64	11.86	$410.43	090	A B M
66740		Destruction ciliary body	5.14	7.27	5.79	0.40	12.81	$443.31	11.33	$392.09	090	A B M
66761		Revision of iris	3.00	5.54	3.62	0.23	8.77	$303.50	6.85	$237.05	010	A B M
66762		Revision of iris	5.38	8.12	6.49	0.41	13.91	$481.37	12.28	$424.96	090	A B M
66770		Removal of inner eye lesion	6.13	8.83	7.31	0.45	15.41	$533.28	13.89	$480.68	090	A B M
66820		Incision secondary cataract	4.01	NA	9.63	0.31	NA	NA	13.95	$482.76	090	A B M
66821		After cataract laser surgery	3.42	6.08	5.37	0.25	9.75	$337.41	9.04	$312.84	090	A B M
66825		Reposition intraocular lens	9.01	NA	14.80	0.70	NA	NA	24.51	$848.20	090	A+ B M
66830		Removal of lens lesion	9.47	NA	10.34	0.73	NA	NA	20.54	$710.81	090	A B M
66840		Removal of lens material	9.18	NA	10.16	0.72	NA	NA	20.06	$694.20	090	A B M
66850		Removal of lens material	10.55	NA	11.45	0.79	NA	NA	22.79	$788.68	090	A B M
66852		Removal of lens material	11.41	NA	11.98	0.89	NA	NA	24.28	$840.24	090	A+ B C+ M
66920		Extraction of lens	10.13	NA	10.75	0.77	NA	NA	21.65	$749.22	090	A+ B C+ M
66930		Extraction of lens	11.61	NA	12.31	0.90	NA	NA	24.82	$858.93	090	A+ B M
66940		Extraction of lens	10.37	NA	11.55	0.79	NA	NA	22.71	$785.91	090	A+ B C+ M
66982		Xcapsl ctrc rmvl cplx wo ecp	10.25	NA	10.54	0.77	NA	NA	21.56	$746.11	090	A B M
66983	CP	Cataract surg w/iol 1 stage	0.00	0.00	0.00	0.00	0.00	$0.00	0.00	$0.00	090	A B M
66984		Xcapsl ctrc rmvl w/o ecp	7.35	NA	7.83	0.56	NA	NA	15.74	$544.70	090	A B M
66985		Insert lens prosthesis	9.98	NA	11.52	0.77	NA	NA	22.27	$770.68	090	A B C+ M
66986		Exchange lens prosthesis	12.26	NA	12.93	0.95	NA	NA	26.14	$904.61	090	A B C+ M
66987	CP	Xcapsl ctrc rmvl cplx w/ecp	0.00	0.00	0.00	0.00	0.00	$0.00	0.00	$0.00	090	A+ B C+ M T+
66988	CP	Xcapsl ctrc rmvl w/ecp	0.00	0.00	0.00	0.00	0.00	$0.00	0.00	$0.00	090	A+ B C+ M T+
66989		Xcpsl ctrc rmvl cplx insj 1+	12.13	NA	11.69	0.93	NA	NA	24.75	$856.50	090	A B M
66990		Ophthalmic endoscope add-on	1.51	NA	0.93	0.11	NA	NA	2.55	$88.25	ZZZ	A
66991		Xcapsl ctrc rmvl insj 1+	9.23	NA	9.84	0.68	NA	NA	19.75	$683.47	090	A B M
66999	CP	Eye surgery procedure	0.00	0.00	0.00	0.00	0.00	$0.00	0.00	$0.00	YYY	A+ B C+ M T+
67005		Partial removal of eye fluid	5.89	NA	7.39	0.44	NA	NA	13.72	$474.80	090	A B C+ M
67010		Partial removal of eye fluid	7.06	NA	8.11	0.55	NA	NA	15.72	$544.01	090	A B C+ M

67015	Release of eye fluid	7.14	NA	9.94	0.56	NA	NA	17.64	$610.45	090	A B C+ M
67025	Replace eye fluid	8.11	12.97	9.50	0.62	21.70	$750.95	18.23	$630.87	090	A B C+ M
67027	Implant eye drug system	11.62	NA	12.00	0.90	NA	NA	24.52	$848.54	090	B C+ M
67028	Injection eye drug	1.44	1.75	1.10	0.11	3.30	$114.20	2.65	$91.71	000	A B M
67030	Incise inner eye strands	6.11	NA	9.68	0.45	NA	NA	16.24	$562.00	090	A B C+ M
67031	Laser surgery eye strands	4.47	6.56	5.45	0.34	11.37	$393.47	10.26	$355.06	090	A B M
67036	Removal of inner eye fluid	12.13	NA	12.85	0.95	NA	NA	25.93	$897.34	090	B C+ M
67039	Laser treatment of retina	13.20	NA	13.51	1.01	NA	NA	27.72	$959.28	090	B C+ M
67040	Laser treatment of retina	14.50	NA	14.32	1.11	NA	NA	29.93	$1035.76	090	B C+ M
67041	Vit for macular pucker	16.33	NA	15.44	1.26	NA	NA	33.03	$1143.04	090	B C+ M
67042	Vit for macular hole	16.33	NA	15.44	1.26	NA	NA	33.03	$1143.04	090	B C+ M
67043	Vit for membrane dissect	17.40	NA	16.10	1.33	NA	NA	34.83	$1205.33	090	B C+ M
67101	Repair detached retina crtx	3.50	5.99	4.45	0.25	9.74	$337.06	8.20	$283.77	010	A B M
67105	Repair detached retina pc	3.39	4.97	4.30	0.25	8.61	$297.96	7.94	$274.77	010	A B M
67107	Repair detached retina	16.00	NA	15.24	1.24	NA	NA	32.48	$1124.01	090	B C+ M
67108	Repair detached retina	17.13	NA	15.93	1.32	NA	NA	34.38	$1189.76	090	B C+ M
67110	Repair detached retina	10.25	14.93	12.48	0.78	25.96	$898.38	23.51	$813.59	090	A B M
67113	Repair retinal detach cplx	19.00	NA	17.96	1.47	NA	NA	38.43	$1329.92	090	B C+ M
67115	Release encircling material	6.11	NA	7.84	0.45	NA	NA	14.40	$498.33	090	A B M
67120	Remove eye implant material	7.10	12.01	8.40	0.56	19.67	$680.70	16.06	$555.78	090	A B C+ M
67121	Remove eye implant material	12.25	NA	12.92	0.95	NA	NA	26.12	$903.91	090	B C+ M
67141	Proph rta dtchmnt crtx dthrm	2.53	5.15	3.54	0.20	7.88	$272.70	6.27	$216.98	010	A B M
67145	Proph rta dtchmnt pc	2.53	4.33	3.54	0.20	7.06	$244.32	6.27	$216.98	010	A B M
67208	Treatment of retinal lesion	7.65	9.25	8.45	0.60	17.50	$605.61	16.70	$577.92	090	A B M
67210	Treatment of retinal lesion	6.36	8.13	7.55	0.50	14.99	$518.75	14.41	$498.68	090	A B M
67218	Treatment of retinal lesion	20.36	NA	18.48	1.55	NA	NA	40.39	$1397.74	090	A B M
67220	Treatment of choroid lesion	6.36	8.58	7.55	0.50	15.44	$534.32	14.41	$498.68	090	A B M
67221	Ocular photodynamic ther	3.45	4.24	2.32	0.25	7.94	$274.77	6.02	$208.33	000	A M

*Please note that these calculations are based on the Medicare 2022 Conversion Factor of $34.6062 and the DRA RVU cap rates at time of publication.

A = assistant-at-surgery restriction

A+ = assistant-at-surgery restriction unless medical necessity established with documentation

B = bilateral surgery adjustment applies

C = cosurgeons payable

C+ = cosurgeons payable if medical necessity established with documentation

CP = carriers may establish RVUs and payment amounts for these services, generally on an individual basis following review of documentation such as an operative report

M = multiple surgery adjustment applies

Me = multiple endoscopy rules may apply

M+ = multiple therapy rules apply

Mtc = multiple diagnostic imaging rules apply

T = team surgeons permitted

T+ = team surgeons payable if medical necessity established with documentation

§ = indicates code is not covered by Medicare

GS = procedure must be performed under the general supervision of a physician

DS = procedure must be performed under the direct supervision of a physician

PS = procedure must be performed under the personal supervision of a physician

DRA = procedure subject to DRA limitation

Relative Value Units

CPT Code and Modifier		Description	Work RVU	Nonfacility Practice Expense RVU	Facility Practice Expense RVU	PLI RVU	Total Non-facility RVUs	Medicare Payment Nonfacility	Total Facility RVUs	Medicare Payment Facility	Global Period	Payment Policy Indicators
67225		Eye photodynamic ther add-on	0.47	0.34	0.29	0.04	0.85	$29.42	0.80	$27.68	ZZZ	A
67227		Dstrj extensive retinopathy	3.50	4.83	3.58	0.25	8.58	$296.92	7.33	$253.66	010	A B M
67228		Treatment x10sv retinopathy	4.39	5.14	4.04	0.34	9.87	$341.56	8.77	$303.50	010	A B M
67229		Tr retinal les preterm inf	16.30	NA	15.93	1.26	NA	NA	33.49	$1158.96	090	A B M
67250		Reinforce eye wall	9.61	NA	16.47	0.73	NA	NA	26.81	$927.79	090	A B C+ M
67255		Reinforce/graft eye wall	8.38	NA	10.92	0.65	NA	NA	19.95	$690.39	090	B C+ M
67299	CP	Eye surgery procedure	0.00	0.00	0.00	0.00	0.00	$0.00	0.00	$0.00	YYY	A+ B C+ M T+
67311		Revise eye muscle	5.93	NA	7.61	0.44	NA	NA	13.98	$483.79	090	A B M
67312		Revise two eye muscles	9.50	NA	9.01	0.73	NA	NA	19.24	$665.82	090	A B C+ M
67314		Revise eye muscle	5.93	NA	9.63	0.44	NA	NA	16.00	$553.70	090	A B M
67316		Revise two eye muscles	10.31	NA	9.48	0.79	NA	NA	20.58	$712.20	090	A+ B M
67318		Revise eye muscle(s)	9.80	NA	9.36	0.75	NA	NA	19.91	$689.01	090	A B C+ M
67320		Revise eye muscle(s) add-on	3.00	NA	4.16	0.23	NA	NA	7.39	$255.74	ZZZ	A
67331		Eye surgery follow-up add-on	2.00	NA	4.85	0.17	NA	NA	7.02	$242.94	ZZZ	A B C+
67332		Rerevise eye muscles add-on	3.50	NA	3.86	0.25	NA	NA	7.61	$263.35	ZZZ	A B C+
67334		Revise eye muscle w/suture	2.06	NA	4.69	0.17	NA	NA	6.92	$239.47	ZZZ	A B C+
67335		Eye suture during surgery	3.23	NA	1.96	0.25	NA	NA	5.44	$188.26	ZZZ	A B C+
67340		Revise eye muscle add-on	5.00	NA	3.08	0.39	NA	NA	8.47	$293.11	ZZZ	
67343		Release eye tissue	8.47	NA	10.28	0.67	NA	NA	19.42	$672.05	090	A B C+ M
67345		Destroy nerve of eye muscle	3.01	3.69	2.87	0.40	7.10	$245.70	6.28	$217.33	010	A B M
67346		Biopsy eye muscle	2.87	NA	2.41	0.22	NA	NA	5.50	$190.33	000	A+ B M
67399	CP	Unlisted px extraocular musc	0.00	0.00	0.00	0.00	0.00	$0.00	0.00	$0.00	YYY	B C+ M T+
67400		Explore/biopsy eye socket	11.20	NA	18.58	0.89	NA	NA	30.67	$1061.37	090	A B C+ M
67405		Explore/drain eye socket	9.20	NA	16.74	0.86	NA	NA	26.80	$927.45	090	A B M
67412		Explore/treat eye socket	10.30	NA	18.35	0.87	NA	NA	29.52	$1021.58	090	A B C+ M
67413		Explore/treat eye socket	10.24	NA	17.49	0.89	NA	NA	28.62	$990.43	090	B M
67414		Explr/decompress eye socket	17.94	NA	23.54	1.81	NA	NA	43.29	$1498.10	090	B C+ M
67415		Aspiration orbital contents	1.76	NA	1.08	0.12	NA	NA	2.96	$102.43	000	A+ B M
67420		Explore/treat eye socket	21.87	NA	27.49	2.01	NA	NA	51.37	$1777.72	090	B C+ M
67430		Explore/treat eye socket	15.29	NA	24.51	1.18	NA	NA	40.98	$1418.16	090	B M
67440		Explore/drain eye socket	14.84	NA	23.79	1.16	NA	NA	39.79	$1376.98	090	B C+ M
67445		Explr/decompress eye socket	19.12	NA	24.36	1.57	NA	NA	45.05	$1559.01	090	B C+ M
67450		Explore/biopsy eye socket	15.41	NA	24.58	1.18	NA	NA	41.17	$1424.74	090	B C+ M

67500		Inject/treat eye socket	1.18	0.95	0.55	0.09	2.22	$76.83	1.82	$62.98	000	A B M
67505		Inject/treat eye socket	1.18	1.26	0.82	0.09	2.53	$87.55	2.09	$72.33	000	A B M
67515		Inject/treat eye socket	0.75	0.70	0.55	0.07	1.52	$52.60	1.37	$47.41	000	A B M
67550		Insert eye socket implant	11.77	NA	19.33	1.00	NA	NA	32.10	$1110.86	090	A B C+ M
67560		Revise eye socket implant	12.18	NA	19.60	1.00	NA	NA	32.78	$1134.39	090	A+ B M
67570		Decompress optic nerve	14.40	NA	23.55	2.93	NA	NA	40.88	$1414.70	090	B C+ M
67599	CP	Orbit surgery procedure	0.00	0.00	0.00	0.00	0.00	$0.00	0.00	$0.00	YYY	B C+ M T+
67700		Drainage of eyelid abscess	1.40	7.06	1.85	0.11	8.57	$296.58	3.36	$116.28	010	A B M
67710		Incision of eyelid	1.07	6.16	1.67	0.09	7.32	$253.32	2.83	$97.94	010	A B M
67715		Incision of eyelid fold	1.27	6.51	1.70	0.17	7.95	$275.12	3.14	$108.66	010	A B M
67800		Remove eyelid lesion	1.41	2.24	1.44	0.11	3.76	$130.12	2.96	$102.43	010	A M
67801		Remove eyelid lesions	1.91	2.70	1.75	0.14	4.75	$164.38	3.80	$131.50	010	A M
67805		Remove eyelid lesions	2.27	3.48	2.28	0.19	5.94	$205.56	4.74	$164.03	010	A M
67808		Remove eyelid lesion(s)	4.60	NA	5.67	0.37	NA	NA	10.64	$368.21	090	A M
67810		Biopsy eyelid & lid margin	1.18	4.26	0.69	0.11	5.55	$192.06	1.98	$68.52	000	A B M
67820		Revise eyelashes	0.32	0.22	0.30	0.02	0.56	$19.38	0.64	$22.15	000	A B M
67825		Revise eyelashes	1.43	2.43	1.98	0.11	3.97	$137.39	3.52	$121.81	010	A B M
67830		Revise eyelashes	1.75	6.19	2.08	0.12	8.06	$278.93	3.95	$136.69	010	A B M
67835		Revise eyelashes	5.70	NA	6.64	0.42	NA	NA	12.76	$441.58	090	A+ B M
67840		Remove eyelid lesion	2.09	6.12	2.29	0.18	8.39	$290.35	4.56	$157.80	010	A B M
67850		Treat eyelid lesion	1.74	4.55	1.90	0.12	6.41	$221.83	3.76	$130.12	010	A B M
67875		Closure of eyelid by suture	1.35	3.97	1.29	0.11	5.43	$187.91	2.75	$95.17	000	A B M
67880		Revision of eyelid	4.60	8.79	5.67	0.37	13.76	$476.18	10.64	$368.21	090	A B M
67882		Revision of eyelid	6.02	10.29	7.11	0.47	16.78	$580.69	13.60	$470.64	090	A B M
67900		Repair brow defect	6.82	11.69	7.21	0.61	19.12	$661.67	14.64	$506.63	090	A B M
67901		Repair eyelid defect	7.59	15.30	8.90	0.62	23.51	$813.59	17.11	$592.11	090	A B M
67902		Repair eyelid defect	9.82	NA	10.45	0.77	NA	NA	21.04	$728.11	090	A B C+ M
67903		Repair eyelid defect	6.51	10.72	6.86	0.54	17.77	$614.95	13.91	$481.37	090	A B C+ M

*Please note that these calculations are based on the Medicare 2022 Conversion Factor of $34.6062 and the DRA RVU cap rates at time of publication.

A = assistant-at-surgery restriction

A+ = assistant-at-surgery restriction unless medical necessity established with documentation

B = bilateral surgery adjustment applies

C = cosurgeons payable

C+ = cosurgeons payable if medical necessity established with documentation

CP = carriers may establish RVUs and payment amounts for these services, generally on an individual basis following review of documentation such as an operative report

M = multiple surgery adjustment applies

Me = multiple endoscopy rules may apply

M+ = multiple therapy rules apply

Mtc = multiple diagnostic imaging rules apply

T = team surgeons permitted

T+ = team surgeons payable if medical necessity established with documentation

§ = indicates code is not covered by Medicare

GS = procedure must be performed under the general supervision of a physician

DS = procedure must be performed under the direct supervision of a physician

PS = procedure must be performed under the personal supervision of a physician

DRA = procedure subject to DRA limitation

Relative Value Units

CPT Code and Modifier		Description	Work RVU	Nonfacility Practice Expense RVU	Facility Practice Expense RVU	PLI RVU	Total Non-facility RVUs	Medicare Payment Nonfacility	Total Facility RVUs	Medicare Payment Facility	Global Period	Payment Policy Indicators
67904		Repair eyelid defect	7.97	13.15	8.59	0.66	21.78	$753.72	17.22	$595.92	090	A B C+ M
67906		Repair eyelid defect	6.93	NA	7.13	0.55	NA	NA	14.61	$505.60	090	A B M
67908		Repair eyelid defect	5.30	10.27	6.81	0.40	15.97	$552.66	12.51	$432.92	090	A B M
67909		Revise eyelid defect	5.57	10.13	6.63	0.50	16.20	$560.62	12.70	$439.50	090	A B M
67911		Revise eyelid defect	7.50	NA	8.07	0.60	NA	NA	16.17	$559.58	090	A B M
67912		Correction eyelid w/implant	6.36	20.14	7.09	0.66	27.16	$939.90	14.11	$488.29	090	A B M
67914		Repair eyelid defect	3.75	10.45	5.42	0.32	14.52	$502.48	9.49	$328.41	090	A B M
67915		Repair eyelid defect	2.03	7.24	3.55	0.17	9.44	$326.68	5.75	$198.99	090	A B M
67916		Repair eyelid defect	5.48	12.18	6.50	0.44	18.10	$626.37	12.42	$429.81	090	A B M
67917		Repair eyelid defect	5.93	12.06	6.77	0.50	18.49	$639.87	13.20	$456.80	090	A B M
67921		Repair eyelid defect	3.47	10.49	5.27	0.25	14.21	$491.75	8.99	$311.11	090	A B M
67922		Repair eyelid defect	2.03	6.94	3.56	0.17	9.14	$316.30	5.76	$199.33	090	A B M
67923		Repair eyelid defect	5.48	12.19	6.51	0.42	18.09	$626.03	12.41	$429.46	090	A B M
67924		Repair eyelid defect	5.93	12.85	6.78	0.47	19.25	$666.17	13.18	$456.11	090	A B M
67930		Repair eyelid wound	3.65	7.01	2.89	0.29	10.95	$378.94	6.83	$236.36	010	A B M
67935		Repair eyelid wound	6.36	10.72	5.82	0.57	17.65	$610.80	12.75	$441.23	090	A B M
67938		Remove eyelid foreign body	1.38	6.73	1.93	0.09	8.20	$283.77	3.40	$117.66	010	A B M
67950		Revision of eyelid	5.99	10.72	6.86	0.54	17.25	$596.96	13.39	$463.38	090	A B C+ M
67961		Revision of eyelid	5.86	10.97	6.79	0.47	17.30	$598.69	13.12	$454.03	090	A+ B M
67966		Revision of eyelid	8.97	13.12	9.21	0.73	22.82	$789.71	18.91	$654.40	090	A B M
67971		Reconstruction of eyelid	10.01	NA	9.97	0.84	NA	NA	20.82	$720.50	090	A B C+ M
67973		Reconstruction of eyelid	13.13	NA	12.55	1.05	NA	NA	26.73	$925.02	090	B C+ M
67974		Reconstruction of eyelid	13.10	NA	12.53	1.04	NA	NA	26.67	$922.95	090	B C+ M
67975		Reconstruction of eyelid	9.35	NA	9.58	0.78	NA	NA	19.71	$682.09	090	A B M
67999	CP	Revision of eyelid	0.00	0.00	0.00	0.00	0.00	$0.00	0.00	$0.00	YYY	A+ B C+ M T+
68020		Incise/drain eyelid lining	1.42	2.02	1.68	0.10	3.54	$122.51	3.20	$110.74	010	A B M
68040		Treatment of eyelid lesions	0.85	0.92	0.49	0.04	1.81	$62.64	1.38	$47.76	000	A B M
68100		Biopsy of eyelid lining	1.35	3.92	1.29	0.11	5.38	$186.18	2.75	$95.17	000	A B M
68110		Remove eyelid lining lesion	1.82	5.06	2.32	0.12	7.00	$242.24	4.26	$147.42	010	A B M
68115		Remove eyelid lining lesion	2.41	7.32	2.68	0.20	9.93	$343.64	5.29	$183.07	010	A B M
68130		Remove eyelid lining lesion	5.10	10.82	6.44	0.39	16.31	$564.43	11.93	$412.85	090	A B M
68135		Remove eyelid lining lesion	1.89	2.55	2.29	0.12	4.56	$157.80	4.30	$148.81	010	A B M
68200		Treat eyelid by injection	0.49	0.69	0.46	0.04	1.22	$42.22	0.99	$34.26	000	A B M

68320		Revise/graft eyelid lining	6.64	14.76	8.43	0.54	21.94	$759.26	15.61	$540.20	090	A B C+ M
68325		Revise/graft eyelid lining	8.63	NA	9.65	0.66	NA	NA	18.94	$655.44	090	A B C+ M
68326		Revise/graft eyelid lining	8.42	NA	9.52	0.66	NA	NA	18.60	$643.68	090	A B M
68328		Revise/graft eyelid lining	9.45	NA	10.13	0.84	NA	NA	20.42	$706.66	090	A+ B M
68330		Revise eyelid lining	5.78	12.16	7.06	0.43	18.37	$635.72	13.27	$459.22	090	A+ B M
68335		Revise/graft eyelid lining	8.46	NA	9.54	0.65	NA	NA	18.65	$645.41	090	A B C+ M
68340		Separate eyelid adhesions	4.97	12.55	6.14	0.40	17.92	$620.14	11.51	$398.32	090	A+ B M
68360		Revise eyelid lining	5.17	10.44	6.28	0.40	16.01	$554.05	11.85	$410.08	090	A B M
68362		Revise eyelid lining	8.61	NA	9.63	0.66	NA	NA	18.90	$654.06	090	A B C+ M
68371		Harvest eye tissue alograft	5.09	NA	6.46	0.39	NA	NA	11.94	$413.20	010	A B M
68399	CP	Eyelid lining surgery	0.00	0.00	0.00	0.00	0.00	$0.00	0.00	$0.00	YYY	A+ B C+ M T+
68400		Incise/drain tear gland	1.74	7.01	1.90	0.12	8.87	$306.96	3.76	$130.12	010	A B M
68420		Incise/drain tear sac	2.35	7.39	2.27	0.20	9.94	$343.99	4.82	$166.80	010	A B M
68440		Incise tear duct opening	0.99	1.96	1.81	0.09	3.04	$105.20	2.89	$100.01	010	A B M
68500		Removal of tear gland	12.77	NA	17.37	0.99	NA	NA	31.13	$1077.29	090	A B M
68505		Partial removal tear gland	12.69	NA	17.32	0.98	NA	NA	30.99	$1072.45	090	A B M
68510		Biopsy of tear gland	4.60	8.42	3.30	0.37	13.39	$463.38	8.27	$286.19	000	A+ B M
68520		Removal of tear sac	8.78	NA	12.13	0.72	NA	NA	21.63	$748.53	090	A+ B M
68525		Biopsy of tear sac	4.42	NA	2.68	0.39	NA	NA	7.49	$259.20	000	A B C+ M
68530		Clearance of tear duct	3.70	8.91	3.33	0.28	12.89	$446.07	7.31	$252.97	010	A B M
68540		Remove tear gland lesion	12.18	NA	15.64	0.95	NA	NA	28.77	$995.62	090	A B C+ M
68550		Remove tear gland lesion	15.16	NA	19.52	1.17	NA	NA	35.85	$1240.63	090	A B M
68700		Repair tear ducts	7.87	NA	8.94	0.61	NA	NA	17.42	$602.84	090	A B M
68705		Revise tear duct opening	2.11	5.53	2.50	0.18	7.82	$270.62	4.79	$165.76	010	A B M
68720		Create tear sac drain	9.96	NA	12.98	0.79	NA	NA	23.73	$821.21	090	B C+ M
68745		Create tear duct drain	9.90	NA	13.18	0.76	NA	NA	23.84	$825.01	090	B C+ M
68750		Create tear duct drain	10.10	NA	14.29	0.85	NA	NA	25.24	$873.46	090	B C+ M
68760		Close tear duct opening	1.78	4.64	2.29	0.12	6.54	$226.32	4.19	$145.00	010	A B M

*Please note that these calculations are based on the Medicare 2022 Conversion Factor of $34.6062 and the DRA RVU cap rates at time of publication.

A = assistant-at-surgery restriction
A+ = assistant-at-surgery restriction unless medical necessity established with documentation
B = bilateral surgery adjustment applies
C = cosurgeons payable
C+ = cosurgeons payable if medical necessity established with documentation
CP = carriers may establish RVUs and payment amounts for these services, generally on an individual basis following review of documentation such as an operative report
M = multiple surgery adjustment applies
Me = multiple endoscopy rules may apply
M+ = multiple therapy rules apply
Mtc = multiple diagnostic imaging rules apply
T = team surgeons permitted
T+ = team surgeons payable if medical necessity established with documentation
§ = indicates code is not covered by Medicare
GS = procedure must be performed under the general supervision of a physician
DS = procedure must be performed under the direct supervision of a physician
PS = procedure must be performed under the personal supervision of a physician
DRA = procedure subject to DRA limitation

Relative Value Units

CPT Code and Modifier		Description	Work RVU	Nonfacility Practice Expense RVU	Facility Practice Expense RVU	PLI RVU	Total Non-facility RVUs	Medicare Payment Nonfacility	Total Facility RVUs	Medicare Payment Facility	Global Period	Payment Policy Indicators
68761		Close tear duct opening	1.41	2.84	1.91	0.09	4.34	$150.19	3.41	$118.01	010	A+ B M
68770		Close tear system fistula	8.29	NA	9.20	0.64	NA	NA	18.13	$627.41	090	A+ B M
68801		Dilate tear duct opening	0.82	1.96	1.40	0.05	2.83	$97.94	2.27	$78.56	010	A B M
68810		Probe nasolacrimal duct	1.54	3.09	2.03	0.11	4.74	$164.03	3.68	$127.35	010	A B M
68811		Probe nasolacrimal duct	1.74	NA	2.02	0.12	NA	NA	3.88	$134.27	010	A B M
68815		Probe nasolacrimal duct	2.70	8.30	3.50	0.22	11.22	$388.28	6.42	$222.17	010	A B M
68816		Probe nl duct w/balloon	2.10	23.97	2.27	0.18	26.25	$908.41	4.55	$157.46	010	A B M
68840		Explore/irrigate tear ducts	1.30	2.50	1.98	0.10	3.90	$134.96	3.38	$116.97	010	A B M
68841		Insj rx elut implt lac canal	0.49	0.58	0.41	0.04	1.11	$38.41	0.94	$32.53	000	A B M
68850		Injection for tear sac x-ray	0.80	0.87	0.64	0.08	1.75	$60.56	1.52	$52.60	000	A B M
68899	CP	Tear duct system surgery	0.00	0.00	0.00	0.00	0.00	$0.00	0.00	$0.00	YYY	A+ B C+ M T+
69000		Drain external ear lesion	1.50	3.87	1.94	0.23	5.60	$193.79	3.67	$127.00	010	A B M
69005		Drain external ear lesion	2.16	4.09	2.26	0.32	6.57	$227.36	4.74	$164.03	010	A B M
69020		Drain outer ear canal lesion	1.53	5.33	2.52	0.22	7.08	$245.01	4.27	$147.77	010	A B M
69100		Biopsy of external ear	0.81	1.98	0.46	0.09	2.88	$99.67	1.36	$47.06	000	A M
69105		Biopsy of external ear canal	0.85	3.43	0.88	0.11	4.39	$151.92	1.84	$63.68	000	A B M
69110		Remove external ear partial	3.53	10.12	5.74	0.51	14.16	$490.02	9.78	$338.45	090	A B M
69120		Removal of external ear	4.14	NA	6.96	0.60	NA	NA	11.70	$404.89	090	A M
69140		Remove ear canal lesion(s)	8.14	NA	17.96	1.16	NA	NA	27.26	$943.37	090	A+ B M
69145		Remove ear canal lesion(s)	2.70	9.34	4.58	0.39	12.43	$430.16	7.67	$265.43	090	A B M
69150		Extensive ear canal surgery	13.61	NA	14.59	2.04	NA	NA	30.24	$1046.49	090	A C+ M
69155		Extensive ear/neck surgery	23.35	NA	21.80	3.32	NA	NA	48.47	$1677.36	090	C+ M
69200		Clear outer ear canal	0.77	1.50	0.51	0.11	2.38	$82.36	1.39	$48.10	000	A B M
69205		Clear outer ear canal	1.21	NA	1.42	0.17	NA	NA	2.80	$96.90	010	A B M
69209		Remove impacted ear wax uni	0.00	0.44	NA	0.01	0.45	$15.57	NA	NA	000	A B M
69210		Remove impacted ear wax uni	0.61	0.70	0.27	0.09	1.40	$48.45	0.97	$33.57	000	A M
69220		Clean out mastoid cavity	0.83	1.35	0.55	0.11	2.29	$79.25	1.49	$51.56	000	A B M
69222		Clean out mastoid cavity	1.45	4.84	2.39	0.21	6.50	$224.94	4.05	$140.16	010	A B M
69300		Revise external ear	6.44	12.02	6.45	0.93	19.39	$671.01	13.82	$478.26	YYY	A+ B M
69310		Rebuild outer ear canal	10.97	NA	21.16	1.64	NA	NA	33.77	$1168.65	090	A B M
69320		Rebuild outer ear canal	17.18	NA	27.35	2.45	NA	NA	46.98	$1625.80	090	B M
69399	CP	Outer ear surgery procedure	0.00	0.00	0.00	0.00	0.00	$0.00	0.00	$0.00	YYY	A+ C+ M T+
69420		Incision of eardrum	1.38	4.14	1.97	0.20	5.72	$197.95	3.55	$122.85	010	A B M

69421	Incision of eardrum	1.78	NA	2.47	0.25	NA	NA	4.50	$155.73	010	A B M
69424	Remove ventilating tube	0.85	2.93	0.82	0.10	3.88	$134.27	1.77	$61.25	000	A B M
69433	Create eardrum opening	1.57	4.25	2.10	0.22	6.04	$209.02	3.89	$134.62	010	A B M
69436	Create eardrum opening	2.01	NA	2.43	0.28	NA	NA	4.72	$163.34	010	A B M
69440	Exploration of middle ear	7.71	NA	11.96	1.09	NA	NA	20.76	$718.42	090	A B M
69450	Eardrum revision	5.69	NA	9.98	0.84	NA	NA	16.51	$571.35	090	A+ B M
69501	Mastoidectomy	9.21	NA	10.77	1.30	NA	NA	21.28	$736.42	090	A B M
69502	Mastoidectomy	12.56	NA	13.87	1.78	NA	NA	28.21	$976.24	090	A+ B M
69505	Remove mastoid structures	13.17	NA	21.98	1.86	NA	NA	37.01	$1280.78	090	A+ B M
69511	Extensive mastoid surgery	13.70	NA	22.22	1.94	NA	NA	37.86	$1310.19	090	A+ B M
69530	Extensive mastoid surgery	20.38	NA	27.05	2.90	NA	NA	50.33	$1741.73	090	B M
69535	Remove part of temporal bone	37.42	NA	36.99	5.28	NA	NA	79.69	$2757.77	090	A B C+ M
69540	Remove ear lesion	1.25	4.94	2.43	0.19	6.38	$220.79	3.87	$133.93	010	A B M
69550	Remove ear lesion	11.15	NA	19.30	1.59	NA	NA	32.04	$1108.78	090	B M
69552	Remove ear lesion	19.81	NA	25.01	2.82	NA	NA	47.64	$1648.64	090	B M
69554	Remove ear lesion	35.97	NA	34.49	5.10	NA	NA	75.56	$2614.84	090	B C+ M
69601	Mastoid surgery revision	13.45	NA	15.12	1.93	NA	NA	30.50	$1055.49	090	A+ B M
69602	Mastoid surgery revision	13.76	NA	16.93	1.95	NA	NA	32.64	$1129.55	090	A+ B M
69603	Mastoid surgery revision	14.20	NA	22.45	2.01	NA	NA	38.66	$1337.88	090	A+ B M
69604	Mastoid surgery revision	14.20	NA	17.13	2.01	NA	NA	33.34	$1153.77	090	A B M
69610	Repair of eardrum	4.47	6.32	3.38	0.64	11.43	$395.55	8.49	$293.81	010	A B M
69620	Repair of eardrum	6.03	15.47	7.84	0.87	22.37	$774.14	14.74	$510.10	090	A B M
69631	Repair eardrum structures	10.05	NA	15.24	1.42	NA	NA	26.71	$924.33	090	A B M
69632	Rebuild eardrum structures	12.96	NA	17.73	1.90	NA	NA	32.59	$1127.82	090	A B M
69633	Rebuild eardrum structures	12.31	NA	17.45	1.80	NA	NA	31.56	$1092.17	090	A B M
69635	Repair eardrum structures	13.51	NA	22.50	2.17	NA	NA	38.18	$1321.26	090	A B M
69636	Rebuild eardrum structures	15.43	NA	24.80	2.18	NA	NA	42.41	$1467.65	090	A+ B M
69637	Rebuild eardrum structures	15.32	NA	25.31	2.62	NA	NA	43.25	$1496.72	090	A+ B M

*Please note that these calculations are based on the Medicare 2022 Conversion Factor of $34.6062 and the DRA RVU cap rates at time of publication.

A = assistant-at-surgery restriction

A+ = assistant-at-surgery restriction unless medical necessity established with documentation

B = bilateral surgery adjustment applies

C = cosurgeons payable

C+ = cosurgeons payable if medical necessity established with documentation

CP = carriers may establish RVUs and payment amounts for these services, generally on an individual basis following review of documentation such as an operative report

M = multiple surgery adjustment applies

Me = multiple endoscopy rules may apply

M+ = multiple therapy rules apply

Mtc = multiple diagnostic imaging rules apply

T = team surgeons permitted

T+ = team surgeons payable if medical necessity established with documentation

§ = indicates code is not covered by Medicare

GS = procedure must be performed under the general supervision of a physician

DS = procedure must be performed under the direct supervision of a physician

PS = procedure must be performed under the personal supervision of a physician

DRA = procedure subject to DRA limitation

Relative Value Units

CPT Code and Modifier		Description	Work RVU	Nonfacility Practice Expense RVU	Facility Practice Expense RVU	PLI RVU	Total Non-facility RVUs	Medicare Payment Nonfacility	Total Facility RVUs	Medicare Payment Facility	Global Period	Payment Policy Indicators
69641		Revise middle ear & mastoid	12.89	NA	16.55	1.84	NA	NA	31.28	$1082.48	090	A B M
69642		Revise middle ear & mastoid	17.06	NA	20.64	2.43	NA	NA	40.13	$1388.75	090	A B M
69643		Revise middle ear & mastoid	15.59	NA	18.90	2.23	NA	NA	36.72	$1270.74	090	A B M
69644		Revise middle ear & mastoid	17.23	NA	25.62	2.46	NA	NA	45.31	$1568.01	090	A B M
69645		Revise middle ear & mastoid	16.71	NA	25.45	2.43	NA	NA	44.59	$1543.09	090	A B M
69646		Revise middle ear & mastoid	18.37	NA	26.16	2.66	NA	NA	47.19	$1633.07	090	A+ B M
69650		Release middle ear bone	9.80	NA	12.91	1.40	NA	NA	24.11	$834.36	090	A B M
69660		Revise middle ear bone	12.03	NA	13.95	1.72	NA	NA	27.70	$958.59	090	A B M
69661		Revise middle ear bone	15.92	NA	17.85	2.23	NA	NA	36.00	$1245.82	090	A+ B M
69662		Revise middle ear bone	15.60	NA	16.76	2.28	NA	NA	34.64	$1198.76	090	A B M
69666		Repair middle ear structures	9.89	NA	12.95	1.40	NA	NA	24.24	$838.85	090	A+ B M
69667		Repair middle ear structures	9.90	NA	12.95	1.40	NA	NA	24.25	$839.20	090	A+ B M
69670		Remove mastoid air cells	11.73	NA	14.95	1.70	NA	NA	28.38	$982.12	090	B M
69676		Remove middle ear nerve	9.69	NA	13.98	1.38	NA	NA	25.05	$866.89	090	A B M
69700		Close mastoid fistula	8.37	NA	10.38	1.18	NA	NA	19.93	$689.70	090	A B M
69705		Nps surg dilat eust tube uni	3.00	81.59	1.69	0.42	85.01	$2941.87	5.11	$176.84	000	A+ Me
69706		Nps surg dilat eust tube bi	4.27	82.88	2.27	0.60	87.75	$3036.69	7.14	$247.09	000	A+ Me
69711		Remove/repair hearing aid	10.62	NA	13.00	1.50	NA	NA	25.12	$869.31	090	B M
69714		Impltj oi implt skl perq esp	8.69	NA	9.30	1.24	NA	NA	19.23	$665.48	090	A B M
69716		Impltj oi implt skl tc esp	9.77	NA	7.42	0.79	NA	NA	17.98	$622.22	090	A B M
69717		Revj/rplcmt oi implt prq esp	8.80	NA	9.35	1.25	NA	NA	19.40	$671.36	090	A B M
69719		Revj/rplcmt oi implt tc esp	9.77	NA	7.42	0.79	NA	NA	17.98	$622.22	090	A B M
69720		Release facial nerve	14.71	NA	18.68	2.17	NA	NA	35.56	$1230.60	090	A+ B C+ M
69725		Release facial nerve	27.64	NA	24.09	3.93	NA	NA	55.66	$1926.18	090	B M
69726		Rmvl oi implt skl perq esp	5.93	NA	5.81	0.50	NA	NA	12.24	$423.58	090	A B M
69727		Rmvl oi implt skl tc esp	7.13	NA	6.27	0.60	NA	NA	14.00	$484.49	090	A B M
69740		Repair facial nerve	16.27	NA	16.07	2.31	NA	NA	34.65	$1199.10	090	B M
69745		Repair facial nerve	17.02	NA	17.53	2.40	NA	NA	36.95	$1278.70	090	B M
69799	CP	Middle ear surgery procedure	0.00	0.00	0.00	0.00	0.00	$0.00	0.00	$0.00	YYY	A+ B C+ M T+
69801		Incise inner ear	2.06	4.49	1.31	0.28	6.83	$236.36	3.65	$126.31	000	A+ B M
69805		Explore inner ear	14.71	NA	13.87	2.08	NA	NA	30.66	$1061.03	090	B M
69806		Explore inner ear	12.63	NA	13.13	1.80	NA	NA	27.56	$953.75	090	A B M
69905		Remove inner ear	11.26	NA	14.69	1.60	NA	NA	27.55	$953.40	090	A B M

69910		Remove inner ear & mastoid	13.91	NA	13.71	1.98	NA	NA	29.60	$1024.34	090	A+ B M
69915		Incise inner ear nerve	22.77	NA	18.75	3.23	NA	NA	44.75	$1548.63	090	B C+ M
69930		Implant cochlear device	17.73	NA	16.05	2.51	NA	NA	36.29	$1255.86	090	A+ B M
69949	CP	Inner ear surgery procedure	0.00	0.00	0.00	0.00	0.00	$0.00	0.00	$0.00	YYY	A+ B C+ M T+
69950		Incise inner ear nerve	27.63	NA	20.25	3.92	NA	NA	51.80	$1792.60	090	B C+ M
69955		Release facial nerve	29.42	NA	24.92	4.19	NA	NA	58.53	$2025.50	090	B C+ M
69960		Release inner ear canal	29.42	NA	22.39	4.19	NA	NA	56.00	$1937.95	090	B C+ M
69970		Remove inner ear lesion	32.41	NA	26.26	4.60	NA	NA	63.27	$2189.53	090	B C+ M
69979	CP	Temporal bone surgery	0.00	0.00	0.00	0.00	0.00	$0.00	0.00	$0.00	YYY	A+ B C+ M T+
69990		Microsurgery add-on	3.46	NA	1.65	1.29	NA	NA	6.40	$221.48	ZZZ	
70010		Contrast x-ray of brain	1.19	NA	0.43	0.10	NA	NA	1.72	$59.52	XXX	A+
70015		Contrast x-ray of brain	1.19	3.85	NA	0.08	5.12	$177.18	NA	NA	XXX	A+
70015-26		Contrast x-ray of brain	1.19	0.43	0.43	0.07	1.69	$58.48	1.69	$58.48	XXX	A+
70015-TC		Contrast x-ray of brain	0.00	3.42	NA	0.01	3.43	$118.70	NA	NA	XXX	A+ PS
70030		X-ray eye for foreign body	0.18	0.77	NA	0.02	0.97	$33.57	NA	NA	XXX	A+
70030-26		X-ray eye for foreign body	0.18	0.07	0.07	0.01	0.26	$9.00	0.26	$9.00	XXX	A+
70030-TC		X-ray eye for foreign body	0.00	0.70	NA	0.01	0.71	$24.57	NA	NA	XXX	A+ GS
70100		X-ray exam of jaw <4views	0.18	0.95	NA	0.02	1.15	$39.80	NA	NA	XXX	A+
70100-26		X-ray exam of jaw <4views	0.18	0.07	0.07	0.01	0.26	$9.00	0.26	$9.00	XXX	A+
70100-TC		X-ray exam of jaw <4views	0.00	0.88	NA	0.01	0.89	$30.80	NA	NA	XXX	A+ GS
70110		X-ray exam of jaw 4/> views	0.25	1.04	NA	0.02	1.31	$45.33	NA	NA	XXX	A+
70110-26		X-ray exam of jaw 4/> views	0.25	0.09	0.09	0.01	0.35	$12.11	0.35	$12.11	XXX	A+
70110-TC		X-ray exam of jaw 4/> views	0.00	0.95	NA	0.01	0.96	$33.22	NA	NA	XXX	A+ GS
70120		X-ray exam of mastoids	0.18	0.96	NA	0.02	1.16	$40.14	NA	NA	XXX	A+
70120-26		X-ray exam of mastoids	0.18	0.07	0.07	0.01	0.26	$9.00	0.26	$9.00	XXX	A+
70120-TC		X-ray exam of mastoids	0.00	0.89	NA	0.01	0.90	$31.15	NA	NA	XXX	A+ GS
70130		X-ray exam of mastoids	0.34	1.51	NA	0.03	1.88	$65.06	NA	NA	XXX	A+
70130-26		X-ray exam of mastoids	0.34	0.13	0.13	0.02	0.49	$16.96	0.49	$16.96	XXX	A+

*Please note that these calculations are based on the Medicare 2022 Conversion Factor of $34.6062 and the DRA RVU cap rates at time of publication.

A = assistant-at-surgery restriction
A+ = assistant-at-surgery restriction unless medical necessity established with documentation
B = bilateral surgery adjustment applies
C = cosurgeons payable
C+ = cosurgeons payable if medical necessity established with documentation
CP = carriers may establish RVUs and payment amounts for these services, generally on an individual basis following review of documentation such as an operative report
M = multiple surgery adjustment applies
Me = multiple endoscopy rules may apply
M+ = multiple therapy rules apply
Mtc = multiple diagnostic imaging rules apply
T = team surgeons permitted
T+ = team surgeons payable if medical necessity established with documentation
§ = indicates code is not covered by Medicare
GS = procedure must be performed under the general supervision of a physician
DS = procedure must be performed under the direct supervision of a physician
PS = procedure must be performed under the personal supervision of a physician
DRA = procedure subject to DRA limitation

Relative Value Units

CPT Code and Modifier		Description	Work RVU	Nonfacility Practice Expense RVU	Facility Practice Expense RVU	PLI RVU	Total Non-facility RVUs	Medicare Payment Nonfacility	Total Facility RVUs	Medicare Payment Facility	Global Period	Payment Policy Indicators
70130-TC		X-ray exam of mastoids	0.00	1.38	NA	0.01	1.39	$48.10	NA	NA	XXX	A+ GS
70134		X-ray exam of middle ear	0.34	1.48	NA	0.02	1.84	$63.68	NA	NA	XXX	A+
70134-26		X-ray exam of middle ear	0.34	0.16	0.16	0.01	0.51	$17.65	0.51	$17.65	XXX	A+
70134-TC		X-ray exam of middle ear	0.00	1.32	NA	0.01	1.33	$46.03	NA	NA	XXX	A+ GS
70140		X-ray exam of facial bones	0.19	0.75	NA	0.02	0.96	$33.22	NA	NA	XXX	A+
70140-26		X-ray exam of facial bones	0.19	0.09	0.09	0.01	0.29	$10.04	0.29	$10.04	XXX	A+
70140-TC		X-ray exam of facial bones	0.00	0.66	NA	0.01	0.67	$23.19	NA	NA	XXX	A+ GS
70150		X-ray exam of facial bones	0.26	1.14	NA	0.02	1.42	$49.14	NA	NA	XXX	A+
70150-26		X-ray exam of facial bones	0.26	0.10	0.10	0.01	0.37	$12.80	0.37	$12.80	XXX	A+
70150-TC		X-ray exam of facial bones	0.00	1.04	NA	0.01	1.05	$36.34	NA	NA	XXX	A+ GS
70160		X-ray exam of nasal bones	0.17	0.95	NA	0.02	1.14	$39.45	NA	NA	XXX	A+
70160-26		X-ray exam of nasal bones	0.17	0.07	0.07	0.01	0.25	$8.65	0.25	$8.65	XXX	A+
70160-TC		X-ray exam of nasal bones	0.00	0.88	NA	0.01	0.89	$30.80	NA	NA	XXX	A+ GS
70170	CP	X-ray exam of tear duct	0.00	0.00	NA	0.00	0.00	$0.00	NA	NA	XXX	A+
70170-26		X-ray exam of tear duct	0.30	0.11	0.11	0.01	0.42	$14.53	0.42	$14.53	XXX	A+
70170-TC	CP	X-ray exam of tear duct	0.00	0.00	NA	0.00	0.00	$0.00	NA	NA	XXX	A+ PS
70190		X-ray exam of eye sockets	0.21	0.91	NA	0.02	1.14	$39.45	NA	NA	XXX	A+
70190-26		X-ray exam of eye sockets	0.21	0.10	0.10	0.01	0.32	$11.07	0.32	$11.07	XXX	A+
70190-TC		X-ray exam of eye sockets	0.00	0.81	NA	0.01	0.82	$28.38	NA	NA	XXX	A+ GS
70200		X-ray exam of eye sockets	0.28	1.15	NA	0.02	1.45	$50.18	NA	NA	XXX	A+
70200-26		X-ray exam of eye sockets	0.28	0.11	0.11	0.01	0.40	$13.84	0.40	$13.84	XXX	A+
70200-TC		X-ray exam of eye sockets	0.00	1.04	NA	0.01	1.05	$36.34	NA	NA	XXX	A+ GS
70210		X-ray exam of sinuses	0.17	0.78	NA	0.02	0.97	$33.57	NA	NA	XXX	A+
70210-26		X-ray exam of sinuses	0.17	0.07	0.07	0.01	0.25	$8.65	0.25	$8.65	XXX	A+
70210-TC		X-ray exam of sinuses	0.00	0.71	NA	0.01	0.72	$24.92	NA	NA	XXX	A+ GS
70220		X-ray exam of sinuses	0.22	0.89	NA	0.02	1.13	$39.11	NA	NA	XXX	A+
70220-26		X-ray exam of sinuses	0.22	0.08	0.08	0.01	0.31	$10.73	0.31	$10.73	XXX	A+
70220-TC		X-ray exam of sinuses	0.00	0.81	NA	0.01	0.82	$28.38	NA	NA	XXX	A+ GS
70240		X-ray exam pituitary saddle	0.19	0.78	NA	0.02	0.99	$34.26	NA	NA	XXX	A+
70240-26		X-ray exam pituitary saddle	0.19	0.07	0.07	0.01	0.27	$9.34	0.27	$9.34	XXX	A+
70240-TC		X-ray exam pituitary saddle	0.00	0.71	NA	0.01	0.72	$24.92	NA	NA	XXX	A+ GS
70250		X-ray exam of skull	0.18	0.87	NA	0.02	1.07	$37.03	NA	NA	XXX	A+
70250-26		X-ray exam of skull	0.18	0.07	0.07	0.01	0.26	$9.00	0.26	$9.00	XXX	A+

70250-TC	X-ray exam of skull	0.00	0.80	NA	0.01	0.81	$28.03	NA	NA	XXX	A+ GS
70260	X-ray exam of skull	0.28	1.04	NA	0.02	1.34	$46.37	NA	NA	XXX	A+
70260-26	X-ray exam of skull	0.28	0.11	0.11	0.01	0.40	$13.84	0.40	$13.84	XXX	A+
70260-TC	X-ray exam of skull	0.00	0.93	NA	0.01	0.94	$32.53	NA	NA	XXX	A+ GS
70300	X-ray exam of teeth	0.10	0.26	NA	0.02	0.38	$13.15	NA	NA	XXX	A+
70300-26	X-ray exam of teeth	0.10	0.04	0.04	0.01	0.15	$5.19	0.15	$5.19	XXX	A+
70300-TC	X-ray exam of teeth	0.00	0.22	NA	0.01	0.23	$7.96	NA	NA	XXX	A+ GS
70310	X-ray exam of teeth	0.16	0.96	NA	0.02	1.14	$39.45	NA	NA	XXX	A+
70310-26	X-ray exam of teeth	0.16	0.06	0.06	0.01	0.23	$7.96	0.23	$7.96	XXX	A+
70310-TC	X-ray exam of teeth	0.00	0.90	NA	0.01	0.91	$31.49	NA	NA	XXX	A+ GS
70320	Full mouth x-ray of teeth	0.22	1.39	NA	0.02	1.63	$56.41	NA	NA	XXX	A+
70320-26	Full mouth x-ray of teeth	0.22	0.09	0.09	0.01	0.32	$11.07	0.32	$11.07	XXX	A+
70320-TC	Full mouth x-ray of teeth	0.00	1.30	NA	0.01	1.31	$45.33	NA	NA	XXX	A+ GS
70328	X-ray exam of jaw joint	0.18	0.84	NA	0.02	1.04	$35.99	NA	NA	XXX	A+
70328-26	X-ray exam of jaw joint	0.18	0.07	0.07	0.01	0.26	$9.00	0.26	$9.00	XXX	A+
70328-TC	X-ray exam of jaw joint	0.00	0.77	NA	0.01	0.78	$26.99	NA	NA	XXX	A+ GS
70330	X-ray exam of jaw joints	0.24	1.34	NA	0.02	1.60	$55.37	NA	NA	XXX	A+
70330-26	X-ray exam of jaw joints	0.24	0.09	0.09	0.01	0.34	$11.77	0.34	$11.77	XXX	A+
70330-TC	X-ray exam of jaw joints	0.00	1.25	NA	0.01	1.26	$43.60	NA	NA	XXX	A+ GS
70332	X-ray exam of jaw joint	0.54	1.99	NA	0.05	2.58	$89.28	NA	NA	XXX	A+
70332-26	X-ray exam of jaw joint	0.54	0.20	0.20	0.04	0.78	$26.99	0.78	$26.99	XXX	A+
70332-TC	X-ray exam of jaw joint	0.00	1.79	NA	0.01	1.80	$62.29	NA	NA	XXX	A+ PS
70336	Magnetic image jaw joint	1.48	6.84	NA	0.10	8.42	$291.38	NA	NA	XXX	A+ Mtc
70336-26	Magnetic image jaw joint	1.48	0.52	0.52	0.08	2.08	$71.98	2.08	$71.98	XXX	A+ Mtc
70336-TC	Magnetic image jaw joint	0.00	6.32	NA	0.02	6.34	$219.40	NA	NA	XXX	A+ Mtc GS
70350	X-ray head for orthodontia	0.17	0.29	NA	0.02	0.48	$16.61	NA	NA	XXX	A+
70350-26	X-ray head for orthodontia	0.17	0.07	0.07	0.01	0.25	$8.65	0.25	$8.65	XXX	A+
70350-TC	X-ray head for orthodontia	0.00	0.22	NA	0.01	0.23	$7.96	NA	NA	XXX	A+ GS

*Please note that these calculations are based on the Medicare 2022 Conversion Factor of $34.6062 and the DRA RVU cap rates at time of publication.

A = assistant-at-surgery restriction
A+ = assistant-at-surgery restriction unless medical necessity established with documentation
B = bilateral surgery adjustment applies
C = cosurgeons payable

C+ = cosurgeons payable if medical necessity established with documentation
CP = carriers may establish RVUs and payment amounts for these services, generally on an individual basis following review of documentation such as an operative report
M = multiple surgery adjustment applies
Me = multiple endoscopy rules may apply

M+ = multiple therapy rules apply
Mtc = multiple diagnostic imaging rules apply
T = team surgeons permitted
T+ = team surgeons payable if medical necessity established with documentation
§ = indicates code is not covered by Medicare

GS = procedure must be performed under the general supervision of a physician
DS = procedure must be performed under the direct supervision of a physician
PS = procedure must be performed under the personal supervision of a physician
DRA = procedure subject to DRA limitation

Relative Value Units

CPT Code and Modifier	Description	Work RVU	Nonfacility Practice Expense RVU	Facility Practice Expense RVU	PLI RVU	Total Non-facility RVUs	Medicare Payment Nonfacility	Total Facility RVUs	Medicare Payment Facility	Global Period	Payment Policy Indicators
70355	Panoramic x-ray of jaws	0.20	0.31	NA	0.02	0.53	$18.34	NA	NA	XXX	A+
70355-26	Panoramic x-ray of jaws	0.20	0.08	0.08	0.01	0.29	$10.04	0.29	$10.04	XXX	A+
70355-TC	Panoramic x-ray of jaws	0.00	0.23	NA	0.01	0.24	$8.31	NA	NA	XXX	A+ GS
70360	X-ray exam of neck	0.18	0.74	NA	0.02	0.94	$32.53	NA	NA	XXX	A+
70360-26	X-ray exam of neck	0.18	0.07	0.07	0.01	0.26	$9.00	0.26	$9.00	XXX	A+
70360-TC	X-ray exam of neck	0.00	0.67	NA	0.01	0.68	$23.53	NA	NA	XXX	A+ GS
70370	Throat x-ray & fluoroscopy	0.32	2.74	NA	0.03	3.09	$97.94	NA	NA	XXX	A+ DRA
70370-26	Throat x-ray & fluoroscopy	0.32	0.10	0.10	0.02	0.44	$15.23	0.44	$15.23	XXX	A+
70370-TC	Throat x-ray & fluoroscopy	0.00	2.64	NA	0.01	2.65	$82.71	NA	NA	XXX	A+ PS DRA
70371	Speech evaluation complex	0.84	2.24	NA	0.05	3.13	$108.32	NA	NA	XXX	A+
70371-26	Speech evaluation complex	0.84	0.31	0.31	0.04	1.19	$41.18	1.19	$41.18	XXX	A+
70371-TC	Speech evaluation complex	0.00	1.93	NA	0.01	1.94	$67.14	NA	NA	XXX	A+ PS
70380	X-ray exam of salivary gland	0.17	0.94	NA	0.02	1.13	$39.11	NA	NA	XXX	A+
70380-26	X-ray exam of salivary gland	0.17	0.06	0.06	0.01	0.24	$8.31	0.24	$8.31	XXX	A+
70380-TC	X-ray exam of salivary gland	0.00	0.88	NA	0.01	0.89	$30.80	NA	NA	XXX	A+ GS
70390	X-ray exam of salivary duct	0.38	3.20	NA	0.03	3.61	$124.93	NA	NA	XXX	A+
70390-26	X-ray exam of salivary duct	0.38	0.14	0.14	0.02	0.54	$18.69	0.54	$18.69	XXX	A+
70390-TC	X-ray exam of salivary duct	0.00	3.06	NA	0.01	3.07	$106.24	NA	NA	XXX	A+ PS
70450	Ct head/brain w/o dye	0.85	2.37	NA	0.05	3.27	$113.16	NA	NA	XXX	A+ Mtc
70450-26	Ct head/brain w/o dye	0.85	0.30	0.30	0.04	1.19	$41.18	1.19	$41.18	XXX	A+ Mtc
70450-TC	Ct head/brain w/o dye	0.00	2.07	NA	0.01	2.08	$71.98	NA	NA	XXX	A+ Mtc GS
70460	Ct head/brain w/dye	1.13	3.41	NA	0.06	4.60	$159.19	NA	NA	XXX	A+ Mtc
70460-26	Ct head/brain w/dye	1.13	0.41	0.41	0.05	1.59	$55.02	1.59	$55.02	XXX	A+ Mtc
70460-TC	Ct head/brain w/dye	0.00	3.00	NA	0.01	3.01	$104.16	NA	NA	XXX	A+ Mtc DS
70470	Ct head/brain w/o & w/dye	1.27	4.06	NA	0.08	5.41	$187.22	NA	NA	XXX	A+ Mtc
70470-26	Ct head/brain w/o & w/dye	1.27	0.46	0.46	0.07	1.80	$62.29	1.80	$62.29	XXX	A+ Mtc
70470-TC	Ct head/brain w/o & w/dye	0.00	3.60	NA	0.01	3.61	$124.93	NA	NA	XXX	A+ Mtc DS
70480	Ct orbit/ear/fossa w/o dye	1.28	3.56	NA	0.08	4.92	$170.26	NA	NA	XXX	A+ Mtc
70480-26	Ct orbit/ear/fossa w/o dye	1.28	0.46	0.46	0.07	1.81	$62.64	1.81	$62.64	XXX	A+ Mtc
70480-TC	Ct orbit/ear/fossa w/o dye	0.00	3.10	NA	0.01	3.11	$107.63	NA	NA	XXX	A+ Mtc GS
70481	Ct orbit/ear/fossa w/dye	1.13	4.43	NA	0.06	5.62	$194.49	NA	NA	XXX	A+ Mtc
70481-26	Ct orbit/ear/fossa w/dye	1.13	0.40	0.40	0.05	1.58	$54.68	1.58	$54.68	XXX	A+ Mtc
70481-TC	Ct orbit/ear/fossa w/dye	0.00	4.03	NA	0.01	4.04	$139.81	NA	NA	XXX	A+ Mtc DS

70482	Ct orbit/ear/fossa w/o&w/dye	1.27	5.25	NA	0.09	6.61	$228.75	NA	NA	XXX	A+ Mtc
70482-26	Ct orbit/ear/fossa w/o&w/dye	1.27	0.45	0.45	0.07	1.79	$61.95	1.79	$61.95	XXX	A+ Mtc
70482-TC	Ct orbit/ear/fossa w/o&w/dye	0.00	4.80	NA	0.02	4.82	$166.80	NA	NA	XXX	A+ Mtc DS
70486	Ct maxillofacial w/o dye	0.85	3.06	NA	0.05	3.96	$137.04	NA	NA	XXX	A+ Mtc
70486-26	Ct maxillofacial w/o dye	0.85	0.31	0.31	0.04	1.20	$41.53	1.20	$41.53	XXX	A+ Mtc
70486-TC	Ct maxillofacial w/o dye	0.00	2.75	NA	0.01	2.76	$95.51	NA	NA	XXX	A+ Mtc GS
70487	Ct maxillofacial w/dye	1.13	3.53	NA	0.06	4.72	$163.34	NA	NA	XXX	A+ Mtc
70487-26	Ct maxillofacial w/dye	1.13	0.40	0.40	0.05	1.58	$54.68	1.58	$54.68	XXX	A+ Mtc
70487-TC	Ct maxillofacial w/dye	0.00	3.13	NA	0.01	3.14	$108.66	NA	NA	XXX	A+ Mtc DS
70488	Ct maxillofacial w/o & w/dye	1.27	4.42	NA	0.08	5.77	$199.68	NA	NA	XXX	A+ Mtc
70488-26	Ct maxillofacial w/o & w/dye	1.27	0.45	0.45	0.07	1.79	$61.95	1.79	$61.95	XXX	A+ Mtc
70488-TC	Ct maxillofacial w/o & w/dye	0.00	3.97	NA	0.01	3.98	$137.73	NA	NA	XXX	A+ Mtc DS
70490	Ct soft tissue neck w/o dye	1.28	3.30	NA	0.08	4.66	$161.26	NA	NA	XXX	A+ Mtc
70490-26	Ct soft tissue neck w/o dye	1.28	0.46	0.46	0.07	1.81	$62.64	1.81	$62.64	XXX	A+ Mtc
70490-TC	Ct soft tissue neck w/o dye	0.00	2.84	NA	0.01	2.85	$98.63	NA	NA	XXX	A+ Mtc GS
70491	Ct soft tissue neck w/dye	1.38	4.29	NA	0.08	5.75	$198.99	NA	NA	XXX	A+ Mtc
70491-26	Ct soft tissue neck w/dye	1.38	0.50	0.50	0.07	1.95	$67.48	1.95	$67.48	XXX	A+ Mtc
70491-TC	Ct soft tissue neck w/dye	0.00	3.79	NA	0.01	3.80	$131.50	NA	NA	XXX	A+ Mtc DS
70492	Ct sft tsue nck w/o & w/dye	1.62	5.19	NA	0.11	6.92	$239.47	NA	NA	XXX	A+ Mtc
70492-26	Ct sft tsue nck w/o & w/dye	1.62	0.57	0.57	0.09	2.28	$78.90	2.28	$78.90	XXX	A+ Mtc
70492-TC	Ct sft tsue nck w/o & w/dye	0.00	4.62	NA	0.02	4.64	$160.57	NA	NA	XXX	A+ Mtc DS
70496	Ct angiography head	1.75	6.70	NA	0.13	8.58	$267.51	NA	NA	XXX	A+ Mtc DRA
70496-26	Ct angiography head	1.75	0.62	0.62	0.09	2.46	$85.13	2.46	$85.13	XXX	A+ Mtc
70496-TC	Ct angiography head	0.00	6.08	NA	0.04	6.12	$182.37	NA	NA	XXX	A+ Mtc DS DRA
70498	Ct angiography neck	1.75	6.69	NA	0.13	8.57	$267.51	NA	NA	XXX	A+ Mtc DRA
70498-26	Ct angiography neck	1.75	0.62	0.62	0.09	2.46	$85.13	2.46	$85.13	XXX	A+ Mtc
70498-TC	Ct angiography neck	0.00	6.07	NA	0.04	6.11	$182.37	NA	NA	XXX	A+ Mtc DS DRA
70540	Mri orbit/face/neck w/o dye	1.35	5.70	NA	0.09	7.14	$247.09	NA	NA	XXX	A+ Mtc

*Please note that these calculations are based on the Medicare 2022 Conversion Factor of $34.6062 and the DRA RVU cap rates at time of publication.

A = assistant-at-surgery restriction
A+ = assistant-at-surgery restriction unless medical necessity established with documentation
B = bilateral surgery adjustment applies
C = cosurgeons payable
C+ = cosurgeons payable if medical necessity established with documentation
CP = carriers may establish RVUs and payment amounts for these services, generally on an individual basis following review of documentation such as an operative report
M = multiple surgery adjustment applies
Me = multiple endoscopy rules may apply
M+ = multiple therapy rules apply
Mtc = multiple diagnostic imaging rules apply
T = team surgeons permitted
T+ = team surgeons payable if medical necessity established with documentation
§ = indicates code is not covered by Medicare
GS = procedure must be performed under the general supervision of a physician
DS = procedure must be performed under the direct supervision of a physician
PS = procedure must be performed under the personal supervision of a physician
DRA = procedure subject to DRA limitation

Relative Value Units

CPT Code and Modifier	Description	Work RVU	Nonfacility Practice Expense RVU	Facility Practice Expense RVU	PLI RVU	Total Non-facility RVUs	Medicare Payment Nonfacility	Total Facility RVUs	Medicare Payment Facility	Global Period	Payment Policy Indicators
70540-26	Mri orbit/face/neck w/o dye	1.35	0.48	0.48	0.07	1.90	$65.75	1.90	$65.75	XXX	A+ Mtc
70540-TC	Mri orbit/face/neck w/o dye	0.00	5.22	NA	0.02	5.24	$181.34	NA	NA	XXX	A+ Mtc GS
70542	Mri orbit/face/neck w/dye	1.62	6.76	NA	0.10	8.48	$293.46	NA	NA	XXX	A+ Mtc
70542-26	Mri orbit/face/neck w/dye	1.62	0.58	0.58	0.08	2.28	$78.90	2.28	$78.90	XXX	A+ Mtc
70542-TC	Mri orbit/face/neck w/dye	0.00	6.18	NA	0.02	6.20	$214.56	NA	NA	XXX	A+ Mtc DS
70543	Mri orbt/fac/nck w/o &w/dye	2.15	8.41	NA	0.14	10.70	$370.29	NA	NA	XXX	A+ Mtc
70543-26	Mri orbt/fac/nck w/o &w/dye	2.15	0.76	0.76	0.10	3.01	$104.16	3.01	$104.16	XXX	A+ Mtc
70543-TC	Mri orbt/fac/nck w/o &w/dye	0.00	7.65	NA	0.04	7.69	$266.12	NA	NA	XXX	A+ Mtc DS
70544	Mr angiography head w/o dye	1.20	5.46	NA	0.09	6.75	$233.59	NA	NA	XXX	A+ Mtc
70544-26	Mr angiography head w/o dye	1.20	0.43	0.43	0.07	1.70	$58.83	1.70	$58.83	XXX	A+ Mtc
70544-TC	Mr angiography head w/o dye	0.00	5.03	NA	0.02	5.05	$174.76	NA	NA	XXX	A+ Mtc GS
70545	Mr angiography head w/dye	1.20	5.83	NA	0.09	7.12	$246.40	NA	NA	XXX	A+ Mtc
70545-26	Mr angiography head w/dye	1.20	0.42	0.42	0.07	1.69	$58.48	1.69	$58.48	XXX	A+ Mtc
70545-TC	Mr angiography head w/dye	0.00	5.41	NA	0.02	5.43	$187.91	NA	NA	XXX	A+ Mtc DS
70546	Mr angiograph head w/o&w/dye	1.48	8.73	NA	0.12	10.33	$357.48	NA	NA	XXX	A+ Mtc
70546-26	Mr angiograph head w/o&w/dye	1.48	0.53	0.53	0.08	2.09	$72.33	2.09	$72.33	XXX	A+ Mtc
70546-TC	Mr angiograph head w/o&w/dye	0.00	8.20	NA	0.04	8.24	$285.16	NA	NA	XXX	A+ Mtc DS
70547	Mr angiography neck w/o dye	1.20	5.48	NA	0.09	6.77	$234.28	NA	NA	XXX	A+ Mtc
70547-26	Mr angiography neck w/o dye	1.20	0.43	0.43	0.07	1.70	$58.83	1.70	$58.83	XXX	A+ Mtc
70547-TC	Mr angiography neck w/o dye	0.00	5.05	NA	0.02	5.07	$175.45	NA	NA	XXX	A+ Mtc GS
70548	Mr angiography neck w/dye	1.50	6.11	NA	0.10	7.71	$266.81	NA	NA	XXX	A+ Mtc
70548-26	Mr angiography neck w/dye	1.50	0.54	0.54	0.08	2.12	$73.37	2.12	$73.37	XXX	A+ Mtc
70548-TC	Mr angiography neck w/dye	0.00	5.57	NA	0.02	5.59	$193.45	NA	NA	XXX	A+ Mtc DS
70549	Mr angiograph neck w/o&w/dye	1.80	8.90	NA	0.13	10.83	$374.79	NA	NA	XXX	A+ Mtc
70549-26	Mr angiograph neck w/o&w/dye	1.80	0.65	0.65	0.09	2.54	$87.90	2.54	$87.90	XXX	A+ Mtc
70549-TC	Mr angiograph neck w/o&w/dye	0.00	8.25	NA	0.04	8.29	$286.89	NA	NA	XXX	A+ Mtc DS
70551	Mri brain stem w/o dye	1.48	4.55	NA	0.10	6.13	$212.14	NA	NA	XXX	A+ Mtc
70551-26	Mri brain stem w/o dye	1.48	0.53	0.53	0.08	2.09	$72.33	2.09	$72.33	XXX	A+ Mtc
70551-TC	Mri brain stem w/o dye	0.00	4.02	NA	0.02	4.04	$139.81	NA	NA	XXX	A+ Mtc GS
70552	Mri brain stem w/dye	1.78	6.59	NA	0.11	8.48	$293.46	NA	NA	XXX	A+ Mtc
70552-26	Mri brain stem w/dye	1.78	0.64	0.64	0.09	2.51	$86.86	2.51	$86.86	XXX	A+ Mtc
70552-TC	Mri brain stem w/dye	0.00	5.95	NA	0.02	5.97	$206.60	NA	NA	XXX	A+ Mtc DS
70553	Mri brain stem w/o & w/dye	2.29	7.57	NA	0.15	10.01	$346.41	NA	NA	XXX	A+ Mtc

70553-26		Mri brain stem w/o & w/dye	2.29	0.82	0.82	0.11	3.22	$111.43	3.22	$111.43	XXX	A+ Mtc
70553-TC		Mri brain stem w/o & w/dye	0.00	6.75	NA	0.04	6.79	$234.98	NA	NA	XXX	A+ Mtc DS
70554		Fmri brain by tech	2.11	9.70	NA	0.15	11.96	$413.89	NA	NA	XXX	A+ Mtc
70554-26		Fmri brain by tech	2.11	0.76	0.76	0.11	2.98	$103.13	2.98	$103.13	XXX	A+ Mtc
70554-TC		Fmri brain by tech	0.00	8.94	NA	0.04	8.98	$310.76	NA	NA	XXX	A+ Mtc DS
70555	CP	Fmri brain by phys/psych	0.00	0.00	NA	0.00	0.00	$0.00	NA	NA	XXX	A+
70555-26		Fmri brain by phys/psych	2.54	0.87	0.87	0.11	3.52	$121.81	3.52	$121.81	XXX	A+
70555-TC	CP	Fmri brain by phys/psych	0.00	0.00	NA	0.00	0.00	$0.00	NA	NA	XXX	A+ DS
70557	CP	Mri brain w/o dye	0.00	0.00	NA	0.00	0.00	$0.00	NA	NA	XXX	A+
70557-26		Mri brain w/o dye	2.90	1.20	1.20	0.57	4.67	$161.61	4.67	$161.61	XXX	A+
70557-TC	CP	Mri brain w/o dye	0.00	0.00	NA	0.00	0.00	$0.00	NA	NA	XXX	A+ GS
70558	CP	Mri brain w/dye	0.00	0.00	NA	0.00	0.00	$0.00	NA	NA	XXX	A+
70558-26		Mri brain w/dye	3.20	1.61	1.61	0.14	4.95	$171.30	4.95	$171.30	XXX	A+
70558-TC	CP	Mri brain w/dye	0.00	0.00	NA	0.00	0.00	$0.00	NA	NA	XXX	A+ DS
70559	CP	Mri brain w/o & w/dye	0.00	0.00	NA	0.00	0.00	$0.00	NA	NA	XXX	A+
70559-26		Mri brain w/o & w/dye	3.20	1.22	1.22	0.25	4.67	$161.61	4.67	$161.61	XXX	A+
70559-TC	CP	Mri brain w/o & w/dye	0.00	0.00	NA	0.00	0.00	$0.00	NA	NA	XXX	A+ DS
71045		X-ray exam chest 1 view	0.18	0.57	NA	0.02	0.77	$26.65	NA	NA	XXX	A+
71045-26		X-ray exam chest 1 view	0.18	0.07	0.07	0.01	0.26	$9.00	0.26	$9.00	XXX	A+
71045-TC		X-ray exam chest 1 view	0.00	0.50	NA	0.01	0.51	$17.65	NA	NA	XXX	A+ GS
71046		X-ray exam chest 2 views	0.22	0.76	NA	0.02	1.00	$34.61	NA	NA	XXX	A+
71046-26		X-ray exam chest 2 views	0.22	0.08	0.08	0.01	0.31	$10.73	0.31	$10.73	XXX	A+
71046-TC		X-ray exam chest 2 views	0.00	0.68	NA	0.01	0.69	$23.88	NA	NA	XXX	A+ GS
71047		X-ray exam chest 3 views	0.27	0.97	NA	0.02	1.26	$43.60	NA	NA	XXX	A+
71047-26		X-ray exam chest 3 views	0.27	0.10	0.10	0.01	0.38	$13.15	0.38	$13.15	XXX	A+
71047-TC		X-ray exam chest 3 views	0.00	0.87	NA	0.01	0.88	$30.45	NA	NA	XXX	A+ GS
71048		X-ray exam chest 4+ views	0.31	1.05	NA	0.02	1.38	$47.76	NA	NA	XXX	A+
71048-26		X-ray exam chest 4+ views	0.31	0.12	0.12	0.01	0.44	$15.23	0.44	$15.23	XXX	A+

*Please note that these calculations are based on the Medicare 2022 Conversion Factor of $34.6062 and the DRA RVU cap rates at time of publication.

A = assistant-at-surgery restriction
A+ = assistant-at-surgery restriction unless medical necessity established with documentation
B = bilateral surgery adjustment applies
C = cosurgeons payable
C+ = cosurgeons payable if medical necessity established with documentation
CP = carriers may establish RVUs and payment amounts for these services, generally on an individual basis following review of documentation such as an operative report
M = multiple surgery adjustment applies
Me = multiple endoscopy rules may apply
M+ = multiple therapy rules apply
Mtc = multiple diagnostic imaging rules apply
T = team surgeons permitted
T+ = team surgeons payable if medical necessity established with documentation
§ = indicates code is not covered by Medicare
GS = procedure must be performed under the general supervision of a physician
DS = procedure must be performed under the direct supervision of a physician
PS = procedure must be performed under the personal supervision of a physician
DRA = procedure subject to DRA limitation

Relative Value Units

CPT Code and Modifier	Description	Work RVU	Nonfacility Practice Expense RVU	Facility Practice Expense RVU	PLI RVU	Total Non-facility RVUs	Medicare Payment Nonfacility	Total Facility RVUs	Medicare Payment Facility	Global Period	Payment Policy Indicators
71048-TC	X-ray exam chest 4+ views	0.00	0.93	NA	0.01	0.94	$32.53	NA	NA	XXX	A+ GS
71100	X-ray exam ribs uni 2 views	0.22	0.86	NA	0.02	1.10	$38.07	NA	NA	XXX	A+
71100-26	X-ray exam ribs uni 2 views	0.22	0.09	0.09	0.01	0.32	$11.07	0.32	$11.07	XXX	A+
71100-TC	X-ray exam ribs uni 2 views	0.00	0.77	NA	0.01	0.78	$26.99	NA	NA	XXX	A+ GS
71101	X-ray exam unilat ribs/chest	0.27	0.97	NA	0.02	1.26	$43.60	NA	NA	XXX	A+
71101-26	X-ray exam unilat ribs/chest	0.27	0.10	0.10	0.01	0.38	$13.15	0.38	$13.15	XXX	A+
71101-TC	X-ray exam unilat ribs/chest	0.00	0.87	NA	0.01	0.88	$30.45	NA	NA	XXX	A+ GS
71110	X-ray exam ribs bil 3 views	0.29	1.00	NA	0.02	1.31	$45.33	NA	NA	XXX	A+
71110-26	X-ray exam ribs bil 3 views	0.29	0.11	0.11	0.01	0.41	$14.19	0.41	$14.19	XXX	A+
71110-TC	X-ray exam ribs bil 3 views	0.00	0.89	NA	0.01	0.90	$31.15	NA	NA	XXX	A+ GS
71111	X-ray exam ribs/chest4/> vws	0.32	1.23	NA	0.02	1.57	$54.33	NA	NA	XXX	A+
71111-26	X-ray exam ribs/chest4/> vws	0.32	0.12	0.12	0.01	0.45	$15.57	0.45	$15.57	XXX	A+
71111-TC	X-ray exam ribs/chest4/> vws	0.00	1.11	NA	0.01	1.12	$38.76	NA	NA	XXX	A+ GS
71120	X-ray exam breastbone 2/>vws	0.20	0.79	NA	0.02	1.01	$34.95	NA	NA	XXX	A+
71120-26	X-ray exam breastbone 2/>vws	0.20	0.07	0.07	0.01	0.28	$9.69	0.28	$9.69	XXX	A+
71120-TC	X-ray exam breastbone 2/>vws	0.00	0.72	NA	0.01	0.73	$25.26	NA	NA	XXX	A+ GS
71130	X-ray strenoclavic jt 3/>vws	0.22	1.00	NA	0.02	1.24	$42.91	NA	NA	XXX	A+
71130-26	X-ray strenoclavic jt 3/>vws	0.22	0.08	0.08	0.01	0.31	$10.73	0.31	$10.73	XXX	A+
71130-TC	X-ray strenoclavic jt 3/>vws	0.00	0.92	NA	0.01	0.93	$32.18	NA	NA	XXX	A+ GS
71250	Ct thorax dx c-	1.08	2.97	NA	0.06	4.11	$142.23	NA	NA	XXX	A+ Mtc
71250-26	Ct thorax dx c-	1.08	0.39	0.39	0.05	1.52	$52.60	1.52	$52.60	XXX	A+ Mtc
71250-TC	Ct thorax dx c-	0.00	2.58	NA	0.01	2.59	$89.63	NA	NA	XXX	A+ Mtc GS
71260	Ct thorax dx c+	1.16	3.95	NA	0.06	5.17	$178.91	NA	NA	XXX	A+ Mtc
71260-26	Ct thorax dx c+	1.16	0.42	0.42	0.05	1.63	$56.41	1.63	$56.41	XXX	A+ Mtc
71260-TC	Ct thorax dx c+	0.00	3.53	NA	0.01	3.54	$122.51	NA	NA	XXX	A+ Mtc DS
71270	Ct thorax dx c-/c+	1.25	4.81	NA	0.09	6.15	$212.83	NA	NA	XXX	A+ Mtc
71270-26	Ct thorax dx c-/c+	1.25	0.45	0.45	0.07	1.77	$61.25	1.77	$61.25	XXX	A+ Mtc
71270-TC	Ct thorax dx c-/c+	0.00	4.36	NA	0.02	4.38	$151.58	NA	NA	XXX	A+ Mtc DS
71271	Ct thorax lung cancer scr c-	1.08	3.11	NA	0.06	4.25	$147.08	NA	NA	XXX	A+ Mtc
71271-26	Ct thorax lung cancer scr c-	1.08	0.39	0.39	0.05	1.52	$52.60	1.52	$52.60	XXX	A+ Mtc
71271-TC	Ct thorax lung cancer scr c-	0.00	2.72	NA	0.01	2.73	$94.47	NA	NA	XXX	A+ Mtc
71275	Ct angiography chest	1.82	6.81	NA	0.13	8.76	$270.97	NA	NA	XXX	A+ Mtc DRA
71275-26	Ct angiography chest	1.82	0.65	0.65	0.09	2.56	$88.59	2.56	$88.59	XXX	A+ Mtc

71275-TC	Ct angiography chest	0.00	6.16	NA	0.04	6.20	$182.37	NA	NA	XXX	A+ Mtc DS DRA
71550	Mri chest w/o dye	1.46	9.20	NA	0.12	10.78	$306.26	NA	NA	XXX	A+ Mtc DRA
71550-26	Mri chest w/o dye	1.46	0.52	0.52	0.08	2.06	$71.29	2.06	$71.29	XXX	A+ Mtc
71550-TC	Mri chest w/o dye	0.00	8.68	NA	0.04	8.72	$234.98	NA	NA	XXX	A+ Mtc GS DRA
71551	Mri chest w/dye	1.73	10.06	NA	0.13	11.92	$412.51	NA	NA	XXX	A+ Mtc
71551-26	Mri chest w/dye	1.73	0.62	0.62	0.09	2.44	$84.44	2.44	$84.44	XXX	A+ Mtc
71551-TC	Mri chest w/dye	0.00	9.44	NA	0.04	9.48	$328.07	NA	NA	XXX	A+ Mtc DS
71552	Mri chest w/o & w/dye	2.26	12.65	NA	0.14	15.05	$485.87	NA	NA	XXX	A+ Mtc DRA
71552-26	Mri chest w/o & w/dye	2.26	0.81	0.81	0.10	3.17	$109.70	3.17	$109.70	XXX	A+ Mtc
71552-TC	Mri chest w/o & w/dye	0.00	11.84	NA	0.04	11.88	$376.17	NA	NA	XXX	A+ Mtc DS DRA
71555	Mri angio chest w or w/o dye	1.81	8.60	NA	0.13	10.54	$364.75	NA	NA	XXX	A+ Mtc
71555-26	Mri angio chest w or w/o dye	1.81	0.63	0.63	0.09	2.53	$87.55	2.53	$87.55	XXX	A+ Mtc
71555-TC	Mri angio chest w or w/o dye	0.00	7.97	NA	0.04	8.01	$277.20	NA	NA	XXX	A+ Mtc DS
72020	X-ray exam of spine 1 view	0.16	0.55	NA	0.02	0.73	$25.26	NA	NA	XXX	A+
72020-26	X-ray exam of spine 1 view	0.16	0.06	0.06	0.01	0.23	$7.96	0.23	$7.96	XXX	A+
72020-TC	X-ray exam of spine 1 view	0.00	0.49	NA	0.01	0.50	$17.30	NA	NA	XXX	A+ GS
72040	X-ray exam neck spine 2-3 vw	0.22	0.94	NA	0.02	1.18	$40.84	NA	NA	XXX	A+
72040-26	X-ray exam neck spine 2-3 vw	0.22	0.09	0.09	0.01	0.32	$11.07	0.32	$11.07	XXX	A+
72040-TC	X-ray exam neck spine 2-3 vw	0.00	0.85	NA	0.01	0.86	$29.76	NA	NA	XXX	A+ GS
72050	X-ray exam neck spine 4/5vws	0.27	1.30	NA	0.02	1.59	$55.02	NA	NA	XXX	A+
72050-26	X-ray exam neck spine 4/5vws	0.27	0.11	0.11	0.01	0.39	$13.50	0.39	$13.50	XXX	A+
72050-TC	X-ray exam neck spine 4/5vws	0.00	1.19	NA	0.01	1.20	$41.53	NA	NA	XXX	A+ GS
72052	X-ray exam neck spine 6/>vws	0.30	1.53	NA	0.02	1.85	$64.02	NA	NA	XXX	A+
72052-26	X-ray exam neck spine 6/>vws	0.30	0.11	0.11	0.01	0.42	$14.53	0.42	$14.53	XXX	A+
72052-TC	X-ray exam neck spine 6/>vws	0.00	1.42	NA	0.01	1.43	$49.49	NA	NA	XXX	A+ GS
72070	X-ray exam thorac spine 2vws	0.20	0.76	NA	0.02	0.98	$33.91	NA	NA	XXX	A+
72070-26	X-ray exam thorac spine 2vws	0.20	0.08	0.08	0.01	0.29	$10.04	0.29	$10.04	XXX	A+
72070-TC	X-ray exam thorac spine 2vws	0.00	0.68	NA	0.01	0.69	$23.88	NA	NA	XXX	A+ GS

*Please note that these calculations are based on the Medicare 2022 Conversion Factor of $34.6062 and the DRA RVU cap rates at time of publication.

A = assistant-at-surgery restriction

A+ = assistant-at-surgery restriction unless medical necessity established with documentation

B = bilateral surgery adjustment applies

C = cosurgeons payable

C+ = cosurgeons payable if medical necessity established with documentation

CP = carriers may establish RVUs and payment amounts for these services, generally on an individual basis following review of documentation such as an operative report

M = multiple surgery adjustment applies

Me = multiple endoscopy rules may apply

M+ = multiple therapy rules apply

Mtc = multiple diagnostic imaging rules apply

T = team surgeons permitted

T+ = team surgeons payable if medical necessity established with documentation

§ = indicates code is not covered by Medicare

GS = procedure must be performed under the general supervision of a physician

DS = procedure must be performed under the direct supervision of a physician

PS = procedure must be performed under the personal supervision of a physician

DRA = procedure subject to DRA limitation

Relative Value Units

CPT Code and Modifier	Description	Work RVU	Nonfacility Practice Expense RVU	Facility Practice Expense RVU	PLI RVU	Total Non-facility RVUs	Medicare Payment Nonfacility	Total Facility RVUs	Medicare Payment Facility	Global Period	Payment Policy Indicators
72072	X-ray exam thorac spine 3vws	0.23	0.92	NA	0.02	1.17	$40.49	NA	NA	XXX	A+
72072-26	X-ray exam thorac spine 3vws	0.23	0.08	0.08	0.01	0.32	$11.07	0.32	$11.07	XXX	A+
72072-TC	X-ray exam thorac spine 3vws	0.00	0.84	NA	0.01	0.85	$29.42	NA	NA	XXX	A+ GS
72074	X-ray exam thorac spine4/>vw	0.25	1.06	NA	0.02	1.33	$46.03	NA	NA	XXX	A+
72074-26	X-ray exam thorac spine4/>vw	0.25	0.09	0.09	0.01	0.35	$12.11	0.35	$12.11	XXX	A+
72074-TC	X-ray exam thorac spine4/>vw	0.00	0.97	NA	0.01	0.98	$33.91	NA	NA	XXX	A+ GS
72080	X-ray exam thoracolmb 2/> vw	0.21	0.81	NA	0.02	1.04	$35.99	NA	NA	XXX	A+
72080-26	X-ray exam thoracolmb 2/> vw	0.21	0.08	0.08	0.01	0.30	$10.38	0.30	$10.38	XXX	A+
72080-TC	X-ray exam thoracolmb 2/> vw	0.00	0.73	NA	0.01	0.74	$25.61	NA	NA	XXX	A+ GS
72081	X-ray exam entire spi 1 vw	0.26	0.99	NA	0.02	1.27	$43.95	NA	NA	XXX	A+
72081-26	X-ray exam entire spi 1 vw	0.26	0.10	0.10	0.01	0.37	$12.80	0.37	$12.80	XXX	A+
72081-TC	X-ray exam entire spi 1 vw	0.00	0.89	NA	0.01	0.90	$31.15	NA	NA	XXX	A+ GS
72082	X-ray exam entire spi 2/3 vw	0.31	1.76	NA	0.03	2.10	$72.67	NA	NA	XXX	A+
72082-26	X-ray exam entire spi 2/3 vw	0.31	0.12	0.12	0.02	0.45	$15.57	0.45	$15.57	XXX	A+
72082-TC	X-ray exam entire spi 2/3 vw	0.00	1.64	NA	0.01	1.65	$57.10	NA	NA	XXX	A+ GS
72083	X-ray exam entire spi 4/5 vw	0.35	1.98	NA	0.02	2.35	$81.32	NA	NA	XXX	A+
72083-26	X-ray exam entire spi 4/5 vw	0.35	0.15	0.15	0.01	0.51	$17.65	0.51	$17.65	XXX	A+
72083-TC	X-ray exam entire spi 4/5 vw	0.00	1.83	NA	0.01	1.84	$63.68	NA	NA	XXX	A+ GS
72084	X-ray exam entire spi 6/> vw	0.41	2.51	NA	0.03	2.95	$102.09	NA	NA	XXX	A+
72084-26	X-ray exam entire spi 6/> vw	0.41	0.17	0.17	0.02	0.60	$20.76	0.60	$20.76	XXX	A+
72084-TC	X-ray exam entire spi 6/> vw	0.00	2.34	NA	0.01	2.35	$81.32	NA	NA	XXX	A+ GS
72100	X-ray exam l-s spine 2/3 vws	0.22	0.95	NA	0.02	1.19	$41.18	NA	NA	XXX	A+
72100-26	X-ray exam l-s spine 2/3 vws	0.22	0.09	0.09	0.01	0.32	$11.07	0.32	$11.07	XXX	A+
72100-TC	X-ray exam l-s spine 2/3 vws	0.00	0.86	NA	0.01	0.87	$30.11	NA	NA	XXX	A+ GS
72110	X-ray exam l-2 spine 4/>vws	0.26	1.25	NA	0.02	1.53	$52.95	NA	NA	XXX	A+
72110-26	X-ray exam l-2 spine 4/>vws	0.26	0.10	0.10	0.01	0.37	$12.80	0.37	$12.80	XXX	A+
72110-TC	X-ray exam l-2 spine 4/>vws	0.00	1.15	NA	0.01	1.16	$40.14	NA	NA	XXX	A+ GS
72114	X-ray exam l-s spine bending	0.30	1.53	NA	0.02	1.85	$64.02	NA	NA	XXX	A+
72114-26	X-ray exam l-s spine bending	0.30	0.12	0.12	0.01	0.43	$14.88	0.43	$14.88	XXX	A+
72114-TC	X-ray exam l-s spine bending	0.00	1.41	NA	0.01	1.42	$49.14	NA	NA	XXX	A+ GS
72120	X-ray bend only l-s spine	0.22	0.98	NA	0.02	1.22	$42.22	NA	NA	XXX	A+
72120-26	X-ray bend only l-s spine	0.22	0.09	0.09	0.01	0.32	$11.07	0.32	$11.07	XXX	A+
72120-TC	X-ray bend only l-s spine	0.00	0.89	NA	0.01	0.90	$31.15	NA	NA	XXX	A+ GS

72125	Ct neck spine w/o dye	1.00	2.97	NA	0.06	4.03	$139.46	NA	NA	XXX	A+ Mtc
72125-26	Ct neck spine w/o dye	1.00	0.36	0.36	0.05	1.41	$48.79	1.41	$48.79	XXX	A+ Mtc
72125-TC	Ct neck spine w/o dye	0.00	2.61	NA	0.01	2.62	$90.67	NA	NA	XXX	A+ Mtc GS
72126	Ct neck spine w/dye	1.22	3.95	NA	0.08	5.25	$181.68	NA	NA	XXX	A+ Mtc
72126-26	Ct neck spine w/dye	1.22	0.43	0.43	0.07	1.72	$59.52	1.72	$59.52	XXX	A+ Mtc
72126-TC	Ct neck spine w/dye	0.00	3.52	NA	0.01	3.53	$122.16	NA	NA	XXX	A+ Mtc DS
72127	Ct neck spine w/o & w/dye	1.27	4.81	NA	0.10	6.18	$213.87	NA	NA	XXX	A+ Mtc
72127-26	Ct neck spine w/o & w/dye	1.27	0.45	0.45	0.08	1.80	$62.29	1.80	$62.29	XXX	A+ Mtc
72127-TC	Ct neck spine w/o & w/dye	0.00	4.36	NA	0.02	4.38	$151.58	NA	NA	XXX	A+ Mtc DS
72128	Ct chest spine w/o dye	1.00	2.96	NA	0.06	4.02	$139.12	NA	NA	XXX	A+ Mtc
72128-26	Ct chest spine w/o dye	1.00	0.36	0.36	0.05	1.41	$48.79	1.41	$48.79	XXX	A+ Mtc
72128-TC	Ct chest spine w/o dye	0.00	2.60	NA	0.01	2.61	$90.32	NA	NA	XXX	A+ Mtc GS
72129	Ct chest spine w/dye	1.22	3.99	NA	0.08	5.29	$183.07	NA	NA	XXX	A+ Mtc
72129-26	Ct chest spine w/dye	1.22	0.44	0.44	0.07	1.73	$59.87	1.73	$59.87	XXX	A+ Mtc
72129-TC	Ct chest spine w/dye	0.00	3.55	NA	0.01	3.56	$123.20	NA	NA	XXX	A+ Mtc DS
72130	Ct chest spine w/o & w/dye	1.27	4.84	NA	0.09	6.20	$214.56	NA	NA	XXX	A+ Mtc
72130-26	Ct chest spine w/o & w/dye	1.27	0.45	0.45	0.07	1.79	$61.95	1.79	$61.95	XXX	A+ Mtc
72130-TC	Ct chest spine w/o & w/dye	0.00	4.39	NA	0.02	4.41	$152.61	NA	NA	XXX	A+ Mtc DS
72131	Ct lumbar spine w/o dye	1.00	2.95	NA	0.06	4.01	$138.77	NA	NA	XXX	A+ Mtc
72131-26	Ct lumbar spine w/o dye	1.00	0.36	0.36	0.05	1.41	$48.79	1.41	$48.79	XXX	A+ Mtc
72131-TC	Ct lumbar spine w/o dye	0.00	2.59	NA	0.01	2.60	$89.98	NA	NA	XXX	A+ Mtc GS
72132	Ct lumbar spine w/dye	1.22	3.95	NA	0.08	5.25	$181.68	NA	NA	XXX	A+ Mtc
72132-26	Ct lumbar spine w/dye	1.22	0.43	0.43	0.07	1.72	$59.52	1.72	$59.52	XXX	A+ Mtc
72132-TC	Ct lumbar spine w/dye	0.00	3.52	NA	0.01	3.53	$122.16	NA	NA	XXX	A+ Mtc DS
72133	Ct lumbar spine w/o & w/dye	1.27	4.80	NA	0.10	6.17	$213.52	NA	NA	XXX	A+ Mtc
72133-26	Ct lumbar spine w/o & w/dye	1.27	0.45	0.45	0.08	1.80	$62.29	1.80	$62.29	XXX	A+ Mtc
72133-TC	Ct lumbar spine w/o & w/dye	0.00	4.35	NA	0.02	4.37	$151.23	NA	NA	XXX	A+ Mtc DS
72141	Mri neck spine w/o dye	1.48	4.41	NA	0.10	5.99	$207.29	NA	NA	XXX	A+ Mtc

*Please note that these calculations are based on the Medicare 2022 Conversion Factor of $34.6062 and the DRA RVU cap rates at time of publication.

A = assistant-at-surgery restriction
A+ = assistant-at-surgery restriction unless medical necessity established with documentation
B = bilateral surgery adjustment applies
C = cosurgeons payable
C+ = cosurgeons payable if medical necessity established with documentation
CP = carriers may establish RVUs and payment amounts for these services, generally on an individual basis following review of documentation such as an operative report
M = multiple surgery adjustment applies
Me = multiple endoscopy rules may apply
M+ = multiple therapy rules apply
Mtc = multiple diagnostic imaging rules apply
T = team surgeons permitted
T+ = team surgeons payable if medical necessity established with documentation
§ = indicates code is not covered by Medicare
GS = procedure must be performed under the general supervision of a physician
DS = procedure must be performed under the direct supervision of a physician
PS = procedure must be performed under the personal supervision of a physician
DRA = procedure subject to DRA limitation

Relative Value Units

CPT Code and Modifier	Description	Work RVU	Nonfacility Practice Expense RVU	Facility Practice Expense RVU	PLI RVU	Total Non-facility RVUs	Medicare Payment Nonfacility	Total Facility RVUs	Medicare Payment Facility	Global Period	Payment Policy Indicators
72141-26	Mri neck spine w/o dye	1.48	0.54	0.54	0.08	2.10	$72.67	2.10	$72.67	XXX	A+ Mtc
72141-TC	Mri neck spine w/o dye	0.00	3.87	NA	0.02	3.89	$134.62	NA	NA	XXX	A+ Mtc GS
72142	Mri neck spine w/dye	1.78	6.79	NA	0.11	8.68	$300.38	NA	NA	XXX	A+ Mtc
72142-26	Mri neck spine w/dye	1.78	0.65	0.65	0.09	2.52	$87.21	2.52	$87.21	XXX	A+ Mtc
72142-TC	Mri neck spine w/dye	0.00	6.14	NA	0.02	6.16	$213.17	NA	NA	XXX	A+ Mtc DS
72146	Mri chest spine w/o dye	1.48	4.40	NA	0.10	5.98	$206.95	NA	NA	XXX	A+ Mtc
72146-26	Mri chest spine w/o dye	1.48	0.53	0.53	0.08	2.09	$72.33	2.09	$72.33	XXX	A+ Mtc
72146-TC	Mri chest spine w/o dye	0.00	3.87	NA	0.02	3.89	$134.62	NA	NA	XXX	A+ Mtc GS
72147	Mri chest spine w/dye	1.78	6.70	NA	0.11	8.59	$297.27	NA	NA	XXX	A+ Mtc
72147-26	Mri chest spine w/dye	1.78	0.64	0.64	0.09	2.51	$86.86	2.51	$86.86	XXX	A+ Mtc
72147-TC	Mri chest spine w/dye	0.00	6.06	NA	0.02	6.08	$210.41	NA	NA	XXX	A+ Mtc DS
72148	Mri lumbar spine w/o dye	1.48	4.42	NA	0.10	6.00	$207.64	NA	NA	XXX	A+ Mtc
72148-26	Mri lumbar spine w/o dye	1.48	0.54	0.54	0.08	2.10	$72.67	2.10	$72.67	XXX	A+ Mtc
72148-TC	Mri lumbar spine w/o dye	0.00	3.88	NA	0.02	3.90	$134.96	NA	NA	XXX	A+ Mtc GS
72149	Mri lumbar spine w/dye	1.78	6.63	NA	0.11	8.52	$294.84	NA	NA	XXX	A+ Mtc
72149-26	Mri lumbar spine w/dye	1.78	0.64	0.64	0.09	2.51	$86.86	2.51	$86.86	XXX	A+ Mtc
72149-TC	Mri lumbar spine w/dye	0.00	5.99	NA	0.02	6.01	$207.98	NA	NA	XXX	A+ Mtc DS
72156	Mri neck spine w/o & w/dye	2.29	7.65	NA	0.13	10.07	$348.48	NA	NA	XXX	A+ Mtc
72156-26	Mri neck spine w/o & w/dye	2.29	0.82	0.82	0.11	3.22	$111.43	3.22	$111.43	XXX	A+ Mtc
72156-TC	Mri neck spine w/o & w/dye	0.00	6.83	NA	0.02	6.85	$237.05	NA	NA	XXX	A+ Mtc DS
72157	Mri chest spine w/o & w/dye	2.29	7.66	NA	0.13	10.08	$348.83	NA	NA	XXX	A+ Mtc
72157-26	Mri chest spine w/o & w/dye	2.29	0.82	0.82	0.11	3.22	$111.43	3.22	$111.43	XXX	A+ Mtc
72157-TC	Mri chest spine w/o & w/dye	0.00	6.84	NA	0.02	6.86	$237.40	NA	NA	XXX	A+ Mtc DS
72158	Mri lumbar spine w/o & w/dye	2.29	7.62	NA	0.13	10.04	$347.45	NA	NA	XXX	A+ Mtc
72158-26	Mri lumbar spine w/o & w/dye	2.29	0.82	0.82	0.11	3.22	$111.43	3.22	$111.43	XXX	A+ Mtc
72158-TC	Mri lumbar spine w/o & w/dye	0.00	6.80	NA	0.02	6.82	$236.01	NA	NA	XXX	A+ Mtc DS
72159	Mr angio spine w/o&w/dye	1.80	8.96	NA	0.13	10.89	$376.86	NA	NA	XXX	A+ Mtc
72159-26	Mr angio spine w/o&w/dye	1.80	0.65	0.65	0.09	2.54	$87.90	2.54	$87.90	XXX	A+ Mtc
72159-TC	Mr angio spine w/o&w/dye	0.00	8.31	NA	0.04	8.35	$288.96	NA	NA	XXX	Mtc DS
72170	X-ray exam of pelvis	0.17	0.64	NA	0.02	0.83	$28.72	NA	NA	XXX	A+
72170-26	X-ray exam of pelvis	0.17	0.07	0.07	0.01	0.25	$8.65	0.25	$8.65	XXX	A+
72170-TC	X-ray exam of pelvis	0.00	0.57	NA	0.01	0.58	$20.07	NA	NA	XXX	A+ GS
72190	X-ray exam of pelvis	0.25	0.99	NA	0.02	1.26	$43.60	NA	NA	XXX	A+

72190-26	X-ray exam of pelvis	0.25	0.10	0.10	0.01	0.36	$12.46	0.36	$12.46	XXX	A+
72190-TC	X-ray exam of pelvis	0.00	0.89	NA	0.01	0.90	$31.15	NA	NA	XXX	A+ GS
72191	Ct angiograph pelv w/o&w/dye	1.81	7.65	NA	0.11	9.57	$269.93	NA	NA	XXX	A+ Mtc DRA
72191-26	Ct angiograph pelv w/o&w/dye	1.81	0.62	0.62	0.09	2.52	$87.21	2.52	$87.21	XXX	A+ Mtc
72191-TC	Ct angiograph pelv w/o&w/dye	0.00	7.03	NA	0.02	7.05	$182.72	NA	NA	XXX	A+ Mtc DS DRA
72192	Ct pelvis w/o dye	1.09	2.97	NA	0.06	4.12	$142.58	NA	NA	XXX	A+ Mtc
72192-26	Ct pelvis w/o dye	1.09	0.39	0.39	0.05	1.53	$52.95	1.53	$52.95	XXX	A+ Mtc
72192-TC	Ct pelvis w/o dye	0.00	2.58	NA	0.01	2.59	$89.63	NA	NA	XXX	A+ Mtc GS
72193	Ct pelvis w/dye	1.16	6.05	NA	0.06	7.27	$238.78	NA	NA	XXX	A+ Mtc DRA
72193-26	Ct pelvis w/dye	1.16	0.42	0.42	0.05	1.63	$56.41	1.63	$56.41	XXX	A+ Mtc
72193-TC	Ct pelvis w/dye	0.00	5.63	NA	0.01	5.64	$182.37	NA	NA	XXX	A+ Mtc DS DRA
72194	Ct pelvis w/o & w/dye	1.22	6.71	NA	0.09	8.02	$241.90	NA	NA	XXX	A+ Mtc DRA
72194-26	Ct pelvis w/o & w/dye	1.22	0.43	0.43	0.07	1.72	$59.52	1.72	$59.52	XXX	A+ Mtc
72194-TC	Ct pelvis w/o & w/dye	0.00	6.28	NA	0.02	6.30	$182.37	NA	NA	XXX	A+ Mtc DS DRA
72195	Mri pelvis w/o dye	1.46	5.70	NA	0.10	7.26	$251.24	NA	NA	XXX	A+ Mtc
72195-26	Mri pelvis w/o dye	1.46	0.53	0.53	0.08	2.07	$71.63	2.07	$71.63	XXX	A+ Mtc
72195-TC	Mri pelvis w/o dye	0.00	5.17	NA	0.02	5.19	$179.61	NA	NA	XXX	A+ Mtc GS
72196	Mri pelvis w/dye	1.73	6.66	NA	0.11	8.50	$294.15	NA	NA	XXX	A+ Mtc
72196-26	Mri pelvis w/dye	1.73	0.62	0.62	0.09	2.44	$84.44	2.44	$84.44	XXX	A+ Mtc
72196-TC	Mri pelvis w/dye	0.00	6.04	NA	0.02	6.06	$209.71	NA	NA	XXX	A+ Mtc DS
72197	Mri pelvis w/o & w/dye	2.20	8.34	NA	0.14	10.68	$369.59	NA	NA	XXX	A+ Mtc
72197-26	Mri pelvis w/o & w/dye	2.20	0.79	0.79	0.10	3.09	$106.93	3.09	$106.93	XXX	A+ Mtc
72197-TC	Mri pelvis w/o & w/dye	0.00	7.55	NA	0.04	7.59	$262.66	NA	NA	XXX	A+ Mtc DS
72198	Mr angio pelvis w/o & w/dye	1.80	8.66	NA	0.13	10.59	$366.48	NA	NA	XXX	A+ Mtc
72198-26	Mr angio pelvis w/o & w/dye	1.80	0.62	0.62	0.09	2.51	$86.86	2.51	$86.86	XXX	A+ Mtc
72198-TC	Mr angio pelvis w/o & w/dye	0.00	8.04	NA	0.04	8.08	$279.62	NA	NA	XXX	A+ Mtc DS
72200	X-ray exam si joints	0.17	0.79	NA	0.02	0.98	$33.91	NA	NA	XXX	A+
72200-26	X-ray exam si joints	0.17	0.06	0.06	0.01	0.24	$8.31	0.24	$8.31	XXX	A+

*Please note that these calculations are based on the Medicare 2022 Conversion Factor of $34.6062 and the DRA RVU cap rates at time of publication.

A = assistant-at-surgery restriction
A+ = assistant-at-surgery restriction unless medical necessity established with documentation
B = bilateral surgery adjustment applies
C = cosurgeons payable
C+ = cosurgeons payable if medical necessity established with documentation
CP = carriers may establish RVUs and payment amounts for these services, generally on an individual basis following review of documentation such as an operative report
M = multiple surgery adjustment applies
Me = multiple endoscopy rules may apply
M+ = multiple therapy rules apply
Mtc = multiple diagnostic imaging rules apply
T = team surgeons permitted
T+ = team surgeons payable if medical necessity established with documentation
§ = indicates code is not covered by Medicare
GS = procedure must be performed under the general supervision of a physician
DS = procedure must be performed under the direct supervision of a physician
PS = procedure must be performed under the personal supervision of a physician
DRA = procedure subject to DRA limitation

Relative Value Units

CPT Code and Modifier	Description	Work RVU	Nonfacility Practice Expense RVU	Facility Practice Expense RVU	PLI RVU	Total Non-facility RVUs	Medicare Payment Nonfacility	Total Facility RVUs	Medicare Payment Facility	Global Period	Payment Policy Indicators
72200-TC	X-ray exam si joints	0.00	0.73	NA	0.01	0.74	$25.61	NA	NA	XXX	A+ GS
72202	X-ray exam si joints 3/> vws	0.23	0.92	NA	0.02	1.17	$40.49	NA	NA	XXX	A+
72202-26	X-ray exam si joints 3/> vws	0.23	0.08	0.08	0.01	0.32	$11.07	0.32	$11.07	XXX	A+
72202-TC	X-ray exam si joints 3/> vws	0.00	0.84	NA	0.01	0.85	$29.42	NA	NA	XXX	A+ GS
72220	X-ray exam sacrum tailbone	0.17	0.78	NA	0.02	0.97	$33.57	NA	NA	XXX	A+
72220-26	X-ray exam sacrum tailbone	0.17	0.07	0.07	0.01	0.25	$8.65	0.25	$8.65	XXX	A+
72220-TC	X-ray exam sacrum tailbone	0.00	0.71	NA	0.01	0.72	$24.92	NA	NA	XXX	A+ GS
72240	Myelography neck spine	0.91	2.49	NA	0.06	3.46	$119.74	NA	NA	XXX	A+
72240-26	Myelography neck spine	0.91	0.34	0.34	0.05	1.30	$44.99	1.30	$44.99	XXX	A+
72240-TC	Myelography neck spine	0.00	2.15	NA	0.01	2.16	$74.75	NA	NA	XXX	A+ PS
72255	Myelography thoracic spine	0.91	2.56	NA	0.06	3.53	$122.16	NA	NA	XXX	A+
72255-26	Myelography thoracic spine	0.91	0.37	0.37	0.05	1.33	$46.03	1.33	$46.03	XXX	A+
72255-TC	Myelography thoracic spine	0.00	2.19	NA	0.01	2.20	$76.13	NA	NA	XXX	A+ PS
72265	Myelography l-s spine	0.83	2.40	NA	0.05	3.28	$113.51	NA	NA	XXX	A+
72265-26	Myelography l-s spine	0.83	0.30	0.30	0.04	1.17	$40.49	1.17	$40.49	XXX	A+
72265-TC	Myelography l-s spine	0.00	2.10	NA	0.01	2.11	$73.02	NA	NA	XXX	A+ PS
72270	Myelogphy 2/> spine regions	1.33	3.58	NA	0.10	5.01	$173.38	NA	NA	XXX	A+
72270-26	Myelogphy 2/> spine regions	1.33	0.55	0.55	0.09	1.97	$68.17	1.97	$68.17	XXX	A+
72270-TC	Myelogphy 2/> spine regions	0.00	3.03	NA	0.01	3.04	$105.20	NA	NA	XXX	A+ PS
72285	Discography cerv/thor spine	1.16	2.57	NA	0.06	3.79	$131.16	NA	NA	XXX	A+
72285-26	Discography cerv/thor spine	1.16	0.44	0.44	0.05	1.65	$57.10	1.65	$57.10	XXX	A+
72285-TC	Discography cerv/thor spine	0.00	2.13	NA	0.01	2.14	$74.06	NA	NA	XXX	A+ PS
72295	X-ray of lower spine disk	0.83	2.47	NA	0.06	3.36	$116.28	NA	NA	XXX	A+
72295-26	X-ray of lower spine disk	0.83	0.31	0.31	0.05	1.19	$41.18	1.19	$41.18	XXX	A+
72295-TC	X-ray of lower spine disk	0.00	2.16	NA	0.01	2.17	$75.10	NA	NA	XXX	A+ PS
73000	X-ray exam of collar bone	0.16	0.78	NA	0.02	0.96	$33.22	NA	NA	XXX	A+
73000-26	X-ray exam of collar bone	0.16	0.07	0.07	0.01	0.24	$8.31	0.24	$8.31	XXX	A+
73000-TC	X-ray exam of collar bone	0.00	0.71	NA	0.01	0.72	$24.92	NA	NA	XXX	A+ GS
73010	X-ray exam of shoulder blade	0.17	0.52	NA	0.02	0.71	$24.57	NA	NA	XXX	A+
73010-26	X-ray exam of shoulder blade	0.17	0.08	0.08	0.01	0.26	$9.00	0.26	$9.00	XXX	A+
73010-TC	X-ray exam of shoulder blade	0.00	0.44	NA	0.01	0.45	$15.57	NA	NA	XXX	A+ GS
73020	X-ray exam of shoulder	0.15	0.47	NA	0.02	0.64	$22.15	NA	NA	XXX	A+
73020-26	X-ray exam of shoulder	0.15	0.06	0.06	0.01	0.22	$7.61	0.22	$7.61	XXX	A+

73020-TC	X-ray exam of shoulder	0.00	0.41	NA	0.01	0.42	$14.53	NA	NA	XXX	A+ GS
73030	X-ray exam of shoulder	0.18	0.83	NA	0.02	1.03	$35.64	NA	NA	XXX	A+
73030-26	X-ray exam of shoulder	0.18	0.08	0.08	0.01	0.27	$9.34	0.27	$9.34	XXX	A+
73030-TC	X-ray exam of shoulder	0.00	0.75	NA	0.01	0.76	$26.30	NA	NA	XXX	A+ GS
73040	Contrast x-ray of shoulder	0.54	3.39	NA	0.05	3.98	$137.73	NA	NA	XXX	A+
73040-26	Contrast x-ray of shoulder	0.54	0.22	0.22	0.04	0.80	$27.68	0.80	$27.68	XXX	A+
73040-TC	Contrast x-ray of shoulder	0.00	3.17	NA	0.01	3.18	$110.05	NA	NA	XXX	A+ PS
73050	X-ray exam of shoulders	0.18	0.65	NA	0.02	0.85	$29.42	NA	NA	XXX	A+
73050-26	X-ray exam of shoulders	0.18	0.08	0.08	0.01	0.27	$9.34	0.27	$9.34	XXX	A+
73050-TC	X-ray exam of shoulders	0.00	0.57	NA	0.01	0.58	$20.07	NA	NA	XXX	A+ GS
73060	X-ray exam of humerus	0.16	0.77	NA	0.02	0.95	$32.88	NA	NA	XXX	A+
73060-26	X-ray exam of humerus	0.16	0.06	0.06	0.01	0.23	$7.96	0.23	$7.96	XXX	A+
73060-TC	X-ray exam of humerus	0.00	0.71	NA	0.01	0.72	$24.92	NA	NA	XXX	A+ GS
73070	X-ray exam of elbow	0.16	0.69	NA	0.02	0.87	$30.11	NA	NA	XXX	A+
73070-26	X-ray exam of elbow	0.16	0.07	0.07	0.01	0.24	$8.31	0.24	$8.31	XXX	A+
73070-TC	X-ray exam of elbow	0.00	0.62	NA	0.01	0.63	$21.80	NA	NA	XXX	A+ GS
73080	X-ray exam of elbow	0.17	0.78	NA	0.02	0.97	$33.57	NA	NA	XXX	A+
73080-26	X-ray exam of elbow	0.17	0.07	0.07	0.01	0.25	$8.65	0.25	$8.65	XXX	A+
73080-TC	X-ray exam of elbow	0.00	0.71	NA	0.01	0.72	$24.92	NA	NA	XXX	A+ GS
73085	Contrast x-ray of elbow	0.54	2.81	NA	0.06	3.41	$118.01	NA	NA	XXX	A+
73085-26	Contrast x-ray of elbow	0.54	0.23	0.23	0.05	0.82	$28.38	0.82	$28.38	XXX	A+
73085-TC	Contrast x-ray of elbow	0.00	2.58	NA	0.01	2.59	$89.63	NA	NA	XXX	A+ PS
73090	X-ray exam of forearm	0.16	0.69	NA	0.02	0.87	$30.11	NA	NA	XXX	A+
73090-26	X-ray exam of forearm	0.16	0.06	0.06	0.01	0.23	$7.96	0.23	$7.96	XXX	A+
73090-TC	X-ray exam of forearm	0.00	0.63	NA	0.01	0.64	$22.15	NA	NA	XXX	A+ GS
73092	X-ray exam of arm infant	0.16	0.77	NA	0.02	0.95	$32.88	NA	NA	XXX	A+
73092-26	X-ray exam of arm infant	0.16	0.06	0.06	0.01	0.23	$7.96	0.23	$7.96	XXX	A+
73092-TC	X-ray exam of arm infant	0.00	0.71	NA	0.01	0.72	$24.92	NA	NA	XXX	A+ GS

*Please note that these calculations are based on the Medicare 2022 Conversion Factor of $34.6062 and the DRA RVU cap rates at time of publication.

A = assistant-at-surgery restriction
A+ = assistant-at-surgery restriction unless medical necessity established with documentation
B = bilateral surgery adjustment applies
C = cosurgeons payable
C+ = cosurgeons payable if medical necessity established with documentation
CP = carriers may establish RVUs and payment amounts for these services, generally on an individual basis following review of documentation such as an operative report
M = multiple surgery adjustment applies
Me = multiple endoscopy rules may apply
M+ = multiple therapy rules apply
Mtc = multiple diagnostic imaging rules apply
T = team surgeons permitted
T+ = team surgeons payable if medical necessity established with documentation
§ = indicates code is not covered by Medicare
GS = procedure must be performed under the general supervision of a physician
DS = procedure must be performed under the direct supervision of a physician
PS = procedure must be performed under the personal supervision of a physician
DRA = procedure subject to DRA limitation

Relative Value Units

CPT Code and Modifier	Description	Work RVU	Nonfacility Practice Expense RVU	Facility Practice Expense RVU	PLI RVU	Total Non-facility RVUs	Medicare Payment Nonfacility	Total Facility RVUs	Medicare Payment Facility	Global Period	Payment Policy Indicators
73100	X-ray exam of wrist	0.16	0.83	NA	0.02	1.01	$34.95	NA	NA	XXX	A+
73100-26	X-ray exam of wrist	0.16	0.07	0.07	0.01	0.24	$8.31	0.24	$8.31	XXX	A+
73100-TC	X-ray exam of wrist	0.00	0.76	NA	0.01	0.77	$26.65	NA	NA	XXX	A+ GS
73110	X-ray exam of wrist	0.17	1.03	NA	0.02	1.22	$42.22	NA	NA	XXX	A+
73110-26	X-ray exam of wrist	0.17	0.07	0.07	0.01	0.25	$8.65	0.25	$8.65	XXX	A+
73110-TC	X-ray exam of wrist	0.00	0.96	NA	0.01	0.97	$33.57	NA	NA	XXX	A+ GS
73115	Contrast x-ray of wrist	0.54	3.54	NA	0.05	4.13	$142.92	NA	NA	XXX	A+
73115-26	Contrast x-ray of wrist	0.54	0.23	0.23	0.04	0.81	$28.03	0.81	$28.03	XXX	A+
73115-TC	Contrast x-ray of wrist	0.00	3.31	NA	0.01	3.32	$114.89	NA	NA	XXX	A+ PS
73120	X-ray exam of hand	0.16	0.75	NA	0.02	0.93	$32.18	NA	NA	XXX	A+
73120-26	X-ray exam of hand	0.16	0.07	0.07	0.01	0.24	$8.31	0.24	$8.31	XXX	A+
73120-TC	X-ray exam of hand	0.00	0.68	NA	0.01	0.69	$23.88	NA	NA	XXX	A+ GS
73130	X-ray exam of hand	0.17	0.90	NA	0.02	1.09	$37.72	NA	NA	XXX	A+
73130-26	X-ray exam of hand	0.17	0.07	0.07	0.01	0.25	$8.65	0.25	$8.65	XXX	A+
73130-TC	X-ray exam of hand	0.00	0.83	NA	0.01	0.84	$29.07	NA	NA	XXX	A+ GS
73140	X-ray exam of finger(s)	0.13	0.97	NA	0.02	1.12	$38.76	NA	NA	XXX	A+
73140-26	X-ray exam of finger(s)	0.13	0.06	0.06	0.01	0.20	$6.92	0.20	$6.92	XXX	A+
73140-TC	X-ray exam of finger(s)	0.00	0.91	NA	0.01	0.92	$31.84	NA	NA	XXX	A+ GS
73200	Ct upper extremity w/o dye	1.00	4.02	NA	0.06	5.08	$159.88	NA	NA	XXX	A+ Mtc DRA
73200-26	Ct upper extremity w/o dye	1.00	0.36	0.36	0.05	1.41	$48.79	1.41	$48.79	XXX	A+ Mtc
73200-TC	Ct upper extremity w/o dye	0.00	3.66	NA	0.01	3.67	$111.09	NA	NA	XXX	A+ Mtc GS DRA
73201	Ct upper extremity w/dye	1.16	5.07	NA	0.06	6.29	$217.67	NA	NA	XXX	A+ Mtc
73201-26	Ct upper extremity w/dye	1.16	0.41	0.41	0.05	1.62	$56.06	1.62	$56.06	XXX	A+ Mtc
73201-TC	Ct upper extremity w/dye	0.00	4.66	NA	0.01	4.67	$161.61	NA	NA	XXX	A+ Mtc DS
73202	Ct uppr extremity w/o&w/dye	1.22	6.58	NA	0.09	7.89	$241.90	NA	NA	XXX	A+ Mtc DRA
73202-26	Ct uppr extremity w/o&w/dye	1.22	0.43	0.43	0.07	1.72	$59.52	1.72	$59.52	XXX	A+ Mtc
73202-TC	Ct uppr extremity w/o&w/dye	0.00	6.15	NA	0.02	6.17	$182.37	NA	NA	XXX	A+ Mtc DS DRA
73206	Ct angio upr extrm w/o&w/dye	1.81	7.39	NA	0.13	9.33	$269.58	NA	NA	XXX	A+ Mtc DRA
73206-26	Ct angio upr extrm w/o&w/dye	1.81	0.62	0.62	0.09	2.52	$87.21	2.52	$87.21	XXX	A+ Mtc
73206-TC	Ct angio upr extrm w/o&w/dye	0.00	6.77	NA	0.04	6.81	$182.37	NA	NA	XXX	A+ Mtc DS DRA
73218	Mri upper extremity w/o dye	1.35	8.21	NA	0.09	9.65	$301.42	NA	NA	XXX	A+ Mtc DRA
73218-26	Mri upper extremity w/o dye	1.35	0.50	0.50	0.07	1.92	$66.44	1.92	$66.44	XXX	A+ Mtc
73218-TC	Mri upper extremity w/o dye	0.00	7.71	NA	0.02	7.73	$234.98	NA	NA	XXX	A+ Mtc GS DRA

73219	Mri upper extremity w/dye	1.62	8.79	NA	0.11	10.52	$364.06	NA	NA	XXX	A+ Mtc
73219-26	Mri upper extremity w/dye	1.62	0.59	0.59	0.09	2.30	$79.59	2.30	$79.59	XXX	A+ Mtc
73219-TC	Mri upper extremity w/dye	0.00	8.20	NA	0.02	8.22	$284.46	NA	NA	XXX	A+ Mtc DS
73220	Mri uppr extremity w/o&w/dye	2.15	10.77	NA	0.14	13.06	$451.96	NA	NA	XXX	A+ Mtc
73220-26	Mri uppr extremity w/o&w/dye	2.15	0.78	0.78	0.10	3.03	$104.86	3.03	$104.86	XXX	A+ Mtc
73220-TC	Mri uppr extremity w/o&w/dye	0.00	9.99	NA	0.04	10.03	$347.10	NA	NA	XXX	A+ Mtc DS
73221	Mri joint upr extrem w/o dye	1.35	4.89	NA	0.10	6.34	$219.40	NA	NA	XXX	A+ Mtc
73221-26	Mri joint upr extrem w/o dye	1.35	0.50	0.50	0.08	1.93	$66.79	1.93	$66.79	XXX	A+ Mtc
73221-TC	Mri joint upr extrem w/o dye	0.00	4.39	NA	0.02	4.41	$152.61	NA	NA	XXX	A+ Mtc GS
73222	Mri joint upr extrem w/dye	1.62	8.24	NA	0.11	9.97	$345.02	NA	NA	XXX	A+ Mtc
73222-26	Mri joint upr extrem w/dye	1.62	0.60	0.60	0.09	2.31	$79.94	2.31	$79.94	XXX	A+ Mtc
73222-TC	Mri joint upr extrem w/dye	0.00	7.64	NA	0.02	7.66	$265.08	NA	NA	XXX	A+ Mtc DS
73223	Mri joint upr extr w/o&w/dye	2.15	10.05	NA	0.14	12.34	$427.04	NA	NA	XXX	A+ Mtc
73223-26	Mri joint upr extr w/o&w/dye	2.15	0.78	0.78	0.10	3.03	$104.86	3.03	$104.86	XXX	A+ Mtc
73223-TC	Mri joint upr extr w/o&w/dye	0.00	9.27	NA	0.04	9.31	$322.18	NA	NA	XXX	A+ Mtc DS
73225	Mr angio upr extr w/o&w/dye	1.73	8.94	NA	0.13	10.80	$373.75	NA	NA	XXX	A+ Mtc
73225-26	Mr angio upr extr w/o&w/dye	1.73	0.63	0.63	0.09	2.45	$84.79	2.45	$84.79	XXX	A+ Mtc
73225-TC	Mr angio upr extr w/o&w/dye	0.00	8.31	NA	0.04	8.35	$288.96	NA	NA	XXX	Mtc DS
73501	X-ray exam hip uni 1 view	0.18	0.77	NA	0.02	0.97	$33.57	NA	NA	XXX	A+
73501-26	X-ray exam hip uni 1 view	0.18	0.08	0.08	0.01	0.27	$9.34	0.27	$9.34	XXX	A+
73501-TC	X-ray exam hip uni 1 view	0.00	0.69	NA	0.01	0.70	$24.22	NA	NA	XXX	A+ GS
73502	X-ray exam hip uni 2-3 views	0.22	1.16	NA	0.02	1.40	$48.45	NA	NA	XXX	A+
73502-26	X-ray exam hip uni 2-3 views	0.22	0.09	0.09	0.01	0.32	$11.07	0.32	$11.07	XXX	A+
73502-TC	X-ray exam hip uni 2-3 views	0.00	1.07	NA	0.01	1.08	$37.37	NA	NA	XXX	A+ GS
73503	X-ray exam hip uni 4/> views	0.27	1.47	NA	0.02	1.76	$60.91	NA	NA	XXX	A+
73503-26	X-ray exam hip uni 4/> views	0.27	0.11	0.11	0.01	0.39	$13.50	0.39	$13.50	XXX	A+
73503-TC	X-ray exam hip uni 4/> views	0.00	1.36	NA	0.01	1.37	$47.41	NA	NA	XXX	A+ GS
73521	X-ray exam hips bi 2 views	0.22	0.99	NA	0.02	1.23	$42.57	NA	NA	XXX	A+

*Please note that these calculations are based on the Medicare 2022 Conversion Factor of $34.6062 and the DRA RVU cap rates at time of publication.

A = assistant-at-surgery restriction
A+ = assistant-at-surgery restriction unless medical necessity established with documentation
B = bilateral surgery adjustment applies
C = cosurgeons payable
C+ = cosurgeons payable if medical necessity established with documentation
CP = carriers may establish RVUs and payment amounts for these services, generally on an individual basis following review of documentation such as an operative report
M = multiple surgery adjustment applies
Me = multiple endoscopy rules may apply
M+ = multiple therapy rules apply
Mtc = multiple diagnostic imaging rules apply
T = team surgeons permitted
T+ = team surgeons payable if medical necessity established with documentation
§ = indicates code is not covered by Medicare
GS = procedure must be performed under the general supervision of a physician
DS = procedure must be performed under the direct supervision of a physician
PS = procedure must be performed under the personal supervision of a physician
DRA = procedure subject to DRA limitation

Relative Value Units

CPT Code and Modifier	Description	Work RVU	Nonfacility Practice Expense RVU	Facility Practice Expense RVU	PLI RVU	Total Non-facility RVUs	Medicare Payment Nonfacility	Total Facility RVUs	Medicare Payment Facility	Global Period	Payment Policy Indicators
73521-26	X-ray exam hips bi 2 views	0.22	0.09	0.09	0.01	0.32	$11.07	0.32	$11.07	XXX	A+
73521-TC	X-ray exam hips bi 2 views	0.00	0.90	NA	0.01	0.91	$31.49	NA	NA	XXX	A+ GS
73522	X-ray exam hips bi 3-4 views	0.29	1.29	NA	0.02	1.60	$55.37	NA	NA	XXX	A+
73522-26	X-ray exam hips bi 3-4 views	0.29	0.12	0.12	0.01	0.42	$14.53	0.42	$14.53	XXX	A+
73522-TC	X-ray exam hips bi 3-4 views	0.00	1.17	NA	0.01	1.18	$40.84	NA	NA	XXX	A+ GS
73523	X-ray exam hips bi 5/> views	0.31	1.50	NA	0.02	1.83	$63.33	NA	NA	XXX	A+
73523-26	X-ray exam hips bi 5/> views	0.31	0.12	0.12	0.01	0.44	$15.23	0.44	$15.23	XXX	A+
73523-TC	X-ray exam hips bi 5/> views	0.00	1.38	NA	0.01	1.39	$48.10	NA	NA	XXX	A+ GS
73525	Contrast x-ray of hip	0.54	3.45	NA	0.06	4.05	$140.16	NA	NA	XXX	A+
73525-26	Contrast x-ray of hip	0.54	0.25	0.25	0.05	0.84	$29.07	0.84	$29.07	XXX	A+
73525-TC	Contrast x-ray of hip	0.00	3.20	NA	0.01	3.21	$111.09	NA	NA	XXX	A+ PS
73551	X-ray exam of femur 1	0.16	0.69	NA	0.02	0.87	$30.11	NA	NA	XXX	A+
73551-26	X-ray exam of femur 1	0.16	0.07	0.07	0.01	0.24	$8.31	0.24	$8.31	XXX	A+
73551-TC	X-ray exam of femur 1	0.00	0.62	NA	0.01	0.63	$21.80	NA	NA	XXX	A+ GS
73552	X-ray exam of femur 2/>	0.18	0.85	NA	0.02	1.05	$36.34	NA	NA	XXX	A+
73552-26	X-ray exam of femur 2/>	0.18	0.07	0.07	0.01	0.26	$9.00	0.26	$9.00	XXX	A+
73552-TC	X-ray exam of femur 2/>	0.00	0.78	NA	0.01	0.79	$27.34	NA	NA	XXX	A+ GS
73560	X-ray exam of knee 1 or 2	0.16	0.84	NA	0.02	1.02	$35.30	NA	NA	XXX	A+
73560-26	X-ray exam of knee 1 or 2	0.16	0.07	0.07	0.01	0.24	$8.31	0.24	$8.31	XXX	A+
73560-TC	X-ray exam of knee 1 or 2	0.00	0.77	NA	0.01	0.78	$26.99	NA	NA	XXX	A+ GS
73562	X-ray exam of knee 3	0.18	1.02	NA	0.02	1.22	$42.22	NA	NA	XXX	A+
73562-26	X-ray exam of knee 3	0.18	0.08	0.08	0.01	0.27	$9.34	0.27	$9.34	XXX	A+
73562-TC	X-ray exam of knee 3	0.00	0.94	NA	0.01	0.95	$32.88	NA	NA	XXX	A+
73564	X-ray exam knee 4 or more	0.22	1.14	NA	0.02	1.38	$47.76	NA	NA	XXX	A+
73564-26	X-ray exam knee 4 or more	0.22	0.09	0.09	0.01	0.32	$11.07	0.32	$11.07	XXX	A+
73564-TC	X-ray exam knee 4 or more	0.00	1.05	NA	0.01	1.06	$36.68	NA	NA	XXX	A+ GS
73565	X-ray exam of knees	0.16	1.03	NA	0.02	1.21	$41.87	NA	NA	XXX	A+
73565-26	X-ray exam of knees	0.16	0.08	0.08	0.01	0.25	$8.65	0.25	$8.65	XXX	A+
73565-TC	X-ray exam of knees	0.00	0.95	NA	0.01	0.96	$33.22	NA	NA	XXX	A+ GS
73580	Contrast x-ray of knee joint	0.54	3.85	NA	0.08	4.47	$154.69	NA	NA	XXX	A+
73580-26	Contrast x-ray of knee joint	0.54	0.23	0.23	0.07	0.84	$29.07	0.84	$29.07	XXX	A+
73580-TC	Contrast x-ray of knee joint	0.00	3.62	NA	0.01	3.63	$125.62	NA	NA	XXX	A+ PS
73590	X-ray exam of lower leg	0.16	0.76	NA	0.02	0.94	$32.53	NA	NA	XXX	A+

73590-26	X-ray exam of lower leg	0.16	0.06	0.06	0.01	0.23	$7.96	0.23	$7.96	XXX	A+
73590-TC	X-ray exam of lower leg	0.00	0.70	NA	0.01	0.71	$24.57	NA	NA	XXX	A+ GS
73592	X-ray exam of leg infant	0.16	0.77	NA	0.02	0.95	$32.88	NA	NA	XXX	A+
73592-26	X-ray exam of leg infant	0.16	0.06	0.06	0.01	0.23	$7.96	0.23	$7.96	XXX	A+
73592-TC	X-ray exam of leg infant	0.00	0.71	NA	0.01	0.72	$24.92	NA	NA	XXX	A+ GS
73600	X-ray exam of ankle	0.16	0.78	NA	0.02	0.96	$33.22	NA	NA	XXX	A+
73600-26	X-ray exam of ankle	0.16	0.06	0.06	0.01	0.23	$7.96	0.23	$7.96	XXX	A+
73600-TC	X-ray exam of ankle	0.00	0.72	NA	0.01	0.73	$25.26	NA	NA	XXX	A+ GS
73610	X-ray exam of ankle	0.17	0.91	NA	0.02	1.10	$38.07	NA	NA	XXX	A+
73610-26	X-ray exam of ankle	0.17	0.07	0.07	0.01	0.25	$8.65	0.25	$8.65	XXX	A+
73610-TC	X-ray exam of ankle	0.00	0.84	NA	0.01	0.85	$29.42	NA	NA	XXX	A+ GS
73615	Contrast x-ray of ankle	0.54	3.42	NA	0.06	4.02	$139.12	NA	NA	XXX	A+
73615-26	Contrast x-ray of ankle	0.54	0.23	0.23	0.05	0.82	$28.38	0.82	$28.38	XXX	A+
73615-TC	Contrast x-ray of ankle	0.00	3.19	NA	0.01	3.20	$110.74	NA	NA	XXX	A+ PS
73620	X-ray exam of foot	0.16	0.66	NA	0.02	0.84	$29.07	NA	NA	XXX	A+
73620-26	X-ray exam of foot	0.16	0.05	0.05	0.01	0.22	$7.61	0.22	$7.61	XXX	A+
73620-TC	X-ray exam of foot	0.00	0.61	NA	0.01	0.62	$21.46	NA	NA	XXX	A+ GS
73630	X-ray exam of foot	0.17	0.84	NA	0.02	1.03	$35.64	NA	NA	XXX	A+
73630-26	X-ray exam of foot	0.17	0.06	0.06	0.01	0.24	$8.31	0.24	$8.31	XXX	A+
73630-TC	X-ray exam of foot	0.00	0.78	NA	0.01	0.79	$27.34	NA	NA	XXX	A+ GS
73650	X-ray exam of heel	0.16	0.68	NA	0.02	0.86	$29.76	NA	NA	XXX	A+
73650-26	X-ray exam of heel	0.16	0.06	0.06	0.01	0.23	$7.96	0.23	$7.96	XXX	A+
73650-TC	X-ray exam of heel	0.00	0.62	NA	0.01	0.63	$21.80	NA	NA	XXX	A+ GS
73660	X-ray exam of toe(s)	0.13	0.72	NA	0.02	0.87	$30.11	NA	NA	XXX	A+
73660-26	X-ray exam of toe(s)	0.13	0.05	0.05	0.01	0.19	$6.58	0.19	$6.58	XXX	A+
73660-TC	X-ray exam of toe(s)	0.00	0.67	NA	0.01	0.68	$23.53	NA	NA	XXX	A+ GS
73700	Ct lower extremity w/o dye	1.00	2.95	NA	0.06	4.01	$138.77	NA	NA	XXX	A+ Mtc
73700-26	Ct lower extremity w/o dye	1.00	0.36	0.36	0.05	1.41	$48.79	1.41	$48.79	XXX	A+ Mtc

*Please note that these calculations are based on the Medicare 2022 Conversion Factor of $34.6062 and the DRA RVU cap rates at time of publication.

A = assistant-at-surgery restriction

A+ = assistant-at-surgery restriction unless medical necessity established with documentation

B = bilateral surgery adjustment applies

C = cosurgeons payable

C+ = cosurgeons payable if medical necessity established with documentation

CP = carriers may establish RVUs and payment amounts for these services, generally on an individual basis following review of documentation such as an operative report

M = multiple surgery adjustment applies

Me = multiple endoscopy rules may apply

M+ = multiple therapy rules apply

Mtc = multiple diagnostic imaging rules apply

T = team surgeons permitted

T+ = team surgeons payable if medical necessity established with documentation

§ = indicates code is not covered by Medicare

GS = procedure must be performed under the general supervision of a physician

DS = procedure must be performed under the direct supervision of a physician

PS = procedure must be performed under the personal supervision of a physician

DRA = procedure subject to DRA limitation

Relative Value Units

CPT Code and Modifier	Description	Work RVU	Nonfacility Practice Expense RVU	Facility Practice Expense RVU	PLI RVU	Total Non-facility RVUs	Medicare Payment Nonfacility	Total Facility RVUs	Medicare Payment Facility	Global Period	Payment Policy Indicators
73700-TC	Ct lower extremity w/o dye	0.00	2.59	NA	0.01	2.60	$89.98	NA	NA	XXX	A+ Mtc GS
73701	Ct lower extremity w/dye	1.16	3.96	NA	0.06	5.18	$179.26	NA	NA	XXX	A+ Mtc
73701-26	Ct lower extremity w/dye	1.16	0.42	0.42	0.05	1.63	$56.41	1.63	$56.41	XXX	A+ Mtc
73701-TC	Ct lower extremity w/dye	0.00	3.54	NA	0.01	3.55	$122.85	NA	NA	XXX	A+ Mtc DS
73702	Ct lwr extremity w/o&w/dye	1.22	4.77	NA	0.09	6.08	$210.41	NA	NA	XXX	A+ Mtc
73702-26	Ct lwr extremity w/o&w/dye	1.22	0.43	0.43	0.07	1.72	$59.52	1.72	$59.52	XXX	A+ Mtc
73702-TC	Ct lwr extremity w/o&w/dye	0.00	4.34	NA	0.02	4.36	$150.88	NA	NA	XXX	A+ Mtc DS
73706	Ct angio lwr extr w/o&w/dye	1.90	8.09	NA	0.13	10.12	$273.74	NA	NA	XXX	A+ Mtc DRA
73706-26	Ct angio lwr extr w/o&w/dye	1.90	0.65	0.65	0.09	2.64	$91.36	2.64	$91.36	XXX	A+ Mtc
73706-TC	Ct angio lwr extr w/o&w/dye	0.00	7.44	NA	0.04	7.48	$182.37	NA	NA	XXX	A+ Mtc DS DRA
73718	Mri lower extremity w/o dye	1.35	5.61	NA	0.09	7.05	$243.97	NA	NA	XXX	A+ Mtc
73718-26	Mri lower extremity w/o dye	1.35	0.48	0.48	0.07	1.90	$65.75	1.90	$65.75	XXX	A+ Mtc
73718-TC	Mri lower extremity w/o dye	0.00	5.13	NA	0.02	5.15	$178.22	NA	NA	XXX	A+ Mtc GS
73719	Mri lower extremity w/dye	1.62	6.57	NA	0.11	8.30	$287.23	NA	NA	XXX	A+ Mtc
73719-26	Mri lower extremity w/dye	1.62	0.58	0.58	0.09	2.29	$79.25	2.29	$79.25	XXX	A+ Mtc
73719-TC	Mri lower extremity w/dye	0.00	5.99	NA	0.02	6.01	$207.98	NA	NA	XXX	A+ Mtc DS
73720	Mri lwr extremity w/o&w/dye	2.15	8.39	NA	0.14	10.68	$369.59	NA	NA	XXX	A+ Mtc
73720-26	Mri lwr extremity w/o&w/dye	2.15	0.77	0.77	0.10	3.02	$104.51	3.02	$104.51	XXX	A+ Mtc
73720-TC	Mri lwr extremity w/o&w/dye	0.00	7.62	NA	0.04	7.66	$265.08	NA	NA	XXX	A+ Mtc DS
73721	Mri jnt of lwr extre w/o dye	1.35	4.88	NA	0.10	6.33	$219.06	NA	NA	XXX	A+ Mtc
73721-26	Mri jnt of lwr extre w/o dye	1.35	0.50	0.50	0.08	1.93	$66.79	1.93	$66.79	XXX	A+ Mtc
73721-TC	Mri jnt of lwr extre w/o dye	0.00	4.38	NA	0.02	4.40	$152.27	NA	NA	XXX	A+ Mtc GS
73722	Mri joint of lwr extr w/dye	1.62	8.26	NA	0.11	9.99	$345.72	NA	NA	XXX	A+ Mtc
73722-26	Mri joint of lwr extr w/dye	1.62	0.60	0.60	0.09	2.31	$79.94	2.31	$79.94	XXX	A+ Mtc
73722-TC	Mri joint of lwr extr w/dye	0.00	7.66	NA	0.02	7.68	$265.78	NA	NA	XXX	A+ Mtc DS
73723	Mri joint lwr extr w/o&w/dye	2.15	10.01	NA	0.14	12.30	$425.66	NA	NA	XXX	A+ Mtc
73723-26	Mri joint lwr extr w/o&w/dye	2.15	0.77	0.77	0.10	3.02	$104.51	3.02	$104.51	XXX	A+ Mtc
73723-TC	Mri joint lwr extr w/o&w/dye	0.00	9.24	NA	0.04	9.28	$321.15	NA	NA	XXX	A+ Mtc DS
73725	Mr ang lwr ext w or w/o dye	1.82	8.60	NA	0.13	10.55	$365.10	NA	NA	XXX	A+ Mtc
73725-26	Mr ang lwr ext w or w/o dye	1.82	0.61	0.61	0.09	2.52	$87.21	2.52	$87.21	XXX	A+ Mtc
73725-TC	Mr ang lwr ext w or w/o dye	0.00	7.99	NA	0.04	8.03	$277.89	NA	NA	XXX	A+ Mtc DS
74018	X-ray exam abdomen 1 view	0.18	0.70	NA	0.02	0.90	$31.15	NA	NA	XXX	A+
74018-26	X-ray exam abdomen 1 view	0.18	0.07	0.07	0.01	0.26	$9.00	0.26	$9.00	XXX	A+

74018-TC	X-ray exam abdomen 1 view	0.00	0.63	NA	0.01	0.64	$22.15	NA	NA	XXX	A+ GS
74019	X-ray exam abdomen 2 views	0.23	0.85	NA	0.02	1.10	$38.07	NA	NA	XXX	A+
74019-26	X-ray exam abdomen 2 views	0.23	0.09	0.09	0.01	0.33	$11.42	0.33	$11.42	XXX	A+
74019-TC	X-ray exam abdomen 2 views	0.00	0.76	NA	0.01	0.77	$26.65	NA	NA	XXX	A+ GS
74021	X-ray exam abdomen 3+ views	0.27	1.00	NA	0.02	1.29	$44.64	NA	NA	XXX	A+
74021-26	X-ray exam abdomen 3+ views	0.27	0.10	0.10	0.01	0.38	$13.15	0.38	$13.15	XXX	A+
74021-TC	X-ray exam abdomen 3+ views	0.00	0.90	NA	0.01	0.91	$31.49	NA	NA	XXX	A+ GS
74022	X-ray exam complete abdomen	0.32	1.15	NA	0.02	1.49	$51.56	NA	NA	XXX	A+
74022-26	X-ray exam complete abdomen	0.32	0.12	0.12	0.01	0.45	$15.57	0.45	$15.57	XXX	A+
74022-TC	X-ray exam complete abdomen	0.00	1.03	NA	0.01	1.04	$35.99	NA	NA	XXX	A+ GS
74150	Ct abdomen w/o dye	1.19	2.98	NA	0.08	4.25	$147.08	NA	NA	XXX	A+ Mtc
74150-26	Ct abdomen w/o dye	1.19	0.43	0.43	0.07	1.69	$58.48	1.69	$58.48	XXX	A+ Mtc
74150-TC	Ct abdomen w/o dye	0.00	2.55	NA	0.01	2.56	$88.59	NA	NA	XXX	A+ Mtc GS
74160	Ct abdomen w/dye	1.27	6.07	NA	0.08	7.42	$244.67	NA	NA	XXX	A+ Mtc DRA
74160-26	Ct abdomen w/dye	1.27	0.46	0.46	0.07	1.80	$62.29	1.80	$62.29	XXX	A+ Mtc
74160-TC	Ct abdomen w/dye	0.00	5.61	NA	0.01	5.62	$182.37	NA	NA	XXX	A+ Mtc DS DRA
74170	Ct abdomen w/o & w/dye	1.40	6.81	NA	0.10	8.31	$250.89	NA	NA	XXX	A+ Mtc DRA
74170-26	Ct abdomen w/o & w/dye	1.40	0.50	0.50	0.08	1.98	$68.52	1.98	$68.52	XXX	A+ Mtc
74170-TC	Ct abdomen w/o & w/dye	0.00	6.31	NA	0.02	6.33	$182.37	NA	NA	XXX	A+ Mtc DS DRA
74174	Ct angio abd&pelv w/o&w/dye	2.20	9.58	NA	0.15	11.93	$412.85	NA	NA	XXX	A+ Mtc
74174-26	Ct angio abd&pelv w/o&w/dye	2.20	0.76	0.76	0.11	3.07	$106.24	3.07	$106.24	XXX	A+ Mtc
74174-TC	Ct angio abd&pelv w/o&w/dye	0.00	8.82	NA	0.04	8.86	$306.61	NA	NA	XXX	A+ Mtc DS
74175	Ct angio abdom w/o & w/dye	1.82	7.65	NA	0.11	9.58	$270.62	NA	NA	XXX	A+ Mtc DRA
74175-26	Ct angio abdom w/o & w/dye	1.82	0.63	0.63	0.09	2.54	$87.90	2.54	$87.90	XXX	A+ Mtc
74175-TC	Ct angio abdom w/o & w/dye	0.00	7.02	NA	0.02	7.04	$182.72	NA	NA	XXX	A+ Mtc DS DRA
74176	Ct abd & pelvis w/o contrast	1.74	3.82	NA	0.10	5.66	$195.87	NA	NA	XXX	Mtc
74176-26	Ct abd & pelvis w/o contrast	1.74	0.62	0.62	0.09	2.45	$84.79	2.45	$84.79	XXX	Mtc
74176-TC	Ct abd & pelvis w/o contrast	0.00	3.20	NA	0.01	3.21	$111.09	NA	NA	XXX	Mtc GS

*Please note that these calculations are based on the Medicare 2022 Conversion Factor of $34.6062 and the DRA RVU cap rates at time of publication.

A = assistant-at-surgery restriction

A+ = assistant-at-surgery restriction unless medical necessity established with documentation

B = bilateral surgery adjustment applies

C = cosurgeons payable

C+ = cosurgeons payable if medical necessity established with documentation

CP = carriers may establish RVUs and payment amounts for these services, generally on an individual basis following review of documentation such as an operative report

M = multiple surgery adjustment applies

Me = multiple endoscopy rules may apply

M+ = multiple therapy rules apply

Mtc = multiple diagnostic imaging rules apply

T = team surgeons permitted

T+ = team surgeons payable if medical necessity established with documentation

§ = indicates code is not covered by Medicare

GS = procedure must be performed under the general supervision of a physician

DS = procedure must be performed under the direct supervision of a physician

PS = procedure must be performed under the personal supervision of a physician

DRA = procedure subject to DRA limitation

Relative Value Units

CPT Code and Modifier		Description	Work RVU	Nonfacility Practice Expense RVU	Facility Practice Expense RVU	PLI RVU	Total Non-facility RVUs	Medicare Payment Nonfacility	Total Facility RVUs	Medicare Payment Facility	Global Period	Payment Policy Indicators
74177		Ct abd & pelv w/contrast	1.82	7.70	NA	0.11	9.63	$333.26	NA	NA	XXX	Mtc
74177-26		Ct abd & pelv w/contrast	1.82	0.66	0.66	0.09	2.57	$88.94	2.57	$88.94	XXX	Mtc
74177-TC		Ct abd & pelv w/contrast	0.00	7.04	NA	0.02	7.06	$244.32	NA	NA	XXX	Mtc DS
74178		Ct abd & pelv 1/> regns	2.01	8.66	NA	0.11	10.78	$373.05	NA	NA	XXX	Mtc
74178-26		Ct abd & pelv 1/> regns	2.01	0.72	0.72	0.09	2.82	$97.59	2.82	$97.59	XXX	Mtc
74178-TC		Ct abd & pelv 1/> regns	0.00	7.94	NA	0.02	7.96	$275.47	NA	NA	XXX	Mtc DS
74181		Mri abdomen w/o dye	1.46	4.60	NA	0.09	6.15	$212.83	NA	NA	XXX	A+ Mtc
74181-26		Mri abdomen w/o dye	1.46	0.52	0.52	0.08	2.06	$71.29	2.06	$71.29	XXX	A+ Mtc
74181-TC		Mri abdomen w/o dye	0.00	4.08	NA	0.01	4.09	$141.54	NA	NA	XXX	A+ Mtc GS
74182		Mri abdomen w/dye	1.73	7.73	NA	0.11	9.57	$331.18	NA	NA	XXX	A+ Mtc
74182-26		Mri abdomen w/dye	1.73	0.62	0.62	0.09	2.44	$84.44	2.44	$84.44	XXX	A+ Mtc
74182-TC		Mri abdomen w/dye	0.00	7.11	NA	0.02	7.13	$246.74	NA	NA	XXX	A+ Mtc DS
74183		Mri abdomen w/o & w/dye	2.20	8.36	NA	0.14	10.70	$370.29	NA	NA	XXX	A+ Mtc
74183-26		Mri abdomen w/o & w/dye	2.20	0.78	0.78	0.10	3.08	$106.59	3.08	$106.59	XXX	A+ Mtc
74183-TC		Mri abdomen w/o & w/dye	0.00	7.58	NA	0.04	7.62	$263.70	NA	NA	XXX	A+ Mtc DS
74185		Mri angio abdom w orw/o dye	1.80	8.68	NA	0.13	10.61	$367.17	NA	NA	XXX	A+ Mtc
74185-26		Mri angio abdom w orw/o dye	1.80	0.62	0.62	0.09	2.51	$86.86	2.51	$86.86	XXX	A+ Mtc
74185-TC		Mri angio abdom w orw/o dye	0.00	8.06	NA	0.04	8.10	$280.31	NA	NA	XXX	A+ Mtc DS
74190	CP	X-ray exam of peritoneum	0.00	0.00	NA	0.00	0.00	$0.00	NA	NA	XXX	A+
74190-26		X-ray exam of peritoneum	0.48	0.14	0.14	0.04	0.66	$22.84	0.66	$22.84	XXX	A+
74190-TC	CP	X-ray exam of peritoneum	0.00	0.00	NA	0.00	0.00	$0.00	NA	NA	XXX	A+ PS
74210		X-ray xm phrnx&/crv esoph c+	0.59	2.34	NA	0.05	2.98	$103.13	NA	NA	XXX	A+
74210-26		X-ray xm phrnx&/crv esoph c+	0.59	0.21	0.21	0.04	0.84	$29.07	0.84	$29.07	XXX	A+
74210-TC		X-ray xm phrnx&/crv esoph c+	0.00	2.13	NA	0.01	2.14	$74.06	NA	NA	XXX	A+ PS
74220		X-ray xm esophagus 1cntrst	0.60	2.36	NA	0.05	3.01	$104.16	NA	NA	XXX	A+
74220-26		X-ray xm esophagus 1cntrst	0.60	0.21	0.21	0.04	0.85	$29.42	0.85	$29.42	XXX	A+
74220-TC		X-ray xm esophagus 1cntrst	0.00	2.15	NA	0.01	2.16	$74.75	NA	NA	XXX	A+ PS
74221		X-ray xm esophagus 2cntrst	0.70	2.64	NA	0.05	3.39	$117.32	NA	NA	XXX	A+
74221-26		X-ray xm esophagus 2cntrst	0.70	0.25	0.25	0.04	0.99	$34.26	0.99	$34.26	XXX	A+
74221-TC		X-ray xm esophagus 2cntrst	0.00	2.39	NA	0.01	2.40	$83.05	NA	NA	XXX	A+ PS
74230		X-ray xm swlng funcj c+	0.53	3.32	NA	0.05	3.90	$134.96	NA	NA	XXX	A+
74230-26		X-ray xm swlng funcj c+	0.53	0.19	0.19	0.04	0.76	$26.30	0.76	$26.30	XXX	A+
74230-TC		X-ray xm swlng funcj c+	0.00	3.13	NA	0.01	3.14	$108.66	NA	NA	XXX	A+ PS

74235	CP	Remove esophagus obstruction	0.00	0.00	NA	0.00	0.00	$0.00	NA	NA	XXX	A+
74235-26		Remove esophagus obstruction	1.19	0.43	0.43	0.07	1.69	$58.48	1.69	$58.48	XXX	A+
74235-TC	CP	Remove esophagus obstruction	0.00	0.00	NA	0.00	0.00	$0.00	NA	NA	XXX	A+ PS
74240		X-ray xm upr gi trc 1cntrst	0.80	2.92	NA	0.05	3.77	$130.47	NA	NA	XXX	A+
74240-26		X-ray xm upr gi trc 1cntrst	0.80	0.29	0.29	0.04	1.13	$39.11	1.13	$39.11	XXX	A+
74240-TC		X-ray xm upr gi trc 1cntrst	0.00	2.63	NA	0.01	2.64	$91.36	NA	NA	XXX	A+ PS
74246		X-ray xm upr gi trc 2cntrst	0.90	3.35	NA	0.05	4.30	$148.81	NA	NA	XXX	A+
74246-26		X-ray xm upr gi trc 2cntrst	0.90	0.32	0.32	0.04	1.26	$43.60	1.26	$43.60	XXX	A+
74246-TC		X-ray xm upr gi trc 2cntrst	0.00	3.03	NA	0.01	3.04	$105.20	NA	NA	XXX	A+ PS
74248		X-ray sm int f-thru std	0.70	1.79	NA	0.05	2.54	$87.90	NA	NA	ZZZ	A+
74248-26		X-ray sm int f-thru std	0.70	0.25	0.25	0.04	0.99	$34.26	0.99	$34.26	ZZZ	A+
74248-TC		X-ray sm int f-thru std	0.00	1.54	NA	0.01	1.55	$53.64	NA	NA	ZZZ	A+ PS
74250		X-ray xm sm int 1cntrst std	0.81	2.90	NA	0.05	3.76	$130.12	NA	NA	XXX	A+
74250-26		X-ray xm sm int 1cntrst std	0.81	0.29	0.29	0.04	1.14	$39.45	1.14	$39.45	XXX	A+
74250-TC		X-ray xm sm int 1cntrst std	0.00	2.61	NA	0.01	2.62	$90.67	NA	NA	XXX	A+ DS
74251		X-ray xm sm int 2cntrst std	1.17	10.28	NA	0.08	11.53	$240.17	NA	NA	XXX	A+ DRA
74251-26		X-ray xm sm int 2cntrst std	1.17	0.42	0.42	0.07	1.66	$57.45	1.66	$57.45	XXX	A+
74251-TC		X-ray xm sm int 2cntrst std	0.00	9.86	NA	0.01	9.87	$182.72	NA	NA	XXX	A+ PS DRA
74261		Ct colonography dx	2.40	10.70	NA	0.13	13.23	$228.05	NA	NA	XXX	A+ Mtc DRA
74261-26		Ct colonography dx	2.40	0.86	0.86	0.11	3.37	$116.62	3.37	$116.62	XXX	A+ Mtc
74261-TC		Ct colonography dx	0.00	9.84	NA	0.02	9.86	$111.43	NA	NA	XXX	A+ Mtc DS DRA
74262		Ct colonography dx w/dye	2.50	12.31	NA	0.15	14.96	$303.84	NA	NA	XXX	A+ Mtc DRA
74262-26		Ct colonography dx w/dye	2.50	0.90	0.90	0.11	3.51	$121.47	3.51	$121.47	XXX	A+ Mtc
74262-TC		Ct colonography dx w/dye	0.00	11.41	NA	0.04	11.45	$182.37	NA	NA	XXX	A+ Mtc DS DRA
74263	§	Ct colonography screening	2.28	18.79	NA	0.12	21.19	$733.31	NA	NA	XXX	
74263-26	§	Ct colonography screening	2.28	0.88	0.88	0.10	3.26	$112.82	3.26	$112.82	XXX	
74263-TC	§	Ct colonography screening	0.00	17.91	NA	0.02	17.93	$620.49	NA	NA	XXX	DS
74270		X-ray xm colon 1cntrst std	1.04	3.63	NA	0.06	4.73	$163.69	NA	NA	XXX	A+

*Please note that these calculations are based on the Medicare 2022 Conversion Factor of $34.6062 and the DRA RVU cap rates at time of publication.

A = assistant-at-surgery restriction
A+ = assistant-at-surgery restriction unless medical necessity established with documentation
B = bilateral surgery adjustment applies
C = cosurgeons payable
C+ = cosurgeons payable if medical necessity established with documentation
CP = carriers may establish RVUs and payment amounts for these services, generally on an individual basis following review of documentation such as an operative report
M = multiple surgery adjustment applies
Me = multiple endoscopy rules may apply
M+ = multiple therapy rules apply
Mtc = multiple diagnostic imaging rules apply
T = team surgeons permitted
T+ = team surgeons payable if medical necessity established with documentation
§ = indicates code is not covered by Medicare
GS = procedure must be performed under the general supervision of a physician
DS = procedure must be performed under the direct supervision of a physician
PS = procedure must be performed under the personal supervision of a physician
DRA = procedure subject to DRA limitation

Relative Value Units

CPT Code and Modifier		Description	Work RVU	Nonfacility Practice Expense RVU	Facility Practice Expense RVU	PLI RVU	Total Non-facility RVUs	Medicare Payment Nonfacility	Total Facility RVUs	Medicare Payment Facility	Global Period	Payment Policy Indicators
74270-26		X-ray xm colon 1cntrst std	1.04	0.37	0.37	0.05	1.46	$50.53	1.46	$50.53	XXX	A+
74270-TC		X-ray xm colon 1cntrst std	0.00	3.26	NA	0.01	3.27	$113.16	NA	NA	XXX	A+ PS
74280		X-ray xm colon 2cntrst std	1.26	5.48	NA	0.08	6.82	$236.01	NA	NA	XXX	A+
74280-26		X-ray xm colon 2cntrst std	1.26	0.45	0.45	0.07	1.78	$61.60	1.78	$61.60	XXX	A+
74280-TC		X-ray xm colon 2cntrst std	0.00	5.03	NA	0.01	5.04	$174.42	NA	NA	XXX	A+ PS
74283		Ther nma rdctj intus/obstrcj	2.02	5.68	NA	0.11	7.81	$270.27	NA	NA	XXX	A+
74283-26		Ther nma rdctj intus/obstrcj	2.02	0.84	0.84	0.10	2.96	$102.43	2.96	$102.43	XXX	A+
74283-TC		Ther nma rdctj intus/obstrcj	0.00	4.84	NA	0.01	4.85	$167.84	NA	NA	XXX	A+ PS
74290		Contrast x-ray gallbladder	0.32	2.31	NA	0.02	2.65	$91.71	NA	NA	XXX	A+
74290-26		Contrast x-ray gallbladder	0.32	0.12	0.12	0.01	0.45	$15.57	0.45	$15.57	XXX	A+
74290-TC		Contrast x-ray gallbladder	0.00	2.19	NA	0.01	2.20	$76.13	NA	NA	XXX	A+ GS
74300	CP	X-ray bile ducts/pancreas	0.00	0.00	NA	0.00	0.00	$0.00	NA	NA	XXX	A+
74300-26		X-ray bile ducts/pancreas	0.27	0.10	0.10	0.02	0.39	$13.50	0.39	$13.50	XXX	A+
74300-TC	CP	X-ray bile ducts/pancreas	0.00	0.00	NA	0.00	0.00	$0.00	NA	NA	XXX	A+ PS
74301	CP	X-rays at surgery add-on	0.00	0.00	NA	0.00	0.00	$0.00	NA	NA	ZZZ	A+
74301-26		X-rays at surgery add-on	0.21	0.08	0.08	0.01	0.30	$10.38	0.30	$10.38	ZZZ	A+
74301-TC	CP	X-rays at surgery add-on	0.00	0.00	NA	0.00	0.00	$0.00	NA	NA	ZZZ	A+ PS
74328	CP	X-ray bile duct endoscopy	0.00	0.00	NA	0.00	0.00	$0.00	NA	NA	XXX	A+
74328-26		X-ray bile duct endoscopy	0.47	0.19	0.19	0.02	0.68	$23.53	0.68	$23.53	XXX	A+
74328-TC	CP	X-ray bile duct endoscopy	0.00	0.00	NA	0.00	0.00	$0.00	NA	NA	XXX	A+ PS
74329	CP	X-ray for pancreas endoscopy	0.00	0.00	NA	0.00	0.00	$0.00	NA	NA	XXX	A+
74329-26		X-ray for pancreas endoscopy	0.47	0.19	0.19	0.02	0.68	$23.53	0.68	$23.53	XXX	A+
74329-TC	CP	X-ray for pancreas endoscopy	0.00	0.00	NA	0.00	0.00	$0.00	NA	NA	XXX	A+ PS
74330	CP	X-ray bile/panc endoscopy	0.00	0.00	NA	0.00	0.00	$0.00	NA	NA	XXX	A+
74330-26		X-ray bile/panc endoscopy	0.56	0.27	0.27	0.02	0.85	$29.42	0.85	$29.42	XXX	A+
74330-TC	CP	X-ray bile/panc endoscopy	0.00	0.00	NA	0.00	0.00	$0.00	NA	NA	XXX	A+ PS
74340	CP	X-ray guide for gi tube	0.00	0.00	NA	0.00	0.00	$0.00	NA	NA	XXX	A+
74340-26		X-ray guide for gi tube	0.54	0.19	0.19	0.04	0.77	$26.65	0.77	$26.65	XXX	A+
74340-TC	CP	X-ray guide for gi tube	0.00	0.00	NA	0.00	0.00	$0.00	NA	NA	XXX	A+ PS
74355	CP	X-ray guide intestinal tube	0.00	0.00	NA	0.00	0.00	$0.00	NA	NA	XXX	A+
74355-26		X-ray guide intestinal tube	0.76	0.28	0.28	0.04	1.08	$37.37	1.08	$37.37	XXX	A+
74355-TC	CP	X-ray guide intestinal tube	0.00	0.00	NA	0.00	0.00	$0.00	NA	NA	XXX	A+ PS
74360	CP	X-ray guide gi dilation	0.00	0.00	NA	0.00	0.00	$0.00	NA	NA	XXX	A+

74360-26		X-ray guide gi dilation	0.54	0.22	0.22	0.04	0.80	$27.68	0.80	$27.68	XXX	A+
74360-TC	CP	X-ray guide gi dilation	0.00	0.00	NA	0.00	0.00	$0.00	NA	NA	XXX	A+ PS
74363	CP	X-ray bile duct dilation	0.00	0.00	NA	0.00	0.00	$0.00	NA	NA	XXX	A+
74363-26		X-ray bile duct dilation	0.88	0.31	0.31	0.04	1.23	$42.57	1.23	$42.57	XXX	A+
74363-TC	CP	X-ray bile duct dilation	0.00	0.00	NA	0.00	0.00	$0.00	NA	NA	XXX	A+ PS
74400		Urography iv +-kub tomog	0.49	3.61	NA	0.03	4.13	$142.92	NA	NA	XXX	A+
74400-26		Urography iv +-kub tomog	0.49	0.17	0.17	0.02	0.68	$23.53	0.68	$23.53	XXX	A+
74400-TC		Urography iv +-kub tomog	0.00	3.44	NA	0.01	3.45	$119.39	NA	NA	XXX	A+ DS
74410		Urography nfs drip&/bolus	0.49	3.75	NA	0.03	4.27	$147.77	NA	NA	XXX	A+
74410-26		Urography nfs drip&/bolus	0.49	0.17	0.17	0.02	0.68	$23.53	0.68	$23.53	XXX	A+
74410-TC		Urography nfs drip&/bolus	0.00	3.58	NA	0.01	3.59	$124.24	NA	NA	XXX	A+ DS
74415		Urography nfs drip&/bls w/nf	0.49	4.20	NA	0.03	4.72	$163.34	NA	NA	XXX	A+
74415-26		Urography nfs drip&/bls w/nf	0.49	0.17	0.17	0.02	0.68	$23.53	0.68	$23.53	XXX	A+
74415-TC		Urography nfs drip&/bls w/nf	0.00	4.03	NA	0.01	4.04	$139.81	NA	NA	XXX	A+ DS
74420		Urography rtrgr +-kub	0.52	1.74	NA	0.03	2.29	$79.25	NA	NA	XXX	A+
74420-26		Urography rtrgr +-kub	0.52	0.18	0.18	0.02	0.72	$24.92	0.72	$24.92	XXX	A+
74420-TC		Urography rtrgr +-kub	0.00	1.56	NA	0.01	1.57	$54.33	NA	NA	XXX	A+ PS
74425		Urography antegrade rs&i	0.51	3.62	NA	0.03	4.16	$143.96	NA	NA	XXX	A+
74425-26		Urography antegrade rs&i	0.51	0.17	0.17	0.02	0.70	$24.22	0.70	$24.22	XXX	A+
74425-TC		Urography antegrade rs&i	0.00	3.45	NA	0.01	3.46	$119.74	NA	NA	XXX	A+ PS
74430		Contrast x-ray bladder	0.32	0.87	NA	0.02	1.21	$41.87	NA	NA	XXX	A+
74430-26		Contrast x-ray bladder	0.32	0.11	0.11	0.01	0.44	$15.23	0.44	$15.23	XXX	A+
74430-TC		Contrast x-ray bladder	0.00	0.76	NA	0.01	0.77	$26.65	NA	NA	XXX	A+ PS
74440		X-ray male genital tract	0.38	2.56	NA	0.02	2.96	$102.43	NA	NA	XXX	A+
74440-26		X-ray male genital tract	0.38	0.13	0.13	0.01	0.52	$18.00	0.52	$18.00	XXX	A+
74440-TC		X-ray male genital tract	0.00	2.43	NA	0.01	2.44	$84.44	NA	NA	XXX	A+ PS
74445	CP	X-ray exam of penis	0.00	0.00	NA	0.00	0.00	$0.00	NA	NA	XXX	A+
74445-26		X-ray exam of penis	1.14	0.39	0.39	0.04	1.57	$54.33	1.57	$54.33	XXX	A+

*Please note that these calculations are based on the Medicare 2022 Conversion Factor of $34.6062 and the DRA RVU cap rates at time of publication.

A = assistant-at-surgery restriction

A+ = assistant-at-surgery restriction unless medical necessity established with documentation

B = bilateral surgery adjustment applies

C = cosurgeons payable

C+ = cosurgeons payable if medical necessity established with documentation

CP = carriers may establish RVUs and payment amounts for these services, generally on an individual basis following review of documentation such as an operative report

M = multiple surgery adjustment applies

Me = multiple endoscopy rules may apply

M+ = multiple therapy rules apply

Mtc = multiple diagnostic imaging rules apply

T = team surgeons permitted

T+ = team surgeons payable if medical necessity established with documentation

§ = indicates code is not covered by Medicare

GS = procedure must be performed under the general supervision of a physician

DS = procedure must be performed under the direct supervision of a physician

PS = procedure must be performed under the personal supervision of a physician

DRA = procedure subject to DRA limitation

Relative Value Units

CPT Code and Modifier		Description	Work RVU	Nonfacility Practice Expense RVU	Facility Practice Expense RVU	PLI RVU	Total Non-facility RVUs	Medicare Payment Nonfacility	Total Facility RVUs	Medicare Payment Facility	Global Period	Payment Policy Indicators
74445-TC	CP	X-ray exam of penis	0.00	0.00	NA	0.00	0.00	$0.00	NA	NA	XXX	A+ PS
74450	CP	X-ray urethra/bladder	0.00	0.00	NA	0.00	0.00	$0.00	NA	NA	XXX	A+
74450-26		X-ray urethra/bladder	0.33	0.12	0.12	0.01	0.46	$15.92	0.46	$15.92	XXX	A+
74450-TC	CP	X-ray urethra/bladder	0.00	0.00	NA	0.00	0.00	$0.00	NA	NA	XXX	A+ PS
74455		X-ray urethra/bladder	0.33	2.83	NA	0.02	3.18	$110.05	NA	NA	XXX	A+
74455-26		X-ray urethra/bladder	0.33	0.11	0.11	0.01	0.45	$15.57	0.45	$15.57	XXX	A+
74455-TC		X-ray urethra/bladder	0.00	2.72	NA	0.01	2.73	$94.47	NA	NA	XXX	A+ PS
74470	CP	X-ray exam of kidney lesion	0.00	0.00	NA	0.00	0.00	$0.00	NA	NA	XXX	A+
74470-26		X-ray exam of kidney lesion	0.54	0.16	0.16	0.04	0.74	$25.61	0.74	$25.61	XXX	A+
74470-TC	CP	X-ray exam of kidney lesion	0.00	0.00	NA	0.00	0.00	$0.00	NA	NA	XXX	A+ PS
74485		Dilation urtr/urt rs&i	0.83	2.72	NA	0.03	3.58	$123.89	NA	NA	XXX	A+
74485-26		Dilation urtr/urt rs&i	0.83	0.28	0.28	0.02	1.13	$39.11	1.13	$39.11	XXX	A+
74485-TC		Dilation urtr/urt rs&i	0.00	2.44	NA	0.01	2.45	$84.79	NA	NA	XXX	A+ PS
74710		X-ray measurement of pelvis	0.34	0.83	NA	0.03	1.20	$41.53	NA	NA	XXX	A+
74710-26		X-ray measurement of pelvis	0.34	0.12	0.12	0.02	0.48	$16.61	0.48	$16.61	XXX	A+
74710-TC		X-ray measurement of pelvis	0.00	0.71	NA	0.01	0.72	$24.92	NA	NA	XXX	A+ GS
74712		Mri fetal sngl/1st gestation	3.00	9.74	NA	0.16	12.90	$380.67	NA	NA	XXX	A+ Mtc DRA
74712-26		Mri fetal sngl/1st gestation	3.00	1.09	1.09	0.12	4.21	$145.69	4.21	$145.69	XXX	A+ Mtc
74712-TC		Mri fetal sngl/1st gestation	0.00	8.65	NA	0.04	8.69	$234.98	NA	NA	XXX	A+ Mtc DS DRA
74713		Mri fetal ea addl gestation	1.85	4.32	NA	0.10	6.27	$216.98	NA	NA	ZZZ	A+
74713-26		Mri fetal ea addl gestation	1.85	0.67	0.67	0.09	2.61	$90.32	2.61	$90.32	ZZZ	A+
74713-TC		Mri fetal ea addl gestation	0.00	3.65	NA	0.01	3.66	$126.66	NA	NA	ZZZ	A+ DS
74740		X-ray female genital tract	0.38	2.53	NA	0.03	2.94	$101.74	NA	NA	XXX	A+
74740-26		X-ray female genital tract	0.38	0.14	0.14	0.02	0.54	$18.69	0.54	$18.69	XXX	A+
74740-TC		X-ray female genital tract	0.00	2.39	NA	0.01	2.40	$83.05	NA	NA	XXX	A+ PS
74742	CP	X-ray fallopian tube	0.00	0.00	NA	0.00	0.00	$0.00	NA	NA	XXX	A+
74742-26		X-ray fallopian tube	0.61	0.22	0.22	0.04	0.87	$30.11	0.87	$30.11	XXX	A+
74742-TC	CP	X-ray fallopian tube	0.00	0.00	NA	0.00	0.00	$0.00	NA	NA	XXX	A+ PS
74775	CP	X-ray exam of perineum	0.00	0.00	NA	0.00	0.00	$0.00	NA	NA	XXX	A+
74775-26		X-ray exam of perineum	0.62	0.22	0.22	0.04	0.88	$30.45	0.88	$30.45	XXX	A+
74775-TC	CP	X-ray exam of perineum	0.00	0.00	NA	0.00	0.00	$0.00	NA	NA	XXX	A+ PS
75557		Cardiac mri for morph	2.35	6.38	NA	0.10	8.83	$305.57	NA	NA	XXX	A+ Mtc
75557-26		Cardiac mri for morph	2.35	0.83	0.83	0.09	3.27	$113.16	3.27	$113.16	XXX	A+ Mtc

75557-TC	Cardiac mri for morph	0.00	5.55	NA	0.01	5.56	$192.41	NA	NA	XXX	A+ Mtc GS
75559	Cardiac mri w/stress img	2.95	8.84	NA	0.12	11.91	$412.16	NA	NA	XXX	A+ Mtc
75559-26	Cardiac mri w/stress img	2.95	1.02	1.02	0.10	4.07	$140.85	4.07	$140.85	XXX	A+ Mtc
75559-TC	Cardiac mri w/stress img	0.00	7.82	NA	0.02	7.84	$271.31	NA	NA	XXX	A+ Mtc DS
75561	Cardiac mri for morph w/dye	2.60	8.87	NA	0.12	11.59	$401.09	NA	NA	XXX	A+ Mtc
75561-26	Cardiac mri for morph w/dye	2.60	0.92	0.92	0.10	3.62	$125.27	3.62	$125.27	XXX	A+ Mtc
75561-TC	Cardiac mri for morph w/dye	0.00	7.95	NA	0.02	7.97	$275.81	NA	NA	XXX	A+ Mtc GS
75563	Card mri w/stress img & dye	3.00	10.45	NA	0.13	13.58	$469.95	NA	NA	XXX	A+ Mtc
75563-26	Card mri w/stress img & dye	3.00	1.04	1.04	0.11	4.15	$143.62	4.15	$143.62	XXX	A+ Mtc
75563-TC	Card mri w/stress img & dye	0.00	9.41	NA	0.02	9.43	$326.34	NA	NA	XXX	A+ Mtc GS
75565	Card mri veloc flow mapping	0.25	1.20	NA	0.01	1.46	$50.53	NA	NA	ZZZ	A+
75565-26	Card mri veloc flow mapping	0.25	0.09	0.09	0.01	0.35	$12.11	0.35	$12.11	ZZZ	A+
75565-TC	Card mri veloc flow mapping	0.00	1.11	NA	0.00	1.11	$38.41	NA	NA	ZZZ	A+ GS
75571	Ct hrt w/o dye w/ca test	0.58	2.43	NA	0.05	3.06	$105.89	NA	NA	XXX	A+ Mtc
75571-26	Ct hrt w/o dye w/ca test	0.58	0.20	0.20	0.04	0.82	$28.38	0.82	$28.38	XXX	A+ Mtc
75571-TC	Ct hrt w/o dye w/ca test	0.00	2.23	NA	0.01	2.24	$77.52	NA	NA	XXX	A+ Mtc DS
75572	Ct hrt w/3d image	1.75	5.17	NA	0.12	7.04	$243.63	NA	NA	XXX	A+ Mtc
75572-26	Ct hrt w/3d image	1.75	0.62	0.62	0.08	2.45	$84.79	2.45	$84.79	XXX	A+ Mtc
75572-TC	Ct hrt w/3d image	0.00	4.55	NA	0.04	4.59	$158.84	NA	NA	XXX	A+ Mtc DS
75573	Ct hrt c+ strux cgen hrt ds	2.55	6.75	NA	0.15	9.45	$306.26	NA	NA	XXX	A+ Mtc DRA
75573-26	Ct hrt c+ strux cgen hrt ds	2.55	0.91	0.91	0.11	3.57	$123.54	3.57	$123.54	XXX	A+ Mtc
75573-TC	Ct hrt c+ strux cgen hrt ds	0.00	5.84	NA	0.04	5.88	$182.72	NA	NA	XXX	A+ Mtc DS DRA
75574	Ct angio hrt w/3d image	2.40	7.51	NA	0.14	10.05	$297.96	NA	NA	XXX	A+ Mtc DRA
75574-26	Ct angio hrt w/3d image	2.40	0.84	0.84	0.10	3.34	$115.58	3.34	$115.58	XXX	A+ Mtc
75574-TC	Ct angio hrt w/3d image	0.00	6.67	NA	0.04	6.71	$182.37	NA	NA	XXX	A+ Mtc DS DRA
75600	Contrast exam thoracic aorta	0.49	5.07	NA	0.10	5.66	$195.87	NA	NA	XXX	A+
75600-26	Contrast exam thoracic aorta	0.49	0.14	0.14	0.08	0.71	$24.57	0.71	$24.57	XXX	A+
75600-TC	Contrast exam thoracic aorta	0.00	4.93	NA	0.02	4.95	$171.30	NA	NA	XXX	A+ PS

*Please note that these calculations are based on the Medicare 2022 Conversion Factor of $34.6062 and the DRA RVU cap rates at time of publication.

A = assistant-at-surgery restriction

A+ = assistant-at-surgery restriction unless medical necessity established with documentation

B = bilateral surgery adjustment applies

C = cosurgeons payable

C+ = cosurgeons payable if medical necessity established with documentation

CP = carriers may establish RVUs and payment amounts for these services, generally on an individual basis following review of documentation such as an operative report

M = multiple surgery adjustment applies

Me = multiple endoscopy rules may apply

M+ = multiple therapy rules apply

Mtc = multiple diagnostic imaging rules apply

T = team surgeons permitted

T+ = team surgeons payable if medical necessity established with documentation

§ = indicates code is not covered by Medicare

GS = procedure must be performed under the general supervision of a physician

DS = procedure must be performed under the direct supervision of a physician

PS = procedure must be performed under the personal supervision of a physician

DRA = procedure subject to DRA limitation

Relative Value Units

CPT Code and Modifier	Description	Work RVU	Nonfacility Practice Expense RVU	Facility Practice Expense RVU	PLI RVU	Total Non-facility RVUs	Medicare Payment Nonfacility	Total Facility RVUs	Medicare Payment Facility	Global Period	Payment Policy Indicators
75605	Contrast exam thoracic aorta	1.14	2.35	NA	0.13	3.62	$125.27	NA	NA	XXX	A+
75605-26	Contrast exam thoracic aorta	1.14	0.33	0.33	0.11	1.58	$54.68	1.58	$54.68	XXX	A+
75605-TC	Contrast exam thoracic aorta	0.00	2.02	NA	0.02	2.04	$70.60	NA	NA	XXX	A+ PS
75625	Contrast exam abdominl aorta	1.44	2.17	NA	0.21	3.82	$132.20	NA	NA	XXX	A+
75625-26	Contrast exam abdominl aorta	1.44	0.36	0.36	0.20	2.00	$69.21	2.00	$69.21	XXX	A+
75625-TC	Contrast exam abdominl aorta	0.00	1.81	NA	0.01	1.82	$62.98	NA	NA	XXX	A+ PS
75630	X-ray aorta leg arteries	2.00	2.51	NA	0.22	4.73	$163.69	NA	NA	XXX	A+
75630-26	X-ray aorta leg arteries	2.00	0.57	0.57	0.21	2.78	$96.21	2.78	$96.21	XXX	A+
75630-TC	X-ray aorta leg arteries	0.00	1.94	NA	0.01	1.95	$67.48	NA	NA	XXX	A+ PS
75635	Ct angio abdominal arteries	2.40	10.20	NA	0.15	12.75	$297.27	NA	NA	XXX	A+ Mtc DRA
75635-26	Ct angio abdominal arteries	2.40	0.81	0.81	0.11	3.32	$114.89	3.32	$114.89	XXX	A+ Mtc
75635-TC	Ct angio abdominal arteries	0.00	9.39	NA	0.04	9.43	$182.37	NA	NA	XXX	A+ Mtc DS DRA
75705	Artery x-rays spine	2.18	4.67	NA	0.41	7.26	$251.24	NA	NA	XXX	A+
75705-26	Artery x-rays spine	2.18	0.82	0.82	0.39	3.39	$117.32	3.39	$117.32	XXX	A+
75705-TC	Artery x-rays spine	0.00	3.85	NA	0.02	3.87	$133.93	NA	NA	XXX	A+ PS
75710	Artery x-rays arm/leg	1.75	2.54	NA	0.23	4.52	$156.42	NA	NA	XXX	A+
75710-26	Artery x-rays arm/leg	1.75	0.47	0.47	0.22	2.44	$84.44	2.44	$84.44	XXX	A+
75710-TC	Artery x-rays arm/leg	0.00	2.07	NA	0.01	2.08	$71.98	NA	NA	XXX	A+ PS
75716	Artery x-rays arms/legs	1.97	2.68	NA	0.23	4.88	$168.88	NA	NA	XXX	A+
75716-26	Artery x-rays arms/legs	1.97	0.55	0.55	0.21	2.73	$94.47	2.73	$94.47	XXX	A+
75716-TC	Artery x-rays arms/legs	0.00	2.13	NA	0.02	2.15	$74.40	NA	NA	XXX	A+ PS
75726	Artery x-rays abdomen	2.05	2.88	NA	0.14	5.07	$175.45	NA	NA	XXX	A+
75726-26	Artery x-rays abdomen	2.05	0.58	0.58	0.12	2.75	$95.17	2.75	$95.17	XXX	A+
75726-TC	Artery x-rays abdomen	0.00	2.30	NA	0.02	2.32	$80.29	NA	NA	XXX	A+ PS
75731	Artery x-rays adrenal gland	1.14	3.29	NA	0.07	4.50	$155.73	NA	NA	XXX	A+
75731-26	Artery x-rays adrenal gland	1.14	0.41	0.41	0.05	1.60	$55.37	1.60	$55.37	XXX	A+
75731-TC	Artery x-rays adrenal gland	0.00	2.88	NA	0.02	2.90	$100.36	NA	NA	XXX	A+ PS
75733	Artery x-rays adrenals	1.31	3.61	NA	0.08	5.00	$173.03	NA	NA	XXX	A+
75733-26	Artery x-rays adrenals	1.31	0.45	0.45	0.04	1.80	$62.29	1.80	$62.29	XXX	A+
75733-TC	Artery x-rays adrenals	0.00	3.16	NA	0.04	3.20	$110.74	NA	NA	XXX	A+ PS
75736	Artery x-rays pelvis	1.14	2.95	NA	0.11	4.20	$145.35	NA	NA	XXX	A+
75736-26	Artery x-rays pelvis	1.14	0.31	0.31	0.09	1.54	$53.29	1.54	$53.29	XXX	A+
75736-TC	Artery x-rays pelvis	0.00	2.64	NA	0.02	2.66	$92.05	NA	NA	XXX	A+ PS

75741		Artery x-rays lung	1.31	2.48	NA	0.10	3.89	$134.62	NA	NA	XXX	A+
75741-26		Artery x-rays lung	1.31	0.37	0.37	0.09	1.77	$61.25	1.77	$61.25	XXX	A+
75741-TC		Artery x-rays lung	0.00	2.11	NA	0.01	2.12	$73.37	NA	NA	XXX	A+ PS
75743		Artery x-rays lungs	1.66	2.63	NA	0.13	4.42	$152.96	NA	NA	XXX	A+
75743-26		Artery x-rays lungs	1.66	0.49	0.49	0.11	2.26	$78.21	2.26	$78.21	XXX	A+
75743-TC		Artery x-rays lungs	0.00	2.14	NA	0.02	2.16	$74.75	NA	NA	XXX	A+ PS
75746		Artery x-rays lung	1.14	2.75	NA	0.10	3.99	$138.08	NA	NA	XXX	A+
75746-26		Artery x-rays lung	1.14	0.35	0.35	0.08	1.57	$54.33	1.57	$54.33	XXX	A+
75746-TC		Artery x-rays lung	0.00	2.40	NA	0.02	2.42	$83.75	NA	NA	XXX	A+ PS
75756		Artery x-rays chest	1.14	3.44	NA	0.13	4.71	$163.00	NA	NA	XXX	A+
75756-26		Artery x-rays chest	1.14	0.36	0.36	0.11	1.61	$55.72	1.61	$55.72	XXX	A+
75756-TC		Artery x-rays chest	0.00	3.08	NA	0.02	3.10	$107.28	NA	NA	XXX	A+ PS
75774		Artery x-ray each vessel	1.01	1.80	NA	0.10	2.91	$100.70	NA	NA	ZZZ	A+
75774-26		Artery x-ray each vessel	1.01	0.27	0.27	0.09	1.37	$47.41	1.37	$47.41	ZZZ	A+
75774-TC		Artery x-ray each vessel	0.00	1.53	NA	0.01	1.54	$53.29	NA	NA	ZZZ	A+ PS
75801	CP	Lymph vessel x-ray arm/leg	0.00	0.00	NA	0.00	0.00	$0.00	NA	NA	XXX	A+
75801-26		Lymph vessel x-ray arm/leg	0.81	0.32	0.32	0.11	1.24	$42.91	1.24	$42.91	XXX	A+
75801-TC	CP	Lymph vessel x-ray arm/leg	0.00	0.00	NA	0.00	0.00	$0.00	NA	NA	XXX	A+ PS
75803	CP	Lymph vessel x-ray arms/legs	0.00	0.00	NA	0.00	0.00	$0.00	NA	NA	XXX	A+
75803-26		Lymph vessel x-ray arms/legs	1.17	0.42	0.42	0.05	1.64	$56.75	1.64	$56.75	XXX	A+
75803-TC	CP	Lymph vessel x-ray arms/legs	0.00	0.00	NA	0.00	0.00	$0.00	NA	NA	XXX	A+ PS
75805	CP	Lymph vessel x-ray trunk	0.00	0.00	NA	0.00	0.00	$0.00	NA	NA	XXX	A+
75805-26		Lymph vessel x-ray trunk	0.81	0.29	0.29	0.04	1.14	$39.45	1.14	$39.45	XXX	A+
75805-TC	CP	Lymph vessel x-ray trunk	0.00	0.00	NA	0.00	0.00	$0.00	NA	NA	XXX	A+ PS
75807	CP	Lymph vessel x-ray trunk	0.00	0.00	NA	0.00	0.00	$0.00	NA	NA	XXX	A+
75807-26		Lymph vessel x-ray trunk	1.17	0.31	0.31	0.08	1.56	$53.99	1.56	$53.99	XXX	A+
75807-TC	CP	Lymph vessel x-ray trunk	0.00	0.00	NA	0.00	0.00	$0.00	NA	NA	XXX	A+ PS
75809		Nonvascular shunt x-ray	0.47	1.94	NA	0.05	2.46	$85.13	NA	NA	XXX	A+

*Please note that these calculations are based on the Medicare 2022 Conversion Factor of $34.6062 and the DRA RVU cap rates at time of publication.

A = assistant-at-surgery restriction
A+ = assistant-at-surgery restriction unless medical necessity established with documentation
B = bilateral surgery adjustment applies
C = cosurgeons payable
C+ = cosurgeons payable if medical necessity established with documentation
CP = carriers may establish RVUs and payment amounts for these services, generally on an individual basis following review of documentation such as an operative report
M = multiple surgery adjustment applies
Me = multiple endoscopy rules may apply
M+ = multiple therapy rules apply
Mtc = multiple diagnostic imaging rules apply
T = team surgeons permitted
T+ = team surgeons payable if medical necessity established with documentation
§ = indicates code is not covered by Medicare
GS = procedure must be performed under the general supervision of a physician
DS = procedure must be performed under the direct supervision of a physician
PS = procedure must be performed under the personal supervision of a physician
DRA = procedure subject to DRA limitation

Relative Value Units

CPT Code and Modifier		Description	Work RVU	Nonfacility Practice Expense RVU	Facility Practice Expense RVU	PLI RVU	Total Non-facility RVUs	Medicare Payment Nonfacility	Total Facility RVUs	Medicare Payment Facility	Global Period	Payment Policy Indicators
75809-26		Nonvascular shunt x-ray	0.47	0.17	0.17	0.04	0.68	$23.53	0.68	$23.53	XXX	A+
75809-TC		Nonvascular shunt x-ray	0.00	1.77	NA	0.01	1.78	$61.60	NA	NA	XXX	A+ PS
75810	CP	Vein x-ray spleen/liver	0.00	0.00	NA	0.00	0.00	$0.00	NA	NA	XXX	A+
75810-26		Vein x-ray spleen/liver	1.14	0.19	0.19	0.08	1.41	$48.79	1.41	$48.79	XXX	A+
75810-TC	CP	Vein x-ray spleen/liver	0.00	0.00	NA	0.00	0.00	$0.00	NA	NA	XXX	A+ PS
75820		Vein x-ray arm/leg	1.05	2.15	NA	0.10	3.30	$114.20	NA	NA	XXX	A+
75820-26		Vein x-ray arm/leg	1.05	0.33	0.33	0.09	1.47	$50.87	1.47	$50.87	XXX	A+
75820-TC		Vein x-ray arm/leg	0.00	1.82	NA	0.01	1.83	$63.33	NA	NA	XXX	A+ PS
75822		Vein x-ray arms/legs	1.48	2.39	NA	0.12	3.99	$138.08	NA	NA	XXX	A+
75822-26		Vein x-ray arms/legs	1.48	0.43	0.43	0.11	2.02	$69.90	2.02	$69.90	XXX	A+
75822-TC		Vein x-ray arms/legs	0.00	1.96	NA	0.01	1.97	$68.17	NA	NA	XXX	A+ PS
75825		Vein x-ray trunk	1.14	2.13	NA	0.13	3.40	$117.66	NA	NA	XXX	A+
75825-26		Vein x-ray trunk	1.14	0.29	0.29	0.12	1.55	$53.64	1.55	$53.64	XXX	A+
75825-TC		Vein x-ray trunk	0.00	1.84	NA	0.01	1.85	$64.02	NA	NA	XXX	A+ PS
75827		Vein x-ray chest	1.14	2.31	NA	0.13	3.58	$123.89	NA	NA	XXX	A+
75827-26		Vein x-ray chest	1.14	0.31	0.31	0.12	1.57	$54.33	1.57	$54.33	XXX	A+
75827-TC		Vein x-ray chest	0.00	2.00	NA	0.01	2.01	$69.56	NA	NA	XXX	A+ PS
75831		Vein x-ray kidney	1.14	2.32	NA	0.10	3.56	$123.20	NA	NA	XXX	A+
75831-26		Vein x-ray kidney	1.14	0.29	0.29	0.09	1.52	$52.60	1.52	$52.60	XXX	A+
75831-TC		Vein x-ray kidney	0.00	2.03	NA	0.01	2.04	$70.60	NA	NA	XXX	A+ PS
75833		Vein x-ray kidneys	1.49	2.72	NA	0.20	4.41	$152.61	NA	NA	XXX	A+
75833-26		Vein x-ray kidneys	1.49	0.40	0.40	0.18	2.07	$71.63	2.07	$71.63	XXX	A+
75833-TC		Vein x-ray kidneys	0.00	2.32	NA	0.02	2.34	$80.98	NA	NA	XXX	A+ PS
75840		Vein x-ray adrenal gland	1.14	2.64	NA	0.06	3.84	$132.89	NA	NA	XXX	A+
75840-26		Vein x-ray adrenal gland	1.14	0.41	0.41	0.05	1.60	$55.37	1.60	$55.37	XXX	A+
75840-TC		Vein x-ray adrenal gland	0.00	2.23	NA	0.01	2.24	$77.52	NA	NA	XXX	A+ PS
75842		Vein x-ray adrenal glands	1.49	3.13	NA	0.10	4.72	$163.34	NA	NA	XXX	A+
75842-26		Vein x-ray adrenal glands	1.49	0.54	0.54	0.08	2.11	$73.02	2.11	$73.02	XXX	A+
75842-TC		Vein x-ray adrenal glands	0.00	2.59	NA	0.02	2.61	$90.32	NA	NA	XXX	A+ PS
75860		Vein x-ray neck	1.14	2.52	NA	0.10	3.76	$130.12	NA	NA	XXX	A+
75860-26		Vein x-ray neck	1.14	0.35	0.35	0.09	1.58	$54.68	1.58	$54.68	XXX	A+
75860-TC		Vein x-ray neck	0.00	2.17	NA	0.01	2.18	$75.44	NA	NA	XXX	A+ PS
75870		Vein x-ray skull	1.14	3.49	NA	0.18	4.81	$166.46	NA	NA	XXX	A+

75870-26		Vein x-ray skull	1.14	0.43	0.43	0.17	1.74	$60.21	1.74	$60.21	XXX	A+
75870-TC		Vein x-ray skull	0.00	3.06	NA	0.01	3.07	$106.24	NA	NA	XXX	A+ PS
75872		Vein x-ray skull epidural	1.14	2.64	NA	0.06	3.84	$132.89	NA	NA	XXX	A+
75872-26		Vein x-ray skull epidural	1.14	0.41	0.41	0.05	1.60	$55.37	1.60	$55.37	XXX	A+
75872-TC		Vein x-ray skull epidural	0.00	2.23	NA	0.01	2.24	$77.52	NA	NA	XXX	A+ PS
75880		Vein x-ray eye socket	0.70	2.47	NA	0.05	3.22	$111.43	NA	NA	XXX	A+
75880-26		Vein x-ray eye socket	0.70	0.25	0.25	0.04	0.99	$34.26	0.99	$34.26	XXX	A+
75880-TC		Vein x-ray eye socket	0.00	2.22	NA	0.01	2.23	$77.17	NA	NA	XXX	A+ PS
75885		Vein x-ray liver w/hemodynam	1.44	2.50	NA	0.10	4.04	$139.81	NA	NA	XXX	A+
75885-26		Vein x-ray liver w/hemodynam	1.44	0.37	0.37	0.09	1.90	$65.75	1.90	$65.75	XXX	A+
75885-TC		Vein x-ray liver w/hemodynam	0.00	2.13	NA	0.01	2.14	$74.06	NA	NA	XXX	A+ PS
75887		Vein x-ray liver w/o hemodyn	1.44	2.57	NA	0.10	4.11	$142.23	NA	NA	XXX	A+
75887-26		Vein x-ray liver w/o hemodyn	1.44	0.40	0.40	0.09	1.93	$66.79	1.93	$66.79	XXX	A+
75887-TC		Vein x-ray liver w/o hemodyn	0.00	2.17	NA	0.01	2.18	$75.44	NA	NA	XXX	A+ PS
75889		Vein x-ray liver w/hemodynam	1.14	2.46	NA	0.08	3.68	$127.35	NA	NA	XXX	A+
75889-26		Vein x-ray liver w/hemodynam	1.14	0.31	0.31	0.07	1.52	$52.60	1.52	$52.60	XXX	A+
75889-TC		Vein x-ray liver w/hemodynam	0.00	2.15	NA	0.01	2.16	$74.75	NA	NA	XXX	A+ PS
75891		Vein x-ray liver	1.14	2.48	NA	0.08	3.70	$128.04	NA	NA	XXX	A+
75891-26		Vein x-ray liver	1.14	0.32	0.32	0.07	1.53	$52.95	1.53	$52.95	XXX	A+
75891-TC		Vein x-ray liver	0.00	2.16	NA	0.01	2.17	$75.10	NA	NA	XXX	A+ PS
75893		Venous sampling by catheter	0.54	2.49	NA	0.05	3.08	$106.59	NA	NA	XXX	A+
75893-26		Venous sampling by catheter	0.54	0.16	0.16	0.04	0.74	$25.61	0.74	$25.61	XXX	A+
75893-TC		Venous sampling by catheter	0.00	2.33	NA	0.01	2.34	$80.98	NA	NA	XXX	A+ PS
75894	CP	X-rays transcath therapy	0.00	0.00	NA	0.00	0.00	$0.00	NA	NA	XXX	A+
75894-26		X-rays transcath therapy	1.31	0.52	0.52	0.24	2.07	$71.63	2.07	$71.63	XXX	A+
75894-TC	CP	X-rays transcath therapy	0.00	0.00	NA	0.00	0.00	$0.00	NA	NA	XXX	A+ PS
75898	CP	Follow-up angiography	0.00	0.00	NA	0.00	0.00	$0.00	NA	NA	XXX	A+
75898-26		Follow-up angiography	1.65	0.66	0.66	0.31	2.62	$90.67	2.62	$90.67	XXX	A+

*Please note that these calculations are based on the Medicare 2022 Conversion Factor of $34.6062 and the DRA RVU cap rates at time of publication.

A = assistant-at-surgery restriction
A+ = assistant-at-surgery restriction unless medical necessity established with documentation
B = bilateral surgery adjustment applies
C = cosurgeons payable
C+ = cosurgeons payable if medical necessity established with documentation
CP = carriers may establish RVUs and payment amounts for these services, generally on an individual basis following review of documentation such as an operative report
M = multiple surgery adjustment applies
Me = multiple endoscopy rules may apply
M+ = multiple therapy rules apply
Mtc = multiple diagnostic imaging rules apply
T = team surgeons permitted
T+ = team surgeons payable if medical necessity established with documentation
§ = indicates code is not covered by Medicare
GS = procedure must be performed under the general supervision of a physician
DS = procedure must be performed under the direct supervision of a physician
PS = procedure must be performed under the personal supervision of a physician
DRA = procedure subject to DRA limitation

Relative Value Units

CPT Code and Modifier		Description	Work RVU	Nonfacility Practice Expense RVU	Facility Practice Expense RVU	PLI RVU	Total Non-facility RVUs	Medicare Payment Nonfacility	Total Facility RVUs	Medicare Payment Facility	Global Period	Payment Policy Indicators
75898-TC	CP	Follow-up angiography	0.00	0.00	NA	0.00	0.00	$0.00	NA	NA	XXX	A+
75901		Remove cva device obstruct	0.49	6.63	NA	0.06	7.18	$248.47	NA	NA	XXX	A+
75901-26		Remove cva device obstruct	0.49	0.15	0.15	0.04	0.68	$23.53	0.68	$23.53	XXX	A+
75901-TC		Remove cva device obstruct	0.00	6.48	NA	0.02	6.50	$224.94	NA	NA	XXX	A+ PS
75902		Remove cva lumen obstruct	0.39	2.37	NA	0.05	2.81	$97.24	NA	NA	XXX	A+
75902-26		Remove cva lumen obstruct	0.39	0.12	0.12	0.04	0.55	$19.03	0.55	$19.03	XXX	A+
75902-TC		Remove cva lumen obstruct	0.00	2.25	NA	0.01	2.26	$78.21	NA	NA	XXX	A+ PS
75956	CP	Xray endovasc thor ao repr	0.00	0.00	NA	0.00	0.00	$0.00	NA	NA	XXX	A+
75956-26		Xray endovasc thor ao repr	7.00	1.52	1.52	1.32	9.84	$340.53	9.84	$340.53	XXX	A+
75956-TC	CP	Xray endovasc thor ao repr	0.00	0.00	NA	0.00	0.00	$0.00	NA	NA	XXX	A+ PS
75957	CP	Xray endovasc thor ao repr	0.00	0.00	NA	0.00	0.00	$0.00	NA	NA	XXX	A+
75957-26		Xray endovasc thor ao repr	6.00	1.29	1.29	1.12	8.41	$291.04	8.41	$291.04	XXX	A+
75957-TC	CP	Xray endovasc thor ao repr	0.00	0.00	NA	0.00	0.00	$0.00	NA	NA	XXX	A+ PS
75958	CP	Xray place prox ext thor ao	0.00	0.00	NA	0.00	0.00	$0.00	NA	NA	XXX	A+
75958-26		Xray place prox ext thor ao	4.00	0.83	0.83	0.76	5.59	$193.45	5.59	$193.45	XXX	A+
75958-TC	CP	Xray place prox ext thor ao	0.00	0.00	NA	0.00	0.00	$0.00	NA	NA	XXX	A+ PS
75959	CP	Xray place dist ext thor ao	0.00	0.00	NA	0.00	0.00	$0.00	NA	NA	XXX	A+
75959-26		Xray place dist ext thor ao	3.50	0.77	0.77	0.65	4.92	$170.26	4.92	$170.26	XXX	A+
75959-TC	CP	Xray place dist ext thor ao	0.00	0.00	NA	0.00	0.00	$0.00	NA	NA	XXX	A+ PS
75970	CP	Vascular biopsy	0.00	0.00	NA	0.00	0.00	$0.00	NA	NA	XXX	A+
75970-26		Vascular biopsy	0.83	0.23	0.23	0.05	1.11	$38.41	1.11	$38.41	XXX	A+
75970-TC	CP	Vascular biopsy	0.00	0.00	NA	0.00	0.00	$0.00	NA	NA	XXX	A+ PS
75984		Xray control catheter change	0.83	2.03	NA	0.05	2.91	$100.70	NA	NA	XXX	A+
75984-26		Xray control catheter change	0.83	0.24	0.24	0.04	1.11	$38.41	1.11	$38.41	XXX	A+
75984-TC		Xray control catheter change	0.00	1.79	NA	0.01	1.80	$62.29	NA	NA	XXX	A+ PS
75989		Abscess drainage under x-ray	1.19	2.14	NA	0.09	3.42	$118.35	NA	NA	XXX	A+
75989-26		Abscess drainage under x-ray	1.19	0.37	0.37	0.08	1.64	$56.75	1.64	$56.75	XXX	A+
75989-TC		Abscess drainage under x-ray	0.00	1.77	NA	0.01	1.78	$61.60	NA	NA	XXX	A+ PS
76000		Fluoroscopy <1 hr phys/qhp	0.30	0.93	NA	0.05	1.28	$44.30	NA	NA	XXX	A+
76000-26		Fluoroscopy <1 hr phys/qhp	0.30	0.11	0.11	0.04	0.45	$15.57	0.45	$15.57	XXX	A+
76000-TC		Fluoroscopy <1 hr phys/qhp	0.00	0.82	NA	0.01	0.83	$28.72	NA	NA	XXX	A+ PS
76010		X-ray nose to rectum	0.18	0.69	NA	0.02	0.89	$30.80	NA	NA	XXX	A+
76010-26		X-ray nose to rectum	0.18	0.07	0.07	0.01	0.26	$9.00	0.26	$9.00	XXX	A+

76010-TC		X-ray nose to rectum	0.00	0.62	NA	0.01	0.63	$21.80	NA	NA	XXX	A+ GS
76080		X-ray exam of fistula	0.54	1.22	NA	0.05	1.81	$62.64	NA	NA	XXX	A+
76080-26		X-ray exam of fistula	0.54	0.16	0.16	0.04	0.74	$25.61	0.74	$25.61	XXX	A+
76080-TC		X-ray exam of fistula	0.00	1.06	NA	0.01	1.07	$37.03	NA	NA	XXX	A+ PS
76098		X-ray exam surgical specimen	0.31	0.87	NA	0.03	1.21	$41.87	NA	NA	XXX	A+
76098-26		X-ray exam surgical specimen	0.31	0.12	0.12	0.02	0.45	$15.57	0.45	$15.57	XXX	A+
76098-TC		X-ray exam surgical specimen	0.00	0.75	NA	0.01	0.76	$26.30	NA	NA	XXX	A+ GS
76100		X-ray exam of body section	0.58	2.06	NA	0.05	2.69	$93.09	NA	NA	XXX	A+
76100-26		X-ray exam of body section	0.58	0.21	0.21	0.04	0.83	$28.72	0.83	$28.72	XXX	A+
76100-TC		X-ray exam of body section	0.00	1.85	NA	0.01	1.86	$64.37	NA	NA	XXX	A+ GS
76120		Cine/video x-rays	0.38	3.05	NA	0.05	3.48	$120.43	NA	NA	XXX	A+
76120-26		Cine/video x-rays	0.38	0.15	0.15	0.04	0.57	$19.73	0.57	$19.73	XXX	A+
76120-TC		Cine/video x-rays	0.00	2.90	NA	0.01	2.91	$100.70	NA	NA	XXX	A+ DS
76125	CP	Cine/video x-rays add-on	0.00	0.00	NA	0.00	0.00	$0.00	NA	NA	ZZZ	A+
76125-26		Cine/video x-rays add-on	0.27	0.10	0.10	0.01	0.38	$13.15	0.38	$13.15	ZZZ	A+
76125-TC	CP	Cine/video x-rays add-on	0.00	0.00	NA	0.00	0.00	$0.00	NA	NA	ZZZ	A+ DS
76145		Med physic dos eval rad exps	0.00	23.50	NA	0.57	24.07	$832.97	NA	NA	XXX	A+
76376		3d render w/intrp postproces	0.20	0.46	NA	0.02	0.68	$23.53	NA	NA	XXX	A+
76376-26		3d render w/intrp postproces	0.20	0.07	0.07	0.01	0.28	$9.69	0.28	$9.69	XXX	A+
76376-TC		3d render w/intrp postproces	0.00	0.39	NA	0.01	0.40	$13.84	NA	NA	XXX	A+ GS
76377		3d render w/intrp postproces	0.79	1.30	NA	0.05	2.14	$74.06	NA	NA	XXX	A+
76377-26		3d render w/intrp postproces	0.79	0.29	0.29	0.04	1.12	$38.76	1.12	$38.76	XXX	A+
76377-TC		3d render w/intrp postproces	0.00	1.01	NA	0.01	1.02	$35.30	NA	NA	XXX	A+ PS
76380		Cat scan follow-up study	0.98	3.06	NA	0.06	4.10	$129.43	NA	NA	XXX	A+ DRA
76380-26		Cat scan follow-up study	0.98	0.32	0.32	0.05	1.35	$46.72	1.35	$46.72	XXX	A+
76380-TC		Cat scan follow-up study	0.00	2.74	NA	0.01	2.75	$82.71	NA	NA	XXX	A+ GS DRA
76390	§	Mr spectroscopy	1.40	10.11	NA	0.09	11.60	$401.43	NA	NA	XXX	
76390-26	§	Mr spectroscopy	1.40	0.54	0.54	0.07	2.01	$69.56	2.01	$69.56	XXX	

*Please note that these calculations are based on the Medicare 2022 Conversion Factor of $34.6062 and the DRA RVU cap rates at time of publication.

A = assistant-at-surgery restriction
A+ = assistant-at-surgery restriction unless medical necessity established with documentation
B = bilateral surgery adjustment applies
C = cosurgeons payable
C+ = cosurgeons payable if medical necessity established with documentation
CP = carriers may establish RVUs and payment amounts for these services, generally on an individual basis following review of documentation such as an operative report
M = multiple surgery adjustment applies
Me = multiple endoscopy rules may apply
M+ = multiple therapy rules apply
Mtc = multiple diagnostic imaging rules apply
T = team surgeons permitted
T+ = team surgeons payable if medical necessity established with documentation
§ = indicates code is not covered by Medicare
GS = procedure must be performed under the general supervision of a physician
DS = procedure must be performed under the direct supervision of a physician
PS = procedure must be performed under the personal supervision of a physician
DRA = procedure subject to DRA limitation

Relative Value Units

CPT Code and Modifier		Description	Work RVU	Nonfacility Practice Expense RVU	Facility Practice Expense RVU	PLI RVU	Total Non-facility RVUs	Medicare Payment Nonfacility	Total Facility RVUs	Medicare Payment Facility	Global Period	Payment Policy Indicators
76390-TC	§	Mr spectroscopy	0.00	9.57	NA	0.02	9.59	$331.87	NA	NA	XXX	GS
76391		Mr elastography	1.10	5.20	NA	0.07	6.37	$220.44	NA	NA	XXX	A+ Mtc
76391-26		Mr elastography	1.10	0.40	0.40	0.05	1.55	$53.64	1.55	$53.64	XXX	A+ Mtc
76391-TC		Mr elastography	0.00	4.80	NA	0.02	4.82	$166.80	NA	NA	XXX	A+ Mtc DS
76496	CP	Fluoroscopic procedure	0.00	0.00	NA	0.00	0.00	$0.00	NA	NA	XXX	A+ PS
76496-26	CP	Fluoroscopic procedure	0.00	0.00	0.00	0.00	0.00	$0.00	0.00	$0.00	XXX	A+
76496-TC	CP	Fluoroscopic procedure	0.00	0.00	NA	0.00	0.00	$0.00	NA	NA	XXX	A+ PS
76497	CP	Ct procedure	0.00	0.00	NA	0.00	0.00	$0.00	NA	NA	XXX	A+ DS
76497-26	CP	Ct procedure	0.00	0.00	0.00	0.00	0.00	$0.00	0.00	$0.00	XXX	A+
76497-TC	CP	Ct procedure	0.00	0.00	NA	0.00	0.00	$0.00	NA	NA	XXX	A+ DS
76498	CP	Mri procedure	0.00	0.00	NA	0.00	0.00	$0.00	NA	NA	XXX	A+ DS
76498-26	CP	Mri procedure	0.00	0.00	0.00	0.00	0.00	$0.00	0.00	$0.00	XXX	A+
76498-TC	CP	Mri procedure	0.00	0.00	NA	0.00	0.00	$0.00	NA	NA	XXX	A+ DS
76499	CP	Radiographic procedure	0.00	0.00	NA	0.00	0.00	$0.00	NA	NA	XXX	A+
76499-26	CP	Radiographic procedure	0.00	0.00	0.00	0.00	0.00	$0.00	0.00	$0.00	XXX	A+
76499-TC	CP	Radiographic procedure	0.00	0.00	NA	0.00	0.00	$0.00	NA	NA	XXX	A+
76506		Echo exam of head	0.63	2.78	NA	0.06	3.47	$120.08	NA	NA	XXX	A+
76506-26		Echo exam of head	0.63	0.23	0.23	0.05	0.91	$31.49	0.91	$31.49	XXX	A+
76506-TC		Echo exam of head	0.00	2.55	NA	0.01	2.56	$88.59	NA	NA	XXX	A+ GS
76510		Oph us dx b-scan&quan a-scan	0.70	1.33	NA	0.02	2.05	$70.94	NA	NA	XXX	A+
76510-26		Oph us dx b-scan&quan a-scan	0.70	0.43	0.43	0.01	1.14	$39.45	1.14	$39.45	XXX	A+
76510-TC		Oph us dx b-scan&quan a-scan	0.00	0.90	NA	0.01	0.91	$31.49	NA	NA	XXX	A+ DS
76511		Oph us dx quan a-scan only	0.64	1.01	NA	0.02	1.67	$57.79	NA	NA	XXX	A+
76511-26		Oph us dx quan a-scan only	0.64	0.38	0.38	0.01	1.03	$35.64	1.03	$35.64	XXX	A+
76511-TC		Oph us dx quan a-scan only	0.00	0.63	NA	0.01	0.64	$22.15	NA	NA	XXX	A+ DS
76512		Oph us dx b-scan	0.56	0.83	NA	0.02	1.41	$48.79	NA	NA	XXX	A+
76512-26		Oph us dx b-scan	0.56	0.32	0.32	0.01	0.89	$30.80	0.89	$30.80	XXX	A+
76512-TC		Oph us dx b-scan	0.00	0.51	NA	0.01	0.52	$18.00	NA	NA	XXX	A+ DS
76513		Oph us dx ant sgm us uni/bi	0.60	1.62	NA	0.02	2.24	$77.52	NA	NA	XXX	A+
76513-26		Oph us dx ant sgm us uni/bi	0.60	0.33	0.33	0.01	0.94	$32.53	0.94	$32.53	XXX	A+
76513-TC		Oph us dx ant sgm us uni/bi	0.00	1.29	NA	0.01	1.30	$44.99	NA	NA	XXX	A+ DS
76514		Echo exam of eye thickness	0.14	0.18	NA	0.02	0.34	$11.77	NA	NA	XXX	A+
76514-26		Echo exam of eye thickness	0.14	0.08	0.08	0.01	0.23	$7.96	0.23	$7.96	XXX	A+

76514-TC	Echo exam of eye thickness	0.00	0.10	NA	0.01	0.11	$3.81	NA	NA	XXX	A+ GS
76516	Echo exam of eye	0.40	0.95	NA	0.02	1.37	$47.41	NA	NA	XXX	A+
76516-26	Echo exam of eye	0.40	0.24	0.24	0.01	0.65	$22.49	0.65	$22.49	XXX	A+
76516-TC	Echo exam of eye	0.00	0.71	NA	0.01	0.72	$24.92	NA	NA	XXX	A+ GS
76519	Echo exam of eye	0.54	1.42	NA	0.02	1.98	$68.52	NA	NA	XXX	A+
76519-26	Echo exam of eye	0.54	0.33	0.33	0.01	0.88	$30.45	0.88	$30.45	XXX	A+
76519-TC	Echo exam of eye	0.00	1.09	NA	0.01	1.10	$38.07	NA	NA	XXX	A+ GS
76529	Echo exam of eye	0.57	1.95	NA	0.02	2.54	$87.90	NA	NA	XXX	A+
76529-26	Echo exam of eye	0.57	0.35	0.35	0.01	0.93	$32.18	0.93	$32.18	XXX	A+
76529-TC	Echo exam of eye	0.00	1.60	NA	0.01	1.61	$55.72	NA	NA	XXX	A+ GS
76536	Us exam of head and neck	0.56	2.76	NA	0.05	3.37	$116.62	NA	NA	XXX	A+
76536-26	Us exam of head and neck	0.56	0.21	0.21	0.04	0.81	$28.03	0.81	$28.03	XXX	A+
76536-TC	Us exam of head and neck	0.00	2.55	NA	0.01	2.56	$88.59	NA	NA	XXX	A+ GS
76604	Us exam chest	0.59	1.10	NA	0.05	1.74	$60.21	NA	NA	XXX	A+ Mtc
76604-26	Us exam chest	0.59	0.19	0.19	0.04	0.82	$28.38	0.82	$28.38	XXX	A+ Mtc
76604-TC	Us exam chest	0.00	0.91	NA	0.01	0.92	$31.84	NA	NA	XXX	A+ Mtc GS
76641	Ultrasound breast complete	0.73	2.32	NA	0.05	3.10	$107.28	NA	NA	XXX	A+ B
76641-26	Ultrasound breast complete	0.73	0.26	0.26	0.04	1.03	$35.64	1.03	$35.64	XXX	A+ B
76641-TC	Ultrasound breast complete	0.00	2.06	NA	0.01	2.07	$71.63	NA	NA	XXX	A+ B GS
76642	Ultrasound breast limited	0.68	1.81	NA	0.05	2.54	$87.90	NA	NA	XXX	A+ B
76642-26	Ultrasound breast limited	0.68	0.24	0.24	0.04	0.96	$33.22	0.96	$33.22	XXX	A+ B
76642-TC	Ultrasound breast limited	0.00	1.57	NA	0.01	1.58	$54.68	NA	NA	XXX	A+ B GS
76700	Us exam abdom complete	0.81	2.67	NA	0.05	3.53	$122.16	NA	NA	XXX	A+ Mtc
76700-26	Us exam abdom complete	0.81	0.29	0.29	0.04	1.14	$39.45	1.14	$39.45	XXX	A+ Mtc
76700-TC	Us exam abdom complete	0.00	2.38	NA	0.01	2.39	$82.71	NA	NA	XXX	A+ Mtc GS
76705	Echo exam of abdomen	0.59	2.00	NA	0.05	2.64	$91.36	NA	NA	XXX	A+ Mtc
76705-26	Echo exam of abdomen	0.59	0.21	0.21	0.04	0.84	$29.07	0.84	$29.07	XXX	A+ Mtc
76705-TC	Echo exam of abdomen	0.00	1.79	NA	0.01	1.80	$62.29	NA	NA	XXX	A+ Mtc GS

*Please note that these calculations are based on the Medicare 2022 Conversion Factor of $34.6062 and the DRA RVU cap rates at time of publication.

A = assistant-at-surgery restriction
A+ = assistant-at-surgery restriction unless medical necessity established with documentation
B = bilateral surgery adjustment applies
C = cosurgeons payable

C+ = cosurgeons payable if medical necessity established with documentation
CP = carriers may establish RVUs and payment amounts for these services, generally on an individual basis following review of documentation such as an operative report
M = multiple surgery adjustment applies
Me = multiple endoscopy rules may apply

M+ = multiple therapy rules apply
Mtc = multiple diagnostic imaging rules apply
T = team surgeons permitted
T+ = team surgeons payable if medical necessity established with documentation
§ = indicates code is not covered by Medicare

GS = procedure must be performed under the general supervision of a physician
DS = procedure must be performed under the direct supervision of a physician
PS = procedure must be performed under the personal supervision of a physician
DRA = procedure subject to DRA limitation

Relative Value Units

CPT Code and Modifier	Description	Work RVU	Nonfacility Practice Expense RVU	Facility Practice Expense RVU	PLI RVU	Total Non-facility RVUs	Medicare Payment Nonfacility	Total Facility RVUs	Medicare Payment Facility	Global Period	Payment Policy Indicators
76706	Us abdl aorta screen aaa	0.55	2.61	NA	0.05	3.21	$111.09	NA	NA	XXX	A+
76706-26	Us abdl aorta screen aaa	0.55	0.19	0.19	0.04	0.78	$26.99	0.78	$26.99	XXX	A+
76706-TC	Us abdl aorta screen aaa	0.00	2.42	NA	0.01	2.43	$84.09	NA	NA	XXX	A+
76770	Us exam abdo back wall comp	0.74	2.48	NA	0.05	3.27	$113.16	NA	NA	XXX	A+ Mtc
76770-26	Us exam abdo back wall comp	0.74	0.26	0.26	0.04	1.04	$35.99	1.04	$35.99	XXX	A+ Mtc
76770-TC	Us exam abdo back wall comp	0.00	2.22	NA	0.01	2.23	$77.17	NA	NA	XXX	A+ Mtc GS
76775	Us exam abdo back wall lim	0.58	1.10	NA	0.05	1.73	$59.87	NA	NA	XXX	A+ Mtc
76775-26	Us exam abdo back wall lim	0.58	0.20	0.20	0.04	0.82	$28.38	0.82	$28.38	XXX	A+ Mtc
76775-TC	Us exam abdo back wall lim	0.00	0.90	NA	0.01	0.91	$31.49	NA	NA	XXX	A+ Mtc GS
76776	Us exam k transpl w/doppler	0.76	3.67	NA	0.06	4.49	$155.38	NA	NA	XXX	A+ Mtc
76776-26	Us exam k transpl w/doppler	0.76	0.27	0.27	0.04	1.07	$37.03	1.07	$37.03	XXX	A+ Mtc
76776-TC	Us exam k transpl w/doppler	0.00	3.40	NA	0.02	3.42	$118.35	NA	NA	XXX	A+ Mtc GS
76800	Us exam spinal canal	1.13	3.07	NA	0.18	4.38	$151.58	NA	NA	XXX	A+
76800-26	Us exam spinal canal	1.13	0.45	0.45	0.17	1.75	$60.56	1.75	$60.56	XXX	A+
76800-TC	Us exam spinal canal	0.00	2.62	NA	0.01	2.63	$91.01	NA	NA	XXX	A+ GS
76801	Ob us < 14 wks single fetus	0.99	2.48	NA	0.05	3.52	$121.81	NA	NA	XXX	A+ GS
76801-26	Ob us < 14 wks single fetus	0.99	0.36	0.36	0.04	1.39	$48.10	1.39	$48.10	XXX	A+
76801-TC	Ob us < 14 wks single fetus	0.00	2.12	NA	0.01	2.13	$73.71	NA	NA	XXX	A+ GS
76802	Ob us < 14 wks addl fetus	0.83	0.95	NA	0.04	1.82	$62.98	NA	NA	ZZZ	A+ GS
76802-26	Ob us < 14 wks addl fetus	0.83	0.31	0.31	0.04	1.18	$40.84	1.18	$40.84	ZZZ	A+
76802-TC	Ob us < 14 wks addl fetus	0.00	0.64	NA	0.00	0.64	$22.15	NA	NA	ZZZ	A+ GS
76805	Ob us >= 14 wks sngl fetus	0.99	3.01	NA	0.05	4.05	$140.16	NA	NA	XXX	A+
76805-26	Ob us >= 14 wks sngl fetus	0.99	0.37	0.37	0.04	1.40	$48.45	1.40	$48.45	XXX	A+
76805-TC	Ob us >= 14 wks sngl fetus	0.00	2.64	NA	0.01	2.65	$91.71	NA	NA	XXX	A+ GS
76810	Ob us >= 14 wks addl fetus	0.98	1.60	NA	0.05	2.63	$91.01	NA	NA	ZZZ	A+
76810-26	Ob us >= 14 wks addl fetus	0.98	0.36	0.36	0.04	1.38	$47.76	1.38	$47.76	ZZZ	A+
76810-TC	Ob us >= 14 wks addl fetus	0.00	1.24	NA	0.01	1.25	$43.26	NA	NA	ZZZ	A+ GS
76811	Ob us detailed sngl fetus	1.90	3.18	NA	0.11	5.19	$179.61	NA	NA	XXX	A+ GS
76811-26	Ob us detailed sngl fetus	1.90	0.72	0.72	0.07	2.69	$93.09	2.69	$93.09	XXX	A+
76811-TC	Ob us detailed sngl fetus	0.00	2.46	NA	0.04	2.50	$86.52	NA	NA	XXX	A+ GS
76812	Ob us detailed addl fetus	1.78	3.91	NA	0.09	5.78	$200.02	NA	NA	ZZZ	A+ GS
76812-26	Ob us detailed addl fetus	1.78	0.68	0.68	0.07	2.53	$87.55	2.53	$87.55	ZZZ	A+
76812-TC	Ob us detailed addl fetus	0.00	3.23	NA	0.02	3.25	$112.47	NA	NA	ZZZ	A+ GS

76813	Ob us nuchal meas 1 gest	1.18	2.30	NA	0.05	3.53	$122.16	NA	NA	XXX	A+ GS
76813-26	Ob us nuchal meas 1 gest	1.18	0.45	0.45	0.04	1.67	$57.79	1.67	$57.79	XXX	A+
76813-TC	Ob us nuchal meas 1 gest	0.00	1.85	NA	0.01	1.86	$64.37	NA	NA	XXX	A+ GS
76814	Ob us nuchal meas add-on	0.99	1.22	NA	0.05	2.26	$78.21	NA	NA	XXX	A+ GS
76814-26	Ob us nuchal meas add-on	0.99	0.38	0.38	0.04	1.41	$48.79	1.41	$48.79	XXX	A+
76814-TC	Ob us nuchal meas add-on	0.00	0.84	NA	0.01	0.85	$29.42	NA	NA	XXX	A+ GS
76815	Ob us limited fetus(s)	0.65	1.74	NA	0.05	2.44	$84.44	NA	NA	XXX	A+
76815-26	Ob us limited fetus(s)	0.65	0.23	0.23	0.04	0.92	$31.84	0.92	$31.84	XXX	A+
76815-TC	Ob us limited fetus(s)	0.00	1.51	NA	0.01	1.52	$52.60	NA	NA	XXX	A+ GS
76816	Ob us follow-up per fetus	0.85	2.39	NA	0.05	3.29	$113.85	NA	NA	XXX	A+
76816-26	Ob us follow-up per fetus	0.85	0.32	0.32	0.04	1.21	$41.87	1.21	$41.87	XXX	A+
76816-TC	Ob us follow-up per fetus	0.00	2.07	NA	0.01	2.08	$71.98	NA	NA	XXX	A+ GS
76817	Transvaginal us obstetric	0.75	1.99	NA	0.05	2.79	$96.55	NA	NA	XXX	A+ GS
76817-26	Transvaginal us obstetric	0.75	0.28	0.28	0.04	1.07	$37.03	1.07	$37.03	XXX	A+
76817-TC	Transvaginal us obstetric	0.00	1.71	NA	0.01	1.72	$59.52	NA	NA	XXX	A+ GS
76818	Fetal biophys profile w/nst	1.05	2.31	NA	0.06	3.42	$118.35	NA	NA	XXX	A+
76818-26	Fetal biophys profile w/nst	1.05	0.40	0.40	0.04	1.49	$51.56	1.49	$51.56	XXX	A+
76818-TC	Fetal biophys profile w/nst	0.00	1.91	NA	0.02	1.93	$66.79	NA	NA	XXX	A+ GS
76819	Fetal biophys profil w/o nst	0.77	1.68	NA	0.05	2.50	$86.52	NA	NA	XXX	A+
76819-26	Fetal biophys profil w/o nst	0.77	0.29	0.29	0.04	1.10	$38.07	1.10	$38.07	XXX	A+
76819-TC	Fetal biophys profil w/o nst	0.00	1.39	NA	0.01	1.40	$48.45	NA	NA	XXX	A+ GS
76820	Umbilical artery echo	0.50	0.82	NA	0.03	1.35	$46.72	NA	NA	XXX	A+
76820-26	Umbilical artery echo	0.50	0.19	0.19	0.02	0.71	$24.57	0.71	$24.57	XXX	A+
76820-TC	Umbilical artery echo	0.00	0.63	NA	0.01	0.64	$22.15	NA	NA	XXX	A+ GS
76821	Middle cerebral artery echo	0.70	1.92	NA	0.03	2.65	$91.71	NA	NA	XXX	A+
76821-26	Middle cerebral artery echo	0.70	0.27	0.27	0.02	0.99	$34.26	0.99	$34.26	XXX	A+
76821-TC	Middle cerebral artery echo	0.00	1.65	NA	0.01	1.66	$57.45	NA	NA	XXX	A+ GS
76825	Echo exam of fetal heart	1.67	6.16	NA	0.09	7.92	$274.08	NA	NA	XXX	A+

*Please note that these calculations are based on the Medicare 2022 Conversion Factor of $34.6062 and the DRA RVU cap rates at time of publication.

A = assistant-at-surgery restriction
A+ = assistant-at-surgery restriction unless medical necessity established with documentation
B = bilateral surgery adjustment applies
C = cosurgeons payable
C+ = cosurgeons payable if medical necessity established with documentation
CP = carriers may establish RVUs and payment amounts for these services, generally on an individual basis following review of documentation such as an operative report
M = multiple surgery adjustment applies
Me = multiple endoscopy rules may apply
M+ = multiple therapy rules apply
Mtc = multiple diagnostic imaging rules apply
T = team surgeons permitted
T+ = team surgeons payable if medical necessity established with documentation
§ = indicates code is not covered by Medicare
GS = procedure must be performed under the general supervision of a physician
DS = procedure must be performed under the direct supervision of a physician
PS = procedure must be performed under the personal supervision of a physician
DRA = procedure subject to DRA limitation

Relative Value Units

CPT Code and Modifier	Description	Work RVU	Nonfacility Practice Expense RVU	Facility Practice Expense RVU	PLI RVU	Total Non-facility RVUs	Medicare Payment Nonfacility	Total Facility RVUs	Medicare Payment Facility	Global Period	Payment Policy Indicators
76825-26	Echo exam of fetal heart	1.67	0.62	0.62	0.05	2.34	$80.98	2.34	$80.98	XXX	A+
76825-TC	Echo exam of fetal heart	0.00	5.54	NA	0.04	5.58	$193.10	NA	NA	XXX	A+ GS
76826	Echo exam of fetal heart	0.83	3.88	NA	0.06	4.77	$165.07	NA	NA	XXX	A+
76826-26	Echo exam of fetal heart	0.83	0.31	0.31	0.04	1.18	$40.84	1.18	$40.84	XXX	A+
76826-TC	Echo exam of fetal heart	0.00	3.57	NA	0.02	3.59	$124.24	NA	NA	XXX	A+ GS
76827	Echo exam of fetal heart	0.58	1.50	NA	0.03	2.11	$73.02	NA	NA	XXX	A+
76827-26	Echo exam of fetal heart	0.58	0.21	0.21	0.02	0.81	$28.03	0.81	$28.03	XXX	A+
76827-TC	Echo exam of fetal heart	0.00	1.29	NA	0.01	1.30	$44.99	NA	NA	XXX	A+ GS
76828	Echo exam of fetal heart	0.56	0.89	NA	0.03	1.48	$51.22	NA	NA	XXX	A+
76828-26	Echo exam of fetal heart	0.56	0.21	0.21	0.02	0.79	$27.34	0.79	$27.34	XXX	A+
76828-TC	Echo exam of fetal heart	0.00	0.68	NA	0.01	0.69	$23.88	NA	NA	XXX	A+ GS
76830	Transvaginal us non-ob	0.69	2.87	NA	0.05	3.61	$124.93	NA	NA	XXX	A+
76830-26	Transvaginal us non-ob	0.69	0.25	0.25	0.04	0.98	$33.91	0.98	$33.91	XXX	A+
76830-TC	Transvaginal us non-ob	0.00	2.62	NA	0.01	2.63	$91.01	NA	NA	XXX	A+ GS
76831	Echo exam uterus	0.72	2.74	NA	0.05	3.51	$121.47	NA	NA	XXX	A+ Mtc
76831-26	Echo exam uterus	0.72	0.27	0.27	0.04	1.03	$35.64	1.03	$35.64	XXX	A+ Mtc
76831-TC	Echo exam uterus	0.00	2.47	NA	0.01	2.48	$85.82	NA	NA	XXX	A+ Mtc PS
76856	Us exam pelvic complete	0.69	2.45	NA	0.05	3.19	$110.39	NA	NA	XXX	A+ Mtc
76856-26	Us exam pelvic complete	0.69	0.25	0.25	0.04	0.98	$33.91	0.98	$33.91	XXX	A+ Mtc
76856-TC	Us exam pelvic complete	0.00	2.20	NA	0.01	2.21	$76.48	NA	NA	XXX	A+ Mtc GS
76857	Us exam pelvic limited	0.50	0.89	NA	0.03	1.42	$49.14	NA	NA	XXX	A+ Mtc
76857-26	Us exam pelvic limited	0.50	0.17	0.17	0.02	0.69	$23.88	0.69	$23.88	XXX	A+ Mtc
76857-TC	Us exam pelvic limited	0.00	0.72	NA	0.01	0.73	$25.26	NA	NA	XXX	A+ Mtc GS
76870	Us exam scrotum	0.64	2.35	NA	0.05	3.04	$105.20	NA	NA	XXX	A+ Mtc
76870-26	Us exam scrotum	0.64	0.23	0.23	0.04	0.91	$31.49	0.91	$31.49	XXX	A+ Mtc
76870-TC	Us exam scrotum	0.00	2.12	NA	0.01	2.13	$73.71	NA	NA	XXX	A+ Mtc GS
76872	Us transrectal	0.69	5.38	NA	0.04	6.11	$143.96	NA	NA	XXX	A+ DRA
76872-26	Us transrectal	0.69	0.24	0.24	0.02	0.95	$32.88	0.95	$32.88	XXX	A+
76872-TC	Us transrectal	0.00	5.14	NA	0.02	5.16	$111.09	NA	NA	XXX	A+ GS DRA
76873	Echograp trans r pros study	1.55	3.57	NA	0.06	5.18	$179.26	NA	NA	XXX	A+
76873-26	Echograp trans r pros study	1.55	0.63	0.63	0.05	2.23	$77.17	2.23	$77.17	XXX	A+
76873-TC	Echograp trans r pros study	0.00	2.94	NA	0.01	2.95	$102.09	NA	NA	XXX	A+ DS
76881	Us compl joint r-t w/img	0.63	1.08	NA	0.03	1.74	$60.21	NA	NA	XXX	A+

76881-26		Us compl joint r-t w/img	0.63	0.24	0.24	0.02	0.89	$30.80	0.89	$30.80	XXX	A+
76881-TC		Us compl joint r-t w/img	0.00	0.84	NA	0.01	0.85	$29.42	NA	NA	XXX	A+ GS
76882		Us lmtd jt/nonvasc xtr strux	0.49	1.15	NA	0.03	1.67	$57.79	NA	NA	XXX	A+
76882-26		Us lmtd jt/nonvasc xtr strux	0.49	0.17	0.17	0.02	0.68	$23.53	0.68	$23.53	XXX	A+
76882-TC		Us lmtd jt/nonvasc xtr strux	0.00	0.98	NA	0.01	0.99	$34.26	NA	NA	XXX	A+ GS
76885		Us exam infant hips dynamic	0.74	3.34	NA	0.06	4.14	$119.05	NA	NA	XXX	A+ DRA
76885-26		Us exam infant hips dynamic	0.74	0.27	0.27	0.04	1.05	$36.34	1.05	$36.34	XXX	A+
76885-TC		Us exam infant hips dynamic	0.00	3.07	NA	0.02	3.09	$82.71	NA	NA	XXX	A+ GS DRA
76886		Us exam infant hips static	0.62	2.36	NA	0.05	3.03	$104.86	NA	NA	XXX	A+
76886-26		Us exam infant hips static	0.62	0.22	0.22	0.04	0.88	$30.45	0.88	$30.45	XXX	A+
76886-TC		Us exam infant hips static	0.00	2.14	NA	0.01	2.15	$74.40	NA	NA	XXX	A+ GS
76932	CP	Echo guide for heart biopsy	0.00	0.00	NA	0.00	0.00	$0.00	NA	NA	YYY	A+
76932-26		Echo guide for heart biopsy	0.67	0.29	0.29	0.09	1.05	$36.34	1.05	$36.34	XXX	A+
76932-TC	CP	Echo guide for heart biopsy	0.00	0.00	NA	0.00	0.00	$0.00	NA	NA	YYY	A+ PS
76936		Echo guide for artery repair	1.99	5.59	NA	0.26	7.84	$271.31	NA	NA	XXX	A+
76936-26		Echo guide for artery repair	1.99	0.57	0.57	0.22	2.78	$96.21	2.78	$96.21	XXX	A+
76936-TC		Echo guide for artery repair	0.00	5.02	NA	0.04	5.06	$175.11	NA	NA	XXX	A+ PS
76937		Us guide vascular access	0.30	0.85	NA	0.02	1.17	$40.49	NA	NA	ZZZ	A+
76937-26		Us guide vascular access	0.30	0.08	0.08	0.02	0.40	$13.84	0.40	$13.84	ZZZ	A+
76937-TC		Us guide vascular access	0.00	0.77	NA	0.00	0.77	$26.65	NA	NA	ZZZ	A+ PS
76940	CP	Us guide tissue ablation	0.00	0.00	NA	0.00	0.00	$0.00	NA	NA	YYY	A+
76940-26		Us guide tissue ablation	2.00	0.68	0.68	0.25	2.93	$101.40	2.93	$101.40	XXX	A+
76940-TC	CP	Us guide tissue ablation	0.00	0.00	NA	0.00	0.00	$0.00	NA	NA	YYY	A+ PS
76941	CP	Echo guide for transfusion	0.00	0.00	NA	0.00	0.00	$0.00	NA	NA	XXX	A+
76941-26		Echo guide for transfusion	1.34	0.51	0.51	0.04	1.89	$65.41	1.89	$65.41	XXX	A+
76941-TC	CP	Echo guide for transfusion	0.00	0.00	NA	0.00	0.00	$0.00	NA	NA	XXX	A+ PS
76942		Echo guide for biopsy	0.67	1.00	NA	0.05	1.72	$59.52	NA	NA	XXX	A+
76942-26		Echo guide for biopsy	0.67	0.19	0.19	0.04	0.90	$31.15	0.90	$31.15	XXX	A+

*Please note that these calculations are based on the Medicare 2022 Conversion Factor of $34.6062 and the DRA RVU cap rates at time of publication.

A = assistant-at-surgery restriction

A+ = assistant-at-surgery restriction unless medical necessity established with documentation

B = bilateral surgery adjustment applies

C = cosurgeons payable

C+ = cosurgeons payable if medical necessity established with documentation

CP = carriers may establish RVUs and payment amounts for these services, generally on an individual basis following review of documentation such as an operative report

M = multiple surgery adjustment applies

Me = multiple endoscopy rules may apply

M+ = multiple therapy rules apply

Mtc = multiple diagnostic imaging rules apply

T = team surgeons permitted

T+ = team surgeons payable if medical necessity established with documentation

§ = indicates code is not covered by Medicare

GS = procedure must be performed under the general supervision of a physician

DS = procedure must be performed under the direct supervision of a physician

PS = procedure must be performed under the personal supervision of a physician

DRA = procedure subject to DRA limitation

Relative Value Units

CPT Code and Modifier		Description	Work RVU	Nonfacility Practice Expense RVU	Facility Practice Expense RVU	PLI RVU	Total Non-facility RVUs	Medicare Payment Nonfacility	Total Facility RVUs	Medicare Payment Facility	Global Period	Payment Policy Indicators
76942-TC		Echo guide for biopsy	0.00	0.81	NA	0.01	0.82	$28.38	NA	NA	XXX	A+ PS
76945	CP	Echo guide villus sampling	0.00	0.00	NA	0.00	0.00	$0.00	NA	NA	XXX	A+
76945-26		Echo guide villus sampling	0.67	0.25	0.25	0.02	0.94	$32.53	0.94	$32.53	XXX	A+
76945-TC	CP	Echo guide villus sampling	0.00	0.00	NA	0.00	0.00	$0.00	NA	NA	XXX	A+ PS
76946		Echo guide for amniocentesis	0.38	0.55	NA	0.02	0.95	$32.88	NA	NA	XXX	A+
76946-26		Echo guide for amniocentesis	0.38	0.14	0.14	0.01	0.53	$18.34	0.53	$18.34	XXX	A+
76946-TC		Echo guide for amniocentesis	0.00	0.41	NA	0.01	0.42	$14.53	NA	NA	XXX	A+ PS
76948		Echo guide ova aspiration	0.67	1.69	NA	0.03	2.39	$82.71	NA	NA	XXX	A+
76948-26		Echo guide ova aspiration	0.67	0.25	0.25	0.02	0.94	$32.53	0.94	$32.53	XXX	A+
76948-TC		Echo guide ova aspiration	0.00	1.44	NA	0.01	1.45	$50.18	NA	NA	XXX	A+ PS
76965		Echo guidance radiotherapy	1.34	1.34	NA	0.05	2.73	$94.47	NA	NA	XXX	A+
76965-26		Echo guidance radiotherapy	1.34	0.57	0.57	0.04	1.95	$67.48	1.95	$67.48	XXX	A+
76965-TC		Echo guidance radiotherapy	0.00	0.77	NA	0.01	0.78	$26.99	NA	NA	XXX	A+ PS
76975	CP	Gi endoscopic ultrasound	0.00	0.00	NA	0.00	0.00	$0.00	NA	NA	XXX	A+
76975-26		Gi endoscopic ultrasound	0.81	0.36	0.36	0.02	1.19	$41.18	1.19	$41.18	XXX	A+
76975-TC	CP	Gi endoscopic ultrasound	0.00	0.00	NA	0.00	0.00	$0.00	NA	NA	XXX	A+ PS
76977		Us bone density measure	0.05	0.14	NA	0.02	0.21	$7.27	NA	NA	XXX	A+
76977-26		Us bone density measure	0.05	0.02	0.02	0.01	0.08	$2.77	0.08	$2.77	XXX	A+
76977-TC		Us bone density measure	0.00	0.12	NA	0.01	0.13	$4.50	NA	NA	XXX	A+ GS
76978		Us trgt dyn mbubb 1st les	1.62	7.21	NA	0.11	8.94	$309.38	NA	NA	XXX	A+ Mtc
76978-26		Us trgt dyn mbubb 1st les	1.62	0.58	0.58	0.09	2.29	$79.25	2.29	$79.25	XXX	A+ Mtc
76978-TC		Us trgt dyn mbubb 1st les	0.00	6.63	NA	0.02	6.65	$230.13	NA	NA	XXX	A+ Mtc PS
76979		Us trgt dyn mbubb ea addl	0.85	5.02	NA	0.05	5.92	$204.87	NA	NA	ZZZ	A+
76979-26		Us trgt dyn mbubb ea addl	0.85	0.31	0.31	0.04	1.20	$41.53	1.20	$41.53	ZZZ	A+
76979-TC		Us trgt dyn mbubb ea addl	0.00	4.71	NA	0.01	4.72	$163.34	NA	NA	ZZZ	A+ PS
76981		Use parenchyma	0.59	2.49	NA	0.05	3.13	$108.32	NA	NA	XXX	A+ Mtc
76981-26		Use parenchyma	0.59	0.22	0.22	0.04	0.85	$29.42	0.85	$29.42	XXX	A+ Mtc
76981-TC		Use parenchyma	0.00	2.27	NA	0.01	2.28	$78.90	NA	NA	XXX	A+ Mtc DS
76982		Use 1st target lesion	0.59	2.18	NA	0.05	2.82	$97.59	NA	NA	XXX	A+ Mtc
76982-26		Use 1st target lesion	0.59	0.22	0.22	0.04	0.85	$29.42	0.85	$29.42	XXX	A+ Mtc
76982-TC		Use 1st target lesion	0.00	1.96	NA	0.01	1.97	$68.17	NA	NA	XXX	A+ Mtc DS
76983		Use ea addl target lesion	0.50	1.30	NA	0.03	1.83	$63.33	NA	NA	ZZZ	A+
76983-26		Use ea addl target lesion	0.50	0.20	0.20	0.02	0.72	$24.92	0.72	$24.92	ZZZ	A+

76983-TC		Use ea addl target lesion	0.00	1.10	NA	0.01	1.11	$38.41	NA	NA	ZZZ	A+ DS
76998	CP	Us guide intraop	0.00	0.00	NA	0.00	0.00	$0.00	NA	NA	XXX	A+
76998-26		Us guide intraop	1.20	0.40	0.40	0.21	1.81	$62.64	1.81	$62.64	XXX	A+
76998-TC	CP	Us guide intraop	0.00	0.00	NA	0.00	0.00	$0.00	NA	NA	XXX	A+ PS
76999	CP	Echo examination procedure	0.00	0.00	NA	0.00	0.00	$0.00	NA	NA	XXX	A+
76999-26	CP	Echo examination procedure	0.00	0.00	0.00	0.00	0.00	$0.00	0.00	$0.00	XXX	A+
76999-TC	CP	Echo examination procedure	0.00	0.00	NA	0.00	0.00	$0.00	NA	NA	XXX	A+
77001		Fluoroguide for vein device	0.38	2.65	NA	0.05	3.08	$106.59	NA	NA	ZZZ	A+
77001-26		Fluoroguide for vein device	0.38	0.12	0.12	0.04	0.54	$18.69	0.54	$18.69	ZZZ	A+
77001-TC		Fluoroguide for vein device	0.00	2.53	NA	0.01	2.54	$87.90	NA	NA	ZZZ	A+ PS
77002		Needle localization by xray	0.54	2.90	NA	0.05	3.49	$120.78	NA	NA	ZZZ	A+
77002-26		Needle localization by xray	0.54	0.22	0.22	0.04	0.80	$27.68	0.80	$27.68	ZZZ	A+
77002-TC		Needle localization by xray	0.00	2.68	NA	0.01	2.69	$93.09	NA	NA	ZZZ	A+ PS
77003		Fluoroguide for spine inject	0.60	2.51	NA	0.05	3.16	$109.36	NA	NA	ZZZ	A+
77003-26		Fluoroguide for spine inject	0.60	0.21	0.21	0.04	0.85	$29.42	0.85	$29.42	ZZZ	A+
77003-TC		Fluoroguide for spine inject	0.00	2.30	NA	0.01	2.31	$79.94	NA	NA	ZZZ	A+ PS
77011		Ct scan for localization	1.21	5.46	NA	0.09	6.76	$233.94	NA	NA	XXX	
77011-26		Ct scan for localization	1.21	0.52	0.52	0.08	1.81	$62.64	1.81	$62.64	XXX	
77011-TC		Ct scan for localization	0.00	4.94	NA	0.01	4.95	$171.30	NA	NA	XXX	PS
77012		Ct scan for needle biopsy	1.50	2.65	NA	0.10	4.25	$147.08	NA	NA	XXX	
77012-26		Ct scan for needle biopsy	1.50	0.48	0.48	0.09	2.07	$71.63	2.07	$71.63	XXX	
77012-TC		Ct scan for needle biopsy	0.00	2.17	NA	0.01	2.18	$75.44	NA	NA	XXX	PS
77013	CP	Ct guide for tissue ablation	0.00	0.00	NA	0.00	0.00	$0.00	NA	NA	XXX	A+
77013-26		Ct guide for tissue ablation	3.99	1.15	1.15	0.21	5.35	$185.14	5.35	$185.14	XXX	A+
77013-TC	CP	Ct guide for tissue ablation	0.00	0.00	NA	0.00	0.00	$0.00	NA	NA	XXX	A+
77014		Ct scan for therapy guide	0.85	2.68	NA	0.05	3.58	$123.89	NA	NA	XXX	
77014-26		Ct scan for therapy guide	0.85	0.42	0.42	0.04	1.31	$45.33	1.31	$45.33	XXX	
77014-TC		Ct scan for therapy guide	0.00	2.26	NA	0.01	2.27	$78.56	NA	NA	XXX	DS

*Please note that these calculations are based on the Medicare 2022 Conversion Factor of $34.6062 and the DRA RVU cap rates at time of publication.

A = assistant-at-surgery restriction
A+ = assistant-at-surgery restriction unless medical necessity established with documentation
B = bilateral surgery adjustment applies
C = cosurgeons payable
C+ = cosurgeons payable if medical necessity established with documentation
CP = carriers may establish RVUs and payment amounts for these services, generally on an individual basis following review of documentation such as an operative report
M = multiple surgery adjustment applies
Me = multiple endoscopy rules may apply
M+ = multiple therapy rules apply
Mtc = multiple diagnostic imaging rules apply
T = team surgeons permitted
T+ = team surgeons payable if medical necessity established with documentation
§ = indicates code is not covered by Medicare
GS = procedure must be performed under the general supervision of a physician
DS = procedure must be performed under the direct supervision of a physician
PS = procedure must be performed under the personal supervision of a physician
DRA = procedure subject to DRA limitation

Relative Value Units

CPT Code and Modifier		Description	Work RVU	Nonfacility Practice Expense RVU	Facility Practice Expense RVU	PLI RVU	Total Non-facility RVUs	Medicare Payment Nonfacility	Total Facility RVUs	Medicare Payment Facility	Global Period	Payment Policy Indicators
77021		Mri guidance ndl plmt rs&i	1.50	11.26	NA	0.07	12.83	$444.00	NA	NA	XXX	
77021-26		Mri guidance ndl plmt rs&i	1.50	0.51	0.51	0.05	2.06	$71.29	2.06	$71.29	XXX	
77021-TC		Mri guidance ndl plmt rs&i	0.00	10.75	NA	0.02	10.77	$372.71	NA	NA	XXX	PS
77022	CP	Mri gdn parnchyma tiss abltj	0.00	0.00	NA	0.00	0.00	$0.00	NA	NA	XXX	A+
77022-26		Mri gdn parnchyma tiss abltj	4.24	1.48	1.48	0.23	5.95	$205.91	5.95	$205.91	XXX	
77022-TC	CP	Mri gdn parnchyma tiss abltj	0.00	0.00	NA	0.00	0.00	$0.00	NA	NA	XXX	A+
77046		Mri breast c- unilateral	1.45	5.16	NA	0.10	6.71	$232.21	NA	NA	XXX	A+ Mtc
77046-26		Mri breast c- unilateral	1.45	0.52	0.52	0.08	2.05	$70.94	2.05	$70.94	XXX	A+ Mtc
77046-TC		Mri breast c- unilateral	0.00	4.64	NA	0.02	4.66	$161.26	NA	NA	XXX	A+ Mtc DS
77047		Mri breast c- bilateral	1.60	5.19	NA	0.10	6.89	$238.44	NA	NA	XXX	A+ Mtc
77047-26		Mri breast c- bilateral	1.60	0.57	0.57	0.08	2.25	$77.86	2.25	$77.86	XXX	A+ Mtc
77047-TC		Mri breast c- bilateral	0.00	4.62	NA	0.02	4.64	$160.57	NA	NA	XXX	A+ Mtc DS
77048		Mri breast c-+ w/cad uni	2.10	8.40	NA	0.12	10.62	$367.52	NA	NA	XXX	A+ Mtc
77048-26		Mri breast c-+ w/cad uni	2.10	0.75	0.75	0.10	2.95	$102.09	2.95	$102.09	XXX	A+ Mtc
77048-TC		Mri breast c-+ w/cad uni	0.00	7.65	NA	0.02	7.67	$265.43	NA	NA	XXX	A+ Mtc DS
77049		Mri breast c-+ w/cad bi	2.30	8.41	NA	0.13	10.84	$375.13	NA	NA	XXX	A+ Mtc
77049-26		Mri breast c-+ w/cad bi	2.30	0.82	0.82	0.11	3.23	$111.78	3.23	$111.78	XXX	A+ Mtc
77049-TC		Mri breast c-+ w/cad bi	0.00	7.59	NA	0.02	7.61	$263.35	NA	NA	XXX	A+ Mtc DS
77053		X-ray of mammary duct	0.36	1.20	NA	0.03	1.59	$55.02	NA	NA	XXX	
77053-26		X-ray of mammary duct	0.36	0.13	0.13	0.02	0.51	$17.65	0.51	$17.65	XXX	
77053-TC		X-ray of mammary duct	0.00	1.07	NA	0.01	1.08	$37.37	NA	NA	XXX	PS
77054		X-ray of mammary ducts	0.45	1.57	NA	0.03	2.05	$70.94	NA	NA	XXX	
77054-26		X-ray of mammary ducts	0.45	0.16	0.16	0.02	0.63	$21.80	0.63	$21.80	XXX	
77054-TC		X-ray of mammary ducts	0.00	1.41	NA	0.01	1.42	$49.14	NA	NA	XXX	PS
77063		Breast tomosynthesis bi	0.60	0.92	NA	0.04	1.56	$53.99	NA	NA	ZZZ	
77063-26		Breast tomosynthesis bi	0.60	0.22	0.22	0.04	0.86	$29.76	0.86	$29.76	ZZZ	
77063-TC		Breast tomosynthesis bi	0.00	0.70	NA	0.00	0.70	$24.22	NA	NA	ZZZ	
77065		Dx mammo incl cad uni	0.81	2.90	NA	0.05	3.76	$130.12	NA	NA	XXX	A+
77065-26		Dx mammo incl cad uni	0.81	0.29	0.29	0.04	1.14	$39.45	1.14	$39.45	XXX	A+
77065-TC		Dx mammo incl cad uni	0.00	2.61	NA	0.01	2.62	$90.67	NA	NA	XXX	A+
77066		Dx mammo incl cad bi	1.00	3.69	NA	0.06	4.75	$164.38	NA	NA	XXX	A+
77066-26		Dx mammo incl cad bi	1.00	0.36	0.36	0.05	1.41	$48.79	1.41	$48.79	XXX	A+
77066-TC		Dx mammo incl cad bi	0.00	3.33	NA	0.01	3.34	$115.58	NA	NA	XXX	A+

77067	Scr mammo bi incl cad	0.76	3.02	NA	0.05	3.83	$132.54	NA	NA	XXX	A+
77067-26	Scr mammo bi incl cad	0.76	0.27	0.27	0.04	1.07	$37.03	1.07	$37.03	XXX	A+
77067-TC	Scr mammo bi incl cad	0.00	2.75	NA	0.01	2.76	$95.51	NA	NA	XXX	A+
77071	X-ray stress view	0.41	1.16	1.16	0.08	1.65	$57.10	1.65	$57.10	XXX	A+ PS
77072	X-rays for bone age	0.19	0.57	NA	0.02	0.78	$26.99	NA	NA	XXX	A+
77072-26	X-rays for bone age	0.19	0.07	0.07	0.01	0.27	$9.34	0.27	$9.34	XXX	A+
77072-TC	X-rays for bone age	0.00	0.50	NA	0.01	0.51	$17.65	NA	NA	XXX	A+ GS
77073	X-rays bone length studies	0.26	1.06	NA	0.03	1.35	$46.72	NA	NA	XXX	A+
77073-26	X-rays bone length studies	0.26	0.11	0.11	0.02	0.39	$13.50	0.39	$13.50	XXX	A+
77073-TC	X-rays bone length studies	0.00	0.95	NA	0.01	0.96	$33.22	NA	NA	XXX	A+ GS
77074	X-rays bone survey limited	0.44	1.48	NA	0.03	1.95	$67.48	NA	NA	XXX	A+
77074-26	X-rays bone survey limited	0.44	0.16	0.16	0.02	0.62	$21.46	0.62	$21.46	XXX	A+
77074-TC	X-rays bone survey limited	0.00	1.32	NA	0.01	1.33	$46.03	NA	NA	XXX	A+ GS
77075	X-rays bone survey complete	0.55	2.38	NA	0.05	2.98	$103.13	NA	NA	XXX	A+
77075-26	X-rays bone survey complete	0.55	0.20	0.20	0.04	0.79	$27.34	0.79	$27.34	XXX	A+
77075-TC	X-rays bone survey complete	0.00	2.18	NA	0.01	2.19	$75.79	NA	NA	XXX	A+ GS
77076	X-rays bone survey infant	0.70	2.45	NA	0.05	3.20	$110.74	NA	NA	XXX	A+
77076-26	X-rays bone survey infant	0.70	0.25	0.25	0.04	0.99	$34.26	0.99	$34.26	XXX	A+
77076-TC	X-rays bone survey infant	0.00	2.20	NA	0.01	2.21	$76.48	NA	NA	XXX	A+ GS
77077	Joint survey single view	0.33	1.04	NA	0.03	1.40	$48.45	NA	NA	XXX	A+
77077-26	Joint survey single view	0.33	0.14	0.14	0.02	0.49	$16.96	0.49	$16.96	XXX	A+
77077-TC	Joint survey single view	0.00	0.90	NA	0.01	0.91	$31.49	NA	NA	XXX	A+ GS
77078	Ct bone density axial	0.25	2.94	NA	0.02	3.21	$94.82	NA	NA	XXX	A+ DRA
77078-26	Ct bone density axial	0.25	0.09	0.09	0.01	0.35	$12.11	0.35	$12.11	XXX	A+
77078-TC	Ct bone density axial	0.00	2.85	NA	0.01	2.86	$82.71	NA	NA	XXX	A+ GS DRA
77080	Dxa bone density axial	0.20	0.88	NA	0.02	1.10	$38.07	NA	NA	XXX	A+
77080-26	Dxa bone density axial	0.20	0.07	0.07	0.01	0.28	$9.69	0.28	$9.69	XXX	A+
77080-TC	Dxa bone density axial	0.00	0.81	NA	0.01	0.82	$28.38	NA	NA	XXX	A+ GS

*Please note that these calculations are based on the Medicare 2022 Conversion Factor of $34.6062 and the DRA RVU cap rates at time of publication.

A = assistant-at-surgery restriction
A+ = assistant-at-surgery restriction unless medical necessity established with documentation
B = bilateral surgery adjustment applies
C = cosurgeons payable
C+ = cosurgeons payable if medical necessity established with documentation
CP = carriers may establish RVUs and payment amounts for these services, generally on an individual basis following review of documentation such as an operative report
M = multiple surgery adjustment applies
Me = multiple endoscopy rules may apply
M+ = multiple therapy rules apply
Mtc = multiple diagnostic imaging rules apply
T = team surgeons permitted
T+ = team surgeons payable if medical necessity established with documentation
§ = indicates code is not covered by Medicare
GS = procedure must be performed under the general supervision of a physician
DS = procedure must be performed under the direct supervision of a physician
PS = procedure must be performed under the personal supervision of a physician
DRA = procedure subject to DRA limitation

Relative Value Units

CPT Code and Modifier	Description	Work RVU	Nonfacility Practice Expense RVU	Facility Practice Expense RVU	PLI RVU	Total Non-facility RVUs	Medicare Payment Nonfacility	Total Facility RVUs	Medicare Payment Facility	Global Period	Payment Policy Indicators
77081	Dxa bone density/peripheral	0.20	0.70	NA	0.02	0.92	$31.84	NA	NA	XXX	A+
77081-26	Dxa bone density/peripheral	0.20	0.08	0.08	0.01	0.29	$10.04	0.29	$10.04	XXX	A+
77081-TC	Dxa bone density/peripheral	0.00	0.62	NA	0.01	0.63	$21.80	NA	NA	XXX	A+ GS
77084	Magnetic image bone marrow	1.60	8.37	NA	0.10	10.07	$313.19	NA	NA	XXX	A+ DRA
77084-26	Magnetic image bone marrow	1.60	0.58	0.58	0.08	2.26	$78.21	2.26	$78.21	XXX	A+
77084-TC	Magnetic image bone marrow	0.00	7.79	NA	0.02	7.81	$234.98	NA	NA	XXX	A+ GS DRA
77085	Dxa bone density study	0.30	1.19	NA	0.02	1.51	$52.26	NA	NA	XXX	A+
77085-26	Dxa bone density study	0.30	0.12	0.12	0.01	0.43	$14.88	0.43	$14.88	XXX	A+
77085-TC	Dxa bone density study	0.00	1.07	NA	0.01	1.08	$37.37	NA	NA	XXX	A+ GS
77086	Fracture assessment via dxa	0.17	0.78	NA	0.02	0.97	$33.57	NA	NA	XXX	A+
77086-26	Fracture assessment via dxa	0.17	0.06	0.06	0.01	0.24	$8.31	0.24	$8.31	XXX	A+
77086-TC	Fracture assessment via dxa	0.00	0.72	NA	0.01	0.73	$25.26	NA	NA	XXX	A+ GS
77089	Tbs dxa cal w/i&r fx risk	0.20	0.97	NA	0.03	1.20	$41.53	NA	NA	XXX	A+
77090	Tbs techl prep&transmis data	0.00	0.06	NA	0.01	0.07	$2.42	NA	NA	XXX	A+ GS
77091	Tbs techl calculation only	0.00	0.82	NA	0.01	0.83	$28.72	NA	NA	XXX	A+ GS
77092	Tbs i&r fx rsk qhp	0.20	0.09	0.09	0.01	0.30	$10.38	0.30	$10.38	XXX	A+
77261	Radiation therapy planning	1.30	0.69	0.69	0.09	2.08	$71.98	2.08	$71.98	XXX	A+
77262	Radiation therapy planning	2.00	1.03	1.03	0.12	3.15	$109.01	3.15	$109.01	XXX	A+
77263	Radiation therapy planning	3.14	1.55	1.55	0.23	4.92	$170.26	4.92	$170.26	XXX	A+
77280	Set radiation therapy field	0.70	7.21	NA	0.05	7.96	$275.47	NA	NA	XXX	A+
77280-26	Set radiation therapy field	0.70	0.37	0.37	0.04	1.11	$38.41	1.11	$38.41	XXX	A+
77280-TC	Set radiation therapy field	0.00	6.84	NA	0.01	6.85	$237.05	NA	NA	XXX	A+
77285	Set radiation therapy field	1.05	12.05	NA	0.06	13.16	$455.42	NA	NA	XXX	A+
77285-26	Set radiation therapy field	1.05	0.57	0.57	0.04	1.66	$57.45	1.66	$57.45	XXX	A+
77285-TC	Set radiation therapy field	0.00	11.48	NA	0.02	11.50	$397.97	NA	NA	XXX	A+
77290	Set radiation therapy field	1.56	11.91	NA	0.09	13.56	$469.26	NA	NA	XXX	A+
77290-26	Set radiation therapy field	1.56	0.78	0.78	0.07	2.41	$83.40	2.41	$83.40	XXX	A+
77290-TC	Set radiation therapy field	0.00	11.13	NA	0.02	11.15	$385.86	NA	NA	XXX	A+
77293	Respirator motion mgmt simul	2.00	10.24	NA	0.13	12.37	$428.08	NA	NA	ZZZ	A+
77293-26	Respirator motion mgmt simul	2.00	0.99	0.99	0.09	3.08	$106.59	3.08	$106.59	ZZZ	A+
77293-TC	Respirator motion mgmt simul	0.00	9.25	NA	0.04	9.29	$321.49	NA	NA	ZZZ	A+
77295	3-d radiotherapy plan	4.29	9.42	NA	0.24	13.95	$482.76	NA	NA	XXX	A+
77295-26	3-d radiotherapy plan	4.29	2.12	2.12	0.17	6.58	$227.71	6.58	$227.71	XXX	A+

77295-TC		3-d radiotherapy plan	0.00	7.30	NA	0.07	7.37	$255.05	NA	NA	XXX	A+
77299	CP	Radiation therapy planning	0.00	0.00	NA	0.00	0.00	$0.00	NA	NA	XXX	A+
77299-26	CP	Radiation therapy planning	0.00	0.00	0.00	0.00	0.00	$0.00	0.00	$0.00	XXX	A+
77299-TC	CP	Radiation therapy planning	0.00	0.00	NA	0.00	0.00	$0.00	NA	NA	XXX	A+
77300		Radiation therapy dose plan	0.62	1.26	NA	0.03	1.91	$66.10	NA	NA	XXX	A+
77300-26		Radiation therapy dose plan	0.62	0.31	0.31	0.02	0.95	$32.88	0.95	$32.88	XXX	A+
77300-TC		Radiation therapy dose plan	0.00	0.95	NA	0.01	0.96	$33.22	NA	NA	XXX	A+
77301		Radiotherapy dose plan imrt	7.99	45.27	NA	0.60	53.86	$1863.89	NA	NA	XXX	A+
77301-26		Radiotherapy dose plan imrt	7.99	3.95	3.95	0.29	12.23	$423.23	12.23	$423.23	XXX	A+
77301-TC		Radiotherapy dose plan imrt	0.00	41.32	NA	0.31	41.63	$1440.66	NA	NA	XXX	A+
77306		Telethx isodose plan simple	1.40	2.81	NA	0.07	4.28	$148.11	NA	NA	XXX	A+
77306-26		Telethx isodose plan simple	1.40	0.69	0.69	0.05	2.14	$74.06	2.14	$74.06	XXX	A+
77306-TC		Telethx isodose plan simple	0.00	2.12	NA	0.02	2.14	$74.06	NA	NA	XXX	A+
77307		Telethx isodose plan cplx	2.90	5.27	NA	0.15	8.32	$287.92	NA	NA	XXX	A+
77307-26		Telethx isodose plan cplx	2.90	1.43	1.43	0.11	4.44	$153.65	4.44	$153.65	XXX	A+
77307-TC		Telethx isodose plan cplx	0.00	3.84	NA	0.04	3.88	$134.27	NA	NA	XXX	A+
77316		Brachytx isodose plan simple	1.40	5.62	NA	0.09	7.11	$246.05	NA	NA	XXX	A+
77316-26		Brachytx isodose plan simple	1.40	0.69	0.69	0.05	2.14	$74.06	2.14	$74.06	XXX	A+
77316-TC		Brachytx isodose plan simple	0.00	4.93	NA	0.04	4.97	$171.99	NA	NA	XXX	A+
77317		Brachytx isodose intermed	1.83	7.42	NA	0.15	9.40	$325.30	NA	NA	XXX	A+
77317-26		Brachytx isodose intermed	1.83	0.91	0.91	0.08	2.82	$97.59	2.82	$97.59	XXX	A+
77317-TC		Brachytx isodose intermed	0.00	6.51	NA	0.07	6.58	$227.71	NA	NA	XXX	A+
77318		Brachytx isodose complex	2.90	10.23	NA	0.20	13.33	$461.30	NA	NA	XXX	A+
77318-26		Brachytx isodose complex	2.90	1.43	1.43	0.11	4.44	$153.65	4.44	$153.65	XXX	A+
77318-TC		Brachytx isodose complex	0.00	8.80	NA	0.09	8.89	$307.65	NA	NA	XXX	A+
77321		Special teletx port plan	0.95	1.74	NA	0.05	2.74	$94.82	NA	NA	XXX	A+
77321-26		Special teletx port plan	0.95	0.47	0.47	0.04	1.46	$50.53	1.46	$50.53	XXX	A+
77321-TC		Special teletx port plan	0.00	1.27	NA	0.01	1.28	$44.30	NA	NA	XXX	A+

*Please note that these calculations are based on the Medicare 2022 Conversion Factor of $34.6062 and the DRA RVU cap rates at time of publication.

A = assistant-at-surgery restriction
A+ = assistant-at-surgery restriction unless medical necessity established with documentation
B = bilateral surgery adjustment applies
C = cosurgeons payable
C+ = cosurgeons payable if medical necessity established with documentation
CP = carriers may establish RVUs and payment amounts for these services, generally on an individual basis following review of documentation such as an operative report
M = multiple surgery adjustment applies
Me = multiple endoscopy rules may apply
M+ = multiple therapy rules apply
Mtc = multiple diagnostic imaging rules apply
T = team surgeons permitted
T+ = team surgeons payable if medical necessity established with documentation
§ = indicates code is not covered by Medicare
GS = procedure must be performed under the general supervision of a physician
DS = procedure must be performed under the direct supervision of a physician
PS = procedure must be performed under the personal supervision of a physician
DRA = procedure subject to DRA limitation

Relative Value Units

CPT Code and Modifier		Description	Work RVU	Nonfacility Practice Expense RVU	Facility Practice Expense RVU	PLI RVU	Total Non-facility RVUs	Medicare Payment Nonfacility	Total Facility RVUs	Medicare Payment Facility	Global Period	Payment Policy Indicators
77331		Special radiation dosimetry	0.87	0.97	NA	0.05	1.89	$65.41	NA	NA	XXX	A+
77331-26		Special radiation dosimetry	0.87	0.43	0.43	0.04	1.34	$46.37	1.34	$46.37	XXX	A+
77331-TC		Special radiation dosimetry	0.00	0.54	NA	0.01	0.55	$19.03	NA	NA	XXX	A+
77332		Radiation treatment aid(s)	0.45	0.65	NA	0.03	1.13	$39.11	NA	NA	XXX	A+
77332-26		Radiation treatment aid(s)	0.45	0.23	0.23	0.02	0.70	$24.22	0.70	$24.22	XXX	A+
77332-TC		Radiation treatment aid(s)	0.00	0.42	NA	0.01	0.43	$14.88	NA	NA	XXX	A+
77333		Radiation treatment aid(s)	0.75	3.31	NA	0.05	4.11	$142.23	NA	NA	XXX	A+
77333-26		Radiation treatment aid(s)	0.75	0.37	0.37	0.04	1.16	$40.14	1.16	$40.14	XXX	A+
77333-TC		Radiation treatment aid(s)	0.00	2.94	NA	0.01	2.95	$102.09	NA	NA	XXX	A+
77334		Radiation treatment aid(s)	1.15	2.44	NA	0.05	3.64	$125.97	NA	NA	XXX	A+
77334-26		Radiation treatment aid(s)	1.15	0.57	0.57	0.04	1.76	$60.91	1.76	$60.91	XXX	A+
77334-TC		Radiation treatment aid(s)	0.00	1.87	NA	0.01	1.88	$65.06	NA	NA	XXX	A+
77336		Radiation physics consult	0.00	2.35	NA	0.08	2.43	$84.09	NA	NA	XXX	A+
77338		Design mlc device for imrt	4.29	8.92	NA	0.26	13.47	$466.15	NA	NA	XXX	A+
77338-26		Design mlc device for imrt	4.29	2.12	2.12	0.17	6.58	$227.71	6.58	$227.71	XXX	A+
77338-TC		Design mlc device for imrt	0.00	6.80	NA	0.09	6.89	$238.44	NA	NA	XXX	A+
77370		Radiation physics consult	0.00	3.75	NA	0.12	3.87	$133.93	NA	NA	XXX	A+
77371	CP	Srs multisource	0.00	0.00	0.00	0.00	0.00	$0.00	0.00	$0.00	XXX	A+
77372		Srs linear based	0.00	28.91	NA	0.18	29.09	$1006.69	NA	NA	XXX	A+
77373		Sbrt delivery	0.00	29.84	NA	0.21	30.05	$1039.92	NA	NA	XXX	A+
77399	CP	External radiation dosimetry	0.00	0.00	NA	0.00	0.00	$0.00	NA	NA	XXX	A+
77399-26	CP	External radiation dosimetry	0.00	0.00	0.00	0.00	0.00	$0.00	0.00	$0.00	XXX	A+
77399-TC	CP	External radiation dosimetry	0.00	0.00	NA	0.00	0.00	$0.00	NA	NA	XXX	A+
77401		Radiation treatment delivery	0.00	1.21	NA	0.01	1.22	$42.22	NA	NA	XXX	A+
77417		Radiology port images(s)	0.00	0.36	NA	0.01	0.37	$12.80	NA	NA	XXX	A+ GS
77423	CP	Neutron beam tx complex	0.00	0.00	0.00	0.00	0.00	$0.00	0.00	$0.00	XXX	A+
77427		Radiation tx management x5	3.37	1.95	1.95	0.25	5.57	$192.76	5.57	$192.76	XXX	
77431		Radiation therapy management	1.81	1.19	1.19	0.12	3.12	$107.97	3.12	$107.97	XXX	A+
77432		Stereotactic radiation trmt	7.92	3.91	3.91	0.60	12.43	$430.16	12.43	$430.16	XXX	A+
77435		Sbrt management	11.87	5.99	5.99	0.89	18.75	$648.87	18.75	$648.87	XXX	A+
77469		Io radiation tx management	5.75	NA	3.13	0.42	NA	NA	9.30	$321.84	XXX	A+
77470		Special radiation treatment	2.03	1.85	NA	0.10	3.98	$137.73	NA	NA	XXX	A+
77470-26		Special radiation treatment	2.03	1.01	1.01	0.09	3.13	$108.32	3.13	$108.32	XXX	A+

77470-TC		Special radiation treatment	0.00	0.84	NA	0.01	0.85	$29.42	NA	NA	XXX	A+
77499	CP	Radiation therapy management	0.00	0.00	NA	0.00	0.00	$0.00	NA	NA	XXX	A+
77499-26	CP	Radiation therapy management	0.00	0.00	0.00	0.00	0.00	$0.00	0.00	$0.00	XXX	A+
77499-TC	CP	Radiation therapy management	0.00	0.00	NA	0.00	0.00	$0.00	NA	NA	XXX	A+
77520	CP	Proton trmt simple w/o comp	0.00	0.00	0.00	0.00	0.00	$0.00	0.00	$0.00	XXX	A+
77522	CP	Proton trmt simple w/comp	0.00	0.00	0.00	0.00	0.00	$0.00	0.00	$0.00	XXX	A+
77523	CP	Proton trmt intermediate	0.00	0.00	0.00	0.00	0.00	$0.00	0.00	$0.00	XXX	A+
77525	CP	Proton treatment complex	0.00	0.00	0.00	0.00	0.00	$0.00	0.00	$0.00	XXX	A+
77600		Hyperthermia treatment	1.31	13.68	NA	0.10	15.09	$522.21	NA	NA	XXX	A+
77600-26		Hyperthermia treatment	1.31	0.70	0.70	0.05	2.06	$71.29	2.06	$71.29	XXX	A+
77600-TC		Hyperthermia treatment	0.00	12.98	NA	0.05	13.03	$450.92	NA	NA	XXX	A+
77605		Hyperthermia treatment	1.84	27.48	NA	0.41	29.73	$1028.84	NA	NA	XXX	A+
77605-26		Hyperthermia treatment	1.84	0.80	0.80	0.34	2.98	$103.13	2.98	$103.13	XXX	A+
77605-TC		Hyperthermia treatment	0.00	26.68	NA	0.07	26.75	$925.72	NA	NA	XXX	A+
77610		Hyperthermia treatment	1.31	19.23	NA	0.12	20.66	$714.96	NA	NA	XXX	A+
77610-26		Hyperthermia treatment	1.31	0.65	0.65	0.05	2.01	$69.56	2.01	$69.56	XXX	A+
77610-TC		Hyperthermia treatment	0.00	18.58	NA	0.07	18.65	$645.41	NA	NA	XXX	A+
77615		Hyperthermia treatment	1.84	30.15	NA	0.19	32.18	$1113.63	NA	NA	XXX	A+
77615-26		Hyperthermia treatment	1.84	0.91	0.91	0.08	2.83	$97.94	2.83	$97.94	XXX	A+
77615-TC		Hyperthermia treatment	0.00	29.24	NA	0.11	29.35	$1015.69	NA	NA	XXX	A+
77620		Hyperthermia treatment	1.56	17.46	NA	0.41	19.43	$672.40	NA	NA	XXX	A+
77620-26		Hyperthermia treatment	1.56	0.58	0.58	0.34	2.48	$85.82	2.48	$85.82	XXX	A+
77620-TC		Hyperthermia treatment	0.00	16.88	NA	0.07	16.95	$586.58	NA	NA	XXX	A+
77750		Infuse radioactive materials	5.00	6.19	NA	0.25	11.44	$395.89	NA	NA	090	A+
77750-26		Infuse radioactive materials	5.00	2.48	2.48	0.20	7.68	$265.78	7.68	$265.78	090	A+
77750-TC		Infuse radioactive materials	0.00	3.71	NA	0.05	3.76	$130.12	NA	NA	090	A+
77761		Apply intrcav radiat simple	3.85	8.05	NA	0.22	12.12	$419.43	NA	NA	090	A+
77761-26		Apply intrcav radiat simple	3.85	1.90	1.90	0.14	5.89	$203.83	5.89	$203.83	090	A+

*Please note that these calculations are based on the Medicare 2022 Conversion Factor of $34.6062 and the DRA RVU cap rates at time of publication.

A = assistant-at-surgery restriction
A+ = assistant-at-surgery restriction unless medical necessity established with documentation
B = bilateral surgery adjustment applies
C = cosurgeons payable
C+ = cosurgeons payable if medical necessity established with documentation
CP = carriers may establish RVUs and payment amounts for these services, generally on an individual basis following review of documentation such as an operative report
M = multiple surgery adjustment applies
Me = multiple endoscopy rules may apply
M+ = multiple therapy rules apply
Mtc = multiple diagnostic imaging rules apply
T = team surgeons permitted
T+ = team surgeons payable if medical necessity established with documentation
§ = indicates code is not covered by Medicare
GS = procedure must be performed under the general supervision of a physician
DS = procedure must be performed under the direct supervision of a physician
PS = procedure must be performed under the personal supervision of a physician
DRA = procedure subject to DRA limitation

Relative Value Units

CPT Code and Modifier		Description	Work RVU	Nonfacility Practice Expense RVU	Facility Practice Expense RVU	PLI RVU	Total Non-facility RVUs	Medicare Payment Nonfacility	Total Facility RVUs	Medicare Payment Facility	Global Period	Payment Policy Indicators
77761-TC		Apply intrcav radiat simple	0.00	6.15	NA	0.08	6.23	$215.60	NA	NA	090	A+
77762		Apply intrcav radiat interm	5.76	9.85	NA	0.31	15.92	$550.93	NA	NA	090	A+
77762-26		Apply intrcav radiat interm	5.76	2.85	2.85	0.22	8.83	$305.57	8.83	$305.57	090	A+
77762-TC		Apply intrcav radiat interm	0.00	7.00	NA	0.09	7.09	$245.36	NA	NA	090	A+
77763		Apply intrcav radiat compl	8.66	13.31	NA	0.44	22.41	$775.52	NA	NA	090	A+
77763-26		Apply intrcav radiat compl	8.66	4.28	4.28	0.33	13.27	$459.22	13.27	$459.22	090	A+
77763-TC		Apply intrcav radiat compl	0.00	9.03	NA	0.11	9.14	$316.30	NA	NA	090	A+
77767		Hdr rdncl skn surf brachytx	1.05	6.16	NA	0.08	7.29	$252.28	NA	NA	XXX	A+
77767-26		Hdr rdncl skn surf brachytx	1.05	0.52	0.52	0.04	1.61	$55.72	1.61	$55.72	XXX	A+
77767-TC		Hdr rdncl skn surf brachytx	0.00	5.64	NA	0.04	5.68	$196.56	NA	NA	XXX	A+
77768		Hdr rdncl skn surf brachytx	1.40	9.11	NA	0.12	10.63	$367.86	NA	NA	XXX	A+
77768-26		Hdr rdncl skn surf brachytx	1.40	0.70	0.70	0.05	2.15	$74.40	2.15	$74.40	XXX	A+
77768-TC		Hdr rdncl skn surf brachytx	0.00	8.41	NA	0.07	8.48	$293.46	NA	NA	XXX	A+
77770		Hdr rdncl ntrstl/icav brchtx	1.95	8.09	NA	0.13	10.17	$351.95	NA	NA	XXX	A+
77770-26		Hdr rdncl ntrstl/icav brchtx	1.95	0.97	0.97	0.08	3.00	$103.82	3.00	$103.82	XXX	A+
77770-TC		Hdr rdncl ntrstl/icav brchtx	0.00	7.12	NA	0.05	7.17	$248.13	NA	NA	XXX	A+
77771		Hdr rdncl ntrstl/icav brchtx	3.80	13.48	NA	0.21	17.49	$605.26	NA	NA	XXX	A+
77771-26		Hdr rdncl ntrstl/icav brchtx	3.80	1.88	1.88	0.12	5.80	$200.72	5.80	$200.72	XXX	A+
77771-TC		Hdr rdncl ntrstl/icav brchtx	0.00	11.60	NA	0.09	11.69	$404.55	NA	NA	XXX	A+
77772		Hdr rdncl ntrstl/icav brchtx	5.40	20.27	NA	0.34	26.01	$900.11	NA	NA	XXX	A+
77772-26		Hdr rdncl ntrstl/icav brchtx	5.40	2.60	2.60	0.20	8.20	$283.77	8.20	$283.77	XXX	A+
77772-TC		Hdr rdncl ntrstl/icav brchtx	0.00	17.67	NA	0.14	17.81	$616.34	NA	NA	XXX	A+
77778		Apply interstit radiat compl	8.78	17.18	NA	0.47	26.43	$914.64	NA	NA	000	A+
77778-26		Apply interstit radiat compl	8.78	4.31	4.31	0.33	13.42	$464.42	13.42	$464.42	000	A+
77778-TC		Apply interstit radiat compl	0.00	12.87	NA	0.14	13.01	$450.23	NA	NA	000	A+ GS
77789		Apply surf ldr radionuclide	1.14	2.70	NA	0.06	3.90	$134.96	NA	NA	000	A+
77789-26		Apply surf ldr radionuclide	1.14	0.58	0.58	0.04	1.76	$60.91	1.76	$60.91	000	A+
77789-TC		Apply surf ldr radionuclide	0.00	2.12	NA	0.02	2.14	$74.06	NA	NA	000	A+
77790		Radiation handling	0.00	0.46	NA	0.01	0.47	$16.26	NA	NA	XXX	A+
77799	CP	Radium/radioisotope therapy	0.00	0.00	NA	0.00	0.00	$0.00	NA	NA	XXX	A+
77799-26	CP	Radium/radioisotope therapy	0.00	0.00	0.00	0.00	0.00	$0.00	0.00	$0.00	XXX	A+
77799-TC	CP	Radium/radioisotope therapy	0.00	0.00	NA	0.00	0.00	$0.00	NA	NA	XXX	A+
78012		Thyroid uptake measurement	0.19	2.15	NA	0.05	2.39	$82.71	NA	NA	XXX	A+

78012-26	Thyroid uptake measurement	0.19	0.06	0.06	0.01	0.26	$9.00	0.26	$9.00	XXX	A+
78012-TC	Thyroid uptake measurement	0.00	2.09	NA	0.04	2.13	$73.71	NA	NA	XXX	A+
78013	Thyroid imaging w/blood flow	0.37	5.08	NA	0.05	5.50	$190.33	NA	NA	XXX	A+
78013-26	Thyroid imaging w/blood flow	0.37	0.13	0.13	0.01	0.51	$17.65	0.51	$17.65	XXX	A+
78013-TC	Thyroid imaging w/blood flow	0.00	4.95	NA	0.04	4.99	$172.68	NA	NA	XXX	A+
78014	Thyroid imaging w/blood flow	0.50	6.19	NA	0.06	6.75	$233.59	NA	NA	XXX	A+
78014-26	Thyroid imaging w/blood flow	0.50	0.17	0.17	0.02	0.69	$23.88	0.69	$23.88	XXX	A+
78014-TC	Thyroid imaging w/blood flow	0.00	6.02	NA	0.04	6.06	$209.71	NA	NA	XXX	A+
78015	Thyroid met imaging	0.67	5.76	NA	0.08	6.51	$225.29	NA	NA	XXX	A+
78015-26	Thyroid met imaging	0.67	0.24	0.24	0.04	0.95	$32.88	0.95	$32.88	XXX	A+
78015-TC	Thyroid met imaging	0.00	5.52	NA	0.04	5.56	$192.41	NA	NA	XXX	A+ GS
78016	Thyroid met imaging/studies	0.82	7.12	NA	0.06	8.00	$276.85	NA	NA	XXX	A+
78016-26	Thyroid met imaging/studies	0.82	0.14	0.14	0.01	0.97	$33.57	0.97	$33.57	XXX	A+
78016-TC	Thyroid met imaging/studies	0.00	6.98	NA	0.05	7.03	$243.28	NA	NA	XXX	A+ GS
78018	Thyroid met imaging body	0.86	7.93	NA	0.09	8.88	$307.30	NA	NA	XXX	A+
78018-26	Thyroid met imaging body	0.86	0.27	0.27	0.04	1.17	$40.49	1.17	$40.49	XXX	A+
78018-TC	Thyroid met imaging body	0.00	7.66	NA	0.05	7.71	$266.81	NA	NA	XXX	A+ GS
78020	Thyroid met uptake	0.60	1.72	NA	0.04	2.36	$81.67	NA	NA	ZZZ	A+
78020-26	Thyroid met uptake	0.60	0.17	0.17	0.02	0.79	$27.34	0.79	$27.34	ZZZ	A+
78020-TC	Thyroid met uptake	0.00	1.55	NA	0.02	1.57	$54.33	NA	NA	ZZZ	A+
78070	Parathyroid planar imaging	0.80	7.41	NA	0.08	8.29	$286.89	NA	NA	XXX	A+
78070-26	Parathyroid planar imaging	0.80	0.26	0.26	0.04	1.10	$38.07	1.10	$38.07	XXX	A+
78070-TC	Parathyroid planar imaging	0.00	7.15	NA	0.04	7.19	$248.82	NA	NA	XXX	A+ GS
78071	Parathyrd planar w/wo subtrj	1.20	8.61	NA	0.10	9.91	$342.95	NA	NA	XXX	A+
78071-26	Parathyrd planar w/wo subtrj	1.20	0.40	0.40	0.05	1.65	$57.10	1.65	$57.10	XXX	A+
78071-TC	Parathyrd planar w/wo subtrj	0.00	8.21	NA	0.05	8.26	$285.85	NA	NA	XXX	A+
78072	Parathyrd planar w/spect&ct	1.60	10.74	NA	0.12	12.46	$431.19	NA	NA	XXX	A+
78072-26	Parathyrd planar w/spect&ct	1.60	0.50	0.50	0.07	2.17	$75.10	2.17	$75.10	XXX	A+

*Please note that these calculations are based on the Medicare 2022 Conversion Factor of $34.6062 and the DRA RVU cap rates at time of publication.

A = assistant-at-surgery restriction
A+ = assistant-at-surgery restriction unless medical necessity established with documentation
B = bilateral surgery adjustment applies
C = cosurgeons payable
C+ = cosurgeons payable if medical necessity established with documentation
CP = carriers may establish RVUs and payment amounts for these services, generally on an individual basis following review of documentation such as an operative report
M = multiple surgery adjustment applies
Me = multiple endoscopy rules may apply
M+ = multiple therapy rules apply
Mtc = multiple diagnostic imaging rules apply
T = team surgeons permitted
T+ = team surgeons payable if medical necessity established with documentation
§ = indicates code is not covered by Medicare
GS = procedure must be performed under the general supervision of a physician
DS = procedure must be performed under the direct supervision of a physician
PS = procedure must be performed under the personal supervision of a physician
DRA = procedure subject to DRA limitation

Relative Value Units

CPT Code and Modifier		Description	Work RVU	Nonfacility Practice Expense RVU	Facility Practice Expense RVU	PLI RVU	Total Non-facility RVUs	Medicare Payment Nonfacility	Total Facility RVUs	Medicare Payment Facility	Global Period	Payment Policy Indicators
78072-TC		Parathyrd planar w/spect&ct	0.00	10.24	NA	0.05	10.29	$356.10	NA	NA	XXX	A+
78075		Adrenal cortex & medulla img	0.74	11.75	NA	0.11	12.60	$436.04	NA	NA	XXX	A+
78075-26		Adrenal cortex & medulla img	0.74	0.27	0.27	0.04	1.05	$36.34	1.05	$36.34	XXX	A+
78075-TC		Adrenal cortex & medulla img	0.00	11.48	NA	0.07	11.55	$399.70	NA	NA	XXX	A+ GS
78099	CP	Endocrine nuclear procedure	0.00	0.00	NA	0.00	0.00	$0.00	NA	NA	XXX	A+
78099-26	CP	Endocrine nuclear procedure	0.00	0.00	0.00	0.00	0.00	$0.00	0.00	$0.00	XXX	A+
78099-TC	CP	Endocrine nuclear procedure	0.00	0.00	NA	0.00	0.00	$0.00	NA	NA	XXX	A+
78102		Bone marrow imaging ltd	0.55	4.28	NA	0.06	4.89	$169.22	NA	NA	XXX	A+
78102-26		Bone marrow imaging ltd	0.55	0.17	0.17	0.02	0.74	$25.61	0.74	$25.61	XXX	A+
78102-TC		Bone marrow imaging ltd	0.00	4.11	NA	0.04	4.15	$143.62	NA	NA	XXX	A+ GS
78103		Bone marrow imaging mult	0.75	4.58	NA	0.05	5.38	$186.18	NA	NA	XXX	A+
78103-26		Bone marrow imaging mult	0.75	0.13	0.13	0.01	0.89	$30.80	0.89	$30.80	XXX	A+
78103-TC		Bone marrow imaging mult	0.00	4.45	NA	0.04	4.49	$155.38	NA	NA	XXX	A+ GS
78104		Bone marrow imaging body	0.80	6.21	NA	0.08	7.09	$245.36	NA	NA	XXX	A+
78104-26		Bone marrow imaging body	0.80	0.26	0.26	0.04	1.10	$38.07	1.10	$38.07	XXX	A+
78104-TC		Bone marrow imaging body	0.00	5.95	NA	0.04	5.99	$207.29	NA	NA	XXX	A+ GS
78110		Plasma volume single	0.19	1.83	NA	0.05	2.07	$71.63	NA	NA	XXX	A+
78110-26		Plasma volume single	0.19	0.03	0.03	0.01	0.23	$7.96	0.23	$7.96	XXX	A+
78110-TC		Plasma volume single	0.00	1.80	NA	0.04	1.84	$63.68	NA	NA	XXX	A+ GS
78111		Plasma volume multiple	0.22	1.93	NA	0.05	2.20	$76.13	NA	NA	XXX	A+
78111-26		Plasma volume multiple	0.22	0.04	0.04	0.01	0.27	$9.34	0.27	$9.34	XXX	A+
78111-TC		Plasma volume multiple	0.00	1.89	NA	0.04	1.93	$66.79	NA	NA	XXX	A+ GS
78120		Red cell mass single	0.23	1.84	NA	0.05	2.12	$73.37	NA	NA	XXX	A+
78120-26		Red cell mass single	0.23	0.04	0.04	0.01	0.28	$9.69	0.28	$9.69	XXX	A+
78120-TC		Red cell mass single	0.00	1.80	NA	0.04	1.84	$63.68	NA	NA	XXX	A+ GS
78121		Red cell mass multiple	0.32	1.95	NA	0.05	2.32	$80.29	NA	NA	XXX	A+
78121-26		Red cell mass multiple	0.32	0.06	0.06	0.01	0.39	$13.50	0.39	$13.50	XXX	A+
78121-TC		Red cell mass multiple	0.00	1.89	NA	0.04	1.93	$66.79	NA	NA	XXX	A+ GS
78122		Blood volume	0.45	2.39	NA	0.05	2.89	$100.01	NA	NA	XXX	A+
78122-26		Blood volume	0.45	0.14	0.14	0.01	0.60	$20.76	0.60	$20.76	XXX	A+
78122-TC		Blood volume	0.00	2.25	NA	0.04	2.29	$79.25	NA	NA	XXX	A+ GS
78130		Red cell survival study	0.61	3.04	NA	0.06	3.71	$128.39	NA	NA	XXX	A+
78130-26		Red cell survival study	0.61	0.11	0.11	0.01	0.73	$25.26	0.73	$25.26	XXX	A+

78130-TC		Red cell survival study	0.00	2.93	NA	0.05	2.98	$103.13	NA	NA	XXX	A+ GS
78140		Red cell sequestration	0.61	2.63	NA	0.05	3.29	$113.85	NA	NA	XXX	A+
78140-26		Red cell sequestration	0.61	0.11	0.11	0.01	0.73	$25.26	0.73	$25.26	XXX	A+
78140-TC		Red cell sequestration	0.00	2.52	NA	0.04	2.56	$88.59	NA	NA	XXX	A+ GS
78185		Spleen imaging	0.40	4.44	NA	0.05	4.89	$169.22	NA	NA	XXX	A+
78185-26		Spleen imaging	0.40	0.07	0.07	0.01	0.48	$16.61	0.48	$16.61	XXX	A+
78185-TC		Spleen imaging	0.00	4.37	NA	0.04	4.41	$152.61	NA	NA	XXX	A+ GS
78191		Platelet survival	0.61	3.04	NA	0.06	3.71	$128.39	NA	NA	XXX	A+
78191-26		Platelet survival	0.61	0.11	0.11	0.01	0.73	$25.26	0.73	$25.26	XXX	A+
78191-TC		Platelet survival	0.00	2.93	NA	0.05	2.98	$103.13	NA	NA	XXX	A+ GS
78195		Lymph system imaging	1.20	8.72	NA	0.10	10.02	$346.75	NA	NA	XXX	A+
78195-26		Lymph system imaging	1.20	0.39	0.39	0.05	1.64	$56.75	1.64	$56.75	XXX	A+
78195-TC		Lymph system imaging	0.00	8.33	NA	0.05	8.38	$290.00	NA	NA	XXX	A+ GS
78199	CP	Blood/lymph nuclear exam	0.00	0.00	NA	0.00	0.00	$0.00	NA	NA	XXX	A+
78199-26	CP	Blood/lymph nuclear exam	0.00	0.00	0.00	0.00	0.00	$0.00	0.00	$0.00	XXX	A+
78199-TC	CP	Blood/lymph nuclear exam	0.00	0.00	NA	0.00	0.00	$0.00	NA	NA	XXX	A+
78201		Liver imaging	0.44	4.91	NA	0.06	5.41	$187.22	NA	NA	XXX	A+
78201-26		Liver imaging	0.44	0.14	0.14	0.02	0.60	$20.76	0.60	$20.76	XXX	A+
78201-TC		Liver imaging	0.00	4.77	NA	0.04	4.81	$166.46	NA	NA	XXX	A+ GS
78202		Liver imaging with flow	0.51	5.42	NA	0.06	5.99	$207.29	NA	NA	XXX	A+
78202-26		Liver imaging with flow	0.51	0.16	0.16	0.02	0.69	$23.88	0.69	$23.88	XXX	A+
78202-TC		Liver imaging with flow	0.00	5.26	NA	0.04	5.30	$183.41	NA	NA	XXX	A+ GS
78215		Liver and spleen imaging	0.49	5.02	NA	0.06	5.57	$192.76	NA	NA	XXX	A+
78215-26		Liver and spleen imaging	0.49	0.17	0.17	0.02	0.68	$23.53	0.68	$23.53	XXX	A+
78215-TC		Liver and spleen imaging	0.00	4.85	NA	0.04	4.89	$169.22	NA	NA	XXX	A+ GS
78216		Liver & spleen image/flow	0.57	3.17	NA	0.06	3.80	$131.50	NA	NA	XXX	A+
78216-26		Liver & spleen image/flow	0.57	0.18	0.18	0.02	0.77	$26.65	0.77	$26.65	XXX	A+
78216-TC		Liver & spleen image/flow	0.00	2.99	NA	0.04	3.03	$104.86	NA	NA	XXX	A+ GS

*Please note that these calculations are based on the Medicare 2022 Conversion Factor of $34.6062 and the DRA RVU cap rates at time of publication.

A = assistant-at-surgery restriction
A+ = assistant-at-surgery restriction unless medical necessity established with documentation
B = bilateral surgery adjustment applies
C = cosurgeons payable
C+ = cosurgeons payable if medical necessity established with documentation
CP = carriers may establish RVUs and payment amounts for these services, generally on an individual basis following review of documentation such as an operative report
M = multiple surgery adjustment applies
Me = multiple endoscopy rules may apply
M+ = multiple therapy rules apply
Mtc = multiple diagnostic imaging rules apply
T = team surgeons permitted
T+ = team surgeons payable if medical necessity established with documentation
§ = indicates code is not covered by Medicare
GS = procedure must be performed under the general supervision of a physician
DS = procedure must be performed under the direct supervision of a physician
PS = procedure must be performed under the personal supervision of a physician
DRA = procedure subject to DRA limitation

Relative Value Units

CPT Code and Modifier	Description	Work RVU	Nonfacility Practice Expense RVU	Facility Practice Expense RVU	PLI RVU	Total Non-facility RVUs	Medicare Payment Nonfacility	Total Facility RVUs	Medicare Payment Facility	Global Period	Payment Policy Indicators
78226	Hepatobiliary system imaging	0.74	8.38	NA	0.09	9.21	$318.72	NA	NA	XXX	A+
78226-26	Hepatobiliary system imaging	0.74	0.25	0.25	0.04	1.03	$35.64	1.03	$35.64	XXX	A+
78226-TC	Hepatobiliary system imaging	0.00	8.13	NA	0.05	8.18	$283.08	NA	NA	XXX	A+ GS
78227	Hepatobil syst image w/drug	0.90	11.38	NA	0.11	12.39	$428.77	NA	NA	XXX	A+
78227-26	Hepatobil syst image w/drug	0.90	0.31	0.31	0.04	1.25	$43.26	1.25	$43.26	XXX	A+
78227-TC	Hepatobil syst image w/drug	0.00	11.07	NA	0.07	11.14	$385.51	NA	NA	XXX	A+ GS
78230	Salivary gland imaging	0.45	4.49	NA	0.06	5.00	$173.03	NA	NA	XXX	A+
78230-26	Salivary gland imaging	0.45	0.16	0.16	0.02	0.63	$21.80	0.63	$21.80	XXX	A+
78230-TC	Salivary gland imaging	0.00	4.33	NA	0.04	4.37	$151.23	NA	NA	XXX	A+ GS
78231	Serial salivary imaging	0.52	2.55	NA	0.05	3.12	$107.97	NA	NA	XXX	A+
78231-26	Serial salivary imaging	0.52	0.09	0.09	0.01	0.62	$21.46	0.62	$21.46	XXX	A+
78231-TC	Serial salivary imaging	0.00	2.46	NA	0.04	2.50	$86.52	NA	NA	XXX	A+ GS
78232	Salivary gland function exam	0.47	2.55	NA	0.05	3.07	$106.24	NA	NA	XXX	A+
78232-26	Salivary gland function exam	0.47	0.08	0.08	0.01	0.56	$19.38	0.56	$19.38	XXX	A+
78232-TC	Salivary gland function exam	0.00	2.47	NA	0.04	2.51	$86.86	NA	NA	XXX	A+ GS
78258	Esophageal motility study	0.74	5.26	NA	0.06	6.06	$209.71	NA	NA	XXX	A+
78258-26	Esophageal motility study	0.74	0.22	0.22	0.02	0.98	$33.91	0.98	$33.91	XXX	A+
78258-TC	Esophageal motility study	0.00	5.04	NA	0.04	5.08	$175.80	NA	NA	XXX	A+ GS
78261	Gastric mucosa imaging	0.69	5.08	NA	0.05	5.82	$201.41	NA	NA	XXX	A+
78261-26	Gastric mucosa imaging	0.69	0.12	0.12	0.01	0.82	$28.38	0.82	$28.38	XXX	A+
78261-TC	Gastric mucosa imaging	0.00	4.96	NA	0.04	5.00	$173.03	NA	NA	XXX	A+ GS
78262	Gastroesophageal reflux exam	0.68	6.20	NA	0.08	6.96	$240.86	NA	NA	XXX	A+
78262-26	Gastroesophageal reflux exam	0.68	0.25	0.25	0.04	0.97	$33.57	0.97	$33.57	XXX	A+
78262-TC	Gastroesophageal reflux exam	0.00	5.95	NA	0.04	5.99	$207.29	NA	NA	XXX	A+ GS
78264	Gastric emptying imag study	0.79	8.48	NA	0.09	9.36	$323.91	NA	NA	XXX	A+
78264-26	Gastric emptying imag study	0.79	0.27	0.27	0.04	1.10	$38.07	1.10	$38.07	XXX	A+
78264-TC	Gastric emptying imag study	0.00	8.21	NA	0.05	8.26	$285.85	NA	NA	XXX	A+ GS
78265	Gastric emptying imag study	0.98	9.99	NA	0.11	11.08	$383.44	NA	NA	XXX	A+
78265-26	Gastric emptying imag study	0.98	0.33	0.33	0.04	1.35	$46.72	1.35	$46.72	XXX	A+
78265-TC	Gastric emptying imag study	0.00	9.66	NA	0.07	9.73	$336.72	NA	NA	XXX	A+ GS
78266	Gastric emptying imag study	1.08	11.23	NA	0.12	12.43	$430.16	NA	NA	XXX	A+
78266-26	Gastric emptying imag study	1.08	0.31	0.31	0.04	1.43	$49.49	1.43	$49.49	XXX	A+
78266-TC	Gastric emptying imag study	0.00	10.92	NA	0.08	11.00	$380.67	NA	NA	XXX	A+ GS

78278		Acute gi blood loss imaging	0.99	8.78	NA	0.09	9.86	$341.22	NA	NA	XXX	A+
78278-26		Acute gi blood loss imaging	0.99	0.34	0.34	0.04	1.37	$47.41	1.37	$47.41	XXX	A+
78278-TC		Acute gi blood loss imaging	0.00	8.44	NA	0.05	8.49	$293.81	NA	NA	XXX	A+ GS
78282	CP	Gi protein loss exam	0.00	0.00	NA	0.00	0.00	$0.00	NA	NA	XXX	A+
78282-26		Gi protein loss exam	0.38	0.07	0.07	0.01	0.46	$15.92	0.46	$15.92	XXX	A+
78282-TC	CP	Gi protein loss exam	0.00	0.00	NA	0.00	0.00	$0.00	NA	NA	XXX	A+ GS
78290		Meckels divert exam	0.68	8.56	NA	0.09	9.33	$322.88	NA	NA	XXX	A+
78290-26		Meckels divert exam	0.68	0.22	0.22	0.04	0.94	$32.53	0.94	$32.53	XXX	A+
78290-TC		Meckels divert exam	0.00	8.34	NA	0.05	8.39	$290.35	NA	NA	XXX	A+ GS
78291		Leveen/shunt patency exam	0.88	6.47	NA	0.08	7.43	$257.12	NA	NA	XXX	A+
78291-26		Leveen/shunt patency exam	0.88	0.32	0.32	0.04	1.24	$42.91	1.24	$42.91	XXX	A+
78291-TC		Leveen/shunt patency exam	0.00	6.15	NA	0.04	6.19	$214.21	NA	NA	XXX	A+ GS
78299	CP	Gi nuclear procedure	0.00	0.00	NA	0.00	0.00	$0.00	NA	NA	XXX	A+
78299-26	CP	Gi nuclear procedure	0.00	0.00	0.00	0.00	0.00	$0.00	0.00	$0.00	XXX	A+
78299-TC	CP	Gi nuclear procedure	0.00	0.00	NA	0.00	0.00	$0.00	NA	NA	XXX	A+
78300		Bone imaging limited area	0.62	5.77	NA	0.08	6.47	$223.90	NA	NA	XXX	A+
78300-26		Bone imaging limited area	0.62	0.22	0.22	0.04	0.88	$30.45	0.88	$30.45	XXX	A+
78300-TC		Bone imaging limited area	0.00	5.55	NA	0.04	5.59	$193.45	NA	NA	XXX	A+ GS
78305		Bone imaging multiple areas	0.83	6.89	NA	0.08	7.80	$269.93	NA	NA	XXX	A+
78305-26		Bone imaging multiple areas	0.83	0.28	0.28	0.04	1.15	$39.80	1.15	$39.80	XXX	A+
78305-TC		Bone imaging multiple areas	0.00	6.61	NA	0.04	6.65	$230.13	NA	NA	XXX	A+ GS
78306		Bone imaging whole body	0.86	7.45	NA	0.08	8.39	$290.35	NA	NA	XXX	A+ M
78306-26		Bone imaging whole body	0.86	0.28	0.28	0.04	1.18	$40.84	1.18	$40.84	XXX	A+ M
78306-TC		Bone imaging whole body	0.00	7.17	NA	0.04	7.21	$249.51	NA	NA	XXX	A+ M GS
78315		Bone imaging 3 phase	1.02	8.68	NA	0.09	9.79	$338.79	NA	NA	XXX	A+
78315-26		Bone imaging 3 phase	1.02	0.34	0.34	0.04	1.40	$48.45	1.40	$48.45	XXX	A+
78315-TC		Bone imaging 3 phase	0.00	8.34	NA	0.05	8.39	$290.35	NA	NA	XXX	A+ GS
78350	§	Bone mineral single photon	0.22	0.69	NA	0.02	0.93	$32.18	NA	NA	XXX	

*Please note that these calculations are based on the Medicare 2022 Conversion Factor of $34.6062 and the DRA RVU cap rates at time of publication.

A = assistant-at-surgery restriction
A+ = assistant-at-surgery restriction unless medical necessity established with documentation
B = bilateral surgery adjustment applies
C = cosurgeons payable
C+ = cosurgeons payable if medical necessity established with documentation
CP = carriers may establish RVUs and payment amounts for these services, generally on an individual basis following review of documentation such as an operative report
M = multiple surgery adjustment applies
Me = multiple endoscopy rules may apply
M+ = multiple therapy rules apply
Mtc = multiple diagnostic imaging rules apply
T = team surgeons permitted
T+ = team surgeons payable if medical necessity established with documentation
§ = indicates code is not covered by Medicare
GS = procedure must be performed under the general supervision of a physician
DS = procedure must be performed under the direct supervision of a physician
PS = procedure must be performed under the personal supervision of a physician
DRA = procedure subject to DRA limitation

Relative Value Units

CPT Code and Modifier		Description	Work RVU	Nonfacility Practice Expense RVU	Facility Practice Expense RVU	PLI RVU	Total Non-facility RVUs	Medicare Payment Nonfacility	Total Facility RVUs	Medicare Payment Facility	Global Period	Payment Policy Indicators
78350-26	§	Bone mineral single photon	0.22	0.09	0.09	0.01	0.32	$11.07	0.32	$11.07	XXX	
78350-TC	§	Bone mineral single photon	0.00	0.60	NA	0.01	0.61	$21.11	NA	NA	XXX	GS
78351	§	Bone mineral dual photon	0.30	NA	0.12	0.02	NA	NA	0.44	$15.23	XXX	
78399	CP	Musculoskeletal nuclear exam	0.00	0.00	NA	0.00	0.00	$0.00	NA	NA	XXX	A+
78399-26	CP	Musculoskeletal nuclear exam	0.00	0.00	0.00	0.00	0.00	$0.00	0.00	$0.00	XXX	A+
78399-TC	CP	Musculoskeletal nuclear exam	0.00	0.00	NA	0.00	0.00	$0.00	NA	NA	XXX	A+
78414	CP	Non-imaging heart function	0.00	0.00	NA	0.00	0.00	$0.00	NA	NA	XXX	A+
78414-26		Non-imaging heart function	0.45	0.17	0.17	0.01	0.63	$21.80	0.63	$21.80	XXX	A+
78414-TC	CP	Non-imaging heart function	0.00	0.00	NA	0.00	0.00	$0.00	NA	NA	XXX	A+ GS
78428		Cardiac shunt imaging	0.78	4.49	NA	0.08	5.35	$185.14	NA	NA	XXX	A+
78428-26		Cardiac shunt imaging	0.78	0.26	0.26	0.04	1.08	$37.37	1.08	$37.37	XXX	A+
78428-TC		Cardiac shunt imaging	0.00	4.23	NA	0.04	4.27	$147.77	NA	NA	XXX	A+ GS
78429	CP	Myocrd img pet 1 std w/ct	0.00	0.00	NA	0.00	0.00	$0.00	NA	NA	XXX	A+
78429-26		Myocrd img pet 1 std w/ct	1.76	0.53	0.53	0.05	2.34	$80.98	2.34	$80.98	XXX	A+
78429-TC	CP	Myocrd img pet 1 std w/ct	0.00	0.00	NA	0.00	0.00	$0.00	NA	NA	XXX	A+ GS
78430	CP	Myocrd img pet rst/strs w/ct	0.00	0.00	NA	0.00	0.00	$0.00	NA	NA	XXX	A+
78430-26		Myocrd img pet rst/strs w/ct	1.67	0.51	0.51	0.05	2.23	$77.17	2.23	$77.17	XXX	A+
78430-TC	CP	Myocrd img pet rst/strs w/ct	0.00	0.00	NA	0.00	0.00	$0.00	NA	NA	XXX	A+ GS
78431	CP	Myocrd img pet rst&strs ct	0.00	0.00	NA	0.00	0.00	$0.00	NA	NA	XXX	A+
78431-26		Myocrd img pet rst&strs ct	1.90	0.63	0.63	0.07	2.60	$89.98	2.60	$89.98	XXX	A+
78431-TC	CP	Myocrd img pet rst&strs ct	0.00	0.00	NA	0.00	0.00	$0.00	NA	NA	XXX	A+ GS
78432	CP	Myocrd img pet 2rtracer	0.00	0.00	NA	0.00	0.00	$0.00	NA	NA	XXX	A+
78432-26		Myocrd img pet 2rtracer	2.07	0.61	0.61	0.07	2.75	$95.17	2.75	$95.17	XXX	A+
78432-TC	CP	Myocrd img pet 2rtracer	0.00	0.00	NA	0.00	0.00	$0.00	NA	NA	XXX	A+ GS
78433	CP	Myocrd img pet 2rtracer ct	0.00	0.00	NA	0.00	0.00	$0.00	NA	NA	XXX	A+
78433-26		Myocrd img pet 2rtracer ct	2.26	0.69	0.69	0.08	3.03	$104.86	3.03	$104.86	XXX	A+
78433-TC	CP	Myocrd img pet 2rtracer ct	0.00	0.00	NA	0.00	0.00	$0.00	NA	NA	XXX	A+ GS
78434	CP	Aqmbf pet rest & rx stress	0.00	0.00	NA	0.00	0.00	$0.00	NA	NA	ZZZ	A+
78434-26		Aqmbf pet rest & rx stress	0.63	0.21	0.21	0.02	0.86	$29.76	0.86	$29.76	ZZZ	A+
78434-TC	CP	Aqmbf pet rest & rx stress	0.00	0.00	NA	0.00	0.00	$0.00	NA	NA	ZZZ	A+ GS
78445		Vascular flow imaging	0.49	5.39	NA	0.09	5.97	$206.60	NA	NA	XXX	A+
78445-26		Vascular flow imaging	0.49	0.19	0.19	0.05	0.73	$25.26	0.73	$25.26	XXX	A+
78445-TC		Vascular flow imaging	0.00	5.20	NA	0.04	5.24	$181.34	NA	NA	XXX	A+ GS

78451		Ht muscle image spect sing	1.38	8.15	NA	0.10	9.63	$333.26	NA	NA	XXX	A+
78451-26		Ht muscle image spect sing	1.38	0.47	0.47	0.05	1.90	$65.75	1.90	$65.75	XXX	A+
78451-TC		Ht muscle image spect sing	0.00	7.68	NA	0.05	7.73	$267.51	NA	NA	XXX	A+ GS
78452		Ht muscle image spect mult	1.62	11.65	NA	0.15	13.42	$464.42	NA	NA	XXX	A+
78452-26		Ht muscle image spect mult	1.62	0.56	0.56	0.07	2.25	$77.86	2.25	$77.86	XXX	A+
78452-TC		Ht muscle image spect mult	0.00	11.09	NA	0.08	11.17	$386.55	NA	NA	XXX	A+ GS
78453		Ht muscle image planar sing	1.00	7.28	NA	0.08	8.36	$289.31	NA	NA	XXX	A+
78453-26		Ht muscle image planar sing	1.00	0.34	0.34	0.04	1.38	$47.76	1.38	$47.76	XXX	A+
78453-TC		Ht muscle image planar sing	0.00	6.94	NA	0.04	6.98	$241.55	NA	NA	XXX	A+ GS
78454		Ht musc image planar mult	1.34	10.81	NA	0.14	12.29	$425.31	NA	NA	XXX	A+
78454-26		Ht musc image planar mult	1.34	0.47	0.47	0.07	1.88	$65.06	1.88	$65.06	XXX	A+
78454-TC		Ht musc image planar mult	0.00	10.34	NA	0.07	10.41	$360.25	NA	NA	XXX	A+ GS
78456		Acute venous thrombus image	1.00	7.80	NA	0.09	8.89	$307.65	NA	NA	XXX	
78456-26		Acute venous thrombus image	1.00	0.35	0.35	0.04	1.39	$48.10	1.39	$48.10	XXX	
78456-TC		Acute venous thrombus image	0.00	7.45	NA	0.05	7.50	$259.55	NA	NA	XXX	
78457		Venous thrombosis imaging	0.77	4.29	NA	0.08	5.14	$177.88	NA	NA	XXX	A+
78457-26		Venous thrombosis imaging	0.77	0.27	0.27	0.04	1.08	$37.37	1.08	$37.37	XXX	A+
78457-TC		Venous thrombosis imaging	0.00	4.02	NA	0.04	4.06	$140.50	NA	NA	XXX	A+ GS
78458		Ven thrombosis images bilat	0.90	4.89	NA	0.08	5.87	$203.14	NA	NA	XXX	A+
78458-26		Ven thrombosis images bilat	0.90	0.33	0.33	0.04	1.27	$43.95	1.27	$43.95	XXX	A+
78458-TC		Ven thrombosis images bilat	0.00	4.56	NA	0.04	4.60	$159.19	NA	NA	XXX	A+ GS
78459	CP	Myocrd img pet single study	0.00	0.00	NA	0.00	0.00	$0.00	NA	NA	XXX	A+
78459-26		Myocrd img pet single study	1.61	0.49	0.49	0.05	2.15	$74.40	2.15	$74.40	XXX	A+
78459-TC	CP	Myocrd img pet single study	0.00	0.00	NA	0.00	0.00	$0.00	NA	NA	XXX	A+ GS
78466		Heart infarct image	0.69	4.76	NA	0.08	5.53	$191.37	NA	NA	XXX	A+
78466-26		Heart infarct image	0.69	0.27	0.27	0.04	1.00	$34.61	1.00	$34.61	XXX	A+
78466-TC		Heart infarct image	0.00	4.49	NA	0.04	4.53	$156.77	NA	NA	XXX	A+ GS
78468		Heart infarct image (ef)	0.80	4.71	NA	0.08	5.59	$193.45	NA	NA	XXX	A+

*Please note that these calculations are based on the Medicare 2022 Conversion Factor of $34.6062 and the DRA RVU cap rates at time of publication.

A = assistant-at-surgery restriction
A+ = assistant-at-surgery restriction unless medical necessity established with documentation
B = bilateral surgery adjustment applies
C = cosurgeons payable
C+ = cosurgeons payable if medical necessity established with documentation
CP = carriers may establish RVUs and payment amounts for these services, generally on an individual basis following review of documentation such as an operative report
M = multiple surgery adjustment applies
Me = multiple endoscopy rules may apply
M+ = multiple therapy rules apply
Mtc = multiple diagnostic imaging rules apply
T = team surgeons permitted
T+ = team surgeons payable if medical necessity established with documentation
§ = indicates code is not covered by Medicare
GS = procedure must be performed under the general supervision of a physician
DS = procedure must be performed under the direct supervision of a physician
PS = procedure must be performed under the personal supervision of a physician
DRA = procedure subject to DRA limitation

Relative Value Units

CPT Code and Modifier		Description	Work RVU	Nonfacility Practice Expense RVU	Facility Practice Expense RVU	PLI RVU	Total Non-facility RVUs	Medicare Payment Nonfacility	Total Facility RVUs	Medicare Payment Facility	Global Period	Payment Policy Indicators
78468-26		Heart infarct image (ef)	0.80	0.27	0.27	0.04	1.11	$38.41	1.11	$38.41	XXX	A+
78468-TC		Heart infarct image (ef)	0.00	4.44	NA	0.04	4.48	$155.04	NA	NA	XXX	A+ GS
78469		Heart infarct image (3d)	0.92	5.29	NA	0.08	6.29	$217.67	NA	NA	XXX	A+
78469-26		Heart infarct image (3d)	0.92	0.32	0.32	0.04	1.28	$44.30	1.28	$44.30	XXX	A+
78469-TC		Heart infarct image (3d)	0.00	4.97	NA	0.04	5.01	$173.38	NA	NA	XXX	A+ GS
78472		Gated heart planar single	0.98	5.42	NA	0.08	6.48	$224.25	NA	NA	XXX	A+
78472-26		Gated heart planar single	0.98	0.34	0.34	0.04	1.36	$47.06	1.36	$47.06	XXX	A+
78472-TC		Gated heart planar single	0.00	5.08	NA	0.04	5.12	$177.18	NA	NA	XXX	A+ GS
78473		Gated heart multiple	1.47	6.65	NA	0.09	8.21	$284.12	NA	NA	XXX	A+
78473-26		Gated heart multiple	1.47	0.49	0.49	0.05	2.01	$69.56	2.01	$69.56	XXX	A+
78473-TC		Gated heart multiple	0.00	6.16	NA	0.04	6.20	$214.56	NA	NA	XXX	A+ GS
78481		Heart first pass single	0.98	4.01	NA	0.08	5.07	$175.45	NA	NA	XXX	A+
78481-26		Heart first pass single	0.98	0.34	0.34	0.04	1.36	$47.06	1.36	$47.06	XXX	A+
78481-TC		Heart first pass single	0.00	3.67	NA	0.04	3.71	$128.39	NA	NA	XXX	A+ GS
78483		Heart first pass multiple	1.47	5.35	NA	0.09	6.91	$239.13	NA	NA	XXX	A+
78483-26		Heart first pass multiple	1.47	0.52	0.52	0.05	2.04	$70.60	2.04	$70.60	XXX	A+
78483-TC		Heart first pass multiple	0.00	4.83	NA	0.04	4.87	$168.53	NA	NA	XXX	A+ GS
78491	CP	Myocrd img pet 1std rst/strs	0.00	0.00	NA	0.00	0.00	$0.00	NA	NA	XXX	A+
78491-26		Myocrd img pet 1std rst/strs	1.56	0.47	0.47	0.05	2.08	$71.98	2.08	$71.98	XXX	A+
78491-TC	CP	Myocrd img pet 1std rst/strs	0.00	0.00	NA	0.00	0.00	$0.00	NA	NA	XXX	A+ GS
78492	CP	Myocrd img pet mlt rst&strs	0.00	0.00	NA	0.00	0.00	$0.00	NA	NA	XXX	A+
78492-26		Myocrd img pet mlt rst&strs	1.80	0.61	0.61	0.07	2.48	$85.82	2.48	$85.82	XXX	A+
78492-TC	CP	Myocrd img pet mlt rst&strs	0.00	0.00	NA	0.00	0.00	$0.00	NA	NA	XXX	A+ GS
78494		Heart image spect	1.19	5.25	NA	0.08	6.52	$225.63	NA	NA	XXX	A+
78494-26		Heart image spect	1.19	0.42	0.42	0.04	1.65	$57.10	1.65	$57.10	XXX	A+
78494-TC		Heart image spect	0.00	4.83	NA	0.04	4.87	$168.53	NA	NA	XXX	A+ GS
78496		Heart first pass add-on	0.50	0.73	NA	0.03	1.26	$43.60	NA	NA	ZZZ	A+
78496-26		Heart first pass add-on	0.50	0.18	0.18	0.02	0.70	$24.22	0.70	$24.22	ZZZ	A+
78496-TC		Heart first pass add-on	0.00	0.55	NA	0.01	0.56	$19.38	NA	NA	ZZZ	A+ GS
78499	CP	Cardiovascular nuclear exam	0.00	0.00	NA	0.00	0.00	$0.00	NA	NA	XXX	A+
78499-26	CP	Cardiovascular nuclear exam	0.00	0.00	0.00	0.00	0.00	$0.00	0.00	$0.00	XXX	A+
78499-TC	CP	Cardiovascular nuclear exam	0.00	0.00	NA	0.00	0.00	$0.00	NA	NA	XXX	A+
78579		Lung ventilation imaging	0.49	4.75	NA	0.06	5.30	$183.41	NA	NA	XXX	A+

78579-26		Lung ventilation imaging	0.49	0.16	0.16	0.02	0.67	$23.19	0.67	$23.19	XXX	A+
78579-TC		Lung ventilation imaging	0.00	4.59	NA	0.04	4.63	$160.23	NA	NA	XXX	A+ GS
78580		Lung perfusion imaging	0.74	5.88	NA	0.08	6.70	$231.86	NA	NA	XXX	A+
78580-26		Lung perfusion imaging	0.74	0.25	0.25	0.04	1.03	$35.64	1.03	$35.64	XXX	A+
78580-TC		Lung perfusion imaging	0.00	5.63	NA	0.04	5.67	$196.22	NA	NA	XXX	A+ GS
78582		Lung ventilat&perfus imaging	1.07	8.25	NA	0.09	9.41	$325.64	NA	NA	XXX	A+
78582-26		Lung ventilat&perfus imaging	1.07	0.36	0.36	0.04	1.47	$50.87	1.47	$50.87	XXX	A+
78582-TC		Lung ventilat&perfus imaging	0.00	7.89	NA	0.05	7.94	$274.77	NA	NA	XXX	A+ GS
78597		Lung perfusion differential	0.75	4.90	NA	0.06	5.71	$197.60	NA	NA	XXX	A+
78597-26		Lung perfusion differential	0.75	0.22	0.22	0.02	0.99	$34.26	0.99	$34.26	XXX	A+
78597-TC		Lung perfusion differential	0.00	4.68	NA	0.04	4.72	$163.34	NA	NA	XXX	A+ GS
78598		Lung perf&ventilat diferentl	0.85	7.67	NA	0.08	8.60	$297.61	NA	NA	XXX	A+
78598-26		Lung perf&ventilat diferentl	0.85	0.27	0.27	0.04	1.16	$40.14	1.16	$40.14	XXX	A+
78598-TC		Lung perf&ventilat diferentl	0.00	7.40	NA	0.04	7.44	$257.47	NA	NA	XXX	A+ GS
78599	CP	Respiratory nuclear exam	0.00	0.00	NA	0.00	0.00	$0.00	NA	NA	XXX	A+
78599-26	CP	Respiratory nuclear exam	0.00	0.00	0.00	0.00	0.00	$0.00	0.00	$0.00	XXX	A+
78599-TC	CP	Respiratory nuclear exam	0.00	0.00	NA	0.00	0.00	$0.00	NA	NA	XXX	A+
78600		Brain image < 4 views	0.44	4.72	NA	0.06	5.22	$180.64	NA	NA	XXX	A+
78600-26		Brain image < 4 views	0.44	0.16	0.16	0.02	0.62	$21.46	0.62	$21.46	XXX	A+
78600-TC		Brain image < 4 views	0.00	4.56	NA	0.04	4.60	$159.19	NA	NA	XXX	A+ GS
78601		Brain image w/flow < 4 views	0.51	5.54	NA	0.06	6.11	$211.44	NA	NA	XXX	A+
78601-26		Brain image w/flow < 4 views	0.51	0.17	0.17	0.02	0.70	$24.22	0.70	$24.22	XXX	A+
78601-TC		Brain image w/flow < 4 views	0.00	5.37	NA	0.04	5.41	$187.22	NA	NA	XXX	A+ GS
78605		Brain image 4+ views	0.53	5.09	NA	0.06	5.68	$196.56	NA	NA	XXX	A+
78605-26		Brain image 4+ views	0.53	0.19	0.19	0.02	0.74	$25.61	0.74	$25.61	XXX	A+
78605-TC		Brain image 4+ views	0.00	4.90	NA	0.04	4.94	$170.95	NA	NA	XXX	A+ GS
78606		Brain image w/flow 4 + views	0.64	8.55	NA	0.09	9.28	$321.15	NA	NA	XXX	A+
78606-26		Brain image w/flow 4 + views	0.64	0.21	0.21	0.04	0.89	$30.80	0.89	$30.80	XXX	A+

*Please note that these calculations are based on the Medicare 2022 Conversion Factor of $34.6062 and the DRA RVU cap rates at time of publication.

A = assistant-at-surgery restriction
A+ = assistant-at-surgery restriction unless medical necessity established with documentation
B = bilateral surgery adjustment applies
C = cosurgeons payable
C+ = cosurgeons payable if medical necessity established with documentation
CP = carriers may establish RVUs and payment amounts for these services, generally on an individual basis following review of documentation such as an operative report
M = multiple surgery adjustment applies
Me = multiple endoscopy rules may apply
M+ = multiple therapy rules apply
Mtc = multiple diagnostic imaging rules apply
T = team surgeons permitted
T+ = team surgeons payable if medical necessity established with documentation
§ = indicates code is not covered by Medicare
GS = procedure must be performed under the general supervision of a physician
DS = procedure must be performed under the direct supervision of a physician
PS = procedure must be performed under the personal supervision of a physician
DRA = procedure subject to DRA limitation

Relative Value Units

CPT Code and Modifier		Description	Work RVU	Nonfacility Practice Expense RVU	Facility Practice Expense RVU	PLI RVU	Total Non-facility RVUs	Medicare Payment Nonfacility	Total Facility RVUs	Medicare Payment Facility	Global Period	Payment Policy Indicators
78606-TC		Brain image w/flow 4 + views	0.00	8.34	NA	0.05	8.39	$290.35	NA	NA	XXX	A+ GS
78608	CP	Brain imaging (pet)	0.00	0.00	NA	0.00	0.00	$0.00	NA	NA	XXX	A+
78608-26		Brain imaging (pet)	1.50	0.47	0.47	0.05	2.02	$69.90	2.02	$69.90	XXX	A+
78608-TC	CP	Brain imaging (pet)	0.00	0.00	NA	0.00	0.00	$0.00	NA	NA	XXX	A+ GS
78609	§	Brain imaging (pet)	1.50	0.58	NA	0.08	2.16	$74.75	NA	NA	XXX	
78609-26	§	Brain imaging (pet)	1.50	0.58	0.58	0.08	2.16	$74.75	2.16	$74.75	XXX	
78610		Brain flow imaging only	0.30	4.61	NA	0.05	4.96	$171.65	NA	NA	XXX	A+
78610-26		Brain flow imaging only	0.30	0.10	0.10	0.01	0.41	$14.19	0.41	$14.19	XXX	A+
78610-TC		Brain flow imaging only	0.00	4.51	NA	0.04	4.55	$157.46	NA	NA	XXX	A+ GS
78630		Cerebrospinal fluid scan	0.68	8.80	NA	0.09	9.57	$331.18	NA	NA	XXX	A+
78630-26		Cerebrospinal fluid scan	0.68	0.23	0.23	0.04	0.95	$32.88	0.95	$32.88	XXX	A+
78630-TC		Cerebrospinal fluid scan	0.00	8.57	NA	0.05	8.62	$298.31	NA	NA	XXX	A+ GS
78635		Csf ventriculography	0.61	8.85	NA	0.09	9.55	$330.49	NA	NA	XXX	A+
78635-26		Csf ventriculography	0.61	0.22	0.22	0.04	0.87	$30.11	0.87	$30.11	XXX	A+
78635-TC		Csf ventriculography	0.00	8.63	NA	0.05	8.68	$300.38	NA	NA	XXX	A+ GS
78645		Csf shunt evaluation	0.57	8.50	NA	0.07	9.14	$316.30	NA	NA	XXX	A+
78645-26		Csf shunt evaluation	0.57	0.18	0.18	0.02	0.77	$26.65	0.77	$26.65	XXX	A+
78645-TC		Csf shunt evaluation	0.00	8.32	NA	0.05	8.37	$289.65	NA	NA	XXX	A+ GS
78650		Csf leakage imaging	0.61	7.19	NA	0.06	7.86	$272.00	NA	NA	XXX	A+
78650-26		Csf leakage imaging	0.61	0.11	0.11	0.01	0.73	$25.26	0.73	$25.26	XXX	A+
78650-TC		Csf leakage imaging	0.00	7.08	NA	0.05	7.13	$246.74	NA	NA	XXX	A+ GS
78660		Nuclear exam of tear flow	0.53	4.69	NA	0.06	5.28	$182.72	NA	NA	XXX	A+
78660-26		Nuclear exam of tear flow	0.53	0.19	0.19	0.02	0.74	$25.61	0.74	$25.61	XXX	A+
78660-TC		Nuclear exam of tear flow	0.00	4.50	NA	0.04	4.54	$157.11	NA	NA	XXX	A+ GS
78699	CP	Nervous system nuclear exam	0.00	0.00	NA	0.00	0.00	$0.00	NA	NA	XXX	A+
78699-26	CP	Nervous system nuclear exam	0.00	0.00	0.00	0.00	0.00	$0.00	0.00	$0.00	XXX	A+
78699-TC	CP	Nervous system nuclear exam	0.00	0.00	NA	0.00	0.00	$0.00	NA	NA	XXX	A+
78700		Kidney imaging morphol	0.45	4.34	NA	0.06	4.85	$167.84	NA	NA	XXX	A+
78700-26		Kidney imaging morphol	0.45	0.15	0.15	0.02	0.62	$21.46	0.62	$21.46	XXX	A+
78700-TC		Kidney imaging morphol	0.00	4.19	NA	0.04	4.23	$146.38	NA	NA	XXX	A+ GS
78701		Kidney imaging with flow	0.49	5.72	NA	0.06	6.27	$216.98	NA	NA	XXX	A+
78701-26		Kidney imaging with flow	0.49	0.17	0.17	0.02	0.68	$23.53	0.68	$23.53	XXX	A+
78701-TC		Kidney imaging with flow	0.00	5.55	NA	0.04	5.59	$193.45	NA	NA	XXX	A+ GS

78707		K flow/funct image w/o drug	0.96	5.54	NA	0.08	6.58	$227.71	NA	NA	XXX	A+
78707-26		K flow/funct image w/o drug	0.96	0.30	0.30	0.04	1.30	$44.99	1.30	$44.99	XXX	A+
78707-TC		K flow/funct image w/o drug	0.00	5.24	NA	0.04	5.28	$182.72	NA	NA	XXX	A+ GS
78708		K flow/funct image w/drug	1.21	3.87	NA	0.10	5.18	$179.26	NA	NA	XXX	A+
78708-26		K flow/funct image w/drug	1.21	0.40	0.40	0.05	1.66	$57.45	1.66	$57.45	XXX	A+
78708-TC		K flow/funct image w/drug	0.00	3.47	NA	0.05	3.52	$121.81	NA	NA	XXX	A+ GS
78709		K flow/funct image multiple	1.41	8.94	NA	0.12	10.47	$362.33	NA	NA	XXX	A+
78709-26		K flow/funct image multiple	1.41	0.46	0.46	0.07	1.94	$67.14	1.94	$67.14	XXX	A+
78709-TC		K flow/funct image multiple	0.00	8.48	NA	0.05	8.53	$295.19	NA	NA	XXX	A+ GS
78725		Kidney function study	0.38	2.90	NA	0.05	3.33	$115.24	NA	NA	XXX	A+
78725-26		Kidney function study	0.38	0.13	0.13	0.01	0.52	$18.00	0.52	$18.00	XXX	A+
78725-TC		Kidney function study	0.00	2.77	NA	0.04	2.81	$97.24	NA	NA	XXX	A+ GS
78730		Urinary bladder retention	0.15	1.98	NA	0.01	2.14	$74.06	NA	NA	ZZZ	A+
78730-26		Urinary bladder retention	0.15	0.07	0.07	0.00	0.22	$7.61	0.22	$7.61	ZZZ	A+
78730-TC		Urinary bladder retention	0.00	1.91	NA	0.01	1.92	$66.44	NA	NA	ZZZ	A+ GS
78740		Ureteral reflux study	0.57	5.55	NA	0.05	6.17	$213.52	NA	NA	XXX	A+
78740-26		Ureteral reflux study	0.57	0.18	0.18	0.01	0.76	$26.30	0.76	$26.30	XXX	A+
78740-TC		Ureteral reflux study	0.00	5.37	NA	0.04	5.41	$187.22	NA	NA	XXX	A+ GS
78761		Testicular imaging w/flow	0.71	5.24	NA	0.08	6.03	$208.68	NA	NA	XXX	A+
78761-26		Testicular imaging w/flow	0.71	0.26	0.26	0.04	1.01	$34.95	1.01	$34.95	XXX	A+
78761-TC		Testicular imaging w/flow	0.00	4.98	NA	0.04	5.02	$173.72	NA	NA	XXX	A+ GS
78799	CP	Genitourinary nuclear exam	0.00	0.00	NA	0.00	0.00	$0.00	NA	NA	XXX	A+
78799-26	CP	Genitourinary nuclear exam	0.00	0.00	0.00	0.00	0.00	$0.00	0.00	$0.00	XXX	A+
78799-TC	CP	Genitourinary nuclear exam	0.00	0.00	NA	0.00	0.00	$0.00	NA	NA	XXX	A+
78800		Rp loclzj tum 1 area 1 d img	0.64	6.46	NA	0.09	7.19	$248.82	NA	NA	XXX	A+
78800-26		Rp loclzj tum 1 area 1 d img	0.64	0.22	0.22	0.05	0.91	$31.49	0.91	$31.49	XXX	A+
78800-TC		Rp loclzj tum 1 area 1 d img	0.00	6.24	NA	0.04	6.28	$217.33	NA	NA	XXX	A+ GS
78801		Rp loclzj tum 2+area 1+d img	0.73	6.99	NA	0.08	7.80	$269.93	NA	NA	XXX	A+

*Please note that these calculations are based on the Medicare 2022 Conversion Factor of $34.6062 and the DRA RVU cap rates at time of publication.

A = assistant-at-surgery restriction
A+ = assistant-at-surgery restriction unless medical necessity established with documentation
B = bilateral surgery adjustment applies
C = cosurgeons payable
C+ = cosurgeons payable if medical necessity established with documentation
CP = carriers may establish RVUs and payment amounts for these services, generally on an individual basis following review of documentation such as an operative report
M = multiple surgery adjustment applies
Me = multiple endoscopy rules may apply
M+ = multiple therapy rules apply
Mtc = multiple diagnostic imaging rules apply
T = team surgeons permitted
T+ = team surgeons payable if medical necessity established with documentation
§ = indicates code is not covered by Medicare
GS = procedure must be performed under the general supervision of a physician
DS = procedure must be performed under the direct supervision of a physician
PS = procedure must be performed under the personal supervision of a physician
DRA = procedure subject to DRA limitation

Relative Value Units

CPT Code and Modifier		Description	Work RVU	Nonfacility Practice Expense RVU	Facility Practice Expense RVU	PLI RVU	Total Non-facility RVUs	Medicare Payment Nonfacility	Total Facility RVUs	Medicare Payment Facility	Global Period	Payment Policy Indicators
78801-26		Rp loclzj tum 2+area 1+d img	0.73	0.23	0.23	0.04	1.00	$34.61	1.00	$34.61	XXX	A+
78801-TC		Rp loclzj tum 2+area 1+d img	0.00	6.76	NA	0.04	6.80	$235.32	NA	NA	XXX	A+ GS
78802		Rp loclzj tum whbdy 1 d img	0.80	7.91	NA	0.08	8.79	$304.19	NA	NA	XXX	A+ M
78802-26		Rp loclzj tum whbdy 1 d img	0.80	0.26	0.26	0.04	1.10	$38.07	1.10	$38.07	XXX	A+ M
78802-TC		Rp loclzj tum whbdy 1 d img	0.00	7.65	NA	0.04	7.69	$266.12	NA	NA	XXX	A+ M GS
78803		Rp loclzj tum spect 1 area	1.09	9.68	NA	0.09	10.86	$375.82	NA	NA	XXX	A+ M
78803-26		Rp loclzj tum spect 1 area	1.09	0.34	0.34	0.04	1.47	$50.87	1.47	$50.87	XXX	A+ M
78803-TC		Rp loclzj tum spect 1 area	0.00	9.34	NA	0.05	9.39	$324.95	NA	NA	XXX	A+ M GS
78804		Rp loclzj tum whbdy 2+d img	1.01	17.36	NA	0.13	18.50	$640.21	NA	NA	XXX	A+
78804-26		Rp loclzj tum whbdy 2+d img	1.01	0.34	0.34	0.04	1.39	$48.10	1.39	$48.10	XXX	A+
78804-TC		Rp loclzj tum whbdy 2+d img	0.00	17.02	NA	0.09	17.11	$592.11	NA	NA	XXX	A+ GS
78808		Iv inj ra drug dx study	0.18	0.99	NA	0.02	1.19	$41.18	NA	NA	XXX	A+
78811	CP	Pet image ltd area	0.00	0.00	NA	0.00	0.00	$0.00	NA	NA	XXX	A+
78811-26		Pet image ltd area	1.54	0.48	0.48	0.07	2.09	$72.33	2.09	$72.33	XXX	A+
78811-TC	CP	Pet image ltd area	0.00	0.00	NA	0.00	0.00	$0.00	NA	NA	XXX	A+ GS
78812	CP	Pet image skull-thigh	0.00	0.00	NA	0.00	0.00	$0.00	NA	NA	XXX	A+
78812-26		Pet image skull-thigh	1.93	0.63	0.63	0.08	2.64	$91.36	2.64	$91.36	XXX	A+
78812-TC	CP	Pet image skull-thigh	0.00	0.00	NA	0.00	0.00	$0.00	NA	NA	XXX	A+ GS
78813	CP	Pet image full body	0.00	0.00	NA	0.00	0.00	$0.00	NA	NA	XXX	A+
78813-26		Pet image full body	2.00	0.58	0.58	0.07	2.65	$91.71	2.65	$91.71	XXX	A+
78813-TC	CP	Pet image full body	0.00	0.00	NA	0.00	0.00	$0.00	NA	NA	XXX	A+ GS
78814	CP	Pet image w/ct lmtd	0.00	0.00	NA	0.00	0.00	$0.00	NA	NA	XXX	A+
78814-26		Pet image w/ct lmtd	2.20	0.72	0.72	0.09	3.01	$104.16	3.01	$104.16	XXX	A+
78814-TC	CP	Pet image w/ct lmtd	0.00	0.00	NA	0.00	0.00	$0.00	NA	NA	XXX	A+ GS
78815	CP	Pet image w/ct skull-thigh	0.00	0.00	NA	0.00	0.00	$0.00	NA	NA	XXX	A+
78815-26		Pet image w/ct skull-thigh	2.44	0.80	0.80	0.10	3.34	$115.58	3.34	$115.58	XXX	A+
78815-TC	CP	Pet image w/ct skull-thigh	0.00	0.00	NA	0.00	0.00	$0.00	NA	NA	XXX	A+ GS
78816	CP	Pet image w/ct full body	0.00	0.00	NA	0.00	0.00	$0.00	NA	NA	XXX	A+
78816-26		Pet image w/ct full body	2.50	0.78	0.78	0.09	3.37	$116.62	3.37	$116.62	XXX	A+
78816-TC	CP	Pet image w/ct full body	0.00	0.00	NA	0.00	0.00	$0.00	NA	NA	XXX	A+ GS
78830		Rp loclzj tum spect w/ct 1	1.49	12.12	NA	0.10	13.71	$474.45	NA	NA	XXX	A+
78830-26		Rp loclzj tum spect w/ct 1	1.49	0.46	0.46	0.05	2.00	$69.21	2.00	$69.21	XXX	A+
78830-TC		Rp loclzj tum spect w/ct 1	0.00	11.66	NA	0.05	11.71	$405.24	NA	NA	XXX	A+ GS

78831		Rp loclzj tum spect 2 areas	1.82	18.00	NA	0.17	19.99	$691.78	NA	NA	XXX	A+
78831-26		Rp loclzj tum spect 2 areas	1.82	0.57	0.57	0.08	2.47	$85.48	2.47	$85.48	XXX	A+
78831-TC		Rp loclzj tum spect 2 areas	0.00	17.43	NA	0.09	17.52	$606.30	NA	NA	XXX	A+ GS
78832		Rp loclzj tum spect w/ct 2	2.12	23.71	NA	0.19	26.02	$900.45	NA	NA	XXX	A+
78832-26		Rp loclzj tum spect w/ct 2	2.12	0.66	0.66	0.09	2.87	$99.32	2.87	$99.32	XXX	A+
78832-TC		Rp loclzj tum spect w/ct 2	0.00	23.05	NA	0.10	23.15	$801.13	NA	NA	XXX	A+ GS
78835		Rp quan meas single area	0.47	2.33	NA	0.03	2.83	$97.94	NA	NA	ZZZ	A+
78835-26		Rp quan meas single area	0.47	0.14	0.14	0.02	0.63	$21.80	0.63	$21.80	ZZZ	A+
78835-TC		Rp quan meas single area	0.00	2.19	NA	0.01	2.20	$76.13	NA	NA	ZZZ	A+ GS
78999	CP	Nuclear diagnostic exam	0.00	0.00	NA	0.00	0.00	$0.00	NA	NA	XXX	A+
78999-26	CP	Nuclear diagnostic exam	0.00	0.00	0.00	0.00	0.00	$0.00	0.00	$0.00	XXX	A+
78999-TC	CP	Nuclear diagnostic exam	0.00	0.00	NA	0.00	0.00	$0.00	NA	NA	XXX	A+
79005		Nuclear rx oral admin	1.80	2.10	NA	0.10	4.00	$138.42	NA	NA	XXX	A+
79005-26		Nuclear rx oral admin	1.80	0.61	0.61	0.08	2.49	$86.17	2.49	$86.17	XXX	A+
79005-TC		Nuclear rx oral admin	0.00	1.49	NA	0.02	1.51	$52.26	NA	NA	XXX	A+
79101		Nuclear rx iv admin	1.96	2.28	NA	0.09	4.33	$149.84	NA	NA	XXX	A+
79101-26		Nuclear rx iv admin	1.96	0.73	0.73	0.07	2.76	$95.51	2.76	$95.51	XXX	A+
79101-TC		Nuclear rx iv admin	0.00	1.55	NA	0.02	1.57	$54.33	NA	NA	XXX	A+
79200		Nuclear rx intracav admin	1.99	1.93	NA	0.04	3.96	$137.04	NA	NA	XXX	A+
79200-26		Nuclear rx intracav admin	1.99	0.35	0.35	0.02	2.36	$81.67	2.36	$81.67	XXX	A+
79200-TC		Nuclear rx intracav admin	0.00	1.58	NA	0.02	1.60	$55.37	NA	NA	XXX	A+
79300	CP	Nuclr rx interstit colloid	0.00	0.00	NA	0.00	0.00	$0.00	NA	NA	XXX	A+
79300-26		Nuclr rx interstit colloid	1.60	0.28	0.28	0.01	1.89	$65.41	1.89	$65.41	XXX	A+
79300-TC	CP	Nuclr rx interstit colloid	0.00	0.00	NA	0.00	0.00	$0.00	NA	NA	XXX	A+
79403		Hematopoietic nuclear tx	2.25	2.38	NA	0.06	4.69	$162.30	NA	NA	XXX	A+
79403-26		Hematopoietic nuclear tx	2.25	0.39	0.39	0.02	2.66	$92.05	2.66	$92.05	XXX	A+
79403-TC		Hematopoietic nuclear tx	0.00	1.99	NA	0.04	2.03	$70.25	NA	NA	XXX	A+
79440		Nuclear rx intra-articular	1.99	1.54	NA	0.04	3.57	$123.54	NA	NA	XXX	A+

*Please note that these calculations are based on the Medicare 2022 Conversion Factor of $34.6062 and the DRA RVU cap rates at time of publication.

A = assistant-at-surgery restriction
A+ = assistant-at-surgery restriction unless medical necessity established with documentation
B = bilateral surgery adjustment applies
C = cosurgeons payable
C+ = cosurgeons payable if medical necessity established with documentation
CP = carriers may establish RVUs and payment amounts for these services, generally on an individual basis following review of documentation such as an operative report
M = multiple surgery adjustment applies
Me = multiple endoscopy rules may apply
M+ = multiple therapy rules apply
Mtc = multiple diagnostic imaging rules apply
T = team surgeons permitted
T+ = team surgeons payable if medical necessity established with documentation
§ = indicates code is not covered by Medicare
GS = procedure must be performed under the general supervision of a physician
DS = procedure must be performed under the direct supervision of a physician
PS = procedure must be performed under the personal supervision of a physician
DRA = procedure subject to DRA limitation

Relative Value Units

CPT Code and Modifier		Description	Work RVU	Nonfacility Practice Expense RVU	Facility Practice Expense RVU	PLI RVU	Total Non-facility RVUs	Medicare Payment Nonfacility	Total Facility RVUs	Medicare Payment Facility	Global Period	Payment Policy Indicators
79440-26		Nuclear rx intra-articular	1.99	0.35	0.35	0.02	2.36	$81.67	2.36	$81.67	XXX	A+
79440-TC		Nuclear rx intra-articular	0.00	1.19	NA	0.02	1.21	$41.87	NA	NA	XXX	A+
79445	CP	Nuclear rx intra-arterial	0.00	0.00	NA	0.00	0.00	$0.00	NA	NA	XXX	A+
79445-26		Nuclear rx intra-arterial	2.40	0.69	0.69	0.11	3.20	$110.74	3.20	$110.74	XXX	A+
79445-TC	CP	Nuclear rx intra-arterial	0.00	0.00	NA	0.00	0.00	$0.00	NA	NA	XXX	A+
79999	CP	Nuclear medicine therapy	0.00	0.00	NA	0.00	0.00	$0.00	NA	NA	XXX	A+
79999-26	CP	Nuclear medicine therapy	0.00	0.00	0.00	0.00	0.00	$0.00	0.00	$0.00	XXX	A+
79999-TC	CP	Nuclear medicine therapy	0.00	0.00	NA	0.00	0.00	$0.00	NA	NA	XXX	A+
80503		Path clin consltj sf 5-20	0.43	0.32	0.20	0.02	0.77	$26.65	0.65	$22.49	XXX	A+
80504		Path clin consltj mod 21-40	0.91	0.58	0.43	0.05	1.54	$53.29	1.39	$48.10	XXX	A+
80505		Path clin consltj high 41-60	1.71	0.98	0.81	0.10	2.79	$96.55	2.62	$90.67	XXX	A+
80506		Path clin consltj prolng svc	0.80	0.41	NA	0.04	1.25	$43.26	NA	NA	ZZZ	A+
83020-26		Hemoglobin electrophoresis	0.37	0.14	0.14	0.02	0.53	$18.34	0.53	$18.34	XXX	A+
84165-26		Protein e-phoresis serum	0.37	0.14	0.14	0.02	0.53	$18.34	0.53	$18.34	XXX	A+
84166-26		Protein e-phoresis/urine/csf	0.37	0.14	0.14	0.02	0.53	$18.34	0.53	$18.34	XXX	A+
84181-26		Western blot test	0.37	0.14	0.14	0.02	0.53	$18.34	0.53	$18.34	XXX	A+
84182-26		Protein western blot test	0.37	0.14	0.14	0.02	0.53	$18.34	0.53	$18.34	XXX	A+
85060		Blood smear interpretation	0.45	NA	0.22	0.04	NA	NA	0.71	$24.57	XXX	A+
85097		Bone marrow interpretation	0.94	1.02	0.41	0.05	2.01	$69.56	1.40	$48.45	XXX	A+
85390-26		Fibrinolysins screen i&r	0.75	0.29	0.29	0.04	1.08	$37.37	1.08	$37.37	XXX	A+
85396		Clotting assay whole blood	0.37	NA	0.18	0.02	NA	NA	0.57	$19.73	XXX	A+
85576-26		Blood platelet aggregation	0.37	0.14	0.14	0.02	0.53	$18.34	0.53	$18.34	XXX	A+
86077		Phys blood bank serv xmatch	0.94	0.56	0.45	0.05	1.55	$53.64	1.44	$49.83	XXX	A+
86078		Phys blood bank serv reactj	0.94	0.56	0.45	0.05	1.55	$53.64	1.44	$49.83	XXX	A+
86079		Phys blood bank serv authrj	0.94	0.56	0.45	0.05	1.55	$53.64	1.44	$49.83	XXX	A+
86153-26		Cell enumeration phys interp	0.69	0.27	0.27	0.04	1.00	$34.61	1.00	$34.61	XXX	A+
86255-26		Fluorescent antibody screen	0.37	0.14	0.14	0.02	0.53	$18.34	0.53	$18.34	XXX	A+
86256-26		Fluorescent antibody titer	0.37	0.14	0.14	0.02	0.53	$18.34	0.53	$18.34	XXX	A+
86320-26		Serum immunoelectrophoresis	0.37	0.14	0.14	0.02	0.53	$18.34	0.53	$18.34	XXX	A+
86325-26		Other immunoelectrophoresis	0.37	0.14	0.14	0.02	0.53	$18.34	0.53	$18.34	XXX	A+
86327-26		Immunoelectrophoresis assay	0.42	0.20	0.20	0.01	0.63	$21.80	0.63	$21.80	XXX	A+
86334-26		Immunofix e-phoresis serum	0.37	0.14	0.14	0.02	0.53	$18.34	0.53	$18.34	XXX	A+
86335-26		Immunfix e-phorsis/urine/csf	0.37	0.14	0.14	0.02	0.53	$18.34	0.53	$18.34	XXX	A+

86485	CP	Skin test candida	0.00	0.00	0.00	0.00	0.00	$0.00	0.00	$0.00	XXX	A+
86486		Skin test nos antigen	0.00	0.17	NA	0.01	0.18	$6.23	NA	NA	XXX	A+
86490		Coccidioidomycosis skin test	0.00	2.47	NA	0.01	2.48	$85.82	NA	NA	XXX	A+
86510		Histoplasmosis skin test	0.00	0.21	NA	0.01	0.22	$7.61	NA	NA	XXX	A+
86580		Tb intradermal test	0.00	0.30	NA	0.01	0.31	$10.73	NA	NA	XXX	A+
87164-26		Dark field examination	0.37	0.18	0.18	0.01	0.56	$19.38	0.56	$19.38	XXX	A+
87207-26		Smear special stain	0.37	0.14	0.14	0.02	0.53	$18.34	0.53	$18.34	XXX	A+
88104		Cytopath fl nongyn smears	0.56	1.39	NA	0.02	1.97	$68.17	NA	NA	XXX	A+
88104-26		Cytopath fl nongyn smears	0.56	0.22	0.22	0.01	0.79	$27.34	0.79	$27.34	XXX	A+
88104-TC		Cytopath fl nongyn smears	0.00	1.17	NA	0.01	1.18	$40.84	NA	NA	XXX	A+
88106		Cytopath fl nongyn filter	0.37	1.58	NA	0.02	1.97	$68.17	NA	NA	XXX	A+
88106-26		Cytopath fl nongyn filter	0.37	0.17	0.17	0.01	0.55	$19.03	0.55	$19.03	XXX	A+
88106-TC		Cytopath fl nongyn filter	0.00	1.41	NA	0.01	1.42	$49.14	NA	NA	XXX	A+
88108		Cytopath concentrate tech	0.44	1.43	NA	0.02	1.89	$65.41	NA	NA	XXX	A+
88108-26		Cytopath concentrate tech	0.44	0.20	0.20	0.01	0.65	$22.49	0.65	$22.49	XXX	A+
88108-TC		Cytopath concentrate tech	0.00	1.23	NA	0.01	1.24	$42.91	NA	NA	XXX	A+
88112		Cytopath cell enhance tech	0.56	1.37	NA	0.02	1.95	$67.48	NA	NA	XXX	A+
88112-26		Cytopath cell enhance tech	0.56	0.23	0.23	0.01	0.80	$27.68	0.80	$27.68	XXX	A+
88112-TC		Cytopath cell enhance tech	0.00	1.14	NA	0.01	1.15	$39.80	NA	NA	XXX	A+
88120		Cytp urne 3-5 probes ea spec	1.20	16.96	NA	0.06	18.22	$630.52	NA	NA	XXX	A+
88120-26		Cytp urne 3-5 probes ea spec	1.20	0.46	0.46	0.02	1.68	$58.14	1.68	$58.14	XXX	A+
88120-TC		Cytp urne 3-5 probes ea spec	0.00	16.50	NA	0.04	16.54	$572.39	NA	NA	XXX	A+
88121		Cytp urine 3-5 probes cmptr	1.00	11.80	NA	0.03	12.83	$444.00	NA	NA	XXX	A+
88121-26		Cytp urine 3-5 probes cmptr	1.00	0.37	0.37	0.02	1.39	$48.10	1.39	$48.10	XXX	A+
88121-TC		Cytp urine 3-5 probes cmptr	0.00	11.43	NA	0.01	11.44	$395.89	NA	NA	XXX	A+
88125		Forensic cytopathology	0.26	0.51	NA	0.02	0.79	$27.34	NA	NA	XXX	A+
88125-26		Forensic cytopathology	0.26	0.13	0.13	0.01	0.40	$13.84	0.40	$13.84	XXX	A+
88125-TC		Forensic cytopathology	0.00	0.38	NA	0.01	0.39	$13.50	NA	NA	XXX	A+

*Please note that these calculations are based on the Medicare 2022 Conversion Factor of $34.6062 and the DRA RVU cap rates at time of publication.

A = assistant-at-surgery restriction
A+ = assistant-at-surgery restriction unless medical necessity established with documentation
B = bilateral surgery adjustment applies
C = cosurgeons payable
C+ = cosurgeons payable if medical necessity established with documentation
CP = carriers may establish RVUs and payment amounts for these services, generally on an individual basis following review of documentation such as an operative report
M = multiple surgery adjustment applies
Me = multiple endoscopy rules may apply
M+ = multiple therapy rules apply
Mtc = multiple diagnostic imaging rules apply
T = team surgeons permitted
T+ = team surgeons payable if medical necessity established with documentation
§ = indicates code is not covered by Medicare
GS = procedure must be performed under the general supervision of a physician
DS = procedure must be performed under the direct supervision of a physician
PS = procedure must be performed under the personal supervision of a physician
DRA = procedure subject to DRA limitation

Relative Value Units

CPT Code and Modifier		Description	Work RVU	Nonfacility Practice Expense RVU	Facility Practice Expense RVU	PLI RVU	Total Non-facility RVUs	Medicare Payment Nonfacility	Total Facility RVUs	Medicare Payment Facility	Global Period	Payment Policy Indicators
88141		Cytopath c/v interpret	0.26	0.38	0.38	0.01	0.65	$22.49	0.65	$22.49	XXX	A+
88160		Cytopath smear other source	0.50	1.58	NA	0.02	2.10	$72.67	NA	NA	XXX	A+
88160-26		Cytopath smear other source	0.50	0.23	0.23	0.01	0.74	$25.61	0.74	$25.61	XXX	A+
88160-TC		Cytopath smear other source	0.00	1.35	NA	0.01	1.36	$47.06	NA	NA	XXX	A+
88161		Cytopath smear other source	0.50	1.64	NA	0.02	2.16	$74.75	NA	NA	XXX	A+
88161-26		Cytopath smear other source	0.50	0.22	0.22	0.01	0.73	$25.26	0.73	$25.26	XXX	A+
88161-TC		Cytopath smear other source	0.00	1.42	NA	0.01	1.43	$49.49	NA	NA	XXX	A+
88162		Cytopath smear other source	0.76	2.54	NA	0.03	3.33	$115.24	NA	NA	XXX	A+
88162-26		Cytopath smear other source	0.76	0.36	0.36	0.01	1.13	$39.11	1.13	$39.11	XXX	A+
88162-TC		Cytopath smear other source	0.00	2.18	NA	0.02	2.20	$76.13	NA	NA	XXX	A+
88172		Cytp dx eval fna 1st ea site	0.69	0.88	NA	0.02	1.59	$55.02	NA	NA	XXX	A+
88172-26		Cytp dx eval fna 1st ea site	0.69	0.32	0.32	0.01	1.02	$35.30	1.02	$35.30	XXX	A+
88172-TC		Cytp dx eval fna 1st ea site	0.00	0.56	NA	0.01	0.57	$19.73	NA	NA	XXX	A+
88173		Cytopath eval fna report	1.39	3.14	NA	0.08	4.61	$159.53	NA	NA	XXX	A+
88173-26		Cytopath eval fna report	1.39	0.60	0.60	0.04	2.03	$70.25	2.03	$70.25	XXX	A+
88173-TC		Cytopath eval fna report	0.00	2.54	NA	0.04	2.58	$89.28	NA	NA	XXX	A+
88177		Cytp fna eval ea addl	0.42	0.41	NA	0.01	0.84	$29.07	NA	NA	ZZZ	A+
88177-26		Cytp fna eval ea addl	0.42	0.20	0.20	0.01	0.63	$21.80	0.63	$21.80	ZZZ	A+
88177-TC		Cytp fna eval ea addl	0.00	0.21	NA	0.00	0.21	$7.27	NA	NA	ZZZ	A+
88182		Cell marker study	0.77	3.49	NA	0.05	4.31	$149.15	NA	NA	XXX	A+
88182-26		Cell marker study	0.77	0.33	0.33	0.01	1.11	$38.41	1.11	$38.41	XXX	A+
88182-TC		Cell marker study	0.00	3.16	NA	0.04	3.20	$110.74	NA	NA	XXX	A+
88184		Flowcytometry/ tc 1 marker	0.00	1.98	NA	0.02	2.00	$69.21	NA	NA	XXX	A+
88185		Flowcytometry/tc add-on	0.00	0.64	NA	0.00	0.64	$22.15	NA	NA	ZZZ	A+
88187		Flowcytometry/read 2-8	0.74	0.26	0.26	0.04	1.04	$35.99	1.04	$35.99	XXX	A+
88188		Flowcytometry/read 9-15	1.20	0.54	0.54	0.08	1.82	$62.98	1.82	$62.98	XXX	A+
88189		Flowcytometry/read 16 & >	1.70	0.65	0.65	0.09	2.44	$84.44	2.44	$84.44	XXX	A+
88199	CP	Cytopathology procedure	0.00	0.00	NA	0.00	0.00	$0.00	NA	NA	XXX	A+
88199-26	CP	Cytopathology procedure	0.00	0.00	0.00	0.00	0.00	$0.00	0.00	$0.00	XXX	A+
88199-TC	CP	Cytopathology procedure	0.00	0.00	NA	0.00	0.00	$0.00	NA	NA	XXX	A+
88291		Cyto/molecular report	0.52	0.41	0.41	0.04	0.97	$33.57	0.97	$33.57	XXX	A+
88299	CP	Cytogenetic study	0.00	0.00	0.00	0.00	0.00	$0.00	0.00	$0.00	XXX	A+
88300		Surgical path gross	0.08	0.35	NA	0.02	0.45	$15.57	NA	NA	XXX	A+

88300-26	Surgical path gross	0.08	0.04	0.04	0.01	0.13	$4.50	0.13	$4.50	XXX	A+
88300-TC	Surgical path gross	0.00	0.31	NA	0.01	0.32	$11.07	NA	NA	XXX	A+
88302	Tissue exam by pathologist	0.13	0.78	NA	0.02	0.93	$32.18	NA	NA	XXX	A+
88302-26	Tissue exam by pathologist	0.13	0.06	0.06	0.01	0.20	$6.92	0.20	$6.92	XXX	A+
88302-TC	Tissue exam by pathologist	0.00	0.72	NA	0.01	0.73	$25.26	NA	NA	XXX	A+
88304	Tissue exam by pathologist	0.22	0.98	NA	0.02	1.22	$42.22	NA	NA	XXX	A+
88304-26	Tissue exam by pathologist	0.22	0.10	0.10	0.01	0.33	$11.42	0.33	$11.42	XXX	A+
88304-TC	Tissue exam by pathologist	0.00	0.88	NA	0.01	0.89	$30.80	NA	NA	XXX	A+
88305	Tissue exam by pathologist	0.75	1.31	NA	0.02	2.08	$71.98	NA	NA	XXX	A+
88305-26	Tissue exam by pathologist	0.75	0.32	0.32	0.01	1.08	$37.37	1.08	$37.37	XXX	A+
88305-TC	Tissue exam by pathologist	0.00	0.99	NA	0.01	1.00	$34.61	NA	NA	XXX	A+
88307	Tissue exam by pathologist	1.59	6.73	NA	0.08	8.40	$290.69	NA	NA	XXX	A+
88307-26	Tissue exam by pathologist	1.59	0.75	0.75	0.04	2.38	$82.36	2.38	$82.36	XXX	A+
88307-TC	Tissue exam by pathologist	0.00	5.98	NA	0.04	6.02	$208.33	NA	NA	XXX	A+
88309	Tissue exam by pathologist	2.80	9.87	NA	0.09	12.76	$441.58	NA	NA	XXX	A+
88309-26	Tissue exam by pathologist	2.80	1.33	1.33	0.05	4.18	$144.65	4.18	$144.65	XXX	A+
88309-TC	Tissue exam by pathologist	0.00	8.54	NA	0.04	8.58	$296.92	NA	NA	XXX	A+
88311	Decalcify tissue	0.24	0.35	NA	0.02	0.61	$21.11	NA	NA	XXX	A+
88311-26	Decalcify tissue	0.24	0.11	0.11	0.01	0.36	$12.46	0.36	$12.46	XXX	A+
88311-TC	Decalcify tissue	0.00	0.24	NA	0.01	0.25	$8.65	NA	NA	XXX	A+
88312	Special stains group 1	0.54	2.75	NA	0.02	3.31	$114.55	NA	NA	XXX	A+
88312-26	Special stains group 1	0.54	0.21	0.21	0.01	0.76	$26.30	0.76	$26.30	XXX	A+
88312-TC	Special stains group 1	0.00	2.54	NA	0.01	2.55	$88.25	NA	NA	XXX	A+
88313	Special stains group 2	0.24	2.12	NA	0.02	2.38	$82.36	NA	NA	XXX	A+
88313-26	Special stains group 2	0.24	0.10	0.10	0.01	0.35	$12.11	0.35	$12.11	XXX	A+
88313-TC	Special stains group 2	0.00	2.02	NA	0.01	2.03	$70.25	NA	NA	XXX	A+
88314	Histochemical stains add-on	0.45	2.43	NA	0.02	2.90	$100.36	NA	NA	XXX	A+
88314-26	Histochemical stains add-on	0.45	0.15	0.15	0.01	0.61	$21.11	0.61	$21.11	XXX	A+

*Please note that these calculations are based on the Medicare 2022 Conversion Factor of $34.6062 and the DRA RVU cap rates at time of publication.

A = assistant-at-surgery restriction
A+ = assistant-at-surgery restriction unless medical necessity established with documentation
B = bilateral surgery adjustment applies
C = cosurgeons payable

C+ = cosurgeons payable if medical necessity established with documentation
CP = carriers may establish RVUs and payment amounts for these services, generally on an individual basis following review of documentation such as an operative report
M = multiple surgery adjustment applies
Me = multiple endoscopy rules may apply

M+ = multiple therapy rules apply
Mtc = multiple diagnostic imaging rules apply
T = team surgeons permitted
T+ = team surgeons payable if medical necessity established with documentation
§ = indicates code is not covered by Medicare

GS = procedure must be performed under the general supervision of a physician
DS = procedure must be performed under the direct supervision of a physician
PS = procedure must be performed under the personal supervision of a physician
DRA = procedure subject to DRA limitation

Relative Value Units

CPT Code and Modifier	Description	Work RVU	Nonfacility Practice Expense RVU	Facility Practice Expense RVU	PLI RVU	Total Non-facility RVUs	Medicare Payment Nonfacility	Total Facility RVUs	Medicare Payment Facility	Global Period	Payment Policy Indicators
88314-TC	Histochemical stains add-on	0.00	2.28	NA	0.01	2.29	$79.25	NA	NA	XXX	A+
88319	Enzyme histochemistry	0.53	3.55	NA	0.03	4.11	$142.23	NA	NA	XXX	A+
88319-26	Enzyme histochemistry	0.53	0.24	0.24	0.01	0.78	$26.99	0.78	$26.99	XXX	A+
88319-TC	Enzyme histochemistry	0.00	3.31	NA	0.02	3.33	$115.24	NA	NA	XXX	A+
88321	Microslide consultation	1.63	1.11	0.71	0.09	2.83	$97.94	2.43	$84.09	XXX	A+
88323	Microslide consultation	1.83	1.44	NA	0.03	3.30	$114.20	NA	NA	XXX	A+
88323-26	Microslide consultation	1.83	0.66	0.66	0.02	2.51	$86.86	2.51	$86.86	XXX	A+
88323-TC	Microslide consultation	0.00	0.78	NA	0.01	0.79	$27.34	NA	NA	XXX	A+
88325	Comprehensive review of data	2.85	1.62	0.95	0.12	4.59	$158.84	3.92	$135.66	XXX	A+
88329	Path consult introp	0.67	0.97	0.32	0.04	1.68	$58.14	1.03	$35.64	XXX	A+
88331	Path consult intraop 1 bloc	1.19	1.77	NA	0.03	2.99	$103.47	NA	NA	XXX	A+
88331-26	Path consult intraop 1 bloc	1.19	0.58	0.58	0.02	1.79	$61.95	1.79	$61.95	XXX	A+
88331-TC	Path consult intraop 1 bloc	0.00	1.19	NA	0.01	1.20	$41.53	NA	NA	XXX	A+
88332	Path consult intraop addl	0.59	0.98	NA	0.02	1.59	$55.02	NA	NA	XXX	A+
88332-26	Path consult intraop addl	0.59	0.28	0.28	0.01	0.88	$30.45	0.88	$30.45	XXX	A+
88332-TC	Path consult intraop addl	0.00	0.70	NA	0.01	0.71	$24.57	NA	NA	XXX	A+
88333	Intraop cyto path consult 1	1.20	1.50	NA	0.03	2.73	$94.47	NA	NA	XXX	A+
88333-26	Intraop cyto path consult 1	1.20	0.56	0.56	0.02	1.78	$61.60	1.78	$61.60	XXX	A+
88333-TC	Intraop cyto path consult 1	0.00	0.94	NA	0.01	0.95	$32.88	NA	NA	XXX	A+
88334	Intraop cyto path consult 2	0.73	0.90	NA	0.01	1.64	$56.75	NA	NA	ZZZ	A+
88334-26	Intraop cyto path consult 2	0.73	0.34	0.34	0.01	1.08	$37.37	1.08	$37.37	ZZZ	A+
88334-TC	Intraop cyto path consult 2	0.00	0.56	NA	0.00	0.56	$19.38	NA	NA	ZZZ	A+
88341	Immunohisto antb addl slide	0.56	2.02	NA	0.01	2.59	$89.63	NA	NA	ZZZ	A+
88341-26	Immunohisto antb addl slide	0.56	0.24	0.24	0.01	0.81	$28.03	0.81	$28.03	ZZZ	A+
88341-TC	Immunohisto antb addl slide	0.00	1.78	NA	0.00	1.78	$61.60	NA	NA	ZZZ	A+
88342	Immunohisto antb 1st stain	0.70	2.24	NA	0.02	2.96	$102.43	NA	NA	XXX	A+
88342-26	Immunohisto antb 1st stain	0.70	0.29	0.29	0.01	1.00	$34.61	1.00	$34.61	XXX	A+
88342-TC	Immunohisto antb 1st stain	0.00	1.95	NA	0.01	1.96	$67.83	NA	NA	XXX	A+
88344	Immunohisto antibody slide	0.77	4.21	NA	0.02	5.00	$173.03	NA	NA	XXX	A+
88344-26	Immunohisto antibody slide	0.77	0.32	0.32	0.01	1.10	$38.07	1.10	$38.07	XXX	A+
88344-TC	Immunohisto antibody slide	0.00	3.89	NA	0.01	3.90	$134.96	NA	NA	XXX	A+
88346	Immunofluor antb 1st stain	0.74	3.74	NA	0.02	4.50	$155.73	NA	NA	XXX	A+
88346-26	Immunofluor antb 1st stain	0.74	0.29	0.29	0.01	1.04	$35.99	1.04	$35.99	XXX	A+

88346-TC	Immunofluor antb 1st stain	0.00	3.45	NA	0.01	3.46	$119.74	NA	NA	XXX	A+
88348	Electron microscopy	1.51	11.76	NA	0.12	13.39	$463.38	NA	NA	XXX	A+
88348-26	Electron microscopy	1.51	0.69	0.69	0.04	2.24	$77.52	2.24	$77.52	XXX	A+
88348-TC	Electron microscopy	0.00	11.07	NA	0.08	11.15	$385.86	NA	NA	XXX	A+
88350	Immunofluor antb addl stain	0.59	2.86	NA	0.02	3.47	$120.08	NA	NA	ZZZ	A+
88350-26	Immunofluor antb addl stain	0.59	0.24	0.24	0.01	0.84	$29.07	0.84	$29.07	ZZZ	A+
88350-TC	Immunofluor antb addl stain	0.00	2.62	NA	0.01	2.63	$91.01	NA	NA	ZZZ	A+
88355	Analysis skeletal muscle	1.85	2.26	NA	0.02	4.13	$142.92	NA	NA	XXX	A+
88355-26	Analysis skeletal muscle	1.85	0.51	0.51	0.01	2.37	$82.02	2.37	$82.02	XXX	A+
88355-TC	Analysis skeletal muscle	0.00	1.75	NA	0.01	1.76	$60.91	NA	NA	XXX	A+
88356	Analysis nerve	2.80	4.31	NA	0.09	7.20	$249.16	NA	NA	XXX	A+
88356-26	Analysis nerve	2.80	0.88	0.88	0.05	3.73	$129.08	3.73	$129.08	XXX	A+
88356-TC	Analysis nerve	0.00	3.43	NA	0.04	3.47	$120.08	NA	NA	XXX	A+
88358	Analysis tumor	0.95	3.11	NA	0.03	4.09	$141.54	NA	NA	XXX	A+
88358-26	Analysis tumor	0.95	0.46	0.46	0.02	1.43	$49.49	1.43	$49.49	XXX	A+
88358-TC	Analysis tumor	0.00	2.65	NA	0.01	2.66	$92.05	NA	NA	XXX	A+
88360	Tumor immunohistochem/manual	0.85	2.67	NA	0.02	3.54	$122.51	NA	NA	XXX	A+
88360-26	Tumor immunohistochem/manual	0.85	0.34	0.34	0.01	1.20	$41.53	1.20	$41.53	XXX	A+
88360-TC	Tumor immunohistochem/manual	0.00	2.33	NA	0.01	2.34	$80.98	NA	NA	XXX	A+
88361	Tumor immunohistochem/comput	0.95	2.56	NA	0.02	3.53	$122.16	NA	NA	XXX	A+
88361-26	Tumor immunohistochem/comput	0.95	0.30	0.30	0.01	1.26	$43.60	1.26	$43.60	XXX	A+
88361-TC	Tumor immunohistochem/comput	0.00	2.26	NA	0.01	2.27	$78.56	NA	NA	XXX	A+
88362	Nerve teasing preparations	2.17	4.25	NA	0.07	6.49	$224.59	NA	NA	XXX	A+
88362-26	Nerve teasing preparations	2.17	1.00	1.00	0.05	3.22	$111.43	3.22	$111.43	XXX	A+
88362-TC	Nerve teasing preparations	0.00	3.25	NA	0.02	3.27	$113.16	NA	NA	XXX	A+
88363	Xm archive tissue molec anal	0.37	0.28	0.17	0.02	0.67	$23.19	0.56	$19.38	XXX	A+
88364	Insitu hybridization (fish)	0.70	3.33	NA	0.02	4.05	$140.16	NA	NA	ZZZ	A+
88364-26	Insitu hybridization (fish)	0.70	0.28	0.28	0.01	0.99	$34.26	0.99	$34.26	ZZZ	A+

*Please note that these calculations are based on the Medicare 2022 Conversion Factor of $34.6062 and the DRA RVU cap rates at time of publication.

A = assistant-at-surgery restriction
A+ = assistant-at-surgery restriction unless medical necessity established with documentation
B = bilateral surgery adjustment applies
C = cosurgeons payable
C+ = cosurgeons payable if medical necessity established with documentation
CP = carriers may establish RVUs and payment amounts for these services, generally on an individual basis following review of documentation such as an operative report
M = multiple surgery adjustment applies
Me = multiple endoscopy rules may apply
M+ = multiple therapy rules apply
Mtc = multiple diagnostic imaging rules apply
T = team surgeons permitted
T+ = team surgeons payable if medical necessity established with documentation
§ = indicates code is not covered by Medicare
GS = procedure must be performed under the general supervision of a physician
DS = procedure must be performed under the direct supervision of a physician
PS = procedure must be performed under the personal supervision of a physician
DRA = procedure subject to DRA limitation

Relative Value Units

CPT Code and Modifier	Description	Work RVU	Nonfacility Practice Expense RVU	Facility Practice Expense RVU	PLI RVU	Total Non-facility RVUs	Medicare Payment Nonfacility	Total Facility RVUs	Medicare Payment Facility	Global Period	Payment Policy Indicators
88364-TC	Insitu hybridization (fish)	0.00	3.05	NA	0.01	3.06	$105.89	NA	NA	ZZZ	A+
88365	Insitu hybridization (fish)	0.88	4.36	NA	0.04	5.28	$182.72	NA	NA	XXX	A+
88365-26	Insitu hybridization (fish)	0.88	0.36	0.36	0.02	1.26	$43.60	1.26	$43.60	XXX	A+
88365-TC	Insitu hybridization (fish)	0.00	4.00	NA	0.02	4.02	$139.12	NA	NA	XXX	A+
88366	Insitu hybridization (fish)	1.24	7.09	NA	0.04	8.37	$289.65	NA	NA	XXX	A+
88366-26	Insitu hybridization (fish)	1.24	0.53	0.53	0.02	1.79	$61.95	1.79	$61.95	XXX	A+
88366-TC	Insitu hybridization (fish)	0.00	6.56	NA	0.02	6.58	$227.71	NA	NA	XXX	A+
88367	Insitu hybridization auto	0.73	2.57	NA	0.02	3.32	$114.89	NA	NA	XXX	A+
88367-26	Insitu hybridization auto	0.73	0.23	0.23	0.01	0.97	$33.57	0.97	$33.57	XXX	A+
88367-TC	Insitu hybridization auto	0.00	2.34	NA	0.01	2.35	$81.32	NA	NA	XXX	A+
88368	Insitu hybridization manual	0.88	3.08	NA	0.03	3.99	$138.08	NA	NA	XXX	A+
88368-26	Insitu hybridization manual	0.88	0.30	0.30	0.01	1.19	$41.18	1.19	$41.18	XXX	A+
88368-TC	Insitu hybridization manual	0.00	2.78	NA	0.02	2.80	$96.90	NA	NA	XXX	A+
88369	M/phmtrc alysishquant/semiq	0.70	2.66	NA	0.02	3.38	$116.97	NA	NA	ZZZ	A+
88369-26	M/phmtrc alysishquant/semiq	0.70	0.22	0.22	0.01	0.93	$32.18	0.93	$32.18	ZZZ	A+
88369-TC	M/phmtrc alysishquant/semiq	0.00	2.44	NA	0.01	2.45	$84.79	NA	NA	ZZZ	A+
88371-26	Protein western blot tissue	0.37	0.18	0.18	0.01	0.56	$19.38	0.56	$19.38	XXX	A+
88372-26	Protein analysis w/probe	0.37	0.14	0.14	0.02	0.53	$18.34	0.53	$18.34	XXX	A+
88373	M/phmtrc alys ishquant/semiq	0.58	1.44	NA	0.01	2.03	$70.25	NA	NA	ZZZ	A+
88373-26	M/phmtrc alys ishquant/semiq	0.58	0.15	0.15	0.01	0.74	$25.61	0.74	$25.61	ZZZ	A+
88373-TC	M/phmtrc alys ishquant/semiq	0.00	1.29	NA	0.00	1.29	$44.64	NA	NA	ZZZ	A+
88374	M/phmtrc alys ishquant/semiq	0.93	8.64	NA	0.02	9.59	$331.87	NA	NA	XXX	A+
88374-26	M/phmtrc alys ishquant/semiq	0.93	0.31	0.31	0.01	1.25	$43.26	1.25	$43.26	XXX	A+
88374-TC	M/phmtrc alys ishquant/semiq	0.00	8.33	NA	0.01	8.34	$288.62	NA	NA	XXX	A+
88375	Optical endomicroscpy interp	0.91	0.44	0.44	0.05	1.40	$48.45	1.40	$48.45	XXX	A+
88377	M/phmtrc alys ishquant/semiq	1.40	10.46	NA	0.04	11.90	$411.81	NA	NA	XXX	A+
88377-26	M/phmtrc alys ishquant/semiq	1.40	0.42	0.42	0.02	1.84	$63.68	1.84	$63.68	XXX	A+
88377-TC	M/phmtrc alys ishquant/semiq	0.00	10.04	NA	0.02	10.06	$348.14	NA	NA	XXX	A+
88380	Microdissection laser	1.14	2.55	NA	0.04	3.73	$129.08	NA	NA	XXX	A+
88380-26	Microdissection laser	1.14	0.41	0.41	0.02	1.57	$54.33	1.57	$54.33	XXX	A+
88380-TC	Microdissection laser	0.00	2.14	NA	0.02	2.16	$74.75	NA	NA	XXX	A+
88381	Microdissection manual	0.53	5.60	NA	0.05	6.18	$213.87	NA	NA	XXX	A+
88381-26	Microdissection manual	0.53	0.15	0.15	0.01	0.69	$23.88	0.69	$23.88	XXX	A+

88381-TC		Microdissection manual	0.00	5.45	NA	0.04	5.49	$189.99	NA	NA	XXX	A+
88387		Tiss exam molecular study	0.62	0.36	NA	0.02	1.00	$34.61	NA	NA	XXX	A+
88387-26		Tiss exam molecular study	0.62	0.14	0.14	0.01	0.77	$26.65	0.77	$26.65	XXX	A+
88387-TC		Tiss exam molecular study	0.00	0.22	NA	0.01	0.23	$7.96	NA	NA	XXX	A+
88388		Tiss ex molecul study add-on	0.45	0.63	NA	0.02	1.10	$38.07	NA	NA	XXX	A+
88388-26		Tiss ex molecul study add-on	0.45	0.22	0.22	0.01	0.68	$23.53	0.68	$23.53	XXX	A+
88388-TC		Tiss ex molecul study add-on	0.00	0.41	NA	0.01	0.42	$14.53	NA	NA	XXX	A+
88399	CP	Surgical pathology procedure	0.00	0.00	NA	0.00	0.00	$0.00	NA	NA	XXX	A+
88399-26	CP	Surgical pathology procedure	0.00	0.00	0.00	0.00	0.00	$0.00	0.00	$0.00	XXX	A+
88399-TC	CP	Surgical pathology procedure	0.00	0.00	NA	0.00	0.00	$0.00	NA	NA	XXX	A+
89049		Chct for mal hyperthermia	1.40	6.41	0.25	0.12	7.93	$274.43	1.77	$61.25	XXX	A+
89060-26		Exam synovial fluid crystals	0.37	0.14	0.14	0.02	0.53	$18.34	0.53	$18.34	XXX	A+
89220		Sputum specimen collection	0.00	0.53	NA	0.02	0.55	$19.03	NA	NA	XXX	A+
89230		Collect sweat for test	0.00	0.06	NA	0.01	0.07	$2.42	NA	NA	XXX	A+
89240	CP	Pathology lab procedure	0.00	0.00	0.00	0.00	0.00	$0.00	0.00	$0.00	XXX	A+
90460		Im admin 1st/only component	0.17	0.31	NA	0.01	0.49	$16.96	NA	NA	XXX	A+
90461		Im admin each addl component	0.15	0.21	NA	0.01	0.37	$12.80	NA	NA	ZZZ	A+
90471		Immunization admin	0.17	0.31	NA	0.01	0.49	$16.96	NA	NA	XXX	A+
90472		Immunization admin each add	0.15	0.21	NA	0.01	0.37	$12.80	NA	NA	ZZZ	A+
90473		Immune admin oral/nasal	0.17	0.31	NA	0.01	0.49	$16.96	NA	NA	XXX	A+
90474		Immune admin oral/nasal addl	0.15	0.21	NA	0.01	0.37	$12.80	NA	NA	ZZZ	A+
90785		Psytx complex interactive	0.33	0.09	0.04	0.01	0.43	$14.88	0.38	$13.15	ZZZ	
90791		Psych diagnostic evaluation	3.84	1.21	0.49	0.12	5.17	$178.91	4.45	$154.00	XXX	
90792		Psych diag eval w/med srvcs	4.16	1.46	0.75	0.17	5.79	$200.37	5.08	$175.80	XXX	
90832		Psytx w pt 30 minutes	1.70	0.48	0.22	0.07	2.25	$77.86	1.99	$68.87	XXX	
90833		Psytx w pt w e/m 30 min	1.50	0.49	0.27	0.07	2.06	$71.29	1.84	$63.68	ZZZ	
90834		Psytx w pt 45 minutes	2.24	0.64	0.29	0.09	2.97	$102.78	2.62	$90.67	XXX	
90836		Psytx w pt w e/m 45 min	1.90	0.62	0.34	0.08	2.60	$89.98	2.32	$80.29	ZZZ	

*Please note that these calculations are based on the Medicare 2022 Conversion Factor of $34.6062 and the DRA RVU cap rates at time of publication.

A = assistant-at-surgery restriction
A+ = assistant-at-surgery restriction unless medical necessity established with documentation
B = bilateral surgery adjustment applies
C = cosurgeons payable
C+ = cosurgeons payable if medical necessity established with documentation
CP = carriers may establish RVUs and payment amounts for these services, generally on an individual basis following review of documentation such as an operative report
M = multiple surgery adjustment applies
Me = multiple endoscopy rules may apply
M+ = multiple therapy rules apply
Mtc = multiple diagnostic imaging rules apply
T = team surgeons permitted
T+ = team surgeons payable if medical necessity established with documentation
§ = indicates code is not covered by Medicare
GS = procedure must be performed under the general supervision of a physician
DS = procedure must be performed under the direct supervision of a physician
PS = procedure must be performed under the personal supervision of a physician
DRA = procedure subject to DRA limitation

Relative Value Units

CPT Code and Modifier		Description	Work RVU	Nonfacility Practice Expense RVU	Facility Practice Expense RVU	PLI RVU	Total Non-facility RVUs	Medicare Payment Nonfacility	Total Facility RVUs	Medicare Payment Facility	Global Period	Payment Policy Indicators
90837		Psytx w pt 60 minutes	3.31	0.94	0.42	0.11	4.36	$150.88	3.84	$132.89	XXX	
90838		Psytx w pt w e/m 60 min	2.50	0.82	0.47	0.10	3.42	$118.35	3.07	$106.24	ZZZ	
90839		Psytx crisis initial 60 min	3.13	0.92	0.44	0.12	4.17	$144.31	3.69	$127.70	XXX	A+
90840		Psytx crisis ea addl 30 min	1.50	0.47	0.25	0.11	2.08	$71.98	1.86	$64.37	ZZZ	A+
90845		Psychoanalysis	2.10	0.62	0.31	0.09	2.81	$97.24	2.50	$86.52	XXX	A+
90846		Family psytx w/o pt 50 min	2.40	0.35	0.33	0.09	2.84	$98.28	2.82	$97.59	XXX	A+
90847		Family psytx w/pt 50 min	2.50	0.35	0.34	0.09	2.94	$101.74	2.93	$101.40	XXX	A+
90849		Multiple family group psytx	0.59	0.41	0.21	0.02	1.02	$35.30	0.82	$28.38	XXX	A+
90853		Group psychotherapy	0.59	0.18	0.08	0.02	0.79	$27.34	0.69	$23.88	XXX	A+
90863	§	Pharmacologic mgmt w/psytx	0.48	0.23	0.19	0.04	0.75	$25.95	0.71	$24.57	XXX	
90865		Narcosynthesis	2.84	1.92	0.70	0.11	4.87	$168.53	3.65	$126.31	XXX	A+
90867	CP	Tcranial magn stim tx plan	0.00	0.00	0.00	0.00	0.00	$0.00	0.00	$0.00	000	A
90868	CP	Tcranial magn stim tx deli	0.00	0.00	0.00	0.00	0.00	$0.00	0.00	$0.00	000	A
90869	CP	Tcran magn stim redetemine	0.00	0.00	0.00	0.00	0.00	$0.00	0.00	$0.00	000	A
90870		Electroconvulsive therapy	2.50	2.52	0.51	0.09	5.11	$176.84	3.10	$107.28	000	A+
90875	§	Psychophysiological therapy	1.20	0.48	0.46	0.10	1.78	$61.60	1.76	$60.91	XXX	
90876	§	Psychophysiological therapy	1.90	1.03	0.73	0.17	3.10	$107.28	2.80	$96.90	XXX	
90880		Hypnotherapy	2.19	0.82	0.34	0.09	3.10	$107.28	2.62	$90.67	XXX	A+
90885	§	Psy evaluation of records	0.97	0.37	0.37	0.09	1.43	$49.49	1.43	$49.49	XXX	
90887	§	Consultation with family	1.48	0.94	0.57	0.11	2.53	$87.55	2.16	$74.75	XXX	
90899	CP	Psychiatric service/therapy	0.00	0.00	0.00	0.00	0.00	$0.00	0.00	$0.00	XXX	A+
90901		Biofeedback train any meth	0.41	0.77	0.13	0.02	1.20	$41.53	0.56	$19.38	000	A+
90912		Bfb training 1st 15 min	0.90	1.44	0.31	0.05	2.39	$82.71	1.26	$43.60	000	A+
90913		Bfb training ea addl 15 min	0.50	0.40	0.17	0.04	0.94	$32.53	0.71	$24.57	ZZZ	A+
90935		Hemodialysis one evaluation	1.48	NA	0.54	0.09	NA	NA	2.11	$73.02	000	A+
90937		Hemodialysis repeated eval	2.11	NA	0.79	0.12	NA	NA	3.02	$104.51	000	A+
90945		Dialysis one evaluation	1.56	NA	0.85	0.10	NA	NA	2.51	$86.86	000	A+
90947		Dialysis repeated eval	2.52	NA	0.93	0.18	NA	NA	3.63	$125.62	000	A+
90951		Esrd serv 4 visits p mo <2yr	23.92	9.21	9.21	1.60	34.73	$1201.87	34.73	$1201.87	XXX	A+
90952	CP	Esrd serv 2-3 vsts p mo <2yr	0.00	0.00	0.00	0.00	0.00	$0.00	0.00	$0.00	XXX	A+
90953	CP	Esrd serv 1 visit p mo <2yrs	0.00	0.00	0.00	0.00	0.00	$0.00	0.00	$0.00	XXX	A+
90954		Esrd serv 4 vsts p mo 2-11	20.86	7.62	7.62	1.36	29.84	$1032.65	29.84	$1032.65	XXX	A+
90955		Esrd srv 2-3 vsts p mo 2-11	10.32	4.46	4.46	0.64	15.42	$533.63	15.42	$533.63	XXX	A+

90956		Esrd srv 1 visit p mo 2-11	6.64	3.16	3.16	0.41	10.21	$353.33	10.21	$353.33	XXX	A+
90957		Esrd srv 4 vsts p mo 12-19	15.46	6.35	6.35	1.00	22.81	$789.37	22.81	$789.37	XXX	A+
90958		Esrd srv 2-3 vsts p mo 12-19	9.87	4.35	4.35	0.62	14.84	$513.56	14.84	$513.56	XXX	A+
90959		Esrd serv 1 vst p mo 12-19	6.19	3.01	3.01	0.39	9.59	$331.87	9.59	$331.87	XXX	A+
90960		Esrd srv 4 visits p mo 20+	6.77	3.26	3.26	0.41	10.44	$361.29	10.44	$361.29	XXX	A+
90961		Esrd srv 2-3 vsts p mo 20+	5.52	2.80	2.80	0.34	8.66	$299.69	8.66	$299.69	XXX	A+
90962		Esrd serv 1 visit p mo 20+	3.57	2.16	2.16	0.22	5.95	$205.91	5.95	$205.91	XXX	A+
90963		Esrd home pt serv p mo <2yrs	12.09	5.06	5.06	0.77	17.92	$620.14	17.92	$620.14	XXX	A+
90964		Esrd home pt serv p mo 2-11	10.25	4.47	4.47	0.65	15.37	$531.90	15.37	$531.90	XXX	A+
90965		Esrd home pt serv p mo 12-19	9.80	4.35	4.35	0.62	14.77	$511.13	14.77	$511.13	XXX	A+
90966		Esrd home pt serv p mo 20+	5.52	2.80	2.80	0.34	8.66	$299.69	8.66	$299.69	XXX	A+
90967		Esrd svc pr day pt <2	0.35	0.15	0.15	0.02	0.52	$18.00	0.52	$18.00	XXX	A+
90968		Esrd svc pr day pt 2-11	0.34	0.15	0.15	0.02	0.51	$17.65	0.51	$17.65	XXX	A+
90969		Esrd svc pr day pt 12-19	0.33	0.15	0.15	0.02	0.50	$17.30	0.50	$17.30	XXX	A+
90970		Esrd svc pr day pt 20+	0.18	0.09	0.09	0.01	0.28	$9.69	0.28	$9.69	XXX	A+
90997		Hemoperfusion	1.84	NA	0.65	0.11	NA	NA	2.60	$89.98	000	A+
90999	CP	Dialysis procedure	0.00	0.00	0.00	0.00	0.00	$0.00	0.00	$0.00	XXX	A+
91010		Esophagus motility study	1.28	5.40	NA	0.09	6.77	$234.28	NA	NA	000	A+
91010-26		Esophagus motility study	1.28	0.56	0.56	0.07	1.91	$66.10	1.91	$66.10	000	A+
91010-TC		Esophagus motility study	0.00	4.84	NA	0.02	4.86	$168.19	NA	NA	000	A+ DS
91013		Esophgl motil w/stim/perfus	0.18	0.59	NA	0.01	0.78	$26.99	NA	NA	ZZZ	A+
91013-26		Esophgl motil w/stim/perfus	0.18	0.08	0.08	0.01	0.27	$9.34	0.27	$9.34	ZZZ	A+
91013-TC		Esophgl motil w/stim/perfus	0.00	0.51	NA	0.00	0.51	$17.65	NA	NA	ZZZ	A+ DS
91020		Gastric motility studies	1.44	6.94	NA	0.07	8.45	$292.42	NA	NA	000	A+
91020-26		Gastric motility studies	1.44	0.65	0.65	0.05	2.14	$74.06	2.14	$74.06	000	A+
91020-TC		Gastric motility studies	0.00	6.29	NA	0.02	6.31	$218.37	NA	NA	000	A+ DS
91022		Duodenal motility study	1.44	3.66	NA	0.06	5.16	$178.57	NA	NA	000	A+
91022-26		Duodenal motility study	1.44	0.65	0.65	0.04	2.13	$73.71	2.13	$73.71	000	A+

*Please note that these calculations are based on the Medicare 2022 Conversion Factor of $34.6062 and the DRA RVU cap rates at time of publication.

A = assistant-at-surgery restriction

A+ = assistant-at-surgery restriction unless medical necessity established with documentation

B = bilateral surgery adjustment applies

C = cosurgeons payable

C+ = cosurgeons payable if medical necessity established with documentation

CP = carriers may establish RVUs and payment amounts for these services, generally on an individual basis following review of documentation such as an operative report

M = multiple surgery adjustment applies

Me = multiple endoscopy rules may apply

M+ = multiple therapy rules apply

Mtc = multiple diagnostic imaging rules apply

T = team surgeons permitted

T+ = team surgeons payable if medical necessity established with documentation

§ = indicates code is not covered by Medicare

GS = procedure must be performed under the general supervision of a physician

DS = procedure must be performed under the direct supervision of a physician

PS = procedure must be performed under the personal supervision of a physician

DRA = procedure subject to DRA limitation

Relative Value Units

CPT Code and Modifier	Description	Work RVU	Nonfacility Practice Expense RVU	Facility Practice Expense RVU	PLI RVU	Total Non-facility RVUs	Medicare Payment Nonfacility	Total Facility RVUs	Medicare Payment Facility	Global Period	Payment Policy Indicators
91022-TC	Duodenal motility study	0.00	3.01	NA	0.02	3.03	$104.86	NA	NA	000	A+ DS
91030	Acid perfusion of esophagus	0.91	3.40	NA	0.06	4.37	$151.23	NA	NA	000	A+
91030-26	Acid perfusion of esophagus	0.91	0.41	0.41	0.04	1.36	$47.06	1.36	$47.06	000	A+
91030-TC	Acid perfusion of esophagus	0.00	2.99	NA	0.02	3.01	$104.16	NA	NA	000	A+ DS
91034	Gastroesophageal reflux test	0.97	4.77	NA	0.08	5.82	$201.41	NA	NA	000	A+
91034-26	Gastroesophageal reflux test	0.97	0.42	0.42	0.07	1.46	$50.53	1.46	$50.53	000	A+
91034-TC	Gastroesophageal reflux test	0.00	4.35	NA	0.01	4.36	$150.88	NA	NA	000	A+ DS
91035	G-esoph reflx tst w/electrod	1.59	12.65	NA	0.12	14.36	$496.95	NA	NA	000	A+
91035-26	G-esoph reflx tst w/electrod	1.59	0.68	0.68	0.11	2.38	$82.36	2.38	$82.36	000	A+
91035-TC	G-esoph reflx tst w/electrod	0.00	11.97	NA	0.01	11.98	$414.58	NA	NA	000	A+ DS
91037	Esoph imped function test	0.97	4.12	NA	0.05	5.14	$177.88	NA	NA	000	A+
91037-26	Esoph imped function test	0.97	0.43	0.43	0.04	1.44	$49.83	1.44	$49.83	000	A+
91037-TC	Esoph imped function test	0.00	3.69	NA	0.01	3.70	$128.04	NA	NA	000	A+ DS
91038	Esoph imped funct test > 1hr	1.10	11.55	NA	0.06	12.71	$439.84	NA	NA	000	A+
91038-26	Esoph imped funct test > 1hr	1.10	0.49	0.49	0.04	1.63	$56.41	1.63	$56.41	000	A+
91038-TC	Esoph imped funct test > 1hr	0.00	11.06	NA	0.02	11.08	$383.44	NA	NA	000	A+ DS
91040	Esoph balloon distension tst	0.97	15.36	NA	0.08	16.41	$567.89	NA	NA	000	A+
91040-26	Esoph balloon distension tst	0.97	0.41	0.41	0.07	1.45	$50.18	1.45	$50.18	000	A+
91040-TC	Esoph balloon distension tst	0.00	14.95	NA	0.01	14.96	$517.71	NA	NA	000	A+ DS
91065	Breath hydrogen/methane test	0.20	2.50	NA	0.02	2.72	$94.13	NA	NA	000	A+
91065-26	Breath hydrogen/methane test	0.20	0.09	0.09	0.01	0.30	$10.38	0.30	$10.38	000	A+
91065-TC	Breath hydrogen/methane test	0.00	2.41	NA	0.01	2.42	$83.75	NA	NA	000	A+
91110	Gi trc img intral esoph-ile	2.24	20.99	NA	0.09	23.32	$807.02	NA	NA	XXX	A+
91110-26	Gi trc img intral esoph-ile	2.24	1.00	1.00	0.08	3.32	$114.89	3.32	$114.89	XXX	A+
91110-TC	Gi trc img intral esoph-ile	0.00	19.99	NA	0.01	20.00	$692.12	NA	NA	XXX	A+
91111	Gi trc img intral esophagus	0.90	27.13	NA	0.05	28.08	$872.77	NA	NA	XXX	A+ DRA
91111-26	Gi trc img intral esophagus	0.90	0.40	0.40	0.04	1.34	$46.37	1.34	$46.37	XXX	A+
91111-TC	Gi trc img intral esophagus	0.00	26.73	NA	0.01	26.74	$826.40	NA	NA	XXX	A+ DRA
91112	Gi wireless capsule measure	2.10	49.66	NA	0.10	51.86	$1794.68	NA	NA	XXX	A+
91112-26	Gi wireless capsule measure	2.10	0.93	0.93	0.09	3.12	$107.97	3.12	$107.97	XXX	A+
91112-TC	Gi wireless capsule measure	0.00	48.73	NA	0.01	48.74	$1686.71	NA	NA	XXX	A+
91113	Gi trc img intral colon i&r	2.41	25.58	NA	0.09	28.08	$933.33	NA	NA	XXX	A+ DRA
91113-26	Gi trc img intral colon i&r	2.41	1.06	1.06	0.08	3.55	$122.85	3.55	$122.85	XXX	A+

91113-TC		Gi trc img intral colon i&r	0.00	24.52	NA	0.01	24.53	$810.48	NA	NA	XXX	A+ DRA
91117		Colon motility 6 hr study	2.45	NA	1.37	0.17	NA	NA	3.99	$138.08	000	A+
91120		Rectal sensation test	0.97	14.85	NA	0.06	15.88	$549.55	NA	NA	XXX	A+
91120-26		Rectal sensation test	0.97	0.40	0.40	0.05	1.42	$49.14	1.42	$49.14	XXX	A+
91120-TC		Rectal sensation test	0.00	14.45	NA	0.01	14.46	$500.41	NA	NA	XXX	A+ DS
91122		Anal pressure record	1.77	6.35	NA	0.11	8.23	$284.81	NA	NA	000	A+
91122-26		Anal pressure record	1.77	0.70	0.70	0.09	2.56	$88.59	2.56	$88.59	000	A+
91122-TC		Anal pressure record	0.00	5.65	NA	0.02	5.67	$196.22	NA	NA	000	A+ DS
91132		Electrogastrography	0.52	13.49	NA	0.03	14.04	$485.87	NA	NA	XXX	A+
91132-26		Electrogastrography	0.52	0.23	0.23	0.02	0.77	$26.65	0.77	$26.65	XXX	A+
91132-TC		Electrogastrography	0.00	13.26	NA	0.01	13.27	$459.22	NA	NA	XXX	A+ GS
91133		Electrogastrography w/test	0.66	13.99	NA	0.03	14.68	$508.02	NA	NA	XXX	A+
91133-26		Electrogastrography w/test	0.66	0.30	0.30	0.02	0.98	$33.91	0.98	$33.91	XXX	A+
91133-TC		Electrogastrography w/test	0.00	13.69	NA	0.01	13.70	$474.10	NA	NA	XXX	A+ PS
91200		Liver elastography	0.21	0.68	NA	0.02	0.91	$31.49	NA	NA	XXX	A+
91200-26		Liver elastography	0.21	0.09	0.09	0.01	0.31	$10.73	0.31	$10.73	XXX	A+
91200-TC		Liver elastography	0.00	0.59	NA	0.01	0.60	$20.76	NA	NA	XXX	A+ GS
91299	CP	Gastroenterology procedure	0.00	0.00	NA	0.00	0.00	$0.00	NA	NA	XXX	A+
91299-26	CP	Gastroenterology procedure	0.00	0.00	0.00	0.00	0.00	$0.00	0.00	$0.00	XXX	A+
91299-TC	CP	Gastroenterology procedure	0.00	0.00	NA	0.00	0.00	$0.00	NA	NA	XXX	A+
92002		Eye exam new patient	0.88	1.61	0.44	0.04	2.53	$87.55	1.36	$47.06	XXX	A+
92004		Eye exam new patient	1.82	2.52	0.90	0.05	4.39	$151.92	2.77	$95.86	XXX	A+
92012		Eye exam establish patient	0.92	1.66	0.52	0.04	2.62	$90.67	1.48	$51.22	XXX	A+
92014		Eye exam&tx estab pt 1/>vst	1.42	2.24	0.76	0.05	3.71	$128.39	2.23	$77.17	XXX	A+
92015	§	Determine refractive state	0.38	0.16	0.15	0.04	0.58	$20.07	0.57	$19.73	XXX	
92018		New eye exam & treatment	2.50	NA	1.42	0.10	NA	NA	4.02	$139.12	XXX	A+
92019		Eye exam & treatment	1.31	NA	0.72	0.05	NA	NA	2.08	$71.98	XXX	A+
92020		Special eye evaluation	0.37	0.44	0.21	0.01	0.82	$28.38	0.59	$20.42	XXX	A+

*Please note that these calculations are based on the Medicare 2022 Conversion Factor of $34.6062 and the DRA RVU cap rates at time of publication.

A = assistant-at-surgery restriction

A+ = assistant-at-surgery restriction unless medical necessity established with documentation

B = bilateral surgery adjustment applies

C = cosurgeons payable

C+ = cosurgeons payable if medical necessity established with documentation

CP = carriers may establish RVUs and payment amounts for these services, generally on an individual basis following review of documentation such as an operative report

M = multiple surgery adjustment applies

Me = multiple endoscopy rules may apply

M+ = multiple therapy rules apply

Mtc = multiple diagnostic imaging rules apply

T = team surgeons permitted

T+ = team surgeons payable if medical necessity established with documentation

§ = indicates code is not covered by Medicare

GS = procedure must be performed under the general supervision of a physician

DS = procedure must be performed under the direct supervision of a physician

PS = procedure must be performed under the personal supervision of a physician

DRA = procedure subject to DRA limitation

Relative Value Units

CPT Code and Modifier	Description	Work RVU	Nonfacility Practice Expense RVU	Facility Practice Expense RVU	PLI RVU	Total Non-facility RVUs	Medicare Payment Nonfacility	Total Facility RVUs	Medicare Payment Facility	Global Period	Payment Policy Indicators
92025	Corneal topography	0.35	0.69	NA	0.02	1.06	$36.68	NA	NA	XXX	A+
92025-26	Corneal topography	0.35	0.20	0.20	0.01	0.56	$19.38	0.56	$19.38	XXX	A+
92025-TC	Corneal topography	0.00	0.49	NA	0.01	0.50	$17.30	NA	NA	XXX	A+
92060	Special eye evaluation	0.69	1.13	NA	0.02	1.84	$63.68	NA	NA	XXX	A+
92060-26	Special eye evaluation	0.69	0.37	0.37	0.01	1.07	$37.03	1.07	$37.03	XXX	A+
92060-TC	Special eye evaluation	0.00	0.76	NA	0.01	0.77	$26.65	NA	NA	XXX	A+ GS
92065	Orthoptic training	0.37	1.16	NA	0.02	1.55	$53.64	NA	NA	XXX	A+
92065-26	Orthoptic training	0.37	0.13	0.13	0.01	0.51	$17.65	0.51	$17.65	XXX	A+
92065-TC	Orthoptic training	0.00	1.03	NA	0.01	1.04	$35.99	NA	NA	XXX	A+ GS
92071	Contact lens fitting for tx	0.61	0.44	0.31	0.02	1.07	$37.03	0.94	$32.53	XXX	A+ B
92072	Fit contac lens for managmnt	1.97	1.72	0.77	0.04	3.73	$129.08	2.78	$96.21	XXX	A+
92081	Visual field examination(s)	0.30	0.65	NA	0.02	0.97	$33.57	NA	NA	XXX	A+
92081-26	Visual field examination(s)	0.30	0.15	0.15	0.01	0.46	$15.92	0.46	$15.92	XXX	A+
92081-TC	Visual field examination(s)	0.00	0.50	NA	0.01	0.51	$17.65	NA	NA	XXX	A+ GS
92082	Visual field examination(s)	0.40	0.94	NA	0.02	1.36	$47.06	NA	NA	XXX	A+
92082-26	Visual field examination(s)	0.40	0.19	0.19	0.01	0.60	$20.76	0.60	$20.76	XXX	A+
92082-TC	Visual field examination(s)	0.00	0.75	NA	0.01	0.76	$26.30	NA	NA	XXX	A+ GS
92083	Visual field examination(s)	0.50	1.32	NA	0.02	1.84	$63.68	NA	NA	XXX	A+
92083-26	Visual field examination(s)	0.50	0.27	0.27	0.01	0.78	$26.99	0.78	$26.99	XXX	A+
92083-TC	Visual field examination(s)	0.00	1.05	NA	0.01	1.06	$36.68	NA	NA	XXX	A+ GS
92100	Serial tonometry exam(s)	0.61	1.87	0.31	0.02	2.50	$86.52	0.94	$32.53	XXX	A+
92132	Cmptr ophth dx img ant segmt	0.30	0.60	NA	0.02	0.92	$31.84	NA	NA	XXX	A+
92132-26	Cmptr ophth dx img ant segmt	0.30	0.16	0.16	0.01	0.47	$16.26	0.47	$16.26	XXX	A+
92132-TC	Cmptr ophth dx img ant segmt	0.00	0.44	NA	0.01	0.45	$15.57	NA	NA	XXX	A+ GS
92133	Cmptr ophth img optic nerve	0.40	0.66	NA	0.02	1.08	$37.37	NA	NA	XXX	A+
92133-26	Cmptr ophth img optic nerve	0.40	0.22	0.22	0.01	0.63	$21.80	0.63	$21.80	XXX	A+
92133-TC	Cmptr ophth img optic nerve	0.00	0.44	NA	0.01	0.45	$15.57	NA	NA	XXX	A+ GS
92134	Cptr ophth dx img post segmt	0.45	0.72	NA	0.02	1.19	$41.18	NA	NA	XXX	A+
92134-26	Cptr ophth dx img post segmt	0.45	0.27	0.27	0.01	0.73	$25.26	0.73	$25.26	XXX	A+
92134-TC	Cptr ophth dx img post segmt	0.00	0.45	NA	0.01	0.46	$15.92	NA	NA	XXX	A+ GS
92136	Ophthalmic biometry	0.54	0.90	NA	0.02	1.46	$50.53	NA	NA	XXX	A+
92136-26	Ophthalmic biometry	0.54	0.33	0.33	0.01	0.88	$30.45	0.88	$30.45	XXX	A+
92136-TC	Ophthalmic biometry	0.00	0.57	NA	0.01	0.58	$20.07	NA	NA	XXX	A+

92145	Corneal hysteresis deter	0.10	0.25	NA	0.02	0.37	$12.80	NA	NA	XXX	A+
92145-26	Corneal hysteresis deter	0.10	0.05	0.05	0.01	0.16	$5.54	0.16	$5.54	XXX	A+
92145-TC	Corneal hysteresis deter	0.00	0.20	NA	0.01	0.21	$7.27	NA	NA	XXX	A+ GS
92201	Opscpy extnd rta draw uni/bi	0.40	0.30	0.24	0.02	0.72	$24.92	0.66	$22.84	XXX	A+
92202	Opscpy extnd on/mac draw	0.26	0.19	0.15	0.01	0.46	$15.92	0.42	$14.53	XXX	A+
92227	Img rta detcj/mntr ds staff	0.00	0.46	NA	0.01	0.47	$16.26	NA	NA	XXX	A+
92228	Img rta detc/mntr ds phy/qhp	0.32	0.56	NA	0.02	0.90	$31.15	NA	NA	XXX	A+
92228-26	Img rta detc/mntr ds phy/qhp	0.32	0.19	0.19	0.01	0.52	$18.00	0.52	$18.00	XXX	A+
92228-TC	Img rta detc/mntr ds phy/qhp	0.00	0.37	NA	0.01	0.38	$13.15	NA	NA	XXX	A+ GS
92229	Img rta detc/mntr ds poc aly	0.00	1.35	NA	0.01	1.36	$47.06	NA	NA	XXX	A+
92230	Eye exam with photos	0.60	2.24	0.31	0.04	2.88	$99.67	0.95	$32.88	XXX	A+
92235	Fluorescein angrph uni/bi	0.75	2.92	NA	0.02	3.69	$127.70	NA	NA	XXX	A+
92235-26	Fluorescein angrph uni/bi	0.75	0.46	0.46	0.01	1.22	$42.22	1.22	$42.22	XXX	A+
92235-TC	Fluorescein angrph uni/bi	0.00	2.46	NA	0.01	2.47	$85.48	NA	NA	XXX	A+ DS
92240	Icg angiography uni/bi	0.80	4.82	NA	0.10	5.72	$197.95	NA	NA	XXX	A+
92240-26	Icg angiography uni/bi	0.80	0.49	0.49	0.09	1.38	$47.76	1.38	$47.76	XXX	A+
92240-TC	Icg angiography uni/bi	0.00	4.33	NA	0.01	4.34	$150.19	NA	NA	XXX	A+ DS
92242	Fluorescein icg angiography	0.95	6.38	NA	0.05	7.38	$255.39	NA	NA	XXX	A+
92242-26	Fluorescein icg angiography	0.95	0.59	0.59	0.04	1.58	$54.68	1.58	$54.68	XXX	A+
92242-TC	Fluorescein icg angiography	0.00	5.79	NA	0.01	5.80	$200.72	NA	NA	XXX	A+ DS
92250	Eye exam with photos	0.40	0.67	NA	0.02	1.09	$37.72	NA	NA	XXX	A+
92250-26	Eye exam with photos	0.40	0.20	0.20	0.01	0.61	$21.11	0.61	$21.11	XXX	A+
92250-TC	Eye exam with photos	0.00	0.47	NA	0.01	0.48	$16.61	NA	NA	XXX	A+ GS
92260	Ophthalmoscopy/dynamometry	0.20	0.37	0.10	0.01	0.58	$20.07	0.31	$10.73	XXX	A+
92265	Eye muscle evaluation	0.81	1.70	NA	0.02	2.53	$87.55	NA	NA	XXX	A+
92265-26	Eye muscle evaluation	0.81	0.50	0.50	0.01	1.32	$45.68	1.32	$45.68	XXX	A+
92265-TC	Eye muscle evaluation	0.00	1.20	NA	0.01	1.21	$41.87	NA	NA	XXX	A+ PS
92270	Electro-oculography	0.81	2.36	NA	0.03	3.20	$110.74	NA	NA	XXX	A+

*Please note that these calculations are based on the Medicare 2022 Conversion Factor of $34.6062 and the DRA RVU cap rates at time of publication.

A = assistant-at-surgery restriction

A+ = assistant-at-surgery restriction unless medical necessity established with documentation

B = bilateral surgery adjustment applies

C = cosurgeons payable

C+ = cosurgeons payable if medical necessity established with documentation

CP = carriers may establish RVUs and payment amounts for these services, generally on an individual basis following review of documentation such as an operative report

M = multiple surgery adjustment applies

Me = multiple endoscopy rules may apply

M+ = multiple therapy rules apply

Mtc = multiple diagnostic imaging rules apply

T = team surgeons permitted

T+ = team surgeons payable if medical necessity established with documentation

§ = indicates code is not covered by Medicare

GS = procedure must be performed under the general supervision of a physician

DS = procedure must be performed under the direct supervision of a physician

PS = procedure must be performed under the personal supervision of a physician

DRA = procedure subject to DRA limitation

Relative Value Units

CPT Code and Modifier		Description	Work RVU	Nonfacility Practice Expense RVU	Facility Practice Expense RVU	PLI RVU	Total Non-facility RVUs	Medicare Payment Nonfacility	Total Facility RVUs	Medicare Payment Facility	Global Period	Payment Policy Indicators
92270-26		Electro-oculography	0.81	0.41	0.41	0.01	1.23	$42.57	1.23	$42.57	XXX	A+
92270-TC		Electro-oculography	0.00	1.95	NA	0.02	1.97	$68.17	NA	NA	XXX	A+ GS
92273		Full field erg w/i&r	0.69	3.01	NA	0.03	3.73	$129.08	NA	NA	XXX	A+
92273-26		Full field erg w/i&r	0.69	0.36	0.36	0.01	1.06	$36.68	1.06	$36.68	XXX	A+
92273-TC		Full field erg w/i&r	0.00	2.65	NA	0.02	2.67	$92.40	NA	NA	XXX	A+ GS
92274		Multifocal erg w/i&r	0.61	1.92	NA	0.02	2.55	$88.25	NA	NA	XXX	A+
92274-26		Multifocal erg w/i&r	0.61	0.32	0.32	0.01	0.94	$32.53	0.94	$32.53	XXX	A+
92274-TC		Multifocal erg w/i&r	0.00	1.60	NA	0.01	1.61	$55.72	NA	NA	XXX	A+ GS
92283		Color vision examination	0.17	1.40	NA	0.02	1.59	$55.02	NA	NA	XXX	A+
92283-26		Color vision examination	0.17	0.08	0.08	0.01	0.26	$9.00	0.26	$9.00	XXX	A+
92283-TC		Color vision examination	0.00	1.32	NA	0.01	1.33	$46.03	NA	NA	XXX	A+ GS
92284		Dark adaptation eye exam	0.24	1.43	NA	0.03	1.70	$58.83	NA	NA	XXX	A+
92284-26		Dark adaptation eye exam	0.24	0.10	0.10	0.01	0.35	$12.11	0.35	$12.11	XXX	A+
92284-TC		Dark adaptation eye exam	0.00	1.33	NA	0.02	1.35	$46.72	NA	NA	XXX	A+ GS
92285		Eye photography	0.05	0.61	NA	0.02	0.68	$23.53	NA	NA	XXX	A+
92285-26		Eye photography	0.05	0.03	0.03	0.01	0.09	$3.11	0.09	$3.11	XXX	A+
92285-TC		Eye photography	0.00	0.58	NA	0.01	0.59	$20.42	NA	NA	XXX	A+ GS
92286		Internal eye photography	0.40	0.73	NA	0.02	1.15	$39.80	NA	NA	XXX	A+
92286-26		Internal eye photography	0.40	0.22	0.22	0.01	0.63	$21.80	0.63	$21.80	XXX	A+
92286-TC		Internal eye photography	0.00	0.51	NA	0.01	0.52	$18.00	NA	NA	XXX	A+ GS
92287		Internal eye photography	0.81	4.48	NA	0.03	5.32	$160.92	NA	NA	XXX	A+ DRA
92287-26		Internal eye photography	0.81	0.50	0.50	0.01	1.32	$45.68	1.32	$45.68	XXX	A+
92287-TC		Internal eye photography	0.00	3.98	NA	0.02	4.00	$115.24	NA	NA	XXX	A+ DRA
92310	§	Contact lens fitting	1.17	1.74	0.45	0.10	3.01	$104.16	1.72	$59.52	XXX	
92311		Contact lens fitting	1.08	2.03	0.43	0.02	3.13	$108.32	1.53	$52.95	XXX	A+
92312		Contact lens fitting	1.26	2.35	0.49	0.02	3.63	$125.62	1.77	$61.25	XXX	A+
92313		Contact lens fitting	0.92	2.03	0.33	0.01	2.96	$102.43	1.26	$43.60	XXX	A+
92314	§	Prescription of contact lens	0.69	1.87	0.27	0.07	2.63	$91.01	1.03	$35.64	XXX	
92315		Rx cntact lens aphakia 1 eye	0.45	1.98	0.15	0.01	2.44	$84.44	0.61	$21.11	XXX	A+
92316		Rx cntact lens aphakia 2 eye	0.68	2.32	0.23	0.01	3.01	$104.16	0.92	$31.84	XXX	A+
92317		Rx corneoscleral cntact lens	0.45	2.10	0.15	0.01	2.56	$88.59	0.61	$21.11	XXX	A+
92325		Modification of contact lens	0.00	1.35	NA	0.01	1.36	$47.06	NA	NA	XXX	A+
92326		Replacement of contact lens	0.00	1.15	NA	0.01	1.16	$40.14	NA	NA	XXX	A+

92340	§	Fit spectacles monofocal	0.37	0.61	0.14	0.04	1.02	$35.30	0.55	$19.03	XXX	
92341	§	Fit spectacles bifocal	0.47	0.65	0.18	0.04	1.16	$40.14	0.69	$23.88	XXX	
92342	§	Fit spectacles multifocal	0.53	0.67	0.20	0.04	1.24	$42.91	0.77	$26.65	XXX	
92352	§	Fit aphakia spectcl monofocl	0.37	0.95	0.14	0.04	1.36	$47.06	0.55	$19.03	XXX	
92353	§	Fit aphakia spectcl multifoc	0.50	1.00	0.19	0.04	1.54	$53.29	0.73	$25.26	XXX	
92354	§	Fit spectacles single system	0.00	0.38	NA	0.01	0.39	$13.50	NA	NA	XXX	
92355	§	Fit spectacles compound lens	0.00	0.59	NA	0.02	0.61	$21.11	NA	NA	XXX	
92358	§	Aphakia prosth service temp	0.00	0.31	NA	0.01	0.32	$11.07	NA	NA	XXX	
92370	§	Repair & adjust spectacles	0.32	0.56	0.12	0.04	0.92	$31.84	0.48	$16.61	XXX	
92371	§	Repair & adjust spectacles	0.00	0.32	NA	0.01	0.33	$11.42	NA	NA	XXX	
92499	CP	Eye service or procedure	0.00	0.00	NA	0.00	0.00	$0.00	NA	NA	XXX	A+
92499-26	CP	Eye service or procedure	0.00	0.00	0.00	0.00	0.00	$0.00	0.00	$0.00	XXX	A+
92499-TC	CP	Eye service or procedure	0.00	0.00	NA	0.00	0.00	$0.00	NA	NA	XXX	A+
92502		Ear and throat examination	1.51	NA	1.17	0.10	NA	NA	2.78	$96.21	000	A+
92504		Ear microscopy examination	0.18	0.67	0.08	0.01	0.86	$29.76	0.27	$9.34	XXX	A+
92507		Speech/hearing therapy	1.30	0.91	NA	0.05	2.26	$78.21	NA	NA	XXX	A+ Mt
92508		Speech/hearing therapy	0.33	0.36	NA	0.01	0.70	$24.22	NA	NA	XXX	A+ Mt
92511		Nasopharyngoscopy	0.61	2.88	0.45	0.04	3.53	$122.16	1.10	$38.07	000	A+ PS
92512		Nasal function studies	0.55	1.25	0.22	0.04	1.84	$63.68	0.81	$28.03	XXX	A+
92516		Facial nerve function test	0.43	1.58	0.20	0.04	2.05	$70.94	0.67	$23.19	XXX	A+
92517		Vemp test i&r cervical	0.80	1.17	0.37	0.05	2.02	$69.90	1.22	$42.22	XXX	A+ DS
92518		Vemp test i&r ocular	0.80	1.05	0.37	0.05	1.90	$65.75	1.22	$42.22	XXX	A+ DS
92519		Vemp tst i&r cervical&ocular	1.20	1.86	0.55	0.08	3.14	$108.66	1.83	$63.33	XXX	A+ DS
92520		Laryngeal function studies	0.75	1.64	0.37	0.04	2.43	$84.09	1.16	$40.14	XXX	A+
92521		Evaluation of speech fluency	2.24	1.59	NA	0.09	3.92	$135.66	NA	NA	XXX	A+ Mt
92522		Evaluate speech production	1.92	1.28	NA	0.09	3.29	$113.85	NA	NA	XXX	A+ Mt
92523		Speech sound lang comprehen	3.84	2.73	NA	0.12	6.69	$231.52	NA	NA	XXX	A+ Mt
92524		Behavral qualit analys voice	1.92	1.23	NA	0.09	3.24	$112.12	NA	NA	XXX	A+ Mt

*Please note that these calculations are based on the Medicare 2022 Conversion Factor of $34.6062 and the DRA RVU cap rates at time of publication.

A = assistant-at-surgery restriction
A+ = assistant-at-surgery restriction unless medical necessity established with documentation
B = bilateral surgery adjustment applies
C = cosurgeons payable
C+ = cosurgeons payable if medical necessity established with documentation
CP = carriers may establish RVUs and payment amounts for these services, generally on an individual basis following review of documentation such as an operative report
M = multiple surgery adjustment applies
Me = multiple endoscopy rules may apply
M+ = multiple therapy rules apply
Mtc = multiple diagnostic imaging rules apply
T = team surgeons permitted
T+ = team surgeons payable if medical necessity established with documentation
§ = indicates code is not covered by Medicare
GS = procedure must be performed under the general supervision of a physician
DS = procedure must be performed under the direct supervision of a physician
PS = procedure must be performed under the personal supervision of a physician
DRA = procedure subject to DRA limitation

Relative Value Units

CPT Code and Modifier	Description	Work RVU	Nonfacility Practice Expense RVU	Facility Practice Expense RVU	PLI RVU	Total Non-facility RVUs	Medicare Payment Nonfacility	Total Facility RVUs	Medicare Payment Facility	Global Period	Payment Policy Indicators
92526	Oral function therapy	1.34	1.12	NA	0.05	2.51	$86.86	NA	NA	XXX	A+ Mt
92537	Caloric vstblr test w/rec	0.60	0.59	NA	0.02	1.21	$41.87	NA	NA	XXX	A+
92537-26	Caloric vstblr test w/rec	0.60	0.30	0.30	0.01	0.91	$31.49	0.91	$31.49	XXX	A+
92537-TC	Caloric vstblr test w/rec	0.00	0.29	NA	0.01	0.30	$10.38	NA	NA	XXX	A+ DS
92538	Caloric vstblr test w/rec	0.30	0.35	NA	0.02	0.67	$23.19	NA	NA	XXX	A+
92538-26	Caloric vstblr test w/rec	0.30	0.16	0.16	0.01	0.47	$16.26	0.47	$16.26	XXX	A+
92538-TC	Caloric vstblr test w/rec	0.00	0.19	NA	0.01	0.20	$6.92	NA	NA	XXX	A+ DS
92540	Basic vestibular evaluation	1.50	1.72	NA	0.05	3.27	$113.16	NA	NA	XXX	A+
92540-26	Basic vestibular evaluation	1.50	0.74	0.74	0.04	2.28	$78.90	2.28	$78.90	XXX	A+
92540-TC	Basic vestibular evaluation	0.00	0.98	NA	0.01	0.99	$34.26	NA	NA	XXX	A+ DS
92541	Spontaneous nystagmus test	0.40	0.33	NA	0.02	0.75	$25.95	NA	NA	XXX	A+
92541-26	Spontaneous nystagmus test	0.40	0.20	0.20	0.01	0.61	$21.11	0.61	$21.11	XXX	A+
92541-TC	Spontaneous nystagmus test	0.00	0.13	NA	0.01	0.14	$4.84	NA	NA	XXX	A+ DS
92542	Positional nystagmus test	0.48	0.36	NA	0.02	0.86	$29.76	NA	NA	XXX	A+
92542-26	Positional nystagmus test	0.48	0.24	0.24	0.01	0.73	$25.26	0.73	$25.26	XXX	A+
92542-TC	Positional nystagmus test	0.00	0.12	NA	0.01	0.13	$4.50	NA	NA	XXX	A+ DS
92544	Optokinetic nystagmus test	0.27	0.24	NA	0.02	0.53	$18.34	NA	NA	XXX	A+
92544-26	Optokinetic nystagmus test	0.27	0.14	0.14	0.01	0.42	$14.53	0.42	$14.53	XXX	A+
92544-TC	Optokinetic nystagmus test	0.00	0.10	NA	0.01	0.11	$3.81	NA	NA	XXX	A+ DS
92545	Oscillating tracking test	0.25	0.23	NA	0.02	0.50	$17.30	NA	NA	XXX	A+
92545-26	Oscillating tracking test	0.25	0.13	0.13	0.01	0.39	$13.50	0.39	$13.50	XXX	A+
92545-TC	Oscillating tracking test	0.00	0.10	NA	0.01	0.11	$3.81	NA	NA	XXX	A+ DS
92546	Sinusoidal rotational test	0.29	3.38	NA	0.03	3.70	$128.04	NA	NA	XXX	A+
92546-26	Sinusoidal rotational test	0.29	0.14	0.14	0.01	0.44	$15.23	0.44	$15.23	XXX	A+
92546-TC	Sinusoidal rotational test	0.00	3.24	NA	0.02	3.26	$112.82	NA	NA	XXX	A+ DS
92547	Supplemental electrical test	0.00	0.31	NA	0.00	0.31	$10.73	NA	NA	ZZZ	A+ DS
92548	Cdp-sot 6 cond w/i&r	0.67	0.74	NA	0.03	1.44	$49.83	NA	NA	XXX	A+
92548-26	Cdp-sot 6 cond w/i&r	0.67	0.31	0.31	0.02	1.00	$34.61	1.00	$34.61	XXX	A+
92548-TC	Cdp-sot 6 cond w/i&r	0.00	0.43	NA	0.01	0.44	$15.23	NA	NA	XXX	A+ DS
92549	Cdp-sot 6 cond w/i&r mct&adt	0.87	0.99	NA	0.02	1.88	$65.06	NA	NA	XXX	A+
92549-26	Cdp-sot 6 cond w/i&r mct&adt	0.87	0.42	0.42	0.01	1.30	$44.99	1.30	$44.99	XXX	A+
92549-TC	Cdp-sot 6 cond w/i&r mct&adt	0.00	0.57	NA	0.01	0.58	$20.07	NA	NA	XXX	A+ DS
92550	Tympanometry & reflex thresh	0.35	0.29	NA	0.02	0.66	$22.84	NA	NA	XXX	A+ DS

92551	§	Pure tone hearing test air	0.00	0.33	NA	0.01	0.34	$11.77	NA	NA	XXX	
92552		Pure tone audiometry air	0.00	0.98	NA	0.01	0.99	$34.26	NA	NA	XXX	A+ DS
92553		Audiometry air & bone	0.00	1.19	NA	0.01	1.20	$41.53	NA	NA	XXX	A+ DS
92555		Speech threshold audiometry	0.00	0.74	NA	0.01	0.75	$25.95	NA	NA	XXX	A+ DS
92556		Speech audiometry complete	0.00	1.17	NA	0.01	1.18	$40.84	NA	NA	XXX	A+ DS
92557		Comprehensive hearing test	0.60	0.47	0.31	0.04	1.11	$38.41	0.95	$32.88	XXX	A+ DS
92562		Loudness balance test	0.00	1.35	NA	0.01	1.36	$47.06	NA	NA	XXX	A+ DS
92563		Tone decay hearing test	0.00	0.93	NA	0.01	0.94	$32.53	NA	NA	XXX	A+ DS
92565		Stenger test pure tone	0.00	0.55	NA	0.01	0.56	$19.38	NA	NA	XXX	A+ DS
92567		Tympanometry	0.20	0.28	0.10	0.01	0.49	$16.96	0.31	$10.73	XXX	A+ DS
92568		Acoustic refl threshold tst	0.29	0.15	0.14	0.02	0.46	$15.92	0.45	$15.57	XXX	A+ DS
92570		Acoustic immitance testing	0.55	0.38	0.28	0.04	0.97	$33.57	0.87	$30.11	XXX	A+ DS
92571		Filtered speech hearing test	0.00	0.83	NA	0.01	0.84	$29.07	NA	NA	XXX	A+ DS
92572		Staggered spondaic word test	0.00	1.20	NA	0.01	1.21	$41.87	NA	NA	XXX	A+ DS
92575		Sensorineural acuity test	0.00	2.03	NA	0.04	2.07	$71.63	NA	NA	XXX	A+ DS
92576		Synthetic sentence test	0.00	1.11	NA	0.01	1.12	$38.76	NA	NA	XXX	A+ DS
92577		Stenger test speech	0.00	0.54	NA	0.01	0.55	$19.03	NA	NA	XXX	A+ DS
92579		Visual audiometry (vra)	0.70	0.62	0.37	0.04	1.36	$47.06	1.11	$38.41	XXX	A+ DS
92582		Conditioning play audiometry	0.00	2.26	NA	0.02	2.28	$78.90	NA	NA	XXX	A+ DS
92583		Select picture audiometry	0.00	1.48	NA	0.01	1.49	$51.56	NA	NA	XXX	A+ DS
92584		Electrocochleography	1.00	2.35	NA	0.05	3.40	$117.66	NA	NA	XXX	A+ DS
92587		Evoked auditory test limited	0.35	0.28	NA	0.02	0.65	$22.49	NA	NA	XXX	A+
92587-26		Evoked auditory test limited	0.35	0.17	0.17	0.01	0.53	$18.34	0.53	$18.34	XXX	A+
92587-TC		Evoked auditory test limited	0.00	0.11	NA	0.01	0.12	$4.15	NA	NA	XXX	A+ DS
92588		Evoked auditory tst complete	0.55	0.43	NA	0.02	1.00	$34.61	NA	NA	XXX	A+
92588-26		Evoked auditory tst complete	0.55	0.28	0.28	0.01	0.84	$29.07	0.84	$29.07	XXX	A+
92588-TC		Evoked auditory tst complete	0.00	0.15	NA	0.01	0.16	$5.54	NA	NA	XXX	A+ DS
92596		Ear protector evaluation	0.00	2.01	NA	0.01	2.02	$69.90	NA	NA	XXX	A+

*Please note that these calculations are based on the Medicare 2022 Conversion Factor of $34.6062 and the DRA RVU cap rates at time of publication.

A = assistant-at-surgery restriction

A+ = assistant-at-surgery restriction unless medical necessity established with documentation

B = bilateral surgery adjustment applies

C = cosurgeons payable

C+ = cosurgeons payable if medical necessity established with documentation

CP = carriers may establish RVUs and payment amounts for these services, generally on an individual basis following review of documentation such as an operative report

M = multiple surgery adjustment applies

Me = multiple endoscopy rules may apply

M+ = multiple therapy rules apply

Mtc = multiple diagnostic imaging rules apply

T = team surgeons permitted

T+ = team surgeons payable if medical necessity established with documentation

§ = indicates code is not covered by Medicare

GS = procedure must be performed under the general supervision of a physician

DS = procedure must be performed under the direct supervision of a physician

PS = procedure must be performed under the personal supervision of a physician

DRA = procedure subject to DRA limitation

Relative Value Units

CPT Code and Modifier		Description	Work RVU	Nonfacility Practice Expense RVU	Facility Practice Expense RVU	PLI RVU	Total Non-facility RVUs	Medicare Payment Nonfacility	Total Facility RVUs	Medicare Payment Facility	Global Period	Payment Policy Indicators
92597		Oral speech device eval	1.26	0.80	NA	0.07	2.13	$73.71	NA	NA	XXX	A+ Mt
92601		Cochlear implt f/up exam <7	2.30	2.43	1.24	0.09	4.82	$166.80	3.63	$125.62	XXX	A+ DS
92602		Reprogram cochlear implt <7	1.30	1.70	0.70	0.05	3.05	$105.55	2.05	$70.94	XXX	A+ DS
92603		Cochlear implt f/up exam 7/>	2.25	2.17	1.19	0.09	4.51	$156.07	3.53	$122.16	XXX	A+ DS
92604		Reprogram cochlear implt 7/>	1.25	1.42	0.66	0.05	2.72	$94.13	1.96	$67.83	XXX	A+ DS
92605	§	Ex for nonspeech device rx	1.75	0.86	0.68	0.12	2.73	$94.47	2.55	$88.25	XXX	
92606	§	Non-speech device service	1.40	0.90	0.54	0.11	2.41	$83.40	2.05	$70.94	XXX	
92607		Ex for speech device rx 1hr	1.85	1.73	NA	0.08	3.66	$126.66	NA	NA	XXX	A+ Mt
92608		Ex for speech device rx addl	0.70	0.71	NA	0.04	1.45	$50.18	NA	NA	ZZZ	A+
92609		Use of speech device service	1.50	1.50	NA	0.07	3.07	$106.24	NA	NA	XXX	A+ Mt
92610		Evaluate swallowing function	1.30	1.15	0.69	0.07	2.52	$87.21	2.06	$71.29	XXX	A+
92611		Motion fluoroscopy/swallow	1.34	1.28	NA	0.09	2.71	$93.78	NA	NA	XXX	A+
92612		Endoscopy swallow (fees) vid	1.27	4.39	0.61	0.08	5.74	$198.64	1.96	$67.83	XXX	A+
92613		Endoscopy swallow (fees) i&r	0.71	0.32	0.32	0.04	1.07	$37.03	1.07	$37.03	XXX	A+
92614		Laryngoscopic sensory vid	1.27	2.97	0.59	0.08	4.32	$149.50	1.94	$67.14	XXX	A+
92615		Laryngoscopic sensory i&r	0.63	0.29	0.29	0.04	0.96	$33.22	0.96	$33.22	XXX	A+
92616		Fees w/laryngeal sense test	1.88	4.40	0.90	0.11	6.39	$221.13	2.89	$100.01	XXX	A+
92617		Fees w/laryngeal sense i&r	0.79	0.36	0.36	0.05	1.20	$41.53	1.20	$41.53	XXX	A+
92618	§	Ex for nonspeech dev rx add	0.65	0.26	0.25	0.05	0.96	$33.22	0.95	$32.88	ZZZ	
92620		Auditory function 60 min	1.50	1.11	0.78	0.08	2.69	$93.09	2.36	$81.67	XXX	A+ DS
92621		Auditory function + 15 min	0.35	0.29	0.19	0.01	0.65	$22.49	0.55	$19.03	ZZZ	A+ DS
92625		Tinnitus assessment	1.15	0.82	0.60	0.05	2.02	$69.90	1.80	$62.29	XXX	A+ DS
92626		Eval aud funcj 1st hour	1.40	1.15	0.74	0.05	2.60	$89.98	2.19	$75.79	XXX	A+ DS
92627		Eval aud funcj ea addl 15	0.33	0.27	0.18	0.01	0.61	$21.11	0.52	$18.00	ZZZ	A+ DS
92640		Aud brainstem implt programg	1.76	1.45	0.95	0.07	3.28	$113.51	2.78	$96.21	XXX	A+
92650	§	Aep scr auditory potential	0.25	0.58	NA	0.02	0.85	$29.42	NA	NA	XXX	A+ DS
92651		Aep hearing status deter i&r	1.00	1.56	NA	0.05	2.61	$90.32	NA	NA	XXX	A+ DS
92652		Aep thrshld est mlt freq i&r	1.50	1.83	NA	0.09	3.42	$118.35	NA	NA	XXX	A+ DS
92653		Aep neurodiagnostic i&r	1.05	1.42	NA	0.07	2.54	$87.90	NA	NA	XXX	A+ DS
92700	CP	Ent procedure/service	0.00	0.00	0.00	0.00	0.00	$0.00	0.00	$0.00	XXX	A+
92920		Prq cardiac angioplast 1 art	9.85	NA	3.43	2.25	NA	NA	15.53	$537.43	000	A+ M
92924		Prq card angio/athrect 1 art	11.74	NA	4.08	2.69	NA	NA	18.51	$640.56	000	A+ M
92928		Prq card stent w/angio 1 vsl	10.96	NA	3.81	2.51	NA	NA	17.28	$598.00	000	A+ M

92933		Prq card stent/ath/angio	12.29	NA	4.26	2.83	NA	NA	19.38	$670.67	000	A+ M
92937		Prq revasc byp graft 1 vsl	10.95	NA	3.80	2.51	NA	NA	17.26	$597.30	000	A+ M
92941		Prq card revasc mi 1 vsl	12.31	NA	4.28	2.83	NA	NA	19.42	$672.05	000	A+ M
92943		Prq card revasc chronic 1vsl	12.31	NA	4.27	2.84	NA	NA	19.42	$672.05	000	A+ M
92950		Heart/lung resuscitation cpr	4.00	5.44	0.99	0.40	9.84	$340.53	5.39	$186.53	000	A+
92953		Temporary external pacing	0.01	NA	0.01	0.01	NA	NA	0.03	$1.04	000	A+
92960		Cardioversion electric ext	2.00	2.46	1.02	0.14	4.60	$159.19	3.16	$109.36	000	A+
92961		Cardioversion electric int	4.34	NA	1.91	0.96	NA	NA	7.21	$249.51	000	
92970		Cardioassist internal	3.51	NA	1.22	0.83	NA	NA	5.56	$192.41	000	A+
92971		Cardioassist external	1.77	NA	0.75	0.41	NA	NA	2.93	$101.40	000	A+
92973		Prq coronary mech thrombect	3.28	NA	1.15	0.75	NA	NA	5.18	$179.26	ZZZ	A+
92974		Cath place cardio brachytx	3.00	NA	1.05	0.68	NA	NA	4.73	$163.69	ZZZ	A+
92975		Dissolve clot heart vessel	6.99	NA	2.41	1.64	NA	NA	11.04	$382.05	000	A+ M
92977		Dissolve clot heart vessel	0.00	1.42	NA	0.11	1.53	$52.95	NA	NA	XXX	A+
92978	CP	Endoluminl ivus oct c 1st	0.00	0.00	NA	0.00	0.00	$0.00	NA	NA	ZZZ	A+
92978-26		Endoluminl ivus oct c 1st	1.80	0.63	0.63	0.34	2.77	$95.86	2.77	$95.86	ZZZ	A+
92978-TC	CP	Endoluminl ivus oct c 1st	0.00	0.00	NA	0.00	0.00	$0.00	NA	NA	ZZZ	A+ PS
92979	CP	Endoluminl ivus oct c ea	0.00	0.00	NA	0.00	0.00	$0.00	NA	NA	ZZZ	A+
92979-26		Endoluminl ivus oct c ea	1.44	0.50	0.50	0.27	2.21	$76.48	2.21	$76.48	ZZZ	A+
92979-TC	CP	Endoluminl ivus oct c ea	0.00	0.00	NA	0.00	0.00	$0.00	NA	NA	ZZZ	A+ PS
92986		Revision of aortic valve	22.60	NA	11.06	5.17	NA	NA	38.83	$1343.76	090	A+ M
92987		Revision of mitral valve	23.38	NA	11.41	5.38	NA	NA	40.17	$1390.13	090	A+ M
92990		Revision of pulmonary valve	18.27	NA	9.47	4.26	NA	NA	32.00	$1107.40	090	A+ M
92997		Pul art balloon repr percut	11.98	NA	4.24	2.44	NA	NA	18.66	$645.75	000	A+ M
92998		Pul art balloon repr percut	5.99	NA	2.02	1.29	NA	NA	9.30	$321.84	ZZZ	A+
93000		Electrocardiogram complete	0.17	0.23	NA	0.02	0.42	$14.53	NA	NA	XXX	A+ GS
93005		Electrocardiogram tracing	0.00	0.17	NA	0.01	0.18	$6.23	NA	NA	XXX	A+ GS
93010		Electrocardiogram report	0.17	0.06	0.06	0.01	0.24	$8.31	0.24	$8.31	XXX	A+

*Please note that these calculations are based on the Medicare 2022 Conversion Factor of $34.6062 and the DRA RVU cap rates at time of publication.

A = assistant-at-surgery restriction

A+ = assistant-at-surgery restriction unless medical necessity established with documentation

B = bilateral surgery adjustment applies

C = cosurgeons payable

C+ = cosurgeons payable if medical necessity established with documentation

CP = carriers may establish RVUs and payment amounts for these services, generally on an individual basis following review of documentation such as an operative report

M = multiple surgery adjustment applies

Me = multiple endoscopy rules may apply

M+ = multiple therapy rules apply

Mtc = multiple diagnostic imaging rules apply

T = team surgeons permitted

T+ = team surgeons payable if medical necessity established with documentation

§ = indicates code is not covered by Medicare

GS = procedure must be performed under the general supervision of a physician

DS = procedure must be performed under the direct supervision of a physician

PS = procedure must be performed under the personal supervision of a physician

DRA = procedure subject to DRA limitation

Relative Value Units

CPT Code and Modifier		Description	Work RVU	Nonfacility Practice Expense RVU	Facility Practice Expense RVU	PLI RVU	Total Non-facility RVUs	Medicare Payment Nonfacility	Total Facility RVUs	Medicare Payment Facility	Global Period	Payment Policy Indicators
93015		Cardiovascular stress test	0.75	1.29	NA	0.05	2.09	$72.33	NA	NA	XXX	A+ DS
93016		Cardiovascular stress test	0.45	0.16	0.16	0.02	0.63	$21.80	0.63	$21.80	XXX	A+ DS
93017		Cardiovascular stress test	0.00	1.02	NA	0.02	1.04	$35.99	NA	NA	XXX	A+ DS
93018		Cardiovascular stress test	0.30	0.11	0.11	0.01	0.42	$14.53	0.42	$14.53	XXX	A+
93024		Cardiac drug stress test	1.17	1.97	NA	0.08	3.22	$111.43	NA	NA	XXX	A+
93024-26		Cardiac drug stress test	1.17	0.41	0.41	0.04	1.62	$56.06	1.62	$56.06	XXX	A+
93024-TC		Cardiac drug stress test	0.00	1.56	NA	0.04	1.60	$55.37	NA	NA	XXX	A+ PS
93025		Microvolt t-wave assess	0.75	2.77	NA	0.04	3.56	$123.20	NA	NA	XXX	A+
93025-26		Microvolt t-wave assess	0.75	0.31	0.31	0.02	1.08	$37.37	1.08	$37.37	XXX	A+
93025-TC		Microvolt t-wave assess	0.00	2.46	NA	0.02	2.48	$85.82	NA	NA	XXX	A+ GS
93040		Rhythm ecg with report	0.15	0.20	NA	0.02	0.37	$12.80	NA	NA	XXX	A+ GS
93041		Rhythm ecg tracing	0.00	0.16	NA	0.01	0.17	$5.88	NA	NA	XXX	A+ GS
93042		Rhythm ecg report	0.15	0.04	0.04	0.01	0.20	$6.92	0.20	$6.92	XXX	A+
93050		Art pressure waveform analys	0.17	0.28	NA	0.02	0.47	$16.26	NA	NA	XXX	A+
93050-26		Art pressure waveform analys	0.17	0.06	0.06	0.01	0.24	$8.31	0.24	$8.31	XXX	A+
93050-TC		Art pressure waveform analys	0.00	0.22	NA	0.01	0.23	$7.96	NA	NA	XXX	A+
93224		Ecg monit/reprt up to 48 hrs	0.39	1.81	NA	0.03	2.23	$77.17	NA	NA	XXX	A+ GS
93225		Ecg monit/reprt up to 48 hrs	0.00	0.56	NA	0.01	0.57	$19.73	NA	NA	XXX	A+ GS
93226		Ecg monit/reprt up to 48 hrs	0.00	1.11	NA	0.01	1.12	$38.76	NA	NA	XXX	A+ GS
93227		Ecg monit/reprt up to 48 hrs	0.39	0.14	0.14	0.01	0.54	$18.69	0.54	$18.69	XXX	A+
93228		Remote 30 day ecg rev/report	0.48	0.23	0.23	0.04	0.75	$25.95	0.75	$25.95	XXX	A+
93229		Remote 30 day ecg tech supp	0.00	26.25	NA	0.10	26.35	$911.87	NA	NA	XXX	A+ GS
93241	CP	Ext ecg>48hr<7d rec scan a/r	0.00	0.00	0.00	0.00	0.00	$0.00	0.00	$0.00	XXX	A+ GS
93242		Ext ecg>48hr<7d recording	0.00	0.41	NA	0.01	0.42	$14.53	NA	NA	XXX	A+ GS
93243	CP	Ext ecg>48hr<7d scan a/r	0.00	0.00	0.00	0.00	0.00	$0.00	0.00	$0.00	XXX	A+ GS
93244		Ext ecg>48hr<7d rev&interpj	0.50	0.19	0.19	0.02	0.71	$24.57	0.71	$24.57	XXX	A+
93245	CP	Ext ecg>7d<15d rec scan a/r	0.00	0.00	0.00	0.00	0.00	$0.00	0.00	$0.00	XXX	A+ GS
93246		Ext ecg>7d<15d recording	0.00	0.41	NA	0.01	0.42	$14.53	NA	NA	XXX	A+ GS
93247	CP	Ext ecg>7d<15d scan a/r	0.00	0.00	0.00	0.00	0.00	$0.00	0.00	$0.00	XXX	A+ GS
93248		Ext ecg>7d<15d rev&interpj	0.55	0.21	0.21	0.02	0.78	$26.99	0.78	$26.99	XXX	A+
93260		Prgrmg dev eval impltbl sys	0.85	1.40	NA	0.05	2.30	$79.59	NA	NA	XXX	A+
93260-26		Prgrmg dev eval impltbl sys	0.85	0.35	0.35	0.04	1.24	$42.91	1.24	$42.91	XXX	A+
93260-TC		Prgrmg dev eval impltbl sys	0.00	1.05	NA	0.01	1.06	$36.68	NA	NA	XXX	A+ DS

93261	Interrogate subq defib	0.74	1.34	NA	0.05	2.13	$73.71	NA	NA	XXX	A+
93261-26	Interrogate subq defib	0.74	0.30	0.30	0.04	1.08	$37.37	1.08	$37.37	XXX	A+
93261-TC	Interrogate subq defib	0.00	1.04	NA	0.01	1.05	$36.34	NA	NA	XXX	A+ DS
93264	Rem mntr wrls p-art prs snr	0.70	0.71	0.28	0.05	1.46	$50.53	1.03	$35.64	XXX	A+
93268	Ecg record/review	0.52	4.91	NA	0.04	5.47	$189.30	NA	NA	XXX	A+ GS
93270	Remote 30 day ecg rev/report	0.00	0.24	NA	0.01	0.25	$8.65	NA	NA	XXX	A+ GS
93271	Ecg/monitoring and analysis	0.00	4.49	NA	0.01	4.50	$155.73	NA	NA	XXX	A+ GS
93272	Ecg/review interpret only	0.52	0.18	0.18	0.02	0.72	$24.92	0.72	$24.92	XXX	A+
93278	Ecg/signal-averaged	0.25	0.58	NA	0.02	0.85	$29.42	NA	NA	XXX	A+
93278-26	Ecg/signal-averaged	0.25	0.10	0.10	0.01	0.36	$12.46	0.36	$12.46	XXX	A+
93278-TC	Ecg/signal-averaged	0.00	0.48	NA	0.01	0.49	$16.96	NA	NA	XXX	A+ GS
93279	Prgrmg dev eval pm/ldls pm	0.65	1.37	NA	0.03	2.05	$70.94	NA	NA	XXX	A+
93279-26	Prgrmg dev eval pm/ldls pm	0.65	0.25	0.25	0.02	0.92	$31.84	0.92	$31.84	XXX	A+
93279-TC	Prgrmg dev eval pm/ldls pm	0.00	1.12	NA	0.01	1.13	$39.11	NA	NA	XXX	A+ DS
93280	Pm device progr eval dual	0.77	1.61	NA	0.05	2.43	$84.09	NA	NA	XXX	A+
93280-26	Pm device progr eval dual	0.77	0.30	0.30	0.04	1.11	$38.41	1.11	$38.41	XXX	A+
93280-TC	Pm device progr eval dual	0.00	1.31	NA	0.01	1.32	$45.68	NA	NA	XXX	A+ DS
93281	Pm device progr eval multi	0.85	1.67	NA	0.05	2.57	$88.94	NA	NA	XXX	A+
93281-26	Pm device progr eval multi	0.85	0.34	0.34	0.04	1.23	$42.57	1.23	$42.57	XXX	A+
93281-TC	Pm device progr eval multi	0.00	1.33	NA	0.01	1.34	$46.37	NA	NA	XXX	A+ DS
93282	Prgrmg eval implantable dfb	0.85	1.55	NA	0.05	2.45	$84.79	NA	NA	XXX	A+
93282-26	Prgrmg eval implantable dfb	0.85	0.34	0.34	0.04	1.23	$42.57	1.23	$42.57	XXX	A+
93282-TC	Prgrmg eval implantable dfb	0.00	1.21	NA	0.01	1.22	$42.22	NA	NA	XXX	A+ DS
93283	Prgrmg eval implantable dfb	1.15	1.78	NA	0.05	2.98	$103.13	NA	NA	XXX	A+
93283-26	Prgrmg eval implantable dfb	1.15	0.46	0.46	0.04	1.65	$57.10	1.65	$57.10	XXX	A+
93283-TC	Prgrmg eval implantable dfb	0.00	1.32	NA	0.01	1.33	$46.03	NA	NA	XXX	A+ DS
93284	Prgrmg eval implantable dfb	1.25	1.91	NA	0.05	3.21	$111.09	NA	NA	XXX	A+
93284-26	Prgrmg eval implantable dfb	1.25	0.50	0.50	0.04	1.79	$61.95	1.79	$61.95	XXX	A+

*Please note that these calculations are based on the Medicare 2022 Conversion Factor of $34.6062 and the DRA RVU cap rates at time of publication.

A = assistant-at-surgery restriction
A+ = assistant-at-surgery restriction unless medical necessity established with documentation
B = bilateral surgery adjustment applies
C = cosurgeons payable
C+ = cosurgeons payable if medical necessity established with documentation
CP = carriers may establish RVUs and payment amounts for these services, generally on an individual basis following review of documentation such as an operative report
M = multiple surgery adjustment applies
Me = multiple endoscopy rules may apply
M+ = multiple therapy rules apply
Mtc = multiple diagnostic imaging rules apply
T = team surgeons permitted
T+ = team surgeons payable if medical necessity established with documentation
§ = indicates code is not covered by Medicare
GS = procedure must be performed under the general supervision of a physician
DS = procedure must be performed under the direct supervision of a physician
PS = procedure must be performed under the personal supervision of a physician
DRA = procedure subject to DRA limitation

Relative Value Units

CPT Code and Modifier	Description	Work RVU	Nonfacility Practice Expense RVU	Facility Practice Expense RVU	PLI RVU	Total Non-facility RVUs	Medicare Payment Nonfacility	Total Facility RVUs	Medicare Payment Facility	Global Period	Payment Policy Indicators
93284-TC	Prgrmg eval implantable dfb	0.00	1.41	NA	0.01	1.42	$49.14	NA	NA	XXX	A+ DS
93285	Prgrmg dev eval scrms ip	0.52	1.30	NA	0.03	1.85	$64.02	NA	NA	XXX	A+
93285-26	Prgrmg dev eval scrms ip	0.52	0.21	0.21	0.02	0.75	$25.95	0.75	$25.95	XXX	A+
93285-TC	Prgrmg dev eval scrms ip	0.00	1.09	NA	0.01	1.10	$38.07	NA	NA	XXX	A+ DS
93286	Peri-px eval pm/ldls pm ip	0.30	1.10	NA	0.02	1.42	$49.14	NA	NA	XXX	A+
93286-26	Peri-px eval pm/ldls pm ip	0.30	0.13	0.13	0.01	0.44	$15.23	0.44	$15.23	XXX	A+
93286-TC	Peri-px eval pm/ldls pm ip	0.00	0.97	NA	0.01	0.98	$33.91	NA	NA	XXX	A+ DS
93287	Peri-px device eval & prgr	0.45	1.16	NA	0.03	1.64	$56.75	NA	NA	XXX	A+
93287-26	Peri-px device eval & prgr	0.45	0.19	0.19	0.02	0.66	$22.84	0.66	$22.84	XXX	A+
93287-TC	Peri-px device eval & prgr	0.00	0.97	NA	0.01	0.98	$33.91	NA	NA	XXX	A+ DS
93288	Interrog evl pm/ldls pm ip	0.43	1.27	NA	0.03	1.73	$59.87	NA	NA	XXX	A+
93288-26	Interrog evl pm/ldls pm ip	0.43	0.16	0.16	0.02	0.61	$21.11	0.61	$21.11	XXX	A+
93288-TC	Interrog evl pm/ldls pm ip	0.00	1.11	NA	0.01	1.12	$38.76	NA	NA	XXX	A+ DS
93289	Interrog device eval heart	0.75	1.41	NA	0.05	2.21	$76.48	NA	NA	XXX	A+
93289-26	Interrog device eval heart	0.75	0.29	0.29	0.04	1.08	$37.37	1.08	$37.37	XXX	A+
93289-TC	Interrog device eval heart	0.00	1.12	NA	0.01	1.13	$39.11	NA	NA	XXX	A+ DS
93290	Interrog dev eval icpms ip	0.43	1.19	NA	0.03	1.65	$57.10	NA	NA	XXX	A+
93290-26	Interrog dev eval icpms ip	0.43	0.17	0.17	0.02	0.62	$21.46	0.62	$21.46	XXX	A+
93290-TC	Interrog dev eval icpms ip	0.00	1.02	NA	0.01	1.03	$35.64	NA	NA	XXX	A+ DS
93291	Interrog dev eval scrms ip	0.37	1.13	NA	0.02	1.52	$52.60	NA	NA	XXX	A+
93291-26	Interrog dev eval scrms ip	0.37	0.15	0.15	0.01	0.53	$18.34	0.53	$18.34	XXX	A+
93291-TC	Interrog dev eval scrms ip	0.00	0.98	NA	0.01	0.99	$34.26	NA	NA	XXX	A+ DS
93292	Wcd device interrogate	0.43	1.08	NA	0.03	1.54	$53.29	NA	NA	XXX	A+
93292-26	Wcd device interrogate	0.43	0.16	0.16	0.02	0.61	$21.11	0.61	$21.11	XXX	A+
93292-TC	Wcd device interrogate	0.00	0.92	NA	0.01	0.93	$32.18	NA	NA	XXX	A+ DS
93293	Pm phone r-strip device eval	0.31	1.08	NA	0.02	1.41	$48.79	NA	NA	XXX	A+
93293-26	Pm phone r-strip device eval	0.31	0.11	0.11	0.01	0.43	$14.88	0.43	$14.88	XXX	A+
93293-TC	Pm phone r-strip device eval	0.00	0.97	NA	0.01	0.98	$33.91	NA	NA	XXX	A+ GS
93294	Rem interrog evl pm/ldls pm	0.60	0.24	0.24	0.04	0.88	$30.45	0.88	$30.45	XXX	A+
93295	Dev interrog remote 1/2/mlt	0.74	0.30	0.30	0.05	1.09	$37.72	1.09	$37.72	XXX	A+
93296	Rem interrog evl pm/ids	0.00	0.68	NA	0.01	0.69	$23.88	NA	NA	XXX	A+ GS
93297	Rem interrog dev eval icpms	0.52	0.21	0.21	0.04	0.77	$26.65	0.77	$26.65	XXX	A+
93298	Rem interrog dev eval scrms	0.52	0.21	0.21	0.04	0.77	$26.65	0.77	$26.65	XXX	A+

93303		Echo transthoracic	1.30	5.32	NA	0.06	6.68	$231.17	NA	NA	XXX	A+
93303-26		Echo transthoracic	1.30	0.47	0.47	0.04	1.81	$62.64	1.81	$62.64	XXX	A+
93303-TC		Echo transthoracic	0.00	4.85	NA	0.02	4.87	$168.53	NA	NA	XXX	A+ GS
93304		Echo transthoracic	0.75	3.90	NA	0.06	4.71	$163.00	NA	NA	XXX	A+
93304-26		Echo transthoracic	0.75	0.27	0.27	0.04	1.06	$36.68	1.06	$36.68	XXX	A+
93304-TC		Echo transthoracic	0.00	3.63	NA	0.02	3.65	$126.31	NA	NA	XXX	A+ GS
93306		Tte w/doppler complete	1.46	4.39	NA	0.07	5.92	$204.87	NA	NA	XXX	A+
93306-26		Tte w/doppler complete	1.46	0.52	0.52	0.05	2.03	$70.25	2.03	$70.25	XXX	A+
93306-TC		Tte w/doppler complete	0.00	3.87	NA	0.02	3.89	$134.62	NA	NA	XXX	A+ GS
93307		Tte w/o doppler complete	0.92	3.17	NA	0.06	4.15	$143.62	NA	NA	XXX	A+
93307-26		Tte w/o doppler complete	0.92	0.33	0.33	0.04	1.29	$44.64	1.29	$44.64	XXX	A+
93307-TC		Tte w/o doppler complete	0.00	2.84	NA	0.02	2.86	$98.97	NA	NA	XXX	A+ GS
93308		Tte f-up or lmtd	0.53	2.38	NA	0.03	2.94	$101.74	NA	NA	XXX	A+
93308-26		Tte f-up or lmtd	0.53	0.18	0.18	0.02	0.73	$25.26	0.73	$25.26	XXX	A+
93308-TC		Tte f-up or lmtd	0.00	2.20	NA	0.01	2.21	$76.48	NA	NA	XXX	A+ GS
93312		Echo transesophageal	2.30	4.73	NA	0.11	7.14	$247.09	NA	NA	XXX	A+
93312-26		Echo transesophageal	2.30	0.75	0.75	0.09	3.14	$108.66	3.14	$108.66	XXX	A+
93312-TC		Echo transesophageal	0.00	3.98	NA	0.02	4.00	$138.42	NA	NA	XXX	A+ PS
93313		Echo transesophageal	0.26	NA	0.05	0.02	NA	NA	0.33	$11.42	XXX	A+ PS
93314		Echo transesophageal	1.85	4.81	NA	0.20	6.86	$237.40	NA	NA	XXX	A+
93314-26		Echo transesophageal	1.85	0.60	0.60	0.18	2.63	$91.01	2.63	$91.01	XXX	A+
93314-TC		Echo transesophageal	0.00	4.21	NA	0.02	4.23	$146.38	NA	NA	XXX	A+ PS
93315	CP	Echo transesophageal	0.00	0.00	NA	0.00	0.00	$0.00	NA	NA	XXX	A+
93315-26		Echo transesophageal	2.69	0.91	0.91	0.09	3.69	$127.70	3.69	$127.70	XXX	A+
93315-TC	CP	Echo transesophageal	0.00	0.00	NA	0.00	0.00	$0.00	NA	NA	XXX	A+ PS
93316		Echo transesophageal	0.60	NA	0.11	0.05	NA	NA	0.76	$26.30	XXX	A+ PS
93317	CP	Echo transesophageal	0.00	0.00	NA	0.00	0.00	$0.00	NA	NA	XXX	A+
93317-26		Echo transesophageal	1.84	0.66	0.66	0.10	2.60	$89.98	2.60	$89.98	XXX	A+

*Please note that these calculations are based on the Medicare 2022 Conversion Factor of $34.6062 and the DRA RVU cap rates at time of publication.

A = assistant-at-surgery restriction
A+ = assistant-at-surgery restriction unless medical necessity established with documentation
B = bilateral surgery adjustment applies
C = cosurgeons payable

C+ = cosurgeons payable if medical necessity established with documentation
CP = carriers may establish RVUs and payment amounts for these services, generally on an individual basis following review of documentation such as an operative report
M = multiple surgery adjustment applies
Me = multiple endoscopy rules may apply

M+ = multiple therapy rules apply
Mtc = multiple diagnostic imaging rules apply
T = team surgeons permitted
T+ = team surgeons payable if medical necessity established with documentation
§ = indicates code is not covered by Medicare

GS = procedure must be performed under the general supervision of a physician
DS = procedure must be performed under the direct supervision of a physician
PS = procedure must be performed under the personal supervision of a physician
DRA = procedure subject to DRA limitation

Relative Value Units

CPT Code and Modifier		Description	Work RVU	Nonfacility Practice Expense RVU	Facility Practice Expense RVU	PLI RVU	Total Non-facility RVUs	Medicare Payment Nonfacility	Total Facility RVUs	Medicare Payment Facility	Global Period	Payment Policy Indicators
93317-TC	CP	Echo transesophageal	0.00	0.00	NA	0.00	0.00	$0.00	NA	NA	XXX	A+ PS
93318	CP	Echo transesophageal intraop	0.00	0.00	NA	0.00	0.00	$0.00	NA	NA	XXX	A+
93318-26		Echo transesophageal intraop	2.15	0.73	0.73	0.12	3.00	$103.82	3.00	$103.82	XXX	A+
93318-TC	CP	Echo transesophageal intraop	0.00	0.00	NA	0.00	0.00	$0.00	NA	NA	XXX	A+ GS
93319		3d echo img cgen car anomal	0.50	1.24	0.18	0.05	1.79	$61.95	0.73	$25.26	ZZZ	A+
93320		Doppler echo exam heart	0.38	1.13	NA	0.02	1.53	$52.95	NA	NA	ZZZ	A+
93320-26		Doppler echo exam heart	0.38	0.13	0.13	0.01	0.52	$18.00	0.52	$18.00	ZZZ	A+
93320-TC		Doppler echo exam heart	0.00	1.00	NA	0.01	1.01	$34.95	NA	NA	ZZZ	A+ GS
93321		Doppler echo exam heart	0.15	0.60	NA	0.01	0.76	$26.30	NA	NA	ZZZ	A+
93321-26		Doppler echo exam heart	0.15	0.05	0.05	0.01	0.21	$7.27	0.21	$7.27	ZZZ	A+
93321-TC		Doppler echo exam heart	0.00	0.55	NA	0.00	0.55	$19.03	NA	NA	ZZZ	A+ GS
93325		Doppler color flow add-on	0.07	0.64	NA	0.00	0.71	$24.57	NA	NA	ZZZ	A+
93325-26		Doppler color flow add-on	0.07	0.02	0.02	0.00	0.09	$3.11	0.09	$3.11	ZZZ	A+
93325-TC		Doppler color flow add-on	0.00	0.62	NA	0.00	0.62	$21.46	NA	NA	ZZZ	A+ GS
93350		Stress tte only	1.46	4.09	NA	0.07	5.62	$194.49	NA	NA	XXX	A+
93350-26		Stress tte only	1.46	0.52	0.52	0.05	2.03	$70.25	2.03	$70.25	XXX	A+
93350-TC		Stress tte only	0.00	3.57	NA	0.02	3.59	$124.24	NA	NA	XXX	A+ DS
93351		Stress tte complete	1.75	5.12	NA	0.11	6.98	$241.55	NA	NA	XXX	
93351-26		Stress tte complete	1.75	0.62	0.62	0.07	2.44	$84.44	2.44	$84.44	XXX	
93351-TC		Stress tte complete	0.00	4.50	NA	0.04	4.54	$157.11	NA	NA	XXX	DS
93352		Admin ecg contrast agent	0.19	0.78	NA	0.02	0.99	$34.26	NA	NA	ZZZ	A+
93355		Echo transesophageal (tee)	4.66	NA	1.63	0.33	NA	NA	6.62	$229.09	XXX	A+
93356		Myocrd strain img spckl trck	0.24	0.87	0.09	0.02	1.13	$39.11	0.35	$12.11	ZZZ	A+
93451		Right heart cath	2.47	24.06	NA	0.47	27.00	$934.37	NA	NA	000	A+ M
93451-26		Right heart cath	2.47	0.92	0.92	0.43	3.82	$132.20	3.82	$132.20	000	A+ M
93451-TC		Right heart cath	0.00	23.14	NA	0.04	23.18	$802.17	NA	NA	000	A+ PS
93452		Left hrt cath w/ventrclgrphy	4.50	22.56	NA	0.90	27.96	$967.59	NA	NA	000	A+ M
93452-26		Left hrt cath w/ventrclgrphy	4.50	1.57	1.57	0.86	6.93	$239.82	6.93	$239.82	000	A+ M
93452-TC		Left hrt cath w/ventrclgrphy	0.00	20.99	NA	0.04	21.03	$727.77	NA	NA	000	A+ PS
93453		R&l hrt cath w/ventriclgrphy	5.99	28.28	NA	1.17	35.44	$1226.44	NA	NA	000	A+ M
93453-26		R&l hrt cath w/ventriclgrphy	5.99	2.11	2.11	1.12	9.22	$319.07	9.22	$319.07	000	A+ M
93453-TC		R&l hrt cath w/ventriclgrphy	0.00	26.17	NA	0.05	26.22	$907.37	NA	NA	000	A+ PS
93454		Coronary artery angio s&i	4.54	22.55	NA	0.93	28.02	$969.67	NA	NA	000	A+ M

93454-26	Coronary artery angio s&i	4.54	1.58	1.58	0.89	7.01	$242.59	7.01	$242.59	000	A+ M
93454-TC	Coronary artery angio s&i	0.00	20.97	NA	0.04	21.01	$727.08	NA	NA	000	A+ PS
93455	Coronary art/grft angio s&i	5.29	24.81	NA	1.05	31.15	$1077.98	NA	NA	000	A+ M
93455-26	Coronary art/grft angio s&i	5.29	1.84	1.84	1.01	8.14	$281.69	8.14	$281.69	000	A+ M
93455-TC	Coronary art/grft angio s&i	0.00	22.97	NA	0.04	23.01	$796.29	NA	NA	000	A+ PS
93456	R hrt coronary artery angio	5.90	27.76	NA	1.15	34.81	$1204.64	NA	NA	000	A+ M
93456-26	R hrt coronary artery angio	5.90	2.07	2.07	1.11	9.08	$314.22	9.08	$314.22	000	A+ M
93456-TC	R hrt coronary artery angio	0.00	25.69	NA	0.04	25.73	$890.42	NA	NA	000	A+ PS
93457	R hrt art/grft angio	6.64	30.00	NA	1.33	37.97	$1314.00	NA	NA	000	A+ M
93457-26	R hrt art/grft angio	6.64	2.32	2.32	1.28	10.24	$354.37	10.24	$354.37	000	A+ M
93457-TC	R hrt art/grft angio	0.00	27.68	NA	0.05	27.73	$959.63	NA	NA	000	A+ PS
93458	L hrt artery/ventricle angio	5.60	25.40	NA	1.12	32.12	$1111.55	NA	NA	000	A+ M
93458-26	L hrt artery/ventricle angio	5.60	1.95	1.95	1.07	8.62	$298.31	8.62	$298.31	000	A+ M
93458-TC	L hrt artery/ventricle angio	0.00	23.45	NA	0.05	23.50	$813.25	NA	NA	000	A+ PS
93459	L hrt art/grft angio	6.35	26.92	NA	1.27	34.54	$1195.30	NA	NA	000	A+ M
93459-26	L hrt art/grft angio	6.35	2.21	2.21	1.22	9.78	$338.45	9.78	$338.45	000	A+ M
93459-TC	L hrt art/grft angio	0.00	24.71	NA	0.05	24.76	$856.85	NA	NA	000	A+ PS
93460	R&l hrt art/ventricle angio	7.10	29.86	NA	1.42	38.38	$1328.19	NA	NA	000	A+ M
93460-26	R&l hrt art/ventricle angio	7.10	2.48	2.48	1.37	10.95	$378.94	10.95	$378.94	000	A+ M
93460-TC	R&l hrt art/ventricle angio	0.00	27.38	NA	0.05	27.43	$949.25	NA	NA	000	A+ PS
93461	R&l hrt art/ventricle angio	7.85	32.88	NA	1.58	42.31	$1464.19	NA	NA	000	A+ M
93461-26	R&l hrt art/ventricle angio	7.85	2.74	2.74	1.51	12.10	$418.74	12.10	$418.74	000	A+ M
93461-TC	R&l hrt art/ventricle angio	0.00	30.14	NA	0.07	30.21	$1045.45	NA	NA	000	A+ PS
93462	L hrt cath trnsptl puncture	3.73	1.57	1.57	0.87	6.17	$213.52	6.17	$213.52	ZZZ	A+
93463	Drug admin & hemodynmic meas	2.00	0.71	0.71	0.17	2.88	$99.67	2.88	$99.67	ZZZ	A+
93464	Exercise w/hemodynamic meas	1.80	4.75	NA	0.12	6.67	$230.82	NA	NA	ZZZ	A+
93464-26	Exercise w/hemodynamic meas	1.80	0.68	0.68	0.11	2.59	$89.63	2.59	$89.63	ZZZ	A+
93464-TC	Exercise w/hemodynamic meas	0.00	4.07	NA	0.01	4.08	$141.19	NA	NA	ZZZ	A+ PS

*Please note that these calculations are based on the Medicare 2022 Conversion Factor of $34.6062 and the DRA RVU cap rates at time of publication.

A = assistant-at-surgery restriction
A+ = assistant-at-surgery restriction unless medical necessity established with documentation
B = bilateral surgery adjustment applies
C = cosurgeons payable
C+ = cosurgeons payable if medical necessity established with documentation
CP = carriers may establish RVUs and payment amounts for these services, generally on an individual basis following review of documentation such as an operative report
M = multiple surgery adjustment applies
Me = multiple endoscopy rules may apply
M+ = multiple therapy rules apply
Mtc = multiple diagnostic imaging rules apply
T = team surgeons permitted
T+ = team surgeons payable if medical necessity established with documentation
§ = indicates code is not covered by Medicare
GS = procedure must be performed under the general supervision of a physician
DS = procedure must be performed under the direct supervision of a physician
PS = procedure must be performed under the personal supervision of a physician
DRA = procedure subject to DRA limitation

Relative Value Units

CPT Code and Modifier		Description	Work RVU	Nonfacility Practice Expense RVU	Facility Practice Expense RVU	PLI RVU	Total Non-facility RVUs	Medicare Payment Nonfacility	Total Facility RVUs	Medicare Payment Facility	Global Period	Payment Policy Indicators
93503		Insert/place heart catheter	2.00	NA	0.39	0.19	NA	NA	2.58	$89.28	000	A+
93505		Biopsy of heart lining	4.12	15.00	NA	0.79	19.91	$689.01	NA	NA	000	A+ M
93505-26		Biopsy of heart lining	4.12	1.75	1.75	0.77	6.64	$229.79	6.64	$229.79	000	A+ M
93505-TC		Biopsy of heart lining	0.00	13.25	NA	0.02	13.27	$459.22	NA	NA	000	A+ PS
93563		Inject congenital card cath	1.11	0.40	0.40	0.19	1.70	$58.83	1.70	$58.83	ZZZ	A+
93564		Inject hrt congntl art/grft	1.13	0.39	0.39	0.25	1.77	$61.25	1.77	$61.25	ZZZ	A+
93565		Inject l ventr/atrial angio	0.86	0.30	0.30	0.20	1.36	$47.06	1.36	$47.06	ZZZ	A+
93566		Inject r ventr/atrial angio	0.86	2.85	0.31	0.18	3.89	$134.62	1.35	$46.72	ZZZ	A+
93567		Inject suprvlv aortography	0.97	2.10	0.34	0.22	3.29	$113.85	1.53	$52.95	ZZZ	A+
93568		Inject pulm art hrt cath	0.88	2.60	0.32	0.20	3.68	$127.35	1.40	$48.45	ZZZ	A+
93571	CP	Heart flow reserve measure	0.00	NA	NA	0.00	NA	NA	NA	NA	ZZZ	A+
93571-26		Heart flow reserve measure	1.38	0.48	0.48	0.25	2.11	$73.02	2.11	$73.02	ZZZ	A+
93571-TC	CP	Heart flow reserve measure	0.00	NA	NA	0.00	NA	NA	NA	NA	ZZZ	A+ PS
93572	CP	Heart flow reserve measure	0.00	NA	NA	0.00	NA	NA	NA	NA	ZZZ	A+
93572-26		Heart flow reserve measure	1.00	0.35	0.35	0.20	1.55	$53.64	1.55	$53.64	ZZZ	A+
93572-TC	CP	Heart flow reserve measure	0.00	NA	NA	0.00	NA	NA	NA	NA	ZZZ	A+ PS
93580		Transcath closure of asd	17.97	NA	6.60	3.97	NA	NA	28.54	$987.66	000	A+ M
93581		Transcath closure of vsd	24.39	NA	8.76	5.72	NA	NA	38.87	$1345.14	000	A+ M
93582		Perq transcath closure pda	12.31	NA	4.25	2.89	NA	NA	19.45	$673.09	000	A+ M
93583		Perq transcath septal reduxn	13.75	NA	4.81	3.16	NA	NA	21.72	$751.65	000	A+ M
93590		Perq transcath cls mitral	21.70	NA	7.91	1.72	NA	NA	31.33	$1084.21	000	C+ M
93591		Perq transcath cls aortic	17.97	NA	6.50	1.41	NA	NA	25.88	$895.61	000	A+ C M T+
93592		Perq transcath closure each	8.00	NA	2.77	0.65	NA	NA	11.42	$395.20	ZZZ	C+
93593	CP	R hrt cath chd nml nt cnj	0.00	0.00	NA	0.00	0.00	$0.00	NA	NA	000	A+ M
93593-26		R hrt cath chd nml nt cnj	3.99	1.42	1.42	0.12	5.53	$191.37	5.53	$191.37	000	A+ M
93593-TC	CP	R hrt cath chd nml nt cnj	0.00	0.00	0.00	0.00	0.00	$0.00	0.00	$0.00	000	A+ PS
93594	CP	R hrt cath chd abnl nt cnj	0.00	0.00	NA	0.00	0.00	$0.00	NA	NA	000	A+ M
93594-26		R hrt cath chd abnl nt cnj	6.10	2.35	2.35	0.27	8.72	$301.77	8.72	$301.77	000	A+ M
93594-TC	CP	R hrt cath chd abnl nt cnj	0.00	0.00	0.00	0.00	0.00	$0.00	0.00	$0.00	000	A+ PS
93595	CP	L hrt cath chd nm/abn nt cnj	0.00	0.00	NA	0.00	0.00	$0.00	NA	NA	000	A+ M
93595-26		L hrt cath chd nm/abn nt cnj	5.50	2.12	2.12	0.25	7.87	$272.35	7.87	$272.35	000	A+ M
93595-TC	CP	L hrt cath chd nm/abn nt cnj	0.00	0.00	0.00	0.00	0.00	$0.00	0.00	$0.00	000	A+ PS
93596	CP	R&l hrt cath chd nml nt cnj	0.00	0.00	NA	0.00	0.00	$0.00	NA	NA	000	A+ M

93596-26		R&l hrt cath chd nml nt cnj	6.84	2.45	2.45	0.22	9.51	$329.10	9.51	$329.10	000	A+ M
93596-TC	CP	R&l hrt cath chd nml nt cnj	0.00	0.00	0.00	0.00	0.00	$0.00	0.00	$0.00	000	A+ PS
93597	CP	R&l hrt cath chd abnl nt cnj	0.00	0.00	NA	0.00	0.00	$0.00	NA	NA	000	A+ M
93597-26		R&l hrt cath chd abnl nt cnj	8.88	3.42	3.42	0.40	12.70	$439.50	12.70	$439.50	000	A+ M
93597-TC	CP	R&l hrt cath chd abnl nt cnj	0.00	0.00	0.00	0.00	0.00	$0.00	0.00	$0.00	000	A+ PS
93598	CP	Car outp meas drg cath chd	0.00	0.00	NA	0.00	0.00	$0.00	NA	NA	ZZZ	A+
93598-26		Car outp meas drg cath chd	1.44	0.56	0.56	0.08	2.08	$71.98	2.08	$71.98	ZZZ	A+
93598-TC	CP	Car outp meas drg cath chd	0.00	0.00	0.00	0.00	0.00	$0.00	0.00	$0.00	ZZZ	A+ PS
93600	CP	Bundle of his recording	0.00	0.00	NA	0.00	0.00	$0.00	NA	NA	000	A+
93600-26		Bundle of his recording	2.12	0.93	0.93	0.40	3.45	$119.39	3.45	$119.39	000	A+
93600-TC	CP	Bundle of his recording	0.00	0.00	NA	0.00	0.00	$0.00	NA	NA	000	A+ PS
93602	CP	Intra-atrial recording	0.00	0.00	NA	0.00	0.00	$0.00	NA	NA	000	A+
93602-26		Intra-atrial recording	2.12	0.88	0.88	0.40	3.40	$117.66	3.40	$117.66	000	A+
93602-TC	CP	Intra-atrial recording	0.00	0.00	NA	0.00	0.00	$0.00	NA	NA	000	A+ PS
93603	CP	Right ventricular recording	0.00	0.00	NA	0.00	0.00	$0.00	NA	NA	000	A+
93603-26		Right ventricular recording	2.12	0.88	0.88	0.40	3.40	$117.66	3.40	$117.66	000	A+
93603-TC	CP	Right ventricular recording	0.00	0.00	NA	0.00	0.00	$0.00	NA	NA	000	A+ PS
93609	CP	Map tachycardia add-on	0.00	0.00	NA	0.00	0.00	$0.00	NA	NA	ZZZ	A+
93609-26		Map tachycardia add-on	4.99	2.15	2.15	0.96	8.10	$280.31	8.10	$280.31	ZZZ	A+
93609-TC	CP	Map tachycardia add-on	0.00	0.00	NA	0.00	0.00	$0.00	NA	NA	ZZZ	A+ PS
93610	CP	Intra-atrial pacing	0.00	0.00	NA	0.00	0.00	$0.00	NA	NA	000	A+
93610-26		Intra-atrial pacing	3.02	1.21	1.21	0.57	4.80	$166.11	4.80	$166.11	000	A+
93610-TC	CP	Intra-atrial pacing	0.00	0.00	NA	0.00	0.00	$0.00	NA	NA	000	A+ PS
93612	CP	Intraventricular pacing	0.00	0.00	NA	0.00	0.00	$0.00	NA	NA	000	A+
93612-26		Intraventricular pacing	3.02	1.18	1.18	0.56	4.76	$164.73	4.76	$164.73	000	A+
93612-TC	CP	Intraventricular pacing	0.00	0.00	NA	0.00	0.00	$0.00	NA	NA	000	A+ PS
93613		Electrophys map 3d add-on	5.23	NA	2.25	1.20	NA	NA	8.68	$300.38	ZZZ	A+
93615	CP	Esophageal recording	0.00	0.00	NA	0.00	0.00	$0.00	NA	NA	000	A+

*Please note that these calculations are based on the Medicare 2022 Conversion Factor of $34.6062 and the DRA RVU cap rates at time of publication.

A = assistant-at-surgery restriction
A+ = assistant-at-surgery restriction unless medical necessity established with documentation
B = bilateral surgery adjustment applies
C = cosurgeons payable
C+ = cosurgeons payable if medical necessity established with documentation
CP = carriers may establish RVUs and payment amounts for these services, generally on an individual basis following review of documentation such as an operative report
M = multiple surgery adjustment applies
Me = multiple endoscopy rules may apply
M+ = multiple therapy rules apply
Mtc = multiple diagnostic imaging rules apply
T = team surgeons permitted
T+ = team surgeons payable if medical necessity established with documentation
§ = indicates code is not covered by Medicare
GS = procedure must be performed under the general supervision of a physician
DS = procedure must be performed under the direct supervision of a physician
PS = procedure must be performed under the personal supervision of a physician
DRA = procedure subject to DRA limitation

Relative Value Units

CPT Code and Modifier		Description	Work RVU	Nonfacility Practice Expense RVU	Facility Practice Expense RVU	PLI RVU	Total Non-facility RVUs	Medicare Payment Nonfacility	Total Facility RVUs	Medicare Payment Facility	Global Period	Payment Policy Indicators
93615-26		Esophageal recording	0.74	0.33	0.33	0.02	1.09	$37.72	1.09	$37.72	000	A+
93615-TC	CP	Esophageal recording	0.00	0.00	NA	0.00	0.00	$0.00	NA	NA	000	A+ PS
93616	CP	Esophageal recording	0.00	0.00	NA	0.00	0.00	$0.00	NA	NA	000	A+
93616-26		Esophageal recording	1.24	0.43	0.43	0.04	1.71	$59.18	1.71	$59.18	000	A+
93616-TC	CP	Esophageal recording	0.00	0.00	NA	0.00	0.00	$0.00	NA	NA	000	A+ PS
93618	CP	Heart rhythm pacing	0.00	0.00	NA	0.00	0.00	$0.00	NA	NA	000	A+
93618-26		Heart rhythm pacing	4.00	1.65	1.65	0.76	6.41	$221.83	6.41	$221.83	000	A+
93618-TC	CP	Heart rhythm pacing	0.00	0.00	NA	0.00	0.00	$0.00	NA	NA	000	A+ PS
93619	CP	Electrophysiology evaluation	0.00	0.00	NA	0.00	0.00	$0.00	NA	NA	000	A+ M
93619-26		Electrophysiology evaluation	7.06	2.99	2.99	1.34	11.39	$394.16	11.39	$394.16	000	A+ M
93619-TC	CP	Electrophysiology evaluation	0.00	0.00	NA	0.00	0.00	$0.00	NA	NA	000	A+ PS
93620	CP	Electrophysiology evaluation	0.00	0.00	NA	0.00	0.00	$0.00	NA	NA	000	A+ M
93620-26		Electrophysiology evaluation	11.32	4.81	4.81	2.18	18.31	$633.64	18.31	$633.64	000	A+ M
93620-TC	CP	Electrophysiology evaluation	0.00	0.00	NA	0.00	0.00	$0.00	NA	NA	000	A+ PS
93621	CP	Electrophysiology evaluation	0.00	0.00	NA	0.00	0.00	$0.00	NA	NA	ZZZ	A+
93621-26		Electrophysiology evaluation	1.50	0.99	0.99	0.28	2.77	$95.86	2.77	$95.86	ZZZ	A+
93621-TC	CP	Electrophysiology evaluation	0.00	0.00	NA	0.00	0.00	$0.00	NA	NA	ZZZ	A+ PS
93622	CP	Electrophysiology evaluation	0.00	0.00	NA	0.00	0.00	$0.00	NA	NA	ZZZ	A+
93622-26		Electrophysiology evaluation	3.10	1.32	1.32	0.60	5.02	$173.72	5.02	$173.72	ZZZ	A+
93622-TC	CP	Electrophysiology evaluation	0.00	0.00	NA	0.00	0.00	$0.00	NA	NA	ZZZ	A+ PS
93623	CP	Stimulation pacing heart	0.00	0.00	NA	0.00	0.00	$0.00	NA	NA	ZZZ	A+
93623-26		Stimulation pacing heart	0.98	1.83	1.83	0.20	3.01	$104.16	3.01	$104.16	ZZZ	A+
93623-TC	CP	Stimulation pacing heart	0.00	0.00	NA	0.00	0.00	$0.00	NA	NA	ZZZ	A+ PS
93624	CP	Electrophysiologic study	0.00	0.00	NA	0.00	0.00	$0.00	NA	NA	000	A+ M
93624-26		Electrophysiologic study	4.55	1.57	1.57	0.90	7.02	$242.94	7.02	$242.94	000	A+ M
93624-TC	CP	Electrophysiologic study	0.00	0.00	NA	0.00	0.00	$0.00	NA	NA	000	A+ PS
93631	CP	Heart pacing mapping	0.00	0.00	NA	0.00	0.00	$0.00	NA	NA	000	A+
93631-26		Heart pacing mapping	7.59	2.50	2.50	1.49	11.58	$400.74	11.58	$400.74	000	A+
93631-TC	CP	Heart pacing mapping	0.00	0.00	NA	0.00	0.00	$0.00	NA	NA	000	A+ PS
93640	CP	Evaluation heart device	0.00	0.00	NA	0.00	0.00	$0.00	NA	NA	000	A+ M
93640-26		Evaluation heart device	3.26	1.34	1.34	0.62	5.22	$180.64	5.22	$180.64	000	A+ M
93640-TC	CP	Evaluation heart device	0.00	0.00	NA	0.00	0.00	$0.00	NA	NA	000	A+ PS
93641	CP	Electrophysiology evaluation	0.00	0.00	NA	0.00	0.00	$0.00	NA	NA	000	A+ M

93641-26		Electrophysiology evaluation	5.67	2.34	2.34	1.09	9.10	$314.92	9.10	$314.92	000	A+ M
93641-TC	CP	Electrophysiology evaluation	0.00	0.00	NA	0.00	0.00	$0.00	NA	NA	000	A+ PS
93642		Electrophysiology evaluation	4.63	4.32	NA	0.92	9.87	$341.56	NA	NA	000	A+ M
93642-26		Electrophysiology evaluation	4.63	1.91	1.91	0.90	7.44	$257.47	7.44	$257.47	000	A+ M
93642-TC		Electrophysiology evaluation	0.00	2.41	NA	0.02	2.43	$84.09	NA	NA	000	A+ PS
93644		Electrophysiology evaluation	3.04	2.57	NA	0.11	5.72	$197.95	NA	NA	000	A+ M
93644-26		Electrophysiology evaluation	3.04	1.05	1.05	0.10	4.19	$145.00	4.19	$145.00	000	A+ M
93644-TC		Electrophysiology evaluation	0.00	1.52	NA	0.01	1.53	$52.95	NA	NA	000	A+ PS
93650		Ablate heart dysrhythm focus	10.24	NA	4.72	2.36	NA	NA	17.32	$599.38	000	A+ M
93653		Compre ep eval tx svt	14.75	NA	6.33	3.41	NA	NA	24.49	$847.51	000	A+ M
93654		Compre ep eval tx vt	19.75	NA	8.44	4.57	NA	NA	32.76	$1133.70	000	A+ M
93655		Ablate arrhythmia add on	5.50	NA	2.37	1.28	NA	NA	9.15	$316.65	ZZZ	A+
93656		Compre ep eval abltj atr fib	19.77	NA	8.51	4.58	NA	NA	32.86	$1137.16	000	A+ M
93657		Tx l/r atrial fib addl	5.50	NA	2.36	1.28	NA	NA	9.14	$316.30	ZZZ	A+
93660		Tilt table evaluation	1.89	2.69	NA	0.11	4.69	$162.30	NA	NA	000	A+ M
93660-26		Tilt table evaluation	1.89	0.73	0.73	0.07	2.69	$93.09	2.69	$93.09	000	A+ M
93660-TC		Tilt table evaluation	0.00	1.96	NA	0.04	2.00	$69.21	NA	NA	000	A+ DS
93662	CP	Intracardiac ecg (ice)	0.00	0.00	NA	0.00	0.00	$0.00	NA	NA	ZZZ	A+
93662-26		Intracardiac ecg (ice)	1.44	1.18	1.18	0.05	2.67	$92.40	2.67	$92.40	ZZZ	A+
93662-TC	CP	Intracardiac ecg (ice)	0.00	0.00	NA	0.00	0.00	$0.00	NA	NA	ZZZ	A+ PS
93668		Peripheral vascular rehab	0.00	0.40	NA	0.01	0.41	$14.19	NA	NA	XXX	A+
93701		Bioimpedance cv analysis	0.00	0.80	NA	0.01	0.81	$28.03	NA	NA	XXX	A+
93702		Bis xtracell fluid analysis	0.00	4.15	NA	0.02	4.17	$144.31	NA	NA	XXX	A+
93724		Analyze pacemaker system	4.88	3.32	NA	0.19	8.39	$290.35	NA	NA	000	A+
93724-26		Analyze pacemaker system	4.88	1.95	1.95	0.18	7.01	$242.59	7.01	$242.59	000	A+
93724-TC		Analyze pacemaker system	0.00	1.37	NA	0.01	1.38	$47.76	NA	NA	000	A+ PS
93740	§	Temperature gradient studies	0.16	0.06	0.06	0.01	0.23	$7.96	0.23	$7.96	XXX	
93745	CP	Set-up cardiovert-defibrill	0.00	0.00	NA	0.00	0.00	$0.00	NA	NA	XXX	A+

*Please note that these calculations are based on the Medicare 2022 Conversion Factor of $34.6062 and the DRA RVU cap rates at time of publication.

A = assistant-at-surgery restriction
A+ = assistant-at-surgery restriction unless medical necessity established with documentation
B = bilateral surgery adjustment applies
C = cosurgeons payable
C+ = cosurgeons payable if medical necessity established with documentation
CP = carriers may establish RVUs and payment amounts for these services, generally on an individual basis following review of documentation such as an operative report
M = multiple surgery adjustment applies
Me = multiple endoscopy rules may apply
M+ = multiple therapy rules apply
Mtc = multiple diagnostic imaging rules apply
T = team surgeons permitted
T+ = team surgeons payable if medical necessity established with documentation
§ = indicates code is not covered by Medicare
GS = procedure must be performed under the general supervision of a physician
DS = procedure must be performed under the direct supervision of a physician
PS = procedure must be performed under the personal supervision of a physician
DRA = procedure subject to DRA limitation

Relative Value Units

CPT Code and Modifier		Description	Work RVU	Nonfacility Practice Expense RVU	Facility Practice Expense RVU	PLI RVU	Total Non-facility RVUs	Medicare Payment Nonfacility	Total Facility RVUs	Medicare Payment Facility	Global Period	Payment Policy Indicators
93745-26	CP	Set-up cardiovert-defibrill	0.00	0.00	0.00	0.00	0.00	$0.00	0.00	$0.00	XXX	A+
93745-TC	CP	Set-up cardiovert-defibrill	0.00	0.00	NA	0.00	0.00	$0.00	NA	NA	XXX	A+ DS
93750		Interrogation vad in person	0.75	0.62	0.31	0.11	1.48	$51.22	1.17	$40.49	XXX	A+
93770	§	Measure venous pressure	0.16	0.06	0.06	0.01	0.23	$7.96	0.23	$7.96	XXX	
93784		Ambl bp mntr w/software	0.38	0.94	NA	0.03	1.35	$46.72	NA	NA	XXX	A+ GS
93786		Ambl bp mntr w/sw rec only	0.00	0.66	NA	0.01	0.67	$23.19	NA	NA	XXX	A+ GS
93788		Ambl bp mntr w/sw a/r	0.00	0.14	NA	0.01	0.15	$5.19	NA	NA	XXX	A+
93790		Ambl bp mntr w/sw i&r	0.38	0.14	0.14	0.01	0.53	$18.34	0.53	$18.34	XXX	A+
93792		Pt/caregiver traing home inr	0.00	1.84	NA	0.04	1.88	$65.06	NA	NA	XXX	A+ GS
93793		Anticoag mgmt pt warfarin	0.18	0.14	NA	0.01	0.33	$11.42	NA	NA	XXX	A+
93797		Cardiac rehab	0.18	0.29	0.07	0.02	0.49	$16.96	0.27	$9.34	000	A+
93798		Cardiac rehab/monitor	0.28	0.46	0.10	0.02	0.76	$26.30	0.40	$13.84	000	A+
93799	CP	Cardiovascular procedure	0.00	0.00	NA	0.00	0.00	$0.00	NA	NA	XXX	A+
93799-26	CP	Cardiovascular procedure	0.00	0.00	0.00	0.00	0.00	$0.00	0.00	$0.00	XXX	A+
93799-TC	CP	Cardiovascular procedure	0.00	0.00	NA	0.00	0.00	$0.00	NA	NA	XXX	A+
93880		Extracranial bilat study	0.80	4.86	NA	0.10	5.76	$199.33	NA	NA	XXX	A+
93880-26		Extracranial bilat study	0.80	0.26	0.26	0.08	1.14	$39.45	1.14	$39.45	XXX	A+
93880-TC		Extracranial bilat study	0.00	4.60	NA	0.02	4.62	$159.88	NA	NA	XXX	A+ GS
93882		Extracranial uni/ltd study	0.50	3.17	NA	0.10	3.77	$130.47	NA	NA	XXX	A+
93882-26		Extracranial uni/ltd study	0.50	0.14	0.14	0.08	0.72	$24.92	0.72	$24.92	XXX	A+
93882-TC		Extracranial uni/ltd study	0.00	3.03	NA	0.02	3.05	$105.55	NA	NA	XXX	A+ GS
93886		Intracranial complete study	0.91	7.09	NA	0.09	8.09	$279.96	NA	NA	XXX	A+
93886-26		Intracranial complete study	0.91	0.39	0.39	0.05	1.35	$46.72	1.35	$46.72	XXX	A+
93886-TC		Intracranial complete study	0.00	6.70	NA	0.04	6.74	$233.25	NA	NA	XXX	A+ GS
93888		Intracranial limited study	0.50	4.26	NA	0.06	4.82	$137.04	NA	NA	XXX	A+ DRA
93888-26		Intracranial limited study	0.50	0.20	0.20	0.04	0.74	$25.61	0.74	$25.61	XXX	A+
93888-TC		Intracranial limited study	0.00	4.06	NA	0.02	4.08	$111.43	NA	NA	XXX	A+ GS DRA
93890		Tcd vasoreactivity study	1.00	7.17	NA	0.08	8.25	$285.50	NA	NA	XXX	A+
93890-26		Tcd vasoreactivity study	1.00	0.43	0.43	0.04	1.47	$50.87	1.47	$50.87	XXX	A+
93890-TC		Tcd vasoreactivity study	0.00	6.74	NA	0.04	6.78	$234.63	NA	NA	XXX	A+ GS
93892		Tcd emboli detect w/o inj	1.15	8.17	NA	0.11	9.43	$171.30	NA	NA	XXX	A+ DRA
93892-26		Tcd emboli detect w/o inj	1.15	0.51	0.51	0.07	1.73	$59.87	1.73	$59.87	XXX	A+
93892-TC		Tcd emboli detect w/o inj	0.00	7.66	NA	0.04	7.70	$111.43	NA	NA	XXX	A+ GS DRA

93893	Tcd emboli detect w/inj	1.15	10.43	NA	0.12	11.70	$171.99	NA	NA	XXX	A+ DRA
93893-26	Tcd emboli detect w/inj	1.15	0.53	0.53	0.08	1.76	$60.91	1.76	$60.91	XXX	A+
93893-TC	Tcd emboli detect w/inj	0.00	9.90	NA	0.04	9.94	$111.09	NA	NA	XXX	A+ GS DRA
93922	Upr/l xtremity art 2 levels	0.25	2.15	NA	0.05	2.45	$84.79	NA	NA	XXX	A+
93922-26	Upr/l xtremity art 2 levels	0.25	0.07	0.07	0.04	0.36	$12.46	0.36	$12.46	XXX	A+
93922-TC	Upr/l xtremity art 2 levels	0.00	2.08	NA	0.01	2.09	$72.33	NA	NA	XXX	A+ GS
93923	Upr/lxtr art stdy 3+ lvls	0.45	3.30	NA	0.09	3.84	$132.89	NA	NA	XXX	A+
93923-26	Upr/lxtr art stdy 3+ lvls	0.45	0.13	0.13	0.07	0.65	$22.49	0.65	$22.49	XXX	A+
93923-TC	Upr/lxtr art stdy 3+ lvls	0.00	3.17	NA	0.02	3.19	$110.39	NA	NA	XXX	A+ GS
93924	Lwr xtr vasc stdy bilat	0.50	4.13	NA	0.11	4.74	$164.03	NA	NA	XXX	A+
93924-26	Lwr xtr vasc stdy bilat	0.50	0.15	0.15	0.07	0.72	$24.92	0.72	$24.92	XXX	A+
93924-TC	Lwr xtr vasc stdy bilat	0.00	3.98	NA	0.04	4.02	$139.12	NA	NA	XXX	A+ GS
93925	Lower extremity study	0.80	6.38	NA	0.11	7.29	$252.28	NA	NA	XXX	A+
93925-26	Lower extremity study	0.80	0.25	0.25	0.07	1.12	$38.76	1.12	$38.76	XXX	A+
93925-TC	Lower extremity study	0.00	6.13	NA	0.04	6.17	$213.52	NA	NA	XXX	A+ GS
93926	Lower extremity study	0.50	3.74	NA	0.07	4.31	$134.96	NA	NA	XXX	A+ DRA
93926-26	Lower extremity study	0.50	0.13	0.13	0.05	0.68	$23.53	0.68	$23.53	XXX	A+
93926-TC	Lower extremity study	0.00	3.61	NA	0.02	3.63	$111.43	NA	NA	XXX	A+ GS DRA
93930	Upper extremity study	0.80	4.98	NA	0.13	5.91	$204.52	NA	NA	XXX	A+
93930-26	Upper extremity study	0.80	0.24	0.24	0.09	1.13	$39.11	1.13	$39.11	XXX	A+
93930-TC	Upper extremity study	0.00	4.74	NA	0.04	4.78	$165.42	NA	NA	XXX	A+ GS
93931	Upper extremity study	0.50	3.17	NA	0.07	3.74	$129.43	NA	NA	XXX	A+
93931-26	Upper extremity study	0.50	0.15	0.15	0.05	0.70	$24.22	0.70	$24.22	XXX	A+
93931-TC	Upper extremity study	0.00	3.02	NA	0.02	3.04	$105.20	NA	NA	XXX	A+ GS
93970	Extremity study	0.70	4.87	NA	0.09	5.66	$195.87	NA	NA	XXX	A+
93970-26	Extremity study	0.70	0.22	0.22	0.07	0.99	$34.26	0.99	$34.26	XXX	A+
93970-TC	Extremity study	0.00	4.65	NA	0.02	4.67	$161.61	NA	NA	XXX	A+ GS
93971	Extremity study	0.45	3.08	NA	0.06	3.59	$124.24	NA	NA	XXX	A+

*Please note that these calculations are based on the Medicare 2022 Conversion Factor of $34.6062 and the DRA RVU cap rates at time of publication.

A = assistant-at-surgery restriction
A+ = assistant-at-surgery restriction unless medical necessity established with documentation
B = bilateral surgery adjustment applies
C = cosurgeons payable
C+ = cosurgeons payable if medical necessity established with documentation
CP = carriers may establish RVUs and payment amounts for these services, generally on an individual basis following review of documentation such as an operative report
M = multiple surgery adjustment applies
Me = multiple endoscopy rules may apply
M+ = multiple therapy rules apply
Mtc = multiple diagnostic imaging rules apply
T = team surgeons permitted
T+ = team surgeons payable if medical necessity established with documentation
§ = indicates code is not covered by Medicare
GS = procedure must be performed under the general supervision of a physician
DS = procedure must be performed under the direct supervision of a physician
PS = procedure must be performed under the personal supervision of a physician
DRA = procedure subject to DRA limitation

Relative Value Units

CPT Code and Modifier		Description	Work RVU	Nonfacility Practice Expense RVU	Facility Practice Expense RVU	PLI RVU	Total Non-facility RVUs	Medicare Payment Nonfacility	Total Facility RVUs	Medicare Payment Facility	Global Period	Payment Policy Indicators
93971-26		Extremity study	0.45	0.14	0.14	0.04	0.63	$21.80	0.63	$21.80	XXX	A+
93971-TC		Extremity study	0.00	2.94	NA	0.02	2.96	$102.43	NA	NA	XXX	A+ GS
93975		Vascular study	1.16	6.71	NA	0.13	8.00	$276.85	NA	NA	XXX	A+
93975-26		Vascular study	1.16	0.38	0.38	0.09	1.63	$56.41	1.63	$56.41	XXX	A+
93975-TC		Vascular study	0.00	6.33	NA	0.04	6.37	$220.44	NA	NA	XXX	A+ GS
93976		Vascular study	0.80	3.89	NA	0.06	4.75	$150.19	NA	NA	XXX	A+ DRA
93976-26		Vascular study	0.80	0.28	0.28	0.04	1.12	$38.76	1.12	$38.76	XXX	A+
93976-TC		Vascular study	0.00	3.61	NA	0.02	3.63	$111.43	NA	NA	XXX	A+ GS DRA
93978		Vascular study	0.80	4.51	NA	0.14	5.45	$188.60	NA	NA	XXX	A+
93978-26		Vascular study	0.80	0.23	0.23	0.10	1.13	$39.11	1.13	$39.11	XXX	A+
93978-TC		Vascular study	0.00	4.28	NA	0.04	4.32	$149.50	NA	NA	XXX	A+ GS
93979		Vascular study	0.50	2.96	NA	0.07	3.53	$122.16	NA	NA	XXX	A+
93979-26		Vascular study	0.50	0.14	0.14	0.05	0.69	$23.88	0.69	$23.88	XXX	A+
93979-TC		Vascular study	0.00	2.82	NA	0.02	2.84	$98.28	NA	NA	XXX	A+ GS
93980		Penile vascular study	1.25	2.13	NA	0.05	3.43	$118.70	NA	NA	XXX	A+
93980-26		Penile vascular study	1.25	0.44	0.44	0.04	1.73	$59.87	1.73	$59.87	XXX	A+
93980-TC		Penile vascular study	0.00	1.69	NA	0.01	1.70	$58.83	NA	NA	XXX	A+ GS
93981		Penile vascular study	0.44	1.60	NA	0.03	2.07	$71.63	NA	NA	XXX	A+
93981-26		Penile vascular study	0.44	0.15	0.15	0.02	0.61	$21.11	0.61	$21.11	XXX	A+
93981-TC		Penile vascular study	0.00	1.45	NA	0.01	1.46	$50.53	NA	NA	XXX	A+ GS
93985		Dup-scan hemo compl bi std	0.80	6.60	NA	0.15	7.55	$261.28	NA	NA	XXX	A+
93985-26		Dup-scan hemo compl bi std	0.80	0.21	0.21	0.11	1.12	$38.76	1.12	$38.76	XXX	A+
93985-TC		Dup-scan hemo compl bi std	0.00	6.39	NA	0.04	6.43	$222.52	NA	NA	XXX	A+ GS
93986		Dup-scan hemo compl uni std	0.50	3.89	NA	0.10	4.49	$136.00	NA	NA	XXX	A+ DRA
93986-26		Dup-scan hemo compl uni std	0.50	0.13	0.13	0.08	0.71	$24.57	0.71	$24.57	XXX	A+
93986-TC		Dup-scan hemo compl uni std	0.00	3.76	NA	0.02	3.78	$111.43	NA	NA	XXX	A+ GS DRA
93990		Doppler flow testing	0.50	3.83	NA	0.11	4.44	$135.66	NA	NA	XXX	A+ DRA
93990-26		Doppler flow testing	0.50	0.11	0.11	0.09	0.70	$24.22	0.70	$24.22	XXX	A+
93990-TC		Doppler flow testing	0.00	3.72	NA	0.02	3.74	$111.43	NA	NA	XXX	A+ GS DRA
93998	CP	Noninvas vasc dx study proc	0.00	0.00	0.00	0.00	0.00	$0.00	0.00	$0.00	XXX	A+ C+ T+
94002		Vent mgmt inpat init day	1.99	NA	0.54	0.17	NA	NA	2.70	$93.44	XXX	A+
94003		Vent mgmt inpat subq day	1.37	NA	0.42	0.11	NA	NA	1.90	$65.75	XXX	A+
94004		Vent mgmt nf per day	1.00	NA	0.33	0.08	NA	NA	1.41	$48.79	XXX	A+

94005	§	Home vent mgmt supervision	1.50	1.05	NA	0.11	2.66	$92.05	NA	NA	XXX	
94010		Breathing capacity tcst	0.17	0.60	NA	0.02	0.79	$27.34	NA	NA	XXX	A+
94010-26		Breathing capacity test	0.17	0.06	0.06	0.01	0.24	$8.31	0.24	$8.31	XXX	A+
94010-TC		Breathing capacity test	0.00	0.54	NA	0.01	0.55	$19.03	NA	NA	XXX	A+ GS
94011		Spirometry up to 2 yrs old	1.75	NA	0.65	0.11	NA	NA	2.51	$86.86	XXX	A+
94012		Spirmtry w/brnchdil inf-2 yr	2.85	NA	1.06	0.20	NA	NA	4.11	$142.23	XXX	A+
94013		Meas lung vol thru 2 yrs	0.41	NA	0.12	0.04	NA	NA	0.57	$19.73	XXX	A+
94014		Patient recorded spirometry	0.52	1.07	NA	0.03	1.62	$56.06	NA	NA	XXX	A+ GS
94015		Patient recorded spirometry	0.00	0.89	NA	0.01	0.90	$31.15	NA	NA	XXX	A+ GS
94016		Review patient spirometry	0.52	0.18	0.18	0.02	0.72	$24.92	0.72	$24.92	XXX	A+
94060		Evaluation of wheezing	0.22	0.91	NA	0.02	1.15	$39.80	NA	NA	XXX	A+
94060-26		Evaluation of wheezing	0.22	0.07	0.07	0.01	0.30	$10.38	0.30	$10.38	XXX	A+
94060-TC		Evaluation of wheezing	0.00	0.84	NA	0.01	0.85	$29.42	NA	NA	XXX	A+ DS
94070		Evaluation of wheezing	0.60	1.19	NA	0.03	1.82	$62.98	NA	NA	XXX	A+
94070-26		Evaluation of wheezing	0.60	0.20	0.20	0.02	0.82	$28.38	0.82	$28.38	XXX	A+
94070-TC		Evaluation of wheezing	0.00	0.99	NA	0.01	1.00	$34.61	NA	NA	XXX	A+ DS
94150	§	Vital capacity test	0.07	0.64	NA	0.02	0.73	$25.26	NA	NA	XXX	
94150-26	§	Vital capacity test	0.07	0.03	0.03	0.01	0.11	$3.81	0.11	$3.81	XXX	
94150-TC	§	Vital capacity test	0.00	0.61	NA	0.01	0.62	$21.46	NA	NA	XXX	GS
94200		Lung function test (mbc/mvv)	0.05	0.38	NA	0.02	0.45	$15.57	NA	NA	XXX	A+
94200-26		Lung function test (mbc/mvv)	0.05	0.03	0.03	0.01	0.09	$3.11	0.09	$3.11	XXX	A+
94200-TC		Lung function test (mbc/mvv)	0.00	0.35	NA	0.01	0.36	$12.46	NA	NA	XXX	A+ GS
94375		Respiratory flow volume loop	0.31	0.80	NA	0.02	1.13	$39.11	NA	NA	XXX	A+
94375-26		Respiratory flow volume loop	0.31	0.10	0.10	0.01	0.42	$14.53	0.42	$14.53	XXX	A+
94375-TC		Respiratory flow volume loop	0.00	0.70	NA	0.01	0.71	$24.57	NA	NA	XXX	A+ GS
94450		Hypoxia response curve	0.40	1.46	NA	0.03	1.89	$65.41	NA	NA	XXX	A+
94450-26		Hypoxia response curve	0.40	0.11	0.11	0.01	0.52	$18.00	0.52	$18.00	XXX	A+
94450-TC		Hypoxia response curve	0.00	1.35	NA	0.02	1.37	$47.41	NA	NA	XXX	A+ DS

*Please note that these calculations are based on the Medicare 2022 Conversion Factor of $34.6062 and the DRA RVU cap rates at time of publication.

A = assistant-at-surgery restriction
A+ = assistant-at-surgery restriction unless medical necessity established with documentation
B = bilateral surgery adjustment applies
C = cosurgeons payable
C+ = cosurgeons payable if medical necessity established with documentation
CP = carriers may establish RVUs and payment amounts for these services, generally on an individual basis following review of documentation such as an operative report
M = multiple surgery adjustment applies
Me = multiple endoscopy rules may apply
M+ = multiple therapy rules apply
Mtc = multiple diagnostic imaging rules apply
T = team surgeons permitted
T+ = team surgeons payable if medical necessity established with documentation
§ = indicates code is not covered by Medicare
GS = procedure must be performed under the general supervision of a physician
DS = procedure must be performed under the direct supervision of a physician
PS = procedure must be performed under the personal supervision of a physician
DRA = procedure subject to DRA limitation

Relative Value Units

CPT Code and Modifier		Description	Work RVU	Nonfacility Practice Expense RVU	Facility Practice Expense RVU	PLI RVU	Total Non-facility RVUs	Medicare Payment Nonfacility	Total Facility RVUs	Medicare Payment Facility	Global Period	Payment Policy Indicators
94452		Hast w/report	0.31	1.12	NA	0.02	1.45	$50.18	NA	NA	XXX	A+
94452-26		Hast w/report	0.31	0.10	0.10	0.01	0.42	$14.53	0.42	$14.53	XXX	A+
94452-TC		Hast w/report	0.00	1.02	NA	0.01	1.03	$35.64	NA	NA	XXX	A+ DS
94453		Hast w/oxygen titrate	0.40	1.54	NA	0.03	1.97	$68.17	NA	NA	XXX	A+
94453-26		Hast w/oxygen titrate	0.40	0.13	0.13	0.02	0.55	$19.03	0.55	$19.03	XXX	A+
94453-TC		Hast w/oxygen titrate	0.00	1.41	NA	0.01	1.42	$49.14	NA	NA	XXX	A+ DS
94610		Surfactant admin thru tube	1.16	NA	0.37	0.09	NA	NA	1.62	$56.06	XXX	A+
94617		Exercise tst brncspsm w/ecg	0.70	1.87	NA	0.03	2.60	$89.98	NA	NA	XXX	A+
94617-26		Exercise tst brncspsm w/ecg	0.70	0.23	0.23	0.01	0.94	$32.53	0.94	$32.53	XXX	A+
94617-TC		Exercise tst brncspsm w/ecg	0.00	1.64	NA	0.02	1.66	$57.45	NA	NA	XXX	A+ GS
94618		Pulmonary stress testing	0.48	0.47	NA	0.03	0.98	$33.91	NA	NA	XXX	A+
94618-26		Pulmonary stress testing	0.48	0.15	0.15	0.02	0.65	$22.49	0.65	$22.49	XXX	A+
94618-TC		Pulmonary stress testing	0.00	0.32	NA	0.01	0.33	$11.42	NA	NA	XXX	A+ GS
94619		Exercise tst brncspsm wo ecg	0.49	1.51	NA	0.03	2.03	$70.25	NA	NA	XXX	A+
94619-26		Exercise tst brncspsm wo ecg	0.49	0.16	0.16	0.01	0.66	$22.84	0.66	$22.84	XXX	A+
94619-TC		Exercise tst brncspsm wo ecg	0.00	1.35	NA	0.02	1.37	$47.41	NA	NA	XXX	A+ GS
94621		Cardiopulm exercise testing	1.42	3.03	NA	0.13	4.58	$158.50	NA	NA	XXX	A+
94621-26		Cardiopulm exercise testing	1.42	0.51	0.51	0.09	2.02	$69.90	2.02	$69.90	XXX	A+
94621-TC		Cardiopulm exercise testing	0.00	2.52	NA	0.04	2.56	$88.59	NA	NA	XXX	A+ DS
94625		Phy/qhp op pulm rhb w/o mntr	0.36	1.50	0.14	0.05	1.91	$66.10	0.55	$19.03	XXX	A+
94626		Phy/qhp op pulm rhb w/mntr	0.56	1.57	0.19	0.04	2.17	$75.10	0.79	$27.34	XXX	A+
94640		Airway inhalation treatment	0.00	0.32	NA	0.01	0.33	$11.42	NA	NA	XXX	A+
94642	CP	Aerosol inhalation treatment	0.00	0.00	0.00	0.00	0.00	$0.00	0.00	$0.00	XXX	A+
94644		Cbt 1st hour	0.00	1.81	NA	0.01	1.82	$62.98	NA	NA	XXX	A+
94645		Cbt each addl hour	0.00	0.46	NA	0.01	0.47	$16.26	NA	NA	XXX	A+
94660		Pos airway pressure cpap	0.76	1.05	0.28	0.07	1.88	$65.06	1.11	$38.41	XXX	A+
94662		Neg press ventilation cnp	0.76	NA	0.22	0.07	NA	NA	1.05	$36.34	XXX	A+
94664		Evaluate pt use of inhaler	0.00	0.49	NA	0.01	0.50	$17.30	NA	NA	XXX	A+ DS
94667		Chest wall manipulation	0.00	0.65	NA	0.02	0.67	$23.19	NA	NA	XXX	A+
94668		Chest wall manipulation	0.00	1.02	NA	0.02	1.04	$35.99	NA	NA	XXX	A+
94669		Mechanical chest wall oscill	0.00	0.53	NA	0.02	0.55	$19.03	NA	NA	XXX	A+
94680		Exhaled air analysis o2	0.26	1.27	NA	0.03	1.56	$53.99	NA	NA	XXX	A+
94680-26		Exhaled air analysis o2	0.26	0.10	0.10	0.02	0.38	$13.15	0.38	$13.15	XXX	A+

94680-TC		Exhaled air analysis o2	0.00	1.17	NA	0.01	1.18	$40.84	NA	NA	XXX	A+ DS
94681		Exhaled air analysis o2/co2	0.20	1.21	NA	0.02	1.43	$49.49	NA	NA	XXX	A+
94681-26		Exhaled air analysis o2/co2	0.20	0.08	0.08	0.01	0.29	$10.04	0.29	$10.04	XXX	A+
94681-TC		Exhaled air analysis o2/co2	0.00	1.13	NA	0.01	1.14	$39.45	NA	NA	XXX	A+ DS
94690		Exhaled air analysis	0.07	1.19	NA	0.02	1.28	$44.30	NA	NA	XXX	A+
94690-26		Exhaled air analysis	0.07	0.03	0.03	0.01	0.11	$3.81	0.11	$3.81	XXX	A+
94690-TC		Exhaled air analysis	0.00	1.16	NA	0.01	1.17	$40.49	NA	NA	XXX	A+ GS
94726		Pulm funct tst plethysmograp	0.26	1.32	NA	0.03	1.61	$55.72	NA	NA	XXX	A+
94726-26		Pulm funct tst plethysmograp	0.26	0.08	0.08	0.01	0.35	$12.11	0.35	$12.11	XXX	A+
94726-TC		Pulm funct tst plethysmograp	0.00	1.24	NA	0.02	1.26	$43.60	NA	NA	XXX	A+ GS
94727		Pulm function test by gas	0.26	1.01	NA	0.02	1.29	$44.64	NA	NA	XXX	A+
94727-26		Pulm function test by gas	0.26	0.08	0.08	0.01	0.35	$12.11	0.35	$12.11	XXX	A+
94727-TC		Pulm function test by gas	0.00	0.93	NA	0.01	0.94	$32.53	NA	NA	XXX	A+ GS
94728		Airwy resist by oscillometry	0.26	0.89	NA	0.02	1.17	$40.49	NA	NA	XXX	A+
94728-26		Airwy resist by oscillometry	0.26	0.09	0.09	0.01	0.36	$12.46	0.36	$12.46	XXX	A+
94728-TC		Airwy resist by oscillometry	0.00	0.80	NA	0.01	0.81	$28.03	NA	NA	XXX	A+ GS
94729		Co/membane diffuse capacity	0.19	1.52	NA	0.02	1.73	$59.87	NA	NA	ZZZ	A+
94729-26		Co/membane diffuse capacity	0.19	0.06	0.06	0.01	0.26	$9.00	0.26	$9.00	ZZZ	A+
94729-TC		Co/membane diffuse capacity	0.00	1.46	NA	0.01	1.47	$50.87	NA	NA	ZZZ	A+ GS
94760		Measure blood oxygen level	0.00	0.06	NA	0.01	0.07	$2.42	NA	NA	XXX	A+ GS
94761		Measure blood oxygen level	0.00	0.09	NA	0.01	0.10	$3.46	NA	NA	XXX	A+ GS
94762		Measure blood oxygen level	0.00	0.77	NA	0.01	0.78	$26.99	NA	NA	XXX	A+ GS
94772	CP	Breath recording infant	0.00	0.00	NA	0.00	0.00	$0.00	NA	NA	XXX	A+
94772-26	CP	Breath recording infant	0.00	0.00	0.00	0.00	0.00	$0.00	0.00	$0.00	XXX	A+
94772-TC	CP	Breath recording infant	0.00	0.00	NA	0.00	0.00	$0.00	NA	NA	XXX	A+ GS
94774	CP	Ped home apnea rec compl	0.00	0.00	0.00	0.00	0.00	$0.00	0.00	$0.00	YYY	A+
94775	CP	Ped home apnea rec hk-up	0.00	0.00	0.00	0.00	0.00	$0.00	0.00	$0.00	YYY	A+
94776	CP	Ped home apnea rec downld	0.00	0.00	0.00	0.00	0.00	$0.00	0.00	$0.00	YYY	A+

*Please note that these calculations are based on the Medicare 2022 Conversion Factor of $34.6062 and the DRA RVU cap rates at time of publication.

A = assistant-at-surgery restriction
A+ = assistant-at-surgery restriction unless medical necessity established with documentation
B = bilateral surgery adjustment applies
C = cosurgeons payable
C+ = cosurgeons payable if medical necessity established with documentation
CP = carriers may establish RVUs and payment amounts for these services, generally on an individual basis following review of documentation such as an operative report
M = multiple surgery adjustment applies
Me = multiple endoscopy rules may apply
M+ = multiple therapy rules apply
Mtc = multiple diagnostic imaging rules apply
T = team surgeons permitted
T+ = team surgeons payable if medical necessity established with documentation
§ = indicates code is not covered by Medicare
GS = procedure must be performed under the general supervision of a physician
DS = procedure must be performed under the direct supervision of a physician
PS = procedure must be performed under the personal supervision of a physician
DRA = procedure subject to DRA limitation

Relative Value Units

CPT Code and Modifier		Description	Work RVU	Nonfacility Practice Expense RVU	Facility Practice Expense RVU	PLI RVU	Total Non-facility RVUs	Medicare Payment Nonfacility	Total Facility RVUs	Medicare Payment Facility	Global Period	Payment Policy Indicators
94777	CP	Ped home apnea rec report	0.00	0.00	0.00	0.00	0.00	$0.00	0.00	$0.00	YYY	A+
94780		Cars/bd tst inft-12mo 60 min	0.48	1.00	0.18	0.04	1.52	$52.60	0.70	$24.22	XXX	A
94781		Cars/bd tst inft-12mo +30min	0.17	0.42	0.06	0.01	0.60	$20.76	0.24	$8.31	ZZZ	A
94799	CP	Pulmonary service/procedure	0.00	0.00	NA	0.00	0.00	$0.00	NA	NA	XXX	A+
94799-26	CP	Pulmonary service/procedure	0.00	0.00	0.00	0.00	0.00	$0.00	0.00	$0.00	XXX	A+
94799-TC	CP	Pulmonary service/procedure	0.00	0.00	NA	0.00	0.00	$0.00	NA	NA	XXX	A+
95004		Percut allergy skin tests	0.01	0.10	NA	0.01	0.12	$4.15	NA	NA	XXX	A+ DS
95012		Exhaled nitric oxide meas	0.00	0.55	NA	0.01	0.56	$19.38	NA	NA	XXX	A+
95017		Perq & icut allg test venoms	0.07	0.18	0.03	0.01	0.26	$9.00	0.11	$3.81	XXX	A+
95018		Perq&ic allg test drugs/biol	0.14	0.46	0.06	0.01	0.61	$21.11	0.21	$7.27	XXX	A+
95024		Icut allergy test drug/bug	0.01	0.23	0.01	0.01	0.25	$8.65	0.03	$1.04	XXX	A+ DS
95027		Icut allergy titrate-airborn	0.01	0.13	NA	0.01	0.15	$5.19	NA	NA	XXX	A+ DS
95028		Icut allergy test-delayed	0.00	0.37	NA	0.01	0.38	$13.15	NA	NA	XXX	A+ DS
95044		Allergy patch tests	0.00	0.14	NA	0.01	0.15	$5.19	NA	NA	XXX	A+ DS
95052		Photo patch test	0.00	0.18	NA	0.01	0.19	$6.58	NA	NA	XXX	A+ DS
95056		Photosensitivity tests	0.00	1.44	NA	0.01	1.45	$50.18	NA	NA	XXX	A+ DS
95060		Eye allergy tests	0.00	1.07	NA	0.01	1.08	$37.37	NA	NA	XXX	A+ PS
95065		Nose allergy test	0.00	0.79	NA	0.01	0.80	$27.68	NA	NA	XXX	A+ PS
95070		Bronchial allergy tests	0.00	1.03	NA	0.02	1.05	$36.34	NA	NA	XXX	A+ DS
95076		Ingest challenge ini 120 min	1.50	1.94	0.59	0.07	3.51	$121.47	2.16	$74.75	XXX	A+
95079		Ingest challenge addl 60 min	1.38	1.04	0.55	0.05	2.47	$85.48	1.98	$68.52	ZZZ	A+
95115		Immunotherapy one injection	0.00	0.27	NA	0.01	0.28	$9.69	NA	NA	XXX	A+
95117		Immunotherapy injections	0.00	0.33	NA	0.01	0.34	$11.77	NA	NA	XXX	A+
95144		Antigen therapy services	0.06	0.43	0.02	0.01	0.50	$17.30	0.09	$3.11	XXX	A+
95145		Antigen therapy services	0.06	0.95	0.02	0.01	1.02	$35.30	0.09	$3.11	XXX	A+
95146		Antigen therapy services	0.06	1.80	0.02	0.01	1.87	$64.71	0.09	$3.11	XXX	A+
95147		Antigen therapy services	0.06	1.73	0.02	0.01	1.80	$62.29	0.09	$3.11	XXX	A+
95148		Antigen therapy services	0.06	2.60	0.02	0.01	2.67	$92.40	0.09	$3.11	XXX	A+
95149		Antigen therapy services	0.06	3.48	0.02	0.01	3.55	$122.85	0.09	$3.11	XXX	A+
95165		Antigen therapy services	0.06	0.39	0.02	0.01	0.46	$15.92	0.09	$3.11	XXX	A+
95170		Antigen therapy services	0.06	0.27	0.02	0.01	0.34	$11.77	0.09	$3.11	XXX	A+
95180		Rapid desensitization	2.01	1.89	0.89	0.09	3.99	$138.08	2.99	$103.47	XXX	A+
95199	CP	Allergy immunology services	0.00	0.00	0.00	0.00	0.00	$0.00	0.00	$0.00	XXX	A+

95249		Cont gluc mntr pt prov eqp	0.00	1.69	NA	0.04	1.73	$59.87	NA	NA	XXX	A+
95250		Cont gluc mntr phys/qhp eqp	0.00	4.34	NA	0.04	4.38	$151.58	NA	NA	XXX	A+
95251		Cont gluc mntr analysis i&r	0.70	0.28	0.28	0.04	1.02	$35.30	1.02	$35.30	XXX	A+
95700	CP	Eeg cont rec w/vid eeg tech	0.00	0.00	0.00	0.00	0.00	$0.00	0.00	$0.00	XXX	A+ GS
95705	CP	Eeg w/o vid 2-12 hr unmntr	0.00	0.00	0.00	0.00	0.00	$0.00	0.00	$0.00	XXX	A+ GS
95706	CP	Eeg wo vid 2-12hr intmt mntr	0.00	0.00	0.00	0.00	0.00	$0.00	0.00	$0.00	XXX	A+ GS
95707	CP	Eeg w/o vid 2-12hr cont mntr	0.00	0.00	0.00	0.00	0.00	$0.00	0.00	$0.00	XXX	A+ GS
95708	CP	Eeg wo vid ea 12-26hr unmntr	0.00	0.00	0.00	0.00	0.00	$0.00	0.00	$0.00	XXX	A+ GS
95709	CP	Eeg w/o vid ea 12-26hr intmt	0.00	0.00	0.00	0.00	0.00	$0.00	0.00	$0.00	XXX	A+ GS
95710	CP	Eeg w/o vid ea 12-26hr cont	0.00	0.00	0.00	0.00	0.00	$0.00	0.00	$0.00	XXX	A+ GS
95711	CP	Veeg 2-12 hr unmonitored	0.00	0.00	0.00	0.00	0.00	$0.00	0.00	$0.00	XXX	A+ GS
95712	CP	Veeg 2-12 hr intmt mntr	0.00	0.00	0.00	0.00	0.00	$0.00	0.00	$0.00	XXX	A+ GS
95713	CP	Veeg 2-12 hr cont mntr	0.00	0.00	0.00	0.00	0.00	$0.00	0.00	$0.00	XXX	A+ GS
95714	CP	Veeg ea 12-26 hr unmntr	0.00	0.00	0.00	0.00	0.00	$0.00	0.00	$0.00	XXX	A+ GS
95715	CP	Veeg ea 12-26hr intmt mntr	0.00	0.00	0.00	0.00	0.00	$0.00	0.00	$0.00	XXX	A+ GS
95716	CP	Veeg ea 12-26hr cont mntr	0.00	0.00	0.00	0.00	0.00	$0.00	0.00	$0.00	XXX	A+ GS
95717		Eeg phys/qhp 2-12 hr w/o vid	2.00	0.85	0.82	0.12	2.97	$102.78	2.94	$101.74	XXX	A+
95718		Eeg phys/qhp 2-12 hr w/veeg	2.50	1.28	1.22	0.20	3.98	$137.73	3.92	$135.66	XXX	A+
95719		Eeg phys/qhp ea incr w/o vid	3.00	1.39	1.35	0.22	4.61	$159.53	4.57	$158.15	XXX	A+
95720		Eeg phy/qhp ea incr w/veeg	3.86	1.96	1.86	0.31	6.13	$212.14	6.03	$208.68	XXX	A+
95721		Eeg phy/qhp>36<60 hr w/o vid	3.86	1.97	1.85	0.29	6.12	$211.79	6.00	$207.64	XXX	A+
95722		Eeg phy/qhp>36<60 hr w/veeg	4.70	2.39	2.25	0.37	7.46	$258.16	7.32	$253.32	XXX	A+
95723		Eeg phy/qhp>60<84 hr w/o vid	4.75	2.40	2.25	0.37	7.52	$260.24	7.37	$255.05	XXX	A+
95724		Eeg phy/qhp>60<84 hr w/veeg	6.00	3.02	2.85	0.45	9.47	$327.72	9.30	$321.84	XXX	A+
95725		Eeg phy/qhp>84 hr w/o vid	5.40	2.82	2.63	0.42	8.64	$299.00	8.45	$292.42	XXX	A+
95726		Eeg phy/qhp>84 hr w/veeg	7.58	3.85	3.63	0.60	12.03	$416.31	11.81	$408.70	XXX	A+
95782		Polysom <6 yrs 4/> paramtrs	2.60	25.04	NA	0.32	27.96	$967.59	NA	NA	XXX	A+
95782-26		Polysom <6 yrs 4/> paramtrs	2.60	0.96	0.96	0.09	3.65	$126.31	3.65	$126.31	XXX	A+

*Please note that these calculations are based on the Medicare 2022 Conversion Factor of $34.6062 and the DRA RVU cap rates at time of publication.

A = assistant-at-surgery restriction
A+ = assistant-at-surgery restriction unless medical necessity established with documentation
B = bilateral surgery adjustment applies
C = cosurgeons payable
C+ = cosurgeons payable if medical necessity established with documentation
CP = carriers may establish RVUs and payment amounts for these services, generally on an individual basis following review of documentation such as an operative report
M = multiple surgery adjustment applies
Me = multiple endoscopy rules may apply
M+ = multiple therapy rules apply
Mtc = multiple diagnostic imaging rules apply
T = team surgeons permitted
T+ = team surgeons payable if medical necessity established with documentation
§ = indicates code is not covered by Medicare
GS = procedure must be performed under the general supervision of a physician
DS = procedure must be performed under the direct supervision of a physician
PS = procedure must be performed under the personal supervision of a physician
DRA = procedure subject to DRA limitation

Relative Value Units

CPT Code and Modifier	Description	Work RVU	Nonfacility Practice Expense RVU	Facility Practice Expense RVU	PLI RVU	Total Non-facility RVUs	Medicare Payment Nonfacility	Total Facility RVUs	Medicare Payment Facility	Global Period	Payment Policy Indicators
95782-TC	Polysom <6 yrs 4/> paramtrs	0.00	24.08	NA	0.23	24.31	$841.28	NA	NA	XXX	A+ GS
95783	Polysom <6 yrs cpap/bilvl	2.83	26.45	NA	0.33	29.61	$1024.69	NA	NA	XXX	A+
95783-26	Polysom <6 yrs cpap/bilvl	2.83	1.05	1.05	0.09	3.97	$137.39	3.97	$137.39	XXX	A+
95783-TC	Polysom <6 yrs cpap/bilvl	0.00	25.40	NA	0.24	25.64	$887.30	NA	NA	XXX	A+ GS
95800	Slp stdy unattended	0.85	3.84	NA	0.05	4.74	$164.03	NA	NA	XXX	A+
95800-26	Slp stdy unattended	0.85	0.31	0.31	0.04	1.20	$41.53	1.20	$41.53	XXX	A+
95800-TC	Slp stdy unattended	0.00	3.53	NA	0.01	3.54	$122.51	NA	NA	XXX	A+ GS
95801	Slp stdy unatnd w/anal	0.85	1.78	NA	0.05	2.68	$92.74	NA	NA	XXX	A+
95801-26	Slp stdy unatnd w/anal	0.85	0.31	0.31	0.04	1.20	$41.53	1.20	$41.53	XXX	A+
95801-TC	Slp stdy unatnd w/anal	0.00	1.47	NA	0.01	1.48	$51.22	NA	NA	XXX	A+ GS
95803	Actigraphy testing	0.90	3.40	NA	0.03	4.33	$149.84	NA	NA	XXX	A+
95803-26	Actigraphy testing	0.90	0.33	0.33	0.02	1.25	$43.26	1.25	$43.26	XXX	A+
95803-TC	Actigraphy testing	0.00	3.07	NA	0.01	3.08	$106.59	NA	NA	XXX	A+ GS
95805	Multiple sleep latency test	1.20	11.00	NA	0.14	12.34	$427.04	NA	NA	XXX	A+
95805-26	Multiple sleep latency test	1.20	0.44	0.44	0.04	1.68	$58.14	1.68	$58.14	XXX	A+
95805-TC	Multiple sleep latency test	0.00	10.56	NA	0.10	10.66	$368.90	NA	NA	XXX	A+ GS
95806	Sleep study unatt&resp efft	0.93	1.71	NA	0.06	2.70	$93.44	NA	NA	XXX	A+
95806-26	Sleep study unatt&resp efft	0.93	0.33	0.33	0.04	1.30	$44.99	1.30	$44.99	XXX	A+
95806-TC	Sleep study unatt&resp efft	0.00	1.38	NA	0.02	1.40	$48.45	NA	NA	XXX	A+ GS
95807	Sleep study attended	1.28	9.79	NA	0.14	11.21	$387.94	NA	NA	XXX	A+
95807-26	Sleep study attended	1.28	0.42	0.42	0.05	1.75	$60.56	1.75	$60.56	XXX	A+
95807-TC	Sleep study attended	0.00	9.37	NA	0.09	9.46	$327.37	NA	NA	XXX	A+ GS
95808	Polysom any age 1-3> param	1.74	17.89	NA	0.18	19.81	$685.55	NA	NA	XXX	A+
95808-26	Polysom any age 1-3> param	1.74	0.75	0.75	0.07	2.56	$88.59	2.56	$88.59	XXX	A+
95808-TC	Polysom any age 1-3> param	0.00	17.14	NA	0.11	17.25	$596.96	NA	NA	XXX	A+ GS
95810	Polysom 6/> yrs 4/> param	2.50	15.27	NA	0.20	17.97	$621.87	NA	NA	XXX	A+
95810-26	Polysom 6/> yrs 4/> param	2.50	0.89	0.89	0.09	3.48	$120.43	3.48	$120.43	XXX	A+
95810-TC	Polysom 6/> yrs 4/> param	0.00	14.38	NA	0.11	14.49	$501.44	NA	NA	XXX	A+ GS
95811	Polysom 6/>yrs cpap 4/> parm	2.60	15.95	NA	0.21	18.76	$649.21	NA	NA	XXX	A+
95811-26	Polysom 6/>yrs cpap 4/> parm	2.60	0.92	0.92	0.09	3.61	$124.93	3.61	$124.93	XXX	A+
95811-TC	Polysom 6/>yrs cpap 4/> parm	0.00	15.03	NA	0.12	15.15	$524.28	NA	NA	XXX	A+ GS
95812	Eeg 41-60 minutes	1.08	9.11	NA	0.09	10.28	$355.75	NA	NA	XXX	A+
95812-26	Eeg 41-60 minutes	1.08	0.53	0.53	0.05	1.66	$57.45	1.66	$57.45	XXX	A+

95812-TC		Eeg 41-60 minutes	0.00	8.58	NA	0.04	8.62	$298.31	NA	NA	XXX	A+ GS
95813		Eeg extnd mntr 61-119 min	1.63	10.96	NA	0.13	12.72	$440.19	NA	NA	XXX	A+
95813-26		Eeg extnd mntr 61-119 min	1.63	0.81	0.81	0.09	2.53	$87.55	2.53	$87.55	XXX	A+
95813-TC		Eeg extnd mntr 61-119 min	0.00	10.15	NA	0.04	10.19	$352.64	NA	NA	XXX	A+ GS
95816		Eeg awake and drowsy	1.08	10.17	NA	0.09	11.34	$392.43	NA	NA	XXX	A+
95816-26		Eeg awake and drowsy	1.08	0.53	0.53	0.05	1.66	$57.45	1.66	$57.45	XXX	A+
95816-TC		Eeg awake and drowsy	0.00	9.64	NA	0.04	9.68	$334.99	NA	NA	XXX	A+
95819		Eeg awake and asleep	1.08	12.13	NA	0.10	13.31	$460.61	NA	NA	XXX	A+
95819-26		Eeg awake and asleep	1.08	0.54	0.54	0.05	1.67	$57.79	1.67	$57.79	XXX	A+
95819-TC		Eeg awake and asleep	0.00	11.59	NA	0.05	11.64	$402.82	NA	NA	XXX	A+
95822		Eeg coma or sleep only	1.08	11.19	NA	0.09	12.36	$427.73	NA	NA	XXX	A+
95822-26		Eeg coma or sleep only	1.08	0.54	0.54	0.05	1.67	$57.79	1.67	$57.79	XXX	A+
95822-TC		Eeg coma or sleep only	0.00	10.65	NA	0.04	10.69	$369.94	NA	NA	XXX	A+
95824	CP	Eeg cerebral death only	0.00	0.00	NA	0.00	0.00	$0.00	NA	NA	XXX	A+
95824-26		Eeg cerebral death only	0.74	0.36	0.36	0.04	1.14	$39.45	1.14	$39.45	XXX	A+
95824-TC	CP	Eeg cerebral death only	0.00	0.00	NA	0.00	0.00	$0.00	NA	NA	XXX	A+ GS
95829		Surgery electrocorticogram	6.20	47.48	NA	0.51	54.19	$1875.31	NA	NA	XXX	A+
95829-26		Surgery electrocorticogram	6.20	3.08	3.08	0.42	9.70	$335.68	9.70	$335.68	XXX	A+
95829-TC		Surgery electrocorticogram	0.00	44.40	NA	0.09	44.49	$1539.63	NA	NA	XXX	A+ GS
95830		Insert electrodes for eeg	1.70	19.65	0.86	0.12	21.47	$743.00	2.68	$92.74	XXX	A+
95836		Ecog impltd brn npgt <30 d	1.98	0.96	0.96	0.19	3.13	$108.32	3.13	$108.32	XXX	A+
95851		Range of motion measurements	0.16	0.44	0.06	0.01	0.61	$21.11	0.23	$7.96	XXX	A+
95852		Range of motion measurements	0.11	0.39	0.04	0.01	0.51	$17.65	0.16	$5.54	XXX	A+
95857		Cholinesterase challenge	0.53	1.30	0.27	0.04	1.87	$64.71	0.84	$29.07	XXX	A+
95860		Muscle test one limb	0.96	2.38	NA	0.05	3.39	$117.32	NA	NA	XXX	A+
95860-26		Muscle test one limb	0.96	0.49	0.49	0.04	1.49	$51.56	1.49	$51.56	XXX	A+
95860-TC		Muscle test one limb	0.00	1.89	NA	0.01	1.90	$65.75	NA	NA	XXX	A+
95861		Muscle test 2 limbs	1.54	3.27	NA	0.09	4.90	$169.57	NA	NA	XXX	A+

*Please note that these calculations are based on the Medicare 2022 Conversion Factor of $34.6062 and the DRA RVU cap rates at time of publication.

A = assistant-at-surgery restriction
A+ = assistant-at-surgery restriction unless medical necessity established with documentation
B = bilateral surgery adjustment applies
C = cosurgeons payable
C+ = cosurgeons payable if medical necessity established with documentation
CP = carriers may establish RVUs and payment amounts for these services, generally on an individual basis following review of documentation such as an operative report
M = multiple surgery adjustment applies
Me = multiple endoscopy rules may apply
M+ = multiple therapy rules apply
Mtc = multiple diagnostic imaging rules apply
T = team surgeons permitted
T+ = team surgeons payable if medical necessity established with documentation
§ = indicates code is not covered by Medicare
GS = procedure must be performed under the general supervision of a physician
DS = procedure must be performed under the direct supervision of a physician
PS = procedure must be performed under the personal supervision of a physician
DRA = procedure subject to DRA limitation

Relative Value Units

CPT Code and Modifier	Description	Work RVU	Nonfacility Practice Expense RVU	Facility Practice Expense RVU	PLI RVU	Total Non-facility RVUs	Medicare Payment Nonfacility	Total Facility RVUs	Medicare Payment Facility	Global Period	Payment Policy Indicators
95861-26	Muscle test 2 limbs	1.54	0.77	0.77	0.08	2.39	$82.71	2.39	$82.71	XXX	A+
95861-TC	Muscle test 2 limbs	0.00	2.50	NA	0.01	2.51	$86.86	NA	NA	XXX	A+
95863	Muscle test 3 limbs	1.87	4.44	NA	0.09	6.40	$221.48	NA	NA	XXX	A+
95863-26	Muscle test 3 limbs	1.87	0.95	0.95	0.08	2.90	$100.36	2.90	$100.36	XXX	A+
95863-TC	Muscle test 3 limbs	0.00	3.49	NA	0.01	3.50	$121.12	NA	NA	XXX	A+
95864	Muscle test 4 limbs	1.99	5.05	NA	0.11	7.15	$247.43	NA	NA	XXX	A+
95864-26	Muscle test 4 limbs	1.99	1.01	1.01	0.10	3.10	$107.28	3.10	$107.28	XXX	A+
95864-TC	Muscle test 4 limbs	0.00	4.04	NA	0.01	4.05	$140.16	NA	NA	XXX	A+
95865	Muscle test larynx	1.57	2.91	NA	0.08	4.56	$157.80	NA	NA	XXX	A+
95865-26	Muscle test larynx	1.57	0.78	0.78	0.07	2.42	$83.75	2.42	$83.75	XXX	A+
95865-TC	Muscle test larynx	0.00	2.13	NA	0.01	2.14	$74.06	NA	NA	XXX	A+
95866	Muscle test hemidiaphragm	1.25	2.60	NA	0.05	3.90	$134.96	NA	NA	XXX	A+
95866-26	Muscle test hemidiaphragm	1.25	0.59	0.59	0.04	1.88	$65.06	1.88	$65.06	XXX	A+
95866-TC	Muscle test hemidiaphragm	0.00	2.01	NA	0.01	2.02	$69.90	NA	NA	XXX	A+
95867	Muscle test cran nerv unilat	0.79	2.39	NA	0.05	3.23	$111.78	NA	NA	XXX	A+
95867-26	Muscle test cran nerv unilat	0.79	0.39	0.39	0.04	1.22	$42.22	1.22	$42.22	XXX	A+
95867-TC	Muscle test cran nerv unilat	0.00	2.00	NA	0.01	2.01	$69.56	NA	NA	XXX	A+
95868	Muscle test cran nerve bilat	1.18	3.04	NA	0.06	4.28	$148.11	NA	NA	XXX	A+
95868-26	Muscle test cran nerve bilat	1.18	0.60	0.60	0.05	1.83	$63.33	1.83	$63.33	XXX	A+
95868-TC	Muscle test cran nerve bilat	0.00	2.44	NA	0.01	2.45	$84.79	NA	NA	XXX	A+
95869	Muscle test thor paraspinal	0.37	2.57	NA	0.03	2.97	$102.78	NA	NA	XXX	A+
95869-26	Muscle test thor paraspinal	0.37	0.19	0.19	0.02	0.58	$20.07	0.58	$20.07	XXX	A+
95869-TC	Muscle test thor paraspinal	0.00	2.38	NA	0.01	2.39	$82.71	NA	NA	XXX	A+
95870	Muscle test nonparaspinal	0.37	2.17	NA	0.03	2.57	$88.94	NA	NA	XXX	A+
95870-26	Muscle test nonparaspinal	0.37	0.18	0.18	0.02	0.57	$19.73	0.57	$19.73	XXX	A+
95870-TC	Muscle test nonparaspinal	0.00	1.99	NA	0.01	2.00	$69.21	NA	NA	XXX	A+
95872	Muscle test one fiber	2.88	3.27	NA	0.13	6.28	$217.33	NA	NA	XXX	A+
95872-26	Muscle test onc fiber	2.88	1.44	1.44	0.12	4.44	$153.65	4.44	$153.65	XXX	A+
95872-TC	Muscle test one fiber	0.00	1.83	NA	0.01	1.84	$63.68	NA	NA	XXX	A+
95873	Guide nerv destr elec stim	0.37	1.89	NA	0.01	2.27	$78.56	NA	NA	ZZZ	A+
95873-26	Guide nerv destr elec stim	0.37	0.19	0.19	0.01	0.57	$19.73	0.57	$19.73	ZZZ	A+
95873-TC	Guide nerv destr elec stim	0.00	1.70	NA	0.00	1.70	$58.83	NA	NA	ZZZ	A+ PS
95874	Guide nerv destr needle emg	0.37	2.01	NA	0.01	2.39	$82.71	NA	NA	ZZZ	A+

95874-26	Guide nerv destr needle emg	0.37	0.19	0.19	0.01	0.57	$19.73	0.57	$19.73	ZZZ	A+
95874-TC	Guide nerv destr needle emg	0.00	1.82	NA	0.00	1.82	$62.98	NA	NA	ZZZ	A+ PS
95875	Limb exercise test	1.10	2.93	NA	0.06	4.09	$141.54	NA	NA	XXX	A+
95875-26	Limb exercise test	1.10	0.56	0.56	0.05	1.71	$59.18	1.71	$59.18	XXX	A+
95875-TC	Limb exercise test	0.00	2.37	NA	0.01	2.38	$82.36	NA	NA	XXX	A+ PS
95885	Musc tst done w/nerv tst lim	0.35	1.56	NA	0.01	1.92	$66.44	NA	NA	ZZZ	A+
95885-26	Musc tst done w/nerv tst lim	0.35	0.18	0.18	0.01	0.54	$18.69	0.54	$18.69	ZZZ	A+
95885-TC	Musc tst done w/nerv tst lim	0.00	1.38	NA	0.00	1.38	$47.76	NA	NA	ZZZ	A+
95886	Musc test done w/n test comp	0.86	2.08	NA	0.04	2.98	$103.13	NA	NA	ZZZ	A+
95886-26	Musc test done w/n test comp	0.86	0.43	0.43	0.04	1.33	$46.03	1.33	$46.03	ZZZ	A+
95886-TC	Musc test done w/n test comp	0.00	1.65	NA	0.00	1.65	$57.10	NA	NA	ZZZ	A+
95887	Musc tst done w/n tst nonext	0.71	1.82	NA	0.04	2.57	$88.94	NA	NA	ZZZ	A+
95887-26	Musc tst done w/n tst nonext	0.71	0.35	0.35	0.04	1.10	$38.07	1.10	$38.07	ZZZ	A+
95887-TC	Musc tst done w/n tst nonext	0.00	1.47	NA	0.00	1.47	$50.87	NA	NA	ZZZ	A+
95905	Motor &/ sens nrve cndj test	0.05	1.07	NA	0.02	1.14	$39.45	NA	NA	XXX	A+
95905-26	Motor &/ sens nrve cndj test	0.05	0.02	0.02	0.01	0.08	$2.77	0.08	$2.77	XXX	A+
95905-TC	Motor &/ sens nrve cndj test	0.00	1.05	NA	0.01	1.06	$36.68	NA	NA	XXX	A+ GS
95907	Nvr cndj tst 1-2 studies	1.00	1.67	NA	0.05	2.72	$94.13	NA	NA	XXX	A+
95907-26	Nvr cndj tst 1-2 studies	1.00	0.51	0.51	0.04	1.55	$53.64	1.55	$53.64	XXX	A+
95907-TC	Nvr cndj tst 1-2 studies	0.00	1.16	NA	0.01	1.17	$40.49	NA	NA	XXX	A+
95908	Nrv cndj tst 3-4 studies	1.25	2.08	NA	0.06	3.39	$117.32	NA	NA	XXX	A+
95908-26	Nrv cndj tst 3-4 studies	1.25	0.64	0.64	0.05	1.94	$67.14	1.94	$67.14	XXX	A+
95908-TC	Nrv cndj tst 3-4 studies	0.00	1.44	NA	0.01	1.45	$50.18	NA	NA	XXX	A+
95909	Nrv cndj tst 5-6 studies	1.50	2.49	NA	0.08	4.07	$140.85	NA	NA	XXX	A+
95909-26	Nrv cndj tst 5-6 studies	1.50	0.76	0.76	0.07	2.33	$80.63	2.33	$80.63	XXX	A+
95909-TC	Nrv cndj tst 5-6 studies	0.00	1.73	NA	0.01	1.74	$60.21	NA	NA	XXX	A+
95910	Nrv cndj test 7-8 studies	2.00	3.22	NA	0.10	5.32	$184.10	NA	NA	XXX	A+
95910-26	Nrv cndj test 7-8 studies	2.00	1.02	1.02	0.09	3.11	$107.63	3.11	$107.63	XXX	A+

*Please note that these calculations are based on the Medicare 2022 Conversion Factor of $34.6062 and the DRA RVU cap rates at time of publication.

A = assistant-at-surgery restriction

A+ = assistant-at-surgery restriction unless medical necessity established with documentation

B = bilateral surgery adjustment applies

C = cosurgeons payable

C+ = cosurgeons payable if medical necessity established with documentation

CP = carriers may establish RVUs and payment amounts for these services, generally on an individual basis following review of documentation such as an operative report

M = multiple surgery adjustment applies

Me = multiple endoscopy rules may apply

M+ = multiple therapy rules apply

Mtc = multiple diagnostic imaging rules apply

T = team surgeons permitted

T+ = team surgeons payable if medical necessity established with documentation

§ = indicates code is not covered by Medicare

GS = procedure must be performed under the general supervision of a physician

DS = procedure must be performed under the direct supervision of a physician

PS = procedure must be performed under the personal supervision of a physician

DRA = procedure subject to DRA limitation

Relative Value Units

CPT Code and Modifier	Description	Work RVU	Nonfacility Practice Expense RVU	Facility Practice Expense RVU	PLI RVU	Total Non-facility RVUs	Medicare Payment Nonfacility	Total Facility RVUs	Medicare Payment Facility	Global Period	Payment Policy Indicators
95910-TC	Nrv cndj test 7-8 studies	0.00	2.20	NA	0.01	2.21	$76.48	NA	NA	XXX	A+
95911	Nrv cndj test 9-10 studies	2.50	3.79	NA	0.11	6.40	$221.48	NA	NA	XXX	A+
95911-26	Nrv cndj test 9-10 studies	2.50	1.26	1.26	0.10	3.86	$133.58	3.86	$133.58	XXX	A+
95911-TC	Nrv cndj test 9-10 studies	0.00	2.53	NA	0.01	2.54	$87.90	NA	NA	XXX	A+
95912	Nrv cndj test 11-12 studies	3.00	4.32	NA	0.13	7.45	$257.82	NA	NA	XXX	A+
95912-26	Nrv cndj test 11-12 studies	3.00	1.49	1.49	0.11	4.60	$159.19	4.60	$159.19	XXX	A+
95912-TC	Nrv cndj test 11-12 studies	0.00	2.83	NA	0.02	2.85	$98.63	NA	NA	XXX	A+
95913	Nrv cndj test 13/> studies	3.56	4.90	NA	0.16	8.62	$298.31	NA	NA	XXX	A+
95913-26	Nrv cndj test 13/> studies	3.56	1.76	1.76	0.14	5.46	$188.95	5.46	$188.95	XXX	A+
95913-TC	Nrv cndj test 13/> studies	0.00	3.14	NA	0.02	3.16	$109.36	NA	NA	XXX	A+
95921	Autonomic nrv parasym inervj	0.90	1.69	NA	0.05	2.64	$91.36	NA	NA	XXX	A+
95921-26	Autonomic nrv parasym inervj	0.90	0.37	0.37	0.04	1.31	$45.33	1.31	$45.33	XXX	A+
95921-TC	Autonomic nrv parasym inervj	0.00	1.32	NA	0.01	1.33	$46.03	NA	NA	XXX	A+ DS
95922	Autonomic nrv adrenrg inervj	0.96	1.99	NA	0.06	3.01	$104.16	NA	NA	XXX	A+
95922-26	Autonomic nrv adrenrg inervj	0.96	0.37	0.37	0.04	1.37	$47.41	1.37	$47.41	XXX	A+
95922-TC	Autonomic nrv adrenrg inervj	0.00	1.62	NA	0.02	1.64	$56.75	NA	NA	XXX	A+ PS
95923	Autonomic nrv syst funj test	0.90	2.80	NA	0.05	3.75	$129.77	NA	NA	XXX	A+
95923-26	Autonomic nrv syst funj test	0.90	0.37	0.37	0.04	1.31	$45.33	1.31	$45.33	XXX	A+
95923-TC	Autonomic nrv syst funj test	0.00	2.43	NA	0.01	2.44	$84.44	NA	NA	XXX	A+ PS
95924	Ans parasymp & symp w/tilt	1.73	2.62	NA	0.11	4.46	$154.34	NA	NA	XXX	A+
95924-26	Ans parasymp & symp w/tilt	1.73	0.71	0.71	0.09	2.53	$87.55	2.53	$87.55	XXX	A+
95924-TC	Ans parasymp & symp w/tilt	0.00	1.91	NA	0.02	1.93	$66.79	NA	NA	XXX	A+
95925	Somatosensory testing	0.54	4.87	NA	0.08	5.49	$189.99	NA	NA	XXX	A+
95925-26	Somatosensory testing	0.54	0.26	0.26	0.04	0.84	$29.07	0.84	$29.07	XXX	A+
95925-TC	Somatosensory testing	0.00	4.61	NA	0.04	4.65	$160.92	NA	NA	XXX	A+
95926	Somatosensory testing	0.54	4.15	NA	0.06	4.75	$164.38	NA	NA	XXX	A+
95926-26	Somatosensory testing	0.54	0.25	0.25	0.02	0.81	$28.03	0.81	$28.03	XXX	A+
95926-TC	Somatosensory testing	0.00	3.90	NA	0.04	3.94	$136.35	NA	NA	XXX	A+
95927	Somatosensory testing	0.54	3.87	NA	0.06	4.47	$154.69	NA	NA	XXX	A+
95927-26	Somatosensory testing	0.54	0.22	0.22	0.02	0.78	$26.99	0.78	$26.99	XXX	A+
95927-TC	Somatosensory testing	0.00	3.65	NA	0.04	3.69	$127.70	NA	NA	XXX	A+
95928	C motor evoked uppr limbs	1.50	5.45	NA	0.10	7.05	$243.97	NA	NA	XXX	A+
95928-26	C motor evoked uppr limbs	1.50	0.74	0.74	0.08	2.32	$80.29	2.32	$80.29	XXX	A+

95928-TC	C motor evoked uppr limbs	0.00	4.71	NA	0.02	4.73	$163.69	NA	NA	XXX	A+
95929	C motor evoked lwr limbs	1.50	5.66	NA	0.09	7.25	$250.89	NA	NA	XXX	A+
95929-26	C motor evoked lwr limbs	1.50	0.75	0.75	0.07	2.32	$80.29	2.32	$80.29	XXX	A+
95929-TC	C motor evoked lwr limbs	0.00	4.91	NA	0.02	4.93	$170.61	NA	NA	XXX	A+
95930	Visual ep test cns w/i&r	0.35	1.57	NA	0.02	1.94	$67.14	NA	NA	XXX	A+
95930-26	Visual ep test cns w/i&r	0.35	0.18	0.18	0.01	0.54	$18.69	0.54	$18.69	XXX	A+
95930-TC	Visual ep test cns w/i&r	0.00	1.39	NA	0.01	1.40	$48.45	NA	NA	XXX	A+
95933	Blink reflex test	0.59	1.89	NA	0.05	2.53	$87.55	NA	NA	XXX	A+
95933-26	Blink reflex test	0.59	0.29	0.29	0.04	0.92	$31.84	0.92	$31.84	XXX	A+
95933-TC	Blink reflex test	0.00	1.60	NA	0.01	1.61	$55.72	NA	NA	XXX	A+
95937	Neuromuscular junction test	0.65	2.49	NA	0.05	3.19	$110.39	NA	NA	XXX	A+
95937-26	Neuromuscular junction test	0.65	0.32	0.32	0.04	1.01	$34.95	1.01	$34.95	XXX	A+
95937-TC	Neuromuscular junction test	0.00	2.17	NA	0.01	2.18	$75.44	NA	NA	XXX	A+
95938	Somatosensory testing	0.86	9.84	NA	0.08	10.78	$373.05	NA	NA	XXX	A+
95938-26	Somatosensory testing	0.86	0.43	0.43	0.04	1.33	$46.03	1.33	$46.03	XXX	A+
95938-TC	Somatosensory testing	0.00	9.41	NA	0.04	9.45	$327.03	NA	NA	XXX	A+
95939	C motor evoked upr&lwr limbs	2.25	13.89	NA	0.15	16.29	$563.73	NA	NA	XXX	A+
95939-26	C motor evoked upr&lwr limbs	2.25	1.12	1.12	0.10	3.47	$120.08	3.47	$120.08	XXX	A+
95939-TC	C motor evoked upr&lwr limbs	0.00	12.77	NA	0.05	12.82	$443.65	NA	NA	XXX	A+
95940	Ionm in operatng room 15 min	0.60	NA	0.31	0.04	NA	NA	0.95	$32.88	XXX	A+ PS
95954	Eeg monitoring/giving drugs	2.45	9.40	NA	0.19	12.04	$416.66	NA	NA	XXX	A+
95954-26	Eeg monitoring/giving drugs	2.45	0.62	0.62	0.11	3.18	$110.05	3.18	$110.05	XXX	A+
95954-TC	Eeg monitoring/giving drugs	0.00	8.78	NA	0.08	8.86	$306.61	NA	NA	XXX	A+ PS
95955	Eeg during surgery	1.01	5.01	NA	0.05	6.07	$210.06	NA	NA	XXX	A+
95955-26	Eeg during surgery	1.01	0.51	0.51	0.04	1.56	$53.99	1.56	$53.99	XXX	A+
95955-TC	Eeg during surgery	0.00	4.50	NA	0.01	4.51	$156.07	NA	NA	XXX	A+ DS
95957	Eeg digital analysis	1.98	5.61	NA	0.13	7.72	$267.16	NA	NA	XXX	A+
95957-26	Eeg digital analysis	1.98	0.91	0.91	0.09	2.98	$103.13	2.98	$103.13	XXX	A+

*Please note that these calculations are based on the Medicare 2022 Conversion Factor of $34.6062 and the DRA RVU cap rates at time of publication.

A = assistant-at-surgery restriction

A+ = assistant-at-surgery restriction unless medical necessity established with documentation

B = bilateral surgery adjustment applies

C = cosurgeons payable

C+ = cosurgeons payable if medical necessity established with documentation

CP = carriers may establish RVUs and payment amounts for these services, generally on an individual basis following review of documentation such as an operative report

M = multiple surgery adjustment applies

Me = multiple endoscopy rules may apply

M+ = multiple therapy rules apply

Mtc = multiple diagnostic imaging rules apply

T = team surgeons permitted

T+ = team surgeons payable if medical necessity established with documentation

§ = indicates code is not covered by Medicare

GS = procedure must be performed under the general supervision of a physician

DS = procedure must be performed under the direct supervision of a physician

PS = procedure must be performed under the personal supervision of a physician

DRA = procedure subject to DRA limitation

Relative Value Units

CPT Code and Modifier		Description	Work RVU	Nonfacility Practice Expense RVU	Facility Practice Expense RVU	PLI RVU	Total Non-facility RVUs	Medicare Payment Nonfacility	Total Facility RVUs	Medicare Payment Facility	Global Period	Payment Policy Indicators
95957-TC		Eeg digital analysis	0.00	4.70	NA	0.04	4.74	$164.03	NA	NA	XXX	A+ GS
95958		Eeg monitoring/function test	4.24	13.94	NA	0.48	18.66	$645.75	NA	NA	XXX	A+
95958-26		Eeg monitoring/function test	4.24	2.02	2.02	0.40	6.66	$230.48	6.66	$230.48	XXX	A+
95958-TC		Eeg monitoring/function test	0.00	11.92	NA	0.08	12.00	$415.27	NA	NA	XXX	A+ PS
95961		Electrode stimulation brain	2.97	6.35	NA	0.31	9.63	$333.26	NA	NA	XXX	A+
95961-26		Electrode stimulation brain	2.97	1.47	1.47	0.29	4.73	$163.69	4.73	$163.69	XXX	A+
95961-TC		Electrode stimulation brain	0.00	4.88	NA	0.02	4.90	$169.57	NA	NA	XXX	A+ PS
95962		Electrode stim brain add-on	3.21	4.43	NA	0.27	7.91	$273.74	NA	NA	ZZZ	A+
95962-26		Electrode stim brain add-on	3.21	1.60	1.60	0.25	5.06	$175.11	5.06	$175.11	ZZZ	A+
95962-TC		Electrode stim brain add-on	0.00	2.83	NA	0.02	2.85	$98.63	NA	NA	ZZZ	A+ PS
95965	CP	Meg spontaneous	0.00	0.00	NA	0.00	0.00	$0.00	NA	NA	XXX	A+
95965-26		Meg spontaneous	7.99	3.80	3.80	0.35	12.14	$420.12	12.14	$420.12	XXX	A+
95965-TC	CP	Meg spontaneous	0.00	0.00	NA	0.00	0.00	$0.00	NA	NA	XXX	A+
95966	CP	Meg evoked single	0.00	0.00	NA	0.00	0.00	$0.00	NA	NA	XXX	A+
95966-26		Meg evoked single	3.99	2.00	2.00	0.19	6.18	$213.87	6.18	$213.87	XXX	A+
95966-TC	CP	Meg evoked single	0.00	0.00	NA	0.00	0.00	$0.00	NA	NA	XXX	A+
95967	CP	Meg evoked each addl	0.00	0.00	NA	0.00	0.00	$0.00	NA	NA	ZZZ	A+
95967-26		Meg evoked each addl	3.49	1.75	1.75	0.17	5.41	$187.22	5.41	$187.22	ZZZ	A+
95967-TC	CP	Meg evoked each addl	0.00	0.00	NA	0.00	0.00	$0.00	NA	NA	ZZZ	A+
95970		Alys npgt w/o prgrmg	0.35	0.17	0.16	0.04	0.56	$19.38	0.55	$19.03	XXX	A+
95971		Alys smpl sp/pn npgt w/prgrm	0.78	0.58	0.31	0.08	1.44	$49.83	1.17	$40.49	XXX	A+
95972		Alys cplx sp/pn npgt w/prgrm	0.80	0.76	0.30	0.09	1.65	$57.10	1.19	$41.18	XXX	A+
95976		Alys smpl cn npgt prgrmg	0.73	0.38	0.36	0.08	1.19	$41.18	1.17	$40.49	XXX	A+
95977		Alys cplx cn npgt prgrmg	0.97	0.50	0.47	0.10	1.57	$54.33	1.54	$53.29	XXX	A+
95980		Io anal gast n-stim init	0.80	NA	0.35	0.19	NA	NA	1.34	$46.37	XXX	A+
95981		Io anal gast n-stim subsq	0.30	0.78	0.17	0.05	1.13	$39.11	0.52	$18.00	XXX	A+
95982		Io ga n-stim subsq w/reprog	0.65	0.97	0.31	0.11	1.73	$59.87	1.07	$37.03	XXX	A+
95983		Alys brn npgt prgrmg 15 min	0.91	0.49	0.46	0.10	1.50	$51.91	1.47	$50.87	XXX	A+
95984		Alys brn npgt prgrmg addl 15	0.80	0.42	0.40	0.09	1.31	$45.33	1.29	$44.64	ZZZ	A+
95990		Spin/brain pump refil & main	0.00	2.65	NA	0.04	2.69	$93.09	NA	NA	XXX	A+
95991		Spin/brain pump refil & main	0.77	2.40	0.32	0.09	3.26	$112.82	1.18	$40.84	XXX	A+
95992		Canalith repositioning proc	0.75	0.49	0.28	0.04	1.28	$44.30	1.07	$37.03	XXX	A+
95999	CP	Neurological procedure	0.00	0.00	0.00	0.00	0.00	$0.00	0.00	$0.00	XXX	A+

96000		Motion analysis video/3d	1.80	NA	0.62	0.09	NA	NA	2.51	$86.86	XXX	A+
96001		Motion test w/ft press meas	2.15	NA	0.96	0.17	NA	NA	3.28	$113.51	XXX	A+
96002		Dynamic surface emg	0.41	NA	0.19	0.04	NA	NA	0.64	$22.15	XXX	A+
96003		Dynamic fine wire emg	0.37	NA	0.11	0.01	NA	NA	0.49	$16.96	XXX	A+
96004		Phys review of motion tests	2.14	0.92	0.92	0.18	3.24	$112.12	3.24	$112.12	XXX	A+
96020	CP	Functional brain mapping	0.00	0.00	NA	0.00	0.00	$0.00	NA	NA	XXX	A+
96020-26		Functional brain mapping	3.43	1.10	1.10	0.12	4.65	$160.92	4.65	$160.92	XXX	A+
96020-TC	CP	Functional brain mapping	0.00	0.00	NA	0.00	0.00	$0.00	NA	NA	XXX	A+ PS
96040	§	Genetic counseling 30 min	0.00	1.35	NA	0.04	1.39	$48.10	NA	NA	XXX	
96105		Assessment of aphasia	1.75	1.04	NA	0.10	2.89	$100.01	NA	NA	XXX	A+
96110	§	Developmental screen w/score	0.00	0.30	NA	0.01	0.31	$10.73	NA	NA	XXX	
96112		Devel tst phys/qhp 1st hr	2.56	1.05	1.01	0.12	3.73	$129.08	3.69	$127.70	XXX	A+
96113		Devel tst phys/qhp ea addl	1.16	0.53	0.42	0.07	1.76	$60.91	1.65	$57.10	ZZZ	A+
96116		Nubhvl xm phys/qhp 1st hr	1.86	0.82	0.44	0.09	2.77	$95.86	2.39	$82.71	XXX	A+
96121		Nubhvl xm phy/qhp ea addl hr	1.71	0.52	0.28	0.08	2.31	$79.94	2.07	$71.63	ZZZ	A+
96125		Cognitive test by hc pro	1.70	1.27	NA	0.09	3.06	$105.89	NA	NA	XXX	A+ Mt
96127		Brief emotional/behav assmt	0.00	0.13	NA	0.01	0.14	$4.84	NA	NA	XXX	A+
96130		Psycl tst eval phys/qhp 1st	2.56	0.84	0.49	0.11	3.51	$121.47	3.16	$109.36	XXX	A+
96131		Psycl tst eval phys/qhp ea	1.96	0.56	0.27	0.09	2.61	$90.32	2.32	$80.29	ZZZ	A+
96132		Nrpsyc tst eval phys/qhp 1st	2.56	1.16	0.42	0.11	3.83	$132.54	3.09	$106.93	XXX	A+
96133		Nrpsyc tst eval phys/qhp ea	1.96	0.93	0.26	0.08	2.97	$102.78	2.30	$79.59	ZZZ	A+
96136		Psycl/nrpsyc tst phy/qhp 1st	0.55	0.71	0.11	0.04	1.30	$44.99	0.70	$24.22	XXX	A+
96137		Psycl/nrpsyc tst phy/qhp ea	0.46	0.69	0.06	0.02	1.17	$40.49	0.54	$18.69	ZZZ	A+
96138		Psycl/nrpsyc tech 1st	0.00	1.01	NA	0.01	1.02	$35.30	NA	NA	XXX	A+
96139		Psycl/nrpsyc tst tech ea	0.00	1.03	NA	0.01	1.04	$35.99	NA	NA	ZZZ	A+
96146		Psycl/nrpsyc tst auto result	0.00	0.05	NA	0.01	0.06	$2.08	NA	NA	XXX	A+
96156		Hlth bhv assmt/reassessment	2.10	0.63	0.32	0.09	2.82	$97.59	2.51	$86.86	XXX	A+
96158		Hlth bhv ivntj indiv 1st 30	1.45	0.42	0.20	0.07	1.94	$67.14	1.72	$59.52	XXX	A+

*Please note that these calculations are based on the Medicare 2022 Conversion Factor of $34.6062 and the DRA RVU cap rates at time of publication.

A = assistant-at-surgery restriction
A+ = assistant-at-surgery restriction unless medical necessity established with documentation
B = bilateral surgery adjustment applies
C = cosurgeons payable
C+ = cosurgeons payable if medical necessity established with documentation
CP = carriers may establish RVUs and payment amounts for these services, generally on an individual basis following review of documentation such as an operative report
M = multiple surgery adjustment applies
Me = multiple endoscopy rules may apply
M+ = multiple therapy rules apply
Mtc = multiple diagnostic imaging rules apply
T = team surgeons permitted
T+ = team surgeons payable if medical necessity established with documentation
§ = indicates code is not covered by Medicare
GS = procedure must be performed under the general supervision of a physician
DS = procedure must be performed under the direct supervision of a physician
PS = procedure must be performed under the personal supervision of a physician
DRA = procedure subject to DRA limitation

Relative Value Units

CPT Code and Modifier		Description	Work RVU	Nonfacility Practice Expense RVU	Facility Practice Expense RVU	PLI RVU	Total Non-facility RVUs	Medicare Payment Nonfacility	Total Facility RVUs	Medicare Payment Facility	Global Period	Payment Policy Indicators
96159		Hlth bhv ivntj indiv ea addl	0.50	0.14	0.06	0.02	0.66	$22.84	0.58	$20.07	ZZZ	A+
96160		Pt-focused hlth risk assmt	0.00	0.08	NA	0.00	0.08	$2.77	NA	NA	ZZZ	
96161		Caregiver health risk assmt	0.00	0.08	NA	0.00	0.08	$2.77	NA	NA	ZZZ	
96164		Hlth bhv ivntj grp 1st 30	0.21	0.07	0.04	0.01	0.29	$10.04	0.26	$9.00	XXX	A+
96165		Hlth bhv ivntj grp ea addl	0.10	0.03	0.02	0.00	0.13	$4.50	0.12	$4.15	ZZZ	A+
96167		Hlth bhv ivntj fam 1st 30	1.55	0.44	0.21	0.07	2.06	$71.29	1.83	$63.33	XXX	A+
96168		Hlth bhv ivntj fam ea addl	0.55	0.16	0.07	0.02	0.73	$25.26	0.64	$22.15	ZZZ	A+
96170	§	Hlth bhv ivntj fam wo pt 1st	1.50	0.71	0.58	0.11	2.32	$80.29	2.19	$75.79	XXX	
96171	§	Hlth bhv ivntj fam w/o pt ea	0.54	0.26	0.21	0.04	0.84	$29.07	0.79	$27.34	ZZZ	
96360		Hydration iv infusion init	0.17	0.82	NA	0.02	1.01	$34.95	NA	NA	XXX	A+
96361		Hydrate iv infusion add-on	0.09	0.28	NA	0.01	0.38	$13.15	NA	NA	ZZZ	A+
96365		Ther/proph/diag iv inf init	0.21	1.75	NA	0.04	2.00	$69.21	NA	NA	XXX	A+
96366		Ther/proph/diag iv inf addon	0.18	0.43	NA	0.01	0.62	$21.46	NA	NA	ZZZ	A+
96367		Tx/proph/dg addl seq iv inf	0.19	0.68	NA	0.02	0.89	$30.80	NA	NA	ZZZ	A+
96368		Ther/diag concurrent inf	0.17	0.42	NA	0.01	0.60	$20.76	NA	NA	ZZZ	A+
96369		Sc ther infusion up to 1 hr	0.21	4.04	NA	0.02	4.27	$147.77	NA	NA	XXX	A+
96370		Sc ther infusion addl hr	0.18	0.26	NA	0.01	0.45	$15.57	NA	NA	ZZZ	A+
96371		Sc ther infusion reset pump	0.00	1.73	NA	0.00	1.73	$59.87	NA	NA	ZZZ	A+
96372		Ther/proph/diag inj sc/im	0.17	0.24	NA	0.01	0.42	$14.53	NA	NA	XXX	A+
96373		Ther/proph/diag inj ia	0.17	0.35	NA	0.01	0.53	$18.34	NA	NA	XXX	A+
96374		Ther/proph/diag inj iv push	0.18	0.96	NA	0.02	1.16	$40.14	NA	NA	XXX	A+
96375		Tx/pro/dx inj new drug addon	0.10	0.36	NA	0.01	0.47	$16.26	NA	NA	ZZZ	A+
96377		Applicaton on-body injector	0.17	0.38	NA	0.01	0.56	$19.38	NA	NA	XXX	A+
96379	CP	Ther/prop/diag inj/inf proc	0.00	0.00	0.00	0.00	0.00	$0.00	0.00	$0.00	XXX	A+
96401		Chemo anti-neopl sq/im	0.21	1.99	NA	0.05	2.25	$77.86	NA	NA	XXX	A+
96402		Chemo hormon antineopl sq/im	0.19	0.77	NA	0.02	0.98	$33.91	NA	NA	XXX	A+
96405		Chemo intralesional up to 7	0.52	1.95	0.28	0.04	2.51	$86.86	0.84	$29.07	000	A M
96406		Chemo intralesional over 7	0.80	3.10	0.44	0.07	3.97	$137.39	1.31	$45.33	000	A M
96409		Chemo iv push sngl drug	0.24	2.80	NA	0.08	3.12	$107.97	NA	NA	XXX	A+
96411		Chemo iv push addl drug	0.20	1.46	NA	0.04	1.70	$58.83	NA	NA	ZZZ	A+
96413		Chemo iv infusion 1 hr	0.28	3.68	NA	0.09	4.05	$140.16	NA	NA	XXX	A+
96415		Chemo iv infusion addl hr	0.19	0.65	NA	0.02	0.86	$29.76	NA	NA	ZZZ	A+
96416		Chemo prolong infuse w/pump	0.21	3.68	NA	0.08	3.97	$137.39	NA	NA	XXX	A+

96417		Chemo iv infus each addl seq	0.21	1.72	NA	0.04	1.97	$68.17	NA	NA	ZZZ	A+
96420		Chemo ia push tecnique	0.17	2.95	NA	0.08	3.20	$110.74	NA	NA	XXX	A+
96422		Chemo ia infusion up to 1 hr	0.17	4.60	NA	0.10	4.87	$168.53	NA	NA	XXX	A+
96423		Chemo ia infuse each addl hr	0.17	2.03	NA	0.05	2.25	$77.86	NA	NA	ZZZ	A+
96425		Chemotherapy infusion method	0.17	4.96	NA	0.11	5.24	$181.34	NA	NA	XXX	A+
96440		Chemotherapy intracavitary	2.12	21.03	1.65	0.12	23.27	$805.29	3.89	$134.62	000	A+
96446		Chemotx admn prtl cavity	0.37	5.31	0.21	0.21	5.89	$203.83	0.79	$27.34	XXX	A+
96450		Chemotherapy into cns	1.53	3.37	0.59	0.12	5.02	$173.72	2.24	$77.52	000	A+
96521		Refill/maint portable pump	0.21	3.81	NA	0.09	4.11	$142.23	NA	NA	XXX	A+
96522		Refill/maint pump/resvr syst	0.21	3.32	NA	0.09	3.62	$125.27	NA	NA	XXX	A+
96523		Irrig drug delivery device	0.04	0.73	NA	0.02	0.79	$27.34	NA	NA	XXX	A+
96542		Chemotherapy injection	0.75	3.11	0.42	0.07	3.93	$136.00	1.24	$42.91	XXX	A+
96549	CP	Chemotherapy unspecified	0.00	0.00	0.00	0.00	0.00	$0.00	0.00	$0.00	XXX	A+
96567		Pdt dstr prmlg les skn	0.00	4.28	NA	0.01	4.29	$148.46	NA	NA	XXX	A+
96570		Photodynmc tx 30 min add-on	1.10	0.32	0.32	0.09	1.51	$52.26	1.51	$52.26	ZZZ	A
96571		Photodynamic tx addl 15 min	0.55	0.16	0.16	0.04	0.75	$25.95	0.75	$25.95	ZZZ	A
96573		Pdt dstr prmlg les phys/qhp	0.48	6.47	NA	0.02	6.97	$241.21	NA	NA	000	A+
96574		Dbrdmt prmlg les w/pdt	1.01	7.46	NA	0.04	8.51	$294.50	NA	NA	000	A+
96900		Ultraviolet light therapy	0.00	0.70	NA	0.01	0.71	$24.57	NA	NA	XXX	A+
96902	§	Trichogram	0.41	0.23	0.16	0.04	0.68	$23.53	0.61	$21.11	XXX	
96904		Whole body photography	0.00	2.11	NA	0.01	2.12	$73.37	NA	NA	XXX	A+
96910		Photochemotherapy with uv-b	0.00	3.48	NA	0.02	3.50	$121.12	NA	NA	XXX	A+
96912		Photochemotherapy with uv-a	0.00	2.99	NA	0.01	3.00	$103.82	NA	NA	XXX	A+
96913		Photochemotherapy uv-a or b	0.00	4.48	NA	0.02	4.50	$155.73	NA	NA	XXX	A+
96920		Laser tx skin < 250 sq cm	1.15	3.47	0.66	0.05	4.67	$161.61	1.86	$64.37	000	A M
96921		Laser tx skin 250-500 sq cm	1.30	3.75	0.74	0.05	5.10	$176.49	2.09	$72.33	000	A M
96922		Laser tx skin >500 sq cm	2.10	4.75	1.19	0.09	6.94	$240.17	3.38	$116.97	000	A M
96931		Rcm celulr subcelulr img skn	0.80	4.26	NA	0.05	5.11	$176.84	NA	NA	XXX	A+ DS

*Please note that these calculations are based on the Medicare 2022 Conversion Factor of $34.6062 and the DRA RVU cap rates at time of publication.

A = assistant-at-surgery restriction
A+ = assistant-at-surgery restriction unless medical necessity established with documentation
B = bilateral surgery adjustment applies
C = cosurgeons payable
C+ = cosurgeons payable if medical necessity established with documentation
CP = carriers may establish RVUs and payment amounts for these services, generally on an individual basis following review of documentation such as an operative report
M = multiple surgery adjustment applies
Me = multiple endoscopy rules may apply
M+ = multiple therapy rules apply
Mtc = multiple diagnostic imaging rules apply
T = team surgeons permitted
T+ = team surgeons payable if medical necessity established with documentation
§ = indicates code is not covered by Medicare
GS = procedure must be performed under the general supervision of a physician
DS = procedure must be performed under the direct supervision of a physician
PS = procedure must be performed under the personal supervision of a physician
DRA = procedure subject to DRA limitation

Relative Value Units

CPT Code and Modifier		Description	Work RVU	Nonfacility Practice Expense RVU	Facility Practice Expense RVU	PLI RVU	Total Non-facility RVUs	Medicare Payment Nonfacility	Total Facility RVUs	Medicare Payment Facility	Global Period	Payment Policy Indicators
96932		Rcm celulr subcelulr img skn	0.00	3.81	NA	0.01	3.82	$132.20	NA	NA	XXX	A+ DS
96933		Rcm celulr subcelulr img skn	0.80	0.45	NA	0.04	1.29	$44.64	NA	NA	XXX	A+
96934		Rcm celulr subcelulr img skn	0.76	2.76	NA	0.04	3.56	$123.20	NA	NA	ZZZ	A+ DS
96935		Rcm celulr subcelulr img skn	0.00	2.32	NA	0.00	2.32	$80.29	NA	NA	ZZZ	A+ DS
96936		Rcm celulr subcelulr img skn	0.76	0.44	NA	0.04	1.24	$42.91	NA	NA	ZZZ	A+
96999	CP	Dermatological procedure	0.00	0.00	0.00	0.00	0.00	$0.00	0.00	$0.00	XXX	A+
97010	§	Hot or cold packs therapy	0.06	0.11	NA	0.01	0.18	$6.23	NA	NA	XXX	
97012		Mechanical traction therapy	0.25	0.16	NA	0.01	0.42	$14.53	NA	NA	XXX	A+ Mt
97014	§	Electric stimulation therapy	0.18	0.18	NA	0.01	0.37	$12.80	NA	NA	XXX	
97016		Vasopneumatic device therapy	0.18	0.16	NA	0.01	0.35	$12.11	NA	NA	XXX	A+ Mt
97018		Paraffin bath therapy	0.06	0.10	NA	0.01	0.17	$5.88	NA	NA	XXX	A+ Mt
97022		Whirlpool therapy	0.17	0.33	NA	0.01	0.51	$17.65	NA	NA	XXX	A+ Mt
97024		Diathermy eg microwave	0.06	0.14	NA	0.01	0.21	$7.27	NA	NA	XXX	A+ Mt
97026		Infrared therapy	0.06	0.12	NA	0.01	0.19	$6.58	NA	NA	XXX	A+ Mt
97028		Ultraviolet therapy	0.08	0.15	NA	0.01	0.24	$8.31	NA	NA	XXX	A+ Mt
97032		Electrical stimulation	0.25	0.17	NA	0.01	0.43	$14.88	NA	NA	XXX	A+ Mt
97033		Electric current therapy	0.26	0.31	NA	0.01	0.58	$20.07	NA	NA	XXX	A+ Mt
97034		Contrast bath therapy	0.21	0.21	NA	0.01	0.43	$14.88	NA	NA	XXX	A+ Mt
97035		Ultrasound therapy	0.21	0.20	NA	0.01	0.42	$14.53	NA	NA	XXX	A+ Mt
97036		Hydrotherapy	0.28	0.72	NA	0.01	1.01	$34.95	NA	NA	XXX	A+ Mt
97039	CP	Physical therapy treatment	0.00	0.00	0.00	0.00	0.00	$0.00	0.00	$0.00	XXX	A+
97110		Therapeutic exercises	0.45	0.40	NA	0.02	0.87	$30.11	NA	NA	XXX	A+ Mt
97112		Neuromuscular reeducation	0.50	0.49	NA	0.02	1.01	$34.95	NA	NA	XXX	A+ Mt
97113		Aquatic therapy/exercises	0.48	0.59	NA	0.02	1.09	$37.72	NA	NA	XXX	A+ Mt
97116		Gait training therapy	0.45	0.40	NA	0.02	0.87	$30.11	NA	NA	XXX	A+ Mt
97124		Massage therapy	0.35	0.52	NA	0.01	0.88	$30.45	NA	NA	XXX	A+ Mt
97129		Ther ivntj 1st 15 min	0.50	0.15	0.15	0.02	0.67	$23.19	0.67	$23.19	XXX	A+
97130		Ther ivntj ea addl 15 min	0.48	0.15	0.14	0.02	0.65	$22.49	0.64	$22.15	ZZZ	A+
97139	CP	Physical medicine procedure	0.00	0.00	0.00	0.00	0.00	$0.00	0.00	$0.00	XXX	A+
97140		Manual therapy 1/> regions	0.43	0.35	NA	0.02	0.80	$27.68	NA	NA	XXX	A+ Mt
97150		Group therapeutic procedures	0.29	0.22	NA	0.01	0.52	$18.00	NA	NA	XXX	A+ Mt
97151	CP	Bhv id assmt by phys/qhp	0.00	0.00	0.00	0.00	0.00	$0.00	0.00	$0.00	XXX	A+
97152	CP	Bhv id suprt assmt by 1 tech	0.00	0.00	0.00	0.00	0.00	$0.00	0.00	$0.00	XXX	A+

97153	CP	Adaptive behavior tx by tech	0.00	0.00	0.00	0.00	0.00	$0.00	0.00	$0.00	XXX	A+
97154	CP	Grp adapt bhv tx by tech	0.00	0.00	0.00	0.00	0.00	$0.00	0.00	$0.00	XXX	A+
97155	CP	Adapt behavior tx phys/qhp	0.00	0.00	0.00	0.00	0.00	$0.00	0.00	$0.00	XXX	A+
97156	CP	Fam adapt bhv tx gdn phy/qhp	0.00	0.00	0.00	0.00	0.00	$0.00	0.00	$0.00	XXX	A+
97157	CP	Mult fam adapt bhv tx gdn	0.00	0.00	0.00	0.00	0.00	$0.00	0.00	$0.00	XXX	A+
97158	CP	Grp adapt bhv tx by phy/qhp	0.00	0.00	0.00	0.00	0.00	$0.00	0.00	$0.00	XXX	A+
97161		Pt eval low complex 20 min	1.54	1.35	NA	0.07	2.96	$102.43	NA	NA	XXX	A+ Mt
97162		Pt eval mod complex 30 min	1.54	1.35	NA	0.07	2.96	$102.43	NA	NA	XXX	A+ Mt
97163		Pt eval high complex 45 min	1.54	1.35	NA	0.07	2.96	$102.43	NA	NA	XXX	A+ Mt
97164		Pt re-eval est plan care	0.96	1.04	NA	0.04	2.04	$70.60	NA	NA	XXX	A+ Mt
97165		Ot eval low complex 30 min	1.54	1.37	NA	0.07	2.98	$103.13	NA	NA	XXX	A+ Mt
97166		Ot eval mod complex 45 min	1.54	1.37	NA	0.07	2.98	$103.13	NA	NA	XXX	A+ Mt
97167		Ot eval high complex 60 min	1.54	1.37	NA	0.07	2.98	$103.13	NA	NA	XXX	A+ Mt
97168		Ot re-eval est plan care	0.96	1.05	NA	0.04	2.05	$70.94	NA	NA	XXX	A+ Mt
97530		Therapeutic activities	0.44	0.64	NA	0.02	1.10	$38.07	NA	NA	XXX	A+ Mt
97533		Sensory integration	0.48	1.41	NA	0.02	1.91	$66.10	NA	NA	XXX	A+ Mt
97535		Self care mngment training	0.45	0.50	NA	0.02	0.97	$33.57	NA	NA	XXX	A+ Mt
97537		Community/work reintegration	0.48	0.44	NA	0.02	0.94	$32.53	NA	NA	XXX	A+ Mt
97542		Wheelchair mngment training	0.48	0.44	NA	0.02	0.94	$32.53	NA	NA	XXX	A+ Mt
97545		Work hardening	0.00	0.00	0.00	0.00	0.00	$0.00	0.00	$0.00	XXX	A+
97546		Work hardening add-on	0.00	0.00	0.00	0.00	0.00	$0.00	0.00	$0.00	ZZZ	A+
97597		Rmvl devital tis 20 cm/<	0.77	2.19	0.22	0.07	3.03	$104.86	1.06	$36.68	000	A+
97598		Rmvl devital tis addl 20cm/<	0.50	0.78	0.17	0.07	1.35	$46.72	0.74	$25.61	ZZZ	A+
97605		Neg press wound tx <=50 cm	0.55	0.68	0.16	0.02	1.25	$43.26	0.73	$25.26	XXX	A+
97606		Neg press wound tx >50 cm	0.60	0.86	0.18	0.02	1.48	$51.22	0.80	$27.68	XXX	A+
97607		Neg press wnd tx <=50 sq cm	0.41	10.98	0.17	0.08	11.47	$396.93	0.66	$22.84	XXX	A+
97608		Neg press wound tx >50 cm	0.46	10.77	0.19	0.09	11.32	$391.74	0.74	$25.61	XXX	A+
97610		Low frequency non-thermal us	0.40	13.14	0.12	0.01	13.55	$468.91	0.53	$18.34	XXX	A+

*Please note that these calculations are based on the Medicare 2022 Conversion Factor of $34.6062 and the DRA RVU cap rates at time of publication.

A = assistant-at-surgery restriction
A+ = assistant-at-surgery restriction unless medical necessity established with documentation
B = bilateral surgery adjustment applies
C = cosurgeons payable
C+ = cosurgeons payable if medical necessity established with documentation
CP = carriers may establish RVUs and payment amounts for these services, generally on an individual basis following review of documentation such as an operative report
M = multiple surgery adjustment applies
Me = multiple endoscopy rules may apply
M+ = multiple therapy rules apply
Mtc = multiple diagnostic imaging rules apply
T = team surgeons permitted
T+ = team surgeons payable if medical necessity established with documentation
§ = indicates code is not covered by Medicare
GS = procedure must be performed under the general supervision of a physician
DS = procedure must be performed under the direct supervision of a physician
PS = procedure must be performed under the personal supervision of a physician
DRA = procedure subject to DRA limitation

Relative Value Units

CPT Code and Modifier		Description	Work RVU	Nonfacility Practice Expense RVU	Facility Practice Expense RVU	PLI RVU	Total Non-facility RVUs	Medicare Payment Nonfacility	Total Facility RVUs	Medicare Payment Facility	Global Period	Payment Policy Indicators
97750		Physical performance test	0.45	0.52	NA	0.02	0.99	$34.26	NA	NA	XXX	A+ Mt
97755		Assistive technology assess	0.62	0.48	NA	0.02	1.12	$38.76	NA	NA	XXX	A+ Mt
97760		Orthotic mgmt&traing 1st enc	0.50	0.92	NA	0.02	1.44	$49.83	NA	NA	XXX	A+ Mt
97761		Prosthetic traing 1st enc	0.50	0.71	NA	0.02	1.23	$42.57	NA	NA	XXX	A+ Mt
97763		Orthc/prostc mgmt sbsq enc	0.48	1.10	NA	0.02	1.60	$55.37	NA	NA	XXX	A+ Mt
97799	CP	Physical medicine procedure	0.00	0.00	0.00	0.00	0.00	$0.00	0.00	$0.00	XXX	A+
97802		Medical nutrition indiv in	0.53	0.53	0.40	0.02	1.08	$37.37	0.95	$32.88	XXX	A+
97803		Med nutrition indiv subseq	0.45	0.47	0.34	0.02	0.94	$32.53	0.81	$28.03	XXX	A+
97804		Medical nutrition group	0.25	0.24	0.19	0.01	0.50	$17.30	0.45	$15.57	XXX	A+
97810		Acupunct w/o stimul 15 min	0.60	0.52	0.28	0.04	1.16	$40.14	0.92	$31.84	XXX	A
97811		Acupunct w/o stimul addl 15m	0.50	0.33	0.24	0.04	0.87	$30.11	0.78	$26.99	ZZZ	A
97813		Acupunct w/stimul 15 min	0.65	0.67	0.30	0.04	1.36	$47.06	0.99	$34.26	XXX	A
97814		Acupunct w/stimul addl 15m	0.55	0.53	0.26	0.04	1.12	$38.76	0.85	$29.42	ZZZ	A
98925		Osteopath manj 1-2 regions	0.46	0.43	0.19	0.04	0.93	$32.18	0.69	$23.88	000	A+
98926		Osteopath manj 3-4 regions	0.71	0.56	0.28	0.04	1.31	$45.33	1.03	$35.64	000	A+
98927		Osteopath manj 5-6 regions	0.96	0.70	0.35	0.05	1.71	$59.18	1.36	$47.06	000	A+
98928		Osteopath manj 7-8 regions	1.21	0.82	0.44	0.07	2.10	$72.67	1.72	$59.52	000	A+
98929		Osteopath manj 9-10 regions	1.46	0.94	0.52	0.09	2.49	$86.17	2.07	$71.63	000	A+
98940		Chiropract manj 1-2 regions	0.46	0.34	0.17	0.01	0.81	$28.03	0.64	$22.15	000	A+
98941		Chiropract manj 3-4 regions	0.71	0.44	0.27	0.01	1.16	$40.14	0.99	$34.26	000	A+
98942		Chiropractic manj 5 regions	0.96	0.54	0.36	0.02	1.52	$52.60	1.34	$46.37	000	A+
98943	§	Chiropract manj xtrspinl 1/>	0.46	0.28	0.18	0.04	0.78	$26.99	0.68	$23.53	XXX	
98960	§	Self-mgmt educ & train 1 pt	0.00	0.81	NA	0.04	0.85	$29.42	NA	NA	XXX	
98961	§	Self-mgmt educ/train 2-4 pt	0.00	0.39	NA	0.01	0.40	$13.84	NA	NA	XXX	
98962	§	Self-mgmt educ/train 5-8 pt	0.00	0.29	NA	0.01	0.30	$10.38	NA	NA	XXX	
98966		Hc pro phone call 5-10 min	0.25	0.12	0.07	0.01	0.38	$13.15	0.33	$11.42	XXX	A+
98967		Hc pro phone call 11-20 min	0.50	0.18	0.12	0.02	0.70	$24.22	0.64	$22.15	XXX	A+
98968		Hc pro phone call 21-30 min	0.75	0.20	0.14	0.04	0.99	$34.26	0.93	$32.18	XXX	A+
98970		Qnhp ol dig assmt&mgmt 5-10	0.25	0.08	0.08	0.01	0.34	$11.77	0.34	$11.77	XXX	A+
98971		Qnhp ol dig assmt&mgmt 11-20	0.44	0.14	0.13	0.02	0.60	$20.76	0.59	$20.42	XXX	A+
98972		Qnhp ol dig assmt&mgmt 21+	0.69	0.20	0.19	0.04	0.93	$32.18	0.92	$31.84	XXX	A+
98975		Rem ther mntr 1st setup&edu	0.00	0.54	NA	0.02	0.56	$19.38	NA	NA	XXX	A+
98976		Rem ther mntr dev sply resp	0.00	1.60	NA	0.01	1.61	$55.72	NA	NA	XXX	A+

98977		Rem ther mntr dv sply mscskl	0.00	1.60	NA	0.01	1.61	$55.72	NA	NA	XXX	A+
98980		Rem ther mntr 1st 20 min	0.62	0.79	0.25	0.04	1.45	$50.18	0.91	$31.49	XXX	A+
98981		Rem ther mntr ea addl 20 min	0.61	0.52	0.25	0.05	1.18	$40.84	0.91	$31.49	ZZZ	A+
99082	CP	Unusual physician travel	0.00	0.00	0.00	0.00	0.00	$0.00	0.00	$0.00	XXX	A+
99091		Collj & interpj data ea 30 d	1.10	0.44	0.44	0.09	1.63	$56.41	1.63	$56.41	XXX	A+
99151		Mod sed same phys/qhp <5 yrs	0.50	1.52	0.19	0.04	2.06	$71.29	0.73	$25.26	XXX	
99152		Mod sed same phys/qhp 5/>yrs	0.25	1.22	0.08	0.04	1.51	$52.26	0.37	$12.80	XXX	
99153		Mod sed same phys/qhp ea	0.00	0.30	NA	0.02	0.32	$11.07	NA	NA	ZZZ	
99155		Mod sed oth phys/qhp <5 yrs	1.90	NA	0.32	0.21	NA	NA	2.43	$84.09	XXX	
99156		Mod sed oth phys/qhp 5/>yrs	1.65	NA	0.40	0.18	NA	NA	2.23	$77.17	XXX	
99157		Mod sed other phys/qhp ea	1.25	NA	0.46	0.11	NA	NA	1.82	$62.98	ZZZ	
99170		Anogenital exam child w imag	1.75	2.93	0.65	0.11	4.79	$165.76	2.51	$86.86	000	A M
99173	§	Visual acuity screen	0.00	0.08	NA	0.01	0.09	$3.11	NA	NA	XXX	
99174	§	Ocular instrumnt screen bil	0.00	0.16	NA	0.01	0.17	$5.88	NA	NA	XXX	
99175		Induction of vomiting	0.00	0.84	NA	0.01	0.85	$29.42	NA	NA	XXX	A+
99177	§	Ocular instrumnt screen bil	0.00	0.13	NA	0.01	0.14	$4.84	NA	NA	XXX	
99183		Hyperbaric oxygen therapy	2.11	0.78	0.78	0.25	3.14	$108.66	3.14	$108.66	XXX	A+
99184		Hypothermia ill neonate	4.50	NA	1.55	0.31	NA	NA	6.36	$220.10	XXX	A+
99188	§	App topical fluoride varnish	0.20	0.13	0.08	0.02	0.35	$12.11	0.30	$10.38	XXX	A+
99195		Phlebotomy	0.00	2.94	NA	0.07	3.01	$104.16	NA	NA	XXX	A+
99199	CP	Special service/proc/report	0.00	0.00	0.00	0.00	0.00	$0.00	0.00	$0.00	XXX	A+
99202		Office o/p new sf 15-29 min	0.93	1.12	0.41	0.09	2.14	$74.06	1.43	$49.49	XXX	A+
99203		Office o/p new low 30-44 min	1.60	1.52	0.67	0.17	3.29	$113.85	2.44	$84.44	XXX	A+
99204		Office o/p new mod 45-59 min	2.60	2.06	1.11	0.24	4.90	$169.57	3.95	$136.69	XXX	A+
99205		Office o/p new hi 60-74 min	3.50	2.66	1.54	0.32	6.48	$224.25	5.36	$185.49	XXX	A+
99211		Off/op est may x req phy/qhp	0.18	0.49	0.07	0.01	0.68	$23.53	0.26	$9.00	XXX	A+
99212		Office o/p est sf 10-19 min	0.70	0.89	0.29	0.07	1.66	$57.45	1.06	$36.68	XXX	A+
99213		Office o/p est low 20-29 min	1.30	1.26	0.55	0.10	2.66	$92.05	1.95	$67.48	XXX	A+

*Please note that these calculations are based on the Medicare 2022 Conversion Factor of $34.6062 and the DRA RVU cap rates at time of publication.

A = assistant-at-surgery restriction
A+ = assistant-at-surgery restriction unless medical necessity established with documentation
B = bilateral surgery adjustment applies
C = cosurgeons payable
C+ = cosurgeons payable if medical necessity established with documentation
CP = carriers may establish RVUs and payment amounts for these services, generally on an individual basis following review of documentation such as an operative report
M = multiple surgery adjustment applies
Me = multiple endoscopy rules may apply
M+ = multiple therapy rules apply
Mtc = multiple diagnostic imaging rules apply
T = team surgeons permitted
T+ = team surgeons payable if medical necessity established with documentation
§ = indicates code is not covered by Medicare
GS = procedure must be performed under the general supervision of a physician
DS = procedure must be performed under the direct supervision of a physician
PS = procedure must be performed under the personal supervision of a physician
DRA = procedure subject to DRA limitation

Relative Value Units

CPT Code and Modifier		Description	Work RVU	Nonfacility Practice Expense RVU	Facility Practice Expense RVU	PLI RVU	Total Non-facility RVUs	Medicare Payment Nonfacility	Total Facility RVUs	Medicare Payment Facility	Global Period	Payment Policy Indicators
99214		Office o/p est mod 30-39 min	1.92	1.71	0.82	0.12	3.75	$129.77	2.86	$98.97	XXX	A+
99215		Office o/p est hi 40-54 min	2.80	2.28	1.24	0.21	5.29	$183.07	4.25	$147.08	XXX	A+
99217		Observation care discharge	1.28	NA	0.70	0.09	NA	NA	2.07	$71.63	XXX	A+
99218		Initial observation care	1.92	NA	0.73	0.18	NA	NA	2.83	$97.94	XXX	A+
99219		Initial observation care	2.60	NA	1.03	0.20	NA	NA	3.83	$132.54	XXX	A+
99220		Initial observation care	3.56	NA	1.36	0.25	NA	NA	5.17	$178.91	XXX	A+
99221		Initial hospital care	1.92	NA	0.78	0.21	NA	NA	2.91	$100.70	XXX	A+
99222		Initial hospital care	2.61	NA	1.08	0.22	NA	NA	3.91	$135.31	XXX	A+
99223		Initial hospital care	3.86	NA	1.58	0.29	NA	NA	5.73	$198.29	XXX	A+
99224		Subsequent observation care	0.76	NA	0.30	0.07	NA	NA	1.13	$39.11	XXX	A+
99225		Subsequent observation care	1.39	NA	0.56	0.10	NA	NA	2.05	$70.94	XXX	A+
99226		Subsequent observation care	2.00	NA	0.80	0.12	NA	NA	2.92	$101.05	XXX	A+
99231		Subsequent hospital care	0.76	NA	0.29	0.07	NA	NA	1.12	$38.76	XXX	A+
99232		Subsequent hospital care	1.39	NA	0.57	0.10	NA	NA	2.06	$71.29	XXX	A+
99233		Subsequent hospital care	2.00	NA	0.82	0.14	NA	NA	2.96	$102.43	XXX	A+
99234		Observ/hosp same date	2.56	NA	0.99	0.22	NA	NA	3.77	$130.47	XXX	A+
99235		Observ/hosp same date	3.24	NA	1.30	0.24	NA	NA	4.78	$165.42	XXX	A+
99236		Observ/hosp same date	4.20	NA	1.61	0.31	NA	NA	6.12	$211.79	XXX	A+
99238		Hospital discharge day	1.28	NA	0.71	0.09	NA	NA	2.08	$71.98	XXX	A+
99239		Hospital discharge day	1.90	NA	1.02	0.12	NA	NA	3.04	$105.20	XXX	A+
99241	§	Office consultation	0.64	0.66	0.24	0.05	1.35	$46.72	0.93	$32.18	XXX	
99242	§	Office consultation	1.34	1.10	0.51	0.11	2.55	$88.25	1.96	$67.83	XXX	
99243	§	Office consultation	1.88	1.46	0.71	0.17	3.51	$121.47	2.76	$95.51	XXX	
99244	§	Office consultation	3.02	1.96	1.14	0.25	5.23	$180.99	4.41	$152.61	XXX	
99245	§	Office consultation	3.77	2.30	1.38	0.31	6.38	$220.79	5.46	$188.95	XXX	
99251	§	Inpatient consultation	1.00	NA	0.32	0.09	NA	NA	1.41	$48.79	XXX	
99252	§	Inpatient consultation	1.50	NA	0.52	0.11	NA	NA	2.13	$73.71	XXX	
99253	§	Inpatient consultation	2.27	NA	0.84	0.20	NA	NA	3.31	$114.55	XXX	
99254	§	Inpatient consultation	3.29	NA	1.23	0.25	NA	NA	4.77	$165.07	XXX	
99255	§	Inpatient consultation	4.00	NA	1.44	0.33	NA	NA	5.77	$199.68	XXX	
99281		Emergency dept visit	0.48	NA	0.11	0.05	NA	NA	0.64	$22.15	XXX	A+
99282		Emergency dept visit	0.93	NA	0.21	0.10	NA	NA	1.24	$42.91	XXX	A+
99283		Emergency dept visit	1.60	NA	0.33	0.18	NA	NA	2.11	$73.02	XXX	A+

99284		Emergency dept visit	2.74	NA	0.54	0.28	NA	NA	3.56	$123.20	XXX	A+
99285		Emergency dept visit	4.00	NA	0.75	0.42	NA	NA	5.17	$178.91	XXX	A+
99291		Critical care first hour	4.50	3.25	1.42	0.41	8.16	$282.39	6.33	$219.06	XXX	A+
99292		Critical care addl 30 min	2.25	1.10	0.72	0.21	3.56	$123.20	3.18	$110.05	ZZZ	A+
99304		Nursing facility care init	1.64	0.82	0.82	0.11	2.57	$88.94	2.57	$88.94	XXX	A+
99305		Nursing facility care init	2.35	1.22	1.22	0.14	3.71	$128.39	3.71	$128.39	XXX	A+
99306		Nursing facility care init	3.06	1.50	1.50	0.20	4.76	$164.73	4.76	$164.73	XXX	A+
99307		Nursing fac care subseq	0.76	0.45	0.45	0.05	1.26	$43.60	1.26	$43.60	XXX	A+
99308		Nursing fac care subseq	1.16	0.74	0.74	0.09	1.99	$68.87	1.99	$68.87	XXX	A+
99309		Nursing fac care subseq	1.55	0.97	0.97	0.10	2.62	$90.67	2.62	$90.67	XXX	A+
99310		Nursing fac care subseq	2.35	1.37	1.37	0.14	3.86	$133.58	3.86	$133.58	XXX	A+
99315		Nursing fac discharge day	1.28	0.72	0.72	0.09	2.09	$72.33	2.09	$72.33	XXX	A+
99316		Nursing fac discharge day	1.90	0.98	0.98	0.11	2.99	$103.47	2.99	$103.47	XXX	A+
99318		Annual nursing fac assessmnt	1.71	0.93	0.93	0.11	2.75	$95.17	2.75	$95.17	XXX	A+
99324		Domicil/r-home visit new pat	1.01	0.50	NA	0.05	1.56	$53.99	NA	NA	XXX	A+
99325		Domicil/r-home visit new pat	1.52	0.67	NA	0.09	2.28	$78.90	NA	NA	XXX	A+
99326		Domicil/r-home visit new pat	2.63	1.20	NA	0.12	3.95	$136.69	NA	NA	XXX	A+
99327		Domicil/r-home visit new pat	3.46	1.66	NA	0.20	5.32	$184.10	NA	NA	XXX	A+
99328		Domicil/r-home visit new pat	4.09	1.92	NA	0.25	6.26	$216.63	NA	NA	XXX	A+
99334		Domicil/r-home visit est pat	1.07	0.61	NA	0.07	1.75	$60.56	NA	NA	XXX	A+
99335		Domicil/r-home visit est pat	1.72	0.93	NA	0.10	2.75	$95.17	NA	NA	XXX	A+
99336		Domicil/r-home visit est pat	2.46	1.29	NA	0.14	3.89	$134.62	NA	NA	XXX	A+
99337		Domicil/r-home visit est pat	3.58	1.77	NA	0.22	5.57	$192.76	NA	NA	XXX	A+
99339	§	Domicil/r-home care supervis	1.25	0.87	NA	0.10	2.22	$76.83	NA	NA	XXX	
99340	§	Domicil/r-home care supervis	1.80	1.17	NA	0.14	3.11	$107.63	NA	NA	XXX	
99341		Home visit new patient	1.01	0.50	NA	0.05	1.56	$53.99	NA	NA	XXX	A+
99342		Home visit new patient	1.52	0.62	NA	0.08	2.22	$76.83	NA	NA	XXX	A+
99343		Home visit new patient	2.53	0.96	NA	0.12	3.61	$124.93	NA	NA	XXX	A+

*Please note that these calculations are based on the Medicare 2022 Conversion Factor of $34.6062 and the DRA RVU cap rates at time of publication.

A = assistant-at-surgery restriction

A+ = assistant-at-surgery restriction unless medical necessity established with documentation

B = bilateral surgery adjustment applies

C = cosurgeons payable

C+ = cosurgeons payable if medical necessity established with documentation

CP = carriers may establish RVUs and payment amounts for these services, generally on an individual basis following review of documentation such as an operative report

M = multiple surgery adjustment applies

Me = multiple endoscopy rules may apply

M+ = multiple therapy rules apply

Mtc = multiple diagnostic imaging rules apply

T = team surgeons permitted

T+ = team surgeons payable if medical necessity established with documentation

§ = indicates code is not covered by Medicare

GS = procedure must be performed under the general supervision of a physician

DS = procedure must be performed under the direct supervision of a physician

PS = procedure must be performed under the personal supervision of a physician

DRA = procedure subject to DRA limitation

Relative Value Units

CPT Code and Modifier		Description	Work RVU	Nonfacility Practice Expense RVU	Facility Practice Expense RVU	PLI RVU	Total Non-facility RVUs	Medicare Payment Nonfacility	Total Facility RVUs	Medicare Payment Facility	Global Period	Payment Policy Indicators
99344		Home visit new patient	3.38	1.60	NA	0.22	5.20	$179.95	NA	NA	XXX	A+
99345		Home visit new patient	4.09	1.93	NA	0.28	6.30	$218.02	NA	NA	XXX	A+
99347		Home visit est patient	1.00	0.53	NA	0.05	1.58	$54.68	NA	NA	XXX	A+
99348		Home visit est patient	1.56	0.75	NA	0.09	2.40	$83.05	NA	NA	XXX	A+
99349		Home visit est patient	2.33	1.23	NA	0.14	3.70	$128.04	NA	NA	XXX	A+
99350		Home visit est patient	3.28	1.62	NA	0.23	5.13	$177.53	NA	NA	XXX	A+
99354		Prolng svc o/p 1st hour	2.33	1.21	0.97	0.17	3.71	$128.39	3.47	$120.08	ZZZ	A+
99355		Prolng svc o/p ea addl 30	1.77	0.80	0.57	0.11	2.68	$92.74	2.45	$84.79	ZZZ	A+
99356		Prolng svc i/p/obs 1st hour	1.71	NA	0.79	0.11	NA	NA	2.61	$90.32	ZZZ	A+
99357		Prolng svc i/p/obs ea addl	1.71	NA	0.80	0.11	NA	NA	2.62	$90.67	ZZZ	A+
99358		Prolong service w/o contact	2.10	0.96	0.96	0.14	3.20	$110.74	3.20	$110.74	XXX	A+
99359		Prolong serv w/o contact add	1.00	0.47	0.47	0.09	1.56	$53.99	1.56	$53.99	ZZZ	A+
99366	§	Team conf w/pat by hc prof	0.82	0.35	0.32	0.08	1.25	$43.26	1.22	$42.22	XXX	
99367	§	Team conf w/o pat by phys	1.10	NA	0.43	0.09	NA	NA	1.62	$56.06	XXX	
99368	§	Team conf w/o pat by hc pro	0.72	NA	0.28	0.07	NA	NA	1.07	$37.03	XXX	
99374	§	Home health care supervision	1.10	0.82	0.43	0.09	2.01	$69.56	1.62	$56.06	XXX	
99375	§	Home health care supervision	1.73	1.14	0.67	0.12	2.99	$103.47	2.52	$87.21	XXX	
99377	§	Hospice care supervision	1.10	0.82	0.43	0.09	2.01	$69.56	1.62	$56.06	XXX	
99378	§	Hospice care supervision	1.73	1.14	0.67	0.12	2.99	$103.47	2.52	$87.21	XXX	
99379	§	Nursing fac care supervision	1.10	0.82	0.43	0.09	2.01	$69.56	1.62	$56.06	XXX	
99380	§	Nursing fac care supervision	1.73	1.14	0.67	0.12	2.99	$103.47	2.52	$87.21	XXX	
99381	§	Init pm e/m new pat infant	1.50	1.60	0.58	0.11	3.21	$111.09	2.19	$75.79	XXX	
99382	§	Init pm e/m new pat 1-4 yrs	1.60	1.63	0.62	0.12	3.35	$115.93	2.34	$80.98	XXX	
99383	§	Prev visit new age 5-11	1.70	1.66	0.66	0.12	3.48	$120.43	2.48	$85.82	XXX	
99384	§	Prev visit new age 12-17	2.00	1.78	0.77	0.18	3.96	$137.04	2.95	$102.09	XXX	
99385	§	Prev visit new age 18-39	1.92	1.75	0.74	0.17	3.84	$132.89	2.83	$97.94	XXX	
99386	§	Prev visit new age 40-64	2.33	1.91	0.90	0.20	4.44	$153.65	3.43	$118.70	XXX	
99387	§	Init pm e/m new pat 65+ yrs	2.50	2.09	0.97	0.21	4.80	$166.11	3.68	$127.35	XXX	
99391	§	Per pm reeval est pat infant	1.37	1.42	0.53	0.11	2.90	$100.36	2.01	$69.56	XXX	
99392	§	Prev visit est age 1-4	1.50	1.47	0.58	0.11	3.08	$106.59	2.19	$75.79	XXX	
99393	§	Prev visit est age 5-11	1.50	1.46	0.58	0.11	3.07	$106.24	2.19	$75.79	XXX	
99394	§	Prev visit est age 12-17	1.70	1.54	0.66	0.12	3.36	$116.28	2.48	$85.82	XXX	
99395	§	Prev visit est age 18-39	1.75	1.56	0.68	0.12	3.43	$118.70	2.55	$88.25	XXX	

99396	§	Prev visit est age 40-64	1.90	1.62	0.73	0.17	3.69	$127.70	2.80	$96.90	XXX	
99397	§	Per pm reeval est pat 65+ yr	2.00	1.79	0.77	0.18	3.97	$137.39	2.95	$102.09	XXX	
99401	§	Preventive counseling indiv	0.48	0.62	0.19	0.04	1.14	$39.45	0.71	$24.57	XXX	
99402	§	Preventive counseling indiv	0.98	0.82	0.38	0.09	1.89	$65.41	1.45	$50.18	XXX	
99403	§	Preventive counseling indiv	1.46	1.00	0.56	0.11	2.57	$88.94	2.13	$73.71	XXX	
99404	§	Preventive counseling indiv	1.95	1.19	0.75	0.17	3.31	$114.55	2.87	$99.32	XXX	
99406		Behav chng smoking 3-10 min	0.24	0.19	0.09	0.02	0.45	$15.57	0.35	$12.11	XXX	A+
99407		Behav chng smoking > 10 min	0.50	0.29	0.20	0.04	0.83	$28.72	0.74	$25.61	XXX	A+
99408	§	Audit/dast 15-30 min	0.65	0.34	0.25	0.05	1.04	$35.99	0.95	$32.88	XXX	
99409	§	Audit/dast over 30 min	1.30	0.59	0.50	0.11	2.00	$69.21	1.91	$66.10	XXX	
99411	§	Preventive counseling group	0.15	0.45	0.06	0.01	0.61	$21.11	0.22	$7.61	XXX	
99412	§	Preventive counseling group	0.25	0.48	0.10	0.02	0.75	$25.95	0.37	$12.80	XXX	
99415		Prolng clin staff svc 1st hr	0.00	0.29	NA	0.01	0.30	$10.38	NA	NA	ZZZ	A+
99416		Prolng clin staff svc ea add	0.00	0.17	NA	0.00	0.17	$5.88	NA	NA	ZZZ	A+
99417	§	Prolng off/op e/m ea 15 min	0.61	0.27	0.24	0.05	0.93	$32.18	0.90	$31.15	XXX	
99421		Ol dig e/m svc 5-10 min	0.25	0.17	0.11	0.02	0.44	$15.23	0.38	$13.15	XXX	A+
99422		Ol dig e/m svc 11-20 min	0.50	0.32	0.21	0.04	0.86	$29.76	0.75	$25.95	XXX	A+
99423		Ol dig e/m svc 21+ min	0.80	0.53	0.34	0.07	1.40	$48.45	1.21	$41.87	XXX	A+
99424		Prin care mgmt phys 1st 30	1.45	0.86	0.63	0.10	2.41	$83.40	2.18	$75.44	XXX	A+
99425		Prin care mgmt phys ea addl	1.00	0.66	0.44	0.08	1.74	$60.21	1.52	$52.60	ZZZ	A+
99426		Prin care mgmt staff 1st 30	1.00	0.75	0.38	0.08	1.83	$63.33	1.46	$50.53	XXX	A+
99427		Prin care mgmt staff ea addl	0.71	0.64	0.27	0.05	1.40	$48.45	1.03	$35.64	ZZZ	A+
99437		Chrnc care mgmt phys ea addl	1.00	0.69	0.43	0.08	1.77	$61.25	1.51	$52.26	ZZZ	A+
99439		Chrnc care mgmt staf ea addl	0.70	0.65	0.30	0.05	1.40	$48.45	1.05	$36.34	ZZZ	A+
99441		Phone e/m phys/qhp 5-10 min	0.70	0.89	0.29	0.05	1.64	$56.75	1.04	$35.99	XXX	A+
99442		Phone e/m phys/qhp 11-20 min	1.30	1.26	0.55	0.09	2.65	$91.71	1.94	$67.14	XXX	A+
99443		Phone e/m phys/qhp 21-30 min	1.92	1.71	0.82	0.12	3.75	$129.77	2.86	$98.97	XXX	A+
99446		Ntrprof ph1/ntrnet/ehr 5-10	0.35	0.15	0.15	0.04	0.54	$18.69	0.54	$18.69	XXX	A+

*Please note that these calculations are based on the Medicare 2022 Conversion Factor of $34.6062 and the DRA RVU cap rates at time of publication.

A = assistant-at-surgery restriction
A+ = assistant-at-surgery restriction unless medical necessity established with documentation
B = bilateral surgery adjustment applies
C = cosurgeons payable
C+ = cosurgeons payable if medical necessity established with documentation
CP = carriers may establish RVUs and payment amounts for these services, generally on an individual basis following review of documentation such as an operative report
M = multiple surgery adjustment applies
Me = multiple endoscopy rules may apply
M+ = multiple therapy rules apply
Mtc = multiple diagnostic imaging rules apply
T = team surgeons permitted
T+ = team surgeons payable if medical necessity established with documentation
§ = indicates code is not covered by Medicare
GS = procedure must be performed under the general supervision of a physician
DS = procedure must be performed under the direct supervision of a physician
PS = procedure must be performed under the personal supervision of a physician
DRA = procedure subject to DRA limitation

Relative Value Units

CPT Code and Modifier	Description	Work RVU	Nonfacility Practice Expense RVU	Facility Practice Expense RVU	PLI RVU	Total Non-facility RVUs	Medicare Payment Nonfacility	Total Facility RVUs	Medicare Payment Facility	Global Period	Payment Policy Indicators
99447	Ntrprof ph1/ntrnet/ehr 11-20	0.70	0.29	0.29	0.07	1.06	$36.68	1.06	$36.68	XXX	A+
99448	Ntrprof ph1/ntrnet/ehr 21-30	1.05	0.45	0.45	0.09	1.59	$55.02	1.59	$55.02	XXX	A+
99449	Ntrprof ph1/ntrnet/ehr 31/>	1.40	0.62	0.62	0.11	2.13	$73.71	2.13	$73.71	XXX	A+
99451	Ntrprof ph1/ntrnet/ehr 5/>	0.70	0.30	0.30	0.05	1.05	$36.34	1.05	$36.34	XXX	A+
99452	Ntrprof ph1/ntrnet/ehr rfrl	0.70	0.30	0.30	0.07	1.07	$37.03	1.07	$37.03	XXX	A+
99453	Rem mntr physiol param setup	0.00	0.54	NA	0.01	0.55	$19.03	NA	NA	XXX	A+
99454	Rem mntr physiol param dev	0.00	1.60	NA	0.01	1.61	$55.72	NA	NA	XXX	A+
99455	Work related disability exam	0.00	0.00	0.00	0.00	0.00	$0.00	0.00	$0.00	XXX	A+
99456	Disability examination	0.00	0.00	0.00	0.00	0.00	$0.00	0.00	$0.00	XXX	A+
99457	Rem physiol mntr 1st 20 min	0.61	0.80	0.25	0.04	1.45	$50.18	0.90	$31.15	XXX	A+
99458	Rem physiol mntr ea addl 20	0.61	0.53	0.25	0.04	1.18	$40.84	0.90	$31.15	ZZZ	A+
99460	Init nb em per day hosp	1.92	NA	0.71	0.12	NA	NA	2.75	$95.17	XXX	A+
99461	Init nb em per day non-fac	1.26	1.35	0.47	0.09	2.70	$93.44	1.82	$62.98	XXX	A+
99462	Sbsq nb em per day hosp	0.84	NA	0.31	0.07	NA	NA	1.22	$42.22	XXX	A+
99463	Same day nb discharge	2.13	NA	0.92	0.12	NA	NA	3.17	$109.70	XXX	A+
99464	Attendance at delivery	1.50	NA	0.56	0.10	NA	NA	2.16	$74.75	XXX	A+
99465	Nb resuscitation	2.93	NA	1.08	0.20	NA	NA	4.21	$145.69	XXX	A+
99466	Ped crit care transport	4.79	NA	1.76	0.32	NA	NA	6.87	$237.74	XXX	A+
99467	Ped crit care transport addl	2.40	NA	0.89	0.17	NA	NA	3.46	$119.74	ZZZ	A+
99468	Neonate crit care initial	18.46	NA	6.80	1.24	NA	NA	26.50	$917.06	XXX	A+
99469	Neonate crit care subsq	7.99	NA	2.95	0.54	NA	NA	11.48	$397.28	XXX	A+
99471	Ped critical care initial	15.98	NA	5.90	1.06	NA	NA	22.94	$793.87	XXX	A+
99472	Ped critical care subsq	7.99	NA	3.11	0.60	NA	NA	11.70	$404.89	XXX	A+
99473	Self-meas bp pt educaj/train	0.00	0.33	NA	0.01	0.34	$11.77	NA	NA	XXX	A+
99474	Self-meas bp 2 readg bid 30d	0.18	0.25	0.07	0.01	0.44	$15.23	0.26	$9.00	XXX	A+
99475	Ped crit care age 2-5 init	11.25	NA	4.40	0.84	NA	NA	16.49	$570.66	XXX	A+
99476	Ped crit care age 2-5 subsq	6.75	NA	2.64	0.50	NA	NA	9.89	$342.26	XXX	A+
99477	Init day hosp neonate care	7.00	NA	2.58	0.45	NA	NA	10.03	$347.10	XXX	A+
99478	Ic lbw inf < 1500 gm subsq	2.75	NA	1.02	0.19	NA	NA	3.96	$137.04	XXX	A+
99479	Ic lbw inf 1500-2500 g subsq	2.50	NA	0.93	0.18	NA	NA	3.61	$124.93	XXX	A+
99480	Ic inf pbw 2501-5000 g subsq	2.40	NA	0.89	0.17	NA	NA	3.46	$119.74	XXX	A+
99483	Assmt & care pln pt cog imp	3.80	4.13	1.65	0.25	8.18	$283.08	5.70	$197.26	XXX	A+
99484	Care mgmt svc bhvl hlth cond	0.61	0.64	0.23	0.04	1.29	$44.64	0.88	$30.45	XXX	A+

99485	§	Suprv interfacilty transport	1.50	NA	0.58	0.11	NA	NA	2.19	$75.79	XXX	
99486	§	Suprv interfac trnsport addl	1.30	NA	0.50	0.11	NA	NA	1.91	$66.10	XXX	
99487		Cplx chrnc care 1st 60 min	1.81	1.96	0.76	0.11	3.88	$134.27	2.68	$92.74	XXX	A+
99489		Cplx chrnc care ea addl 30	1.00	0.97	0.41	0.07	2.04	$70.60	1.48	$51.22	ZZZ	A+
99490		Chrnc care mgmt staff 1st 20	1.00	0.78	0.42	0.07	1.85	$64.02	1.49	$51.56	XXX	A+
99491		Chrnc care mgmt phys 1st 30	1.50	0.89	0.64	0.10	2.49	$86.17	2.24	$77.52	XXX	A+
99492		1st psyc collab care mgmt	1.88	2.45	0.73	0.11	4.44	$153.65	2.72	$94.13	XXX	A+
99493		Sbsq psyc collab care mgmt	2.05	2.13	0.82	0.12	4.30	$148.81	2.99	$103.47	XXX	A+
99494		1st/sbsq psyc collab care	0.82	0.97	0.35	0.05	1.84	$63.68	1.22	$42.22	ZZZ	A+
99495		Trans care mgmt 14 day disch	2.78	3.07	1.21	0.19	6.04	$209.02	4.18	$144.65	XXX	A+
99496		Trans care mgmt 7 day disch	3.79	4.11	1.63	0.24	8.14	$281.69	5.66	$195.87	XXX	A+
99497		Advncd care plan 30 min	1.50	0.87	0.65	0.10	2.47	$85.48	2.25	$77.86	XXX	A+
99498		Advncd care plan addl 30 min	1.40	0.65	0.63	0.09	2.14	$74.06	2.12	$73.37	ZZZ	A+
99499	CP	Unlisted e&m service	0.00	0.00	0.00	0.00	0.00	$0.00	0.00	$0.00	XXX	A+

*Please note that these calculations are based on the Medicare 2022 Conversion Factor of $34.6062 and the DRA RVU cap rates at time of publication.

A = assistant-at-surgery restriction
A+ = assistant-at-surgery restriction unless medical necessity established with documentation
B = bilateral surgery adjustment applies
C = cosurgeons payable
C+ = cosurgeons payable if medical necessity established with documentation
CP = carriers may establish RVUs and payment amounts for these services, generally on an individual basis following review of documentation such as an operative report
M = multiple surgery adjustment applies
Me = multiple endoscopy rules may apply
M+ = multiple therapy rules apply
Mtc = multiple diagnostic imaging rules apply
T = team surgeons permitted
T+ = team surgeons payable if medical necessity established with documentation
§ = indicates code is not covered by Medicare
GS = procedure must be performed under the general supervision of a physician
DS = procedure must be performed under the direct supervision of a physician
PS = procedure must be performed under the personal supervision of a physician
DRA = procedure subject to DRA limitation

Alphanumeric Coded Services (Level 2)

CPT Code and Modifier		Description	Work RVU	Nonfacility Practice Expense RVU	Facility Practice Expense RVU	PLI RVU	Total Non-facility RVUs	Medicare Payment Nonfacility	Total Facility RVUs	Medicare Payment Facility	Global Period	Payment Policy Indicators
A2001	CP	Innovamatrix ac, per sq cm	0.00	0.00	0.00	0.00	0.00	$0.00	0.00	$0.00	XXX	
A2002	CP	Mirragen adv wnd mat per sq	0.00	0.00	0.00	0.00	0.00	$0.00	0.00	$0.00	XXX	
A2004	CP	Xcellistem, per sq cm	0.00	0.00	0.00	0.00	0.00	$0.00	0.00	$0.00	XXX	
A2005	CP	Microlyte matrix, per sq cm	0.00	0.00	0.00	0.00	0.00	$0.00	0.00	$0.00	XXX	
A2006	CP	Novosorb synpath per sq cm	0.00	0.00	0.00	0.00	0.00	$0.00	0.00	$0.00	XXX	
A2007	CP	Restrata, per sq cm	0.00	0.00	0.00	0.00	0.00	$0.00	0.00	$0.00	XXX	
A2008	CP	Theragenesis, per sq cm	0.00	0.00	0.00	0.00	0.00	$0.00	0.00	$0.00	XXX	
A2009	CP	Symphony, per sq cm	0.00	0.00	0.00	0.00	0.00	$0.00	0.00	$0.00	XXX	
A2010	CP	Apis, per square centimeter	0.00	0.00	0.00	0.00	0.00	$0.00	0.00	$0.00	XXX	
A4641	CP	Radiopharm dx agent noc	0.00	0.00	0.00	0.00	0.00	$0.00	0.00	$0.00	XXX	A+
A4642	CP	In111 satumomab	0.00	0.00	0.00	0.00	0.00	$0.00	0.00	$0.00	XXX	A+
A4890		Repair/maint cont hemo equip	0.00	0.00	0.00	0.00	0.00	$0.00	0.00	$0.00	XXX	A+
A9500	CP	Tc99m sestamibi	0.00	0.00	0.00	0.00	0.00	$0.00	0.00	$0.00	XXX	A+
A9501	CP	Technetium tc-99m teboroxime	0.00	0.00	0.00	0.00	0.00	$0.00	0.00	$0.00	XXX	A+
A9502	CP	Tc99m tetrofosmin	0.00	0.00	0.00	0.00	0.00	$0.00	0.00	$0.00	XXX	A+
A9503	CP	Tc99m medronate	0.00	0.00	0.00	0.00	0.00	$0.00	0.00	$0.00	XXX	A+
A9504	CP	Tc99m apcitide	0.00	0.00	0.00	0.00	0.00	$0.00	0.00	$0.00	XXX	A+
A9505	CP	Tl201 thallium	0.00	0.00	0.00	0.00	0.00	$0.00	0.00	$0.00	XXX	A+
A9507	CP	In111 capromab	0.00	0.00	0.00	0.00	0.00	$0.00	0.00	$0.00	XXX	A+
A9508	CP	I131 iodobenguate, dx	0.00	0.00	0.00	0.00	0.00	$0.00	0.00	$0.00	XXX	A+
A9509	CP	Iodine i-123 sod iodide mil	0.00	0.00	0.00	0.00	0.00	$0.00	0.00	$0.00	XXX	A+
A9510	CP	Tc99m disofenin	0.00	0.00	0.00	0.00	0.00	$0.00	0.00	$0.00	XXX	A+
A9512	CP	Tc99m pertechnetate	0.00	0.00	0.00	0.00	0.00	$0.00	0.00	$0.00	XXX	A+
A9516	CP	Iodine i-123 sod iodide mic	0.00	0.00	0.00	0.00	0.00	$0.00	0.00	$0.00	XXX	A+
A9517	CP	I131 iodide cap, rx	0.00	0.00	0.00	0.00	0.00	$0.00	0.00	$0.00	XXX	A+
A9521	CP	Tc99m exametazime	0.00	0.00	0.00	0.00	0.00	$0.00	0.00	$0.00	XXX	A+
A9524	CP	I131 serum albumin, dx	0.00	0.00	0.00	0.00	0.00	$0.00	0.00	$0.00	XXX	A+
A9526	CP	Nitrogen n-13 ammonia	0.00	0.00	0.00	0.00	0.00	$0.00	0.00	$0.00	XXX	A+
A9527	CP	Iodine i-125 sodium iodide	0.00	0.00	0.00	0.00	0.00	$0.00	0.00	$0.00	XXX	A+
A9528	CP	Iodine i-131 iodide cap, dx	0.00	0.00	0.00	0.00	0.00	$0.00	0.00	$0.00	XXX	A+
A9529	CP	I131 iodide sol, dx	0.00	0.00	0.00	0.00	0.00	$0.00	0.00	$0.00	XXX	A+
A9530	CP	I131 iodide sol, rx	0.00	0.00	0.00	0.00	0.00	$0.00	0.00	$0.00	XXX	A+

A9531	CP	I131 max 100uci	0.00	0.00	0.00	0.00	0.00	$0.00	0.00	$0.00	XXX	A+
A9532	CP	I125 serum albumin, dx	0.00	0.00	0.00	0.00	0.00	$0.00	0.00	$0.00	XXX	A+
A9536	CP	Tc99m depreotide	0.00	0.00	0.00	0.00	0.00	$0.00	0.00	$0.00	XXX	A+
A9537	CP	Tc99m mebrofenin	0.00	0.00	0.00	0.00	0.00	$0.00	0.00	$0.00	XXX	A+
A9538	CP	Tc99m pyrophosphate	0.00	0.00	0.00	0.00	0.00	$0.00	0.00	$0.00	XXX	A+
A9539	CP	Tc99m pentetate	0.00	0.00	0.00	0.00	0.00	$0.00	0.00	$0.00	XXX	A+
A9540	CP	Tc99m maa	0.00	0.00	0.00	0.00	0.00	$0.00	0.00	$0.00	XXX	A+
A9541	CP	Tc99m sulfur colloid	0.00	0.00	0.00	0.00	0.00	$0.00	0.00	$0.00	XXX	A+
A9542	CP	In111 ibritumomab, dx	0.00	0.00	0.00	0.00	0.00	$0.00	0.00	$0.00	XXX	A+
A9543	CP	Y90 ibritumomab, rx	0.00	0.00	0.00	0.00	0.00	$0.00	0.00	$0.00	XXX	A+
A9546	CP	Co57/58	0.00	0.00	0.00	0.00	0.00	$0.00	0.00	$0.00	XXX	A+
A9547	CP	In111 oxyquinoline	0.00	0.00	0.00	0.00	0.00	$0.00	0.00	$0.00	XXX	A+
A9548	CP	In111 pentetate	0.00	0.00	0.00	0.00	0.00	$0.00	0.00	$0.00	XXX	A+
A9550	CP	Tc99m gluceptate	0.00	0.00	0.00	0.00	0.00	$0.00	0.00	$0.00	XXX	A+
A9551	CP	Tc99m succimer	0.00	0.00	0.00	0.00	0.00	$0.00	0.00	$0.00	XXX	A+
A9552	CP	F18 fdg	0.00	0.00	0.00	0.00	0.00	$0.00	0.00	$0.00	XXX	A+
A9553	CP	Cr51 chromate	0.00	0.00	0.00	0.00	0.00	$0.00	0.00	$0.00	XXX	A+
A9554	CP	I125 iothalamate, dx	0.00	0.00	0.00	0.00	0.00	$0.00	0.00	$0.00	XXX	A+
A9555	CP	Rb82 rubidium	0.00	0.00	0.00	0.00	0.00	$0.00	0.00	$0.00	XXX	A+
A9556	CP	Ga67 gallium	0.00	0.00	0.00	0.00	0.00	$0.00	0.00	$0.00	XXX	A+
A9557	CP	Tc99m bicisate	0.00	0.00	0.00	0.00	0.00	$0.00	0.00	$0.00	XXX	A+
A9558	CP	Xe133 xenon 10mci	0.00	0.00	0.00	0.00	0.00	$0.00	0.00	$0.00	XXX	A+
A9559	CP	Co57 cyano	0.00	0.00	0.00	0.00	0.00	$0.00	0.00	$0.00	XXX	A+
A9560	CP	Tc99m labeled rbc	0.00	0.00	0.00	0.00	0.00	$0.00	0.00	$0.00	XXX	A+
A9561	CP	Tc99m oxidronate	0.00	0.00	0.00	0.00	0.00	$0.00	0.00	$0.00	XXX	A+
A9562	CP	Tc99m mertiatide	0.00	0.00	0.00	0.00	0.00	$0.00	0.00	$0.00	XXX	A+
A9563	CP	P32 na phosphate	0.00	0.00	0.00	0.00	0.00	$0.00	0.00	$0.00	XXX	A+
A9564	CP	P32 chromic phosphate	0.00	0.00	0.00	0.00	0.00	$0.00	0.00	$0.00	XXX	A+

*Please note that these calculations are based on the Medicare 2022 Conversion Factor of $34.6062 and the DRA RVU cap rates at time of publication.

A = assistant-at-surgery restriction

A+ = assistant-at-surgery restriction unless medical necessity established with documentation

B = bilateral surgery adjustment applies

C = cosurgeons payable

C+ = cosurgeons payable if medical necessity established with documentation

CP = carriers may establish RVUs and payment amounts for these services, generally on an individual basis following review of documentation such as an operative report

M = multiple surgery adjustment applies

Me = multiple endoscopy rules may apply

M+ = multiple therapy rules apply

Mtc = multiple diagnostic imaging rules apply

T = team surgeons permitted

T+ = team surgeons payable if medical necessity established with documentation

§ = indicates code is not covered by Medicare

GS = procedure must be performed under the general supervision of a physician

DS = procedure must be performed under the direct supervision of a physician

PS = procedure must be performed under the personal supervision of a physician

DRA = procedure subject to DRA limitation

Alphanumeric Coded Services (Level 2)

CPT Code and Modifier		Description	Work RVU	Nonfacility Practice Expense RVU	Facility Practice Expense RVU	PLI RVU	Total Non-facility RVUs	Medicare Payment Nonfacility	Total Facility RVUs	Medicare Payment Facility	Global Period	Payment Policy Indicators
A9566	CP	Tc99m fanolesomab	0.00	0.00	0.00	0.00	0.00	$0.00	0.00	$0.00	XXX	A+
A9567	CP	Technetium tc-99m aerosol	0.00	0.00	0.00	0.00	0.00	$0.00	0.00	$0.00	XXX	A+
A9568	CP	Technetium tc99m arcitumomab	0.00	0.00	0.00	0.00	0.00	$0.00	0.00	$0.00	XXX	A+
A9569	CP	Technetium tc-99m auto wbc	0.00	0.00	0.00	0.00	0.00	$0.00	0.00	$0.00	XXX	A+
A9570	CP	Indium in-111 auto wbc	0.00	0.00	0.00	0.00	0.00	$0.00	0.00	$0.00	XXX	A+
A9571	CP	Indium in-111 auto platelet	0.00	0.00	0.00	0.00	0.00	$0.00	0.00	$0.00	XXX	A+
A9572	CP	Indium in-111 pentetreotide	0.00	0.00	0.00	0.00	0.00	$0.00	0.00	$0.00	XXX	A+
A9580	CP	Sodium fluoride f-18	0.00	0.00	0.00	0.00	0.00	$0.00	0.00	$0.00	XXX	A+
A9586	CP	Florbetapir f18	0.00	0.00	0.00	0.00	0.00	$0.00	0.00	$0.00	YYY	
A9600	CP	Sr89 strontium	0.00	0.00	0.00	0.00	0.00	$0.00	0.00	$0.00	XXX	A+
A9699	CP	Radiopharm rx agent noc	0.00	0.00	0.00	0.00	0.00	$0.00	0.00	$0.00	XXX	A+
G0076		Care manag h vst new pt 20 m	1.01	0.50	NA	0.05	1.56	$53.99	NA	NA	XXX	A+
G0077		Care manag h vst new pt 30 m	1.52	0.62	NA	0.08	2.22	$76.83	NA	NA	XXX	A+
G0078		Care manag h vst new pt 45 m	2.53	0.96	NA	0.12	3.61	$124.93	NA	NA	XXX	A+
G0079		Care manag h vst new pt 60 m	3.38	1.60	NA	0.22	5.20	$179.95	NA	NA	XXX	A+
G0080		Care manag h vst new pt 75 m	4.09	1.93	NA	0.28	6.30	$218.02	NA	NA	XXX	A+
G0081		Care man h v ext pt 20 mi	1.00	0.53	NA	0.05	1.58	$54.68	NA	NA	XXX	A+
G0082		Care man h v ext pt 30 m	1.56	0.75	NA	0.09	2.40	$83.05	NA	NA	XXX	A+
G0083		Care man h v ext pt 45 m	2.33	1.23	NA	0.14	3.70	$128.04	NA	NA	XXX	A+
G0084		Care man h v ext pt 60 m	3.28	1.62	NA	0.23	5.13	$177.53	NA	NA	XXX	A+
G0085		Care man h v ext pt 75 m	4.09	1.93	NA	0.28	6.30	$218.02	NA	NA	XXX	A+
G0086		Care man home care plan 30 m	1.25	0.87	NA	0.10	2.22	$76.83	NA	NA	XXX	A+
G0087		Care man home care plan 60 m	1.80	1.17	NA	0.14	3.11	$107.63	NA	NA	XXX	A+
G0101		Ca screen;pelvic/breast exam	0.45	0.63	0.29	0.08	1.16	$40.14	0.82	$28.38	XXX	A+
G0102		Prostate ca screening; dre	0.18	0.49	0.07	0.01	0.68	$23.53	0.26	$9.00	XXX	
G0104		Ca screen;flexi sigmoidscope	0.84	4.72	0.69	0.11	5.67	$196.22	1.64	$56.75	000	A M
G0105		Colorectal scrn; hi risk ind	3.26	6.66	1.74	0.40	10.32	$357.14	5.40	$186.87	000	A M
G0105-53		Colorectal scrn; hi risk ind	1.63	3.33	0.87	0.20	5.16	$178.57	2.70	$93.44	000	A M
G0106		Colon ca screen;barium enema	1.26	5.48	NA	0.08	6.82	$236.01	NA	NA	XXX	A+
G0106-26		Colon ca screen;barium enema	1.26	0.45	0.45	0.07	1.78	$61.60	1.78	$61.60	XXX	A+
G0106-TC		Colon ca screen;barium enema	0.00	5.03	NA	0.01	5.04	$174.42	NA	NA	XXX	A+ PS
G0108		Diab manage trn per indiv	0.90	0.67	NA	0.05	1.62	$56.06	NA	NA	XXX	A+

G0109		Diab manage trn ind/group	0.25	0.20	NA	0.01	0.46	$15.92	NA	NA	XXX	A+
G0117		Glaucoma scrn hgh risk direc	0.45	1.38	NA	0.02	1.85	$64.02	NA	NA	XXX	A+
G0118		Glaucoma scrn hgh risk direc	0.17	1.06	NA	0.01	1.24	$42.91	NA	NA	XXX	A+
G0120		Colon ca scrn; barium enema	1.26	5.48	NA	0.08	6.82	$236.01	NA	NA	XXX	A+
G0120-26		Colon ca scrn; barium enema	1.26	0.45	0.45	0.07	1.78	$61.60	1.78	$61.60	XXX	A+
G0120-TC		Colon ca scrn; barium enema	0.00	5.03	NA	0.01	5.04	$174.42	NA	NA	XXX	A+
G0121		Colon ca scrn not hi rsk ind	3.26	6.66	1.74	0.41	10.33	$357.48	5.41	$187.22	000	A M
G0121-53		Colon ca scrn not hi rsk ind	1.63	3.33	0.87	0.21	5.17	$178.91	2.71	$93.78	000	A M
G0122	§	Colon ca scrn; barium enema	0.99	8.96	NA	0.07	10.02	$346.75	NA	NA	XXX	
G0122-26	§	Colon ca scrn; barium enema	0.99	0.38	0.38	0.05	1.42	$49.14	1.42	$49.14	XXX	
G0122-TC	§	Colon ca scrn; barium enema	0.00	8.58	NA	0.02	8.60	$297.61	NA	NA	XXX	
G0124		Screen c/v thin layer by md	0.26	0.38	0.38	0.01	0.65	$22.49	0.65	$22.49	XXX	A+
G0127		Trim nail(s)	0.17	0.51	0.04	0.01	0.69	$23.88	0.22	$7.61	000	A M
G0128		Corf skilled nursing service	0.00	0.25	NA	0.01	0.26	$9.00	NA	NA	XXX	A+
G0130		Single energy x-ray study	0.22	0.83	NA	0.02	1.07	$37.03	NA	NA	XXX	A+
G0130-26		Single energy x-ray study	0.22	0.09	0.09	0.01	0.32	$11.07	0.32	$11.07	XXX	A+
G0130-TC		Single energy x-ray study	0.00	0.74	NA	0.01	0.75	$25.95	NA	NA	XXX	A+ GS
G0141		Scr c/v cyto,autosys and md	0.26	0.38	0.38	0.01	0.65	$22.49	0.65	$22.49	XXX	A+
G0166		Extrnl counterpulse, per tx	0.00	3.17	NA	0.04	3.21	$111.09	NA	NA	XXX	
G0168		Wound closure by adhesive	0.31	3.39	0.07	0.07	3.77	$130.47	0.45	$15.57	000	A M
G0179		Md recertification hha pt	0.45	0.71	NA	0.04	1.20	$41.53	NA	NA	XXX	A+
G0180		Md certification hha patient	0.67	0.83	NA	0.05	1.55	$53.64	NA	NA	XXX	A+
G0181		Home health care supervision	1.73	1.22	NA	0.11	3.06	$105.89	NA	NA	XXX	A+
G0182		Hospice care supervision	1.73	1.26	NA	0.11	3.10	$107.28	NA	NA	XXX	A+
G0186	CP	Dstry eye lesn,fdr vssl tech	0.00	0.00	0.00	0.00	0.00	$0.00	0.00	$0.00	YYY	A+ B C+ M T+
G0237		Therapeutic procd strg endur	0.00	0.29	NA	0.01	0.30	$10.38	NA	NA	XXX	A+
G0238		Oth resp proc, indiv	0.00	0.29	NA	0.01	0.30	$10.38	NA	NA	XXX	A+
G0239		Oth resp proc, group	0.00	0.37	NA	0.01	0.38	$13.15	NA	NA	XXX	A+

*Please note that these calculations are based on the Medicare 2022 Conversion Factor of $34.6062 and the DRA RVU cap rates at time of publication.

A = assistant-at-surgery restriction
A+ = assistant-at-surgery restriction unless medical necessity established with documentation
B = bilateral surgery adjustment applies
C = cosurgeons payable
C+ = cosurgeons payable if medical necessity established with documentation
CP = carriers may establish RVUs and payment amounts for these services, generally on an individual basis following review of documentation such as an operative report
M = multiple surgery adjustment applies
Me = multiple endoscopy rules may apply
M+ = multiple therapy rules apply
Mtc = multiple diagnostic imaging rules apply
T = team surgeons permitted
T+ = team surgeons payable if medical necessity established with documentation
§ = indicates code is not covered by Medicare
GS = procedure must be performed under the general supervision of a physician
DS = procedure must be performed under the direct supervision of a physician
PS = procedure must be performed under the personal supervision of a physician
DRA = procedure subject to DRA limitation

Alphanumeric Coded Services (Level 2)

CPT Code and Modifier		Description	Work RVU	Nonfacility Practice Expense RVU	Facility Practice Expense RVU	PLI RVU	Total Non-facility RVUs	Medicare Payment Nonfacility	Total Facility RVUs	Medicare Payment Facility	Global Period	Payment Policy Indicators
G0245		Initial foot exam pt lops	0.88	0.99	0.27	0.05	1.92	$66.44	1.20	$41.53	XXX	A+
G0246		Followup eval of foot pt lop	0.45	0.66	0.12	0.02	1.13	$39.11	0.59	$20.42	XXX	A+
G0247		Routine footcare pt w lops	0.50	1.97	0.11	0.02	2.49	$86.17	0.63	$21.80	ZZZ	A+
G0248		Demonstrate use home inr mon	0.00	1.87	NA	0.04	1.91	$66.10	NA	NA	XXX	A+ GS
G0249		Provide inr test mater/equip	0.00	1.39	NA	0.01	1.40	$48.45	NA	NA	XXX	A+ GS
G0250		Md inr test revie inter mgmt	0.18	0.05	NA	0.01	0.24	$8.31	NA	NA	XXX	A+
G0252-26	§	Pet imaging initial dx	1.50	0.58	0.58	0.08	2.16	$74.75	2.16	$74.75	XXX	
G0268		Removal of impacted wax md	0.61	0.84	0.28	0.09	1.54	$53.29	0.98	$33.91	000	A M
G0270		Mnt subs tx for change dx	0.45	0.47	0.34	0.02	0.94	$32.53	0.81	$28.03	XXX	A+
G0271		Group mnt 2 or more 30 mins	0.25	0.24	0.19	0.01	0.50	$17.30	0.45	$15.57	XXX	A+
G0276		Pild/placebo control clin tr	7.17	NA	3.03	0.78	NA	NA	10.98	$379.98	000	C+ M
G0277		Hbot, full body chamber, 30m	0.00	5.20	NA	0.02	5.22	$180.64	NA	NA	XXX	A+
G0278		Iliac art angio,cardiac cath	0.25	NA	0.09	0.07	NA	NA	0.41	$14.19	ZZZ	A+
G0279		Tomosynthesis, mammo	0.60	0.92	NA	0.04	1.56	$53.99	NA	NA	ZZZ	
G0279-26		Tomosynthesis, mammo	0.60	0.22	0.22	0.04	0.86	$29.76	0.86	$29.76	ZZZ	
G0279-TC		Tomosynthesis, mammo	0.00	0.70	NA	0.00	0.70	$24.22	NA	NA	ZZZ	
G0281		Elec stim unattend for press	0.18	0.17	NA	0.01	0.36	$12.46	NA	NA	XXX	A+ Mt
G0283		Elec stim other than wound	0.18	0.17	NA	0.01	0.36	$12.46	NA	NA	XXX	A+ Mt
G0288		Recon, cta for surg plan	0.00	0.99	NA	0.10	1.09	$37.72	NA	NA	XXX	A+ GS
G0289		Arthro, loose body + chondro	1.48	NA	0.74	0.29	NA	NA	2.51	$86.86	ZZZ	A+ B
G0296		Visit to determ ldct elig	0.52	0.28	0.20	0.04	0.84	$29.07	0.76	$26.30	XXX	A+
G0329		Electromagntic tx for ulcers	0.06	0.25	NA	0.01	0.32	$11.07	NA	NA	XXX	A+ Mt
G0339	CP	Robot lin-radsurg com, first	0.00	0.00	0.00	0.00	0.00	$0.00	0.00	$0.00	XXX	A+
G0340	CP	Robt lin-radsurg fractx 2-5	0.00	0.00	0.00	0.00	0.00	$0.00	0.00	$0.00	XXX	A+
G0341		Percutaneous islet celltrans	6.98	43.36	1.28	0.72	51.06	$1766.99	8.98	$310.76	000	A+ C+ M
G0342		Laparoscopy islet cell trans	11.92	NA	7.60	3.01	NA	NA	22.53	$779.68	090	C+ M
G0343		Laparotomy islet cell transp	19.85	NA	12.13	5.03	NA	NA	37.01	$1280.78	090	C+ M
G0372		Md service required for pmd	0.17	0.08	0.08	0.01	0.26	$9.00	0.26	$9.00	XXX	A+
G0396		Alcohol/subs interv 15-30mn	0.65	0.34	0.25	0.05	1.04	$35.99	0.95	$32.88	XXX	A+
G0397		Alcohol/subs interv >30 min	1.30	0.59	0.50	0.11	2.00	$69.21	1.91	$66.10	XXX	A+
G0398	CP	Home sleep test/type 2 porta	0.00	0.00	NA	0.00	0.00	$0.00	NA	NA	XXX	A+
G0398-26	CP	Home sleep test/type 2 porta	0.00	0.00	0.00	0.00	0.00	$0.00	0.00	$0.00	XXX	A+

G0398-TC	CP	Home sleep test/type 2 porta	0.00	0.00	NA	0.00	0.00	$0.00	NA	NA	XXX	A+
G0399	CP	Home sleep test/type 3 porta	0.00	0.00	NA	0.00	0.00	$0.00	NA	NA	XXX	A+
G0399-26	CP	Home sleep test/type 3 porta	0.00	0.00	0.00	0.00	0.00	$0.00	0.00	$0.00	XXX	A+
G0399-TC	CP	Home sleep test/type 3 porta	0.00	0.00	NA	0.00	0.00	$0.00	NA	NA	XXX	A+
G0400	CP	Home sleep test/type 4 porta	0.00	0.00	NA	0.00	0.00	$0.00	NA	NA	XXX	A+
G0400-26	CP	Home sleep test/type 4 porta	0.00	0.00	0.00	0.00	0.00	$0.00	0.00	$0.00	XXX	A+
G0400-TC	CP	Home sleep test/type 4 porta	0.00	0.00	NA	0.00	0.00	$0.00	NA	NA	XXX	A+
G0402		Initial preventive exam	2.60	2.13	1.13	0.17	4.90	$169.57	3.90	$134.96	XXX	A+
G0403		Ekg for initial prevent exam	0.17	0.23	NA	0.02	0.42	$14.53	NA	NA	XXX	A+
G0404		Ekg tracing for initial prev	0.00	0.17	NA	0.01	0.18	$6.23	NA	NA	XXX	A+
G0405		Ekg interpret & report preve	0.17	0.06	0.06	0.01	0.24	$8.31	0.24	$8.31	XXX	A+
G0406		Inpt/tele follow up 15	0.76	NA	0.29	0.07	NA	NA	1.12	$38.76	XXX	A+
G0407		Inpt/tele follow up 25	1.39	NA	0.57	0.10	NA	NA	2.06	$71.29	XXX	A+
G0408		Inpt/tele follow up 35	2.00	NA	0.82	0.14	NA	NA	2.96	$102.43	XXX	A+
G0409		Corf related serv 15 mins ea	0.00	0.32	NA	0.01	0.33	$11.42	NA	NA	XXX	A+
G0412		Open tx iliac spine uni/bil	10.45	NA	8.93	2.17	NA	NA	21.55	$745.76	090	C M
G0413		Pelvic ring fracture uni/bil	15.73	NA	12.61	3.23	NA	NA	31.57	$1092.52	090	C M
G0414		Pelvic ring fx treat int fix	14.65	NA	12.13	3.00	NA	NA	29.78	$1030.57	090	C M
G0415		Open tx post pelvic fxcture	20.93	NA	15.37	4.36	NA	NA	40.66	$1407.09	090	C M
G0416		Prostate biopsy, any mthd	3.60	6.65	NA	0.11	10.36	$358.52	NA	NA	XXX	A+
G0416-26		Prostate biopsy, any mthd	3.60	1.46	1.46	0.07	5.13	$177.53	5.13	$177.53	XXX	A+
G0416-TC		Prostate biopsy, any mthd	0.00	5.19	NA	0.04	5.23	$180.99	NA	NA	XXX	A+
G0420		Ed svc ckd ind per session	2.12	1.04	NA	0.12	3.28	$113.51	NA	NA	XXX	A+
G0421		Ed svc ckd grp per session	0.50	0.25	NA	0.04	0.79	$27.34	NA	NA	XXX	A+
G0422		Intens cardiac rehab w/exerc	1.71	1.51	1.51	0.21	3.43	$118.70	3.43	$118.70	XXX	A+
G0423		Intens cardiac rehab no exer	1.71	1.51	1.51	0.21	3.43	$118.70	3.43	$118.70	XXX	A+
G0425		Inpt/ed teleconsult30	1.92	NA	0.78	0.21	NA	NA	2.91	$100.70	XXX	A+
G0426		Inpt/ed teleconsult50	2.61	NA	1.08	0.22	NA	NA	3.91	$135.31	XXX	A+

*Please note that these calculations are based on the Medicare 2022 Conversion Factor of $34.6062 and the DRA RVU cap rates at time of publication.

A = assistant-at-surgery restriction
A+ = assistant-at-surgery restriction unless medical necessity established with documentation
B = bilateral surgery adjustment applies
C = cosurgeons payable
C+ = cosurgeons payable if medical necessity established with documentation
CP = carriers may establish RVUs and payment amounts for these services, generally on an individual basis following review of documentation such as an operative report
M = multiple surgery adjustment applies
Me = multiple endoscopy rules may apply
M+ = multiple therapy rules apply
Mtc = multiple diagnostic imaging rules apply
T = team surgeons permitted
T+ = team surgeons payable if medical necessity established with documentation
§ = indicates code is not covered by Medicare
GS = procedure must be performed under the general supervision of a physician
DS = procedure must be performed under the direct supervision of a physician
PS = procedure must be performed under the personal supervision of a physician
DRA = procedure subject to DRA limitation

Alphanumeric Coded Services (Level 2)

CPT Code and Modifier		Description	Work RVU	Nonfacility Practice Expense RVU	Facility Practice Expense RVU	PLI RVU	Total Non-facility RVUs	Medicare Payment Nonfacility	Total Facility RVUs	Medicare Payment Facility	Global Period	Payment Policy Indicators
G0427		Inpt/ed teleconsult70	3.86	NA	1.58	0.29	NA	NA	5.73	$198.29	XXX	A+
G0429		Dermal filler injection(s)	1.19	1.56	0.68	0.11	2.86	$98.97	1.98	$68.52	000	A+ M
G0438		Ppps, initial visit	2.60	2.13	NA	0.17	4.90	$169.57	NA	NA	XXX	A+
G0439		Ppps, subseq visit	1.92	1.80	NA	0.11	3.83	$132.54	NA	NA	XXX	A+
G0442		Annual alcohol screen 15 min	0.18	0.36	0.08	0.01	0.55	$19.03	0.27	$9.34	XXX	A+
G0443		Brief alcohol misuse counsel	0.45	0.28	0.20	0.04	0.77	$26.65	0.69	$23.88	XXX	A+
G0444		Depression screen annual	0.18	0.35	0.08	0.01	0.54	$18.69	0.27	$9.34	XXX	A+
G0445		High inten beh couns std 30m	0.45	0.31	0.18	0.04	0.80	$27.68	0.67	$23.19	XXX	A+
G0446		Intens behave ther cardio dx	0.45	0.28	0.20	0.04	0.77	$26.65	0.69	$23.88	XXX	A+
G0447		Behavior counsel obesity 15m	0.45	0.28	0.19	0.04	0.77	$26.65	0.68	$23.53	XXX	A+
G0451		Devlopment test interpt&rep	0.00	0.30	NA	0.01	0.31	$10.73	NA	NA	XXX	A+
G0452		Molecular pathology interpr	0.93	0.44	NA	0.05	1.42	$49.14	NA	NA	XXX	A+
G0452-26		Molecular pathology interpr	0.93	0.36	0.36	0.04	1.33	$46.03	1.33	$46.03	XXX	A+
G0452-TC		Molecular pathology interpr	0.00	0.08	NA	0.01	0.09	$3.11	NA	NA	XXX	A+
G0453		Cont intraop neuro monitor	0.60	NA	0.30	0.05	NA	NA	0.95	$32.88	XXX	A+
G0454		Md document visit by npp	0.18	0.07	0.07	0.01	0.26	$9.00	0.26	$9.00	XXX	A+
G0455		Fecal microbiota prep instil	1.34	2.38	0.61	0.12	3.84	$132.89	2.07	$71.63	000	A+
G0459		Telehealth inpt pharm mgmt	0.95	NA	0.22	0.05	NA	NA	1.22	$42.22	XXX	
G0460	CP	Autolog prp not diab ulcer	0.00	0.00	0.00	0.00	0.00	$0.00	0.00	$0.00	XXX	A M
G0465	CP	Autolog prp diab wound ulcer	0.00	0.00	0.00	0.00	0.00	$0.00	0.00	$0.00	XXX	A M
G0473		Group behave couns 2-10	0.23	0.13	0.10	0.01	0.37	$12.80	0.34	$11.77	XXX	
G0498	CP	Chemo extend iv infus w/pump	0.00	0.00	0.00	0.00	0.00	$0.00	0.00	$0.00	YYY	A+
G0500		Mod sedat endo service >5yrs	0.10	1.55	0.04	0.02	1.67	$57.79	0.16	$5.54	XXX	
G0506		Comp asses care plan ccm svc	0.87	0.87	0.37	0.07	1.81	$62.64	1.31	$45.33	ZZZ	A+
G0508		Crit care telehea consult 60	4.00	NA	1.74	0.34	NA	NA	6.08	$210.41	XXX	
G0509		Crit care telehea consult 50	3.86	NA	1.43	0.29	NA	NA	5.58	$193.10	XXX	
G0513		Prolong prev svcs, first 30m	1.17	0.64	0.52	0.09	1.90	$65.75	1.78	$61.60	ZZZ	A+
G0514		Prolong prev svcs, addl 30m	1.17	0.64	0.52	0.09	1.90	$65.75	1.78	$61.60	ZZZ	A+
G0516		Insert drug del implant, >=4	1.82	4.04	0.90	0.11	5.97	$206.60	2.83	$97.94	000	A+ M
G0517		Remove drug implant	2.10	4.37	1.01	0.12	6.59	$228.05	3.23	$111.78	000	A+ M
G0518		Remove w insert drug implant	3.55	7.84	1.55	0.24	11.63	$402.47	5.34	$184.80	000	A+ M
G2000		Blinded conv. tx mdd clin tr	0.00	0.00	0.00	0.00	0.00	$0.00	0.00	$0.00	YYY	A+

G2001		Post d/c h vst new pt 20 m	1.01	0.50	NA	0.05	1.56	$53.99	NA	NA	XXX	A+
G2002		Post-d/c h vst new pt 30 m	1.52	0.62	NA	0.08	2.22	$76.83	NA	NA	XXX	A+
G2003		Post-d/c h vst new pt 45 m	2.53	0.96	NA	0.12	3.61	$124.93	NA	NA	XXX	A+
G2004		Post-d/c h vst new pt 60 m	3.38	1.60	NA	0.22	5.20	$179.95	NA	NA	XXX	A+
G2005		Post-d/c h vst new pt 75 m	4.09	1.93	NA	0.28	6.30	$218.02	NA	NA	XXX	A+
G2006		Post-d/c h vst ext pt 20 m	1.00	0.53	NA	0.05	1.58	$54.68	NA	NA	XXX	A+
G2007		Post-d/c h vst ext pt 30 m	1.56	0.75	NA	0.09	2.40	$83.05	NA	NA	XXX	A+
G2008		Post-d/c h vst ext pt 45 m	2.33	1.23	NA	0.14	3.70	$128.04	NA	NA	XXX	A+
G2009		Post-d/c h vst ext pt 60 m	3.28	1.62	NA	0.23	5.13	$177.53	NA	NA	XXX	A+
G2010		Remot image submit by pt	0.18	0.16	0.08	0.01	0.35	$12.11	0.27	$9.34	XXX	A+
G2011		Alcohol/sub misuse assess	0.33	0.12	0.12	0.04	0.49	$16.96	0.49	$16.96	XXX	A+
G2012		Brief check in by md/qhp	0.25	0.15	0.10	0.02	0.42	$14.53	0.37	$12.80	XXX	A+
G2013		Post-d/c h vst ext pt 75 m	4.09	1.93	NA	0.28	6.30	$218.02	NA	NA	XXX	A+
G2014		Post-d/c care plan overs 30m	1.25	0.87	NA	0.10	2.22	$76.83	NA	NA	XXX	A+
G2015		Post-d/c care plan overs 60m	1.80	1.17	NA	0.14	3.11	$107.63	NA	NA	XXX	A+
G2066	CP	Inter devc remote 30d	0.00	0.00	0.00	0.00	0.00	$0.00	0.00	$0.00	XXX	A+ GS
G2082		Visit esketamine 56m or less	0.70	22.48	0.27	0.09	23.27	$805.29	1.06	$36.68	XXX	A+
G2083		Visit esketamine, > 56m	0.70	32.29	0.27	0.09	33.08	$1144.77	1.06	$36.68	XXX	A+
G2086		Off base opioid tx 70min	7.06	4.10	1.86	0.34	11.50	$397.97	9.26	$320.45	XXX	A+
G2087		Off base opioid tx, 60 m	6.89	2.85	1.12	0.27	10.01	$346.41	8.28	$286.54	XXX	A+
G2088		Off base opioid tx, add30	0.82	0.93	0.27	0.04	1.79	$61.95	1.13	$39.11	ZZZ	A+
G2170	CP	Avf by tissue w thermal e	0.00	0.00	0.00	0.00	0.00	$0.00	0.00	$0.00	YYY	C+ M
G2171	CP	Avf use magnetic/art/ven	0.00	0.00	0.00	0.00	0.00	$0.00	0.00	$0.00	YYY	C+ M
G2212		Prolong outpt/office vis	0.61	0.30	0.27	0.05	0.96	$33.22	0.93	$32.18	XXX	A+
G2213		Initiat med assist tx in er	1.30	0.59	0.49	0.11	2.00	$69.21	1.90	$65.75	ZZZ	A+
G2214		Init/sub psych care m 1st 30	0.77	0.97	0.31	0.05	1.79	$61.95	1.13	$39.11	XXX	A+
G2250		Remot img sub by pt, non e/m	0.18	0.16	0.08	0.01	0.35	$12.11	0.27	$9.34	XXX	A+
G2251		Brief chkin, 5-10, non-e/m	0.25	0.15	0.10	0.02	0.42	$14.53	0.37	$12.80	XXX	A+

*Please note that these calculations are based on the Medicare 2022 Conversion Factor of $34.6062 and the DRA RVU cap rates at time of publication.

A = assistant-at-surgery restriction
A+ = assistant-at-surgery restriction unless medical necessity established with documentation
B = bilateral surgery adjustment applies
C = cosurgeons payable
C+ = cosurgeons payable if medical necessity established with documentation
CP = carriers may establish RVUs and payment amounts for these services, generally on an individual basis following review of documentation such as an operative report
M = multiple surgery adjustment applies
Me = multiple endoscopy rules may apply
M+ = multiple therapy rules apply
Mtc = multiple diagnostic imaging rules apply
T = team surgeons permitted
T+ = team surgeons payable if medical necessity established with documentation
§ = indicates code is not covered by Medicare
GS = procedure must be performed under the general supervision of a physician
DS = procedure must be performed under the direct supervision of a physician
PS = procedure must be performed under the personal supervision of a physician
DRA = procedure subject to DRA limitation

Alphanumeric Coded Services (Level 2)

CPT Code and Modifier		Description	Work RVU	Nonfacility Practice Expense RVU	Facility Practice Expense RVU	PLI RVU	Total Non-facility RVUs	Medicare Payment Nonfacility	Total Facility RVUs	Medicare Payment Facility	Global Period	Payment Policy Indicators
G2252		Brief chkin by md/qhp, 11-20	0.50	0.27	0.23	0.04	0.81	$28.03	0.77	$26.65	XXX	A+
G6001		Echo guidance radiotherapy	0.58	4.69	NA	0.03	5.30	$183.41	NA	NA	XXX	A+
G6001-26		Echo guidance radiotherapy	0.58	0.32	0.32	0.02	0.92	$31.84	0.92	$31.84	XXX	A+
G6001-TC		Echo guidance radiotherapy	0.00	4.37	NA	0.01	4.38	$151.58	NA	NA	XXX	A+
G6002		Stereoscopic x-ray guidance	0.39	1.76	NA	0.02	2.17	$75.10	NA	NA	XXX	A+
G6002-26		Stereoscopic x-ray guidance	0.39	0.19	0.19	0.01	0.59	$20.42	0.59	$20.42	XXX	A+
G6002-TC		Stereoscopic x-ray guidance	0.00	1.57	NA	0.01	1.58	$54.68	NA	NA	XXX	A+
G6003		Radiation treatment delivery	0.00	4.34	NA	0.01	4.35	$150.54	NA	NA	XXX	A+
G6004		Radiation treatment delivery	0.00	3.90	NA	0.01	3.91	$135.31	NA	NA	XXX	A+
G6005		Radiation treatment delivery	0.00	3.90	NA	0.01	3.91	$135.31	NA	NA	XXX	A+
G6006		Radiation treatment delivery	0.00	3.90	NA	0.01	3.91	$135.31	NA	NA	XXX	A+
G6007		Radiation treatment delivery	0.00	7.19	NA	0.01	7.20	$249.16	NA	NA	XXX	A+
G6008		Radiation treatment delivery	0.00	5.37	NA	0.01	5.38	$186.18	NA	NA	XXX	A+
G6009		Radiation treatment delivery	0.00	5.36	NA	0.01	5.37	$185.84	NA	NA	XXX	A+
G6010		Radiation treatment delivery	0.00	5.33	NA	0.01	5.34	$184.80	NA	NA	XXX	A+
G6011		Radiation treatment delivery	0.00	7.11	NA	0.02	7.13	$246.74	NA	NA	XXX	A+
G6012		Radiation treatment delivery	0.00	7.10	NA	0.02	7.12	$246.40	NA	NA	XXX	A+
G6013		Radiation treatment delivery	0.00	7.12	NA	0.02	7.14	$247.09	NA	NA	XXX	A+
G6014		Radiation treatment delivery	0.00	7.08	NA	0.02	7.10	$245.70	NA	NA	XXX	A+
G6015		Radiation tx delivery imrt	0.00	10.79	NA	0.05	10.84	$375.13	NA	NA	XXX	A+
G6016		Delivery comp imrt	0.00	10.79	NA	0.01	10.80	$373.75	NA	NA	XXX	A+
G6017	CP	Intrafraction track motion	0.00	0.00	0.00	0.00	0.00	$0.00	0.00	$0.00	YYY	A+
G9148		Medical home level 1	0.00	0.00	0.00	0.00	0.00	$0.00	0.00	$0.00	XXX	
G9149		Medical home level ii	0.00	0.00	0.00	0.00	0.00	$0.00	0.00	$0.00	XXX	
G9150		Medical home level iii	0.00	0.00	0.00	0.00	0.00	$0.00	0.00	$0.00	XXX	
G9151		Mapcp demo state	0.00	0.00	0.00	0.00	0.00	$0.00	0.00	$0.00	XXX	
G9152		Mapcp demo community	0.00	0.00	0.00	0.00	0.00	$0.00	0.00	$0.00	XXX	
G9153		Mapcp demo physician	0.00	0.00	0.00	0.00	0.00	$0.00	0.00	$0.00	XXX	
G9156		Evaluation for wheelchair	0.00	0.00	0.00	0.00	0.00	$0.00	0.00	$0.00	XXX	
G9157		Transesoph doppl cardiac mon	2.20	NA	0.39	0.19	NA	NA	2.78	$96.21	XXX	
G9187		Bpci home visit	0.18	1.13	NA	0.04	1.35	$46.72	NA	NA	XXX	
G9481		Remote e/m new pt 10mins	0.48	0.00	0.00	0.07	0.55	$19.03	0.55	$19.03	XXX	A+

G9482		Remote e/m new pt 20mins	0.93	0.00	0.00	0.09	1.02	$35.30	1.02	$35.30	XXX	A+
G9483		Remote e/m new pt 30mins	1.42	0.00	0.00	0.17	1.59	$55.02	1.59	$55.02	XXX	A+
G9484		Remote e/m new pt 45mins	2.43	0.00	0.00	0.24	2.67	$92.40	2.67	$92.40	XXX	A+
G9485		Remote e/m new pt 60mins	3.17	0.00	0.00	0.32	3.49	$120.78	3.49	$120.78	XXX	A+
G9486		Remote e/m est. pt 10mins	0.48	0.00	0.00	0.07	0.55	$19.03	0.55	$19.03	XXX	A+
G9487		Remote e/m est. pt 15mins	0.97	0.00	0.00	0.10	1.07	$37.03	1.07	$37.03	XXX	A+
G9488		Remote e/m est. pt 25mins	1.50	0.00	0.00	0.12	1.62	$56.06	1.62	$56.06	XXX	A+
G9489		Remote e/m est. pt 40mins	2.11	0.00	0.00	0.21	2.32	$80.29	2.32	$80.29	XXX	A+
G9490		Cmmi mod home visit	0.18	1.13	NA	0.03	1.34	$46.37	NA	NA	XXX	
G9678	CP	Oncology care model service	0.00	0.00	0.00	0.00	0.00	$0.00	0.00	$0.00	XXX	
G9685		Acute nursing facility care	3.86	1.58	1.58	0.29	5.73	$198.29	5.73	$198.29	XXX	A+
G9868		Cmmi asyntelehealth <10min	0.80	0.00	0.00	0.00	0.80	$27.68	0.80	$27.68	XXX	
G9869		Cmmi asyntelehealth 10-20min	1.07	0.00	0.00	0.00	1.07	$37.03	1.07	$37.03	XXX	
G9870		Cmmi asyntelehealth >20min	1.34	0.00	0.00	0.00	1.34	$46.37	1.34	$46.37	XXX	
G9978		Remote e/m new pt 10mins	0.48	0.29	0.29	0.07	0.84	$29.07	0.84	$29.07	XXX	A+
G9979		Remote e/m new pt 20mins	0.93	0.41	0.41	0.09	1.43	$49.49	1.43	$49.49	XXX	A+
G9980		Remote e/m new pt 30 mins	1.42	0.67	0.67	0.17	2.26	$78.21	2.26	$78.21	XXX	A+
G9981		Remote e/m new pt 45mins	2.43	1.11	1.11	0.24	3.78	$130.81	3.78	$130.81	XXX	A+
G9982		Remote e/m new pt 60mins	3.17	1.54	1.54	0.32	5.03	$174.07	5.03	$174.07	XXX	A+
G9983		Remote e/m est. pt 10mins	0.48	0.29	0.29	0.07	0.84	$29.07	0.84	$29.07	XXX	A+
G9984		Remote e/m est. pt 15mins	0.97	0.55	0.55	0.10	1.62	$56.06	1.62	$56.06	XXX	A+
G9985		Remote e/m est. pt 25mins	1.50	0.82	0.82	0.12	2.44	$84.44	2.44	$84.44	XXX	A+
G9986		Remote e/m est. pt 40mins	2.11	1.24	1.24	0.21	3.56	$123.20	3.56	$123.20	XXX	A+
G9987		Bpci advanced in home visit	0.18	1.13	1.13	0.04	1.35	$46.72	1.35	$46.72	XXX	
P3001		Screening pap smear by phys	0.26	0.38	0.38	0.01	0.65	$22.49	0.65	$22.49	XXX	A+
Q0035		Cardiokymography	0.17	0.32	NA	0.02	0.51	$17.65	NA	NA	XXX	A+
Q0035-26		Cardiokymography	0.17	0.06	0.06	0.01	0.24	$8.31	0.24	$8.31	XXX	A+
Q0035-TC		Cardiokymography	0.00	0.26	NA	0.01	0.27	$9.34	NA	NA	XXX	A+ GS

*Please note that these calculations are based on the Medicare 2022 Conversion Factor of $34.6062 and the DRA RVU cap rates at time of publication.

A = assistant-at-surgery restriction
A+ = assistant-at-surgery restriction unless medical necessity established with documentation
B = bilateral surgery adjustment applies
C = cosurgeons payable
C+ = cosurgeons payable if medical necessity established with documentation
CP = carriers may establish RVUs and payment amounts for these services, generally on an individual basis following review of documentation such as an operative report
M = multiple surgery adjustment applies
Me = multiple endoscopy rules may apply
M+ = multiple therapy rules apply
Mtc = multiple diagnostic imaging rules apply
T = team surgeons permitted
T+ = team surgeons payable if medical necessity established with documentation
§ = indicates code is not covered by Medicare
GS = procedure must be performed under the general supervision of a physician
DS = procedure must be performed under the direct supervision of a physician
PS = procedure must be performed under the personal supervision of a physician
DRA = procedure subject to DRA limitation

Alphanumeric Coded Services (Level 2)

CPT Code and Modifier		Description	Work RVU	Nonfacility Practice Expense RVU	Facility Practice Expense RVU	PLI RVU	Total Non-facility RVUs	Medicare Payment Nonfacility	Total Facility RVUs	Medicare Payment Facility	Global Period	Payment Policy Indicators
Q0091		Obtaining screen pap smear	0.37	0.86	0.14	0.04	1.27	$43.95	0.55	$19.03	XXX	A+
Q0092		Set up port xray equipment	0.00	0.68	0.68	0.01	0.69	$23.88	0.69	$23.88	XXX	A+
Q3001	CP	Brachytherapy radioelements	0.00	0.00	0.00	0.00	0.00	$0.00	0.00	$0.00	XXX	A+
R0070	CP	Transport portable x-ray	0.00	0.00	0.00	0.00	0.00	$0.00	0.00	$0.00	XXX	A+
R0075	CP	Transport port x-ray multipl	0.00	0.00	0.00	0.00	0.00	$0.00	0.00	$0.00	XXX	A+
V5299		Hearing service	0.00	0.00	0.00	0.00	0.00	$0.00	0.00	$0.00	XXX	A+

*Please note that these calculations are based on the Medicare 2022 Conversion Factor of $34.6062 and the DRA RVU cap rates at time of publication.

A = assistant-at-surgery restriction

A+ = assistant-at-surgery restriction unless medical necessity established with documentation

B = bilateral surgery adjustment applies

C = cosurgeons payable

C+ = cosurgeons payable if medical necessity established with documentation

CP = carriers may establish RVUs and payment amounts for these services, generally on an individual basis following review of documentation such as an operative report

M = multiple surgery adjustment applies

Me = multiple endoscopy rules may apply

M+ = multiple therapy rules apply

Mtc = multiple diagnostic imaging rules apply

T = team surgeons permitted

T+ = team surgeons payable if medical necessity established with documentation

§ = indicates code is not covered by Medicare

GS = procedure must be performed under the general supervision of a physician

DS = procedure must be performed under the direct supervision of a physician

PS = procedure must be performed under the personal supervision of a physician

DRA = procedure subject to DRA limitation

List of Geographic Practice Cost Indices for Each Medicare Locality

The following list presents the geographic practice cost indices (GPCIs) for 2022 for each Medicare payment locality. Because each component of the Medicare payment schedule (physician work, practice costs, and professional liability insurance) is adjusted for geographic cost differences, three GPCI values are provided for each locality.

Chapter 7 discusses GPCIs in detail. In addition, Chapters 8 and 10 explain how GPCIs are combined with the relative value units and conversion factor to calculate the full payment–schedule amount for each service in a locality.

GPCIs

Geographic Practice Cost Indices by State and Medicare Locality, 2022

Contractor	State	Locality	Locality Name	Work GPCI*	PE GPCI	MP GPCI
10112	AL	00	Alabama	1.000	0.888	0.921
02102	AK	01	Alaska**	1.500	1.118	0.614
03102	AZ	00	Arizona	1.000	0.951	0.857
07102	AR	13	Arkansas	1.000	0.847	0.465
01112	CA	54	Bakersfield	1.036	1.065	0.726
01112	CA	55	Chico	1.027	1.065	0.597
01182	CA	71	El Centro	1.027	1.065	0.620
01112	CA	56	Fresno	1.027	1.065	0.597
01112	CA	57	Hanford-Corcoran	1.027	1.065	0.597
01182	CA	18	Los Angeles-Long Beach-Anaheim (Los Angeles Cnty)	1.048	1.175	0.757
01182	CA	26	Los Angeles-Long Beach-Anaheim (Orange Cnty)	1.048	1.175	0.757
01112	CA	58	Madera	1.027	1.065	0.597
01112	CA	59	Merced	1.027	1.065	0.597
01112	CA	60	Modesto	1.027	1.065	0.597
01112	CA	51	Napa	1.044	1.220	0.504
01112	CA	07	San Francisco-Oakland-Berkeley (Alameda/Contra Costa Cnty)	1.077	1.329	0.458
01182	CA	17	Oxnard-Thousand Oaks-Ventura	1.027	1.179	0.726
01112	CA	61	Redding	1.027	1.065	0.597
01112	CA	62	Riverside-San Bernardino-Ontario	1.027	1.065	0.955
01112	CA	63	Sacramento-Roseville-Folsom	1.038	1.081	0.597
01112	CA	64	Salinas	1.064	1.133	0.597
01182	CA	72	San Diego-Chula Vista-Carlsbad	1.037	1.160	0.620
01112	CA	05	San Francisco-Oakland-Berkeley (San Francisco Cnty)	1.077	1.329	0.458
01112	CA	52	San Francisco-Oakland-Berkeley (Marin Cnty)	1.077	1.329	0.504
01112	CA	65	San Jose-Sunnyvale-Santa Clara (San Benito Cnty)	1.096	1.383	0.597
01182	CA	73	San Luis Obispo-Paso Robles	1.027	1.089	0.597
01112	CA	06	San Francisco-Oakland-Berkeley (San Mateo Cnty)	1.077	1.329	0.458
01112	CA	09	San Jose-Sunnyvale-Santa Clara (Santa Clara Cnty)	1.096	1.383	0.414
01112	CA	66	Santa Cruz-Watsonville	1.045	1.205	0.597
01182	CA	74	Santa Maria-Santa Barbara	1.041	1.175	0.597
01112	CA	67	Santa Rosa-Petaluma	1.045	1.177	0.597
01112	CA	68	Stockton	1.027	1.065	0.597
01112	CA	53	Vallejo	1.044	1.220	0.504
01112	CA	69	Visalia	1.027	1.065	0.597
01112	CA	70	Yuba City	1.027	1.065	0.597
01112	CA	75	Rest of California	1.027	1.065	0.597
04112	CO	01	Colorado	1.001	1.047	0.767
13102	CT	00	Connecticut	1.037	1.114	0.934
12202	DC	01	DC + MD/VA Suburbs	1.054	1.236	1.294

GPCIs

Geographic Practice Cost Indices by State and Medicare Locality, 2022

Contractor	State	Locality	Locality Name	Work GPCI*	PE GPCI	MP GPCI
12102	DE	01	Delaware	1.005	1.022	0.927
09102	FL	03	Fort Lauderdale	1.000	1.001	1.860
09102	FL	04	Miami	1.000	1.023	2.629
09102	FL	99	Rest of Florida	1.000	0.939	1.435
10212	GA	01	Atlanta	1.000	0.998	0.904
10212	GA	99	Rest of Georgia	1.000	0.878	0.904
01212	HI	01	Hawaii, Guam	1.010	1.143	0.675
02202	ID	00	Idaho	1.000	0.877	0.416
06102	IL	16	Chicago	1.011	1.044	1.871
06102	IL	12	East St. Louis	1.000	0.942	1.661
06102	IL	15	Suburban Chicago	1.006	1.062	1.504
06102	IL	99	Rest of Illinois	1.000	0.912	1.182
08102	IN	00	Indiana	1.000	0.900	0.465
05102	IA	00	Iowa	1.000	0.907	0.425
05202	KS	00	Kansas	1.000	0.908	0.458
15102	KY	00	Kentucky	1.000	0.869	0.827
07202	LA	01	New Orleans	1.000	0.927	1.528
07202	LA	99	Rest of Louisiana	1.000	0.872	1.307
14112	ME	03	Southern Maine	1.000	0.997	0.652
14112	ME	99	Rest of Maine	1.000	0.898	0.652
12302	MD	01	Baltimore/Surr. Cntys	1.028	1.096	1.313
12302	MD	99	Rest of Maryland	1.011	1.037	1.070
14212	MA	01	Metropolitan Boston	1.049	1.203	0.842
14212	MA	99	Rest of Massachusetts	1.026	1.061	0.842
08202	MI	01	Detroit	1.000	0.997	1.622
08202	MI	99	Rest of Michigan	1.000	0.911	0.979
06202	MN	00	Minnesota	1.000	1.013	0.353
07302	MS	00	Mississippi	1.000	0.842	0.671
05302	MO	02	Metropolitan Kansas City	1.000	0.955	0.890
05302	MO	01	Metropolitan St. Louis	1.000	0.976	0.889
05302	MO	99	Rest of Missouri	1.000	0.852	0.828
03202	MT	01	Montana***	1.000	1.000	0.977
05402	NE	00	Nebraska	1.000	0.908	0.235
01312	NV	00	Nevada***	1.005	1.000	1.351
14312	NH	40	New Hampshire	1.000	1.038	0.917
12402	NJ	01	Northern NJ	1.049	1.199	0.959
12402	NJ	99	Rest of New Jersey	1.037	1.141	0.959
04212	NM	05	New Mexico	1.000	0.896	1.166
13202	NY	01	Manhattan	1.056	1.203	2.031
13202	NY	02	NYC Suburbs/Long Island	1.046	1.223	2.702

(continued)

GPCIs

Geographic Practice Cost Indices by State and Medicare Locality, 2022

Contractor	State	Locality	Locality Name	Work GPCI*	PE GPCI	MP GPCI
13202	NY	03	Poughkpsie/N NYC Suburbs	1.027	1.105	1.646
13292	NY	04	Queens	1.056	1.228	2.661
13282	NY	99	Rest of New York	1.000	0.955	0.752
11502	NC	00	North Carolina	1.000	0.928	0.819
03302	ND	01	North Dakota***	1.000	1.000	0.431
15202	OH	00	Ohio	1.000	0.913	1.094
04312	OK	00	Oklahoma	1.000	0.881	0.782
02302	OR	01	Portland	1.022	1.063	0.535
02302	OR	99	Rest of Oregon	1.000	0.947	0.535
12502	PA	01	Metropolitan Philadelphia	1.022	1.083	1.199
12502	PA	99	Rest of Pennsylvania	1.000	0.939	0.888
09202	PR	20	Puerto Rico	1.000	1.008	0.986
14412	RI	01	Rhode Island	1.021	1.048	0.981
11202	SC	01	South Carolina	1.000	0.903	0.695
03402	SD	02	South Dakota***	1.000	1.000	0.347
10312	TN	35	Tennessee	1.000	0.892	0.492
04412	TX	31	Austin	1.000	1.059	0.539
04412	TX	20	Beaumont	1.000	0.944	0.550
04412	TX	09	Brazoria	1.032	1.023	0.550
04412	TX	11	Dallas	1.023	1.026	0.546
04412	TX	28	Fort Worth	1.016	0.995	0.539
04412	TX	15	Galveston	1.032	1.026	0.550
04412	TX	18	Houston	1.032	1.029	0.900
04412	TX	99	Rest of Texas	1.000	0.955	0.584
03502	UT	09	Utah	1.000	0.919	0.799
14512	VT	50	Vermont	1.000	1.001	0.569
11302	VA	00	Virginia	1.000	0.995	0.897
09202	VI	50	Virgin Islands	1.000	1.008	0.986
02402	WA	02	Seattle (King Cnty)	1.036	1.194	0.776
02402	WA	99	Rest of Washington	1.000	1.014	0.744
11402	WV	16	West Virginia	1.000	0.858	1.198
06302	WI	00	Wisconsin	1.000	0.942	0.296
03602	WY	21	Wyoming***	1.000	1.000	0.841

*The Consolidated Appropriations Act, 2021, (the Act) that was signed into law on December 27, 2020, extended the 1.0 work GPCI floor through December 31, 2023, as required by Section 101 of the Act.

** Work GPCI reflects a 1.5 floor for Alaska established by MIPPA.

*** PE GPCI reflects a 1.0 floor for frontier states established by the ACA.

RVUs for Anesthesiology Services

Anesthesiologists' services had been compensated according to a "relative value guide" before the implementation of the Medicare payment schedule. This approach has continued with some modifications.

Anesthesia Base Units

Medicare payments for anesthesiology services are based on the American Society of Anesthesiologists (ASA) Relative Value Guide with some of the basic units adjusted by the Centers for Medicare & Medicaid Services (CMS). Two hundred and seventy-six anesthesia codes correspond to the anesthesia services for more than 4000 surgical, endoscopic, and radiological procedures. Each service is assigned a base unit. The base unit reflects the complexity of the service, and includes work provided before and after reportable anesthesia time. The base units also cover usual preoperative and postoperative visits, administering fluids and blood that are part of the anesthesia care, and monitoring procedures.

Because the base units reflect all but the time required for the procedure, they are added to a time factor for each service an anesthesiologist provides. Under the 1991 Final Rule, anesthesia time starts when the physician begins to prepare the patient for induction and ends when the patient is placed under postoperative supervision when the anesthesiologist is no longer in attendance. Time for each procedure is divided into 15-minute increments and is assigned a unit value of one and is added to the base units. The time units account for the time from continuous hands-on-care to transfer of the patient to post-anesthesia care personnel. Currently, each 15 minutes of time is equal to one time-unit according to CMS. The sum of the base and time units are then multiplied by the geographically adjusted dollar–anesthesiology conversion factor to arrive at the final payment for each service. For example, on January 1, 2022, Medicare would allow $236.83 in Montana for anesthesia for intraperitoneal procedures in the upper abdomen (code 00790), which takes one hour.

CPT code 00790 in Montana

(7 base units + 4 time units) × 21.53 = $236.83

The 2022 list of geographically adjusted dollar values is provided after the following anesthesia base-unit table.

Because the resource-based relative value scale (RBRVS) payment system continues to use the uniform relative value guide, CMS did not need to rescale the guide to conform with the RBRVS, but it only needed to establish a separate conversion factor for anesthesiology that would appropriately integrate payments for these services with payments for services on the Harvard scale. To compute this conversion factor, CMS determined the difference between the average payment under the old base and time unit system and the average payment that would result from using Harvard work relative value units (RVUs) for 19 anesthesia services surveyed by Harvard. The 1992 anesthesiology conversion factor represented a reduction of 42% in the work component of anesthesiology services, but an overall reduction from the 1991 conversion factor of 29% across all components. The anesthesia work–RVUs for 1997 were increased by 22.76% as a result of the five-year review, which translated into a 15.95% increase in the anesthesia conversion factor. As a result of the second five-year review efforts, CMS has announced an increase to the work portion of the anesthesia conversion factor of 2.10%, effective in 2003.

In 2007, at the request of CMS, RUC reviewed the work of the post-induction anesthesia period, considered how increases in the work of pre- and post-anesthesia services would affect all anesthesia services, and determined how and whether to apply the E/M update to anesthesia procedures. After this review, RUC determined that the work of anesthesia services is undervalued by approximately 32%. As a result of this review, CMS agreed with RUC's recommendations and increased the work of anesthesia services by 32% in 2008.

Comparing Anesthesia Values to RBRVS Values

Comparing anesthesia values to physician work values is not a straightforward process. In Medicare RBRVS, physician relative values are comprised of three components—physician work, practice expense, and professional liability insurance (PLI)—and are calculated for each code. In the Anesthesia Medicare Payment Schedule, physician work, practice expense, and professional liability insurance components are calculated as a fraction of each anesthesia unit and applied globally across all anesthesia codes. Therefore, the anesthesia base units include all three components. To begin to place the anesthesia values on the same scale as the physician work relative values, the anesthesia base units must be combined with standard time units and then reduced by a percentage that reflects the practice expense and PLI components in the anesthesia values. For 2022, the percentage of the anesthesia units allocated to physician work is 0.776 (PE = 0.161, PLI = 0.063) and is set by CMS and updated annually. Thus, for every anesthesia procedure, the fraction of the total base and time units attributed to physician work is fixed, and the calculated physician work for a given anesthesia code varies with the total base and time units of the procedure.

It is necessary to include physician time and adjust the units to reflect only the work portion of the units, in order to compare anesthesia values on the same scale as the RBRVS. The current formula (published by CMS in the 1994 *Federal Register*) for converting anesthesia values on the same scale as physician work relative values is as follows:

Anesthesia units × *(Anesthesia CF/Payment schedule CF)* × 0.776 *(Anesthesia work fraction) = RVUs*

The following table lists the base units *for 276 anesthesia services.*

Anesthesiology Base Units

CPT Code	2022 Base Units	Long Descriptor
00100	5	Anesthesia for procedures on salivary glands, including biopsy
00102	6	Anesthesia for procedures involving plastic repair of cleft lip
00103	5	Anesthesia for reconstructive procedures of eyelid (eg, blepharoplasty, ptosis surgery)
00104	4	Anesthesia for electroconvulsive therapy
00120	5	Anesthesia for procedures on external, middle, and inner ear including biopsy; not otherwise specified
00124	4	Anesthesia for procedures on external, middle, and inner ear including biopsy; otoscopy
00126	4	Anesthesia for procedures on external, middle, and inner ear including biopsy; tympanotomy
00140	5	Anesthesia for procedures on eye; not otherwise specified
00142	4	Anesthesia for procedures on eye; lens surgery
00144	6	Anesthesia for procedures on eye; corneal transplant
00145	6	Anesthesia for procedures on eye; vitreoretinal surgery
00147	4	Anesthesia for procedures on eye; iridectomy
00148	4	Anesthesia for procedures on eye; ophthalmoscopy
00160	5	Anesthesia for procedures on nose and accessory sinuses; not otherwise specified
00162	7	Anesthesia for procedures on nose and accessory sinuses; radical surgery
00164	4	Anesthesia for procedures on nose and accessory sinuses; biopsy, soft tissue
00170	5	Anesthesia for intraoral procedures, including biopsy; not otherwise specified
00172	6	Anesthesia for intraoral procedures, including biopsy; repair of cleft palate
00174	6	Anesthesia for intraoral procedures, including biopsy; excision of retropharyngeal tumor
00176	7	Anesthesia for intraoral procedures, including biopsy; radical surgery
00190	5	Anesthesia for procedures on facial bones or skull; not otherwise specified
00192	7	Anesthesia for procedures on facial bones or skull; radical surgery (including prognathism)
00210	11	Anesthesia for intracranial procedures; not otherwise specified
00211	10	Anesthesia for intracranial procedures; craniotomy or craniectomy for evacuation of hematoma
00212	5	Anesthesia for intracranial procedures; subdural taps
00214	9	Anesthesia for intracranial procedures; burr holes, including ventriculography
00215	9	Anesthesia for intracranial procedures; cranioplasty or elevation of depressed skull fracture, extradural (simple or compound)
00216	15	Anesthesia for intracranial procedures; vascular procedures
00218	13	Anesthesia for intracranial procedures; procedures in sitting position
00220	10	Anesthesia for intracranial procedures; cerebrospinal fluid shunting procedures
00222	6	Anesthesia for intracranial procedures; electrocoagulation of intracranial nerve
00300	5	Anesthesia for all procedures on the integumentary system, muscles and nerves of head, neck, and posterior trunk, not otherwise specified
00320	6	Anesthesia for all procedures on esophagus, thyroid, larynx, trachea and lymphatic system of neck; not otherwise specified, age 1 year or older
00322	3	Anesthesia for all procedures on esophagus, thyroid, larynx, trachea and lymphatic system of neck; needle biopsy of thyroid
00326	7	Anesthesia for all procedures on the larynx and trachea in children younger than 1 year of age
00350	10	Anesthesia for procedures on major vessels of neck; not otherwise specified
00352	5	Anesthesia for procedures on major vessels of neck; simple ligation
00400	3	Anesthesia for procedures on the integumentary system on the extremities, anterior trunk and perineum; not otherwise specified

(continued)

Anesthesiology Base Units

CPT Code	2022 Base Units	Long Descriptor
00402	5	Anesthesia for procedures on the integumentary system on the extremities, anterior trunk and perineum; reconstructive procedures on breast (eg, reduction or augmentation mammoplasty, muscle flaps)
00404	5	Anesthesia for procedures on the integumentary system on the extremities, anterior trunk and perineum; radical or modified radical procedures on breast
00406	13	Anesthesia for procedures on the integumentary system on the extremities, anterior trunk and perineum; radical or modified radical procedures on breast with internal mammary node dissection
00410	4	Anesthesia for procedures on the integumentary system on the extremities, anterior trunk and perineum; electrical conversion of arrhythmias
00450	5	Anesthesia for procedures on clavicle and scapula; not otherwise specified
00454	3	Anesthesia for procedures on clavicle and scapula; biopsy of clavicle
00470	6	Anesthesia for partial rib resection; not otherwise specified
00472	10	Anesthesia for partial rib resection; thoracoplasty (any type)
00474	13	Anesthesia for partial rib resection; radical procedures (eg, pectus excavatum)
00500	15	Anesthesia for all procedures on esophagus
00520	6	Anesthesia for closed chest procedures; (including bronchoscopy) not otherwise specified
00522	4	Anesthesia for closed chest procedures; needle biopsy of pleura
00524	4	Anesthesia for closed chest procedures; pneumocentesis
00528	8	Anesthesia for closed chest procedures; mediastinoscopy and diagnostic thoracoscopy not utilizing 1 lung ventilation
00529	11	Anesthesia for closed chest procedures; mediastinoscopy and diagnostic thoracoscopy utilizing 1 lung ventilation
00530	4	Anesthesia for permanent transvenous pacemaker insertion
00532	4	Anesthesia for access to central venous circulation
00534	7	Anesthesia for transvenous insertion or replacement of pacing cardioverter-defibrillator
00537	10	Anesthesia for cardiac electrophysiologic procedures including radiofrequency ablation
00539	18	Anesthesia for tracheobronchial reconstruction
00540	12	Anesthesia for thoracotomy procedures involving lungs, pleura, diaphragm, and mediastinum (including surgical thoracoscopy); not otherwise specified
00541	15	Anesthesia for thoracotomy procedures involving lungs, pleura, diaphragm, and mediastinum (including surgical thoracoscopy); utilizing 1 lung ventilation
00542	15	Anesthesia for thoracotomy procedures involving lungs, pleura, diaphragm, and mediastinum (including surgical thoracoscopy); decortication
00546	15	Anesthesia for thoracotomy procedures involving lungs, pleura, diaphragm, and mediastinum (including surgical thoracoscopy); pulmonary resection with thoracoplasty
00548	17	Anesthesia for thoracotomy procedures involving lungs, pleura, diaphragm, and mediastinum (including surgical thoracoscopy); intrathoracic procedures on the trachea and bronchi
00550	10	Anesthesia for sternal debridement
00560	15	Anesthesia for procedures on heart, pericardial sac, and great vessels of chest; without pump oxygenator
00561	25	Anesthesia for procedures on heart, pericardial sac, and great vessels of chest; with pump oxygenator, younger than 1 year of age
00562	20	Anesthesia for procedures on heart, pericardial sac, and great vessels of chest; with pump oxygenator, age 1 year or older, for all noncoronary bypass procedures (eg, valve procedures) or for re-operation for coronary bypass more than 1 month after original operation
00563	25	Anesthesia for procedures on heart, pericardial sac, and great vessels of chest; with pump oxygenator with hypothermic circulatory arrest

Anesthesiology Base Units

CPT Code	2022 Base Units	Long Descriptor
00566	25	Anesthesia for direct coronary artery bypass grafting; without pump oxygenator
00567	18	Anesthesia for direct coronary artery bypass grafting; with pump oxygenator
00580	20	Anesthesia for heart transplant or heart/lung transplant
00600	10	Anesthesia for procedures on cervical spine and cord; not otherwise specified
00604	13	Anesthesia for procedures on cervical spine and cord; procedures with patient in the sitting position
00620	10	Anesthesia for procedures on thoracic spine and cord, not otherwise specified
00625	13	Anesthesia for procedures on the thoracic spine and cord, via an anterior transthoracic approach; not utilizing 1 lung ventilation
00626	15	Anesthesia for procedures on the thoracic spine and cord, via an anterior transthoracic approach; utilizing 1 lung ventilation
00630	8	Anesthesia for procedures in lumbar region; not otherwise specified
00632	7	Anesthesia for procedures in lumbar region; lumbar sympathectomy
00635	4	Anesthesia for procedures in lumbar region; diagnostic or therapeutic lumbar puncture
00640	3	Anesthesia for manipulation of the spine or for closed procedures on the cervical, thoracic or lumbar spine
00670	13	Anesthesia for extensive spine and spinal cord procedures (eg, spinal instrumentation or vascular procedures)
00700	4	Anesthesia for procedures on upper anterior abdominal wall; not otherwise specified
00702	4	Anesthesia for procedures on upper anterior abdominal wall; percutaneous liver biopsy
00730	5	Anesthesia for procedures on upper posterior abdominal wall
00731	5	Anesthesia for upper gastrointestinal endoscopic procedures, endoscope introduced proximal to duodenum; not otherwise specified
00732	6	Anesthesia for upper gastrointestinal endoscopic procedures, endoscope introduced proximal to duodenum; endoscopic retrograde cholangiopancreatography (ercp)
00750	4	Anesthesia for hernia repairs in upper abdomen; not otherwise specified
00752	6	Anesthesia for hernia repairs in upper abdomen; lumbar and ventral (incisional) hernias and/or wound dehiscence
00754	7	Anesthesia for hernia repairs in upper abdomen; omphalocele
00756	7	Anesthesia for hernia repairs in upper abdomen; transabdominal repair of diaphragmatic hernia
00770	15	Anesthesia for all procedures on major abdominal blood vessels
00790	7	Anesthesia for intraperitoneal procedures in upper abdomen including laparoscopy; not otherwise specified
00792	13	Anesthesia for intraperitoneal procedures in upper abdomen including laparoscopy; partial hepatectomy or management of liver hemorrhage (excluding liver biopsy)
00794	8	Anesthesia for intraperitoneal procedures in upper abdomen including laparoscopy; pancreatectomy, partial or total (eg, Whipple procedure)
00796	30	Anesthesia for intraperitoneal procedures in upper abdomen including laparoscopy; liver transplant (recipient)
00797	11	Anesthesia for intraperitoneal procedures in upper abdomen including laparoscopy; gastric restrictive procedure for morbid obesity
00800	4	Anesthesia for procedures on lower anterior abdominal wall; not otherwise specified
00802	5	Anesthesia for procedures on lower anterior abdominal wall; panniculectomy
00811	4	Anesthesia for lower intestinal endoscopic procedures, endoscope introduced distal to duodenum; not otherwise specified
00812	3	Anesthesia for lower intestinal endoscopic procedures, endoscope introduced distal to duodenum; screening colonoscopy

(*continued*)

Anesthesiology Base Units

CPT Code	2022 Base Units	Long Descriptor
00813	5	Anesthesia for combined upper and lower gastrointestinal endoscopic procedures, endoscope introduced both proximal to and distal to the duodenum
00820	5	Anesthesia for procedures on lower posterior abdominal wall
00830	4	Anesthesia for hernia repairs in lower abdomen; not otherwise specified
00832	6	Anesthesia for hernia repairs in lower abdomen; ventral and incisional hernias
00834	5	Anesthesia for hernia repairs in the lower abdomen not otherwise specified, younger than 1 year of age
00836	6	Anesthesia for hernia repairs in the lower abdomen not otherwise specified, infants younger than 37 weeks gestational age at birth and younger than 50 weeks gestational age at time of surgery
00840	6	Anesthesia for intraperitoneal procedures in lower abdomen including laparoscopy; not otherwise specified
00842	4	Anesthesia for intraperitoneal procedures in lower abdomen including laparoscopy; amniocentesis
00844	7	Anesthesia for intraperitoneal procedures in lower abdomen including laparoscopy; abdominoperineal resection
00846	8	Anesthesia for intraperitoneal procedures in lower abdomen including laparoscopy; radical hysterectomy
00848	8	Anesthesia for intraperitoneal procedures in lower abdomen including laparoscopy; pelvic exenteration
00851	6	Anesthesia for intraperitoneal procedures in lower abdomen including laparoscopy; tubal ligation/ transection
00860	6	Anesthesia for extraperitoneal procedures in lower abdomen, including urinary tract; not otherwise specified
00862	7	Anesthesia for extraperitoneal procedures in lower abdomen, including urinary tract; renal procedures, including upper one-third of ureter, or donor nephrectomy
00864	8	Anesthesia for extraperitoneal procedures in lower abdomen, including urinary tract; total cystectomy
00865	7	Anesthesia for extraperitoneal procedures in lower abdomen, including urinary tract; radical prostatectomy (suprapubic, retropubic)
00866	10	Anesthesia for extraperitoneal procedures in lower abdomen, including urinary tract; adrenalectomy
00868	10	Anesthesia for extraperitoneal procedures in lower abdomen, including urinary tract; renal transplant (recipient)
00870	5	Anesthesia for extraperitoneal procedures in lower abdomen, including urinary tract; cystolithotomy
00872	7	Anesthesia for lithotripsy, extracorporeal shock wave; with water bath
00873	5	Anesthesia for lithotripsy, extracorporeal shock wave; without water bath
00880	15	Anesthesia for procedures on major lower abdominal vessels; not otherwise specified
00882	10	Anesthesia for procedures on major lower abdominal vessels; inferior vena cava ligation
00902	5	Anesthesia for; anorectal procedure
00904	7	Anesthesia for; radical perineal procedure
00906	4	Anesthesia for; vulvectomy
00908	6	Anesthesia for; perineal prostatectomy
00910	3	Anesthesia for transurethral procedures (including urethrocystoscopy); not otherwise specified
00912	5	Anesthesia for transurethral procedures (including urethrocystoscopy); transurethral resection of bladder tumor(s)
00914	5	Anesthesia for transurethral procedures (including urethrocystoscopy); transurethral resection of prostate
00916	5	Anesthesia for transurethral procedures (including urethrocystoscopy); post-transurethral resection bleeding
00918	5	Anesthesia for transurethral procedures (including urethrocystoscopy); with fragmentation, manipulation and/or removal of ureteral calculus
00920	3	Anesthesia for procedures on male genitalia (including open urethral procedures); not otherwise specified
00921	3	Anesthesia for procedures on male genitalia (including open urethral procedures); vasectomy, unilateral or bilateral

Anesthesiology Base Units

CPT Code	2022 Base Units	Long Descriptor
00922	6	Anesthesia for procedures on male genitalia (including open urethral procedures); seminal vesicles
00924	4	Anesthesia for procedures on male genitalia (including open urethral procedures); undescended testis, unilateral or bilateral
00926	4	Anesthesia for procedures on male genitalia (including open urethral procedures); radical orchiectomy, inguinal
00928	6	Anesthesia for procedures on male genitalia (including open urethral procedures); radical orchiectomy, abdominal
00930	4	Anesthesia for procedures on male genitalia (including open urethral procedures); orchiopexy, unilateral or bilateral
00932	4	Anesthesia for procedures on male genitalia (including open urethral procedures); complete amputation of penis
00934	6	Anesthesia for procedures on male genitalia (including open urethral procedures); radical amputation of penis with bilateral inguinal lymphadenectomy
00936	8	Anesthesia for procedures on male genitalia (including open urethral procedures); radical amputation of penis with bilateral inguinal and iliac lymphadenectomy
00938	4	Anesthesia for procedures on male genitalia (including open urethral procedures); insertion of penile prosthesis (perineal approach)
00940	3	Anesthesia for vaginal procedures (including biopsy of labia, vagina, cervix or endometrium); not otherwise specified
00942	4	Anesthesia for vaginal procedures (including biopsy of labia, vagina, cervix or endometrium); colpotomy, vaginectomy, colporrhaphy, and open urethral procedures
00944	6	Anesthesia for vaginal procedures (including biopsy of labia, vagina, cervix or endometrium); vaginal hysterectomy
00948	4	Anesthesia for vaginal procedures (including biopsy of labia, vagina, cervix or endometrium); cervical cerclage
00950	5	Anesthesia for vaginal procedures (including biopsy of labia, vagina, cervix or endometrium); culdoscopy
00952	4	Anesthesia for vaginal procedures (including biopsy of labia, vagina, cervix or endometrium); hysteroscopy and/or hysterosalpingography
01112	5	Anesthesia for bone marrow aspiration and/or biopsy, anterior or posterior iliac crest
01120	6	Anesthesia for procedures on bony pelvis
01130	3	Anesthesia for body cast application or revision
01140	15	Anesthesia for interpelviabdominal (hindquarter) amputation
01150	10	Anesthesia for radical procedures for tumor of pelvis, except hindquarter amputation
01160	4	Anesthesia for closed procedures involving symphysis pubis or sacroiliac joint
01170	8	Anesthesia for open procedures involving symphysis pubis or sacroiliac joint
01173	12	Anesthesia for open repair of fracture disruption of pelvis or column fracture involving acetabulum
01200	4	Anesthesia for all closed procedures involving hip joint
01202	4	Anesthesia for arthroscopic procedures of hip joint
01210	6	Anesthesia for open procedures involving hip joint; not otherwise specified
01212	10	Anesthesia for open procedures involving hip joint; hip disarticulation
01214	8	Anesthesia for open procedures involving hip joint; total hip arthroplasty
01215	10	Anesthesia for open procedures involving hip joint; revision of total hip arthroplasty
01220	4	Anesthesia for all closed procedures involving upper two-thirds of femur
01230	6	Anesthesia for open procedures involving upper two-thirds of femur; not otherwise specified
01232	5	Anesthesia for open procedures involving upper two-thirds of femur; amputation

(*continued*)

Anesthesiology Base Units

CPT Code	2022 Base Units	Long Descriptor
01234	8	Anesthesia for open procedures involving upper two-thirds of femur; radical resection
01250	4	Anesthesia for all procedures on nerves, muscles, tendons, fascia, and bursae of upper leg
01260	3	Anesthesia for all procedures involving veins of upper leg, including exploration
01270	8	Anesthesia for procedures involving arteries of upper leg, including bypass graft; not otherwise specified
01272	4	Anesthesia for procedures involving arteries of upper leg, including bypass graft; femoral artery ligation
01274	6	Anesthesia for procedures involving arteries of upper leg, including bypass graft; femoral artery embolectomy
01320	4	Anesthesia for all procedures on nerves, muscles, tendons, fascia, and bursae of knee and/or popliteal area
01340	4	Anesthesia for all closed procedures on lower one-third of femur
01360	5	Anesthesia for all open procedures on lower one-third of femur
01380	3	Anesthesia for all closed procedures on knee joint
01382	3	Anesthesia for diagnostic arthroscopic procedures of knee joint
01390	3	Anesthesia for all closed procedures on upper ends of tibia, fibula, and/or patella
01392	4	Anesthesia for all open procedures on upper ends of tibia, fibula, and/or patella
01400	4	Anesthesia for open or surgical arthroscopic procedures on knee joint; not otherwise specified
01402	7	Anesthesia for open or surgical arthroscopic procedures on knee joint; total knee arthroplasty
01404	5	Anesthesia for open or surgical arthroscopic procedures on knee joint; disarticulation at knee
01420	3	Anesthesia for all cast applications, removal, or repair involving knee joint
01430	3	Anesthesia for procedures on veins of knee and popliteal area; not otherwise specified
01432	6	Anesthesia for procedures on veins of knee and popliteal area; arteriovenous fistula
01440	8	Anesthesia for procedures on arteries of knee and popliteal area; not otherwise specified
01442	8	Anesthesia for procedures on arteries of knee and popliteal area; popliteal thromboendarterectomy, with or without patch graft
01444	8	Anesthesia for procedures on arteries of knee and popliteal area; popliteal excision and graft or repair for occlusion or aneurysm
01462	3	Anesthesia for all closed procedures on lower leg, ankle, and foot
01464	3	Anesthesia for arthroscopic procedures of ankle and/or foot
01470	3	Anesthesia for procedures on nerves, muscles, tendons, and fascia of lower leg, ankle, and foot; not otherwise specified
01472	5	Anesthesia for procedures on nerves, muscles, tendons, and fascia of lower leg, ankle, and foot; repair of ruptured Achilles tendon, with or without graft
01474	5	Anesthesia for procedures on nerves, muscles, tendons, and fascia of lower leg, ankle, and foot; gastrocnemius recession (eg, Strayer procedure)
01480	3	Anesthesia for open procedures on bones of lower leg, ankle, and foot; not otherwise specified
01482	4	Anesthesia for open procedures on bones of lower leg, ankle, and foot; radical resection (including below knee amputation)
01484	4	Anesthesia for open procedures on bones of lower leg, ankle, and foot; osteotomy or osteoplasty of tibia and/or fibula
01486	7	Anesthesia for open procedures on bones of lower leg, ankle, and foot; total ankle replacement
01490	3	Anesthesia for lower leg cast application, removal, or repair
01500	8	Anesthesia for procedures on arteries of lower leg, including bypass graft; not otherwise specified
01502	6	Anesthesia for procedures on arteries of lower leg, including bypass graft; embolectomy, direct or with catheter
01520	3	Anesthesia for procedures on veins of lower leg; not otherwise specified

Anesthesiology Base Units

CPT Code	2022 Base Units	Long Descriptor
01522	5	Anesthesia for procedures on veins of lower leg; venous thrombectomy, direct or with catheter
01610	5	Anesthesia for all procedures on nerves, muscles, tendons, fascia, and bursae of shoulder and axilla
01620	4	Anesthesia for all closed procedures on humeral head and neck, sternoclavicular joint, acromioclavicular joint, and shoulder joint
01622	4	Anesthesia for diagnostic arthroscopic procedures of shoulder joint
01630	5	Anesthesia for open or surgical arthroscopic procedures on humeral head and neck, sternoclavicular joint, acromioclavicular joint, and shoulder joint; not otherwise specified
01634	9	Anesthesia for open or surgical arthroscopic procedures on humeral head and neck, sternoclavicular joint, acromioclavicular joint, and shoulder joint; shoulder disarticulation
01636	15	Anesthesia for open or surgical arthroscopic procedures on humeral head and neck, sternoclavicular joint, acromioclavicular joint, and shoulder joint; interthoracoscapular (forequarter) amputation
01638	10	Anesthesia for open or surgical arthroscopic procedures on humeral head and neck, sternoclavicular joint, acromioclavicular joint, and shoulder joint; total shoulder replacement
01650	6	Anesthesia for procedures on arteries of shoulder and axilla; not otherwise specified
01652	10	Anesthesia for procedures on arteries of shoulder and axilla; axillary-brachial aneurysm
01654	8	Anesthesia for procedures on arteries of shoulder and axilla; bypass graft
01656	10	Anesthesia for procedures on arteries of shoulder and axilla; axillary-femoral bypass graft
01670	4	Anesthesia for all procedures on veins of shoulder and axilla
01680	3	Anesthesia for shoulder cast application, removal or repair, not otherwise specified
01710	3	Anesthesia for procedures on nerves, muscles, tendons, fascia, and bursae of upper arm and elbow; not otherwise specified
01712	5	Anesthesia for procedures on nerves, muscles, tendons, fascia, and bursae of upper arm and elbow; tenotomy, elbow to shoulder, open
01714	5	Anesthesia for procedures on nerves, muscles, tendons, fascia, and bursae of upper arm and elbow; tenoplasty, elbow to shoulder
01716	5	Anesthesia for procedures on nerves, muscles, tendons, fascia, and bursae of upper arm and elbow; tenodesis, rupture of long tendon of biceps
01730	3	Anesthesia for all closed procedures on humerus and elbow
01732	3	Anesthesia for diagnostic arthroscopic procedures of elbow joint
01740	4	Anesthesia for open or surgical arthroscopic procedures of the elbow; not otherwise specified
01742	5	Anesthesia for open or surgical arthroscopic procedures of the elbow; osteotomy of humerus
01744	5	Anesthesia for open or surgical arthroscopic procedures of the elbow; repair of nonunion or malunion of humerus
01756	6	Anesthesia for open or surgical arthroscopic procedures of the elbow; radical procedures
01758	5	Anesthesia for open or surgical arthroscopic procedures of the elbow; excision of cyst or tumor of humerus
01760	7	Anesthesia for open or surgical arthroscopic procedures of the elbow; total elbow replacement
01770	6	Anesthesia for procedures on arteries of upper arm and elbow; not otherwise specified
01772	6	Anesthesia for procedures on arteries of upper arm and elbow; embolectomy
01780	3	Anesthesia for procedures on veins of upper arm and elbow; not otherwise specified
01782	4	Anesthesia for procedures on veins of upper arm and elbow; phlebography
01810	3	Anesthesia for all procedures on nerves, muscles, tendons, fascia, and bursae of forearm, wrist, and hand
01820	3	Anesthesia for all closed procedures on radius, ulna, wrist, or hand bones
01829	3	Anesthesia for diagnostic arthroscopic procedures on the wrist

(*continued*)

Anesthesiology Base Units

CPT Code	2022 Base Units	Long Descriptor
01830	3	Anesthesia for open or surgical arthroscopic/endoscopic procedures on distal radius, distal ulna, wrist, or hand joints; not otherwise specified
01832	6	Anesthesia for open or surgical arthroscopic/endoscopic procedures on distal radius, distal ulna, wrist, or hand joints; total wrist replacement
01840	6	Anesthesia for procedures on arteries of forearm, wrist, and hand; not otherwise specified
01842	6	Anesthesia for procedures on arteries of forearm, wrist, and hand; embolectomy
01844	6	Anesthesia for vascular shunt, or shunt revision, any type (eg, dialysis)
01850	3	Anesthesia for procedures on veins of forearm, wrist, and hand; not otherwise specified
01852	4	Anesthesia for procedures on veins of forearm, wrist, and hand; phlebography
01860	3	Anesthesia for forearm, wrist, or hand cast application, removal, or repair
01916	5	Anesthesia for diagnostic arteriography/venography
01920	7	Anesthesia for cardiac catheterization including coronary angiography and ventriculography (not to include Swan-Ganz catheter)
01922	7	Anesthesia for non-invasive imaging or radiation therapy
01924	5	Anesthesia for therapeutic interventional radiological procedures involving the arterial system; not otherwise specified
01925	7	Anesthesia for therapeutic interventional radiological procedures involving the arterial system; carotid or coronary
01926	8	Anesthesia for therapeutic interventional radiological procedures involving the arterial system; intracranial, intracardiac, or aortic
01930	5	Anesthesia for therapeutic interventional radiological procedures involving the venous/lymphatic system (not to include access to the central circulation); not otherwise specified
01931	7	Anesthesia for therapeutic interventional radiological procedures involving the venous/lymphatic system (not to include access to the central circulation); intrahepatic or portal circulation (eg, transvenous intrahepatic portosystemic shunt[s] [tips])
01932	6	Anesthesia for therapeutic interventional radiological procedures involving the venous/lymphatic system (not to include access to the central circulation); intrathoracic or jugular
01933	7	Anesthesia for therapeutic interventional radiological procedures involving the venous/lymphatic system (not to include access to the central circulation); intracranial
01937	4	Anesthesia for percutaneous image-guided injection, drainage or aspiration procedures on the spine or spinal cord; cervical or thoracic
01938	4	Anesthesia for percutaneous image-guided injection, drainage or aspiration procedures on the spine or spinal cord; lumbar or sacral
01939	4	Anesthesia for percutaneous image-guided destruction procedures by neurolytic agent on the spine or spinal cord; cervical or thoracic
01940	4	Anesthesia for percutaneous image-guided destruction procedures by neurolytic agent on the spine or spinal cord; lumbar or sacral
01941	5	Anesthesia for percutaneous image-guided neuromodulation or intravertebral procedures (eg, kyphoplasty, vertebroplasty) on the spine or spinal cord; cervical or thoracic
01942	5	Anesthesia for percutaneous image-guided neuromodulation or intravertebral procedures (eg, kyphoplasty, vertebroplasty) on the spine or spinal cord; lumbar or sacral
01951	3	Anesthesia for second- and third-degree burn excision or debridement with or without skin grafting, any site, for total body surface area (tbsa) treated during anesthesia and surgery; less than 4% total body surface area
01952	5	Anesthesia for second- and third-degree burn excision or debridement with or without skin grafting, any site, for total body surface area (tbsa) treated during anesthesia and surgery; between 4% and 9% of total body surface area

Anesthesiology Base Units

CPT Code	2022 Base Units	Long Descriptor
01953	1	Anesthesia for second- and third-degree burn excision or debridement with or without skin grafting, any site, for total body surface area (tbsa) treated during anesthesia and surgery; each additional 9% total body surface area or part thereof (list separately in addition to code for primary procedure)
01958	5	Anesthesia for external cephalic version procedure
01960	5	Anesthesia for vaginal delivery only
01961	7	Anesthesia for cesarean delivery only
01962	8	Anesthesia for urgent hysterectomy following delivery
01963	8	Anesthesia for cesarean hysterectomy without any labor analgesia/anesthesia care
01965	4	Anesthesia for incomplete or missed abortion procedures
01966	4	Anesthesia for induced abortion procedures
01967	5	Neuraxial labor analgesia/anesthesia for planned vaginal delivery (this includes any repeat subarachnoid needle placement and drug injection and/or any necessary replacement of an epidural catheter during labor)
01968	2	Anesthesia for cesarean delivery following neuraxial labor analgesia/anesthesia (list separately in addition to code for primary procedure performed)
01969	5	Anesthesia for cesarean hysterectomy following neuraxial labor analgesia/anesthesia (list separately in addition to code for primary procedure performed)
01990	7	Physiological support for harvesting of organ(s) from brain-dead patient
01991	3	Anesthesia for diagnostic or therapeutic nerve blocks and injections (when block or injection is performed by a different physician or other qualified health care professional); other than the prone position
01992	5	Anesthesia for diagnostic or therapeutic nerve blocks and injections (when block or injection is performed by a different physician or other qualified health care professional); prone position
01996	3	Daily hospital management of epidural or subarachnoid continuous drug administration
01999	0	Unlisted anesthesia procedure(s)

+ = Add-on code

Geographically Adjusted Dollar Anesthesia Conversion Factors, 2022

Contractor	State	Locality	Locality Name	Anesthesia Conversion Factor*
10112	AL	0	ALABAMA	21.07
2102	AK	1	ALASKA	29.81
3102	AZ	0	ARIZONA	21.2
7102	AR	13	ARKANSAS	20.3
1112	CA	54	BAKERSFIELD	22.02
1112	CA	55	CHICO	21.69
1182	CA	71	EL CENTRO	21.72
1112	CA	56	FRESNO	21.69
1112	CA	57	HANFORD-CORCORAN	21.69
1182	CA	18	LOS ANGELES-LONG BEACH-ANAHEIM (LOS ANGELES CNTY)	22.64
1182	CA	26	LOS ANGELES-LONG BEACH-ANAHEIM (ORANGE CNTY)	22.64
1112	CA	58	MADERA	21.69
1112	CA	59	MERCED	21.69
1112	CA	60	MODESTO	21.69
1112	CA	51	NAPA	22.39
1112	CA	7	SAN FRANCISCO-OAKLAND-BERKELEY (ALAMEDA/CONTRA COSTA CNTY)	23.26
1182	CA	17	OXNARD-THOUSAND OAKS-VENTURA	22.26
1112	CA	61	REDDING	21.69
1112	CA	62	RIVERSIDE-SAN BERNARDINO-ONTARIO	22.18
1112	CA	63	SACRAMENTO-ROSEVILLE-FOLSOM	21.93
1112	CA	64	SALINAS	22.55
1182	CA	72	SAN DIEGO-CHULA VISTA-CARLSBAD	22.22
1112	CA	5	SAN FRANCISCO-OAKLAND-BERKELEY (SAN FRANCISCO CNTY)	23.26
1112	CA	52	SAN FRANCISCO-OAKLAND-BERKELEY (MARIN CNTY)	23.32
1112	CA	65	SAN JOSE-SUNNYVALE-SANTA CLARA (SAN BENITO CNTY)	23.95
1182	CA	73	SAN LUIS OBISPO-PASO ROBLES	21.78
1112	CA	6	SAN FRANCISCO-OAKLAND-BERKELEY (SAN MATEO CNTY)	23.26
1112	CA	9	SAN JOSE-SUNNYVALE-SANTA CLARA (SANTA CLARA CNTY)	23.7
1112	CA	66	SANTA CRUZ-WATSONVILLE	22.48
1182	CA	74	SANTA MARIA-SANTA BARBARA	22.31
1112	CA	67	SANTA ROSA-PETALUMA	22.38
1112	CA	68	STOCKTON	21.69
1112	CA	53	VALLEJO	22.39
1112	CA	69	VISALIA	21.69
1112	CA	70	YUBA CITY	21.69
1112	CA	75	REST OF CALIFORNIA	21.69
4112	CO	1	COLORADO	21.43

Geographically Adjusted Dollar Anesthesia Conversion Factors, 2022

Contractor	State	Locality	Locality Name	Anesthesia Conversion Factor*
13102	CT	0	CONNECTICUT	22.49
12202	DC	1	DC + MD/VA SUBURBS	23.68
12102	DE	1	DELAWARE	21.62
9102	FL	3	FORT LAUDERDALE	22.73
9102	FL	4	MIAMI	23.86
9102	FL	99	REST OF FLORIDA	21.94
10212	GA	1	ATLANTA	21.42
10212	GA	99	REST OF GEORGIA	21.01
1212	HI	1	HAWAII, GUAM	21.78
2202	ID	0	IDAHO	20.34
6102	IL	16	CHICAGO	23.08
6102	IL	12	EAST ST. LOUIS	22.26
6102	IL	15	SUBURBAN CHICAGO	22.56
6102	IL	99	REST OF ILLINOIS	21.5
8102	IN	0	INDIANA	20.49
5102	IA	0	IOWA	20.46
5202	KS	0	KANSAS	20.51
15102	KY	0	KENTUCKY	20.87
7202	LA	1	NEW ORLEANS	22.03
7202	LA	99	REST OF LOUISIANA	21.53
14112	ME	3	SOUTHERN MAINE	21.08
14112	ME	99	REST OF MAINE	20.74
12302	MD	1	BALTIMORE/SURR. CNTYS	22.79
12302	MD	99	REST OF MARYLAND	21.97
14212	MA	1	METROPOLITAN BOSTON	22.87
14212	MA	99	REST OF MASSACHUSETTS	21.99
8202	MI	1	DETROIT	22.4
8202	MI	99	REST OF MICHIGAN	21.22
6202	MN	0	MINNESOTA	20.73
7302	MS	0	MISSISSIPPI	20.57
5302	MO	2	METROPOLITAN KANSAS CITY	21.26
5302	MO	1	METROPOLITAN ST. LOUIS	21.33
5302	MO	99	REST OF MISSOURI	20.81
3202	MT	1	MONTANA	21.53
5402	NE	0	NEBRASKA	20.2
1312	NV	0	NEVADA	22.12
14312	NH	40	NEW HAMPSHIRE	21.58

(continued)

Geographically Adjusted Dollar Anesthesia Conversion Factors, 2022

Contractor	State	Locality	Locality Name	Anesthesia Conversion Factor*
12402	NJ	1	NORTHERN NJ	23.02
12402	NJ	99	REST OF NEW JERSEY	22.62
4212	NM	5	NEW MEXICO	21.43
13202	NY	1	MANHATTAN	24.6
13202	NY	2	NYC SUBURBS/LONG ISLAND	25.42
13202	NY	3	POUGHKPSIE/N NYC SUBURBS	23.26
13292	NY	4	QUEENS	25.55
13282	NY	99	REST OF NEW YORK	21.07
11502	NC	0	NORTH CAROLINA	21.07
3302	ND	1	NORTH DAKOTA	20.79
15202	OH	0	OHIO	21.39
4312	OK	0	OKLAHOMA	20.85
2302	OR	1	PORTLAND	21.52
2302	OR	99	REST OF OREGON	20.75
12502	PA	1	METROPOLITAN PHILADELPHIA	22.49
12502	PA	99	REST OF PENNSYLVANIA	21.2
9202	PR	20	PUERTO RICO	21.57
14412	RI	1	RHODE ISLAND	22.05
11202	SC	1	SOUTH CAROLINA	20.81
3402	SD	2	SOUTH DAKOTA	20.68
10312	TN	35	TENNESSEE	20.5
4412	TX	31	AUSTIN	21.14
4412	TX	20	BEAUMONT	20.76
4412	TX	9	BRAZORIA	21.57
4412	TX	11	DALLAS	21.42
4412	TX	28	FORT WORTH	21.19
4412	TX	15	GALVESTON	21.58
4412	TX	18	HOUSTON	22.06
4412	TX	99	REST OF TEXAS	20.84
3502	UT	9	UTAH	21.01
14512	VT	50	VERMONT	20.98
11302	VA	0	VIRGINIA	21.41
9202	VI	50	VIRGIN ISLANDS	21.57
2402	WA	2	SEATTLE (KING CNTY)	22.53
2402	WA	99	REST OF WASHINGTON	21.26
11402	WV	16	WEST VIRGINIA	21.34
6302	WI	0	WISCONSIN	20.4
3602	WY	21	WYOMING	21.35

Appendices

Appendix A

Glossary

Achieving a Better Life Experience (ABLE) Act of 2014 Signed into law on December 19, 2014, this Act accelerated annual target adjustments for relative values of misvalued services compared to those originally set by the Protecting Access to Medicare Act (PAMA) of 2014. The ABLE Act increased the target reduction to 1% for 2016 and kept the target reduction at 0.5% for 2017 and 2018.

Actual charge The physician's billed or submitted charge, which is the amount Medicare will pay if it is lower than the Medicare payment-schedule amount.

Affordable Care Act (ACA) The ACA was signed into law by President Barack Obama on March 23, 2010. This Act provides several stipulations including: (1) extending the 1.0 work geographic practice cost index (GPCI) floor to December 31, 2010; (2) raising practice expense GPCIs in low-cost areas by reflecting only half of the geographic wage and rent cost differences in their calculation; (3) extending the current 5% bonus payment for specified psychiatry services; (4) increasing payments for bone density tests; (5) extending the exceptions process for Medicare therapy caps to December 31, 2010; (6) extending a provision allowing independent laboratories to bill for the technical component of physician pathology services; and (7) extending incentive payments under the Physician Quality Reporting System (PQRS) and puts in place payment reductions for failure to participate in the PQRS beginning in 2015 (the PQRS program was bundled into the merit-based incentive payment system [MIPS] in 2019). In addition to these provisions, this Act also announced the creation of an incentive payment to primary care physicians, including family medicine, internal medicine, and geriatric medicine, for which primary care services accounted for at least 60% of their Medicare allowed charges. These physicians were eligible for a 10% bonus payment for these services from January 1, 2011–December 31, 2015. Furthermore, this Act also provides that general surgeons who perform major procedures (with a 010 or 090 day global service period) in a health professional shortage area (HPSA) were eligible for a 10% bonus payment for these services from January 1, 2011–December 31, 2015.

AMA/Specialty Society RVS Update Committee (RUC) RUC was established by the AMA and national medical specialty societies in 1991, and it makes annual recommendations to the Centers for Medicare & Medicaid Services (CMS) on the work RVUs to be assigned to new and revised Current Procedural Terminology (CPT®) codes, as they are adopted by the AMA CPT Editorial Panel.

American Taxpayer Relief Act of 2012 Signed into law on January 2, 2013, this Act prevented a scheduled payment cut of 25.5% from taking effect on January 1, 2013. This new law provided a zero-percent update through December 31, 2013.

Approved amount The full Medicare payment amount that a physician or other health care professional is allowed to receive for a service provided to a Medicare beneficiary; the Medicare program pays 80% and the patient the remaining 20%. Payments to physicians who do not participate in Medicare are calculated based on 95% of the payment schedule; the physician's charges are limited to 115% of this amount.

Assignment When a physician accepts the Medicare approved amount (including the 80% Medicare payment and 20% patient copayment) as payment in full, it is called "accepting assignment." The physician submits a claim to Medicare directly and collects only the appropriate deductible and the 20% copayment from the patient.

Balance bill That portion of a physician's charge exceeding the Medicare approved amount, which is billed to the patient. When a physician balance bills, the patient is responsible for the amount of the physician's charge that exceeds the Medicare approved amount up to the limiting charge, as well as the 20% copayment. Only nonparticipating physicians may balance bill their Medicare patients.

Balanced Budget Act of 1997 Legislation signed by President Bill Clinton on August 5, 1997, significantly changing the Medicare program. The legislation created a Medicare + Choice program that expanded beneficiaries' health plan options, extended Medicare coverage to some preventive medicine services, and changed the system for annual updates to physician payments. (Chapter 1 summarizes key provisions of the legislation.)

Baseline adjustment A 6.5% reduction to the conversion factor (CF) to maintain budget neutrality that was adopted in the 1991 Final Rule to account for volume increases due to patient demand, physician responses to the RBRVS payment system, and other factors projected by CMS. This adjustment replaced an initial 10% "behavioral offset" proposed in the NPRM that reflected anticipated increases in physician services. CMS adopted the term *baseline adjustment* because of concerns of the AMA and others that the term *behavioral offset* was misleading. Such offsets are again included in the budget-neutrality adjustments in 1999.

Behavioral offset A reduction in the CF proposed in the NPRM to compensate for CMS assumption that physicians would increase the volume of services in response to decreases in payment. The NPRM included a 10% volume or "behavioral" offset in 1992 payments, but it was replaced in the 1991 Final Rule with a 6.5% baseline adjustment to maintain budget neutrality during the full transition period. Behavioral offsets also were applied to the CFs in 1997 (–0.9%), 1998 (–0.1%), 1999 (–0.28%), 2000 (–0.12%), 2001 (–0.14%), and 2002 (–0.18%). In 2003, a behavioral offset of –0.49% was applied to the practice expense RVUs. A behavioral offset was not applied in 2004–2013.

Bipartisan Budget Act of 2018 Signed into law on February 9, 2018, this Act amended the positive annual payment updates to the Medicare Program of 0.5% for 2019 to 0.25% for 2019. The Act also extended the work GPCI floor of 1.0 through December 31, 2019.

Budget neutrality A provision of the Omnibus Budget Reconciliation Act of 1989, the legislation that established the Medicare RBRVS payment system, that specifies any changes in RVUs resulting from changes in medical practice, coding, new data, or addition of new services cannot cause Medicare Part B expenditures to differ by more than $20 million from the spending level that would occur in the absence of such changes. To ensure Medicare Part B spending does not differ by more than $20 million, CMS has the regulatory authority to adjust the payment system accordingly. CMS has implemented numerous methods of budget-neutrality adjustments since 1993, including uniform reductions to work RVUs, adjustments to the CF, modification of the MEI weights, and application of a negative adjustor to all work RVUs. The AMA and RUC advocate for any budget-neutrality adjustment deemed necessary to be made to the CF, rather than the work relative values. Despite objections, in 2008, CMS achieved budget neutrality by applying a –11.94 adjustment (0.08806 adjustor) to all work RVUs. However, for 2009, the work adjustor was eliminated through the Medicare Improvement for Patients and Providers Act of 2008, and budget neutrality was achieved through an adjustment to the CF.

Centers for Medicare & Medicaid Services (CMS) Formerly known as the Health Care Financing Administration (HCFA), the agency within the Department of Health and Human Services (HHS) that administers the Medicare program.

Consolidated Appropriations Act, 2021 The Consolidated Appropriations Act, 2021, (the Act) that was signed into law on December 27, 2020, included provisions that offset most of the –10.2% budget-neutrality adjustment that was slated to take effect for Medicare-covered services provided as of January 1, 2021. The Act delayed implementation of HCPCS add-on code G2211 (visit complexity inherent to evaluation and management services) until calendar year (CY) 2024. The Act also provided a one-year 3.75% increase in the Medicare Physician Fee Schedule (MFS) payments for CY 2021. Moreover, the Act suspended the 2% payment adjustment (sequestration) through March 31, 2021 (which was subsequently suspended through the end of 2021) and reinstated the 1.0 floor on the work GCPI through CY 2023.

Continuing Extension Act of 2010 Signed into law on April 15, 2010, this Act was the third time in 2010 that the 21% reduction to the CF was postponed. This Act extended the postponement of the reduction by again applying a zero-percent update to the 2010 CF from April 1, 2010, through May 31, 2010.

Contractor A private contractor to the CMS that administers claims processing and payment for Medicare Part B services.

Conversion factor (CF) The factor that transforms the geographically adjusted relative value for a service into a dollar amount under the physician payment schedule.

Continuing Appropriations Act, 2021, and Other Extensions Act This Act provided Medicare extenders, which included extension of the work geographic index floor under the Medicare program through December 11, 2020. It amended Section 1848(e)(1)(E) of the Social Security Act (SSA) (42 U.S.C. §1395w–4(e)(1)(E)), as amended by section 3801 of the Coronavirus Aid, Relief, and Economic Security (CARES) Act (Public Law 116–136), by striking "December 1, 2020" and inserting "December 12, 2020," such that the SSA now reads, "After calculating the work geographic index in subparagraph (A)(iii), for purposes of payment for services furnished on or after January 1, 2004, and before December 12, 2020, the Secretary shall increase the work geographic index to 1.00 for any locality for which such work geographic index is less than 1.00."

Coronavirus Aid, Relief, and Economic Security (CARES) Act In March 2020, the CARES Act was signed into law, the third and largest major legislative initiative to address coronavirus 2019 (COVID-19). Among many other provisions, the CARES Act provided health and human services extenders, which included Medicare provisions to extend the work geographic index floor of 1.0 from May 23, 2020, through December 1, 2020. It amended Section 1848(e)(1)(E) of the SSA (42 U.S.C. §1395w–4(e)(1)(E)) by striking "May 23, 2020" and inserting "December 1, 2020."

Current Procedural Terminology (CPT®) System for coding procedures and physician services developed by the AMA to file claims with Medicare and other third-party payers; Healthcare Common Procedural Coding System (HCPCS) Level I codes.

Customary charge The physician's median charge for a service that is based on data collected during the July–June period preceding the current calendar year. One of the factors considered in determining a physician's Medicare payment under the CPR system.

Customary, prevailing, and reasonable (CPR) The payment system used to determine physician payment under the Medicare program before implementation of Medicare RBRVS payment system on January 1, 1992. The CPR system paid the lowest of the physician's actual charge for a service, physician's customary charge, or prevailing charge in the locality. Because of the diversity in physicians' charges for the same services, the CPR system allowed for wide variation in Medicare payment levels across specialties and geographic areas. (The CPR system is described in Chapter 1.)

Department of Defense Appropriation Act of 2010 Signed into law on December 19, 2009, this Act applied a zero-percent update to the 2010 CF from January 1, 2010, through February 28, 2010.

Deductible A specified amount of covered medical expenses a beneficiary must pay before receiving benefits.

Deficit Reduction Act (DRA) Effective January 1, 2007, CMS implemented policy that will affect payment for various imaging services in the payment schedule, including X ray, ultrasound, nuclear medicine, magnetic resonance imaging, computed tomography, and fluoroscopy, but excluding diagnostic and screening mammography (see Appendix D in the MFS Final Rule for a complete list of all affected services). Carrier-priced services will also be affected by the DRA because these services are within the statutory definition of imaging services and are within the statutory definition of a physician payment schedule service. The DRA states that payment for the technical component of imaging services paid under the MFS should be capped at the outpatient prospective payment system (OPPS) payment amount for the same imaging services. It is important to note that payment for an individual service, which is affected by the DRA, will only be capped if the MFS technical component–payment amount exceeds the OPPS payment amount.

Department of Health and Human Services (HHS) Department within the US government that is responsible for administering health and social welfare programs.

Evaluation and Management (E/M) services Patient E/M services that a physician provides during a patient's office, hospital, or other visit or consultation. New codes for visits and consultations, developed by the AMA CPT Editorial Panel and adopted by CMS for implementation under the Medicare program beginning January 1, 1992, improved the coding uniformity for these services and their appropriateness for use in an RBRVS-based payment schedule. The E/M codes were originally based on type of history, examination, and medical decision making (MDM). On November 1, 2019, CMS finalized a historic provision in the 2020 MFS Final Rule. This provision included revisions to the code descriptors and documentation standards for CPT E/M office visit codes 99202-99215. Code 99201 has been deleted. These revisions directly addressed the continuing problem of administrative burden for physicians in nearly every specialty across the country. With these landmark changes, as approved by the CPT Editorial Panel, documentation for

E/M office visits will now be centered around how physicians think and take care of patients by allowing physicians to choose whether his or her documentation is based on MDM or total time. (See Chapter 10.)

Final Notice A portion of the November 25, 1992, *Federal Register* containing a summary of the comments received on the 1991 "interim" relative values, a description of the CMS refinement methodology, and a table of the resulting 1993 relative values for physician services.

Final Rule A portion of the *Federal Register* that contains a summary of the final regulations for implementing the Medicare RBRVS payment schedule for a particular year. It generally includes updated RVUs for all physician services, payable under the payment schedule, revised payment rules, analyses of comments on the previous proposed rule and CMS' response, updated GPCIs, and an impact analysis of the new rules on physicians and beneficiaries.

Five-Year Review A review process mandated by OBRA 89 requiring CMS to conduct a review of all work relative values no less often than every 5 years. Activities for the first five-year review were initiated in 1995 and included work RVUs for all codes on the 1995 RBRVS payment schedule. Final RVUs were published by CMS in the 1996 Final Rule, effective for the 1997 Medicare RVS. The second five-year review began in 2000, with changes implemented in 2002. The third five-year review began in 2005, with changes implemented in 2007. The fourth five-year review began in 2010, with changes to be implemented in 2012. In the 2012 Final Rule, CMS states that the agency will be replacing separate five-year reviews with an ongoing annual review of potentially misvalued codes. The AMA/Specialty Society RUC played a key role in each of these review processes.

Further Consolidated Appropriations Act, 2020 This Act provided for extension of the work geographic index floor under the Medicare program. It extended the work GPCI floor to 1.0 from January 1, 2020, through May 22, 2020. This section extends the application of the current floor for the work GPCI, which applies to localities for which the work GPCI is less than 1.0, through May 22, 2020.

Geographic adjustment factor (GAF) The adjustment made to a service included in the RBRVS to account for geographic cost differences across Medicare localities, which are based on GPCIs.

Geographic practice cost index (GPCI) Indices reflecting differences across geographic areas in physicians' resource costs relative to the national average. Payments under the Medicare physician fee schedule are adjusted geographically for three factors to reflect differences in the cost of resources needed to produce physician services: physician work, practice expense, and professional liability insurance (PLI). Three distinct GPCIs—cost of living (physician work), practice costs, and PLI—are used to calculate the payment schedule amount for a service in a Medicare locality. (The list of GPCIs is available in Part 5.)

GPCI Floor The floor applies to the work geographic index as established under Section 1848(e)(1)(E) of the SSA (42 U.S.C. §1395w–4(e)(1)(E)). As of January 1, 2004, the Secretary will increase the work geographic index to 1.0 for any locality for which such work geographic index is less than 1.0. The floor continues to be extended annually through legislation.

Global charge The sum of the professional component and technical component of a procedure when provided and billed by the same physician. (See Chapter 11.)

Global service A payment concept defined by Medicare as a surgical "package" that includes all intraoperative and follow-up services, as well as some preoperative services, associated with the surgery for which the surgeon receives a single payment. The initial evaluation or consultation is excluded from the global package under the Medicare payment schedule. (See Chapter 11.)

Healthcare Common Procedure Coding System (HCPCS) Coding system required for billing Medicare, which is based on CPT code sets, but supplemented with additional codes for nonphysician services.

Health professional shortage areas (HPSAs) Urban or rural areas identified by the Public Health Service (PHS) as medically underserved. The PHS may also designate population groups and public nonprofit medical facilities as medically underserved. Physicians in designated HPSAs who furnish covered services to Medicare patients receive a 10% bonus payment in addition to the payment-schedule amount.

Limiting charge Statutory limit on the amount a nonparticipating physician can charge for services to Medicare patients. The limiting charge replaced the maximum allowable actual charge (MAAC), effective January 1, 1991. The limiting charge in 1993 and subsequent years is 115% of the Medicare approved amount for nonparticipating physicians. (See Chapter 9.)

Locality Geographic areas defined by CMS and used to establish payment amounts for physician services. CMS fundamentally revised the methodology for establishing localities effective for 1997 payments, reducing the number to 89 from 211. The new methodology increased the number of statewide localities and generally combined others into counties and groups of counties. Beginning in CY 2017, PAMA required that the areas used for payment in California must be Metropolitan Statistical Areas (MSAs) as defined by the Office of Management and Budget (OMB). Pursuant to the implementation of the new MSA-based locality structure for California, the total number of localities increased from 89 to 112 in CY 2017.

Maximum allowable actual charge (MAAC) Under the CPR system, a limit on the amount nonparticipating physicians could charge their Medicare patients above the Medicare approved amount. MAACs were different for each physician because they were based on the individual physician's customary charges. During a transition period from January 1, 1991, through December 31, 1992, MAACs were phased out and replaced by limiting charges.

Medicare Access and Children's Health Insurance Program (CHIP) Reauthorization Act (MACRA) of 2015 On April 16, 2015, MACRA was made into law and made several signification changes to the Medicare Program, including the following: (1) permanently repealed the sustainable growth rate (SGR) formula; (2) provided positive annual payment updates of 0.5% that started from July 1, 2015, and lasting through 2019; (3) extended CHIP for two years; (4) consolidated former quality reporting programs into MIPS; (5) extended the 1.0 physician work GPCI floor through December 31, 2017; and (6) provided a pathway to new payment models, including bonuses to mitigate risk- and technical-assistance funding for small practices.

Medicare economic index (MEI) An index introduced in 1976 that is intended to measure the annual growth in physicians' practice costs and general inflation in the cost of operating a medical practice. Under the Medicare payment schedule, the MEI is a factor in updating the CF. Under the CPR payment system, the MEI was a limitation on increases in a physician's prevailing charges.

Medicare Improvements for Patients and Providers Act (MIPPA) of 2008 On July 15, 2008, MIPPA of 2008 was made into law and made several significant changes to the Medicare Program, including the following: (1) an 18-month Medicare physician payment fix, stopping the 10.6% Medicare physician cut on July 1, 2008, and the 5.4% cut on January 1, 2009, continuing the June 2008 rates through December 31, 2008, and providing an additional 1.1% update for 2009; (2) a requirement that budget-neutrality adjustments be applied to the CF rather than the work relative values; (3) expansion of the coverage of the Medicare preventative services by extending the eligibility period for beneficiaries from six months to one year and waiving the initial preventive physical examination from the Medicare beneficiary's deductible; (4) provision of a 2% bonus payment in 2009 and 2010 for e-prescribing by eligible professionals, including physicians and other practitioners (this bonus payment will ultimately become a reduction in payment for eligible professionals who do not successfully e-prescribe by 2012); (5) increased incentive payments for PQRI to 2.0% for 2009; and (6) extension of the work GPCI floor of 1.0 through 2009 and provision of a 1.5 work GPCI for Alaska.

Medicare and Medicaid Extenders Act of 2010 Signed into law December 15, 2010, this Act provides a one-year freeze on the Medicare CF for 2011 established by the Preservation of Access to Care for Medicare Beneficiaries and Pension Relief Act and avoided a 25% reduction to the CF that was set to take effect on January 1, 2011. Further provisions of this Act include: (1) extending the work GPCI floor of 1.0, created in the Medicare Prescription Drug, Improvement and Modernization Act (MMA) of 2003 through December 31, 2011; (2) extending the exceptions process for Medicare therapy caps through December 31, 2011; (3) extending the payment for the technical component of certain physician pathology services; and (4) extending the mental health add-on payment of 5% for certain mental health services through December 31, 2011.

Medicare, Medicaid, and SCHIP Benefits Improvement and Protection Act (BIPA) of 2000 Legislation enacted on December 21, 2000, provides for revisions to policies applicable to the physician payment schedule. This legislation created Medicare coverage changes for several services, including enhancements to screening mammography, pelvic examinations, colonoscopy, and telehealth; new coverage for screening for glaucoma; and new coverage for medical nutrition therapy performed by registered dietitians and nutrition professionals.

Medicare, Medicaid, and SCHIP Extension Act of 2007 This legislation enacted in December 2007 postponed for six months the 10.1% cut in the Medicare CF that was slated to occur on January 1, 2008. This legislation provided a 0.5% increase in the CF from January through June 2008. In addition, this legislation authorized an additional 1.5% bonus for Medicare physician quality reporting initiative (PQRI) activities through December 31, 2008, and extends the 1.0 floor for work geographic adjustment and the physician scarcity bonus through June 30, 2008. Furthermore, the legislation extended the therapy cap exceptions, pathology billing exception, and premium assistance for some low-income seniors through June 30, 2008.

Medicare payment schedule A payment schedule adopted by CMS for payment of physician services effective January 1, 1992, replacing the CPR system. This payment schedule is based on the resource costs of physician work, practice overhead, and PLI with adjustments for differences in geographic practice costs. The payment schedule for a service includes both the 80% that Medicare pays and the patient's 20% copayment.

Medicare Prescription Drug, Improvement, and Modernization Act (MMA) of 2003 This legislation was signed into law on December 8, 2003, which includes the most comprehensive changes to the Medicare program since its inception. The MMA created the Medicare prescription drug benefit, added many new preventive benefits, expanded the private sector options for Medicare, and restored the Medicare CF to 1.5% increases in 2004 and 2005.

Medicare volume performance standard (MVPS) A spending goal for Medicare Part B services before to 1998. It was established either by Congress, based on recommendations submitted by the Department of Health and Human Services and Physician Payment Review Commission (PPRC), or by a statutory default formula if Congress chose not to act. The MVPS was intended to encompass all factors contributing to the growth in Medicare spending for physicians' services, including changes in payment levels, size and age composition of Medicare patients, technology, utilization patterns, and access to care.

A CF update default formula became automatically effective if Congress failed to act by October 31 of each year. It was linked to changes in the MEI, as adjusted for the amount by which actual expenditures the preceding year were greater or less than the MVPS-established goals.

Medicare Payment Advisory Commission (MedPAC) A commission created by the Balanced Budget Act of 1997 to advise Congress on Medicare payment policies and other issues affecting Medicare and the broader health system. It merges the roles of the PPRC and the Prospective Payment Assessment Commission, which previously provided Congress with analysis and advice on policy issues affecting Medicare Parts B and A, respectively.

Merit-based incentive payment system (MIPS) MIPS, established by MACRA, combines parts of the PQRS, the value-based modifier (VM) and the Medicare electronic health record (EHR) incentive program into one single program based on quality, resource use, clinical practice improvement, and meaningful use of certified EHR technology.

Middle Class Tax Relief and Job Creation Act of 2012 Signed on February 22, 2012, this Act postponed reductions to Medicare physician payment rates and extended current Medicare payment rates through December 31, 2012. The estimated cost of this provision was $17.3 billion, over 11 years.

Model payment schedule A payment schedule that CMS developed in 1990 as required in OBRA 89. The narrative portion of the model payment schedule included the statutory requirements of OBRA 89, as well as technical and policy issues not prescribed by statute; preliminary estimates of the relative values for approximately 1400 services studied under Phase I of the Harvard study; and preliminary GPCIs for all Medicare localities.

Nonparticipating physician A physician who has not signed a participation agreement with Medicare, and is therefore, not obligated to accept the Medicare approved amount as payment in full for all cases. Their Medicare patients are billed directly, including the balance of the charge that is not covered by the Medicare approved amount, but this balance cannot exceed the limiting charge. Nonparticipating physicians may still accept assignment on a case-by-case basis.

Notice of Proposed Rulemaking (NPRM) The proposed rules to implement the Medicare payment schedule and relative values. First published by Medicare for public comment on June 5, 1991.

OBRA 89 (Omnibus Budget Reconciliation Act of 1989) The congressional legislation created Medicare physician payment reform that provided for a payment schedule based on an RBRVS, which included three components: physician work, practice expense, and PLI costs.

OBRA 93 The congressional legislation that included several revisions to Medicare physician payment under the RBRVS. These provisions include the elimination of payment reductions for "new" physicians, the repeal of the ban on payment for interpretation of electrocardiograms, and several changes to the default payment update and MVPS.

Participating physician A physician who has signed a participation agreement with Medicare; the physician is bound by the agreement to accept assignment on all Medicare claims for the calendar year.

Pathway for SGR Reform Act of 2013 This Act averted a pending 24% scheduled-payment cut and replaced it with a 0.5% increase until April 1, 2014. In addition, this Act extended the 1.0 GPCI floor and therapy cap extensions process through March 31, 2014.

Pay-for-Performance A reimbursement model that compensates physicians for meeting selected quality and efficiency targets. Physician pay-for-performance programs provide some form of compensation to physicians for making progress toward or achieving standard benchmarks, as defined by the program.

Physician Quality Reporting System (PQRS) On December 20, 2006, President George W. Bush signed the Tax Relief and Health Care Act (TRHCA) of 2006, which authorized the CMS to establish and implement PQRS, a physician quality reporting system, including an incentive payment for eligible physicians, who satisfactorily report data on quality measures for covered services furnished to

Medicare beneficiaries. PQRS has since been bundled into the MIPS program.

Physician Payment Review Commission (PPRC) An advisory body created by Congress in 1986 to recommend Medicare reforms in physician payment methods. The PPRC's charge was broadened to include recommendations for health system reforms to the private as well as public sectors. Its functions were subsumed by a new MedPAC, which was created under the Balanced Budget Act of 1997. MedPAC merges the roles of the PPRC and the Prospective Payment Assessment Commission.

Physician Payment and Therapy Relief Act of 2010 Signed into law on November 30, 2010, this Act maintained the 2010 CF established by the Preservation of Access to Care for Medicare Beneficiaries and Pension Relief Act from December 1–31, 2010. The cost ($1 billion over 10 years) of this one-month postponement will be paid for by changes in Medicare reimbursement for outpatient therapy services.

Physician work The physician's individual effort in providing a service, which includes time, technical difficulty of the procedure, severity of patient's condition, and the physical and mental effort required to provide the service; one of three resource cost components included in the formula for computing payment amounts under the Medicare payment schedule.

Practice expense One of three resource-cost components included in the formula to compute Medicare payment-schedule amount. There are direct and indirect practice resources involved in furnishing each service. Direct-expense categories include clinical labor, medical supplies, and medical equipment. Indirect expenses include physician practice overhead, including rent, staff salaries and benefits, administrative labor, office expense, and all other expenses.

Preservation of Access to Care for Medicare Beneficiaries and Pension Relief Act of 2010 Signed into law by President Barack Obama on June 25, 2010, this Act replaced the 21% Medicare physician payment cut to the 2010 CF that took effect June 1, 2010, with a retroactive 2.2% payment update to the 2010 CF from June 1, 2010, through November 30, 2010.

Prevailing charge One of the factors under the CPR system that is used to determine physician payment for a particular service. The prevailing charge for a service was an amount set high enough to cover the physician's full customary charges in a locality, whose billings accounted for at least 75% of the charges for that service. Increases in prevailing charges were capped by increases in the MEI.

Primary care services Under the Primary Care Incentive Payment Program, which ended on December 31, 2015, CMS restricted its definition of primary care services to the following: office or other outpatient services (99201–99215); initial, subsequent, discharge, and other nursing facility E/M services (99304–99318); new and established patient domiciliary, rest home or custodial care E/M services (99324–99337); and domiciliary, rest home or home care plan oversight services (99339–99340).

Professional component In coding for physician services, that portion of the service that denotes the physician's work and the associated overhead and PLI costs.

Professional liability insurance (PLI) Insurance to protect a physician against professional liability; one of three resource-cost components included in the formula developed by CMS for computing Medicare payment-schedule amounts.

Protecting Access to Medicare Act (PAMA) of 2014 This Act postponed the imminent 24% Medicare physician payment cut for 12 months, from March 31, 2014, until April 1, 2015. In addition, this Act extended the 1.0 work GPCI floor through March 31, 2015. PAMA also sets an annual target for reductions in physician payment schedule spending, from adjustments to relative values of misvalued codes. Later that year, the ABLE Act of 2014 accelerated those targets, increasing the target to 1% for 2016 and keeping it at 0.5% for 2017 and 2018.

Protecting Medicare and American Farmers from Sequester Cuts Act of 2021 Signed into law by President Joe Biden on December 10, 2021, this Act diverted Medicare cuts that would have further compounded the growing financial instability of physician practices due to the significant reduction in revenue caused by the severe acute respiratory syndrome coronavirus 2 (SARS-CoV-2) (coronavirus disease 2019 [COVID-19]) public health emergency (PHE). This law results in the following: (1) A delay in resuming the 2% Medicare sequester for three months (January 1–March 31, 2022), followed by a reduction to 1% for three months (April 1–June 30, 2022); (2) A 1-year increase in the MFS of 3% (0.75% less than the CF boost provided for 2021); (3) A 1-year delay in the cuts to the clinical laboratory fee schedule; and (4) A 1-year delay in the Medicare radiation oncology demonstration. In addition, the law will erase the 4% Medicare Pay-As-You-Go (PAYGO) cut and prevent any additional PAYGO cuts through 2022.

Relative value scale (RVS) An index of physicians' services ranked according to "value," with *value* defined according to the basis for the scale. In a charge-based RVS, services are ranked according to the average payment for the service or some other charge basis. A resource-based RVS ranks services according to the relative costs of the resources required to provide them.

Relative value unit (RVU) The unit of measure for Medicare RBRVS. The RVUs must be multiplied by a dollar-CF to become payment amounts.

Resource-based practice expense A methodology for determining practice expense relative values based on physicians' practice overhead costs, including rent, staff salaries, and medical equipment and supplies. The Balanced Budget Act of 1997 contained provisions mandating development of resource-based practice expense relative values to be fully implemented on January 1, 2002.

Resource-based relative value scale (RBRVS) An RVS based on the resource costs of providing physician services; adopted in OBRA 89 as the basis for physician payment for Medicare Part B services effective January 1, 1992. The relative value of each service is the sum of RVUs representing physician work, practice expense, and PLI adjusted for each locality by a geographic adjustment factor and converted into dollar payment amounts by a CF.

Social Security Act Amendments of 1994 Technical corrections legislation, adopted by Congress, which contains several provisions relative to Medicare RBRVS. These provisions include development of resource-based practice expense relative values, CMS authority to enforce balance billing requirements, study of needed data refinements to update GPCIs, and development and refinement of relative values for the full range of pediatric services.

Specialty differential Under the CPR system, some Medicare carriers paid different amount to physicians, according to specialty, for providing the same service. OBRA 89 required that such payment differentials be eliminated.

Sustainable growth rate (SGR) A system for determining annual CF updates, which replaced the MVPS system under the provisions of the Balanced Budget Act of 1997. The SGR update was based on volume growth in real per capita gross domestic product (GDP). Like the MVPS, the SGR reflected changes in inflation, Medicare beneficiary enrollment, real GDP, and spending because of legislative and regulatory requirements. It did not rely on historical patterns of growth in volume and intensity of physician services, however, as did the MVPS; rather, it used projected growth in real GDP per capita. The SGR was constructed so that projected spending would match growth targets by the end of each year. The SGR was permanently repealed by MACRA.

Tax Relief and Health Care Act of 2006 Legislation enacted on December 20, 2006, set the 2007 CF for physician payment at the same level as in 2006 ($37.8975), reversing the statutorily mandated 5.0% negative update. This legislation extended the 1.0 floor on work GPCIs and the therapy cap exceptions process through December 31, 2007. Furthermore, the legislation authorized the establishment of a physician quality reporting system by CMS. CMS established and titled the statutory program, the PQRS. The PQRS establishes a financial incentive for eligible professionals to participate in a voluntary quality reporting program. Eligible professionals who successfully report a designated set of quality measures on claims for dates of service from July 1 to December 31, 2007, earned a bonus payment, subject to a cap of 1.5% of total allowed charges for covered Medicare MFS services.

Technical component In coding for physician services, the portion of a service or procedure that includes cost of equipment, supplies, and technician salary. Payment for the technical component of a service is composed of relative values for practice expense and PLI.

Temporary Extension Act of 2010 Signed into law on March 2, 2010, this Act further delayed the scheduled 21% Medicare payment reduction for physician services by applying a zero-percent update to the 2010 CF from March 1–31, 2010.

Temporary Payroll Tax Cut Continuation Act of 2011 Signed into law on December 23, 2011, this Act replaced the anticipated 27% Medicare physician-payment cut, with a two-month freeze to the Medicare CF. This Act was effective January 1, 2012, through February 29, 2012.

Transition asymmetry The effect of payments for E/M services increasing at a faster rate than the decrease in payments for other services during the 1992 through 1995 transition to the full-payment schedule, causing total outlays in 1992 to exceed what they would have been, had the CPR system been retained. To allow payments for services during the transition period to increase and decrease at about the same rate and maintain budget neutrality, CMS made a one-time 5.5% reduction to the adjusted historical payment basis (AHPB).

Transition offset To maintain budget neutrality during the transition to the full-payment schedule, given the transition asymmetry, a 5.5% adjustment was adopted in the 1991 Final Rule and applied to the AHPB, instead of the CF, as proposed in the NPRM. By applying this adjustment to the AHPB, permanent cuts to the CF were prevented.

Appendix B

Directory of Resources

This directory includes the names, addresses, and websites of national organizations, medical societies, Medicare Part B contractors, and Centers for Medicare & Medicaid Services (CMS) regional offices. Note that such information changes over time. For example, Medicare Part B contractors occasionally change their field-office locations and Medicare contracts with new contractors from time to time. The CMS regional offices should be able to provide updated contact information in such cases.

American Medical Association

Physicians with general questions or who are looking for up-to-date coding information should use the following address and telephone numbers:

American Medical Association
330 N Wabash Avenue
Suite 39300
Chicago, IL 60611
312 464-5000

Unified Service Center
(for AMA members only)
800 262-3211

CPT® Network and CPT® KnowledgeBase for Coding Inquiries

Quickly research a database of commonly asked questions, use the knowledge base, view clinical examples (vignettes) and submit an electronic inquiry directly to CPT experts.

CPT® Network is an Internet-based system that provides members and subscribers the tools to quickly research a database of commonly asked questions and clinical examples. If the answer to a specific question cannot be found in the database, authorized users have the capability to submit an electronic inquiry using a standardized form directly to Current Procedural Terminology (CPT®) coding experts on staff. CPT Network is one of the benefits of AMA membership in which AMA members and their authorized users are entitled to complimentary service, including six free electronic inquiries per year. CPT Network is also available as a subscription-based service for nonmembers and nonphysicians. A number of different packages are available for purchase. CPT Network is available at https://www.ama-assn.org/practice-management/cpt/need-coding-resources.

Medicare Payment Advisory Commission (MedPAC)

Physicians may contact MedPac via phone, email, or its web site to obtain copies of MedPAC reports.

Medicare Payment Advisory Commission
425 I Street, NW, Suite 701
Washington, DC 20001
202 220-3700
info@medpac.gov
http://www.medpac.gov

Medical Societies

State medical associations and national medical specialty societies can offer assistance on Medicare physician payment questions. Many societies have well-established liaisons with Medicare insurance carriers. Medical society staff may, therefore, have firsthand information about how to approach the problems that physicians may experience. The following list contains contact information for the state and national specialty societies. Physicians should request that their inquiries be routed to the appropriate staff.

State Medical Societies

Alabama
Medical Association of the State of Alabama
Mark Jackson, Executive Director
19 S. Jackson Street
PO Box 1900
Montgomery, AL 36104
staff@alamedical.org
www.alamedical.org

Alaska
Alaska State Medical Association
Pam Ventgen, Executive Director
4107 Laurel Street
Anchorage, AK 99508
www.asmadocs.org

Arizona
Arizona Medical Association
Libby McDannell, Chief Executive Officer
2401 W. Peoria Avenue, Suite 130
Phoenix, AZ 85029
www.azmed.org

Arkansas
Arkansas Medical Society
David Wroten, Executive Vice President
10 Corporate Hill Drive, Suite 300
Little Rock, AR 72205
ams@arkmed.org
www.arkmed.org

California
California Medical Association
Dustin Corcoran, Executive Vice President/CEO
1201 K Street, Suite 200
Sacramento, CA 95814
memberservice@cmadocs.org
www.cmadocs.org

Colorado
Colorado Medical Society
Bryan Campbell, Executive Director
7351 Lowry Boulevard, Suite 110
Denver, CO 80230
www.cms.org

Connecticut
Connecticut State Medical Society
Robert Russo, MD, Executive Director/Government Relations
127 Washington Avenue, East Bldg., Lower Level
North Haven, CT 06473
membership@csms.org
www.csms.org

Delaware
Medical Society of Delaware
Mark B. Thompson, Executive Director
900 Prides Crossing
Newark, DE 19713
www.medicalsocietyofdelaware.org

District of Columbia
Medical Society of the District of Columbia
Robert Hay, Jr., Executive Vice President
1250 23rd Street, NW, Suite 270
Washington, DC 20037
www.msdc.org

Florida
Florida Medical Association
Jeff Scott, Chief Executive Officer
1430 Piedmont Drive East
Tallahassee, FL 32308
membership@flmedical.org
www.flmedical.org

Georgia
Medical Association of Georgia
Jeremy T. Bonfini, Executive Director and CEO
1849 The Exchange, Suite 200
Atlanta, GA 30339
www.mag.org

Guam
Guam Medical Society
Stephanie Taitano, Executive Secretary
2214 Ary Drive
Dededo, GU 96929
guammedicalsociety@gmail.com

Hawaii
Hawaii Medical Association
Marc Alexander, Executive Director
1360 S Beretania Street, #200
Honolulu, HI 96816
www.hawaiimedicalassociation.org

Idaho
Idaho Medical Association
Susie Pouliot, Chief Executive Officer
305 W Jefferson, PO Box 2668
Boise, ID 83702
mail@idmed.org
www.idmed.org

Illinois
Illinois State Medical Society
Alexander R. Lerner, Executive Vice President/CEO
20 N Michigan Avenue, Suite 700
Chicago, IL 60602
info@isms.org
www.isms.org

Indiana
Indiana State Medical Association
Julie Reed, JD, Executive Vice President
322 Canal Walk
Indianapolis, IN 46202-3268
www.ismanet.org

Iowa
Iowa Medical Society
Mike Flesher, Chief Executive Officer
515 E. Locust Street, Suite 400
Des Moines, IA 50309
info@iowamedical.org
www.iowamedical.org

Kansas
Kansas Medical Society
Rachelle Colombo, Executive Director
623 SW 10th Avenue
Topeka, KS 66612
www.kmsonline.org

Kentucky
Kentucky Medical Association
Patrick T. Padgett, Executive Director
9300 Shelbyville Road, Suite 850
Louisville, KY 40222
www.kyma.org

Louisiana
Louisiana State Medical Society
Jeff Williams, Executive Vice President
6767 Perkins Road, Suite 100
Baton Rouge, LA 70808
www.lsms.org

Maine
Maine Medical Association
Andrew MacLean, JD, Executive Vice President
PO Box 190
Manchester, ME 04351
info@mainemed.com
www.mainemed.com

Maryland
MedChi, The Maryland State Medical Society
Gene Ransom III, Chief Executive Officer
1211 Cathedral Street
Baltimore, MD 21201
members@medchi.org
www.medchi.org

Massachusetts
Massachusetts Medical Society
Lois Dehls Cornell, Executive Vice President
860 Winter Street
Waltham, MA 02451-1411
info@massmed.org
www.massmed.org

Michigan
Michigan State Medical Society
Julie L. Novak, Chief Executive Officer
120 W Saginaw Street
East Lansing, MI 48823
msms@msms.org
www.msms.org

Minnesota
Minnesota Medical Association
Janet Silversmith, Chief Executive Officer
3433 Broadway Street, NE
Minneapolis, MN 55413
mma@mnmed.org
www.mnmed.org

Mississippi
Mississippi State Medical Association

Claude Brunson, MD, Executive Director
408 W Parkway Place
PO Box 2548
Ridgeland, MS 39158
www.msmaonline.com

Missouri
Missouri State Medical Association
Jeff Howell, Executive Vice President
113 Madison Street, PO Box 1028
Jefferson City, MO 65102
www.msma.org

Montana
Montana Medical Association
Jean Branscum, Executive Director
2021 Eleventh Avenue, Suite 1
Helena, MT 59601
mma@mmaoffice.org
www.mmaoffice.org

Nebraska
Nebraska Medical Association
Amy Reynoldson, Executive Vice President
1045 Lincoln Mall, Suite 200
Lincoln, NE 68508-2966
www.nebmed.org

Nevada
Nevada State Medical Association
Jaron Hildebrand, Executive Director
5345 Kietzke Lane, Suite 100
Reno, NV 89511
admin@nvdoctors.org
www.nvdoctors.org

New Hampshire
New Hampshire Medical Society
James G. Potter, Executive Vice President
7 N. State Street
Concord, NH 03301-4018
NHMedicalSociety@nhms.org
www.nhms.org

New Jersey
Medical Society of New Jersey
Lawrence Downs, Esq., Executive Officer
2 Princess Road
Lawrenceville, NJ 08648-2302
www.msnj.org

New Mexico
New Mexico Medical Society
Anne Jung, Executive Director
316 Osuna NE, Building 501
Albuquerque, NM 87107
info@nmms.org
www.nmms.org

New York
Medical Society of the State of New York
Troy Oechsner, Executive Vice President
865 Merrick Avenue
Westbury, NY 11590
www.mssny.org

North Carolina
North Carolina Medical Society
Chip Baggett, Executive Vice President/CEO
222 N. Person Street, PO Box 27167
Raleigh, NC 27601-1067
www.ncmedsoc.org

North Dakota
North Dakota Medical Association
Courtney Koebele, JD, Executive Director
1622 E Interstate Avenue, Suite A
Bismarck, ND 58503
staff@ndmed.org
www.ndmed.org

Ohio
Ohio State Medical Association
Todd Baker, Executive Director
5115 Parkcenter Avenue, Suite 200
Dublin, OH 43017
info@osma.org
www.osma.org

Oklahoma
Oklahoma State Medical Association
Wes Glinsmann, Executive Director
313 NE 50th Street, Suite A
Oklahoma City, OK 73105
www.okmed.org

Oregon
Oregon Medical Association
Bryan Boehringer, Chief Executive Officer
11740 SW 68th Parkway, Suite 100
Portland, OR 97223-9038
oma@theoma.org
www.theoma.org

Pennsylvania
Pennsylvania Medical Society
Marty Raniowski, Executive Vice President
400 Winding Creek Blvd
Mechanicsburg, PA 17150
www.pamedsoc.org
stat@pamedsoc.org

Puerto Rico
Puerto Rico Medical Association
Ricardo Marrero Santiago, Executive Director
PO Box 9387
San Juan, PR 00908-9387
associacionmedical1902@gmail.com

Rhode Island
Rhode Island Medical Society
Newell E. Warde, PhD, Executive Director
405 Promenade Street, Suite A
Providence, RI 02908
www.rimed.org

South Carolina
South Carolina Medical Association
Richele Taylor, General Counsel/SVP
132 Westpark Blvd, PO Box 11188
Columbia, SC 29211
www.scmedical.org

South Dakota
South Dakota State Medical Association
Barbara Smith, Chief Executive Officer
2600 W. 49th Street, Suite 200
Sioux Falls, SD 57105
membership@sdsma.org
www.sdsma.org

Tennessee
Tennessee Medical Association
Russ Miller, Chief Executive Officer
701 Bradford Avenue
Nashville, TN 37204
info@tnmed.org
www.tnmed.org

Texas
Texas Medical Association
Michael Darrouzet, Executive Vice President/CEO
401 W 15th Street
Austin, TX 78701-1680
knowledge@texmed.org
www.texmed.org

Utah
Utah Medical Association
Michelle McOmber, Executive Vice President/CEO
310 East 4500 South, Suite 500
Salt Lake City, UT 84107-4250
info@utahmed.org
www.utahmed.org

Vermont
Vermont Medical Society
Jessa Barnard, Esq., Executive Director
134 Main Street, PO Box 1457
Montpelier, VT 05601
www.vtmd.org

Virgin Islands
Virgin Islands Medical Society
Cora L. E. Christian, MD, Executive Secretary/Treasurer
PO Box 5986
St Croix, VI 00823
www.vimipro.org

Virginia
Medical Society of Virginia
Melina Davis, Executive Vice President
2924 Emerywood Pkwy, Suite 300
Richmond, VA 23294
www.msv.org

Washington
Washington State Medical Association
Jennifer Hanscom, Executive Director/CEO
2001 6th Avenue, Suite 2700
Seattle, WA 98121
wsma@wsma.org
www.wsma.org

West Virginia
West Virginia State Medical Association
John Law, Interim Executive Director
2018 Kanawha Blvd. E.
Charleston, WV 25311
info@wvsma.org
www.@wvsma.com

Wisconsin
Wisconsin Medical Society
Clyde Bud Chumbley, Chief Executive Officer
2450 Rimrock Road
Madison, WI 53713
membership@wismed.org
www.wisconsinmedicalsociety.org

Wyoming
Wyoming Medical Society
Sheila Bush, Executive Director
122 E. 17th Street
Cheyenne, WY 82001
info@wyomed.org
www.wyomed.org

National Medical Specialty and Other Societies

Academy of Physicians in Clinical Research
Barbara Arango, Executive Director
Two Woodfield Lake, Suite 350
1100 E. Woodfield Lake
Schaumburg, IL 60173
www.apcrnet.org

Aerospace Medical Association
Jeffery Sventik, Executive Director
320 S. Henry Street
Alexandria, VA 22314-3579
www.asma.org

American Academy of Allergy, Asthma, and Immunology
Rebecca Brandt, CAE, Executive Director
555 E Wells Street, Suite 1100
Milwaukee, WI 53202-3823
www.aaaai.org

American Academy of Child and Adolescent Psychiatry
Heidi B. Fordi, Executive Director
3615 Wisconsin Avenue NW
Washington, DC 20016
www.aacap.org

American Academy of Cosmetic Surgery
Victoria Ceh, Executive Director
225 W. Wacker Drive, Suite 650
Chicago, IL 60606
www.cosmeticsurgery.org

American Academy of Dermatology
Elizabeth Usher, MD, Chief Executive Officer
9500 W Bryn Mawr Avenue
Rosemont, IL 60018-5216
www.aad.org

American Academy of Facial Plastic and Reconstructive Surgery
Steven J. Jurich, Executive Vice President/CEO
310 S Henry Street
Alexandria, VA 22314
www.aafprs.org

American Academy of Family Physicians
R. Shawn Martin, Executive Vice President
11400 Tomahawk Creek Parkway
Leawood, KS 66211
www.aafp.org

American Academy of Hospice and Palliative Medicine
Wendy-Jo Toyama, MBA, CAE, Chief Executive Officer
8735 W. Higgins Road, Suite 300
Chicago, IL 60631
www.aahpm.org

American Academy of Insurance Medicine
Ellyn Holhman, AAIM Secretariat
100-32 Colonnade Road
Ottawa, ON K2E 7J6
Canada
www.aaimedicine.org

American Academy of Neurology
Mary Post, MBA, CAE, Executive Director
201 Chicago Avenue
St Paul, MN 55415
www.aan.com

American Academy of Ophthalmology
David W. Parke, II, MD, Executive Vice President/CEO
655 Beach Street
San Francisco, CA 94109-7424
www.aao.org

American Academy of Orthopaedic Surgeons
Thomas Arend, Chief Executive Officer
9400 West Higgins Road
Rosemont, IL 60018
www.aaos.org

American Academy of Otolaryngic Allergy
Jami Lucas, Executive Director/CEO
11130 Sunrise Valley Drive, Suite 100
Reston, VA 20191
www.aaoallergy.org

American Academy of Otolaryngology Head and Neck Surgery, Inc.
James C. Denneny, III, MD, Executive Vice President/CEO
1650 Diagonal Road
Alexandria, VA 22314
www.entnet.org

American Academy of Pain Medicine
Dana Boyte, Executive Administrator
1705 Edgewater Drive, Suite 7778
Orlando, FL 32804
www.painmed.org

American Academy of Pediatrics
Mark Del Monte, Interim Executive Director/CEO
345 Park Blvd
Itasca, IL 60143
www.aap.org

American Academy of Physical Medicine and Rehabilitation
Thomas E. Stautzenbach, Executive Director
9700 W. Bryn Mawr Avenue, Suite 200
Rosemont, IL 60018
www.aapmr.org

American Academy of Psychiatry and the Law
Jacquelyn T. Coleman, Chief Executive Officer
One Regency Drive
PO Box 30
Bloomfield, CT 06002
www.aapl.org

American Academy of Sleep Medicine
Steve Van Hout, Executive Director
2510 N Frontage Road
Darien, IL 60561
www.aasmnet.org

American Association for Geriatric Psychiatry
Christopher N. Wood, Executive Director
6728 Old McLean Village Drive
McLean, VA 22101
www.aagponline.org

American Association for Hand Surgery
Sarah Boardman, Executive Director
500 Cummings Center, Suite 4400
Beverly, MA 01915
www.handsurgery.org

American Association of Hip and Knee Surgeons
Michael Zarski, JD, Executive Director
9400 W Higgins Road, Suite 230
Rosemont, IL 60018-4206
www.aahks.org

American Association for Thoracic Surgery
Adam Silva, Director of Administration
800 Cummings Center, Suite 350-V
Beverly, MA 01915
www.aats.org

American Association of Clinical Endocrinologists
Paul Markowski, Chief Executive Officer
245 Riverside Ave, Suite 200
Jacksonville, FL 32202-4933
www.aace.com

American Association of Clinical Urologists, Inc.
Barbara Arango, Executive Director
1100 East Woodfield Road, Suite 350
Schaumburg, IL 60173-4950
www.aacuweb.org

American Association of Neuromuscular & Electrodiagnostic Medicine
Shirlyn A. Adkins, JD, Executive Director
2621 Superior Drive NW
Rochester, MN 55901
www.aanem.org

American Association of Physicians of Indian Origin
Vijaya Kodali, Manager
600 Enterprise Drive, Suite 108
Oak Brook, IL 60523
www.aapiusa.org

American Association of Gynecologic Laparoscopists
Linda Michels, Executive Director
6757 Katella Avenue
Cypress, CA 90630-5105
www.aagl.org

American Association of Neurological Surgeons
Kathleen Craig, Executive Director
5550 Meadowbrook Drive
Rolling Meadows, IL 60008
www.aans.org

American Association of Plastic Surgeons
Aurelia Alger, JD, Executive Secretary
500 Cummings Ctr, Suite 4550
Beverly, MA 01915
www.aaps1921.org

American Association of Public Health Physicians
Ryung Suh, MD, President
1605 Pebble Beach Blvd
Green Cove Springs, FL 32043
www.aaphp.org
membership@aaphp.org

American Clinical Neurophysiology Society
Megan M. Hille, CAE, CMP, Executive Director
555 E. Wells Street, Suite 1100
Milwaukee, WI 53202
www.acns.org

American College of Allergy, Asthma, and Immunology
James R. Slawny, Executive Director
85 W. Algonquin Road, Suite 550
Arlington Heights, IL 60005
www.acaai.org

American College of Cardiology
Cathleen Gates, Chief Executive Officer
2400 N Street NW
Washington, DC 20037
www.acc.org

American College of Chest Physicians
Robert A. Musacchio, PhD, Executive Vice President/CEO
2595 Patriot Blvd

Glenview, IL 60026
www.chestnet.org

American College of Emergency Physicians
Sue Sedory, JD, Executive Director
4950 W. Royal Lane
Irving, TX 75063
www.acep.org

American College of Gastroenterology
Bradley C. Stillman, Executive Director
6400 Goldsboro Road, Suite 450
Bethesda, MD 20817
www.gi.org

American College of Legal Medicine
Theodore Kanellakes, Executive Director
515 North Dearborn
Chicago, IL 60654
www.aclm.org

American College of Medical Genetics & Genomics
Muenke Maximilian, MD, FACMG, Executive Director
7101 Wisconsin Avenue, Suite 1101
Bethesda, MD 20814-3998
www.acmg.net

American College of Medical Quality
Amy Thomasson, Executive Director
225 West Wacker Drive, Suite 650
Chicago, IL 60606
www.acmq.org

American College of Mohs Surgery
Mary Riordan, Executive Director
555 East Wells Street, Suite 1100
Milwaukee, WI 53202
www.mohscollege.org

American College of Nuclear Medicine
Virginia Pappas, Chief Executive Director
1850 Samuel Morse Drive
Reston, VA 20190
www.snm.org

American Congress of Obstetricians and Gynecologists
Maureen G. Phipps, MD, MPH, Executive Vice-President
409 12th Street SW
Washington, DC 20024-2188
www.acog.org

American College of Occupational and Environmental Medicine
Bruce C. Williams, Executive Director
25 Northwest Point Blvd. #700
Elk Grove Village, IL 60007-1030
www.acoem.org

American Association for Physician Leadership
Peter B. Angood, MD, Chief Executive Officer/President
400 N. Ashley Drive, Suite 400
Tampa, FL 33609
www.physicianleadership.org

American College of Physicians
Darilyn V. Moyer, MD, Executive Vice President/CEO
190 N Independence Mall West
Philadelphia, PA 19106-1572
www.acponline.org

American College of Preventive Medicine
Donna Grande, MGA Chief Executive Officer
1200 First Street, NE
Washington, DC 20002
www.acpm.org

American College of Radiation Oncology
Shannon Bozarth, Interim Executive Director
2001 6th Avenue, Suite 2700
Seattle, WA 98121
www.acro.org

American College of Radiology
William T. Thorwarth, Jr, MD, Chief Executive Officer
1891 Preston White Drive
Reston, VA 20191-4397
www.acr.org

American College of Rheumatology
Steven Echard, Executive Vice President
2200 Lake Blvd NE
Atlanta, GA 30319
www.rheumatology.org

American College of Surgeons
David Hoyt, MD, Executive Director
633 N. St Clair Street
Chicago, IL 60611-3211
www.facs.org

American Gastroenterological Association
Thomas J. Serena, Executive Vice President
4930 Delray Avenue
Bethesda, MD 20814-2513
www.gastro.org

American Geriatrics Society
Nancy Lundebjerg, Chief Executive Officer
Empire State Building
40 Fulton Street, 18th FL
New York, NY 10038
www.americangeriatrics.org

American Institute of Ultrasound in Medicine
Glynis V. Harvey, CAE, Chief Executive Director
14750 Sweitzer Lane, Suite 100
Laurel, MD 20707-5906
www.aium.org

AMDA–The Society for Post-Acute and Long-Term Care Medicine
Christopher E. Laxton, CAE, Executive Director
10500 Little Patuxent Parkway, Suite 210
Columbia, MD 21044
www.amda.com

American Medical Group Association
Jerry Penso, MD, President/Chief Executive Officer
1 Prince Street, Suite 100
Alexandria, VA 22314-3430
www.amga.org

American Medical Women's Association
Eliza Lo Chin, MD, MPH Executive Director
1100 E. Woodfield Road, Suite 350
Schaumburg, IL 60173
www.amwa-doc.org

American Orthopaedic Association
Kristin O. Glavin, JD, Executive Director
9400 W. Higgins Road, Suite 205
Rosemont, IL 60018-4975
www.aoassn.org

American Orthopaedic Foot and Ankle Society
Elaine M. Leighton, MPH, Executive Director
9400 W. Higgins, Suite 220
Rosemont, IL 60018
www.aofas.org

American Osteopathic Association
Kevin Klauer, DO, Executive Director
142 E Ontario Street, 18th Floor
Chicago, IL 60611
www.osteopathic.org

American Psychiatric Association
Saul Levin, MD, Executive Vice President
800 Maine Avenue, SW, Suite 900
Washington, DC 20024
www.psych.org

American Society for Aesthetic Plastic Surgery, Inc.
Sue Dykema, CAE, Executive Director
11262 Monarch Street
Garden Grove, CA 92841
www.surgery.org

American Society for Dermatologic Surgery, Inc.
Katherine J. Duerdoth CAE, Executive Director
5550 Meadowbrook Drive, Suite 120
Rolling Meadows, IL 60008
www.asds.net

American Society for Gastrointestinal Endoscopy
Donald Palmisano, Jr., JD, CAE, Chief Executive Officer
3300 Woodcreek Drive
Downers Grove, IL 60515
www.asge.org

American Society for Metabolic and Bariatric Surgery
Georgeann Mallory, Executive Director
100 SW 75 Street, Suite 201
Gainesville, FL 32607
www.asmbs.org

American Society for Radiation Oncology
Laura Thevenot, Chief Executive Officer
251 18th Street South, 8th Floor
Arlington, VA 22202
www.astro.org

American Society for Reconstructive Microsurgery
Krista A. Greco, Executive Director
20 North Michigan Avenue, Suite 700
Chicago, IL 60602
www.microsurg.org

American Society for Reproductive Medicine
Vickie Gamble, MPPM, Interim Chief Executive Officer
1209 Montgomery Highway
Birmingham, AL 35216-2809
www.asrm.org

American Society for Surgery of the Hand
Mark C. Anderson, CAE, Chief Executive Officer
822 W. Washington Blvd
Chicago, IL 60607
www.hand-surg.org
info@assh.org

American Society of Abdominal Surgeons
Diane Pothier, CEO/Executive Secretary & Treasurer
203 Middlesex Turnpike, Suite 4
Melrose, MA 02176
www.abdominalsurg.org

American Society of Addiction Medicine
Julia Chang, Executive Vice President/CEO
11400 Rockville Pike, Suite 200
Rockville, MD 20852
www.asam.org

American Society of Anesthesiologists
Paul Pomerantz, Chief Executive Officer
1061 American Lane
Schaumburg, IL 60173
www.asahq.org

American Society Breast Surgeons
Jane Schuster, Executive Director
10330 Old Columbia Road, Suite 100
Columbia, MD 20146
www.breastsurgeons.org

American Society of Cataract and Refractive Surgery
Stephen H. Speares, Executive Director
12587 Fair Lakes Circle
Fairfax, VA 22033
www.ascrs.org

American Society of Clinical Oncology
Clifford A. Hudis, MD, Chief Executive Officer
2318 Mill Road, Suite 800
Alexandria, VA 22314
executiveoffice@asco.org
www.asco.org

American Society of Colon and Rectal Surgeons
David Westman, Executive Director
2549 Waukegan Road, Suite 210
Bannockburn, IL 60015
www.fascrs.org

American Society of Cytopathology
Elizabeth Jenkins, Executive Director
100 W. 10 Street, Suite 605
Wilmington, DE 19801
www.cytopathology.org

American Society of Dermatopathology
Leah Smith, Executive Director
111 W. Jackson, Blvd. Suite 1412
Chicago, IL 60604
www.asdp.org

American Society of Echocardiography
Robin Wiegerinki, Executive Director
2530 Meridian Parkway, Suite 201
Durham, NC 27713
www.asecho.org

American Society of General Surgeons
JoLayne Devers, Executive Director
750 Main Street, Suite 201
Mendota Heights, MN 55118
www.theasgs.org

American Society of Hematology
Martha L. Liggett, Esq. Executive Director
2021 L Street NW, Suite 900
Washington, DC 20036
www.hematology.org

American Society of Maxillofacial Surgeons
Stan Alger, Executive Director
500 Cummings Center, Suite 4400
Beverly, MA 01915
www.maxface.org

American Society of Neuroimaging
Leslie Thomas, Executive Director
5841 Cedar Lake Road
Minneapolis, MN 55416
www.asnaweb.org

American Society of Neuroradiology
Mary Beth Hepp, MBA Executive Director/CEO
800 Enterprise Drive, Suite 205
Oak Brook, IL 60523
www.asnr.org

American Society of Ophthalmic Plastic and Reconstructive Surgery, Inc.
Tisha Kehn, Executive Director
1043 Grand Avenue, Suite 132
Minneapolis, MN 55105
www.asoprs.org

American Society of Plastic Surgeons
Michael D. Costelloe, JD, Executive Director
444 E Algonquin Road
Arlington Heights, IL 60005
www.plasticsurgery.org

American Society of Retina Specialists
Jill Blim, Executive Vice President
20 N. Wacker Drive, Suite 2030
Chicago, IL 60606
www.asrs.org

American Society of Transplant Surgeons
Maggie Kebler-Bullock, CFRE, Executive Director
1401 South Clark Street, Suite 1120
Arlington, VA 22202
www.asts.org

American Thoracic Society
Karen J. Collishaw, MPP, CAE, Executive Director
25 Broadway, 4th Floor
New York, NY 10004
www.thoracic.org

American Urological Association
Michael Sheppard, CPA, Executive Director
1000 Corporate Blvd.
Linthicum, MD 21090
www.auanet.org

American Vein and Lymphatic Society
Dean J. Bender, Executive Director
434 W. Ontario Street, Suite 200
Chicago, IL 60654
www.phlebology.org

AMSUS–The Society of Federal Health Professionals
John M. Cho, MD, Executive Director
12154 Darnestown Road, #506
Gaithersburg, MD 20878-2206
www.amsus.org

Association of University Radiologists
Stephanie Taylor, Account Executive
820 Jorie Blvd
Oak Brook, IL 60523
www.aur.org

College of American Pathologists
Stephen Myers, Chief Executive Officer
325 Waukegan Road
Northfield, IL 60093-2750
www.cap.org

Congress of Neurological Surgeons
Regina Shupak, Chief Executive Officer
10 North Martingale Road, Suite 190
Schaumburg, IL 60173
www.neurosurgeon.org

Eye and Contact Lens Association
Carol Goddard, Director
4582 South Ulster Street, Suite 201
Denver, CO 80237
www.clao.org

GLMA: Health Professionals Advancing LGBT Equality
Hector Vargas, JD, Executive Director
1133 19th Street, Suite 302
Washington, DC 20036
www.glma.org

Heart Rhythm Society
Patricia Blake, FASAE, CAE, CEO
1325 G Street NW, Suite 400
Washington, DC 20005
www.hrsonline.org
info@hrsonline.org

Infectious Diseases Society of America
Chris Busky, Executive Vice President
4040 Wilson Blvd, Suite 300
Arlington, VA 22203
www.idsociety.org

International Academy of Independent Medical Evaluators
Gayle Whitmer, Executive Director
1061 E. Main Street, Suite 300
East Dundee, IL 60118
www.iaime.org

International College of Surgeons–US Section
Nick Rebel, Executive Director
1516 N Lake Shore Drive
Chicago, IL 60610
www.ficsonline.org

International Society of Hair Restoration Surgery
Victoria Ceh, MPA, Executive Director

1932 S. Halsted Street
Chicago, IL 60608
www.ishrs.org

International Society for the Advancement of Spine Surgery
Karin Best, Executive Officer
301 S. County Farm Road
Wheaton, IL 60187
info@ISASS.org
www.isass.org

National Association of Medical Examiners
Denise McNally, Executive Director
15444 Chinnereth Est
Savannah, MO 64485
www.thename.org

National Medical Association
Martin Hanlette, JD, Executive Director
8403 Colesville Road, Suite 820
Silver Spring, MD 20910
www.nmanet.org

North American Neuro-Ophthalmology Society
Toma Ossian, Executive Director
5841 Cedar Lake Road, Suite 204
Minneapolis, MN 55416
www.nanosweb.org

North American Neuromodulation Society
Chris Welber, Executive Director
8735 W Higgins Road, Suite 300
Chicago, IL 60631
www.neuromodulation.org

North American Spine Society
Eric J. Muehlbauer, Executive Director
7075 Veterans Blvd
Burr Ridge, IL 60527
www.spine.org

Obesity Medicine Association
Chris Packard, Interim Executive Director
7173 S. Havana Street, Suite 600-130
Centennial, CO 80112
www.obesitymedicine.org

Radiological Society of North America
Mark G. Watson, CAE, Executive Director
820 Jorie Blvd
Oak Brook, IL 60523
www.rsna.org

Renal Physicians Association
Dale Singer, MHA, Executive Director
1700 Rockville Pike, Suite 220
Rockville, MD 20852
www.renalmd.org

Society for Cardiovascular Angiography and Interventions
Francesca Dea, Executive Director
1100 17th Street, NW
Washington, DC 20036
www.scai.org

Society for Investigative Dermatology, Inc.
Jim Rumsey, Executive Director
526 E. Superior Ave, Suite 340
Cleveland, OH 44114
www.sidnet.org

Society for Vascular Surgery
Kenneth Slaw, PhD, Executive Director
9400 W. Higgins Road, Suite 315
Rosemont, IL 60018
www.vascularweb.org

Society of American Gastrointestinal Endoscopic Surgeons
Sallie Matthews, Executive Director
11300 West Olympic Blvd., Suite 600
Los Angeles, CA 90064
www.sages.org

Society of Critical Care Medicine
David J. Martin, Executive Vice President/CEO
500 Midway Drive
Mount Prospect, IL 60056
www.sccm.org

Society of Hospital Medicine
Eric Howell, MD, MHM, Chief Executive Officer
1500 Spring Garden, Suite 501
Philadelphia, PA 19130
www.hospitalmedicine.org

Society of Interventional Radiology
Keith Hume, Executive Director
3975 Fair Ridge Drive
Suite 400 North
Fairfax, VA 22033
info@sirweb.org
www.sirweb.org

Society of Laparoendoscopic Surgeons
Raymond Lanzafame, MD, Executive Director
7330 SW 62nd Place, Suite 410
Miami, FL 33143
www.sls.org

Society of Laparoscopic and Robotic Surgeons
Raymond Lanzafame, MD, Executive Director
7330 SW 62nd Place, Suite 410
Miami, FL 33143
www.sls.org

Society of Nuclear Medicine and Molecular Imaging
Virginia Pappas, Executive Director
1850 Samuel Morse Dr.
Reston, VA 20190
www.snmmi.org

Society of Thoracic Surgeons
Elaine Weiss, CEO/Executive Director
633 N. Saint Clair Street, Suite 2320
Chicago, IL 60611
www.sts.org

The Endocrine Society
Kate Fryer, Chief Executive Office
2055 L Street, NW, Suite 600
Washington, DC 20036
www.endo-society.org

Eye and Contact Lens Association, Inc
Carol Goddard, Director
4582 South Ulster
Denver, CO 80237
eyes@clao.org
www.clao.org

The Triological Society
Myles L. Pensak, MD, Executive Vice President
13930 Gold Circle, Suite 103
Omaha, NE 68144
info@triological.org
www.triological.org

United States and Canadian Academy of Pathology
David Kaminsky, MD, Executive Vice President
936 Broad Street, Suite 106
Augusta, GA 30901
executivevp@uscap.org
www.uscap.org

Undersea and Hyperbaric Medical Society
John S. Peters, Executive Director
631 US Highway 1, Suite 307
North Palm Beach, FL 33408
www.uhms.org

Medicare Administrative Contractors (MACs)

The following lists MACs by state. Physicians may need to contact their MAC for specific information on payment policies and procedures that is not provided in *Medicare RBRVS: The Physicians' Guide.*

The number of insurance companies that contract with Medicare for claims processing has declined in recent years, as several companies have chosen not to renew their Medicare contracts. As a result, a single contractor will process claims from more than one state.

The Centers for Medicare & Medicaid Services (CMS) can be reached at medicare.gov and a nationwide toll-free beneficiary call number 1-800 MEDICARE (1-800-633-4227) that is available throughout the United States, Puerto Rico, Guam, American Samoa, and Northern Mariana Islands. This number provides Medicare beneficiaries with another tool that they can use to answer questions about Medicare and their Medicare health plan options.

Callers can talk to a customer service representative in English or Spanish 24 hours a day, 7 days a week. Following is a listing of some of the information that is available:

- Receive general information and printed materials on Medicare and the Medicare health plan options in your area as well as plan quality and satisfaction information. The Medicare Plan Finder can help you narrow down your Medicare health plan choices and choose the plan that's best for you.
- Receive information on the Medicare-approved drug discount card sponsors. The Medicare Prescription Drug Plan Finder tool on medicare.gov compares discounted drug prices, prescription drug plans, as well as enrollment fees and other program features.
- Find out the names of Medicare providers and suppliers in your area.
- Find out specific Medicare coverage information.
- Receive the Medicare & You handbook, which is available in print, as an audiocassette for the hearing impaired, large print, or Braille versions. Print and audiocassette versions are available in English or Spanish.
- Request various Medicare publications.
- Un-enroll from Medicare + Choice organizations (managed care plans).
- Obtain phone numbers for the Social Security Administration (SSA), your local state health insurance assistance program (SHIP), state Medicaid office, and more.
- Other sources for Medicare information include the following:
  - ☐ SSA (1-800-772-1213) to apply for Medicare.
  - ☐ SHIP for free, unbiased health insurance counseling and assistance.
  - ☐ Your Medicare carrier or intermediary for specific Medicare claim information and Medicare coverage issues or to report suspected fraud and abuse.

Callers with access to a teletypewriter (TTY) or telecommunications device for the deaf (TDD), can call 877-486-2048.

Alabama
Contractor medical directors: Lisa Banker; Gabriel Blen-Willner, MD; Miguel Brito, MD; Angella Charnot-Katsikas, MD; Michelle Denetto, MD; Harry Feliciano, MD, MPH; Leland Garrett, Jr., MD; Shan R. Mull, MD, MHA, FAAFP, FACHE; Maria Lanez, MD; Jason Stroud, MD, MS; Judith Volkar, MD
Palmetto GBA
www.palmettogba.com

Alaska
Contractor medical directors: Smitha Ballyamanda, MD; RaeAnn Capehart, MD; Laurence Clark, MD, FACP; Anitra Graves, MD; Peter Goldzweig, DO; Janet Lawrence, MD; Arthur N. Lurvey, MD; Fred Mamuya, MD, PhD; Eileen M. Moynihan, MD, FACR, FACP; Gary Oakes, MD, FAAFP; Ann Marie Sun, MD; Richard Whitten, MD
Noridian Healthcare Solutions, LLC
www.noridianmedicare.com

Arizona
Contractor medical directors: RaeAnn Capehart, MD; Laurence Clark, MD, FACP; Anitra Graves, MD; Peter Goldzweig, DO; Janet Lawrence, MD; Arthur N. Lurvey, MD; Eileen M. Moynihan, MD, FACR, FACP; Gary Oakes, MD, FAAFP; Ann Marie Sun, MD; Richard Whitten, MD
Noridian Healthcare Solutions, LLC
www.noridianmedicare.com

Arkansas
Contractor medical directors: Andrew Bloschichak, MD, MBA; Patrick Mann, MD; Jyme Schafer, MD
Novatis Solutions, Inc.
www.novatis-solutions.com

California
Contractor medical directors: Laurence Clark, MD, FACP; Peter Goldzweig, DO; Anitra Graves, MD; Janet Lawrence, MD; Arthur N. Lurvey, MD; Eileen M. Moynihan, MD, FACR, FACP; Ann Marie Sun, MD; Richard Whitten, MD
Noridian Healthcare Solutions, LLC
www.noridianmedicare.com

Colorado
Contractor medical directors: Andrew Bloschichak, MD, MBA; Patrick Mann, MD; Jyme Schafer, MD
Novatis Solutions, Inc.
www.novatis-solutions.com

Connecticut
Contractor medical directors: Olatokunbo Awodele, MD, MPH; Stephen Boren, MD, MBA; Carolyn Cummingham, MD; Marc Duerdan, MD; Greg McKinney, MD, MBA
National Government Services
www.ngsmedicare.com

Delaware
Contractor medical directors: Andrew Bloschichak, MD, MBA; Patrick Mann, MD; Jyme Schafer, MD
Novatis Solutions, Inc.
www.novatis-solutions.com

District of Columbia
Contractor medical directors: Andrew Bloschichak, MD, MBA; Patrick Mann, MD; Jyme Schafer, MD
Novatis Solutions, Inc.
www.novatis-solutions.com

Florida
Contractor medical directors: Alicia Campbell, MD; Jaun L. Schaening-Perez, MD
First Coast Service Options, Inc.
www.fcso.com

Georgia
Contractor medical directors:
Lisa Banker; Gabriel Blen-Willner, MD; Miguel Brito, MD; Michelle DeNetto, MD; Harry Feliciano, MD, MPH; Leland Garrett, Jr., MD; Maria Lanez, MD
Palmetto GBA
www.palmettogba.com

Hawaii
Contractor medical directors:
Laurence Clark, MD, FACP; Peter Goldzweig, DO; Anitra Graves, MD; Janet Lawrence, MD; Arthur N. Lurvey, MD; Eileen M. Moynihan, MD, FACR, FACP; Ann Marie Sun, MD, Richard Whitten, MD
Noridian Healthcare Solutions, LLC
www.noridianmedicare.com

Idaho
Contractor medical directors:
Smith Ballymanda, MD; Laurence Clark, MD, FACP; Peter Goldzweig, DO; Anitra Graves, MD; Janet Lawrence, MD; Arthur N. Lurvey, MD; Eileen M. Moynihan, MD, FACR, FACP; Gary Oakes, MD, FAAFP; Ann Marie Sun, MD; Richard Whitten, MD
Noridian Healthcare Solutions, LLC
www.noridianmedicare.com

Illinois
Contractor medical directors:
Olatokunbo Awodele, MD, MPH; Stephen Boren, MD, MBA; Carolyn Cummingham, MD; Marc Duerdan, MD; Greg McKinney, MD, MBA
National Government Services
www.ngsmedicare.com

Indiana
Contractor medical directors:
Robert Kettler, MD; Tameika Lewis, MD; Denise Nachodsky, MD; Ella Noel, DO, FACO; Barry Whites, MD
Wisconsin Physician Services Corporation
www.wpsic.com

Iowa
Contractor medical directors:
Robert Kettler, MD; Tameika Lewis, MD; Denise Nachodsky, MD; Ella Noel, DO, FACOI; Barry Whites, MD
Wisconsin Physician Services Corporation
www.wpsic.com

Kansas
Contractor medical directors:
Robert Kettler, MD; Tameika Lewis, MD; Denise Nachodsky, MD; Ella Noel, DO, FACOI; Barry Whites, MD
Wisconsin Physician Services Corporation
www.wpsic.com

Kentucky
Contractor medical directors:
Earl Berman, MD, FACP, MAIPS-L; Meredith Loveless, MD, FACOG; Neil Sandler, MD
CGS Administrators, LLC
www.cgsmedical.com

Louisiana
Contractor medical directors:
Andrew Bloschichak, MD, MBA; Patrick Mann, MD; Jyme Schafer, MD
Novatis Solutions, Inc.
www.novatis-solutions.com

Maine
Contractor medical directors:
Olatokundo Awodele, MD; Stephen Boren, MD, MBA; Carolyn Cunningham, MD; Marc Duerdan, MD; Greg McKinney, MD, MBA
National Government Services
www.ngsmedicare.com

Maryland
Contractor medical directors:
Andrew Bloschichak, MD, MBA; Patrick Mann, MD; Jyme Schafer, MD
Novatis Solutions, Inc.
www.novatis-solutions.com

Massachusetts
Contractor medical directors:
Olatokunbo Awodele, MD, MPH; Stephen Boren, MD, MBA; Carolyn Cunningham, MD; Marc Duerdan, MD; Greg McKinney, MD, MBA
National Government Services
www.ngsmedicare.com

Michigan
Contractor medical directors:
Robert Kettler, MD; Tameika Lewis, MD; Denise Nachodsky, MD; Ella Noel, DO, FACOI; Barry Whites, MD
Wisconsin Physician Services Corporation
www.wpsic.com

Minnesota
Contractor medical directors:
Olatokunbo Awodele, MD, MPH; Stephen Boren, MD, MBA; Carolyn Cunningham, MD; Marc Duerden, MD, Greg McKinney, MD, MBA
National Government Services
www.ngsmedicare.com

Mississippi
Contractor medical directors:
Andrew Bloschichak, MD, MBA; Patrick Mann, MD; Jyme Schafer, MD
Novatis Solutions, Inc.
www.novatis-solutions.com

Missouri
Contractor medical directors:
Robert Kettler, MD; Tameika Lewis, MD; Denise Nachodsky, MD; Ella Noel, DO, FACO; Barry Whites, MD
Wisconsin Physician Services Corporation
www.wpsic.com

Montana
Contractor medical directors:
Smitha Ballyamanda, MD; Raehart Capehart, MD; Laurence Clark, MD, FACP; Peter Goldzweig, DO; Anitra Graves, MD; Janet Lawrence, MD; Arthur N. Lurvey, MD; Fred Mamuya, MD, PhD; Eileen M. Moynihan, MD, FACR, FACP; Gary Oakes, MD, FAAFP; Ann Marie Sun, MD; Richard Whitten, MD
Noridian Healthcare Solutions, LLC
www.noridianmedicare.com

Nebraska
Contractor medical directors:
Robert Kettler, MD; Tameika Lewis, MD; Denise Nachodsky, MD; Ella Noel, DO, FACO; Barry Whites, MD
Wisconsin Physician Services Corporation
www.wpsic.com

Nevada
Contractor medical directors:
Smitha Ballyamanda, MD; Raeann Capehart, MD; Laurence Clark, MD, FACP; Peter Goldzweig, DO; Anitra Graves, MD; Janet Lawrence, MD; Arthur N. Lurvey, MD; Fred Mamuya, MD, PhD; Eileen M. Moynihan, MD, FACR, FACP; Ann Marie Sun, MD; Richard Whitten, MD
Noridian Healthcare Solutions, LLC
www.noridianmedicare.com

New Hampshire
Contractor medical directors:
Olatokunbo Awodele, MD, MPH; Stephen Boren, MD, MBA; Carolyn Cunningham, MD; Marc Duerdan, MD; Greg McKinney, MD, MBA
National Government Services
www.ngsmedicare.com

New Jersey
Contractor medical directors:
Andrew Bloschichak, MD, MBA; Patrick Mann, MD; Jyme Schafer, MD
Novatis Solutions, Inc.
www.novatis-solutions.com

New Mexico
Contractor medical directors:
Andrew Bloschichak, MD, MBA; Patrick Mann, MD; Jyme Schafer, MD
Novatis Solutions, Inc.
www.novatis-solutions.com

New York
Contractor medical directors:
Olatokunbo Awodele, MD, MPH; Stephen Boren, MD, MBA; Carolyn Cunningham, MD; Marc Duerdan, MD; Greg McKinney, MD, MBA
National Government Services
www.ngsmedicare.com

North Carolina
Contractor medical directors:
Lisa Banker; Miguel Brito, MD; Angella Charnot-Katsikas, MD; Michelle DeNetto, MD; Harry Feliciano, MD, MPH; Leland Garrett, Jr., MD; Maria Brito, MD; Maria Lanez, MD; Shan R. Mull, MD, MHA, FAAFP, FACHE; Jason Stroud, MD, MS; Judith Volkar, MD
Palmetto GBA
www.palmettogba.com

North Dakota
Contractor medical directors:
Smitha Ballyamanda, MD; RaeAnn Capehart, MD;

Laurence Clark, MD, FACP; Peter Goldzweig, DO; Anitra Graves, MD; Janet Lawrence, MD; Arthur N. Lurvey, MD; Fred Mamuya, MD, PhD; Eileen M. Moynihan, MD, FACR, FACP; Gary Oakes, MD, FAAFP; Ann Marie Sun, MD; Richard Whitten, MD
Noridian Healthcare Solutions, LLC
www.noridianmedicare.com

Ohio
Contractor medical directors: Earl Berman, MD, FACP, MAIPS-L; Meredith Loveless, MD, FACOG; Neil Sandler, MD
CGS Administrators, LLC
www.cgsmedicare.com

Oklahoma
Contractor medical directors: Andrew Bloschichak, MD, MBA; Patrick Mann, MD; Jyme Schafer, MD
Novatis Solutions, Inc.
www.novatis-solutions.com

Oregon
Contractor medical directors: Smitha Ballyamanda, MD; RaeAnn Capehart, MD; Laurence Clark, MD, FACP; Peter Goldzweig, DO; Anitra Graves, MD; Janet Lawrence, MD; Arthur N. Lurvey, MD; Fred Mamuya, MD, PhD; Eileen M. Moynihan, MD, FACR, FACP; Gary Oakes, MD, FAAFP; Ann Marie Sun, MD; Richard Whitten, MD
Noridian Healthcare Solutions, LLC
www.noridianmedicare.com

Pennsylvania
Contractor medical directors: Andrew Bloschichak, MD, MBA; Patrick Mann, MD; Jyme Schafer, MD
Novatis Solutions, Inc.
www.novatis-solutions.com

Puerto Rico
Contractor medical directors: Alicia Campbell, MD; Juan L. Schaening-Perez, MD
First Coast Service Options, Inc.
www.fcso.com

Rhode Island
Contractor medical directors: Olatokunbo Awodele, MD, MPH; Stephen Boren, MD, MBA; Carolyn Cunningham, MD; Marc Duerdan, MD; Greg McKinney, MD, MBA
National Government Services
www.ngsmedicare.com

South Carolina
Contractor medical directors: Lisa Banker; Miguel Brito, MD; Angella Charnot-Katsikas, MD; Michelle DeNetto, MD; Harry Feliciano, MD, MPH; Leland Garrett, Jr., MD; Maria Brito, MD; Maria Lanez, MD; Shan R. Mull, MD, MHA, FAAFP, FACHE; Jason Stroud, MD, MS; Judith Volkar, MD
Palmetto GBA
www.palmettogba.com

South Dakota
Contractor medical directors: Smitha Ballyamanda, MD; RaeAnn Capehart, MD; Laurence Clark, MD, FACP; Peter Goldzweig, DO; Anitra Graves, MD; Janet Lawrence, MD; Arthur N. Lurvey, MD; Fred Mamuya, MD, PhD; Eileen M. Moynihan, MD, FACR, FACP; Gary Oakes, MD, FAAFP; Ann Marie Sun, MD; Richard Whitten, MD
Noridian Healthcare Solutions, LLC
www.noridianmedicare.com

Tennessee
Contractor medical directors: Lisa Banker; Gabriel Blen-Willner, MD; Miguel Brito, MD; Angella Charnot-Katsikas, MD; Michelle DeNetto, MD; Harry Feliciano, MD, MPH; Leland Garrett, Jr., MD; Maria Lanez, MD; Shan R. Mull, MD, MHA, FAAFP, FACHE; Jason Stroud, MD, MS; Judith Volkar, MD
Palmetto GBA
www.palmettogba.com

Texas
Contractor medical directors: Andrew Bloschichak, MD, MBA; Patrick Mann, MD; Jyme Schafer, MD
Novatis Solutions, Inc.
www.novatis-solutions.com

Utah
Contractor medical directors: Smitha Ballyamanda, MD; RaeAnn Capehart, MD; Laurence Clark, MD, FACP; Peter Goldzweig, DO; Anitra Graves, MD; Janet Lawrence, MD; Arthur N. Lurvey, MD; Fred Mamuya, MD, PhD; Eileen M. Moynihan, MD, FACR, FACP; Gary Oakes, MD, FAAFP; Ann Marie Sun, MD; Richard Whitten, MD
Noridian Healthcare Solutions, LLC
www.noridianmedicare.com

Vermont
Contractor medical directors: Olatokunbo Awodele, MD, MPH; Stephen Boren, MD, MBA; Carolyn Cunningham, MD; Marc Duerdan, MD; Greg McKinney, MD, MBA
National Government Services
www.ngsmedicare.com

Virginia
Contractor medical directors: Lisa Banker; Miguel Brito, MD; Angella Charnot-Katsikas, MD; Michelle DeNetto, MD; Harry Feliciano, MD, MPH; Leland Garrett, Jr., MD; Maria Brito, MD; Maria Lanez, MD; Shan R. Mull, MD, MHA, FAAFP, FACHE; Jason Stroud, MD, MS; Judith Volkar, MD
Palmetto GBA
www.palmettogba.com

Virgin Islands
Contractor medical directors: Alicia Campbell, MD; Juan L. Schaening-Perez, MD
First Coast Service Options, Inc.
www.fcso.com

Washington
Contractor medical directors: Smitha Ballyamanda, MD; RaeAnn Capehart, MD; Clark, MD, FACP; Peter Goldzweig, DO; Anitra Graves, MD; Janet Lawrence, MD; Arthur N. Lurvey, MD; Fred Mamuya, MD, PhD; Eileen M. Moynihan, MD, FACR, FACP; Gary Oakes, MD, FAAFP; Ann Marie Sun, MD; Richard Whitten, MD
Noridian Healthcare Solutions, LLC
www.noridianmedicare.com

West Virginia
Contractor medical directors: Lisa Banker; Miguel Brito, MD; Angella Charnot-Katsikas, MD; Michelle DeNetto, MD; Harry Feliciano, MD, MPH; Leland Garrett, Jr., MD; Maria Brito, MD; Maria Lanez, MD; Shan R. Mull, MD, MHA, FAAFP, FACHE; Jason Stroud, MD, MS; Judith Volkar, MD
Palmetto GBA
www.palmettogba.com

Wisconsin
Contractor medical directors: Olatokunbo Awodele, MD, MPH; Stephen Boren, MD, MBA; Carolyn Cunningham, MD; Greg McKinney, MD, MBA
National Government Services
www.ngsmedicare.com

Wyoming
Contractor medical directors: Smitha Ballyamanda, MD; RaeAnn Capehart, MD; Laurence Clark, MD, FACP; Peter Goldzweig, DO; Anitra Graves, MD; Janet Lawrence, MD; Arthur N. Lurvey, MD; Fred Mamuya, MD, PhD; Eileen M. Moynihan, MD, FACR, FACP; Gary Oakes, MD, FAAFP; Ann Marie Sun, MD; Richard Whitten, MD
Noridian Healthcare Solutions, LLC
www.noridianmedicare.com

Durable Medical Equipment Contractors

DME MAC Jurisdiction A
The states included in DME MAC Jurisdiction A are: Connecticut, Delaware, District of Columbia, Maine, Maryland, Massachusetts, New Hampshire, New Jersey, New York, Pennsylvania, Rhode Island, and Vermont.
Contractor medical director: Smitha M. Ballyamanda, MD, CAQSM
Noridian Healthcare, LLC
DMEMDs@noridian.com
www.medicarenhic.com

DME MAC Jurisdiction B
The states included in DME MAC Jurisdiction B are: Illinois, Indiana, Kentucky, Michigan, Minnesota, Ohio, and Wisconsin.
Contractor medical director: Neil Sandler, MD
CGS Administrators, LLC
www.cgsmedicare.com

DME MAC Jurisdiction C
The states included in DME MAC Jurisdiction C are: Alabama, Arkansas, California, Florida, Georgia, Louisiana, Mississippi, New Mexico, North Carolina, Oklahoma, Puerto Rico, South Carolina, Tennessee, Texas, US Virgin Islands, Virginia, and West Virginia.
Contractor medical director: Sunil V. Lalla, MD, FACS, CPC
CGS Administrators, LLC
www.cgsmedicare.com

DME MAC Jurisdiction D
The states included in DME MAC Jurisdiction D are: Alaska, American Samoa, Arizona, Colorado, Guam, Hawaii, Idaho, Iowa, Kansas, Missouri, Montana, Nebraska, Nevada, North Dakota, Northern Mariana Islands, Oregon, South Dakota, Utah, Washington, and Wyoming.
Contractor medical director: Peter J. Gurk, MD, CPE, CHCQM
Noridian Healthcare Solutions, LLC
www.med.noridian.com

Centers for Medicare & Medicaid Services (CMS) Regional Offices

In situations in which the appropriate medical society liaison or a Medicare contractor is unable to provide adequate information, questions can be directed to the appropriate CMS regional office. A list of regional offices is available at https://www.cms.gov/Medicare/Coding/ICD10/CMS-Regional-Offices. This listing provides addresses and phone numbers of the 10 CMS regional offices across the country.

Region I: Boston
Connecticut, Maine, Massachusetts, New Hampshire, Rhode Island, and Vermont
Associate Regional Administrator, CMS Program Operations
John F. Kennedy Federal Building
15 New Sudbury Street, Room 2325
Boston, MA 02203-0003
617 565-1188
ROBOSORA@cms.hhs.gov

Region II: New York
New Jersey, New York, Puerto Rico, and Virgin Islands
Associate Regional Administrator, CMS Program Operations
Jacob K. Javits Federal Building
26 Federal Plaza, Room 3811
New York, NY 10278-0063
212 616-2205
RONYCORA@cms.hhs.gov

Region III: Philadelphia
Delaware, District of Columbia, Maryland, Pennsylvania, Virginia, and West Virginia
Associate Regional Administrator
801 Market Street
Suite 9400
Philadelphia, PA 19107-3134
215 861-4140
ROPHIORA@cms.hhs.gov

Region IV: Atlanta
Alabama, Florida, Georgia, Kentucky, Mississippi, North Carolina, South Carolina, and Tennessee
Associate Regional Administrator, CMS Program Operations
Atlanta Federal Center
61 Forsyth Street SW
Suite 4T20
Atlanta, GA 30303
404 562-7150
ROATLORA@cms.hhs.gov

Region V: Chicago
Indiana, Illinois, Michigan, Minnesota, Ohio, and Wisconsin
Associate Regional Administrator, CMS Program Operations
233 N Michigan Avenue, Suite 600
Chicago, IL 60601
312 886-6432
ROCHIORA@cms.hhs.gov

Region VI: Dallas
Arkansas, Louisiana, Oklahoma, New Mexico, and Texas
Associate Regional Administrator, CMS Program Operations
1301 Young Street, Room 714
Dallas, TX 75202
214 767-6401
RODALORA@cms.hhs.gov

Region VII: Kansas City
Iowa, Kansas, Missouri, and Nebraska
Associate Regional Administrator, CMS Program Operations
Richard Bolling Federal Building
601 E 12th Street, Room 355
Kansas City, MO 64106
816 426-5233
ROKCMORA@cms.hhs.gov

Region VIII: Denver
Colorado, Montana, North Dakota, South Dakota, Wyoming, and Utah
Associate Regional Administrator, CMS Program Operations
Office of the Regional Administrator
1961 Stout Street, Room 08-148
Denver, CO 80294
303 844-2111
ROEAORA@cms.hhs.gov

Region IX: San Francisco
Arizona, California, Nevada, Commonwealth of Northern Marianas Islands, Guam, Hawaii, and American Samoa
Associate Regional Administrator, CMS Program Operations
90–7th Street, Suite 5-300
San Francisco, CA 94103
415 744-3501
ROSFOORA@cms.hhs.gov

Region X: Seattle
Alaska, Idaho, Oregon, and Washington
Office of the Regional Administrator
701 Fifth Avenue, Suite 1600
Seattle, WA 98104
206 615-2306
ROSEA_ORA2@cms.hhs.gov

Index

Note: Page references followed by "*f*" and "*t*" denote figures and tables, respectively. Significant changes for 2022 are highlighted on the inside front (IFC) and inside back cover (IBC) and are included in this index, which are denoted with *IFC* and *IBC*.

A

AAFP (American Academy of Family Physicians), 39
AAP (American Academy of Pediatrics), 34, 37–38
AAPM (Advanced Alternative Payment Model), 173–174
AARP (American Association of Retired Persons), 13
Abdominal aortic aneurysm (AAA), 156, *156t*
Abt Associates, Inc, 30, 37, 38, 47
Abuse. *See* Fraud and abuse
Achieving a Better Life Experience (ABLE) Act of 2014, 21, 82, 540
ACOG (American College of Obstetricians and Gynecologists), 39
ACS (American Community Survey), 73–74, 76
Access to care
  AMA advocacy efforts in 2021, 161–164
  LGBTQ+ health, 163–164
  maternal health and mortality, 164
  prior authorization, 162
Actual charge, defined, 540
Addiction medicine, practice expenses, *54t*
Adjusted historical payment basis (AHPB), 17
Administrative burden, 135–136
Advanced Alternative Payment Model (AAPM), 173–174
Advanced care planning, 143–144
Advanced diagnostic laboratory tests (ADLTs), 124
Advanced heart failure, transplant cardiology, *54t*
Advanced imaging services, 82
Affordable Care Act of 2010
  Centers for Medicare and Medicaid Innovation created by, 173
  changes to HIPAA standards by, 171, 172
  defined, 540
  discontinuance of PPAC by, 11
  on equipment utilization, 64
  on incentive payments, 78, 174
  Medicare beneficiary income thresholds frozen by, 179
  moving physicians away from fee-for-service systems, 173
  on multiple procedure payment reduction, 122
  on nurse midwives, 131
  on pay for performance, 173
  on physical and occupational therapy, 129
  practice expense GPCI for "frontier" states, 74, 75
  practice management issues, 172
  premium subsidy increases, 161
  preventive services coverage, (Modifier 33), 107–108
  on psychiatric therapeutic procedures and psychotherapy, 133–134, 150
  value modifier and, 173
  on work GPCI floor, 14, 75
AHPB (adjusted historical payment basis), 17
AIDS/HIV screening, *159t*
Alaska, work GPCI floor for, 74, 75, 524
Alcohol misuse screening and counseling, *157t*
Allergen immunotherapy, 151
Allergy and immunology, practice expense data, *44t, 52t, 54t*
Allied health professions
  on advisory committees for RUC and CPT, 31
  Medicare Part B payment to, 22–23
  RBRVS payment rules and policies,126–134
Alternative Payment Models (APMs), 84, 92, 173–175, *IBC*
AMA. *See* American Medical Association
AMA/Specialty Society RVS Update Committee (RUC)
  Administrative Subcommittee, 31
  Advisory Committee (specialty society input), 31–32
  annual work value redistributions, 32, 42
  budget-neutrality adjustments policy and, 80–84, *83t*
  CMS acceptance rates for recommendations by, *36t*
  coding changes, work relative values for 2022, *IFC*
  COVID-19 vaccine payment rate for 2022, *IFC*
  CPEP practice expense data, recommendations on, 61
  CPT coding recommendations by year, *36t*
  defined, 540
  direct practice expense input data, 62–63
  E/M office visit revisions, 136
  facilitation committees, 32
  five-year review processes, recommendations from, 37–42
  future plans, 42
  general description of recommendations and results by year, 33–37
  Health Care Professionals Advisory Committee (HCPAC), 31, 128
  history and results of recommendations (CPT 1993–CPT 2022), *36t*
  misvalued services identified by, 32, 35–39, 82
  multidisciplinary work groups, 37–38
  payment for all preventive vaccines, 127-128
  potentially misvalued services, *IBC*
  Practice Expense Advisory Committee (PEAC), 31, 59–60
  practice expense codes and relative values reviewed by, 61–62
  Practice Expense Review Committee (PERC), 32, 62
  Practice Expense Subcommittee, 31
  process for developing recommendations, 31–36
  Professional Liability Insurance Workgroup, 31

AMA/Specialty Society RVS Update Committee (RUC) (*continued*)
publication of voting records, 33
recommendations for 2022, 36–37 *36t*, 127-128
Relativity Assessment Workgroup, 32, 35, 42
Research Subcommittee, 31
resource-based practice expenses refinement, 60–64
role in five-year review process, 37
RVS update process, 27, 31–37
structure of, 31–33
survey instruments, 33
Ambulances, national place of service codes and payment rates for, 197
Ambulatory surgical centers, national place of service code and payment rate for, 197
American Academy of Family Physicians (AAFP), 39
American Academy of Otolaryngology-Head and Neck Surgery, 130
American Academy of Pediatrics (AAP), 34, 37–38
American Association for Vascular Surgery, 39
American Association of Oral and Maxillofacial Surgeons, 43
American Association of Retired Persons (AARP), 13
American Chiropractic Association, 43
American College of Obstetricians and Gynecologists (ACOG), 39, 154
American College of Surgeons, 39
American Community Survey (ACS), 73–74, 76
American Medical Association (AMA). *See also* AMA/Specialty Society RVS Update Committee (RUC); CPT codes; Socioeconomic Monitoring System (SMS)
advocacy efforts in 2021, 161–166
balance billing limits and policy, 9, 177
blueprint for Medicare physician payment reform (1988–1989), 9–10
Board of Trustees report on RBRVS, 8
budget-neutrality adjustments policy and, 80–84, *83t*
Center for Health Policy Research, 76
contact information, 548
conversion factor for 2022 and impact of the pandemic on physician finances, *IFC*, 16, 84, 89–99
correct coding initiative, 151
Council on Legislation evaluation of Harvard RBRVS study, 8
Council on Medical Service evaluation of Harvard RBRVS study, 8
COVID-19 Resource Center, 166
COVID-19 responses, actions in 2021, 161
direct practice expense input data, 62–63
E/M documentation guidelines, 137–139
expenditure target opposition from, 9, 13
fee schedule concept, defined, 2–3, 79
five-year review process preferred approach, 37
fraud and abuse control account, 151
geographic adjustments policy, 14
geographic variation reduction, 71
global period data reporting, 169–170
Harvard RBRVS study and, 5, 7–9
Medicare approved amount as payment in full, 5
Medicare physician payment system change (1989), 9, 12–13
NPRM, 18, 19
payment-for-service systems, 4, 87, 177
payment gap between procedures and visits, 5
payment reform monitoring program, 19
payment schedule concept, defined, 2–3, 79
physician DRGs and mandatory capitation/assignment, 4
Physician Masterfile, 7, 63
physician pay cuts, 20, 21
physician payment reform, 9, 12–13
practice expense methodology, 48
practice expense pilot survey, 63–64
primary care incentive payment policy, 174–175
proposal to reduce administrative burden, 135–136
RBRVS development proposal from, 1985, 5
RBRVS policy formulation and, 8–9
resource-based practice expense refinement, 61
RUC support from, 42
RVS update process, 27, 31–37, *36t*
RVU adjustments to ensure budget neutrality opposed by, 98
SGR modifications and repeal, 21
specialty payment differentials, 9
telehealth information resources, 115
value-based care initiatives, 173
work adjustor policy, 16
American Medical Group Association, 190, *190f*
American Optometric Association, 43
American Podiatric Medical Association, 43
American Recovery and Reinvestment Act (ARRA) of 2009, 171, 172
American Rescue Plan Act of 2021 (ARPA), 161
American Society for General Surgeons, 39
American Society of Anesthesiologists (ASA), 39, 525, 526
American Society of Clinical Oncology, 62
American Speech-Language-Hearing Association (ASHA), 130
American Taxpayer Relief Act of 2012
conversion factor and, 21
defined, 540
on multiple procedure payment reduction, 122
on physical and occupational therapy, 129
replacement of 2013 SGR cut, *97t*, 98
on work GPCI floor, 14
AMGA. *See* American Medical Group Association
Anesthesia services
anesthesiologist assistants, mean practice expenses per hour in patient care, *54t*
base units for, 525, 527–535

comparison of ASA values to RBRVS values, 526
computation of payments for, 46
conversion factor by payer type, 184–186, *183f, 186f*
conversion factor for 2022, 84
generally decreased payments under RBRVS, 169
geographically adjusted conversion factors, 536–538
hospital-based physician DRGs for, 6
practice expense data, *52t, 54t*
practice expense ratios for 1989, *45t*
professional liability component and, 66, 68
RVU adjustments for, 38–39, 41
by surgeon (Modifier 47), 108
teaching anesthesiologists, 118
unusual (Modifier 23), 107
Aneurysm, abdominal aortic, 156, *156t*
Annual wellness visits (AWVs), 152, *156t*
Antigen services, 127
Anti-racism, 163
Aortic aneurysm, abdominal, 156, *156t*
Apheresis, therapeutic, 161
APMs (Alternative Payment Models), 92, 173–174, *IBC*
Approved amount (Medicare), 4, 5, 9, 87–89, *89t*, 541
Appropriate use criteria, 115
ARRA (American Recovery and Reinvestment Act of 2009), 171, 172
ASA (American Society of Anesthesiologists), 39, 525, 526
ASHA (American Speech-Language-Hearing Association), 130
Assignment
acceptance of, 87–89, 166–175176
defined, 541
mandatory, 4, 15, 87
Assistant-at-surgery services, 106, 110–111, 112, 193–194
Assisted living facilities, national place of service code and payment rate for, 196
Attending physicians, 22
Audiology, 22, *52t, 54t,* 130
Audit of practice management, 170–171
Auxiliary personnel, 23
Average wholesale price (AWP), 19, 126
AWVs (annual wellness visits), 152, *156t*

B

BAAs (business associate agreements), 172
Balance billing, 87–89. *See also* Limiting charges
AMA policy (1988–1989), 9
compliance monitoring, 89
defined, 541
Medicare approved amount and, 4
Medicare private contracting and, 10
Medicare reform proposals, 13
OBRA 89 on, 15
patient limits for, 12
PPRC views on, 9
Balanced Budget Act (BBA) of 1997
defined, 541
on expenditure targets and performance adjustment, 94–95
fraud and abuse provisions in, 151
mammography screening provision, 151, 153
Medicare program changes and, 9–10
pelvic examination provision, 155
on practice expense data collection, 14
practice restrictions lifted by, 23, 126
on preventive services coverage, 151, 155
on private contracting, 10, 19–20, 176–177
on resourced-based professional liability insurance RVUs, 68
on SGR as replacement for MVPS, 15, 94–95
on SGR system, 94–95
Balanced Budget Refinement Act (BBRA) of 1999, 94, 95, 129
Barium enema, 154, *157t*
Baseline adjustment, defined, 541
BBA. *See* Balanced Budget Act of 1997
Behavioral health, 58, 126, 145–146, 150
Behavioral offset, 18, 19, 541
Behavioral therapy
cardiovascular disease, *157t*
obesity counseling, *159t*
Bilateral procedures, 108, 193
Billing procedures, 165, 170–171
BIPA. *See* Medicare, Medicaid, and SCHIP Benefits Improvement and Protection Act of 2000
Bipartisan Budget Act of 2018, 15, 75, 82, 129, 541
Birthing centers, national place of service code and payment rate for, 197
Blood clotting factors, 127
Blood tests, 153
BLS (Bureau of Labor Statistics), 73, 74, 76, 93, *IBC*
Bone mass measurements, *157t*
Braun, Peter, 7
Breast biopsy, cross-specialty RVS process for, 29
Breast cancer, mammography screening for, 40, 153, *159t*
Budget neutrality. *See also* Conversion factor (CF); Expenditure targets
83t, 98
adjustments to physician work (1992–2022), 80–84, *83t*
CMS payment schedule adjustments, 98
conversion factor reductions significant for 2021, 2022, *100t*
defined, 541
Medicare conversion factor and, 98
OBRA 89 provisions and subsequent adjustments, 16
practice expense RVU adjustments, 51
professional liability RVU calculations, 67–68
work adjustor elimination and, 98

Bulletin of the American College of Surgeons, 8
Bundled services
CPT-4 code rebundling, 104
critical care, 148–149
ECG transport, 122
glaucoma screening, 155
in global surgical package, 102, 104
hospital DRGs and, 4
initial evaluation and consultation by surgeon, 102
misvalued services, 42
moderate (conscious) sedation, 105–106
physician care plan oversight, 139
pulse oximetry, 150
therapeutic apheresis, 161
transitional care management, 140–141
unbundling, 104
ventilator management on same day as E/M service, 150
work RVUs for, 31, 35
Bureau of Labor Statistics (BLS), 73, 74, 76, 93, *IBC*
Business associate agreements (BAAs), 172

C

California Medical Association, RVS developed by, 4
California Medicare payment localities, 77
Cancer drugs, oral, 127
Cancer screening
breast (mammography), 40, 153, *159t*
cervical, 154–155, *157t*
colorectal, 153–154, *157t*
lung, *159t*
pelvic examinations, 155, *157t*
prostate, *160t*
Capitation-based systems, 4, 6
Cardiac electrophysiology, practice expenses, *54t*
Cardiac rehabilitation, intensive, practice expenses, *55t*
Cardiology, *52t, 54t*
Cardiothoracic surgery
misvalued codes for review, 38
practice expense data, *52t, 54t*
reevaluation of services, 30
RVU adjustments for, 40, 41
Cardiovascular disease, *44t, 157t*
Cardiovascular screening blood tests, 153, *157t*
CARES Act of 2020. *See* Coronavirus Aid, Relief, and Economic Security (CARES) Act of 2020
Carpal tunnel decompression, 28
Carrier medical directors (CMDs), 7, 30, 37
Cataract surgery, RVU adjustments for, 41
CBO (Congressional Budget Office), 21, 97
CCI (correct coding initiative), 151
CCM (chronic care management), 36, 142–143
CDC. *See* Centers for Disease Control (CDC)
CDLTs (clinical diagnostic laboratory tests), 124
Center for Health Economics Research, 72
Centers for Medicare & Medicaid Innovation, 173
Centers for Medicare & Medicaid Services (CMS)
acceptance rates for RUC recommendations, *36t*
AMA advocacy during the COVID-19 pandemic, 161, 168
annual call for RVU comments, 42
on behavioral offset, 18, 19
bottom-up practice expense approach, 49, 57–60
budget-neutrality adjustments policy and, 80–84, *83t*
CMS-1500 claim form, 106
completion of Medicare RBRVS, 31
comprehensive limiting charge compliance program, 89
conversion factor adjustments, 98
correct coding initiative, 151
COVID-19 vaccine payment rate for 2022, *IFC*
defined, 541
on E/M documentation guidelines, 137–139
goals for practice expense data and methodology, 61–63
GPCI modifications (2013), 76
Harvard RBRVS study and, 5
historical payment basis determined by, 17
Medicare physician payment reform recommendations, 12
Medicare telehealth, *IFC*
MEI rebasing (from 2000 to 2006 base years), 26
MEI revisions by (2014), 26
model payment schedule and, 18
in monitoring balance billing compliance, 89
multi-specialty practice expense surveys, 63–64
new patients as defined by, 19, 147
Notice of Proposed Rulemaking (1991), 18, 19
obstetrical services refinement by, 39
payment schedule adjustments to ensure budget neutrality, 98
practice expense methodology and refinement, 47–64
professional liability insurance RVU calculations, 66–68
professional liability insurance RVU methodologies, 2005 through 2020, 68–70
publication of RUC recommendations, 33
Quality Payment Program, 173–174
reaction to Phase I of Harvard RBRVS study, 8
refinement panel organized by, 35
regional offices directory, 559
resource-based practice expenses refinement, 60–64
RVS refinement process, 27–28, 30–31
RVU rescaling by, 16
specialty practice expense ratios for 1989, *44t–45t*
Technical Advisory Panel review of MEI, 93
top-down practice expense approach, 49, 57
transition policies (1991–1992), 19
work RVUs refinement process, 7, 27–28, 30–31, *36t*, 80–84, *83t*
Certified nurse midwives (CNMs), 23, *54t*, 131, *132t*
Certified registered nurse anesthetists (CRNAs), 23, 133
Cerumen removal, RVU adjustments for, 41

Cervical cancer screening, 154–155, *157t*
CF. *See* Conversion factor
Charge-based practice expense RVUs, 43, 49, 51, 60, 65
Charge-based relative value scale, 4–5
Chemotherapy, 127
Chicago, example of locally adjusted payment schedule, 80, *80t*
Chiropractic services, 22, *45t, 52t, 54t,* 128
Chronic care management (CCM), 36, 142–143
Claims-editing packages, 185–186, *185f, 186f*
Claims filing, 170, 172
CLCCP (Comprehensive Limiting Charge Compliance Program), 89, 176
Clerical payroll, mean practice expenses per hour spent in patient care, *52t–53t*
Clinical decision support mechanism, 119
Clinical diagnostic laboratory tests (CDLTs), 124
Clinical laboratory
  interpretation services, 124–125
  payment schedule (CLFS), 123–124
  practice expense data, *54t*
Clinical nurse specialists (CNSs), 23, 121, 126, 131, *132t*
Clinical pathology consultations, 124
Clinical practice expert panels (CPEPs)
  practice expense study, 47–51, *50f*
  quality improvement of data from, 61, 63
  Technical Expert Group, 47
Clinical psychologists, 23, *52t, 54t,* 133
Clinical social workers (CSWs), 23, *52t, 55t,* 133
Clinical staff, labor pricing update for 2022, *IBC*, 64
Clinics, independent, national place of service codes and payment rates for, 197
CMDs (carrier medical directors), 7, 30, 37
CMS. *See* Centers for Medicare & Medicaid Services
CNMs (certified nurse midwives), 23, 131, *132t*
CNSs. *See* Clinical nurse specialists
COBRA (Consolidated Omnibus Budget Reconciliation Act of 1985), 6, 7
Code editing packages, 185–186, *185f, 186f*
Cognitive impairment, coverage of primary care services for, 146
Coinsurance and deductibles
  advanced laboratory test waiver of coinsurance and deductible, 124
  balance billing, 87–89
  defined, 542
  example of payment for participating and nonparticipating physicians, *89t*
  Medicare coinsurance (20%), 4, 9, 15, 79, 169, 171
  Medicare Part B deductible, 87
  Medigap and other supplemental policies, 88, 170–171, 177, 178
  out-of-pocket payments, 87–88, *89t,* 178
  waivers for specified preventive services, 151–156, *156t–160t*, 160
College of American Pathologists, 123
Colonoscopy and colorectal cancer screening, 153–154, *157t*, 193–194
Colorectal surgery, 41, *52t, 54t*
Community mental health centers, national place of service code and payment rate for, 198
Competition, economic, 6, 166
Comprehensive inpatient rehabilitation facilities, national place of service code and payment rate for, 198
Comprehensive Limiting Charge Compliance Program (CLCCP), 89, 176
Comprehensive outpatient rehabilitation facilities, national place of service code and payment rate for, 199
Computed tomography, low-dose, *159t*
Computerized provider order entry (CPOE), 171
Congenital abnormalities, 111
Congressional Budget Office (CBO), 21, 97
Congress (US). *See* US Congress
Consolidated Appropriations Act of 2016, 122, 123
Consolidated Appropriations Act, 2021, 15, 16, 73, *83t,* 84, 98–99, *100t,* 165, 524, 541
Consolidated Appropriations Resolution of 2003, 20, *97t*
Consolidated Consulting Group, Inc, 29–30
Consolidated Omnibus Budget Reconciliation Act (COBRA) of 1985, 6, 7
Consultation services
  clinical, 124
  generally increased payments under RBRVS, 169
  interprofessional, 144–145
  payment lag issues with CPR, 3
  RBRVS payment rules and policies, 139
  RVU adjustments for, 38
  RVU refinement process (1992), 30–31
  surgical, 102
  telephone and Internet, 144–145
Continuing Appropriations Act, 2021, and Other Extensions Act, 73, 75, 542
Continuing Extension Act of 2010, 20, 97, *97t,* 541
Contracting, private. *See* Private contracting
Contractors, defined, 542
Conversion factor (CF)
  AMA advocacy in 2022 (pandemic effects on physician finances), 16
  anesthesia services, 84, 184–186, *183f, 186f*
  budget-neutrality adjustments, reductions, 13, 16, 80–84, *83t, 97t, 98–99, 100t*
  calculating Medicare physician payment schedule, 79–80, *80t, 83t,* 84–86
  calculation for 1992, 17
  calculation for 2022, *IFC*
  CMS budget-neutrality adjustments, 98
  cuts blocked for 2004–2006, 96
  description of, 4, 542
  establishing charges under RBRVS, 177–179, *178t*
  Final Rule (1991) and CF for 1992, 19

Conversion factor (CF) (*continued*)
freeze on, 96
full unadjusted Medicare payment schedule, 70
geographically adjusted, 536–538
historical payment basis and, 17
history (1992-2022), *100t*
legislation on (2010-2019), 20–21, 540–542, 544–546
Medicare, 85-86
Medicare expenditure targets and, 9, 83t, 86, 98
postponement of reductions, 21
proposed reduction in *NPRM,* 18
SGR repeal, 92–93
separate MVPS targets for surgical and nonsurgical services, 94
stabilization by MACRA, 92–93
temporary fixes from 2007–2015, 21, 96–98, *97t*
update for 2022, IFC, 16, 98–99, *100t*
updates to, 13, 91–100
use by third-party payer type, 182–185, *183f, 186f*
Copayments. *See* Coinsurance and deductibles
Coronary artery bypass surgery, 29, 30
Coronavirus Aid, Relief, and Economic Security (CARES) Act of 2020, 73, 75, 542
Coronavirus pandemic. *See* COVID-19 pandemic
Correct coding initiative (CCI), 151
Correctional facilities, national place of service code and payment rate for, 195
Cost control measures, distortions to physician payments due to, 5
Cost-of-living GPCI, 73
Co-surgeon (codes C and C1), explanatory note for list of RVUs, 193
COVID-19 pandemic
AMA advocacy and policy recommendations, *IFC*, 161, 166
AMA resource center, 166
CARES Act of 2020, 73, 75
CPT code 99072, *IFC*, 36
E/M services via telephone, 114
expanded roles for physician assistants and nurses, 131
Medicare MIPS payments and, 162
Medicare telehealth and, *IFC*
MVPs (MIPS Value Pathways), 174
telehealth expansion during, 115
vaccine administration payment rate for 2022, *IFC*, 127
CPEPs. *See* Clinical practice expert panels
CPOE (computerized provider order entry), 171
CPR charges. *See* Customary, prevailing, and reasonable charges
CPT. *See also* Evaluation and management (E/M) services
annual updates by AMA, 31
coding system used in RBRVS, 28
defined, 542
establishment as coding system for Medicare, 101
film technology changes, 62
history of RUC recommendations (CPT 1993–CPT 2022), *36t*
physician and nonphysician advisory committee, 31
CPT codes
alphanumeric coded services, 510–520
anesthesiology base units, 525, 527–535
audio-only telemedicine service, CPT Appendix P, 113
changes for 2022, *IFC*
CMS website on data collection for global periods, 169–170
code 00790, in Montana anesthesia payment, 525–526
code 99024, postoperative service data, 169
code 99072, for use in pandemic, *IFC*, 36, 127
code 99213, direct and indirect costs calculation for 2022, 57–59
code 99442, telehealth in 2022, *IFC*
critical care services, update for 2022, *IBC*
codes 99444 and 98969 eliminated, 114
codes for principal care management, 143
codes for telehealth and telemedicine, 114
list of RVUs by, 192–194, 200–520
moderate sedation, 105–106
modifiers, 106–114
nonphysician practitioners, 127–134
office visits, revisions in 2021, 114–115, 135, 136, 137, 170, *IBC*
professional liability insurance RVUs, 67
remote therapeutic monitoring (98975–98981), 116, *IBC*
RUC yearly recommendations, *36t*
specialty risk factor, 67
Tier 1 and Tier 2 for molecular pathology, 123–124
vignettes for, 28
CPT Editorial Panel, 31–41, 101, 116–122, 129–142, 150
E/M office visit revisions, 136
telehealth/telemedicine E/M CPT codes eliminated and added, 114
CPT-4 codes, rebundling of, 104
CPT modifiers, 104, 106–114, 185–186, *185t, 186t. See also headings beginning with* Modifier
CPT Network, 548
Craniotomy, RVU adjustments for, 41
Critical care services, 38, 148–149, *IBC*
CRNAs (certified registered nurse anesthetists), 23, *54t*, 128, 133
CSWs (clinical social workers), 23, 52*t*, 133
Current Procedural Terminology. *See* CPT
Custodial care facilities, national place of service code and payment rate for, 197
Customary, prevailing, and reasonable (CPR) charges
basis of Medicare payment to physicians, 3–6
defined, 542
Medicare definitions of, 3
prevailing charge adjustment (1992), 16–17
reform options, 3–5
transition period to RBRVS payment system, 168
Customary charges, defined, 3, 542

D

"Dear Doctor" letter, 88, 176
Deductibles. *See* Coinsurance and deductibles
Deficit Reduction Act of 2005
  code DRA, explanatory note for list of RVUs, 194
  conversion factor and, 96
  defined, 542
  on imaging caps to OPPS, 122–123
  on physical and occupational therapy, 129
  replacement of 2006 SGR cut, *97t*
Dentistry, 22
Department of ___. *See specific name of department*
Department of Defense Appropriation Act of 2010, 20, 97, *97t*, 542
Depression screening, *158t*
Dermatology, 40, *45t, 52t, 54t*
Diabetes prevention, *159t*
Diabetes screening, 153, *158t*
Diabetes self-management training, *158t*
Diagnosis-related groups (DRGs), 3–6
Diagnostic imaging, 60–61, 120–122, 194
Diagnostic laboratories, practice expense ratios for 1989, *45t*
Diagnostic mammography, RVU adjustments for, 40
Diagnostic radiology, *54t*
Diagnostic tests, 112, 110, 120–124
Diagnostic x-ray, practice expense ratios for 1989, *45t*
Dietitians, registered, 23, *56t*, 134
Digital imaging, migration from film to, 62
Direct supervision (DS), explanatory note for list of RVUs, 193
Discontinued procedure (Modifier 53), 109
Distinct procedural service (Modifier 59), 110
DME (durable medical equipment), 125, 178, 558
DME, prosthetics, orthotics, and other supplies (DME-POS), 125
DME regional carriers (DMERC), 125
Dollar conversion factor. *See* Conversion factor (CF)
Domiciliary care services, 140
DRGs (diagnosis-related groups), 3–6
Drug overdose epidemic, 162-163
Drugs
  average wholesale price for, 19, 126
  incident to physician's service, 88, 126–128
  limiting charge, 88
  Medicare Part D coverage of, 10, 127
  physician administered, 21
  RBRVS payment rules and policies, 126–127
Due process, 176
Durable medical equipment (DME), 125, 178, 558

E

Economic competition, 6, 166
EFT (electronic funds transfer), 172
Electrocardiograms (ECGs), 18, 19, 122, 160
Electroencephalograms (EEGs), 30
Electronic claims, 171
Electronic data interchange, 168
Electronic funds transfer (EFT), 172
Electronic health records (EHRs), 144–145, 171, 172, 173
Electronic mail, 114–115, 144–145
Electronic remittance advice, 172
E-mail, 114–115, 144–145
Emergency department services, 38, *52t, 54t,* 149, 160
Emergency room in hospitals, national place of service code and payment rate for, 197
Employee wage data, 73, 73–74, 76
Employment worksite, national place of service code and payment rate for, 196
E/M services. *See* Evaluation and management services
Endocrinology, practice expense data, *52t, 54t*
Endoscopy, 104–105, 193–194
End-stage renal disease (ESRD), 160–161
national place of service codes and payment rates for, 199
EOMB (Explanation of Medicare Benefits), 89, 151, 176
e-prescribing systems, 171
Equipment, medical. *See* Medical equipment
Evaluation and management (E/M) services, 134–144
  administrative burden, 135–136
  defined, 542–543
  documentation guidelines, 137–139
  generally increased payments under RBRVS, 169
  increases for mid- to upper-level visits, 30–31
  office visit revisions for 2022, 135, 136, 137, 170, *IBC*
  prolonged, 140, 144, 146
  psychotherapy, 133–134
  RBRVS payment rules and policies, 134–144
  reporting, 139–144, 146–147, 150
  RUC recommendations and results, 38, 40, 59–60
  RVU adjustments and refinements, 30–31, 40
  same-day (Modifier 25), 107, 169
  staff knowledge of new guidelines, 170
  telemedicine and telehealth, 114-116
  telephone communications, 113–115, 136, 144–145
  in third five-year review process, 38
  unrelated postoperative (Modifier 24), 107
  visit complexity code G2211 implementation delayed, *83t*
Expenditure targets, 9, 13, 94–98. *See also* Sustainable growth rate (SGR)
Explanation of Medicare Benefits (EOMB), 89, 151, 176

F

Family practice, 17, *44t, 52t, 54t*, 68
FDA. *See* Food and Drug Administration (FDA)
Fecal occult blood test (FOBT), 153, *157t*
Federally qualified health centers, national place of service code and payment rate for, 197

Federal Register, 7, 18
Federal Trade Commission (FTC), 4, 5
Fee-for-service systems, 10, 173
Fee schedule, 2–3, 77. *See also* Physician fee (payment) schedule
Final Notice, defined, 543
Final Rule, defined, 543
Final Rule (1991), 19, 30, 43
Final Rule (1994), 31, 37
Final Rule (1998), 14
Final Rule (2001), 39
Final Rule (2003), 160
Final Rule (2004), 38
Final Rule (2005), 55
Final Rule (2006), 31, 40, 134, 156
Final Rule (2007), 16
Final Rule (2008), 38
Final Rule (2011), 41
Final Rule (2022), 84
Five-Year Review Compelling Evidence Standards, 37, 38
Five-Year Review Identification Workgroup, 31, 42
Five-year review process, *36t*, 37–42
  defined, 543
  identification of misvalued services in, 31
  OBRA 89 in establishment of, 31
Flexible sigmoidoscopy, 154, 154, *157t*
Florida, GPCI shortcomings in, 75
Flu vaccines, 127, *158t*
FOBT (fecal occult blood test), 153, *157t*
Fracture treatment, RVU adjustments for, 40
Fraud and abuse, 151, 178
FTC (Federal Trade Commission), 4, 5
Further Consolidated Appropriations Act, 2020, 73, 75, 543

G

GAF (geographic adjustment factor), 19, 74–75, 76, 543
GAO (General Accounting Office), 48–49, 76
Gastroenterology, practice expense data, *44t, 52t, 54t*
G codes
  colorectal cancer screening (G0106), 154
  end-stage renal disease, 160–161
  global surgical package, 169
  initial preventive physical exam, G0402, 152
  moderate (conscious) sedation, 105–106
  nonphysician online digital assessments (G2061–G2063), 114
  physician-provided chemotherapy, 126–127
  principal care management, 143
  telehealth, 114, 115
  virtual check-in codes, *IFC,* 115
  visit complexity code G2211 implementation delayed, *83t*
GDP (gross domestic product), 95, 96
General Accounting Office (GAO), 49, 76
General internal medicine, practice expense ratios for 1989, *44t*
General practice, practice expense data, *44t, 52t, 54t*
General supervision (GS), explanatory note for list of RVUs, 193
General surgery
  incentive payments for services in HPSAs, 77–78
  misvalued codes for review, 38
  practice expense data, *52t, 54t*
  practice expense ratios for 1989, *44t*
  RVU adjustments for, 39, 41
Geographic adjustment factor (GAF), 19, 74–75, 76, 543
Geographic adjustments, 14–15, 69, 71–75
Geographically adjusted dollar anesthesia conversion factors, 536–538
Geographically adjusted payment, 13
Geographic practice cost indices (GPCIs), 71–76
  in calculating Medicare physician payment schedule, 79–80, *80t, 84–86*
  CMS modifications (2013), 76
  composite index, 74
  cost-of-living, 73
  cost share weights for work, practice expense, and PLI GPCIs, 75
  data for, 19
  defined, 543
  evaluation of, 76
  floor, 14–15, 20, 73, 524, 543
  GAO validity study, 76
  Institute of Medicine review of methodology, 76
  legislative provisions for, 14–15
  list of, for each Medicare locality, 521–524
  Medicare payment locality methodology, 76–78
  need to improve data sources for, 76
  phase-in of adjustments to, 72–75
  practice expense, 72–74, 79–80, *80t*, 84–86
  professional liability insurance, 74–76, 79–80, *80t*, 84–86
  revisions, updates (1995–2022), 72–75
  variations in, 74
  work GPCI extension, 15, 72–73, 74, 75, 524
Geographic variations, 71–78
  AMA blueprint for Medicare physician payment reform (1988–1989), 9
  AMA policy on reducing, 71
  CPR payment issues and (1970s), 3
  GPCI variations, 74
  Medicare payment localities and, 76–78, 521–524
  Medicare physician payment schedule, 71–78
  OBRA 89 on, 13, 71–72
  PPRC recommendations on, 9
  practice expense GPCIs, 74
  RBRVS payment system standardization and, 17–18, 168, 169

Geriatrics
  practice expense data, *44t, 52t,* 53, *54t*
  psychiatry, *54t*
Glaucoma screening, 155, *158t*
Global charge, defined, 543
Global period, explanatory note for list of RVUs, 193
Global service, defined, 543
Global surgical package
  budget-neutrality adjustments, 16
  CMS informational website on data collection, 169–170
  defining, 101–104
  duration of global period, 104
  Final Rule (1991), 19
  practice management under RBRVS payment system, 169–170
  RBRVS payment rules and policies, 101–104
  reporting guidelines, 169–170
  RVU adjustments for, 39
Glossary of terms, 540–547
GPCIs. *See* Geographic practice cost indices
Gross domestic product (GDP), 95, 96
Group homes, national place of service code and payment rate for, 196
Gun violence, 163
Gynecologist/oncologist, mean practice expenses per hour in patient care, *54t*
Gynecology, 41, *44t, 53t, 55t*

H

Habilitative services (Modifier 96), 113
Hand surgery, practice expense data, *44t, 52t, 54t*
Harvard RBRVS study, 6–9
  AMA policy and role in, 5, 7–9
  credibility enhanced by involvement of organized medicine, 7
  critical role in Medicare physician payment, 26
  cross-specialty process in, 28–29
  exploratory study prior to, 7
  national survey of physician work in, 28
  phases I through IV, 7–9, 13, 27, 29
  physicians' practice costs in, 13
  physician work component of, 7, 26–30
  representative national sample of physicians for, 7
  reviews of, 29–30
  Technical Consulting Groups in, 7, 27–29
  on unreliability of charge data, 5
HCPAC. *See* Health Care Professionals Advisory Committee
HCPCS codes. *See also* G codes
  alphanumeric list of RVUs by, 510–520
  colorectal cancer screening, 153–154
  defined, 543
  J codes, 127
  medical nutrition therapy, 134
  molecular pathology, 123–124
  nonphysician online digital assessments, 114
  physician care plan oversight services, 139
  portable X-ray service, 120
  practice expenses for supplies, equipment and drugs, 64, 125–127
  psychotherapy, 133–134
  telehealth, 114–115
  virtual check-in codes, *IFC*
  visit complexity code G2211 implementation delayed, *83t*
HCV (hepatitis C virus) screening, *159t*
Health and Human Services Department (HHS)
  annual report on limiting charge violations, 89
  COBRA directive on developing RBRVS, 6, 7
  on code set uniformity for claims, 172
  defined, 542
  E/M documentation burden and, 137
  fraud and abuse control program requirements, 151
  model payment schedule from, 18
  Office of Inspector General, 178
  on privacy and security of health information, 172
Health care access. *See* Access to care
Healthcare Common Procedure Coding System. *See* HCPCS codes
Health Care Financing Administration. *See* Centers for Medicare & Medicaid Services (CMS)
Health care fraud and abuse. *See* Fraud and abuse
Health Care Professionals Advisory Committee (HCPAC), 31–34, 101, 128, 130, 156
Health centers, federally qualified, walk-in, national place of service codes and payment rates for, 197
Health clinics
  rural, national place of service codes and payment rates for, 199
  walk-in retail, national place of service codes and payment rates for, 196
Health information, privacy and security of, 164–165, 172
Health information technology, 166, 171, 172
Health Insurance Portability and Accountability Act (HIPAA) of 1996, 151, 171, 172
Health maintenance organizations (HMOs), 3, 4, 6, 10
Health plan identifiers, 172
Health policy research, 166
Health professional shortage areas (HPSAs), 77–78, 175, 543
Heart failure/transplant cardiology, *54t*
Hematology, practice expenses, *55t*
Hematopoietic cell transplantation, *53t, 55t*
Hemodialysis, cross-specialty RVS process for, 29
Hepatitis B immunization, 128, *158t*

Hepatitis B virus (HBV) screening, *159t*
Hepatitis C virus (HCV) screening, *159t*
Hernia repair, in RVS refinement process (1992), 30
HHS. *See* Health and Human Services Department
HIPAA. *See* Health Insurance Portability and Accountability Act of 1996
Historical payment basis, 17
HIV/AIDS screening, *159t*
HMOs. *See* Health maintenance organizations
Home care services, 30, 139–140
Homeless shelters, national place of service code and payment rate for, 195
Homes, national place of service code and payment rate for, 196
Hospice, national place of service code and payment rate for, 197
Hospitalists, practice expense data, *53t, 55t*
Hospitals
  emergency department services, 38, *52t*, *54t*, 149, 160, 197
  emergency department x-rays and ECGs, 160
  inpatient services, 2, 5
  national place of service codes and payment rates for, 196
  observation care services, 149–150
  observation visits, 41
  provider-based and teaching physicians, off-campus departments, 117–118
Housing and Urban Development Department (HUD), 73, 76
HPSAs (health professional shortage areas), 77–78, 175, 543
Hsiao, William C., 7
Human papillomavirus (HPV) screening, 155, *157t*

I

ICD-9, ICD-10 and ICD-10-CM, 107, 110, 172
Imaging services, 60–61, 169
Immigration, 163
Immunizations, 126, 127, 128, *158t, 160t*
Immunosuppressive therapy, 127
Immunotherapy, allergen, 151
Incentive payments. *See also* Merit-based incentive payment system (MIPS)
  e-prescribing, 171
  for Medicare participating physicians, 87–88
  primary care, 174–175
  purchase and meaningful use of EHRs, 171, 173
  Quality Payment Program, 173–174
  in shortage areas, 77–78, 175
  for surgeons in shortage areas, 77–78, 175
Incident-to services, 23, 88, 125–126
Independent clinics, national place of service code and payment rate for, 197
Independent diagnostic testing facilities, practice expense data, *53t, 55t*
Independent laboratories, *52t,* 123, 199
Indian Health Service, national place of service codes and payment rates for, 195
Infants, procedures on (Modifier 63), 111
Infectious disease medicine, practice expense data, *55t*
Influenza vaccines, 127, 128, *158t*
Information resources
  CMS regional offices, 559
  CMS website on global surgery data collection, 169–170
  durable medical equipment contractors, 558
  medical specialty societies, 550–554
  Medicare administrative contractors by state, 555–557
  Medicare Parts A and B for 2022, 179
  state medical associations, 549–550
  telehealth, 115
Initial preventive physical examinations (IPPEs), 152, *156t*
Inpatient hospitals, national place of service code and payment rate for, 196
Inpatient psychiatric facilities, national place of service code and payment rate for, 198
Institute of Medicine (IOM), 76
Insurance, health. *See* Health insurance
Intensity work per unit of time (IWPUT), 31
Intensive cardiac rehabilitation, mean practice expenses per hour in patient care, *54t*
Interest rates, 60–61
Intermediate care facilities (individuals with intellectual disabilities), 198
Internal medicine, 17, *44t, 53t, 55t*
Internet consultations, 144–145
Internist (journal), 8
Interoperability promotion, 172
Interprofessional consultations, 144–145
Interventional cardiology, mean practice expenses per hour in patient care, *54t*
Interventional pain management, *53t, 55t*
Interventional radiology, *53t, 55t*
Intraservice work, 28–30. *See also* Physician work component of RBRVS
IOM (Institute of Medicine), 76
IPPEs (initial preventive physical examinations), 152, *156t*
IWPUT (intensity work per unit of time), 31

J

J codes, 127
JIL Systems, Inc, 72
Journal of the American Medical Association (JAMA), 8

K

Kidney disease, end-stage, 160–161
national place of service codes and payment rates for, 199
KPMG Consulting, 66
Kyl-Archer Bill (proposed), 177

L

Laboratories
  alternative platform testing (Modifier 92), 113
  clinical, 124–125
  independent, *53t,* 123, 199
  mean practice expenses per hour spent in patient care, *53t*
  reference (Modifier 90), 112
  repeat clinical diagnostic test (Modifier 91), 112
Laboratory tests, 124–125
Labor costs, 57, 58, *IBC*
Laminectomy, CPT code for, 28
Laryngology, practice expense ratios for 1989, *44t*
Larynx removal, in RVS refinement process (1992), 30
LDCT (low-dose computed tomography), *159t*
Legislation. *See specific names of legislative acts*
Lesion excision and destruction, RVU adjustments for, 40
LGBTQ+ health, 163-164
Limited license practitioners, 31, 126–134
Limiting charges. *See also* Balance billing
  AMA policy on, 15, 176
  Comprehensive Limiting Charge Compliance Program, 89, 176
  defined, 543
  explaining to patients, 179
  impact of, 169
  limiting charge exception report, 89, 176
  monitoring compliance with, 176
  nonparticipating physicians, 175
  in physician fee (payment) schedule, 88–89
Linear accelerator, 64
Loans, SBA maximum interest rates for, 60, 62
Locality, defined, 543–544
Local public health clinics, national place of service code and payment rate for, 199
Lodging, temporary, national place of service codes and payment rates for, 196
Low-dose computed tomography (LDCT), *159t*
Low osmolar contrast media (LOCM), 120
Lung cancer screening, *159t*

M

MAACs. *See* Maximum allowable actual charges
MACRA. *See* Medicare Access and Children's Health Insurance Program Reauthorization Act of 2015
Magnitude estimation, 28, 29, 137, 138
"Malpractice" GPCI, 74
"Malpractice" RVUs, 192
Mammography, 40, *55t*, 153, *159t*
Mammography Quality Standards Act (MQSA) of 1992, 40
Mammography screening center, mean practice expenses per hour in patient care, *54t*
Mandated services (Modifier32), 107
Mandatory assignment, 4, 15, 87–88
Manipulative therapy, *45t, 53t,* 128
Mass immunization centers, national place of service code and payment rate for, 198
Maternal health, 164
Maxillofacial surgery, practice expense data, *55t*
Maximum allowable actual charges (MAACs), 13, 15, 87, 88, 175, 544
Meaningful use, 171, 173
Medicaid. *See also* Centers for Medicare & Medicaid Services (CMS)
  AMA advocacy during the COVID-19 pandemic, 161, 166
  Centers for Medicare and Medicaid Innovation, 173
  mandatory assignment, 88
  survey on use of RBRVS payment system, 181–185, *181f–186f*, 186
Medical decision making (MDM), 115, 136–137, 141
Medical equipment
  cost computation, 60
  durable, 125, 178, 558
  mean practice expenses per hour spent in patient care, *52t*
  practice expense GPCI component for, 72–74
  pricing updates, 64
  sliding scale approach for interest rates in cost computation, 60–61
  utilization rate for, 64
Medical Group Management Association, 190, *190f*
Medical liability reform, 166
Medically unlikely edits (MUEs), 104
Medical nutrition therapy (MNT), *55t,* 134, 151, 155–156, *159t*
Medical oncology, practice expense data, *53t, 55t*
Medical savings accounts (MSAs), 10
Medical societies. *See* Medical specialty societies; State medical associations
Medical specialties. *See also specific specialties*
  average practice expense RVUs, 50–51
  cross-specialty process, 28–29
  E/M services documentation guidelines, 137–139
  in Harvard RBRVS study, 7, 26–30
  indirect practice expense per hour, *54t–56t*
  mean practice expenses per hour spent in patient care, *52t–53t*
  multi-specialty practice expense surveys, 63–64
  payment gap between visits and procedures, 5, 169

Medical specialties (*continued*)
practice expense cost pools, steps for calculating, 49–50, *50f*, 57
practice expense ratios for 1989, *44t–45t*
professional liability insurance RVU calculations, 65–68
risk factors and professional liability insurance, 66-67, 68
supplemental practice expense data submission guidelines, 63
three-year average of professional liability claims, 66
Medical specialty societies, contact information for, 550–554
Medical toxicology, practice expense data, *53t, 55t*
Medicare. *See also* Centers for Medicare & Medicaid Services (CMS)
AMA advocacy efforts in 2021, 161-166
Centers for Medicare & Medicaid Innovation, 173
conversion factor for 2022, 58, 59, *83t*, 86, 98–99, *100t*
copayments, 87, 171, 178
deductibles, 87, 88, 171, 178
diabetes prevention program, 159*t*
health maintenance organizations as payment reform option, 3, 4
mental health add-on payments, 20
new patients, initial preventive physical examination, 152
private contracting, 89, 176–177
Private Health Plan Option, 6
Quality Payment Program, 173, 174, *IBC*
reform efforts, 9–20
as secondary payer, 151
spending percentages for hospital and physician services, 5
supplemental insurance policies, 88, 170–171
target recapture, 21
therapy caps, 20
Medicare Access and Children's Health Insurance Program Reauthorization Act (MACRA) of 2015
on alternative payment model, 173
AMA information resources on website, 174
annual payment updates of 0.5%, 179
conversion factor and, 21, 92–93, *97t*, 98
defined, 544
global surgical package valuation, 169
on Medicare opt-out affidavits, 177
Medicare physician payments for 2022, 174
Medicare's Quality Payment Program, 173, 174, *IBC*
moving physicians away from fee for service, 173
on pay for performance, 173
penalties with quality programs, 173
on physical and occupational therapy, 129–130
physician payment greater under, 92–93, *93f*
private contracting provisions in, 177
on quality and value-based care, 173
repeal of SGR by, 15–16, 21, 92–93, *97t*, 98
in stabilization of Medicare physician pay, 92–93, *93f*
transition of global postoperative period to zero days, 169
on work GPCI floor, 15, 75
Medicare administrative contractors, directory by state, 555–557
Medicare Advantage, 10
Medicare and Medicaid Extenders Act of 2010
conversion factor legislation and, 21
defined, 544
on independent laboratories, 123
on physical and occupational therapy, 129
on psychiatric therapy procedures and psychotherapy, 133–134, 150
replacement of 2011 SGR cut, *97t*, 98
technical component pathology services and, 123
on work GPCI floor, 14, 21, 75
Medicare Beneficiary Freedom to Contract Act (proposed), 177
Medicare carriers
medical directors, 7, 30, 37
payment policies standardized for, 168
return of incomplete claims, 170
screening of all unassigned claims, 89
Medicare economic index (MEI)
budget-neutrality adjustments and, 80–84, *83t*
changes to price proxies and cost components of, 93
CMS revisions to (2014), 26
defined, 544
distortion of charges by, 5
example using 2015 data, 93–94, *93t*
GPCI components based on 2006 data, 76
productivity adjustments, 93
proxy for inflation from 1976 to 2015, 93
purpose of, 3
rebasing from 2000 to 2006 base years, 26
rescaling of RVUs, 98
review by CMS Technical Advisory Panel, 93
SGR expenditure targets and, 94
Medicare ePrescribing Incentive Program, 171
Medicare Improvements for Patients and Providers Act (MIPPA) of 2008
on bonus payments for shortage areas, 78
on budget-neutrality adjustment applied to conversion factor, 16, 81
conversion factor provisions in, 20
defined, 544
on HPSA and scarcity bonus areas, 78
on initial preventive physical examination, 152
Medicare ePrescribing Incentive Program, 171
on physical and occupational therapy, 129
on physician payment fix, 20
on psychiatric therapy procedures and psychotherapy, 133–134, 150
replacement of 2008 SGR cut, 97, *97t*

on speech language pathology services, 130
on work GPCI floor, 14, 75
Medicare, Medicaid, and SCHIP Benefits Improvement and Protection Act (BIPA) of 2000
defined, 544
glaucoma screening provision, 155
mammography screening provision, 151, 153
on medical nutrition therapy, 134, 155–156
pelvic examination provision, 155
on preventive services benefits, 151
on qualified independent laboratories, 123
replacement of 2008 SGR cut, 96–97, *97t*
Medicare, Medicaid, and SCHIP Extension Act of 2007, 14, 544
Medicare/Medicaid Meaningful Use of Electronic Health Record program, 171
Medicare Modernization Act. *See* Medicare Prescription Drug, Improvement, and Modernization Act (MMA) of 2003
Medicare Part A
cost containment, DRGs and prospective payment (PPS), 2, 3, 4, 5
physicians' services in hospitals or nursing facilities, 22
website, 179
Medicare Part B, 101-161
beneficiary out-of-pocket payments, deductibles, 87–88, *89t*, 178
drug coverage, 126–127
information, website, 179
premiums for 2022, 178-179, *179t*
Medigap and other supplemental policies, 88, 170–171, 177, 178
nonphysician services covered by, 22–23
payment amounts to participating, nonparticipating physicians, *89t*
premiums for, 178–179, *179t*
preventive services coverage, 151–156, *156t–160t*
Medicare Part C, 9
Medicare Part D, 10, 127
Medicare Participating Physicians/Supplier Agreement, 88, 176
Medicare participation
advantages and disadvantages, 175–176
agreement form, 88, 176
defined, 545
nonparticipation, 85–86, 169, 175–176, 545
opt-out affidavits, 176, 177
PAR Program, 87–89, *89t*
payment differential, 88, 169
physician decision making regarding, 84–88, 175–176
rates of physician participation (2009-2019), 88
Medicare Payment Advisory Commission (MedPAC)
contact information, 548
defined, 545
formation of, 11
multi-specialty practice expense surveys, 63–64
opinion regarding professional liability insurance RVUs, 66
Medicare payment localities
bonus payments for health professional shortage areas, 77–78
example of payment schedule calculation, 80, *80t*
geographically adjusted dollar anesthesia conversion factors, 536–538
list of geographic practice cost indices for, 521–524
methodology for defining, 76–77
Medicare payment policy indicators, explanatory notes in list of RVUs, 192–194
Medicare payment schedule, 79–86, 192–193
defined, 544
full, for 2022, 84–86
Medicare payment system under RBRVS. *See* RBRVS payment rules and policies; RBRVS payment system
Medicare + Choice, 9, 10
Medicare Prescription Drug, Improvement, and Modernization Act (MMA) of 2003
on bonus payments for shortage areas, 77
on chiropractic services, 128
conversion factor cut blocked by, 20, 96
on cost-of-living GPCI, 73
defined, 545
on GAO validity study of GPCIs, 76
on gross domestic product component of SGR, 96
on HPSA and scarcity bonus areas, 77–78
on Medicare Advantage as replacement for Medicare + Choice, 9–10
on physical and occupational therapy, 129
Physician Practice Information Survey and, 63
on prescription drug coverage, 20, 126
on preventive services/screening benefits, 151–152
on private fee-for-service, 10
replacement of 2004 SGR cut, *97t*
on work GPCI floor, 14, 72–73, 75
Medicare Preservation and Restoration Act (proposed), 177
Medicare reimbursement. *See* RBRVS payment rules and policies; RBRVS payment system
Medicare volume performance standard (MVPS), 13, 15–16, 92, 94, 95, 545
Medigap policies, 88, 170–171, 177, 178
MedPAC. *See* Medicare Payment Advisory Commission
MEI. *See* Medicare economic index
Mental health services, 20
national place of service codes and payment rates for, 198
telehealth, *IFC*, 114–115
Merit-based incentive payment system (MIPS), 16, 94, 162, 174–175, 545, *IBC*
MGMA. *See* Medical Group Management Association

Middle Class Tax Relief and Job Creation Act of 2012
conversion factor and, 21
defined, 545
replacement of 2012 SGR cut, *97t,* 98
on work GPCI floor, 14, 75
Midwives, 23, 131, *132t*
Military treatment facilities, national place of service code and payment rate for, 197
MIPPA. *See* Medicare Improvements for Patients and Providers Act of 2008
MIPS. *See* Merit-based incentive payment system
Misvalued services, 31, 32, 35–39, 42, 82, *IBC*
MMA. *See* Medicare Prescription Drug, Improvement, and Modernization Act of 2003
MNT. *See* Medical nutrition therapy
Mobile units, national place of service code and payment rate for, 196
Model payment schedule, 18, 545
Moderate (conscious) sedation, 105–106
Modifier 22 (increased procedural services), 106–107
Modifier 23 (unusual anesthesia), 107
Modifier 24 (unrelated postoperative E/M service), 102, 107
Modifier 25 (same-day, separately identifiable E/M services), 102, 107, 149, 169
Modifier 26 (professional component), 107
Modifier 32 (mandated services), 107
Modifier 33 (preventive services), 107–108
Modifier 47 (anesthesia by surgeon), 108
Modifier 50 (bilateral procedure), 108
Modifier 51 (multiple procedures), 108
Modifier 52 (reduced services), 108–109
Modifier 53 (discontinued procedure), 109
Modifier 54 (surgical care only), 109–110
Modifier 55 (postoperative management only), 109–110
Modifier 56 (preoperative management only), 109–110
Modifier 57 (decision for surgery), 102, 110
Modifier 58 (postoperative staged or related procedure or service), 102, 110
Modifier 59 (distinct procedural service), 110
Modifier 62 (two surgeons), 110–111
Modifier 63 (procedure on infant less than 4 kg), 111
Modifier 66 (surgical team), 111
Modifier 76 (repeat procedure or service by same health professional), 111
Modifier 77 (repeat procedure by another health professional), 102, 112
Modifier 78 (unplanned return to operating room), 102, 112
Modifier 79 (unrelated postoperative procedure/service by same health professional), 112
Modifier 80 (assistant surgeon), 112
Modifier 81 (minimum assistant surgeon), 112
Modifier 82 (assistant surgeon when resident surgeon unavailable), 112
Modifier 90 (reference (outside) laboratory), 112
Modifier 91 (repeat clinical diagnostic laboratory test), 112
Modifier 92 (alternative laboratory platform testing), 113
Modifier 93 (synchronous telemedicine service, audio-only), 113
CPT codes, audio-only telemedicine service in CPT Appendix P, 113
Modifier 95 (synchronous telemedicine service), 113
Modifier 96 (habilitative services), 113
Modifier 97 (rehabilitative services), 113
Modifier 99 (multiple modifiers), 113
Modifier AQ, 78, 175
Modifier CQ, 130
Modifier FS (split or shared visits), *IBC*
Modifier KX, 129–130
Modifiers
local, payment levels unaffected, 113
professional and technical component, 119–123
Mohs surgery, RVU adjustments for, 40
Molecular pathology, 123–124
Montana
CPT code 00790 (anesthesiology service), 525–526
practice expense GPCI floor for, 74, 75
MQSA (Mammography Quality Standards Act of 1992), 40
MSAs (medical savings accounts), 10
MUEs (medically unlikely edits), 104
Multianalyte assays, 124
Multiple procedure payment reduction (MPPR), 82, *83t,* 122–123
MVPs (MIPS Value Pathways, for quality improvement), 174
MVPS. *See* Medicare volume performance standard

N

National Correct Coding Initiative (NCCI), 104
National medical specialty societies. *See* Medical specialty societies
National place of service codes, 194–199
National provider identifier (NPI), 174
National Uniform Claim Committee (NUCC), 106
NCCI. *See* National Correct Coding Initiative (NCC1)
Nephrology, practice expense data, *44t, 53t, 55t*
Neurology, practice expense data, *45t, 53t, 55t*
Neuropsychiatry, *55t*
Neurosurgery, 41, *44t, 53t, 55t*
Nevada, practice expense GPCI floor for, 74, 75
New England Journal of Medicine, 8
New patients, 19, 147
New physicians, 18, 117
New York, GPCI shortcomings in, 74
The New York Times, 8
Nonparticipating physicians, 85–86, 169, 175–176, 545
Nonphysician practitioners
on advisory committees for RUC and CPT, 31

clinical staff, mean practice expenses per hour spent in patient care, *52t–55t*
incentive payments for, 174
labor costs, 64
payment for services, 22–23, 126–134
specialties not included in SMS, 63
work pools, 55–58
Non-residential substance abuse treatment facilities, 198
Non-residential opioid treatment facility, national place of service codes and payment rates for, 198
North Dakota, practice expense GPCI floor for, 74, 75
Notice of Proposed Rulemaking (NPRM), 18, 19, 30, 101, 545
Notices of privacy practices (NPPs), 172
NPI (national provider identifier), 174
NUCC (National Uniform Claim Committee), 106
Nuclear medicine, practice expense data, *45t, 53t, 55t*
Nurse anesthetists, 23, 133
Nurse midwives, 23, *54t*, 131, *132t*
Nurse practitioners (NPs), 23, 121, 126, 130–131, *132t*
Nurse specialists, clinical, 23, 121, 126, 130–131, *132t*
Nursing facility services and care, 30, 140, 197
Nutrition therapy. *See* Medical nutrition therapy (MNT)

O

Obesity screenings and counseling, *159t*
OBRA 86 (Omnibus Budget Reconciliation Act of 1986), 7
OBRA 89. *See* Omnibus Budget Reconciliation Act of 1989
OBRA 90. *See* Omnibus Budget Reconciliation Act of 1990
OBRA 93. *See* Omnibus Budget Reconciliation Act of 1993
Observation care services, 149–150
Obstetric care and services, 30, 39, *44t, 53t, 55t*
Occupational therapy, 23, *45t, 55t,* 128–130
Off-campus outpatient hospitals, national place of service code and payment rate for, 196
Office-based services, adjustment to allocation of indirect practice expense, 59–60
Office expense, mean practice expenses per hour spent in patient care, *52t–53t*
Office management practices, audit of, 170–171
Office rental data, 73, 76
Offices, national place of service code and payment rate for, 196
Office visits
discussion of payment during, 179
E/M changes for 2022 (Modifier FS), *IBC*
E/M revisions in effect as of 2021, 135, 136, 137, 170
gap between payments for procedures and, 5, 169
patient code 99213 for, 19
payment lag issues with CPR, 3
RVU adjustments for, 38
RVU refinement process (1992), 31
Ohio Medicine (journal), 8
Omnibus Budget Reconciliation Act of 1986 (OBRA 86), 7
Omnibus Budget Reconciliation Act of 1989 (OBRA 89)
balance billing limits and, 13, 15
budget neutrality and, 13, 16, 98
congressional subcommittee proposals on, 12–13
on conversion factor updates, 13, 94
defined, 545
on five-year review of RBRVS, 31, 34
on five-year transition (1992–1997), 13, 17–18
on geographic adjustments and GPCIs, 14, 71–72, 79
Medicare reform proposals and, 12–13
on Medicare volume performance standard, 13, 15
model payment schedule and, 18
ongoing updates to RBRVS, 31
practice cost method in, 13–14
practice expense method, 43–47
professional liability insurance RVUs and, 16, 65
on radiology payment, 22
on RBRVS-based physician payment schedule, 13
on separate surgical and nonsurgical MVPS targets and conversion factors, 94
on standardization process for RBRVS, 16–18
transition asymmetry, *17f*
transition to new system (1992–1997), 17–19
on uniform coding system for Medicare, 101
Omnibus Budget Reconciliation Act of 1990 (OBRA 90)
on five-year reviews of relative values, 37
statutory provisions of, 19
on three-year GPCI updates, 72–73
Omnibus Budget Reconciliation Act of 1993 (OBRA 93)
on antigen services, 127
on conversion factor for primary care services, 94
defined, 545
ECG payment restoration in, 19
on new physician payment, 117
on oral cancer drug off-label uses, 127
on performance standard factor, 94
practice expense component revisions, 46–47
on primary care services MVPS created, 94
On-campus outpatient hospitals, national place of service code and payment rate for, 196
Oncology services, *53t. See also* Cancer screening
Online E/M services, RBRVS payment rules and policies for, 114–116
Ophthalmology, 41, *44t, 53t, 55t*
Opioid treatment facilities, national place of service codes and payment rates for, 198
OPPS (outpatient prospective payment system), 119, 122–123
Optometry, 22, *45t, 53, 55t*
Oral cancer drugs, 127
Oral surgery, practice expense data, *45t, 53t, 55t*
Orthopedic surgery, 40–41, *44t, 53t, 55t*
Osteopathic manipulative therapy, *45t, 53t, 56t*, 128
Osteopathy, 22

Osteoporosis drugs, 127
Other place of service, national place of service code and payment rate for, 199
Otolaryngology, 41, *44t, 53t, 56t*
Otology, practice expense ratios for 1989, *44t*
Outpatient hospital, national place of service codes and payment rates for, 196
Outpatient prospective payment system (OPPS), 119, 122–123
Oximetry, pulse, 150

P

PACS (picture archiving and communication system), 62, 171
Pain management, *53t, 55t, 56t,* 104
PAMA. *See* Protecting Access to Medicare Act of 2014
Pandemic, 2020–2022. *See* COVID-19 pandemic
Pap (Papanicolau) test, 149, 155, *157t*
PAR (physician participation) Program, 87–88, *89t*
Participating Physician Program, 15, 87–88, *89t*
Participating physicians. *See* Medicare participation
PAs. *See* Physician assistants
Pathologic anatomy (clinical), practice expense ratios for 1989, *45t*
Pathology services
  clinical consultation services, 124
  hospital-based physician DRGs for, 6
  molecular, 123–124
  practice expense data, *53t, 56t*
  practice expense ratios for 1989, *45t*
  RBRVS payment rules and policies, 123–125
  RVU adjustments for, 41
Pathway for Sustainable Growth Rate (SGR) Reform Act of 2013
  conversion factor and, 21
  defined, 545
  replacement of 2014 SGR cut, *97t,* 98
  on work GPCI floor, 14–15, 75
Patient health information, privacy and security of, 164–165, 172
Patient office visit code 99213, 19
Patient-physician relationship, 19, 115, 147, 179
Patients
  advanced lab test waiver of coinsurance and deductible, 124
  balance billing, 87–89
  coinsurance and deductible waivers for specified preventive services, 151–156, *156t–160t*, 160
  discussing payment with, 179
  example of payment for participating and nonparticipating physicians, *89t*
  Medigap and other supplemental policies, 88, 170–171, 177, 178
  Medicare coinsurance (20%), 4, 9, 10, 79, 169, 171
  Medicare Part B deductible, 87
  new, 19, 147
  out-of-pocket payments, 87–88, *89t,* 178
  payment amounts to participating, nonparticipating physicians, 89
  relationships established via telehealth, 114
Pay-for-performance (PFP), 172–173, 546
Payment-for-service systems, 4, 6, 8, 10, 87, 177
Payment schedule. *See* Physician fee (payment) schedule; RBRVS payment system
PCM (principal care management) services, 143
PEAC (Practice Expense Advisory Committee), 31, 61–62
Pediatric services
  practice expense data, *44t, 53t, 56t*
  work RVUs for, 31, 34, 38
Pelvic examinations, 149–155, *157t*
PERC (Practice Expense Review Committee), 32, 62
Performance adjustment, 94–98. *See also* Medicare volume performance standard (MVPS)
Performance standard factor, 94
Performance threshold, 174
Peripheral vascular disease or surgery, *44t, 56t*
Personal health records (PHRs), 171
Personal supervision (PS), explanatory note for list of RVUs, 193–194
PFFS (private fee-for-service), 10
PFP (pay-for-performance), 172–173, 545
Pharmacies, national place of service code and payment rate for, 195
PHS (Public Health Service), 77
Physical examinations, initial preventive, 152, *156t*
Physical medicine and rehabilitation, practice expense data, *45t, 53t, 56t*
Physical therapy
  code Mt, explanatory note for list of RVUs, 193
  practice expense data, *53t, 56t*
  practice expense ratios for 1989, *45t*
  RBRVS coverage, 23, 128–130
Physician assistants (PAs), 23, 121, 128, 130–131, *132t*
Physician burnout and wellness, 165–166
Physician care plan oversight services, 139
Physician fee (payment) schedule, 79–86
  budget neutrality history (1989–2022), 80–84, *83t*
  CMS adjustments to, 98
  customary, prevailing and reasonable (CPR) charges as early basis for, 3
  establishing charges under RBRVS, 177–179
  example of locally adjusted payment schedule, 80, *80t*
  explanatory notes for list of RVUs, 192–194
  fee schedule concept, defined, 2–3, 79
  formula for calculating, 79–80, *80t*
  full Medicare payment schedule, 79–80

full unadjusted Medicare payment schedule components, 70
geographic variations, 71–78
key factors in, 79–80, *80t*
model payment schedule (1990), 18
payment reform options (mid-1980s), 3–5
payment schedule concept, defined, 2–3, 79
publishing of RVS update process results and final values, 33
traditional payment methodologies, 10
usual, customary and reasonable (UCR) charges, 3
worksheets on impact of payment system on individual practices, 84–86
Physician Masterfile, 7, 63
Physician participation (PAR) Program, 87–89, *89t*
Physician Payment and Therapy Relief Act of 2010, 20–21, 82, *97t,* 98, 546
Physician Payment Review Commission (PPRC)
adoption of RBRVS recommendation from, 6
concerns with OBRA 89 practice expense method, 46
defined, 546
establishment of, 6
Harvard RBRVS study, 9, 29
international study of physician payment by, 6
on mandatory assignment, 15
Medicare physician payment reform recommendations from, 12
on resource-based practice expenses, 46, 47
on resource-based professional liability insurance RVUs, 66
Physician payment under Medicare. *See* Balance billing; Customary, prevailing, and reasonable (CPR) charges; Evaluation and management (E/M) services; Primary care services; RBRVS payment rules and policies; RBRVS payment system; *specific specialties and names of procedures/treatments*
Physician Practice Information Survey, 63, 74, 93
Physician Quality Reporting System (PQRS), 173, 546
Physicians
attending, 22
"new," 18, 19, 117
non-Medicare use of RBRVS, 180–190
nonparticipating, 85–86, 169, 175–176, 545
participating, 84–85, 87–89, *89t,* 175–176, 545
productivity of, 93, 190, *190f*
provider-based and teaching, 22, 117–118
survey of RBRVS use by payers, 185–190, *185t, 186t, 186f, 187f, 188t, 189t, 190f*
wellness and burnout, 165–166
Physician work, defined, 27–28, 546
Physician work component of RBRVS, 26–42. *See also* Relative value units — physician work component
annual update, 168
assignment of relative values, 26
budget-neutrality adjustments to (1992–2022), 80–84, *83t*
combining practice expense, PLI RVUs and, 70
cross-specialty process, 28–29
elements of physician work, 27–28
explanatory note for list of RVUs, 192
future plans, 42
GPCIs, 72–73
in Harvard RBRVS study, 7, 27–30
intensity per unit of time factor, 29
intraservice work, 28–30
magnitude estimation to obtain work ratings, 28, 29
OBRA 89 and, 13
percentage of total relative value of services, 25, 26, *26f*
preservice and postservice work, 28, 29
relative value sources and updating, 27–36
RVS refinement process (1992), 27, 30–31
RVU service totals as combination of practice expense, PLI and, 70
work adjustor elimination, 98
Physician work GPCI, 72–73
Physiologic monitoring, remote, 36, 115–116
Physiotherapy, practice expense ratios for 1989, *45t*
Picture archiving and communication system (PACS), 62, 171
Place of employment worksite, national place of service codes and payment rates for, 196
Place of service (POS) codes, 194–199
Plastic surgery, 40, *44t, 53t, 56t*, 68
Pneumococcal pneumonia vaccines, 127, 128, 160*t*
Podiatry, 22, *45t, 53t, 56t*
Portable x-ray service, *56t*, 120
Post-induction period procedure anesthesia (PIPPA), 41
Postoperative care and services
complications following surgery, 103
consultation by nonsurgeons, 147–148
CPT code 99024 for, 169
days of care included in payment for global surgical package, 193
management (Modifier 55), 109–110
pain management, 104
proposed transition of global period, 169
staged unrelated procedure (Modifier 58), 110
by surgeon, 103
unrelated E/M service (Modifier 24), 107
unrelated procedure (Modifier 79), 112
Postservice work, 28, 29
PPAC (Practicing Physician's Advisory Council), 11
PPOs (preferred provider organizations), 10
PPRC. *See* Physician Payment Review Commission
PPS (prospective payment system), 2, 5
PQRS (Physician Quality Reporting System), 173, 545
Practice cost and expense data. *See also* Geographic practice cost indices (GPCIs); Practice expense component of RBRVS; Relative value units—practice expense component

Practice cost and expense data (*continued*)
in AMA blueprint for Medicare physician payment reform (1988–1989), 9
AMA pilot survey, 63–64
Balanced Budget Act on, 14
casting supplies, 125
GPCI floor for frontier states, 74, 524
Harvard study on, 13
mean practice expenses per hour spent in patient care, *52t–53t*
Medicare economic index for measurement of, 3
OBRA 89 provisions for, 13–14
RVU component compared with practice expense GPCI, 72–73
SMS data, 43, 47, 49, 50, 51–52, 57, 63
supply, equipment, and clinical labor pricing updates, 64
yearly RUC recommendations, 34–35
Practice Expense Advisory Committee (PEAC), 31, 59–60
Practice expense component of RBRVS, 43–64. *See also* Relative value units—practice expense component
allocation adjustment of indirect expenses, 59–60
allocation approach, *50f*
AMA pilot survey, 63–64
bottom-up approach, 49, 57–60
budget-neutrality adjustments, 51
code 99213, direct and indirect costs calculation for 2022, 57–59
code Mt, explanatory note for list of RVUs, 193
combining work, PLI RVUs and, 70
cost allocation methodology, 47–50, *50f, 52f–56f, 57*–62, 64
data from AMA Socioeconomic Monitoring System, 43, 47, 49, 50, 51–52, 57, 63
defined, 546
direct and indirect costs, 47–52, *52t–56t, 59*–60
explanatory note for list of RVUs, 192
mean practice expenses per hour spent in patient care, *52t–53t*
medical equipment cost computation, 60
migration from film to digital practice inputs, 62
multi-specialty surveys, 63–64
OBRA 89 method, 43–46
OBRA 93 revisions, 46–47
opposition to CMS Medicare methodology, 48
percentage of total relative value of services, 25, 26, *26f*
per-hour calculation example, 51–52
Physician Practice Information Survey, 63
ratios for 1989 by specialty, *44t–45t*
resource-based, 47–52, 60–64
RVU methodology (2007–2022), 57–60
RVU service totals as combination of work, PLI and, 70
specialty cost pools, steps for calculation of, 49–51, *50f*, 57
survey on direct and indirect costs, 47
top-down approach, 49, 55
Practice Expense Review Committee (PERC), 31, 59
Practice management
audit of office practices, 170–171
claim filing, 170, 172, 185–186
discussing payment with patients, 179
electronic health records, 171
establishing charges under RBRVS, 177–179
implications of RBRVS for physicians, 168–179
incentive payments, 174–175
incomplete claims, 170
Medicare participation decision, 175–176
office management practices, 170–171
private contracting, 176–177
value-based health care, 173–174
Practicing Physician's Advisory Council (PPAC), 11
Preferred provider organizations (PPOs), 10
Premiums, for Medicare Part B, 178–179, *179t*
Preoperative clearance, 147
Preservation of Access to Care for Medicare Beneficiaries and Pension Relief Act of 2010, 20, 82, 97–98, *97t*, 546
Preservice work, 28, 29
Prevailing charges, 3, 5, 16–17, 546. *See also* Customary, prevailing, and reasonable (CPR) charges
Preventive medicine, practice expense data, *56t*
Preventive services
Modifier 33, 107–108
payment policy changes to, 127–128, 151–160, *156t–160t*
prolonged, 33, 82, 140, 144, 146
waiver of coinsurance and deductibles, 151, *156t–160t*
Primary care services
bonus payment for health professional shortage areas, 77–78
concerns with OBRA 89 practice expense method, 46
defined, 546
dissatisfaction with CPR (1970s and 1980s), 3
incentive payments for, 174–175
postoperative consultation by nonsurgeons, 147–148
preoperative medical clearance, 147
preventive services, 151-160, *156t–160t*
RBRVS adoption and, 9
RBRVS payment rules and policies, 141–145
Principal care management (PCM) services, 143
Prisons, national place of service code and payment rate for, 195
Privacy of health information, 164–165, 172
Private contracting, 10, 19–20, 176–177
Private fee-for-service (PFFS), 10
Private Health Plan Option, 6
Procedural services, distinct (Modifier 59), 110
Procedural services, increased (Modifier 22), 106–107
Procedures. *See also specific procedures*
payment gap between visits and, 5, 169
repeat, by another health physician (Modifier 77), 112

repeat, by same physician (Modifier 76), 111
Proctology, practice expense ratios for 1989, *44t*
Productivity, 93, 190, *190f*
Professional component, 119–125
advanced imaging services, 82
code Mtc, explanatory note for list of RVUs, 194
defined, 546
Modifier 26, 107
pathology services, 123–125
radiology services, 119–120
Professional liability insurance component of RBRVS, 65–70. *See also* Relative value units —professional liability insurance component
in AMA blueprint for Medicare physician payment reform (1988–1989), 9
charge-based, 65–66
CMS methodology and five-year reviews, 68–70
defined, 546
examples of, 65–66
explanatory note for list of RVUs, 192
five-year review/update requirement, 66
geographic adjustment, 69
GPCI for, 66, 69, 74, 76
percentage of total relative value of services, 25, 26, *26f*
premium data, 66–69, 93
relative values in OBRA 89, 16
resource-based, 66–68, 168
RUC recommendations, 35
RUC workgroup on, 31
RVU calculations, 65–68, 70
specialty-weighted risk factor, 67, 69, 70
updates to (2005, 2010, 2015), 66
Professional liability premium, 69
Professional liability reform, 166
Prolonged services, 33, 82, 140, 144, 146
Promoting Interoperability Programs, 172
Prospective payment system (PPS), 2, 5
Prostate cancer screening, *160t*
Protecting Access to Medicare Act of 2014 (PAMA)
on advanced diagnostic laboratory tests and clinical diagnostic laboratory tests, 124
California Medicare payment localities and, 77
conversion factor and, 21, 98
defined, 546
physician payment cut postponed by, 179
on proprietary laboratory analyses, 123–124
replacement of 2014 SGR cut, *97t*, 98
target recapture and, 21
on work GPCI floor, 15, 75
Protecting Medicare and American Farmers from Sequester Cuts Act of 2021, *IFC*, 16, 84, 99, 546
Provider Relief Fund, 161
Psychiatric facilities
national place of service codes and payment rates for, 198
partial hospitalization facilities, place of service code, 198
Psychiatric residential treatment centers, national place of service codes and payment rates for, 198
Psychiatry services
collaborative care management, 36, 145–146
practice expense data, *53t, 56t*
practice expense ratios for 1989, *45t*
RVU adjustments for, 39
updated work RVUs, 35, 36
Psychologists, clinical, 23, *56t*, 133–134
Psychotherapy, 35, 39, 133–134, 150
Public health
COVID-19 pandemic, 161, 166
drug overdose epidemic, 162–163
flavored tobacco products, 164
gun violence, 163
threat of racism, 163
Public health clinics, national place of service code and payment rate for, 199
Public Health Service (PHS), 77
Puerto Rico, GPCI for, 74, 75
Pulmonary disease, practice expense data, *44t, 53t, 56t*
Pulse oximetry, 150
Purchased diagnostic tests, 121–122
Purchased services, 72, 76

Q

Quality improvement, MIPS Value Pathways, 174
Quality of care, 172–175
Quality Payment Program (QPP), 173–174, *IBC*
Quality standards, for mammography, 40

R

Racism and bias, 163
Radiation oncology, *53t, 56t*
Radiation therapy services, *45t*, 120
Radiology services
diagnostic tests, 121–122
emergency department x-rays and ECGs, 160
hospital-based physician DRGs for, 6
integration of payment schedule into cross-specialty RBRVS, 22
interventional, *53t, 55t*
interventional procedures, 119–120
mean practice expenses per hour spent in patient care, *53t*
portable, *55t*, 120
practice expense ratios for 1989, *45t*
RBRVS payment rules and policies, 119–120
RVU adjustments for, 41

RBRVS. *See* Resource-based relative value scale
RBRVS payment rules and policies, 91, 101–166
  assistants-at-surgery, 106, 110–111, 112, 193–194, 185, *185*t, *186*t
  CPT modifiers, 104, 106-114, 185, *185t, 186t*
  drugs, 126–127
  durable medical equipment, 125
  E/M codes, 134–151
  emergency department x-rays and ECGs, 160
  end-stage renal disease, 160–161
  fraud and abuse initiatives, 151
  global surgical package, major procedures, 101–104, 169–170, 173
  incident-to services, 125–126
  issues in 2022, 162
  interprofessional consultations, 144–145
  medically unlikely edits, 104
  minor surgery and nonincisional procedures (endoscopies), 104–105
  moderate (conscious) sedation services, 105–106
  new physicians, 117
  nonphysicians, 127–134
  off-campus provider-based hospital departments, 119
  pathology services, 123–125
  preventive services, 151–160, *156t–160t*
  primary care services, 134, 146–151
  professional and technical component services, 119–124
  provider-based and teaching physicians, 117–118
  psychiatric collaborative care management, 145–146
  radiology services, 119–120
  remote physiologic monitoring, 115–116
  remote therapeutic monitoring, 116
  supplies, 125
  survey of RBRVS use by payers, 185–190
  telemedicine, 114–116, 144–145
  telephone and online E/M services, 113, 114, 115, 144–145
  therapeutic apheresis, 161
  use by non-Medicare payers, 180–190
  vaccine administration, 127–128
RBRVS payment system. *See also* Conversion factor (CF); Geographic practice cost indices (GPCIs); Incentive payments; Physician work component of RBRVS; Practice expense component of RBRVS; Professional liability insurance component of RBRVS; RBRVS payment rules and policies
  adjustments to physician work (1992-2022), *83t*
  AMA proposal and Harvard study, 5
  audit of office practices, 170–171
  budget neutrality and, 80–84, *83t*
  in calculating Medicare physician payment schedule, 79–80, *80t*
  changes for 2021, 162
  CMS completion of, 31
  distinction between payment schedule and fee schedule, 79
  electronic and health IT applications, 171
  establishing charges under, 177–179
  frequency of payment schedule updates, 186, *187f*
  full phase-in (January 1, 1996), 2
  geographic payment variations, 168, 169
  global surgical packages, 101–104 169–170
  history and development of, 1–11
  impact on physicians' practices, 84–86, 167–190
  issues in 2022, 162
  legislation creating, 12–21
  limiting charges, 169
  major components of, 25, 26*f*
  method of providing physicians with payment schedules, 186, *187f*
  national standard payment schedule, 168–169, 177–178
  non-Medicare use of, 180–190
  nonphysician services covered by, 22–23
  opinions about, 186–189
  for physician productivity/compensation, 190, *190f*
  physician services not covered by, 22
  practice management implications, 168–179
  scope of, 22–23
  staff knowledge of new payment policies and revisions, 170
  standardization of Medicare carrier payment policies, 168, 169
  survey data on non-Medicare use of, 180–190
  transition begins (January 1, 1992), 2
  transition period from CPR system, 168
  worksheets on impact of payment system on individual practices, 84–86
Reasonable charges, 3. *See also* Customary, prevailing, and reasonable (CPR) charges
Reconstructive surgery, *53t*
Reduced services (Modifier 52), 108–109
Registered dietitians, 23, *56t,* 134
Rehabilitation facilities, national place of service codes and payment rates for, 198
Rehabilitative services (Modifier 97), 113
Relative value scale (RVS). *See also* Conversion factor (CF); Resource-based relative value scale (RBRVS)
  AMA/Specialty Society update process, 31–36
  charge-based, 4–5
  cross-specialty process in Harvard study, 28–29
  defined, 546–547
  Medicare physician payment reform option (mid-1980s), 3–5, 25
  refinement process (1992), 27, 30–31
Relative value units (RVUs). *See also* Relative value units—physician work component; Relative value units—practice expense component; Relative value units—professional liability insurance component
  anesthesiology services, 525–535
  annual rescaling of, 16

assignment to nonsurveyed services, 29
budget-neutrality adjustments, 16
calculating Medicare physician payment schedule, 79–80, *80t*
combining work, practice expense, and PLI, 70
defined, 547
E/M code refinement, 30–31
explanatory information for list of RVUs, payment schedule, and payment policy indicators, 192–194
final values published in November each year, 33
five-year reviews, 37–42
future plans of RUC and, 42
Harvard RBRVS study use of, 7
list of, by CPT code, 200–520
Medicare noncovered services, 31
non-Medicare-covered services frequently allowed by other payers, 192
no relative value assigned (denoted by "0.00") in list of RVUs, 192
pediatric services, 31, 34, 37–38
rescaling to match revised MEI, 98
RUC recommendations and results from five-year reviews, 37–41
RVS refinement process (1992), 30–31
service totals as combination of work, practice expense, and PLI, 70
transition to resource-based, 168
yearly recommendations from RUC, 33–37, *36t*
Relative value units—physician work component, 192
adjustments to, 168
assignment of, 26
budget-neutrality adjustments (1992–2022), 80–84, *83t*
calculating Medicare physician payment schedule, 79–80, *80t*
combining work, practice expense, and PLI, 70
explanatory note, 192
for noncovered services, 31
RVS refinement process (1992), 30–31
service totals as combination of work, practice expense, and PLI, 70
time considerations in, 27–28
updating, 33–36
use for physician productivity/compensation, 185–186, 190, *190f*
Relative value units—practice expense component, 192
adjusted direct RVUs, 55
in calculating Medicare physician payment schedule, 79–80, *80t*
charge-based, 43
code 99213, direct and indirect costs calculation for 2022, 57–59
combining work, practice expense, and PLI, 70
comparison with practice expense GPCI, 73–74
equipment calculations, 60
explanatory note, 192
labor calculations, 57–58
methodology for calculations, 47–60, 168
office-based services, adjustment to allocation of indirect practice expense, 59–60
service totals as combination of work, practice expense, and PLI, 70
supplies calculations, 56
Relative value units—professional liability insurance component, 65–70, 192
in calculating Medicare physician payment schedule, 67–68, 79–80, *80t*
charge-based and resource-based RVUs, 65-68
CMS review (2005 through 2020), 68–70
combining work, practice expense, and PLI, 70
concerns regarding methodology, 68–70
data used for charge-based PLI, 65–66, 69
explanatory note, 192
methodology for calculations, 66–68
service totals as combination of work, practice expense, and PLI, 70
Relativity Assessment Workgroup, 32, 35, 42, *IBC*
Remote physiologic monitoring, 115–116
Remote therapeutic monitoring, 116, *IBC*
Rental data, 73, 76
Residential substance abuse treatment facilities, national place of service code and payment rate for, 198
Resource-based practice expenses, 43–64, 547
Resource-based relative value scale (RBRVS). *See also* Physician work component of RBRVS; Practice expense component of RBRVS; Professional liability insurance component of RBRVS; RBRVS payment system; Relative value units (RVUs)
AMA blueprint for payment reform (1988–1989), 9
AMA proposal for development of, 5
COBRA authorization for development of, 6
CPT coding system and, 28
data use (non-Medicare) 180–190
defined, 4, 547
final values published in November each year, 33
geographic adjustments and, 12, 14–15
government interest in, 5–6
Harvard study on, 6–9, 13
legislative activity since 1991, 19–21
narrowing of specialty and geographic differences, 12
OBRA 89 physician payment reform provisions, 13–14
physicians' services covered by Part A in, 22
PPRC recommendation for, 6
practice expense refinement, 60–64
single cross-specialty RBRVS determined by single conversion factor, 22
standardization process, 17–18
survey of RBRVS use by payers, 185–190
update mechanism, 31–36

Retail health clinic, walk-in, national place of service codes and payment rates for, 196
Rheumatology, practice expense data, *53t, 56t*
Rhinology, practice expense ratios for 1989, *44t*
Roentgenology, practice expense ratios for 1989, *45t*
Roper, William R., 8
RUC. *See* AMA/Specialty Society RVS Update Committee
Rural areas, 3, 9, 71–72, 76, 77–78
Rural health clinics, national place of service code and payment rate for, 199
RVS. *See* Relative value scale
RVUs. *See also* Relative value units

S

SARS-CoV-2. *See* COVID-19 pandemic
SBA (Small Business Administration), 60, 62
Schools, national place of service code and payment rate for, 195
Scope of practice, 165
Screening tests, 151–160, *156t–160t*
Security of health information, 172
Sedation, moderate (conscious), 105–106
Sequestration. *See* Statutory PAYGO
Severe acute respiratory syndrome coronavirus 2 (SARS-CoV-2). *See* COVID-19 pandemic
Sexually transmitted infections (STIs) screening and counseling, *160t*
SGR. *See* Sustainable growth rate
Shortage areas. *See* Health professional shortage areas (HPSAs)
Sigmoidoscopy, 154, *157t*
Single drug price (SDP), 126
Skilled nursing facilities, national place of service code and payment rate for, 197
Sleep medicine, practice expense data, *53t, 56t*
Slide preparation facilities, *56t*
SLPs (speech language pathologists), 22, 130
Small Business Administration (SBA), 60, 62
Smoking and smoking cessation, *160t, 164*
SNPs (special needs plans), 10
Social Security Act Amendments of 1994, 37, 47, 171, 176, 547
Social workers, clinical, 23, *52t, 55t,* 134
Society for Thoracic Surgery, 40
Society for Vascular Surgery, 39
Socioeconomic Monitoring System (SMS)
  Core Survey, 43
  geographic variations data, 72
  nonphysician specialties not included in, 63
  practice expense data, 43, 47, 49–56, 63
  Soft Tissue Tumor and Bone Workgroup, 40
South Dakota, practice expense GPCI floor for, 74, 75
Special needs plans (SNPs), 10
Specialties, medical. *See* Medical specialties
Specialty differentials, 9, 13, 16–17, 547
Specialty societies
  contact information for, 550–554
  E/M documentation guidelines for, 136–139
  in five-year review process, 37, 38
  Harvard RBRVS study contributions from, 7
  input through RUC Advisory Committee, 31
  review panels in 1992 RVS refinement process, 29–30
  RUC survey instruments for, 33
Speech language pathologists (SLPs), 22, *56t*, 130
Sports medicine, practice expense data, *56t*
"Stacking" codes for molecular pathology, 124
Standby surgical teams, 150
Stason, William, 7
State medical associations, contact information for, 549–550
State public health clinics, national place of service code and payment rate for, 199
Statutory PAYGO, sequestration, 16, 84, 98–99
Stimulus law (American Recovery and Reinvestment Act of 2009), 171–172
STIs (sexually transmitted infections), *160t*
Substance abuse treatment facilities, 198
Supervision of diagnostic tests, 121
Supplies
  incident to physician's service, 125–126
  mean practice expenses per hour spent in patient care, *52t–53t*
  practice expense GPCI component for, 73
  pricing updates, 64
  RBRVS payment rules and policies, 125
Surgery. *See also* Global surgical package; Postoperative care and services
  anesthesia by surgeon (Modifier 47), 108
  assistant-at-surgery services, 106, 110–111, 112, 193–194
  bilateral procedures (Modifier 50), 108
  charge-based RVS, 4–5
  code M (multiple surgery rule), explanatory note for list of RVUs, 193
  codes T and T+ (surgical team), explanatory note for list of RVUs, 193
  CPT modifiers, 108–112
  data on preoperative and postoperative services, 169
  decision for (Modifier 57), 110
  discontinued procedure (Modifier 53), 109
  generally decreased payments under RBRVS, 169
  global surgical package, 101–104, 169–170, 173
  incentive payments for shortage areas, 77–78, 175
  for infants less than 4 kg (Modifier 63), 111

initial evaluation or consultation by surgeon, 102
intraoperative services, 103
minor and nonincisional procedures, 104–105
multiple procedures (Modifier 51), 108
payment gap between procedures and visits, 5, 169
practice expense ratios for 1989, *44t*
preoperative management only (Modifier 56), 109–110
preoperative medical clearance, 147
preoperative visits by surgeon, 102–103
RBRVS payment rules and policies, 101–104
second five-year review process, 38
standardization of RBRVS and, 18
standby surgical teams, 150
surgical care only (Modifier 54), 109–110
surgical team (Modifier 66), 111
two surgeons (Modifier 62), 110–111
unplanned return to operating room (Modifier 78), 112
Sustainable growth rate (SGR). *See also* Expenditure targets
Balanced Budget Act and, 94–95
cuts, deficits (2002-2015), 95–98, *97t*
defined, 547
physician-administered drugs and, 21
reform efforts and repeal of, 15–16, 20–21, 92–93, *97t*, 98
replacement of MVPS by, 15–16
targets for 2010–2014, *95t*

T

Target recapture, 21
Tax Relief and Health Care Act (TRHCA) of 2006, 14, 98, *97t,* 127, 173, 547
TCM (transitional care management services), 35, 36, 140–141, 175
Teaching physicians, 22, 117–118
Technical component
code Mtc, explanatory note for list of RVUs, 194
defined, 547
liability risk factor, 67
pathology services, 123–124
radiology services, 119–123
Technical Consulting Groups (TCGs), 7, 27–29
Technical Expert Group (TEG), 47
Technology
electronic health records, 144–145, 171, 173
e-mail, 114, 115, 144–145
new technology, 32, 42
payment rates and, 3
Telehealth/telemedicine services, *IFC,* 114–115
national place of service codes and payment rates for, 195
virtual check-in codes G2012, G2251, G2252, *IFC,* 115
Telephone consultations and services, 113, 114, 115, 144–145
E/M documentation, 136
virtual check-in codes G2012, G2251, G2252, *IFC,* 115
Temporary Extension Act of 2010, 20, 97, *97t,* 547
Temporary lodging, national place of service code and payment rate for, 196
Temporary Payroll Tax Cut Continuation Act of 2011
defined, 547
on physical and occupational therapy, 129
replacement of 2012 SGR cut, *97t,* 98
on work GPCI floor, 14, 21, 75
Terminology, glossary definitions and descriptions, 540–547
Texas, GPCI shortcomings in, 75
Therapeutic apheresis, 161
Third-party payers, survey on use of RBRVS payment system by, 180–190
Thoracic surgery, *44t, 56t*
Time factors, 27–29, 136
Tobacco use addiction, *160t*, 164
Todd, James S., 8, 15
Tomography, computed, low-dose, *159t*
Toxicology, mean practice expenses per hour spent in patient care, *54t*
Transitional care management services (TCM), 35, 36, 140–141, 175
Transition asymmetry, 17*f,* 547
Transition offset, defined, 547
Transplant cardiology, *54t*
TRHCA. *See* Tax Relief and Health Care Act of 2006
Tribal facilities, national place of service codes and payment rates for, 195
TRICARE, use of RBRVS payment system by, 181–186, *181f–186f*, 186
Two surgeons (Modifier 62), 110–111

U

UCR (usual, customary, and reasonable) charges, 3
Ultrasound abdominal aortic aneurysm, 156, *156t*
Unbundling, 104
Unplanned return to operating room (Modifier 78), 112
Urban areas, geographic payment differences in, 72, 74
Urban Institute, 72
Urgent care facilities, national place of service code and payment rate for, 196
Urology, 41, *44t, 53t, 56t*
US Census Bureau, 73
US Centers for Disease Control and Prevention. *See* Centers for Disease Control (CDC)

US Centers for Medicare & Medicaid Services. *See* Centers for Medicare & Medicaid Services (CMS)
US Congress. *See also specific names of legislative acts*
  budget neutrality legislation, 80–84, *83t*
  COBRA authorization for RBRVS development, 6
  conversion factor updates, 94, 95, 96
  cuts blocked for 2004–2006, 96
  House Energy and Commerce Committee, 12, 13
  House Ways and Means Committee, 12, 13
  legislation creating Medicare RBRVS, 12–21
  legislation replacing SGR cuts since 2002, 95–98, *97t*
  legislative initiatives to detect fraud and abuse, 151
  Medicare Payment Advisory Commission formed by, 11
  physician payment reform legislation adopted by (1989), 2
  RBRVS legislation since 1991, 19–21
  Senate Finance Committee, 12, 13
  subcommittee proposals for OBRA 89, 12, 13
US Federal Trade Commission, 4, 5
US Food and Drug Administration. See Food and Drug Administration (FDA)
Usual, customary, and reasonable (UCR) charges, 3

V

Vaccine administration, payment, for SARS-CoV-2 CPT codes, *IFC*, 127–128
Vaccinations, 126, 127, *158t–160t*
Vaginal cancer screening, 154–155, *157t*
Valuation methods. *See* Relative value scale (RVS); Resource-based relative value scale (RBRVS)
Value-based health care,173–174
Value modifier (VM), 173
Value Pathways, 174
Vascular surgery, 38, 39, 41, *53t, 56t*
Ventilator management, 150
Virgin Islands, 74
Virtual check-in codes, *IFC*, 115
Visits. *See* Office visits
Volume performance standard. *See* Medicare volume performance standard (MVPS)

W

Walk-in retail health clinics, national place of service code and payment rate for, 196
Websites. *See* Information resources
Weight loss therapy, *159t*
"Welcome to Medicare: Physical Examination," 152, *156t*
Wellness and burnout, physician, 165–166
Wellness visits, annual, 152, *156t*
Work adjustor, 16
Work component. *See* Physician work component of RBRVS; Relative value units—physician work component
Workers' compensation, RBRVS uses, 181–185, *181f–186f*, 186
Worksheets, determining impact of Medicare payment system on individual practices, 84–86
Worksite, national place of service code and payment rate for, 196
Wyoming, practice expense GPCI floor for, 74, 75

X

X-rays. *See* Radiology services